AACN
PROCEDURE
MANUAL
FOR
CRITICAL
CARE

THIRD EDITION

AACN PROCEDURE MANUAL FOR CRITICAL CARE

Edited by:

ROCHELLE LOGSTON BOGGS, MS, RN, CCRN, CS

Trauma/Critical Care Clinical Nurse Specialist
Surgical, Trauma, Critical Care Associates
Parkersburg, West Virginia

MARIBETH WOOLDRIDGE-KING, MS, RN, CNAA

Assistant Director of Nursing Practice
Memorial Sloan-Kettering Cancer Center
New York, New York

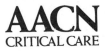

AMERICAN ASSOCIATION OF CRITICAL-CARE NURSES

W. B. SAUNDERS COMPANY *A Division of Harcourt Brace & Company*
Philadelphia, London, Toronto, Montreal, Sydney, Tokyo

W.B. SAUNDERS COMPANY
A Division of
Harcourt Brace & Company

The Curtis Center
Independence Square West
Philadelphia, PA 19106

Library of Congress Cataloging-in-Publication Data

AACN procedure manual for critical care / edited by Rochelle Logston Boggs. Maribeth Wooldridge-King,
  American Association of Critical Care Nurses.—3rd ed.
       p.   cm.
     ISBN 0-7216-3073-1
     1. Intensive care nursing—Handbooks, manuals, etc.   I. Boggs, Rochelle Logston.   II. Wooldridge-
King, Maribeth.   III. American Association of Critical Care Nurses.
RT120.I5A17   1993
616′.028—dc20   91-46858
                                                                                                        CIP

AACN PROCEDURE MANUAL FOR CRITICAL CARE   ISBN   0–7216–3073–1

Printed in the United States of America.

Last digit is the print number: 9   8   7   6   5   4   3

To my colleagues, who
daily practice in the demanding
specialty of critical care nursing.
RLB

To Dan,
for his support,
patience and love.
MWK

CONTRIBUTORS

THOMAS BAKER, RN

Nurse Manager, Hyperbaric Medicine Department, Maryland Institute for Emergency Medical Services Systems
Baltimore, Maryland

GAIL BENNETT, MSN, RN, CIC

Executive Director, ICP Associates
Rome, Georgia

ROCHELLE LOGSTON BOGGS, MS, RN, CCRN, CS

Trauma Critical Care Clinical Nurse Specialist, Surgical Trauma and Critical Care Associates; Clinical Director, Good Samaritan Clinic, Inc.; Adjunct Clinical Faculty, West Virginia University School of Nursing
Parkersburg, West Virginia

JERRI BRYANT, MPH, RN, CIC

Adjunct Assistant Professor, Cleveland State University; Clinical Epidemiologist, Cleveland Clinic Foundation
Cleveland, Ohio

ELAINE SAYRE CAPPADONA, BSN, RN, CCRN

Staff Nurse—Critical Care, Camden Clark Memorial Hospital
Parkersburg, West Virginia

SUSAN L. COLLINS, MSN, RN

Adjunct Clinical Faculty, West Virginia University School of Nursing; Trauma Clinical Nurse Specialist, West Virginia University Hospitals, Inc.
Morgantown, West Virginia

JEAN A. CROSS, MSN, RN, CCRN

Clinical Faculty—Acute and Critical Care Nursing, Frances Payne Botton School of Nursing, Case Western Reserve University; Clinical Nurse Specialist—Cardiac ICU, University Hospitals of Cleveland
Cleveland, Ohio

NANCY A. DODD, MSN, RN, CCRN

Clinical Instructor, University of Pennsylvania School of Nursing; Clinical Nurse Specialist—Surgical Intensive Care Unit, Hospital of the University of Pennsylvania
Philadelphia, Pennsylvania

PHYLLIS M. DUBENDORF, MSN, RN

Clinical Nurse Specialist—Intermediate Neurosensory Care Unit,
Thomas Jefferson University Hospital
Philadelphia, Pennsylvania

SANDRA ENGSTROM, BSN, RN, CCRN

Staff Nurse—Adult Critical Care, Tacoma General Hospital
Tacoma, Washington

JANE A. FISHER, RN, CCRN

Staff Nurse, Tacoma General Hospital
Tacoma, Washington

BARBARA A. GILL, MN, RN

Adjunct Faculty, Graduate School of Nursing, University of Kansas, Kansas City, Kansas;
Fellow, The Annenberg Washington Program
Washington, D.C.

MARIE SCOTTO GIORDANO, MS, RN

Adjunct Faculty, School of Nursing at City College, CUNY
New York, New York

MARGARET T. GOLDBERG, MSN, RN, CETN

Enterostomal Therapist, Crozer Chester Medical Center
Upland, Pennsylvania

SANDRA K. GOODNOUGH-HANNEMAN, PhD, RN

Clinical Professor, Graduate Program, College of Nursing, Texas Woman's University;
Pulmonary Critical Care Consultant, St. Luke's Episcopal Hospital; Nursing Research Consultant, Hermann Hospital, Houston, Texas; National Nursing Advisor, Pulmonary Center
of Excellence, Humana Hospital
Clear Lake, Texas

JAN M. HEADLEY, BS, RN

Critical Care Educational Consultant, Trabuco Canyon, California; Senior Education Consultant to Baxter Healthcare Corporation, Edwards Critical Care Division
Irvine, California

ANN N. HOTTER, RN, MSN, CCRN, CS

Clinical Nurse Specialist, Critical Care, St. Mary's Hospital—Mayo Foundation
Rochester, Minnesota

ANN LOUISE JONES, MSN, RN, CS

Cardiothoracic Clinical Specialist, Surgical Associates—Dr. R. Herman Playforth
Lexington, Kentucky

TERRY JONES, MSN, RN, CCRN

Critical Care Coordinator—Department of Nursing Education, Parkland Memorial Hospital
Dallas, Texas

ROBERTA KAPLOW, MA, RN, CCRN

Nurse Clinician, Special Care Unit, Memorial Sloan-Kettering Cancer Center
New York, New York

LESLIE S. KERN, MN, RN

Assistant Clinical Professor, UCLA School of Nursing, Los Angeles;
Research Specialist, AACN
Aliso Viejo, California

AILEEN R. KILLEN, MS, RN, CNOR

Director of Nursing, Perioperative Service, The Hospital for Special Surgery
New York, New York

BARBARA J. KNOPP, MSN, RN

Associate Professor of Nursing, West Virginia University-Parkersburg; Pediatric Staff Nurse,
St. Joseph Hospital
Parkersburg, West Virginia

DENISE M. LAWRENCE, MS, RN, CCRN, CS

Trauma Clinical Nurse Specialist, Hartford Hospital
Hartford, Connecticut

ALICE B. LUCAS, BSN, RN

Vascular Access Nurse Clinician, Memorial Sloan-Kettering Cancer Center
New York, New York

DEBRA J. LYNN-MCHALE, MSN, RN, CCRN, CS

Clinical Instructor, Thomas Jefferson University; Clinical Nurse Specialist, Surgical Cardiac
Care Unit, Thomas Jefferson University Hospital
Philadelphia, Pennsylvania

ELLEN STRAUSS MCERLEAN, MSN, RN, CCRN

Clinical Faculty Member, Case Western Reserve University and Ohio State University;
Clinical Nurse Specialist, Department of Cardiothoracic Nursing,
The Cleveland Clinic Foundation
Cleveland, Ohio

JOYCE MCGRORY, BSN, RN, CCRN

Nursing Care Coordinator, Surgical Cardiac Care Unit,
Thomas Jefferson University Hospital
Philadelphia, Pennsylvania

MARY GERKIN MCKINLEY, MSN, RN, CCRN

Adjunct Faculty Assistant Professor, West Liberty State College, West Liberty,
West Virginia; Clinical Nurse Specialist—Critical Care, Ohio Valley Medical Center
Wheeling, West Virginia

CAROL MIKOLS, MSN, RNCS, CETN

Clinical Nurse Specialist—Ostomy and Wound Care, Sinai Hospital
Detroit, Michigan

VICKIE ANN MIRACLE, MSN, RN, CCRN

Research Assistant, Jewish Hospital, Heart and Lung Institute
Louisville, Kentucky

ANN MARIE MORAN, MSN, RN, CCRN

Clinical Nurse Specialist, Surgical Intensive Care Unit, Neuroscience/Trauma,
Hospital of the University of Pennsylvania
Philadelphia, Pennsylvania

SHARON GREICHEN O'GRADY, MN, RN

Clinical Education Consultant, Nellcor Inc.
Hayward, California

ALLEN J. ORSI, MSN, RN, CCRN, CS

Doctoral Candidate and Research Assistant, University of Pennsylvania, School of Nursing;
Staff Nurse, Surgical Intensive Care Unit, Hospital of the University of Pennsylvania
Philadelphia, Pennsylvania

ROSALINE PARSON, RN, CCRN

Assistant Nurse Manager, Surgical Trauma ICU, Orlando Regional Medical Center
Orlando, Florida

KAREN PAYTON, RN, CCRN

Senior Staff RN, Neuroscience ICU, Orlando Regional Medical Center
Orlando, Florida

JACQUELINE C. PE, MA, RN, CCRN

Education Specialist, Mt. Sinai Hospital
New York, New York

SUZANNE S. PREVOST, MSN, RN, CCRN

Assistant Professor, Northwestern State University; Clinical Nurse Specialist, Veterans
Administration Medical Center
Shreveport, Louisiana

ANDREA QUINN, MS, RN, CCRN, CS

Clinical Nurse Specialist—Surgical Nursing, Yale-New Haven Hospital
New Haven, Connecticut

CHARLENE RANDALL, BSN, RN, CETN

Enterostomal Therapy Nurse, St. Luke's Episcopal Hospital, Texas Medical Center
Houston, Texas

CATHERINE FREISMUTH ROBINSON, MS, RN, CEN, CCRN

Adjunct Faculty—Assistant Professor, West Liberty State College, West Liberty, West
Virginia; Clinical Nurse Specialist, Emergency Services/Trauma, Ohio Valley Medical
Center
Wheeling, West Virginia

JANICE A. ROBINSON, MS, RN, CS, CNN

CNS-Care Manager, Nephrology, Harper Hospital
Detroit, Michigan

KATHRYN J. ROBINSON, MA, BSN, RN, CNA, CNN

Clinical Coordinator—Transplant, Harper Hospital
Detroit, Michigan

MARCIA A. RYDER, BS, RN, CNSN, CRNI, PHN

Nursing Consultant, Vascular Access and Infusion Therapy Specialist
San Mateo, California

NANCY TOMASELLI, MSN, RN, CETN

Joint Appointment, College of Allied Health Sciences, Thomas Jefferson University; ET Clinical Nurse Specialist, Thomas Jefferson University Hospital; ET CNS Consultant: Jefferson Park Hospital, Magee Rehabilitation Center, Will's Eye Hospital, Philadelphia, Pennsylvania; Alfred I. Dupont Institute
Wilmington, Delaware

CAROLYN D. VIALL, MSN, RN, CNSN

Clinical Specialist, Caremark Inc., Affiliate Baxter Healthcare Corporation
Warrensville, Ohio

CAMILLA BETH WALKER, BSN, RN, CCRN

Medicine Specialty Educator, Department of Nursing Education,
Parkland Memorial Hospital
Dallas, Texas

BETH LOUISE WHITTAKER, MAS, BSN, RN

Clinical Nurse Specialist—Discharge Planning, Maryland Institute for
Emergency Medical Services Systems
Baltimore, Maryland

DEBORAH THALMAN WIGAL, MA, BSN, RN

Director of Health Education, Mid-Ohio Valley Health Department; Adjunct Faculty, West Virginia University
Parkersburg, West Virginia

MARLOT A. WIGGINTON, MN, RN, CCRN

Adjunct Faculty, University of Louisville School of Nursing; Clinical Nurse Specialist—Critical Care, Norton Hospital
Louisville, Kentucky

MARCELLA WYERS WILL, BSN, RN

Education Coordinator, St. Joseph's Hospital
Parkersburg, West Virginia

SANDI WIND, RN, CETN

Clinical Instructor, Hannemann University, School of Health Sciences and Humanities; Enterostomal Therapy Nurse, Hannemann University; Enterostomal Therapy Nurse Consultant, St. Agnes Medical Center
Philadelphia, Pennsylvania

MARIBETH WOOLDRIDGE-KING, MS, RN, CNAA

Assistant Director of Nursing, Memorial Sloan-Kettering Cancer Center
New York, New York

PREFACE

The *AACN Procedure Manual for Critical Care* has undergone a rebirth in its 3rd edition. Entitled *Methods in Critical Care* in the first edition and developing into the *AACN Procedure Manual for Critical Care* in the second, the book in its third edition has been greatly expanded in scope. The independent aspect of nursing practice within the critical care environment has been delineated and emphasized. Great care and thought has been given to specific skills included, taking into account the rapidly changing technologies, the diversity of protocols and equipment in urban vs. rural settings, and the different philosophies in critical care throughout the world.

We have taken the skills in critical care and placed them within the context of the nursing process as the accepted and universal approach to patient care. Specific guidelines for patient and family education have also been included with the growing emphasis on a patient's right to know and to make decisions regarding care and treatment.

The 3rd edition of the *AACN Procedure Manual for Critical Care* continues to address the fundamentals in the care of the critically ill patient, as well as those skills considered to be on the cutting edge of critical care practice. Readers are encouraged to refer to *AACN's Clinical Reference for Critical Care Nurses* and *AACN's Core Curriculum for Critical Care Nursing* as adjunct references on the nursing management of diseases and complications unique to the critically ill.

The book is divided into units using a systems approach. It has been our experience that most critical care nurses use body systems to structure their patient assessment, and so we hope that this approach will facilitate the use of this text as an efficient reference.

Each unit then is divided into chapters which categorize the skills related to that body system. The skill itself then becomes part of the implementation within the nursing process.

CHAPTER FORMAT

Each chapter contains: an overview of basic concepts pertinent to all the skills within that chapter; behavioral objectives; key terms; numerically referenced skills; references; and bibliography.

Assessment guidelines relevant to all the skills begin each chapter. The purpose of each skill is listed along with the prerequisite knowledge and skills.

At the conclusion of each skill is a list of references, bibliography, and a performance checklist. The performance checklist will prove an invaluable evaluation tool for the nurse educator, preceptor, and administrator. Additionally, for the critical care orientee or the experienced nurse unfamiliar with a particular subject matter, the expectations for attaining mastery of performance are clearly arranged and identified. Each chapter was laid out in this manner to facilitate use of the text by nurse educators both within the hospital setting and in schools of nursing. The nurse administrator will find this format allows quick reference to support and evaluate the staff in daily practice and also to provide specific guidelines for the more complex process of standard and policy formulation.

SKILL FORMAT

The skills are numbered, with related topics grouped together. Because nursing has moved beyond mere task-orientation, the nursing process provides the structure for the content within each skill.

The skill content is then separated into: assessment, nursing diagnosis, planning (patient goals), implementation, evaluation, expected outcomes, unexpected outcomes, documentation, and patient and family education. This approach also lends itself to formulating a patient care plan.

A tabular format is used for the skill content, divided into three columns: steps, rationale, and special considerations. The logical sequence of events or the "how" in each section is listed under the "steps" column. The rationale column provides the "why" for the performance in each step. Special considerations address a multitude of variables, including contraindications, age-specific variations, research results or any other helpful tips for efficient performance of a step.

A glossary stating the definition of key terms is listed.

SUMMARY

Skills are but one aspect within critical-care nursing. Underlying this text is our belief that the critical care experience lies within a continuum of a patient's illness: from symptom onset to discharge or demise. We believe that the nurse cares for the "whole": a patient and his family, with a watchful eye toward the patient's quality of life and productivity upon returning to society. We therefore stress both the independent and the collaborative nature of nursing practice in hopes of identifying and clarifying our professional role in providing high-quality and holistic care to the critically ill.

RLB
MWK

ACKNOWLEDGMENTS

When we started this book we had no idea how much time, effort, and dedication it would absorb from our lives. For quite some time our families, friends, and personal interests have been put on the back burner to see this through to its completion. It is for us the attainment of a long-dreamt personal and professional goal. Many people supported us through this process and without them the book would not be a reality.

First and foremost, we recognize our contributors for their formidable knowledge base and clinical expertise; without them this book would not have come to be. They suffered through our seemingly endless requests for clarifications, modifications, permission requests, re-writes, illustrations and photographs, and pleas to meet deadlines. To the end, each one remained gracious and a model of professional excellence.

To our reviewers go our kudos for their thought-provoking comments, suggestions, questions—and for being timely. Their content expertise and critical analysis supported our efforts to provide an up-to-date, research-based description of critical care nursing skills.

Ellen French, Publications Director at AACN, and the entire AACN staff have been most supportive throughout the book's entire history, from its inception as a proposal in 1988 all the way to its printing. They never lost sight of our vision and endeavored to make that vision become a reality. Our warm thanks and enduring appreciation.

Thomas Eoyang, our editor at W. B. Saunders Company wore a variety of hats throughout this project: cheerleader, advocate, mediator, taskmaster, quarterback, and supporter. Certainly an unenviable position, but one that he accomplishes with integrity, sincerity, and an incredible attention to detail. He never failed to get back to us ASAP and that was greatly appreciated. His assistant, Terri Fortiner, is also commended for her sunny disposition and ability to organize the tremendous paper trail.

To Jenni Teachout and Judy Morgan, whose secretarial skills have remained invaluable.

To keep the book a reasonable and affordable length, it underwent several major and painful content cuts. The results of this agonizing process resulted in the exclusion of the work of the following authors: Jane Foreman and Nancy Scanzello. We sincerely appreciate their dedication and devotion to our concept and apologize for this mutual disappointment.

Last but not least, we thank our dear husbands, Joseph Boggs and Daniel King, who wondered if this project was ever going to be finished. They covered for us for the four long years it has taken to complete this work. To our children: Zak, Kyle, Ryan and Colleen, thank you for all your smiles and hugs which always got us over the rough humps. And to our two children to be, may they see our vision of critical care nursing in this work of art.

REVIEWERS

MARY ANN BARTON, BSN, RN, OCN

CPS Advanced Infusion Systems
Mountain View, California

CHERYL RAE BRUMFIELD, BSN, RN, CNA

Camden-Clark Memorial Hospital
Parkersburg, West Virginia

CHERYL BUNGARD, RN, CRTT

Glasrock Home Health Care
Parkersburg, West Virginia

HARRIET W. BUSS, MSN, RN, CCRN

Nash General Hospital
Rocky Mount, North Carolina

EVELYN BUTERA, MS, RN, CNN

Northwest Kidney Centers
Seattle, Washington

JOANNE L. CAHILL, MS, RN, CCRN

Allegheny General Hospital
Pittsburgh, Pennsylvania

CAROL L. DAAKE, MSN, RN

St. Louis University
St. Louis, Missouri

ANN MARIE DENTE-CASSIDY, MSN, RN, CCRN

Nursing Magazine
Spring City, Pennsylvania

BARBARA J. DREW, PhD, RN, CCRN

University of California, San Francisco
San Francisco, California

DENNIS M. DRISCOLL, MS, RN, CCRN, CEN

U.S. Army Institute of Surgical Research
Ft. Sam Houston, Texas

KENDRA ELLIS, BSN, RN, CCRN, CEN

Parkland Memorial Hospital
Dallas, Texas

NANCY EVANS, MSN, RN, CNSN

Hospital of the University
of Pennsylvania
Philadelphia, Pennsylvania

PATRICIA WALSH FELMLY, MSN, RN, CCRN

Kaiser Permanente Medical Center
Honolulu, Hawaii

ANNA GAWLINSKI, MSN, RN, CCRN

UCLA Medical Center
Los Angeles, California

MARSHA HALFMAN, MSN, RN

Consultant, Cardiovascular Nursing
Scottsdale, Arizona

J. KEITH HAMPTON, MSN, RN, CS

The University of Minnesota Hospital and Clinic
Minneapolis, Minnesota

KATHLEEN T. HASSE, BSN, RN, CEN

Camden-Clark Memorial Hospital
Parkersburg, West Virginia

ELIZABETH A. HENNEMAN, MS, RN, CCRN

UCLA Medical Center
Los Angeles, California

APRIL L. HICKEY, MSN, RN, CCRN, CNRN

Parkland Memorial Hospital
Dallas, Texas

O. LEE HICKMAN, BS, RRT

Camden-Clark Memorial Hospital
Parkersburg, West Virginia

MARCIA J. HILL, MSN, RN

The Methodist Hospital
Houston, Texas

DONNA D. IGNATAVICIUS, MS, RNC

Mcqueen Gibbs Willis School of Nursing
Easton, Maryland

MARGUERITE MCMILLAN JACKSON, MS, CIC, FAAN

UCSD Medical Center
San Diego, California

MARIANNE GENGE JAGMIN, MS, RN, CS, ONC

Rush-Presbyterian-St. Luke's Medical Center
Chicago, Illinois

BRENDA BRADLEY JOHANSSON, BSN, RN, CNRN, CCRN

Enloe Hospital
Chico, California

DEBORAH G. KLEIN, MSN, RN, CCRN, CS

MetroHealth Medical Center
Cleveland, Ohio

LINDA S. KNOX, MSN, RN, CNSN

Hospital of the University of Pennsylvania
Philadelphia, Pennsylvania

DEIRDRE A. KRAUSE, PhD, ARNP, CCRN

Health Education and Consultation
Loxahatchee, Florida

JOANNE M. KRUMBERGER, MSN, RN, CCRN

Clement J. Zablocki Veterans Affairs Medical
    Center
Milwaukee, Wisconsin

ANN BUTLER MAHER, MS, RN, ONC

County College of Morris
Randolph, New Jersey

MICHAELENE P. MIRR, PhD, RN, CCRN

University of Wisconsin—Eau Claire
Eau Claire, Wisconsin

SARA R. NEAGLEY, MA, RN

The Milton S. Hershey Medical Center of the
    Pennsylvania State University
Hershey, Pennsylvania

MARY LOU NOLL, PhD, RN, CCRN

University of Central Florida
Orlando, Florida

DIANE M. NORKOOL, MN, RN

Virginia Mason Hospital
Seattle, Washington

NARAYANA N. REDDY, MD

Pulmonary Intensivist
Parkersburg, West Virginia

LAUREN SAUL, MSN, RN, CCRN

Shadyside Hospital
Pittsburgh, Pennsylvania

DOROTHY B. SMITH, MS, RN, ET, OCN

University of Texas M. D. Anderson Cancer
    Center
Houston, Texas

SUSAN L. SMITH, MN, RN, CCRN

Emory University Hospital
Atlanta, Georgia

JOAN A. SNYDER, MS, RN

Trauma Systems Consultant
Alexandria, Virginia

MARILYN SAWYER SOMMERS, PhD, RN, CCRN

University of Cincinnati
Cincinnati, Ohio

NANCY A. STOTTS, EdD, RN

University of California, San Francisco
San Francisco, California

MARITA G. TITLER, PhD, RN

University of Iowa Hospital and Clinics
Iowa City, Iowa

KATHRYN T. VON RUEDEN, MS, RN, CCRN, FCCN

Maryland Institute for Emergency Medical
    Services Systems
Baltimore, Maryland

TERRY WILLEY, MN, RN, CETN

Emory University Hospital
Atlanta, Georgia

CONTENTS

Unit III THE NEUROLOGIC SYSTEM

Unit IV THE GASTROINTESTINAL SYSTEM

Unit V   THE RENAL SYSTEM

Unit VI   THE MUSCULOSKELETAL SYSTEM

Unit XII   ORGAN PROCUREMENT

UNIT I

THE PULMONARY SYSTEM

AIRWAY MANAGEMENT

BEHAVIORAL OBJECTIVES

At the completion of this chapter, the nurse will be able to

- Define the key terms.
- Describe methods for managing the upper airway.
- Discuss the indications for endotracheal intubation.
- Discuss the indications for endotracheal tube care.
- Discuss the indications for suctioning.
- Discuss the indications for tracheotomy.
- Discuss the indications for tracheostomy tube care.
- Describe the methods of tracheal tube cuff management.
- Describe methods for managing the lower airway.
- Demonstrate the skills listed.

The top priority in airway management is to promote adequate ventilation to life-sustaining organs. When patients present with airway problems, the key to their successful management is immediate problem identification and intervention. The method of choice for airway maintenance depends on the nature of the airway obstruction, the hemodynamic status of the patient, the expertise of the nurse, the availability of supplies and equipment, the presence of facial injuries, and the presence of cervical spine injuries.

This chapter focuses on those procedures necessary for the emergency management and continued care of a patient's airway.

KEY TERMS

artificial airway	intubation
airway adjunct	lower airway
bronchus	mandible
carina	translaryngeal
endotracheal tube	upper airway
extubation	vallecula

SKILLS

1-1 Insertion of Oropharyngeal Airway
1-2 Insertion of Nasopharyngeal Airway
1-3 Oropharyngeal and Nasopharyngeal Suctioning
1-4 Tracheobronchial Suctioning
1-5 Endotracheal Intubation and Tube Care
1-6 Endotracheal or Tracheostomy Tube Suctioning
1-7 Tracheal Tube Cuff Care
1-8 Extubation and Decannulation
1-9 Tracheotomy and Tracheostomy Tube Care

GUIDELINES

The following assessment guidelines assist the nurse in formulating a nursing diagnosis and an individualized plan of care to maintain a patent airway:

1. Know the patient's baseline respiratory assessment.
2. Know the patient's baseline vital signs.
3. Know the patient's baseline hemodynamic status.
4. Know the patient's medical history.

5. Know the patient's current medical treatment.
6. Know the therapeutic goals for the patient.
7. Perform systematic respiratory assessments in a timely fashion.
8. Determine appropriate intervention for assessed findings.
9. Become adept with equipment used for airway maintenance.

SKILL 1-1

Insertion of Oropharyngeal Airway

An oral airway is usually made of a hard, curved piece of plastic. Oral airways are inserted through the open mouth with the posterior tip resting in the patient's pharynx. The oral airway is placed over the tongue. The curvature or body of the airway displaces the tongue forward from the posterior pharyngeal wall, a common site of airway obstruction. Oral airways facilitate suctioning of the pharynx and prevent patients from biting their tongues, grinding their teeth, or occluding their endotracheal or oral gastric tubes. The oral airway has four parts: flange, body, tip, and channel (Fig. 1–1). The flange protrudes from the mouth and rests on the lips. This design protects against aspiration into the airway. The body is the part that curves over the tongue. The tip is the distal-most part of the airway toward the base of the tongue. The channel enables passage of a suction catheter through a central core in the Guedel airway or down side channels in the Berman airway.

Oral airways are manufactured in a variety of lengths and width for adults and children and infants (Table 1–1). An alternative method used to select the size of an oral airway is to measure the airway by placing the flange alongside the patient's lips and oral airway tip alongside the angle of the jaw (Fig. 1–2). Improperly sized airways can cause airway obstruction if they are too small and tongue displacement against the oropharynx if they are too large.

Purpose

The nurse inserts an oral airway to

1. Relieve airway obstruction. Causes of airway obstruction include but are not limited to hypopharyngeal relaxation (especially in the unconscious patient), aspiration of foreign substances into the airway, injuries to the upper and lower airways, presence of mucus or other body fluid, and laryngeal spasms.
2. Provide short-term maintenance of an airway.
3. Facilitate removal of tracheobronchial secretions.
4. Facilitate artificial ventilation.
5. Simulate the effect of a bite block.
6. Prevent damage to the tongue and soft tissues of the mouth.

Prerequisite Knowledge and Skills

Prior to inserting an oral airway, the nurse should understand

1. Principles of aseptic technique.
2. Anatomy and physiology of the upper and lower airway.
3. Principles of airway resistance.
4. Concept of anxiety.
5. Concept of fear.
6. Anatomic differences between adults and children.
7. Proper insertion techniques.

The nurse should be able to perform

1. Proper handwashing technique (Skill 35–5).
2. Universal precautions (Skill 35–1).
3. Vital signs assessment.
4. Respiratory assessment (inspection, palpation, percussion, and auscultation).
5. Maneuvers necessary to open the airway (i.e., head tilt with anterior displacement of the mandible, chin lift, and jaw thrust).
6. Oxygen administration via face mask, hood, or nasal cannula (Skills 2–1 and 2–2).
7. Suctioning techniques (Skill 1–3).

Assessment

1. Observe for signs and symptoms of upper airway compromise or obstruction resulting from anatomic displacement of the tongue and other.

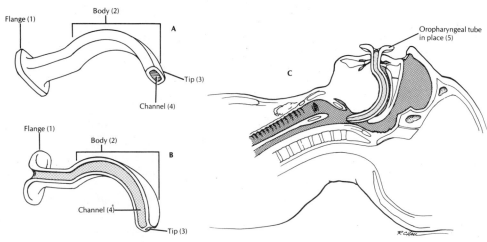

Flange (1)
Body (2)
A
Tip (3)
Channel (4)

Flange (1)
Body (2)
B
Channel (4)
Tip (3)

C

Oropharyngeal tube in place (5)

FIGURE 1–1. Oropharyngeal airways: (*A*) Guedel airway, (*B*) Berman airway, (*C*) properly inserted oropharyngeal tube. (Reproduced with permmission from D. H. Eubanks and R. C. Bone, *Comprehensive Respiratory Care: A Learning System*, 2nd Ed. St. Louis, Mosby, 1990, p. 548.)

TABLE 1–1 ORAL AIRWAY SIZING BY AGE

Age	Size
Premature neonate	000
Newborn	00
Infant	0
1–3 years	1
3–8 years	2
9–18 years, large child, small adult	3
Medium adult	4
Large adult	5,6

a. Soft tissues of the hypopharyngeal. Signs and symptoms include stridor, crowing, gasping respiration, and snoring (definitive signs); tachycardia or irregular pulse rate and diaphoresis (early signs); and circumoral cyanosis, bradycardia, diminished or absent breath sounds, chest excursion, and unconsciousness (late signs). **Rationale:** Relaxation of the tongue and other soft tissues of the hypopharyngeal region may result in their falling backward into the airway causing partial or complete blockage, especially in the unconscious or comatose supine patient. In children, the oral cavity is small in proportion to the tongue, which can result in obstruction (Moloney-Harman 1991).

b. Increased or excessive mucus or other body fluids. Signs and symptoms include gurgling with respiratory cycle, wheezes, crackles, increased amount of oral secretions or excretions, excessive drooling, tachycardia, dyspnea, and tachypnea, damaged or traumatized airway tissue (early signs); and acute dyspnea, physical evidence of vomitus in the mouth, hypoxemia, PaO_2 less than 60 mmHg, bradycardia, and irregular heart rate and failure (late signs). **Rationale:** Mucus, blood, and gastric contents can

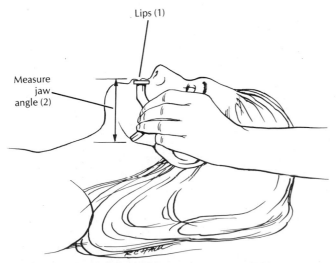

Lips (1)

Measure jaw angle (2)

FIGURE 1–2. Alternative method for selecting the size of an oropharyngeal airway. (Reproduced with permission from D. H. Eubanks and R. C. Bone, *Comprehensive Respiratory Care: A Learning System*, 2d Ed. St. Louis, Mosby, 1990, p. 552.)

diminish or impede gas flow to the lower airway, thus increasing the work of breathing. Inspissated secretions occur more frequently with the inhalation of unhumidified gases or inadequate fluid intake.

c. Aspiration of solid objects, gases, or liquids. Signs and symptoms include stridor, gurgling with respiratory cycle, gasping respiration, physical evidence of foreign body or soot around the mouth or nostrils, reddening and swelling in the trachea, tachycardia or irregular pulse rate, and diaphoresis (early signs); and circumoral cyanosis, hypoxemia PaO_2 less than 60 mmHg, bradycardia, and unconsciousness (late signs). **Rationale:** Most aspirated substances cause immediate and severe spasms of the larynx, trachea, and bronchi. Foreign objects such as food particles, dentures, chewing gum, undersized oral airways, or any other objects that can fit into the mouth can diminish or stop the forward gas flow to the lower airway. Liquids and gases such as toxic constituents of smoke produce tracheal and noncardiac edema (Herndon et al., 1984) and reduce bacterial clearance and mucociliary transport, which can lead to airway obstruction or infection. (Weigelt and McCormack, 1988).

d. Spasms of the larynx, trachea, and bronchi. Signs and symptoms include stridor, crowing, gasping respirations, and snoring (definitive signs); bradycardia, irregular pulse, feeling of weakness, and fainty feeling (early signs); and cyanosis, hypoxemia PaO_2 less than 60 mmHg, and unconsciousness (late signs). **Rationale:** Spasms decrease the likelihood that foreign bodies will be expelled. Artificial stimulation of the cough reflex stimulates vagal activity, evidenced by bradycardia.

2. Observe for signs and symptoms of inadequate breathing patterns, including dyspnea, shallow respirations, and intercostal and suprasternal retractions. **Rationale:** Respiratory distress is a late sign of potential upper airway obstruction.

Special Considerations During Assessment

Patients at increased risk for the development of upper airway obstruction include infants, children, elderly, and adults with colds and influenza, loss of consciousness, coma, seizure disorders, neuromuscular disease, trauma, and secretory tumors of the upper airway.

Nursing Diagnoses

1. Impaired gas exchange related to partial or complete airway obstruction. **Rationale:** The presence of soft tissue, mucus, blood, gastric fluid, inhaled toxic constituents, or solid objects can diminish or stop gas flow to the lower airways.

2. Ineffective airway clearance related to retained se-

cretions and tracheal edema. **Rationale:** Secretions, especially mucoid in character, are sticky and tend to accumulate in pools or pockets along the upper airway, resulting in partial or complete obstruction. Tracheal edema reduces bacterial clearance and mucociliary transport (Weigelt and McCormack, 1988).

3. Potential for infection related to retained secretions. **Rationale:** Pooled secretions provide an ideal medium for bacterial and microorganism growth.

Planning

1. Individualize the following goals for inserting an oropharyngeal airway.
   a. Secure and maintain a patent airway. **Rationale:** Optimal airway management includes prevention of partial and complete occlusion and removal of solid objects, gases, or liquids.
   b. Maintain adequate fluid hydration and humidification. **Rationale:** Inspissated secretions occur more frequently with the inhalation of unhumidified gases or inadequate fluid intake.
2. Prepare all necessary equipment and supplies. **Rationale:** Assembly of all the necessary equipment and supplies facilitates quick and efficient oral airway insertion and minimizes the risk of complications.
   a. Appropriately sized oral airway (see Table 1–1 or Fig. 1–2).
   b. Exam gloves.
   c. Tongue depressor.
   d. Tape.
   e. Suction equipment, if needed (see Skill 1–3).
   f. Goggles, glasses, or face mask.
3. Prepare the patient and family.
   a. Explain the purpose of the airway and the procedure to conscious patients or to the family of unconscious patients. **Rationale:** Communication and explanation for therapy are cited as an important need of patients and families (Parker et al., 1984; Viner, 1988).
   b. Discuss the sensory experiences associated with oral airway insertion, including inability to clench teeth together, presence of hard plastic airway in mouth, inability to freely move tongue, and possibly gagging. **Rationale:** Knowledge of anticipated sensory experiences reduces anxiety and distress (Johnson et al., 1978; Viner, 1988).
   c. Position patient. (1) Semi-Fowler's or supine position is preferred unless contraindicated (used most often for conscious patients). **Rationale:** Promotes patient and nurse comfort and provides easy access to oral cavity. (2) Hyperextend the patient's neck through use of the head-tilt, chin-lift, or jaw-thrust technique (used primarily in unconscious patients). **Rationale:** Airway obstructions can result from posterior displacement of the tongue and epiglottis.
   d. Remove any foreign substances from the mouth. **Rationale:** Removal ensures that objects will not be advanced farther into the airway, thus decreasing the chance of creating a partial or complete obstruction.

Implementation

Steps	Rationale	Special Considerations
1. Wash hands; don exam gloves.	Reduces transmission of microorganisms; universal precautions.	Goggles, glasses, and/or face masks are worn in the presence of copious secretions.
2. Ask the patient to open his or her mouth or open mouth using the crossed-finger technique (Fig. 1–3).	Provides access to oral cavity. Provides leverage to open a tightly closed mouth.	*Caution:* Use great care to prevent injury to your fingers should patient be having a seizure.
3. Insert oral airway.		
a. Hold oral airway with curved end up (Fig. 1–4*A*).	Provides patent upper airway and prevents posterior tongue displacement.	Remove the airway immediately if the patient gags, gasps for air, or begins breathing irregularly.
b. Advance oral airway over the base of the tongue until the flange is parallel with the patient's nose.	Positions airway appropriately.	A tongue depressor may assist in tongue control during insertion.
c. Rotate the tip 180 degrees; the tip should be pointed down (Fig. 1–4*B*).	Provides for open pathway from the mouth to the pharynx.	
4. Recheck the size and position of the oral airway.	Proper placement and size are essential for securing and maintaining a patent airway.	When the oral airway is properly sized, the flange should rest against the patient's lips (see Fig. 1–2). Gagging may indicate that the airway is too long.

Table continues on following page

Steps	Rationale	Special Considerations
5. *Consider* securing the airway.	Taping is indicated to prevent expulsion of airway. *Not* taping is indicated in situations where the patient needs to be able to cough out the airway if he or she begins to gag to prevent stimulation of vomiting and aspiration (i.e., postanesthesia or semiconscious patient).	Note individual institutional policies. Use care not to tape over air channel.
6. Suction secretions if needed.	Maintains patent airway; pooled secretions provide a medium for bacterial growth.	Universal precautions. Use of goggles, glasses, and/or face masks.
7. Reassess patient's respiratory status.	Validates the effectiveness of the oral airway.	
8. Discard gloves in appropriate receptacle.	Reduces transmission of microorganisms. Universal precautions.	
9. Wash hands.	Reduces transmission of microorganisms.	
10. Reposition the oral airway every 1 to 2 hours.	Pressure of the flange on the lips may produce ulcers and necrosis.	Apply water-soluble jelly, petrolatum, or lip balm to the lips to prevent mucosal drying and cracking.
11. Provide meticulous mouth care every 4 to 8 hours or as needed.	Prevents secretion encrustations, mouth infections, and airway port occlusions.	
12. Remove the oral airway every 24 hours or as needed, clean, and reinsert.	Allows for inspection of the lips and oral cavity and enables complete oral hygiene.	

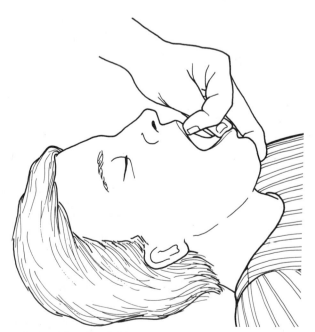

FIGURE 1–3. Crossed-finger technique for opening the mouth. (Reproduced with permission from L. D. Kersten, *Comprehensive Respiratory Nursing: A Decision-Making Approach.* Philadelphia, Saunders, 1989, p. 631.)

Evaluation

Compare patient's vital signs and respiratory assessment before and after the procedure. **Rationale:** Identifies patient response to oral airway insertion.

Expected Outcomes

1. Improvement of respiratory status as evidenced by respiratory rate between 8 and 20 breaths per minute, bilateral breath sounds and decreased cyanosis, unlabored breathing patterns, and lack of gurgling in the throat. **Rationale:** Cleared airways allow for better gas exchange.

2. Short-term patent airway. **Rationale:** Oral airway reduces the incidence of anatomic displacement of the tongue and soft tissues and facilitates removal of tracheobronchial secretions.

Unexpected Outcomes

1. Airway obstruction. **Rationale:** Inappropriate airway sizes can cause impaction of the epiglottis into the larynx if too large and aspiration of the oral device into the airway if too small (Eubanks and Bone, 1990).

2. Pulmonary aspiration. **Rationale:** Inappropriate patient positioning, copious secretions, and gagging promote further movement of secretions, foreign bodies, and solids into the lower airways.

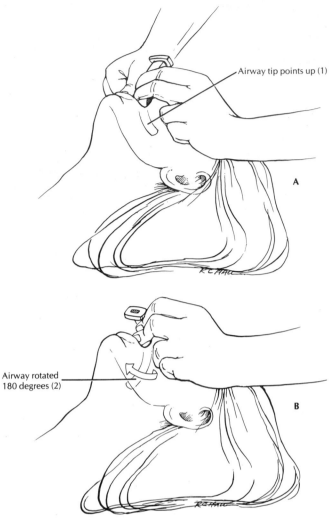

Airway tip points up (1)

A

Airway rotated
180 degrees (2)

B

FIGURE 1–4. **Insertion of an oropharyngeal airway. (A) Advance airway with curved end up. (B) Rotate airway 180 degrees. (Reproduced with permission from D. H. Eubanks and R. C. Bone, *Comprehensive Respiratory Care: A Learning System*, 2d Ed. St. Louis, Mosby, 1990, p. 551.)**

3. Trauma to the lips and oral cavity. **Rationale:** Improper or rough insertion techniques can result in tooth damage or loss, and lacerations to the roof of the mouth. Improper lip, mouth, and tube care can result in pressure sores, cracked lips, and stomatitis.

4. Inability to insert oral airway. **Rationale:** Combative and seizing patients may be difficult to control, or the nurse may be unable to open the patient's mouth.

Documentation

Documentation in the patient record should include respiratory and vital signs assessments before and after procedure; size of oral airway; nursing care given; expected and unexpected outcomes; date, time, and frequency with which the procedure is performed. **Rationale:** Documents nursing actions and patient responses; serves as a legal document of the series of events.

Patient/Family Education

1. Evaluate patient's need for long-term airway maintenance. **Rationale:** Oropharyngeal airways are generally used for temporary maintenance (Eubanks and Bone, 1990; Kersten, 1989).

2. Assess level of understanding of patient and significant others regarding condition and rationale for oropharyngeal airway insertion. **Rationale:** Identification of misconceptions regarding patient's condition, necessity for airway insertion, predicted outcomes, and potential risks allows for additional communication and clarification.

3. Provide frequent communication to patient and significant others regarding patient's condition and progress. **Rationale:** Communication regarding patient's condition, prognosis, progress, and expected outcome is cited as an important need of patients and families (Hickey, 1990; Viner, 1988).

Performance Checklist
Skill 1–1: Insertion of Oropharyngeal Airway

Critical Behaviors	Complies	
	yes	no
1. Wash hands; don gloves.		
2. Open patient's mouth.		
3. Insert oral airway.		
4. Recheck oral airway size and position.		
5. Secure oral airway.		
6. Suction secretions as needed.		
7. Reassess patient.		
8. Discard gloves.		
9. Wash hands.		

Table continues on following page

Critical Behaviors	Complies	
	yes	no
10. Document procedure in patient record.		
11. Reposition oral airway every 1 to 2 hours.		
12. Provide mouth care every 4 to 8 hours.		
13. Remove and clean oral airway every 24 hours.		

SKILL 1–2

Insertion of Nasopharyngeal Airway

The nasopharyngeal airway is a flexible piece of rubber. It is passed through the nose and follows the posterior nasal and oropharyngeal walls to the base of the tongue (Fig. 1–5). The nasopharyngeal airway is most commonly used to facilitate pulmonary toileting in the postanesthesia recovery period and in those situations when the patient is semiconscious. Insertion of the nasopharyngeal airway in an alert patient may stimulate the gag reflex, causing retching and vomiting. The advantages of the nasopharyngeal airway include increased comfort and tolerance in the conscious and pediatric patient, stable airway positioning for long periods of time, decreased incidence of gag-reflex stimulation, ability of insertion in clenched-jaw situations, and minimal incidence of mucosal trauma during frequent suctioning. The nasopharyngeal airway has three parts: flange, cannula, and bevel (tip) (see Fig. 1–5). The flange is the wide, trumpet-like end that prevents further slippage into the airway. The hollow shaft of the cannula permits airflow into the hypopharynx. The bevel, or tip, is the opening at the distal end of the tube. When properly inserted, the tip can be seen resting posterior to the base of the tongue (Fig. 1–6). A nasopharyngeal airway is *contraindicated* when the patient has a history of taking warfarin or heparin, if the patient is prone to epistaxis, if the patient has obstructed nasal passageways, or in the event of facial or head trauma where basilar skull fracture or cranial vault communication is suspected.

Purpose

The nurse inserts a nasopharyngeal airway to

1. Maintain a patent airway to the hypopharynx.
2. Provide for long-term maintenance of an airway.
3. Facilitate removal of tracheobronchial secretions.
4. Avert tissue trauma associated with repeated suctioning.
5. Relieve airway obstruction, especially in mandibular-type injuries that result in jaw immobility and/or soft-tissue obstruction, i.e., jaw wiring, trismus, pain, edema, jaw spasms, or mechanical impairment such as temporomandibular joint fractures and zygomatic fractures (Gotta, 1988).
6. Facilitate passage of a fiberoptic bronchoscope (selected occasions).
7. Tamponade small bleeding blood vessels in the nasal mucosa (selected occasions).

Prerequisite Knowledge and Skills

Prior to inserting a nasopharyngeal airway, the nurse should understand

1. Principles of aseptic technique.

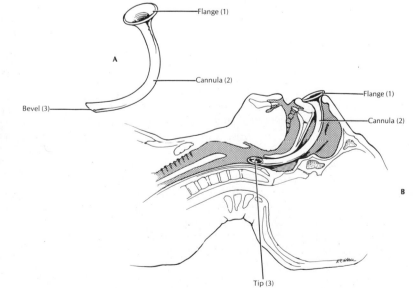

FIGURE 1–5. Nasopharyngeal airways: (A) airway parts, (B) proper placement. (Reproduced with permission from D. H. Eubanks and R. C. Bone, *Comprehensive Respiratory Care: A Learning System*, 2d Ed. St. Louis, Mosby, 1990, p. 548.)

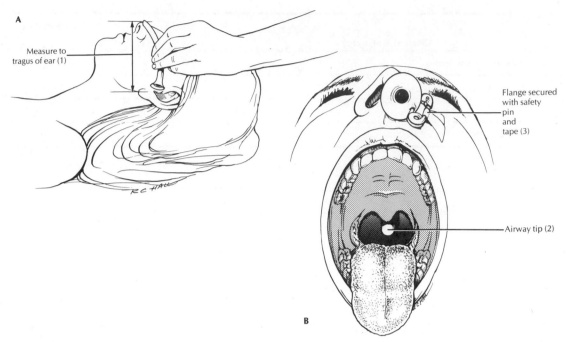

FIGURE 1–6. *(A)* Estimating nasopharyngeal airway size. *(B)* Nasopharyngeal airway position after insertion. (Reproduced with permission from D. H. Eubanks and R. C. Bone, *Comprehensive Respiratory Care: A Learning System*, 2d Ed. St. Louis, Mosby, 1990, p. 552.)

2. Anatomy and physiology of the upper and lower airways.
3. Principles of airway resistance.
4. Concepts of fear and anxiety.
5. Proper insertion technique

The nurse should be able to perform

1. Proper handwashing technique (see Skill 35–5).
2. Universal precautions (see Skill 35–1).
3. Vital signs assessment.
4. Respiratory assessment (inspection, palpation, percussion, and auscultation).
5. Maneuvers necessary to open the airway (i.e., head tilt, chin tilt, and jaw thrust).
6. Oxygen administration via face mask, hood, or cannula (see Skills 2–1 and 2–2).
7. Suctioning technique (see Skill 1–3).

Assessment

1. Observe for signs and symptoms of upper airway compromise or obstruction, including stridor, crowing, gasping respirations, snoring, and gurgling with respiratory cycle (definitive signs); tachycardia, or irregular pulse rate and diaphoresis (early signs); and bradycardia, especially in the pediatric population, circumoral cyanosis, diminished or absent breath sounds, chest excursion, hypoxemia, PaO_2 less than 60 mmHg, and unconsciousness (late signs). **Rationale:** Partial or complete obstruction of the upper airway can diminish or impede gas flow to the lower airway, which is evidenced by physical signs and symptoms.
2. Observe for signs and symptoms of inadequate breathing patterns, including dyspnea, shallow respirations, and intercostal and suprasternal retractions. **Rationale:** Respiratory distress is a late sign of upper airway obstruction.
3. Estimate the size of patient's external naris opening. **Rationale:** Allows the nurse to "narrow down" a range of airway sizes (Table 1–2).

Special Considerations During Assessment

Patients at increased risk for the development of upper airway obstruction include patients sustaining head, neck, or maxillofacial trauma, and infants, children, elderly, and adults with colds or influenza, loss of consciousness, coma, seizure disorders, neuromuscular disease, and secretory tumors of the upper airway.

Nursing Diagnoses

1. Impaired gas exchange related to partial or complete airway obstruction. **Rationale:** Nasal and/or upper airway obstruction can diminish or impede forward gas flow to the lower airway.
2. Ineffective airway clearance related to retained secretions. **Rationale:** Secretions, especially mucoid in

TABLE 1–2 NASOPHARYNGEAL AIRWAY SIZING

Approximate Body Weight	Size, mm
<100 lbs	5–6 (small)
101–150 lbs	7–8 (medium)
>151 lbs	9–10 (large)

character, are sticky and tend to accumulate along the upper airway, resulting in a potential for partial or complete obstruction.

3. Potential for infection related to retained secretions. **Rationale:** Nasal airway device prevents normal sinus drainage. Pooled secretions provide an ideal medium for organism growth.

4. Potential for injury to the nasal and hypopharyngeal mucosa from repeated suction catheter passes. **Rationale:** Repeated irritation can result in mucosal edema, bleeding, and loss of ciliary function.

Planning

1. Individualize the following goals for inserting a nasopharyngeal airway.
   a. Secure and maintain a patent airway. **Rationale:** Optimal airway management includes prevention of partial and complete occlusion.
   b. Facilitate removal of secretions. **Rationale:** Retained secretions increase the potential for airway obstruction and pulmonary infections. *Special consideration:* Aging results in a diminishing mucociliary clearance.

2. Prepare all necessary equipment and supplies. **Rationale:** Assembly of all the necessary equipment and supplies facilitates quick and safe insertion of the nasopharyngeal airway.
   a. Appropriately sized nasal airway (see Table 1–2). The external diameter of the nasopharyngeal airway should be slightly smaller than the patient's external naris opening. The length of the nasopharyngeal airway is determined by measuring the distance between the naris and the tip of the ipsilateral earlobe and adding 1 in. (2.5 cm) (Fig. 1–7). **Rationale:** Inappropriately sized nasopharyngeal tube may result in increased airway resistance, limited airflow (tube too small), kinking and mucosal trauma, gagging, vomiting, and gastic distension (tube too large). *Special consideration:* Some manufacturers provide nasopharyngeal airways shaped specifically for the right and left nares.
   b. Exam gloves.
   c. Water-soluble lubricant.
   d. Tape.
   e. Safety pin (large).
   f. Suction equipment.
   g. Flashlight.

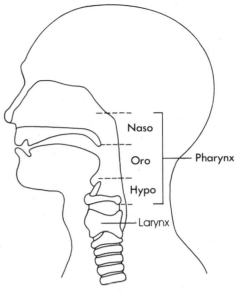

FIGURE 1–7. Anatomy of the upper respiratory tract. (Reproduced with permission from D. H. Dail, Anatomy of Respiratory System, in K. M. Moser and R. G. Spragg (Eds.), *Respiratory Emergencies*, 2d Ed. St. Louis, Mosby, 1982.)

   h. Tongue depressor.
   i. Cotton swabs and topical anesthetic (optional).

3. Prepare the patient and family.
   a. Explain the purpose of the airway and the necessity of the procedure to conscious patients and/or to the family of the unconscious patient. **Rationale:** Communication and explanation for therapy are cited as an important need of patients and families (Parker et al., 1984; Viner, 1988); relieves anxiety and encourages communication.
   b. Position patient. Unless contraindicated, a supine or high Fowler's position is acceptable. **Rationale:** Promotes patient and nurse comfort and provides easy access to external nares.
   c. Identify a patent nasal passageway. With finger pressure, occlude one nostril. Feel for air movement under the open nostril. Patency also can be assessed by inspection with a flashlight of each naris. **Rationale:** Promotes smooth, quick, unobstructed airway insertion.
   d. Remove loose-fitting dentures and any foreign objects from the mouth. **Rationale:** Removal ensures that objects will not be advanced farther into the airway during insertion.

Implementation

Steps	Rationale	Special Considerations
1. Wash hands; don exam gloves.	Reduces transmission of microorganisms; universal precautions.	For copious secretions don goggles, glasses, and/or face masks.
2. Prepare the nasopharyngeal airway.		
a. Inspect for smooth edges.	Decreases chances of mucosal trauma during insertion.	
b. Generously lubricate the tip and outer cannula with water-soluble lubricant.	Decreases incidence of trauma by preventing friction against dry mucosal membrane.	
3. Remove excess secretions from naris.	Allows for visual inspection of naris; removes possible source of obstruction; removes medium source for organism growth.	Nasopharyngeal and nasotracheal suctioning are contraindicated in patients with actual or potential maxillofacial and skull injuries.
4. (Optional) For anticipated difficult insertion (i.e., nasal polyps, septal deviation), apply topical anesthetic to cotton swabs, insert as far as possible, and coat the nasal passageway.	Topical anesthetics with a vasoconstrictor help shrink nasal mucosa and decrease incidence of trauma and bleeding. Vasoconstrictor property acts on capillaries to decrease bleeding.	Check institutional policies, or check with physician or pharmacist for topical anesthetic usage and indications.
5. Gently slide airway into nostril. Guide it medially and downward along the nasal passageway.	Following the natural contour of the nasal passageway decreases incidence of trauma.	If resistance is encountered, rotate the tube and continue gentle forward pressure. *Do not* force should resistance continue. Withdraw tube and try the other nostril. While inserting, if the patient experiences increasing dyspnea and respiratory embarrassment, consider removal of the tube.
6. Verify patency of airway. Feel for air movement over the flange. Auscultate breath sounds bilaterally.	Optimal airway positioning allows for forward gas flow, removal of secretions, and possible prevention of airway occlusion.	The conscious patient will need to exhale with his or her mouth closed.
7. Ask patient to open mouth or hold patient's mouth open. Control tongue with a tongue depressor. Illuminate oral cavity and visualize tip of nasopharyngeal airway behind uvula (see Fig. 1–6).	Verifying location of airway in pharynx verifies proper airway positioning. Allows for inspection of posterior pharynx for excessive bleeding or mucus.	
8. Secure airway with a safety pin through the flange and tape in place (see Fig. 1–6).	Minimizes dislodgement, removal, and deeper penetration into the nasopharynx.	Make sure the safety pin remains closed to avoid pricking and trauma.
9. Suction secretions as needed.	Maintains patent airway.	Recheck flange for proper position.
10. Reassess patient's respiratory status.	Indicates effectiveness of the nasal airway.	
11. Discard gloves in appropriate receptacle.	Reduces transmission of microorganisms. Universal precautions.	
12. Wash hands.	Reduces transmission of microorganisms.	
13. Remove and clean nasal airway daily. If possible, alternate nostrils every 24 hours.	Allows for inspection of external naris and part of the nasal cavity. Removes accumulated secretions and microorganisms. Prevents pressure necrosis.	

Evaluation

Compare patient's respiratory status before and after nasal airway insertion. **Rationale:** Identifies patient response to nasopharyngeal airway insertion.

Expected Outcomes

1. Improvement of respiratory status as evidenced by respiratory rate between 8 and 20 breaths per minute, unlabored breathing patterns, and lack of gurgling, stridor, crowing, snoring, and gasping respirations. **Rationale:** Cleared airways allow for forward gas flow.

2. Long-term patent airway. **Rationale:** Artificial airway maintains patency from external naris to hypopharynx.

3. Diminished mucosal edema/trauma related to frequent suction passes. **Rationale:** Nasopharyngeal airway insertion reduces mucosal irritation (Eubanks and Bone, 1990; Kersten, 1989; Miracle and Allnutt, 1990).

Unexpected Outcomes

1. Inability to pass nasopharyngeal airway. **Rationale:** Nasopharyngeal edema, septal deviations, and enlarged turbinates/polyps may obstruct passageway.

2. Airway obstruction. **Rationale:** Inappropriate airway sizes can result in kinking of tube, mucosal trauma and edema, gagging, vomiting, and possibly gastric aspiration.

3. Head and/or ear pain. **Rationale:** Nasal airway placement predisposes patient to sinusitis and otitis media. Communication of the right and left eustachian tube and sinuses with the nasopharynx allows for direct microorganism migration.

4. Epistaxis. **Rationale:** Bleeding can occur with dry mucosal tissue or mucosal blood vessel injury during insertion.

5. Naris and nasal mucosal ulceration. **Rationale:** Pressure necrosis results from improper positioning and lack of continual care.

Documentation

Documentation in the patient record should include respiratory and vital signs assessment before and after procedure; size of nasopharyngeal airway; nursing care given; expected and unexpected outcomes; date, time, and frequency with which procedure is performed. **Rationale:** Documents nursing actions and patient responses; serves as a legal document of the series of events.

Patient/Family Education

1. Assess level of understanding of patient and significant others regarding condition and rationale for nasopharyngeal airway. **Rationale:** Identification of misconceptions regarding patient's condition, necessity for airway insertion, predicted outcomes, and potential risks allows for additional communication and clarification.

2. Frequently communicate to patient and significant others the patient's condition, progress, prognosis, and expected outcomes. **Rationale:** Frequent updates regarding patient condition, progress, prognosis, and expected outcomes are cited as important needs of patients and families (Hickey, 1990; Viner, 1988).

Performance Checklist
Skill 1–2: Insertion of Nasopharyngeal Airway

Critical Behaviors	Complies	
	yes	no
1. Wash hands; don gloves.		
2. Prepare nasal airway: a. Inspect airway. b. Lubricate airway.		
3. Remove secretions from naris.		
4. (Optional) Apply topical anesthetic.		
5. Insert nasal airway.		
6. Verify airway patency.		
7. Verify proper airway position.		
8. Secure nasal airway.		
9. Suction secretions as needed.		
10. Reassess patient's respiratory status.		
11. Discard gloves.		
12. Wash hands.		
13. Document procedure in patient record.		
14. Remove and clean airway daily.		

SKILL 1–3

Oropharyngeal and Nasopharyngeal Suctioning

Oropharyngeal and nasopharyngeal suctioning is indicated in patients who cannot mobilize secretions in the upper airway, i.e., pharynx, nasal cavity, and larynx (see Fig. 1–7). Suctioning of the pharynx is also indicated prior to endotracheal and tracheostomy tube cuff deflation to prevent aspiration of secretions into the lower respiratory tract (see Skill 1–6).

Emphasis on suctioning techniques is important to minimize the complications of hypoxia and mucosal injury (Jung and Gottlieb, 1976), i.e., atelectasis, mucus stasis, and mucosal hemorrhage and erosion (Table 1–3).

Purpose

The nurse performs oropharyngeal and nasopharyngeal suctioning to

1. Remove excess oral and nasal secretions.
2. Prevent pulmonary aspiration of oral and nasal secretions, blood, and gastric fluids.
3. Stimulate cough reflex.

TABLE 1–3 TECHNICAL CONSIDERATIONS REGARDING SUCTIONING

Technique	Rationale
1. Suction "as needed" rather than on a routine basis.	Unnecessary and repeated episodes result in subatmospheric intrapulmonary pressure, increase the risk of atelectasis, and cause airway trauma.
2. Suction duration is less than 15 seconds.	Decreases incidence of severe hypoxemia.
3. Preoxygenate prior to each suction pass.	Decreases incidence of severe hypoxemia.
4. Rest 2 to 3 minutes prior to each suction pass.	Provides time for oxygen to flow through airways; promotes patient comfort.
5. Apply intermittent negative suction upon catheter withdrawal.	Suction application during advancement increases the risk of panic reactions, mucosal trauma, and hypoxemia. Continuous suctioning increases the incidence of mucosal stripping.
6. Withdraw catheter slowly in a continuous, rotating effort.	Decreases the incidence of mucosal invagination into the catheter ports.
7. Select appropriate catheter size and length.	Decreases hypoxemia and mucosal trauma; assists in effective secretion removal.

Prerequisite Knowledge and Skills

Prior to oropharyngeal and nasopharyngeal suctioning, the nurse should understand

1. Principles of aseptic technique.
2. Anatomy and physiology of the upper and lower airways.
3. Principles of airway management.
4. Principles of airway resistance.
5. Principles of gas exchange.
6. Principles of coughing.
7. Proper suction technique.

The nurse should be able to perform

1. Proper handwashing technique (see Skill 35–5).
2. Universal precautions (see Skill 35–1).
3. Vital signs assessment.
4. Respiratory assessment (inspection, palpation, percussion, and auscultation).
5. Oxygen administration via face mask, hood, or nasal cannula (see Skills 2–1 and 2–2).
6. Oral and nasal airway insertion (see Skills 1–1 and 1–2).
7. Cardiopulmonary assessment.

Assessment

1. Observe for signs and symptoms of upper airway compromise or obstruction, including stridor, crowing, gasping respiration, snoring, and gurgling with respiratory cycle (definitive signs); tachycardia or irregular pulse rate and diaphoresis (early signs); and bradycardia, circumoral cyanosis, diminished or absent breath sounds, chest excursion, hypoxemia, PaO_2 less than 60 mmHg, and unconsciousness (late signs). **Rationale:** Partial or complete obstruction of the upper airway can diminish or impede gas flow to the lower airway, which is evidenced by physical signs and symptoms.

2. Observe for signs and symptoms of inadequate breathing patterns, including dyspnea, shallow respirations, and intercostal and suprasternal retractions. **Rationale:** Respiratory distress is a late sign of upper airway obstruction.

3. Assess patient's ability to cough up secretions. **Rationale:** Impaired cough reflex may be present during postoperative recovery period or as a result of lung disease, retained excessive lung secretions, central nervous system depression, lung cancer, neuromuscular disease, lung surgery, presence of an artificial airway, and immobility.

Nursing Diagnoses

1. Ineffective airway clearance related to retained secretions. **Rationale:** Secretions, especially mucoid in character, are sticky and tend to accumulate along the upper airway, creating a potential for partial or complete airway obstruction.

2. Ineffective airway clearance related to diminished cough reflex. **Rationale:** Altered ability to deep breathe and clear mucus occurs with chest and postoperative

pain, anesthesia, sedative and analgesic therapy, immobility, severe obstructive lung disease, oral and nasal airway placement, and central nervous system disease.

Planning

1. Individualize the following goals for performing oropharyngeal and nasopharyngeal suctioning:
   a. Establish and maintain a patent airway. **Rationale:** Retained secretions provide for potential partial or complete airway obstruction.
   b. Facilitate removal of airway secretions. **Rationale:** Removal of secretions reduces the risk of partial or complete airway obstruction.
   c. Prevent mucus stasis. **Rationale:** Generation of effective cough reflex assists in the mobilization of secretions.
2. Prepare all necessary equipment and supplies. **Rationale:** Assembly of equipment and supplies promotes adherence to aseptic technique and facilitates quick and efficient completion of oropharyngeal and nasopharyngeal suctioning. Institutions may have prepackaged suction kits that contain many of these items.
   a. Portable or wall suction apparatus.
   b. Connecting tube, 6 ft.
   c. Sterile suction catheters.
   d. One sterile and one nonsterile glove (or 2 sterile gloves, see institutional policies).
   e. Sterile cup with sterile water or normal saline, approximately 100 ml.
   f. Sterile towel or drape.
   g. Water-soluble lubricant.
   h. Self-inflating resuscitation bag connected to oxygen flowmeter at 15 L/min.
   i. Oropharyngeal and/or nasopharyngeal airway device.
3. Prepare the patient and family.
   a. Explain the purpose and necessity of oropharyngeal and nasopharyngeal suctioning to conscious patient or to family of unconscious patients. **Rationale:** Communication and explanation for therapy encourage cooperation, minimize risk and anxiety, and are an important need of patients and families (Parker et al., 1984; Viner, 1988).
   b. Position patient. Unless contraindicated, in a semi-Fowler's. **Rationale:** Promotes comfort, provides easy access, and decreases incidence of gastric secretion aspiration.
   c. Explain the importance of coughing and deep breathing to patient and family. **Rationale:** Coughing facilitates the mobilization of secretions.

Implementation

Steps	Rationale	Special Considerations
1. Wash hands.	Reduces transmission of microorganisms.	
2. Turn on suction apparatus and set vacuum regulator to appropriate negative pressure.	Significant hypoxia and mucosal damage can result from excessive negative pressure.	

	Wall setting mmHg	Portable setting inches of H_2O
Infant under 1 yr.	60–80	3–5
Child 1–8 yrs.	80–120	5–10
Adult	120–150	10–15
Over 75 yrs.	80–120	5–10

(Eubanks and Bone, 1990; Kacmarek, Mack, and Dimas, 1990)
Suction manometer setting for recommended amounts of negative pressure.

Steps	Rationale	Special Considerations
3. Select appropriately sized suction catheter.	Correct size allows for easy, safe insertion.	
a. Straight catheter is generally recommended for oropharyngeal and nasopharyngeal suctioning.	Is less traumatic to insert.	*Do not* use catheters with Aero-flo O-shaped tip for nasal insertion. Aero-flo O-shaped catheter tips can impede nasal insertion (Fig. 1–8).
b. Select appropriate catheter diameter.	Atelectasis and hypoxemia occur with catheters that are too large.	For infants/newborns use a bulb syringe. Specific steps regarding bulb-syringe manipulation can be found in Perry and Potter (1985).
	Airway resistance is increased with catheters that are too small (Rindfleisch and Tyler, 1983).	General recommendations

	Catheter size
Children under 10 yrs.	10 (French)
Adults	14 (French)
Over 75 yrs.	10 (French)

Table continues on following page

Steps	Rationale	Special Considerations
4. Secure one end of connecting tube to suction machine and place the other end in a convenient location within reach.	Prepares suction apparatus.	
5. Open sterile catheter package on a clean surface using the inside of the wrapping as a sterile field.	Prepares catheter and prevents transmission of microorganisms.	
6. Set up the sterile solution container or sterile basin on the sterile field. Be careful not to touch the inside of the container. Fill with approximately 100 ml of normal saline or sterile water.	Maintains sterility.	Prepackaged suction kits may be used. Check institutional preferences.
7. Open lubricant and squeeze onto sterile catheter package without touching package.	Maintain sterility while preparing the lubricant.	
8. Provide 3 hyperinflation, hyperoxygenation breaths with a bag valve mask connected to a manual resuscitation bag attached to 100% oxygen.	Decreases the incidence of hypoxemia.	Hyperinflation and hyperoxygenation should be carried out prior to *each* suction pass.
9. Don sterile glove.	Allows nurse to maintain sterility. Protects nurse against herpetic whitlow and cross-contamination among patients (Kersten, 1989).	In the event that one nonsterile glove is used, apply the nonsterile glove to the nondominant hand and the sterile glove to the dominant hand. Handle all nonsterile items with the nondominant hand.
10. Pick up suction catheter, being careful to avoid touching the nonsterile surfaces. With the nondominant hand, pick up connecting tubing and secure the suction catheter to the connecting tubing.	Maintains catheter sterility.	The dominant hand should not come into contact with the connecting tubing.
11. Check equipment for proper functioning by suctioning a small amount of sterile saline from the container.	Validates equipment function.	
12. Coat the distal 6 to 8 cm of catheter with water-soluble lubricant.	Provides ease of catheter insertion.	
13. Leave catheter air vent open.	Decreased tissue trauma, hypoxemia, and anxiety during catheter advancement.	
14. For suctioning:		
a. Nasopharyngeal approach:	*Note:* Because nasopharynx is considered cleaner than oropharynx, it should be suctioned first.	
(1) Identify patent nasal passageway (see Skill 1–2).	Promotes smooth, quick, unobstructed airway insertion.	
(2) Gently insert the catheter through the patent nostril, guiding it medially and downward along the passageway (use same technique when going through nasopharyngeal airway) (see Skill 1–2).	Incidence of trauma is decreased when the natural contour of the nasal passageway is followed.	*Do not* apply suction during catheter advancement.

Table continues on following page

Steps	Rationale	Special Considerations
b. Oropharynx approach:		
(1) Gently insert catheter into mouth and advance catheter tip 3 to 4 in. into secretions of the pharynx. When an oropharyngeal Berman-type tube is used, suction catheter is advanced down either side channel. With a Guedel-type tube, the suction catheter is advanced through the central passageway (see Fig. 1–1).	Positions catheter in the oropharynx.	*Do not* apply suction during catheter advancement.
(2) For infants and small children, a bulb syringe is used to suction the upper airway.	Exerts gentle, controlled pressure, which minimizes mucosal trauma.	
15. Slowly withdraw the suction catheter while rotating it back and forth between dominant thumb and forefinger. Apply intermittent suction of the air vent during withdrawal.	Continuous suction can cause severe hypoxemia and mucosal trauma (Sackner et al., 1973; Czarnik et al., 1991).	
16. Rinse catheter and connecting tubing with sterile water or saline.	Promotes patent suctioning channel. Prevents blockage of suction catheter. Minimizes colonization of the respiratory tract from the connecting tube setup (Cunningham and Sergent, 1983).	
17. Suction both sides of mouth and pharynx.	Secretions coughed up may pool in mouth.	
18. Repeat steps 14 through 17 to clear oropharynx and nasopharynx.	Promotes removal of additional secretions.	Provide 1 to 2 minutes of rest and when necessary supplemental oxygen between passes. Hyperoxygenation and hyperinflation should be carried out between passes.
19. Monitor patient's ECG tracing and heart rate between suction passes.	Aspirated volume at the catheter tip can result in laryngospasms and/or hypoxemia, which may lead to dysrhythmias.	
20. Dispose of catheter and gloves.	Reduces transmission of microorganisms.	
a. Coil catheter around fingers of dominant hand. Pull glove off inside out with catheter coiled inside. Pull off other glove in the same manner.		
b. Discard into appropriate receptacle.	Universal precautions.	
21. Reposition patient.	Provides comfort; communicates caring attitude.	
22. Reassess patient's respiratory status.	Indicates need for artificial airway or emergency intervention.	
23. Discard remainder of supplies in appropriate receptacle.	Reduces transmission of microorganisms. Universal precautions.	
24. Wash hands.	Reduces transmission of microorganisms.	

Table continues on following page

Steps	Rationale	Special Considerations
25. Dispose of suction cannisters and connecting tubing every 24 hours and set up new system.	Decreases incidence of organism colonization and subsequent pulmonary contamination.	Check individual institutional policies.

Evaluation

Compare patient's respiratory status and vital signs assessment before and after suctioning. **Rationale:** Identifies the effects of suctioning.

Expected Outcomes

1.   Removal of secretions in the upper airway. **Rationale:** Patient breathes easier as cleared airways allow for forward gas flow.

2.   Improvement of respiratory status, as evidenced by respiratory rate between 8 and 20 breaths per minute and lack of gurgling, stridor, crowing, snoring, and gasping respirations. **Rationale:** Cleared airways allow for forward gas flow.

3.   Patient coughs up secretions. **Rationale:** Sudden blast of expelled air mobilizes large-airway secretions.

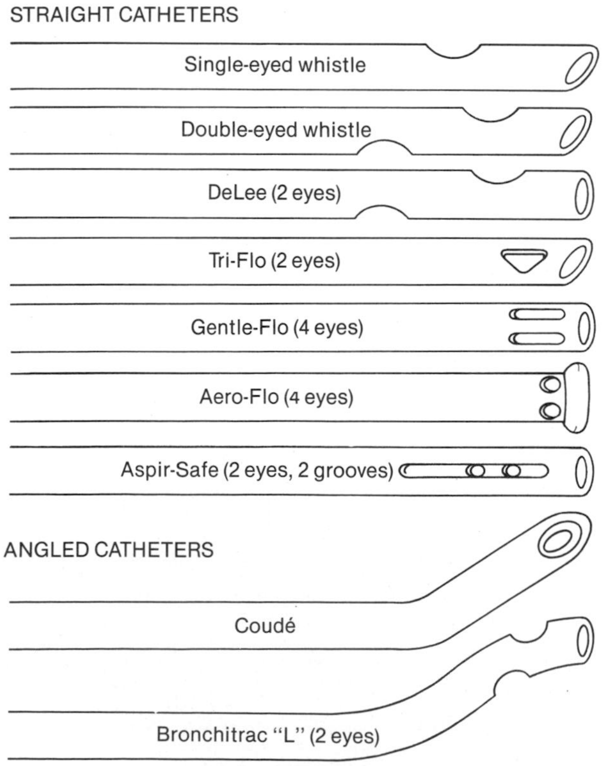

Unexpected Outcomes

1.   Atelectasis. **Rationale:** Repeated suction passes causes a subatmospheric intrapulmonic pressure which when severe results in segmental atelectasis.

2.   Bloody secretions. **Rationale:** Continuous suctioning upon catheter withdrawal can cause the catheter tip to denude the ciliated epithelial mucosa, resulting in mucosal hemorrhage and erosions (Sackner et al., 1973).

3.   Pneumonia. **Rationale:** Multiple catheter passes increase the incidence of bacterial colonization.

4.   Hypoxemia. **Rationale:** Extension and repeated suction passes increase the chance for hypoxemia, which results in cardiac-induced problems, e.g., tachycardia, irregular rhythms, and bradycardia.

5.   Inability to pass suction catheter. **Rationale:** Mucosal edema, foreign objects, soft tissue, and encrusted secretions may present as a partial or complete obstruction.

Documentation

Documentation in the patient record should include respiratory, cardiac, and vital signs assessment before and after procedure; type and size of suction catheter used; nursing care given; expected and unexpected outcomes; date, time, and frequency with which procedure is performed; and color, odor, amount, and description of secretions. **Rationale:** Documents nursing actions and patient responses; serves as a legal document of the series of events.

Patient/Family Education

1.   Assess level of understanding of patient and significant others regarding condition and rationale for suctioning. **Rationale:** Identification of misconceptions regarding patient's condition, necessity for suctioning, predicted outcomes, and potential risks allows for additional communication and clarification.

2.   Frequently communicate to patient and significant others the patient's condition, progress, prognosis, and expected outcomes. **Rationale:** Frequent updates regarding patient condition, prognosis, progress, and expected outcomes are cited as important needs of patients and families (Hickey, 1990; Viner, 1988).

STRAIGHT CATHETERS

Single-eyed whistle

Double-eyed whistle

DeLee (2 eyes)

Tri-Flo (2 eyes)

Gentle-Flo (4 eyes)

Aero-Flo (4 eyes)

Aspir-Safe (2 eyes, 2 grooves)

ANGLED CATHETERS

Coudé

Bronchitrac "L" (2 eyes)

FIGURE 1–8. Types and distal-tip configurations of straight and angled suction catheters. (Reprinted with permission from L. D. Kersten, *Comprehensive Respiratory Nursing: A Decision-Making Approach*. Philadelphia, Saunders, 1989, p. 689.)

Performance Checklist
Skill 1–3: Oropharyngeal and Nasopharyngeal Suctioning

Critical Behaviors	Complies yes	no
1. Wash hands.		
2. Turn on suction apparatus and set vacuum regulator.		
3. Select catheter.		
4. Secure connecting tube to suction machine.		
5. If appropriate, open sterile catheter.		
6. Set up sterile solution container.		
7. Open lubricant.		
8. Provide for hyperinflation and hyperoxygenation.		
9. Don gloves.		
10. Pick up suction catheter.		
11. Check equipment functioning.		
12. Lubricate catheter.		
13. Select catheter approach.		
14. Insert catheter into pharynx.		
15. Apply intermittent suction upon withdrawal.		
16. Rinse catheter and connecting tubing.		
17. Suction both sides of mouth and pharynx.		
18. Monitor ECG tracing.		
19. Repeat steps 14 through 17 of skill.		
20. Dispose of gloves.		
21. Reposition patient.		
22. Discard supplies.		
23. Reassess patient.		
24. Wash hands.		
25. Document procedure in patient record.		
26. Discard suction cannisters and connecting tubing every 24 hours.		

SKILL 1–4

Tracheobronchial Suctioning

Tracheobronchial suctioning is indicated in the presence of audible lower airway secretions, crackles, and wheezes in the chest. Also referred to as *blind tracheal suctioning*, it is used in the management of tracheobronchial secretions prior to more aggressive and invasive methods of tracheobronchial secretion removal such as endotracheal intubation and suctioning. Other management techniques include turning, coughing, and deep breathing and are encouraged prior to lower airway secretion removal.

Suctioning damages tracheal epithelium (Czarnik et al., 1991; Flunk, 1985; Landa et al., 1980; Plum and Dunning, 1956; Rosen and Hillard, 1962). The degree of damage is influenced by the continuous or intermittent application of negative suction. One study indicated that continuous suctioning resulted in hemorrhage, edema, and ulceration, whereas intermittent suctioning resulted in moderately damaged mucosa, minimal edema, and no ulceration (Plum and Dunning, 1956). Since both methods cause damage, the use of *routine suctioning* (suctioning every one to two hours) is contraindicated (Kersten, 1989; Czarnik et al., 1991). The number of suction passes should be kept to a minimum, with the need for each pass carefully evaluated (see Table 1–3).

In either case, tracheobronchial suctioning may be anxiety provoking and induce life-threatening dysrhythmias, initiate hypoxemia, and promote bacterial colonization.

Purpose

The nurse performs nasal and/or oral tracheal suctioning to

1. Maintain a patent lower airway by removing secretions.
2. Stimulate deep cough reflex.
3. Obtain sputum specimens.
4. Prevent pulmonary aspiration of blood and gastric fluids.

Prerequisite Knowledge and Skills

Prior to nasal and/or oral tracheal suctioning, the nurse should understand

1. Principles of aseptic technique.
2. Anatomy and physiology of the upper and lower respiratory system.
3. Principles of gas exchange.
4. Principles of airway resistance.
5. Indications for suctioning.
6. Contraindications for suctioning.
7. Principles of coughing.
8. Principles of airway management.
9. Proper suctioning technique.

The nurse should be able to perform

1. Proper handwashing technique (see Skill 35–5).
2. Universal precautions (see Skill 35–1).
3. Vital signs assessment.
4. Respiratory assessment (inspection, palpation, percussion, and auscultation).
5. Oxygen administration techniques (see Skills 2–1 and 2–2).
6. Oral and nasal airway insertion (see Skills 1–1 and 1–2).
7. Oral and nasal pharyngeal suctioning techniques (see Skill 1–3).

Assessment

1. Observe for signs and symptoms of lower airway obstruction, including presence of audible secretions, crackles and wheezes, tachycardia or irregular pulse rate, and diaphoresis (early signs); and bradycardia, circumoral cyanosis, restlessness, diminished breath sounds, decreasing level of consciousness, PaO_2 less than 60 mmHg, and $PaCO_2$ greater than 45 mmHg (late signs). **Rationale:** Partial or complete obstruction of the lower airway can diminish or stop gas flow to the bronchopulmonary segments of the right and left lungs.
2. Observe patient for contraindications of tracheobronchial suctioning, including refractory hypoxemia, irritable myocardium evidenced by cardiac dysrhythmias, severe hypertension, and increased intracranial pressure. **Rationale:** Prolonged suctioning diminishes oxygen supply, disrupts normal ventilation, and in the presence of fragile pathologic conditions, may lead to worsening or irreversible states.
3. Observe for signs and symptoms of inadequate breathing patterns, including dyspnea, shallow respirations, and intercostal and suprasternal retractions. **Rationale:** Respiratory distress is a late sign of lower airway obstruction.
4. Assess the need for repeated suctioning. **Rationale:** Repeated suctioning of tracheobronchial tree results in subatmospheric intrapulmonic pressure and predisposes patient to segmental and lobular atelectasis.
5. Observe for signs of atelectasis, including decreased breath sounds on auscultation, increasing peak inspiratory pressure, localized dullness to percussion, decreased compliance, decreased PaO_2, and localized consolidation on chest radiograph. **Rationale:** Suctioning techniques, hypoventilation, and conditions resulting in airway obstruction are amenable to nursing interventions (Goodnough et al., 1986).

Nursing Diagnoses

1. Ineffective airway clearance related to retained secretions. **Rationale:** Secretions, especially mucoid in nature, are sticky and tend to accumulate along upper and lower airways, creating a potential for partial or complete airway obstruction.
2. Ineffective airway clearance related to diminished cough reflex. **Rationale:** Altered ability to deep breathe and clear mucus occurs with chest and postoperative pain, anesthesia, sedative and analgesic therapy, immobility, severe obstructive lung disease, airway placement, and central nervous system disease.
3. Impaired gas exchange related to accumulation of related secretions. **Rationale:** Secretions hinder forward gas flow and diffusion across alveolar membrane.

Planning

1. Individualize the following goals for performing tracheobronchial suctioning:
   a. Establish and maintain a patent airway. **Rationale:** Retained secretions provide for potential partial or complete airway obstruction, inhibiting forward gas flow to bronchopulmonary segments of the right and left lungs.
   b. Facilitate removal of airway secretions. **Rationale:** Removal of secretions reduces the chances for partial or complete airway obstruction.
   c. Promote optimal oxygenation. **Rationale:** Suctioning removes secretions, which improves oxygenation.

d. Collect uncontaminated tracheobronchial specimen. **Rationale:** Tracheobronchial specimens decrease the likelihood for salivary contamination and inaccurate laboratory results.

2. Prepare all necessary equipment and supplies. **Rationale:** Assembly of equipment and supplies facilitates quick and efficient completion of tracheobronchial suctioning. *Note:* Institutions may have prepackaged suction kits that contain most of these supplies.
   a. Sterile disposable suction catheters of appropriate size.
   b. One sterile glove and one nonsterile glove or two sterile gloves (see institutional policy).
   c. Sterile cup with sterile water or normal saline, approximately 100 ml.
   d. Portable or wall suction apparatus.
   e. Connecting tube, 6 ft.
   f. Sterile towel or drape.
   g. Water-soluble lubricant.
   h. Oropharyngeal and/or nasopharyngeal airway device.
   i. Oxygen delivery systems, including self-inflating resuscitation bag connected to oxygen flowmeter at 15 L/min (see Skill 4–2).
   j. Goggles, glasses, and mask.

3. Prepare the patient and family.
   a. Explain the purpose and necessity of tracheobronchial suctioning. **Rationale:** Communication and explanation for therapy encourage cooperation, minimize risk and anxiety, and are an important need of patients and families (Parker et al., 1984; Viner, 1988).
   b. Position patient in semi-Fowler's position, head neutral, and choose patent naris. **Rationale:** Promotes general relaxation, oxygenation, and ventilation; reduces stimulation of gag reflex and risk of aspiration; encourages catheter advancement toward the trachea.

4. Prepare for additional personnel to assist with hyperoxygenation and hyperinflation preoxygenation. **Rationale:** Two hands are necessary to properly activate the self-inflating resuscitation bag. "Double teaming" reduces the incidence of unintentional extubation (Pesiri et al., 1990).

Implementation

Steps	Rationale	Special Considerations
1. Wash hands.	Reduces transmission of microorganisms.	
2. Turn on suction apparatus and set vacuum regulator to appropriate negative pressure.	Excessive negative pressures may lead to microatelectasis around the catheter tip.	Suction manometer setting for recommended amounts of negative pressure.

	Wall setting mmHg	Portable setting inches of H_2O
Infant under 1 yr.	60–80	3–5
Child age 1–8 yrs.	80–120	5–10
Adult	120–150	10–15
Over 75 yrs.	80–120	5–10

(Eubanks and Bone, 1990; Kacmarek, Mack, and Dimas, 1990)

Steps	Rationale	Special Considerations
3. Select appropriate style and size of suction catheter.	Allows for easy insertion. Atelectasis and hypoxemia occur with catheters that are too large. Airway resistance is increased with catheters that are too small (Rindfleisch and Tyler, 1983).	Catheter diameter, general recommendations

	Catheter size
Newborn/infant 18 mos.	6–8 (French)
Children	10–12 (French)
Adult	12–16 (French)
Over 75 yrs.	10–14 (French)

Steps	Rationale	Special Considerations
a. Straight catheter, soft red rubber, is generally preferred for tracheostomy suctioning (see Fig. 1–8).	Soft tip produces less mucosal trauma.	
b. Angled catheters increase the chance for successful passes to the left mainstem bronchus (see Fig. 1–8).	The left mainstem bronchus continues off the trachea at about a 40- to 60-degree angle.	When advanced down through the trachea, the Bronchitrac L-angled catheter automatically enters the left mainstem bronchus.

Table continues on following page

Steps	Rationale	Special Considerations
4. Secure one end of connecting tube to suction machine and place the other end in a convenient location within reach.	Prepares suction apparatus.	
5. Open sterile catheter package on a clean surface using the inside of the wrapping as a sterile field.	Prepares catheter and prevents transmission of microorganisms.	
6. Set up the sterile solution container or sterile basin on the sterile field. Be careful not to touch the inside of the container. Fill with approximately 100 ml of normal sterile saline or sterile water.	Prepares catheter flush solution.	Unwrap and open suction kit, if used in institution, according to package instructions.
7. Open lubricant and squeeze onto sterile catheter package without touching package.	Maintains sterility.	
8. Hyperoxygenate and hyperventilate the patient:		
a. Insert nasal prong into patent nostril and/or position oxygen mask over the mouth (see Skill 2–2).	Decreases incidence of hypoxemia.	
b. If conscious, ask the patient to begin slow, deep breathing	Assists in drawing oxygen into lungs.	Continue for 2 to 3 minutes.
c. If the patient is unable to assist, ask additional person to hold and help seal the oxygen mask to the patient's nose and mouth and hold the patient's hand.	Caring touch provides reassurance; protective touch prevents the patient from grabbing at the suction catheter (Estabrooks, 1989).	
9. Don gloves. Apply nonsterile gloves to nondominant hand and sterile glove to dominant hand.	Protects against cross-contamination among patients.	Handle nonsterile items with the nondominant hand.
10. Pick up suction catheter, being careful to avoid touching the nonsterile surfaces. With the nondominant hand, pick up connecting tubing. Secure the suction catheter to the connecting tubing.	Maintains catheter sterility.	Dominant hand should not come into contact with connecting tubing.
11. Check equipment for proper functioning by suctioning a small amount of sterile saline from the container.	Validates equipment function.	
12. Coat the distal 6 to 8 cm of catheter with water-soluble lubricant.	Provides ease of catheter insertion.	
13. With nondominant hand, remove oxygen delivery device (assistant can do this).	Allows for catheter entrance into nose or mouth.	
14. Advance catheter into the pharynx:		
a. Advance through the nose, inferiorly and medially.	Helps to avoid catheter coiling in mouth.	*Do not* force catheter.
b. As catheter passes down the back of the nasopharynx, ask patient to stick out tongue.	Helps to visualize catheter location.	*Do not* apply suction during insertion, since chances for tracheal mucosal or tearing are increased.
15. Advance catheter into tracheobroncheal tree:		

Table continues on following page

Steps	Rationale	Special Considerations
a. Continue to advance 1 to 2 inches (2.5 to 5 cm) with each inspiration in a downward slant until obstruction is met or the catheter tip stimulates a cough. Upon cough, quickly slide catheter into the trachea. Provide patient reassurance when cough/gag reflex is stimulated.	Glottis is open during inspiration. Gag reflex stimulation can increase anxiety.	General guidelines for insertion depths Adults — 20–24 cm Children — 14–20 cm Infants — 8–14 cm
b. Listen briefly for breath sounds at catheter air vent valve prior to applying suctioning.	Verifies tracheal entry, especially in the absence of cough reflex.	
c. To advance catheter into the left bronchus, turn patient's head to the right while inserting.	Decreases the angle from the trachea into lung.	
d. To advance catheter into the right bronchus, turn patient's head to the left while inserting.	Allows for quick, smooth catheter advancement.	Right mainstem bronchus appears as a short extension of the trachea with a 25-degree angle on the vertical axis.
16. Occlude air-vent valve intermittently with dominant hand and withdraw catheter in one smooth, uninterrupted motion, rotating the catheter between thumb and forefinger of dominant hand.	Allows secretions to be drawn up into catheter while minimizing tracheal mucosal tearing.	*Do not* apply suction for longer than 5 seconds at any one time for a total time of up to 15 seconds.
17. Allow patient to rest. Provide hyperinflation and hyperventilation breaths between suction attempts; return to step 8 using an assistant as necessary.	Recovery to baseline PaO_2 takes 1 to 5 minutes.	
a. When possible, resting can occur with the suction catheter near the epiglottis.	Eliminates need for repeated upper airway advancement and reduces incidence of mucosal trauma.	
b. Should catheter need to be withdrawn, rinse catheter and connecting tubing until cleared with sterile saline or water.	Patients experiencing hypoxemia and unbearable discomfort will need complete catheter withdrawal.	
18. Repeat steps 15 through 17 to clear trachea of secretions.	Maintains patent airway.	Allow 2 to 3 minutes between suction catheter passes.
19. Monitor patient's ECG tracing and heart rate throughout suction passes.	Aspirated volume at the catheter tip can result in laryngospasms and in hypoxemia induced dysrhythmias.	
20. When the tracheobronchial tree is cleared of secretions, perform oral and nasopharyngeal suctioning (see Skill 1–3).	Clears upper airway secretions. This sequence allows suctioning to be carried from a sterile to nonsterile area.	
21. To dispose of catheter and gloves, coil catheter around fingers of dominant hand, pull glove off inside out with catheter coiled inside, and pull off other glove in the same manner.	Reduces transmission of microorganisms.	
22. Reposition patient.	Promotes comfort; communicates caring attitude.	
23. Discard remainder of supplies in appropriate receptacle.	Reduces transmission of microorganisms. Universal precautions.	
24. Wash hands.	Reduces transmission of microorganisms.	

Table continues on following page

Steps	Rationale	Special Considerations
25. Reassess patient's respiratory status.	Determines need for artificial airway or emergency intervention.	
26. Dispose of suction cannisters and connecting tubing every 24 hours and set up new system.	Decreases incidence of organism colonization and subsequent pulmonary contamination.	Check individual institutional policies.

Evaluation

Compare patient's respiratory status and vital signs assessment before and after suctioning. **Rationale:** Identifies the effects of suctioning.

Expected Outcomes

1. Removal of obvious upper airway secretions and lower airway secretions. **Rationale:** Patient breathes easier as cleared airways allow for improved gas exchange.
2. Improved respiratory status, as evidenced by respiratory rate between 8 and 20 breaths per minute, lack of audible secretions, bronchial fremitus, circumoral cyanosis, and improving level of consciousness, normalization of heart rate, and increased depth of respiration. **Rationale:** Cleared airways allow for forward gas flow and reduce the work of breathing.
3. Patient coughs up secretions. **Rationale:** Sudden blasts of expelled air mobilize large-airway secretions.

Unexpected Outcomes

1. Hypoxemia. **Rationale:** Repeated suctioning causes subatmospheric intrapulmonic pressure, which can result in atelectasis, hypoxia, and cardiopulmonary compromise.
2. Bloody secretions. **Rationale:** Continuous suctioning upon catheter withdrawal can cause denuding of the ciliated epithelial mucosa, resulting in mucosal hemorrhage and erosion (Sackner et al., 1973).
3. Pneumonia. **Rationale:** Multiple catheter passes increase the incidence of bacterial colonization.
4. Inability to pass catheter. **Rationale:** Mucosal edema, foreign objects, soft tissue swelling, and en-

crusted secretions may present as a partial or complete obstruction.

Documentation

Documentation in the patient record should include respiratory, cardiac, and vital signs assessment before and after suctioning; act of suctioning; routes used to suction; type and size of catheter used; amount, color, consistency, and odor of secretions obtained; patient's response to suctioning; expected and unexpected outcomes; date, time, and frequency with which suctioning is performed. **Rationale:** Documents nursing actions and patient responses; serves as a legal document of the series of events.

Patient/Family Education

1. Assess level of understanding of patient and significant others regarding condition and rationale for suctioning. **Rationale:** Identification of misconceptions regarding patient's condition, necessity for suctioning, predicted outcomes, and potential risks allows for additional communication and clarification, as well as reduction of patient/family anxiety.
2. Frequently communicate to patient and significant others the patient's condition, progress, prognosis, and expected outcomes. **Rationale:** Frequent updates regarding patient condition, prognosis, progress, and expected outcomes are cited as important needs of patients and families (Hickey, 1990; Viner, 1988).

Performance Checklist
Skill 1–4: Tracheobronchial Suctioning

Critical Behaviors	Complies	
	yes	no
1. Wash hands.		
2. Turn on suction apparatus and set vacuum regulator.		
3. Select catheter.		
4. Secure connecting tube to suction machine.		
5. If appropriate, open sterile catheter.		
6. Set up sterile solution container.		
7. Open lubricant.		

Table continues on following page

Critical Behaviors	Complies	
	yes	no
8. Hyperoxygenate and hyperinflate.		
9. Don gloves.		
10. Pick up suction catheter.		
11. Check equipment functioning.		
12. Lubricate catheter.		
13. Remove oxygen delivery device.		
14. Advance catheter into pharynx.		

15. Advance catheter into tracheobroncheal tree:
  a. Advance 1 to 2 in (2.5 to 5 cm) with inspiration.
  b. Assess breath sounds.
  c. Advance to left bronchus.
  d. Advance to right bronchus.		

16. Apply intermittent suction.		
17. Allow for resting and reoxygenation.		
18. Repeat steps 14 or 15 through 17.		
19. Monitor patient's cardiac status.		
20. Perform oral and nasopharyngeal suctioning.		
21. Dispose of catheter and gloves.		
22. Reposition patient.		
23. Discard all supplies.		
24. Wash hands.		
25. Reassess respiratory status.		
26. Document procedure in patient record.		
27. Discard suction cannisters and connecting tubing every 24 hours.		

SKILL 1–5

Endotracheal Intubation and Tube Care

Endotracheal intubation is considered for conditions or problems leading to respiratory failure (Table 1–4). Intubation is performed only as an alternative to more conservative methods of establishing an airway and has been tolerated without sequelae for up to 3 weeks (Stauffer et al., 1981).

The terminology of endotracheal intubation originates from the technique involving placement of the tube under direct visualization through the vocal cords. If the route of intubation is through the mouth, it is called *oral tracheal intubation*, and the tube is referred to as an *orotracheal tube*. If intubation is carried out through the nose, it is called *nasal tracheal intubation*, and the tube is referred to as a *nasotracheal tube*. The advantages and disadvantages of orotracheal versus nasotracheal intubation are summarized in Table 1–5.

The most widely used type of endotracheal tube is made of soft plastic (polyvinyl chloride, PVC) or silicone rubber, is disposable, and is designed for one-time use. The tube material contains plasticizers for flexibility, heat stabilizers to affect thermolability, color pigments, and antioxidants to decrease the deterioration due to constant

TABLE 1–4 INDICATIONS FOR TRACHEAL INTUBATION

Cardiopulmonary arrest
Trauma (especially head, neck, and chest)
Cardiovascular impairment (strokes, tumors, infection, emboli, trauma)
Neurologic impairment (drugs, poisons, myasthenia gravis)
Pulmonary impairment (infections, tumors, pneumothorax, COPD, trauma, pneumonia, poisons)
Surgery requiring general anesthesia

TABLE 1–5 ADVANTAGES AND DISADVANTAGES OF OROTRACHEAL VERSUS NASOTRACHEAL INTUBATION

	Advantages	Disadvantages
Orotracheal intubation	Easier and quicker to perform, and the patient usually requires less sedation. Avoids nasal and paranasal complications associated with nasal intubation. Permits passage of a larger-diameter tube, which in turn decreases turbulent airflow, decreases airway resistance, and increases V_A. Large diameter facilitates secretion management and passage of a fiberoptic bronchoscope. Oral tube permits deeper tracheal suctioning because it usually is shorter than a nasal tube. Oral tubes tend to kink less than nasal tubes.	May not be possible in patients with limited neck mobility. Oral tube is less stable and less comfortable for the patient. More nursing supervision may be necessary to monitor the patient and prevent accidental extubation. Limits access to the mouth for oropharyngeal hygiene. Impairs ability to swallow and communicate. Patients tend to gag more. May stimulate increased salivation, which tends to loosen the tape securing the tube and contribute to pooling of secretions above the cuff.
Nasotracheal intubation	Once in place, the nasal tube causes less discomfort and anxiety than the orotracheal tube. Leaves the mouth more accessible for oropharyngeal hygiene. The patient is likely to demonstrate fewer oral complications and to gag less. Stable position of tube permits increased patient activity with less risk of accidental extubation. Permits swallowing of secretions and small amounts of liquid and communication through use of the lips. May cause less laryngeal injury and fewer posterior glottic ulcers than an oral tube. Reasons are related to the nasal tube's smaller diameter. Also, with its straighter alignment in the throat, it centers better in the glottis and hence exerts less pressure on the posterior glottis.	Nasotracheal intubation is more difficult to perform than orotracheal intubation. May cause nasal hemorrhage during insertion and purulent nasal discharge or sinusitis after several days. Smaller-diameter tube may be necessary for passage through the nares. The nares require a smaller diameter than the larynx. Increased airway resistance and decreased V_A may result from the nasal tube's small diameter, its tendency to accumulate encrusted secretions, and its tendency to kink. Longer tube length may limit the depth and extent of tracheal suctioning of secretions. It also may contribute to increased airway resistance.

Source: Reproduced by permission from L. Kersten, *Comprehensive Respiratory Nursing: A Decision-Making Approach*. Philadelphia, Saunders, 1989, p. 640.

oxygen flow (Berlauk, 1986). The parts of an endotracheal tube are shown in Figure 1–9. The proximal end of the tube is that part which exits the mouth or nose. It has a standard 15-mm "male" adapter (universal adapter) that connects the endotracheal tube to either a resuscitation bag, a mechanical ventilator, or other respiratory devices. The shaft is the long, hollow, curved passageway that allows for gas flow and connects proximal and distal tube ends. Depth markings, usually in centimeters, help the caregiver to gauge and maintain the tube's position. The shaft usually has a radiopaque line that extends to the distal tip. This assists in tip location during radiographic procedures. The bevel is the opening at the distal end of the tube that facilitates tube insertion. The angle of the bevel is generally 45 degrees for oral tubes and 30 degrees for the nasal tubes. The hole adjacent to the bevel, Murphy's eye, ensures (left and right directional) airflow at the carina. The cuff is an inflatable "balloon" at the distal end of the tube.

When inflated with air, it presses against the tracheal walls to prevent air leakage from the lungs and aspiration from the stomach (see Skill 1–6). The pilot balloon indicates the presence of air in the cuff. It is useful in determining whether or not the cuff-inflating system is intact. The one-way valve allows for air to be injected, with a syringe into the cuff. There are three classifications for endotracheal tube size: the Magill and the French (which are becoming obsolete), and the metric. The metric system measures the tube's *internal* diameter and is regarded as the modern sizing method (Eubanks and Bone, 1990). Sizes range from 2.5 mm (newborns) to 11.5 mm (large adults). In children under eight years of age, uncuffed endotracheal tubes are recommended, as the circular narrowing of the cricoid cartilage serves as a "functional" cuff. A guide for selecting the correct endotracheal tube size from children to adults is found in Table 1–6. A quick "rule of thumb" guide for selecting tube size is to select a tube with an *outside* diameter that

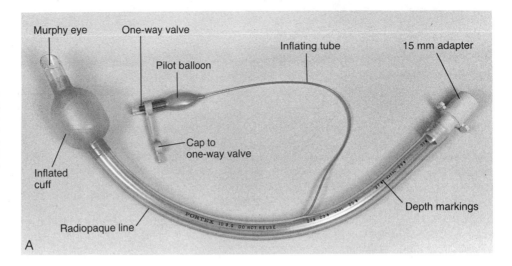

FIGURE 1–9. Parts of endotracheal tube (soft-cuffed tube by Smiths Industries Medical Systems, Co., Valencia, Calif.). (Reproduced with permission from L. D. Kersten, *Comprehensive Respiratory Nursing: A Decision-Making Approach*. Philadelphia, Saunders, 1989, p. 637.)

matches the diameter of the patient's little finger (Eubanks and Bone, 1990).

Purpose

The nurse performs endotracheal intubation to

1. Maintain airway patency.
2. Protect the airway from aspiration.
3. Facilitate the clearance of secretions.
4. Initiate positive-pressure mechanical ventilation.
5. Facilitate ventilation and oxygenation.
6. Provide a route for emergency medications (i.e., naloxone, epinephrine, lidocaine, atropine).

The nurse performs endotracheal tube care to

1. Prevent buccal, oropharyngeal, and tracheal mucosa trauma from the tube and the cuff.
2. Provide oral hygiene.
3. Promote ventilation.

TABLE 1–6   GUIDE FOR ENDOTRACHEAL TUBE SIZES, INFANT TO ADULT

Age	Internal (Tube) Size, mm
Premature	2.5*
Newborn	3.0*
6 months	3.5*
18 months	4.0*
3 years	4.5*
5 years	5.0*
6 years	5.5*
8 years	6.0*
12 years	6.5
16 years (small adults)	7.0
Small adult builds	7.5–8.0
Average adult builds	8.0–8.5
Large adult builds	8.5–9.0
Very large adult builds	10.0–11.5

*Indicates cuffless endotracheal tube is recommended.

Prerequisite Knowledge and Skills

Prior to performing endotracheal tube intubation and care, the nurse should understand

1. Principles of aseptic technique.
2. Anatomy and physiology of the respiratory system.
3. Principles of airway resistance.
4. Physical properties with regard to airflow and artificial airway diameter.
5. Principles of gas exchange.
6. Indications for intubation.
7. Complications of intubation.
8. Concepts of anxiety and fear.
9. Verbal and nonverbal communication strategies.
10. Principles of chest radiograph interpretation.
11. Principles of arterial blood gas analysis.
12. Principles of ventilator management.

The nurse should be able to perform

1. Proper handwashing technique (see Skill 35–5).
2. Universal precautions (see Skill 35–1).
3. Vital signs assessment.
4. Respiratory assessment (inspection, palpation, percussion, and auscultation).
5. Maneuvers necessary to open the airway (i.e., head tilt, chin tilt, and jaw thrust).
6. Oxygen administration (see Skills 2–1 and 2–2) and ventilation via manual resuscitator bag (see Skill 4–2).
7. Basic cardiopulmonary life support.
8. Confirmation of endotracheal tube placement.
9. Measurement of tube cuff pressure (see Skill 1–7).
10. Endotracheal suctioning (see Skill 1–6).
11. Nasopharyngeal and oropharyngeal suctioning (see Skill 1–3).
12. Oral hygiene.
13. Oral and nasal airway and bite-block insertion (see Skills 1–1 and 1–2).

Assessment

Intubation

1. Observe for signs and symptoms of respiratory compromise and failure, including tachypnea, dyspnea, central cyanosis, restlessness, confusion, agitation, and tachycardia (definitive signs); shallow respirations, chest-abdominal dyssynchrony, asterixis, headache, lethargy, apnea, and rising arterial blood pressure (early signs); and atrial and/or ventricular dysrhythmias, bradycardia and/or falling arterial blood pressure, adventitious breath sounds, respiratory and/or metabolic acidosis, physical evidence of vomitus, hypoxemia, PaO_2 less than 60 mmHg, $PaCO_2$ greater than 50 mmHg, and pH less than 7.30 (late signs). **Rationale:** Physical signs and symptoms result when there is a problem with oxygenation and ventilation. The lungs are unable to meet the metabolic demands of the body.
2. Assess patient's ability to mobilize secretions. **Rationale:** Impaired cough reflex may be present during postoperative recovery period, lung disease, retained lung secretions, central nervous system depression, lung cancer, neuromuscular disease, lung surgery, presence of artificial airway, and immobility.
3. Identify the need for premedication. **Rationale:** Medications sedate agitated patients, provide temporary paralysis, and reduce salivation and bronchial secretions. Adequate sedation decreases the likelihood of unintentional extubation (Pesiri et al., 1990).

Endotracheal Tube Care

Observe for signs and symptoms requiring endotracheal tube care, including excessive secretions; soiled ties or tape; biting or kinking of the tube; pressure areas to the naris, corner of mouth, or tongue; loose ties; and tube riding in and out of mouth. **Rationale:** Pooled secretions provide a medium for microorganism growth. Soiled ties are a source for microorganism growth, are unsightly, and convey lack of oral hygiene. Pressure areas occur when capillaries within the mucosa are subjected to constant pressure and trauma. Loose ties allow for accidental extubation.

Nursing Diagnoses

Intubation

1. Ineffective airway clearance related to retained secretions. **Rationale:** Secretions, especially mucoid in nature, are sticky and tend to accumulate along upper and lower airways, creating a potential for partial or complete airway obstruction.
2. Ineffective airway clearance related to diminished cough reflex. **Rationale:** Altered ability to deep breathe and clear mucus occurs with chest and postoperative pain, anesthesia, sedative and analgesic therapy, immobility, severe obstructive lung disease, airway placement, and central nervous system disease.
3. Potential for suffocation related to airway obstruction and mechanical inability to ventilate. **Rationale:** Physical signs and symptoms result when gas flow is impeded.

Endotracheal Tube Care

1. Potential for injury to orotracheal and nasotracheal mucosa related to endotracheal intubation. **Rationale:** Injury can result in mucosal bleeding, edema, and loss of ciliary function. Injury can occur with improper tube size and type. Nasal pressure sore formation is likely, since the nasal tube cannot be rotated from side to side and constant pressure impairs capillary blood flow. Common sites of pressure-induced injury include corners of mouth, naris opening, larynx, and tracheal wall.
2. Impaired gas exchange related to improper endotracheal tube placement. **Rationale:** Right mainstem bronchus intubation impairs left lung gas exchange.
3. Impaired verbal communication related to endotracheal tube placement. **Rationale:** The intubated awake patient will be unable to speak as the endotracheal tube passes between the vocal cords, when properly placed.
4. Potential for infection related to nasotracheal tube placement. **Rationale:** Nasotracheal intubation impairs sinus drainage, predisposing patient to sinusitis and otitis media.

Planning

Intubation

1. Individualize the following goals for performing endotracheal intubation.
   a. Establish and maintain a patent airway. **Rationale:** Intubation is performed as a last resort when conservative methods of airway management have failed (i.e., head tilt, chin tilt, jaw thrust, nasal and oropharyngeal airways).
   b. Facilitate removal of secretions. **Rationale:** Retained secretions increase the potential for airway obstruction, pulmonary, sinus, and ear infections, and are potential causes of partial or complete airway obstruction.
   c. Maintain sterile technique to test cuff and pilot balloon for patency. **Rationale:** Decreases the incidence of inserting a defective tube.

Endotracheal Tube Care

2. Individualize the following goals for endotracheal tube care.
   a. Maintain correct tube placement. **Rationale:** Unintentional extubation and tube manipulation can occur with ineffective restraining of tube and patient, inadequate securing of the tube, inadequate sedation, incorrect tube size and length, improper support of respiratory tubing, under-inflation of endotracheal cuff, and prolonged intubation (Pesiri et al., 1990).
   b. Prevent mucosal pressure sores. **Rationale:** Constant pressure and irritation of the mucosal tissue can result in capillary and cellular damage.
3. Prepare all necessary equipment and supplies. **Rationale:** Assembly of necessary equipment and sup-

plies facilitates quick and efficient endotracheal insertion. *Special considerations:* Remove headboard from bed. **Rationale:** Promotes easy access to the head of the patient.

INTUBATION

a. Soft-cuff endotracheal tube with 15-mm adaptor (standard).
b. Stylet. (Insert into selected tube, making sure stylet does not protrude from endotracheal tube tip.)
c. Laryngoscope handle. (Make sure batteries in handle are functional.)
d. Laryngoscope blades. Two types of blades in a variety of sizes are used, the MacIntosh (curved) and the Miller (straight). (Make sure the small lightbulb in the blade illuminates.)
e. Yankauer pharyngeal suction tip.
f. Topical anesthetic.
g. Luer-tip syringe (10 cc) for cuff inflation. (Fill syringe with 10 cc of air and attach to one-way valve of the pilot balloon.)
h. Portable or wall suction apparatus.
i. Self-inflating resuscitation bag with mask connected to 100% oxygen.
j. Oropharyngeal airway or bite block.
k. Tongue depressor.
l. Oxygen source and connecting tubes.
m. Suctioning equipment (see Skill 1–3).
n. Items for taping: one inch adhesive tape, tincture of benzoin, "skin" scissors or twill tape.
o. Swivel adapter.
p. Lubricant and/or Silicone spray.
q. Magill forceps.
r. Sterile gloves.

TUBE CARE

a. Suctioning equipment (see Skill 1–3).
b. Mouthwash with low alcohol content.
c. Soft toothbrush and toothpaste.
d. Toothette (sponge on a stick).
e. Twill tape.
f. Scissors.

4. Secure additional personnel to assist with endotracheal intubation and tube care. For *intubation*, at least three people are necessary: (1) person properly credentialed in intubation, (2) person to manage the airway, provide supplemental oxygen, and set up respiratory modalities for postintubation use, and (3) person to attend to patient needs, establish IV access, give medications, and assist with airway care. **Rationale:** Provides for a quick, safe, and possibly less traumatic insertion. For *tube care*, at least two persons are necessary: (1) person to activate the self-inflating resuscitation bag and stabilize endotracheal

tube, and (2) person to suction tube, provide oral care, and tape and secure tube. **Rationale:** Prevents inadvertent extubation (Goodnough et al., 1986). "Double teaming" decreases the likelihood of unintentional extubation (Pesiri et al., 1990).

5. Prepare the patient and family for intubation or tube care.
a. Position the patient for intubation. Patient should be supine with the head *slightly* extended and neck flexed. This is achieved by placing several towels under the patient's neck in order to elevate it a few inches above the bed. **Rationale:** When the head is placed in "sniffing" position, the mouth, pharynx, and trachea are aligned, and visualization of the larynx is accomplished (Fig. 1–10).
b. Position the patient for tube care. Position patient in a semi-Fowler's or supine position. **Rationale:** Promotes patient comfort and provides easy access for health care provider.
c. Explain the purpose and necessity of endotracheal intubation and/or tube care to both patient and family. **Rationale:** Communication and explanation for therapy encourage cooperation, minimize risk and anxiety, and are a continually stated patient and family need (Parker et al., 1984; Viner, 1988).
d. Premedicate patient as necessary. **Rationale:** Medication administration allows for a more controlled intubation and reduces the likelihood of laryngospasms, insertion trauma, and improper tube placement.

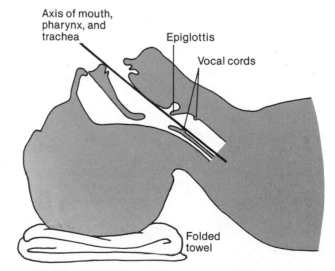

FIGURE 1–10. Neck hyperextension in the sniffing position aligns the axis of the mouth, pharynx, and trachea before endotracheal intubation. (Reprinted with permission from L. D. Kersten, *Comprehensive Respiratory Nursing: A Decision-Making Approach.* Philadelphia, Saunders, 1989, p. 642.)

Implementation

Steps	Rationale	Special Considerations
Intubation, General Setup		
1. Wash hands.	Reduces transmission of microorganisms.	
2. Insert oropharyngeal airway with nasotracheal intubation (see Skill 1–1).	Assists in upper airway patency.	
3. Connect Yankauer suction catheter to connecting tube.	Prepares for oropharyngeal suctioning.	
4. Suction oropharynx.	Removes secretions, diminishes patient's need to cough during the procedure, reduces incidence of aspiration.	
5. Using a self-inflating resuscitation bag with attached mask connected to 100% oxygen. Provide 3 hyperinflation (1½ × tidal volume), hyperoxygenation breaths.	Hyperoxygenation with hyperinflation protects against hypoxemia (Goodnough, 1985) (see Table 4–2).	Therapeutic bagging before and after endotracheal intubation and suctioning provides hyperinflation and/or supplemental oxygenation (Goodnough, 1985; Schumann and Parsons, 1985; Bostick and Wendelgass, 1987; Chulay, 1988).
6. Don gloves.	Reduces transmission of microorganisms.	
Orotracheal Intubation		
1. Open patient's jaw widely, using crossed-finger technique (see Fig. 1–3). Spray pharynx with topical anesthetic.	Provides access to oral cavity. Provides more leverage to open a tightly closed mouth. Topical anesthetic most often used with alert patients.	
2. With blade locked in place and light illuminated, grasp laryngoscope in the left hand.	Prepares for quick, efficient blade placement.	Intubation attempts must not last longer than 30 seconds in order to avoid further hypoxemia and/or cardiopulmonary arrest.
3. Insert the blade in the right side of mouth and advance it inward and toward midline past the base of the tongue (Fig. 1–11).	Displaces the tongue to the left and increases visualization of uvula and epiglottis (Fig. 1–12).	Avoid pressure on the lips and teeth.
4. Once the epiglottis is seen:		
a. *For straight blade:* Advance the blade tip just under the epiglottis and exert upward and outward (at 45-degree angle) traction on the laryngoscope handle.	Exposes the glottic opening.	*Do not* use the upper teeth as a fulcrum.
b. *For curved blade:* Advance blade tip into vallecula and exert upward and outward traction on the laryngoscope handle (Fig. 1–13).	Exposes the glottic opening.	*Do not* use the upper teeth as a fulcrum.
5. Lift laryngoscope handle until vocal cords are seen.	Identifies correct pathway for tube insertion.	Gentle cricoid pressure may aid in visualization of vocal cords and decrease incidence of gastric distension and pulmonary aspiration.
6. Grasp the endotracheal tube with right hand, curved part of tube downward.	Right hand is free to place tube; assists with easy passage.	

Table continues on following page

Steps	Rationale	Special Considerations
7. Gently pass the tube alongside the mouth, down to, and through the vocal cords (Fig. 1–14) until the cuff is no longer visible (Fig. 1–15).	Ensures proper placement of the endotracheal tube.	In infants under 6 months, pass tip of tube no more than 1 cm past cords.
8. Hold tube firmly in place with hand; withdraw laryngoscope; withdraw stylet.	Provides tube stabilization. Decreases incidence of inadvertent extubation (Goodnough et al., 1986).	
9. Inflate cuff according to manufacturer's recommendation (volumes generally vary from 5 to 10 ml) (see Skill 1–6).	Inflation volumes vary among manufacturers and different tube sizes. Mucosal ischemia occurs when lateral wall pressure exceeds capillary perfusion pressure, resulting in decreased mucosal blood flow.	*Keep inflating pressures less than 20 mmHg (24.5 cmH$_2$O). Arterial vessels occlude at 20 to 25 mmHg. Venous vessels occlude at 18 to 20 mmHg. Lymphatic channels occlude at 5 to 8 mmHg. These values are based on a normal arterial blood pressure. For infants and children 8 and under, endotracheal tubes are not cuffed (Table 1–6).*
10. Assess endotracheal tube placement during manual bagging.		
a. Auscultate lung bases and apices for bilateral breath sounds.	*Assists* in verifying correct tube placement.	
b. Inspect for bilateral symmetrical chest expansion.	Absence may indicate right mainstem bronchus intubation.	Improper insertion may result in gastric distension and/or vomiting.
c. Auscultate over epigastrium.	Assesses possible esophageal and/or gastric intubation.	
11. If unequal sounds are heard or are absent, deflate the cuff and		
a. Withdraw tube 1 to 2 cm.	In correct position, the tube tip should rest 5 cm above the carina (Kersten, 1989, p. 644). Right mainstem intubation is more common due to the anatomic position of the right mainstem bronchi.	Malpositioned endotracheal tube is defined as the tube tip less than 2 cm or greater than 8 cm above the carina (Goodnough et al., 1986).
b. Remove tube immediately if esophageal intubation is suspected (e.g., air leak, increasing abdominal distension, deteriorating arterial blood gases) and begin again with step 7.	Inappropriate tube placement in the esophagus diverts gas flow and increases hypoxemia.	
12. Secure endotracheal tube (as securing institutionally varies, check individual policy manual):		
a. Double over a 2-ft piece of twill tape. Tie tape around the tube, bringing frayed ends through the loop below the mark of tube emergence.	Decreases incidence of unintentional extubation (Pesiri et al., 1990).	Locate mark of emergence from mouth or naris; document for future tube placement. (Check the graduated markings on the tube's outer surface.)
b. Pull tape ends in opposite direction to circle around and behind neck.	Provides for circumferential securing of the tube.	
c. Gently pull tape to snug down against skin.	Decreases the incidence for tube movement.	Tincture of Benzoin applied to the skin directly under twill tape will help secure tape.

Table continues on following page

Steps	Rationale	Special Considerations
d. Tie in secure knot at side of patient's neck.	Secures tube.	Take care to make knot *snug* not *tight*. Tight ties may obstruct venous outflow.
13. Suction endotracheal tube (see Skill 1–9).	Removes secretions.	
14. Using swivel adapter, connect patient to humidified oxygen source or mechanical ventilator.	Adapter reduces motion of the tube in the patient's mouth and trachea. Decreases incidence of unintentional extubation (Pesiri et al., 1990).	
15. Discard supplies in appropriate receptacle.	Reduces transmission of microorganisms. Universal precautions.	
16. Wash hands.	Reduces transmission of microorganisms.	
17. Expedite chest radiograph.	Confirms and documents actual tube position.	
18. Check breath sounds.	Assists in determining tube location.	
Nasotracheal Intubation (Blind Technique)		
1. Follow steps 1 to 6 under *General Setup* and 1 to 6 under *Orotracheal Intubation*.	Initial steps necessary to initiate nasotracheal intubation.	
2. Insert nasotracheal tube into patient's nose parallel to hard palate.	Introduces tube into airway channel.	Withdraw tube and extend patient's head further if tube does not advance downward into the pharynx.
3. Advance the tube blindly until the sound of exhalation is at maximal intensity.	Tube is located just superior to the trachea.	
4. Continue to advance the tube during *inspiration*. Magill forceps may assist in this step.	Facilitates forward movement of the tube through the glottic opening. Endotracheal tubes manufactured with a ring pull at the proximal end of the tube assist curving the distal tube tip for ease of advancement.	
5. Follow steps 8 to 18 under *Orotracheal Intubation*.	Allows for completion of orotracheal intubation.	
Tube Care		
1. Wash hands.	Reduces transmission of microorganisms.	
2. Suction endotracheal tube and nasal or oral pharyngeal airway and oral cavity (see Skills 1–3 and 1–6).	Removes secretions. Suctioning the endotracheal tube prior to the pharyngeal area assists in decreasing cross contamination.	Maintaining the endotracheal tube free of secretions decreases the work of breathing (Habib, 1989).
3. Prepare twill tape. Cut 2-ft piece of tape and double over.	Ensures necessary supplies are available for quick execution of procedure.	
4. Don gloves.	Reduces transmission of microorganisms. Universal precautions.	
5. Remove oral airway or bite block.	Allows access to skin and mucosa for assessment and hygiene.	
6. Person 1 holds tube firmly in place while Person 2 cuts and removes soiled twill tape.	Allows for rotation of tube to opposite side of mouth. "Double teaming" decreases the incidence of	

Table continues on following page

Steps	Rationale	Special Considerations
	unintentional extubation (Pesiri et al., 1990).	
7. Clean mouth and gums with mouthwash solution or peroxide on sponge-tipped catheters.	Allows for assessment of skin and mucosa. Promotes oral hygiene and reduces risk of infection to oral mucosa and gums.	Avoid using lemon-glycerine swabs due to their drying effect on the mucosa.
8. Brush teeth and gums with gentle motion.	Promotes oral hygiene and reduces risk of infection to gums and tooth decay.	
9. Rotate orotracheal tube to opposite side of mouth.	Reduces incidence of pressure sore formation.	Be careful not to inadvertently adjust tube depth.
10. Repeat steps 7 and 8 of tube care on opposite side of mouth.		
11. Secure endotracheal tube with twill tape (see steps 11a and 11b under *Orotracheal Intubation*).	Decreases incidence of unintentional extubation (Pesiri et al., 1990).	Institutions may vary as to techniques used for taping.
12. Clean oral airway in warm soapy water and rinse well.	Promotes hygiene.	
13. Reinsert oral airway (see Skill 1–1).	Prevents occlusion of orotracheal tube.	May leave out if patient is not biting or fighting endotracheal tube.
14. Apply lubricant to lips.	Prevents drying, cracking, and excoriation.	
15. Discard supplies in appropriate receptacle.	Reduces transmission of microorganisms. Universal precautions.	
16. Wash hands.	Reduces transmission of microorganisms.	
17. Check breath sounds.	Ensures that the endotracheal tube is in the proper place.	

Evaluation

Compare patient assessment before and after intubation and tube care. **Rationale:** Identifies patient responses.

Expected Outcomes
Intubation and Tube Care

1. Artificial airway established. **Rationale:** Endotracheal tube is patent and secure.
2. Improvement in respiratory status, as evidenced by respiratory rate between 8 and 20 breaths per minute, even, deep, symmetrical chest expansion, PaO_2 between 80 and 100 mmHg, $PaCO_2$ between 35 and 45 mmHg, pH 7.35 to 7.45, and O_2 saturation at 95% or greater. **Rationale:** Proper oxygenation and ventilation assist in meeting the metabolic demands of the body.
3. Removal of secretions. **Rationale:** Lower-airway channel allows for hypopharyngeal secretion removal.
4. Inability to vocalize. **Rationale:** Endotracheal tube passes through the vocal cords, making verbal communication impossible. If the patient can talk with the tube in, the position is incorrect. Notify the physician immediately and prepare for re-intubation.
5. Secured and properly positioned endotracheal tube. **Rationale:** Intubation was executed successfully.

Unexpected Outcomes
Intubation and Tube Care

1. Prolonged apnea, increasing hypoxemia, and/or cardiopulmonary arrest. **Rationale:** Intubation procedure must be performed within 30 seconds.
2. Dislodged or broken teeth. **Rationale:** Improper techniques, where the upper and lower teeth are used as a fulcrum, may result in tooth and gum damage.
3. Accidental intubation of esophagus or right mainstem bronchus. **Rationale:** Improper insertion technique and tube mobility increase the likelihood of improper tube position.
4. Cardiac dysrhythmias. **Rationale:** Hypoxemia and vagal stimulation affect heart rate and rhythm.
5. Necrosis of oral and nasal mucosa. **Rationale:** Improper tube care and oral hygiene.

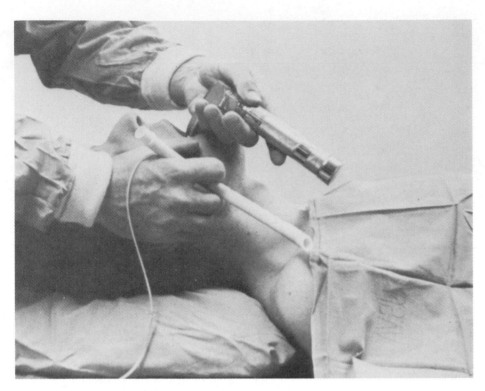

FIGURE 1–11. Technique of orotracheal intubation. Laryngoscope blade is inserted into oral cavity from right, pushing tongue to the left as it is introduced.

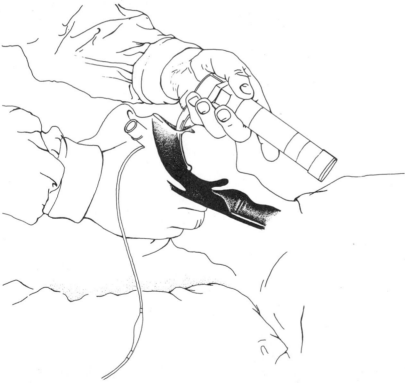

6. Unintentional extubation. **Rationale:** Failure to secure tube allows for dislodgement. Causative factors include improper patient sedation, ineffective patient restraints, inadequate securing devices, underinflation of cuff, and improper tubing support (Pesiri et al., 1990) (see also Table 1–7).

7. Leaking airway cuff. **Rationale:** Defective cuff de-

creases the effectiveness for airway management and/or mechanical ventilation and results in $\downarrow V_T$.

Documentation

Documentation in the patient record should include

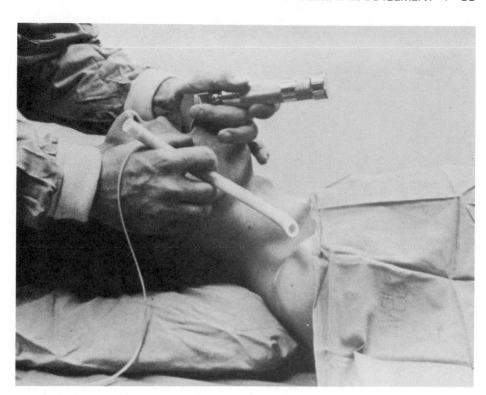

FIGURE 1–12. Blade is advanced into oropharynx, and laryngoscope is lifted to expose the epiglottis.

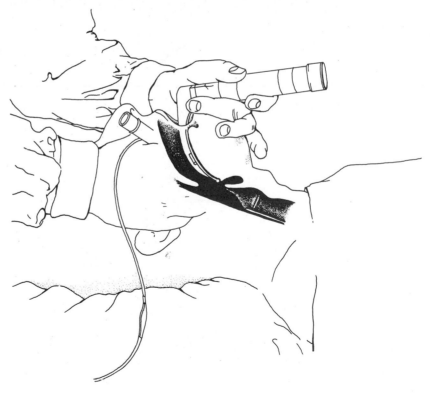

respiratory and vital signs assessment before and after procedure; route of intubation; size (diameter) and length (mark of emergence) of the tube; persons assisting with the procedure; nursing care given; use of medications; measurements of cuff pressures; expected and un-expected outcomes; date, time, and frequency with which procedure is performed. **Rationale:** Documents nursing actions and patient responses; serves as a legal document of the series of events.

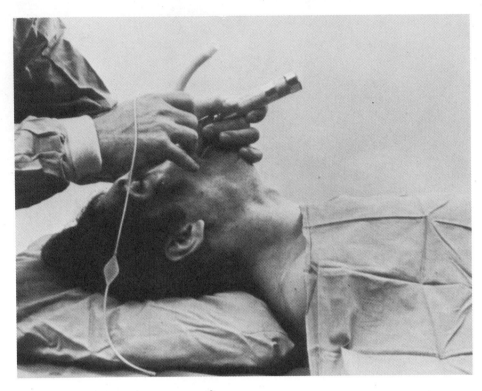

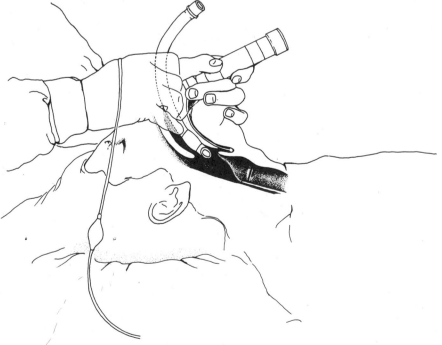

FIGURE 1–13. Tip of blade is placed in vallecula, and laryngoscope is lifted further to expose glottis. The tube is inserted through the right side of the mouth.

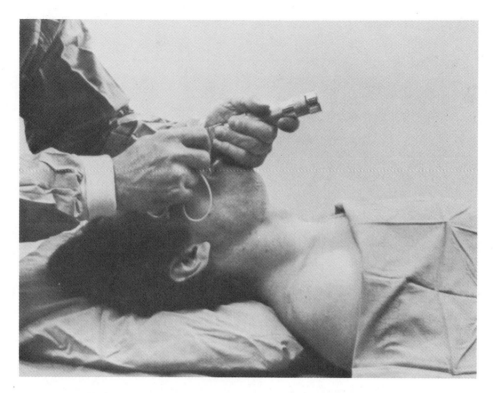

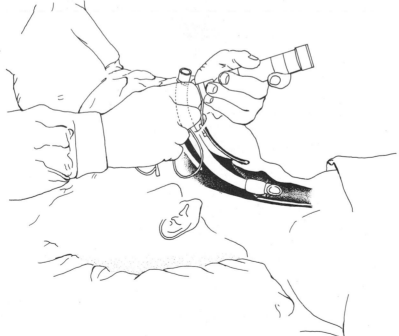

FIGURE 1–14. Tube is advanced through vocal cords into trachea.

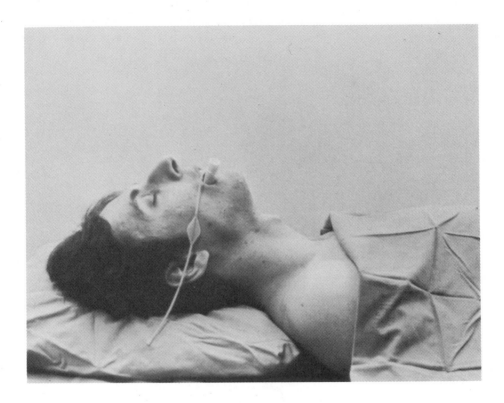

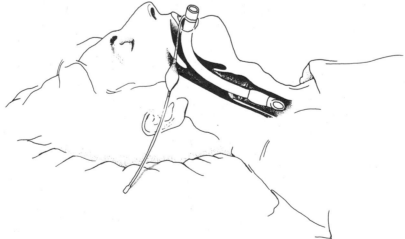

FIGURE 1–15.   Tube is positioned so that cuff is below vocal cords, and laryngoscope is removed.

TABLE 1–7 NURSING ACTIONS THAT DECREASE THE INCIDENCE OF UNINTENTIONAL EXTUBATIONS

Sedate patient as needed.

Use paralytic agents as ordered.

Maintain adequate use of restraints.

Utilize tracheal tube fixation devices.

Maintain correct tube length at 2 in. (5 cm) beyond the fixation device.

Maintain adequate tracheal cuff volume.

Monitor tracheal cuff pressures at least every 8 hours.

Provide ventilator tubing support.

Drain off ventilator tubing condensation.

Activate ventilator alarms.

Provide "swivel adaptor" application between tube and ventilator.

Utilize at least two nurses for mouth and tube care.

Provide emotional reinforcement–psychological comfort measures, including verbal communication, tactile stimulation, decreasing overstimulation.

Provide physical measures for comfort: patient positioning, adequate oxygenation.

Provide education regarding calming and comfort to family and patient.

Patient/Family Education

1. Assess level of understanding of patient and significant others regarding condition and rationale for endotracheal intubation and tube care. **Rationale:** Identification of misconceptions regarding patient's condition, necessity for airway insertion, predicted outcome, and potential risks allows for additional communication and clarification.

2. Frequently communicate to patient and significant others the patient's inability to speak, condition, progress, prognosis, and expected outcomes. **Rationale:** Frequent updates regarding patient's condition, prognosis, progress, and expected outcomes are continually cited as important needs of patients and families (Hickey, 1990; Viner, 1988).

3. Explain how patient and significant others can best communicate. **Rationale:** Encourages an environment of caring and trust.

4. Instruct family on how to perform direct patient care activities such as pharyngeal suctioning and oral hygiene. **Rationale:** Significant others express the need to assist in patient care (O'Neill-Norris and Grove, 1986).

Performance Checklist
Skill 1–5: Endotracheal Intubation and Tube Care

Critical Behaviors	Complies	
	yes	no
Intubation, General Setup		
1. Wash hands.		
2. Place oropharyngeal airway with nasotracheal intubation.		
3. Connect suction catheter to connecting tube.		
4. Suction oropharynx.		
5. Deliver with self-inflating resuscitation bag connected to 100% oxygen 3 hyperinflation (1½ tidal volume) and hyperoxygenation breaths.		
6. Don gloves.		
Orotracheal Intubation		
1. Open jaw with crossed-finger technique.		
2. Lock blade and position laryngoscope in left hand.		
3. Insert blade into mouth.		
4. Visualize epiglottis: a. Use straight blade to advance tip under epiglottis. b. Use curved blade to advance tip into vallecula.		
5. Lift up on laryngoscope handle to visualize vocal cords.		
6. Grasp endotracheal tube with right hand, curved part downward.		
7. Pass cuff through vocal cords (noncuffed tube used in children 8 years and under).		
8. Hold tube and withdraw laryngoscope and stylet.		
9. Inflate cuff on cuffed tube.		

Table continues on following page

Critical Behaviors	Complies	
	yes	no
10. Assess respiratory status: a. Auscultate bilateral lung bases and apices. b. Inspect for symmetrical chest expansion. c. Auscultate over epigastrium.		
11. If breath sounds are absent or unequal: a. Deflate cuff. b. Withdraw tube 1 to 2 cm, checking breath sounds for presence and equality. c. Withdraw tube with esophageal intubation. d. Begin again with step 7.		
12. Secure endotracheal tube.		
13. Suction endotracheal tube.		
14. Attach swivel adapter and connect to humidified oxygen source or mechanical ventilator.		
15. Discard supplies.		
16. Wash hands.		
17. Order chest radiograph.		
18. Check for breath sounds.		
19. Document procedure in patient record.		
NASOTRACHEAL INTUBATION (BLIND TECHNIQUE) 1. Follow steps 1 to 6 under *General Setup* and 1 to 6 under *Orotracheal Intubation*.		
2. Insert nasotracheal tube.		
3. Blindly advance tube.		
4. Advance tube during inspiration through glottis.		
5. Follow steps 8 to 18 under *Orotracheal Intubation*.		
TUBE CARE 1. Wash hands.		
2. Suction endotracheal tube, nasal and oropharyngeal airway, and oral cavity.		
3. Prepare twill tape or other securing device determined on an institutional basis.		
4. Don gloves.		
5. Remove oral airway.		
6. Person 1 stabilizes tube with one hand; Person 2 cuts soiled tape and removes.		
7. Clean mouth and gums.		
8. Brush teeth.		
9. Reposition orotracheal tube to opposite side of mouth.		
10. Repeat steps 7 and 8 on opposite side.		
11. Secure tube.		
12. Clean airway.		
13. Reinsert oral airway.		
14. Apply lubricant to lips.		
15. Discard gloves.		
16. Wash hands.		

Table continues on following page

Critical Behaviors	Complies	
	yes	no
17. Check breath sounds		
18. Document procedure in patient record.		

SKILL 1–6

Endotracheal or Tracheostomy Tube Suctioning

Endotracheal or tracheostomy tube suctioning is performed by passing a sterile catheter through either the endotracheal tube or the tracheostomy tube into the trachea and proximal portions of the mainstem bronchi. Suctioning assists in the aspiration of accumulated secretions.

Endotracheal or tracheostomy tubes reduce a patient's ability to cough. These artificial airways increase secretion formation in the lower tracheobronchial tree. The accumulated secretions enhance the possibility for airway obstruction, atelectasis, tracheobronchitis, and bronchopneumonia. For this reason, it is important to adhere to those suctioning principles which improve effectiveness and efficiency while reducing side effects.

Principles of suctioning include systemic hydration, humidification of inspired air, postural drainage, sterile technique, tube lavaging with normal sterile saline, the act of suctioning, and pre- and postsuctioning hyperoxygenation and hyperinflation. Systemic hydration and humidification of inspired air, along with lavaging, assist in thinning out secretions for easier aspiration and expectoration. Postural drainage facilitates the mobilization of secretions to airways within reach of the suction catheter. Sterile technique is paramount to reduce the incidence of infections. The technique of aspirating the lower airway must be performed safely and effectively, with frequency depending on clinical judgment, not set routines. Pre-and postsuctioning hyperoxygenation and hyperinflation with either a manual resuscitation bag or a mechanical ventilator allow suctioning to be safely performed without seriously reducing arterial oxygen levels.

Closed-system suctioning is designed to prevent or reduce arterial oxygen desaturation, hypotension, and bradycardia. The use of closed system suctioning has been associated with a reduced risk of contamination *from* the patient (Noll, 1991), and a lower incidence of patient related nosocomial and candida type of infections (Baker, 1989). For this method, a catheter is enclosed in a sleeve arrangement and left attached to an artificial airway. The seal near the catheter tip maintains positive end-expiratory pressure (PEEP) during suctioning. However, little investigational evidence is available to support the closed-system method over the open-system method.

When properly instituted, endotracheal or tracheostomy suctioning can improve gas exchange and alleviate respiratory distress, promote comfort, and decrease anxiety.

Purpose

The nurse performs endotracheal and tracheostomy suctioning to

1. Maintain a patent airway.
2. Reduce the work of breathing through the removal of secretions.
3. Stimulate the cough reflex.
4. Prevent pulmonary aspiration of blood and gastric fluids.
5. Prevent infection and atelectasis.

Prerequisite Knowledge and Skills

Prior to performing endotracheal or tracheostomy suctioning, the nurse should understand

1. Principles of aseptic technique.
2. Universal precautions (see Skill 35–1).
3. Anatomy and physiology of the upper and lower respiratory systems.
4. Principles of gas exchange.
5. Principles of airway resistance.
6. Indications for suctioning.
7. Contraindications for suctioning.
8. Principles of coughing.
9. Principles of artificial airway management.
10. Suctioning procedures.

The nurse should be able to perform

1. Proper handwashing technique (see Skill 35–5).
2. Vital signs assessment.
3. Oxygen administration via a manual resuscitator bag (see Skill 4–2).
4. Respiratory system assessment (inspection, palpation, percussion, and auscultation).
5. Oral airway insertion (see Skills 1–1 and 1–2).
6. Oral and nasopharyngeal suctioning techniques (see Skill 1–3).

Assessment

1. Observe for signs and symptoms of lower airway obstruction, including secretions in airway, inspiratory wheezes, expiratory crackles, restlessness, ineffective coughing, decreased level of consciousness, decreased breath sounds, tachypnea, tachycardia or bradycardia, cyanosis, hypertension or hypotension, and shallow respirations. **Rationale:** Physical signs and symptoms result from lower airway obstruction.
2. Monitor the peak airway pressures on the venti-

lator. **Rationale:** Accumulation of secretions, the presence of a mucus plug, and biting or kinking of the endotracheal tube will cause elevated peak airway pressures and cause the ventilator's high-pressure alarm to be triggered.

3. Assess patient for contraindications of endotracheal suctioning, including refractory hypoxemia, irritable myocardium evidenced by cardiac dysrhythmias, severe hypertension, and increased intracranial pressure. **Rationale:** Prolonged suctioning diminishes oxygen supply, disrupts normal ventilation, and in the presence of fragile pathologic conditions, may lead to worsening or irreversible status.

4. Observe for signs and symptoms of inadequate breathing patterns, including dyspnea, shallow respirations, and intercostal and suprasternal retractions, frequent triggering of ventilator alarms, increased respiratory rate. **Rationale:** Respiratory distress is a late sign of lower airway obstruction.

5. Assess the need for suctioning. **Rationale:** Repeated suctioning of the lower airway results in subatmospheric intrapulmonic pressure and predisposes patient to segmental and lobular atelectasis.

6. Assess for signs of atelectasis, including decreased breath sounds on auscultation, increasing peak inspiratory pressure, localized dullness to percussion, decreased compliance, decreased PaO_2, and localized consolidation on chest radiograph. **Rationale:** Suctioning techniques, hypoventilation, and conditions resulting in airway obstruction are amenable to nursing interventions (Goodnough et al., 1986).

Nursing Diagnoses

1. Impaired gas exchange related to accumulated secretions. **Rationale:** Presence of secretions in the lower airway decreases the exchange of respiratory gases across alveoli.

2. Potential for infection related to retained secretions and invasive type of procedure. **Rationale:** Retained secretions create a favorable medium for the growth of microorganisms.

3. Ineffective airway clearance related to retained secretions and inability to cough. **Rationale:** Secretions, especially mucoid in nature, are sticky and tend to accumulate along upper and lower airway tracts, creating a potential for partial or complete airway obstruction.

Planning

1. Individualize the following goals for performing endotracheal or tracheostomy tube suctioning:
   a. Establish and maintain patent airway. **Rationale:** Retained secretions reduce the amount of inhaled oxygen and inhibit gas exchange in the bronchopulmonary segments of the right and left lungs.
   b. Facilitate removal of airway secretions. **Rationale:** Removal of airway secretions reduces the potential for pulmonary infection and partial or complete airway obstruction.
   c. Promote optimal oxygenation. **Rationale:** Suctioning removes secretions, which improves oxygenation.

2. Prepare all necessary equipment and supplies. **Rationale:** Assembly of all the necessary equipment at the bedside ensures that suctioning will be completed quickly and efficiently.
   a. Suction catheter of appropriate size. **Rationale:** Catheter should not be any larger than one-half the diameter of the endotracheal or tracheostomy tube.

   Appropriate suction catheter size for patient can be attained by using the following conversion equations:

   To convert French size (Fr) to millimeters
   $$mm = \frac{Fr - 2}{4}$$

   To convert millimeters to French size (Fr)
   $$Fr = (4)(mm) + 2$$

   b. Water-soluble lubricant or 1 or 2 of the 3-ml sterile saline lavage containers.
   c. One sterile and one nonsterile glove.
   d. Sterile solution container or sterile basin.
   e. Sterile normal saline (at least 100 cc).
   f. Source of suction (wall mounted or portable).
   g. Flowmeter for oxygen, at 15 L/min (see Skill 4–2).
   h. Connecting tube, 6 ft.
   i. Oxygen delivery systems, including self-inflating resuscitation bag connected to 100% oxygen flow.
   j. Goggles or glasses, and mask.

3. Prepare the patient and family.
   a. Explain the purpose of endotracheal/tracheostomy tube suctioning. **Rationale:** Minimizes risk and reduces anxiety.
   b. Explain patient's participation and importance of coughing during procedure. **Rationale:** Encourages cooperation and facilitates the removal of secretions.
   c. Assist the patient in achieving a position that is comfortable for the patient and nurse, generally semi-Fowler's or Fowler's. **Rationale:** Promotes comfort, oxygenation, ventilation, and reduces strain.

4. Secure additional personnel to assist with hyperoxygenation and hyperinflation. **Rationale:** Two hands are necessary to properly activate the self-inflating resuscitation bag. "Double teaming" reduces the incidence of unintentional extubation (Pesiri et al., 1990).

Implementation

Steps	Rationale	Special Considerations
1. Wash hands.	Reduces transmission of microorganisms.	
2. Don goggles or glasses, and mask.	Universal precautions.	Check institutional policies.
3. Turn on suction apparatus and set vacuum regulator to appropriate negative pressure.	Significant hypoxia and damage to the tracheal mucosa can result from excessive negative pressure.	Suction manometer setting for recommended amounts of negative pressure.
4. Secure one end of connecting tube to suction machine, and place the other end in a convenient location within reach.	Prepares suction apparatus.	
5. Open sterile catheter package on a clean surface, using the inside of the wrapping as a sterile field.	Prepares catheter and prevents transmission of microorganisms.	
6. Set up the sterile solution container or sterile field. Be careful not to touch the inside of the container. Fill with approximately 100 ml of normal sterile saline and/or water.	Prepares catheter flush solution.	
7. Don sterile glove(s).	Maintains sterility. Universal precautions.	In the event that one sterile glove and one nonsterile glove are used, apply the nonsterile glove to the nondominant hand and the sterile glove to the dominant hand. Handle all nonsterile items with the nondominant hand.
8. Pick up suction catheter, being careful to avoid touching nonsterile surfaces. With the nondominant hand, pick up connecting tubing. Secure the suction catheter to the connecting tubing.	Maintains catheter sterility. Connects the suction catheter and the connecting tubing.	The dominant hand should not come into contact with the connecting tubing.
9. Check equipment for proper functioning by suctioning a small amount of sterile saline from the container.	Ensures equipment function.	
10. Remove or open oxygen or humidity device connected to the patient with nondominant hand or have second person to disconnect device.	Opens the artificial airway for catheter entrance. "Double teaming" reduces the chance for unintentional extubation and dislodgement (Pesiri et al., 1990).	
11. Replace oxygen delivery device or reconnect the patient to the ventilator. Hyperoxygenate and hyperventilate via 3 breaths (1½ × tidal volume) by manually "bagging" patient or pressing "manual sigh" on the ventilator.	Hyperoxygenation with 100% O_2 is used to offset hypoxemia during interrupted oxygenation and ventilation. Preoxygenation offsets volume and O_2 gas loss out the suction catheter.	Three hyperinflation breaths are generally adequate. However, four to six hyperinflation breaths may be utilized in the unstable or severely compromised patient. Patients receiving positive end-expiratory pressure (PEEP) ventilation should be suctioned through an adaptor (closed system suction method).

Special Considerations for Step 3:

	Wall setting mmHg	Portable setting inches of H_2O
Infant under 1 yr.	60–80	3–5
Child age 1 to 8 yrs.	80–120	5–10
Adult	120–150	10–15
Over 75 yrs.	80–120	5–10

(Eubanks and Bone, 1990; Kacmarek, Mack, and Dimas, 1990)

Table continues on following page

Steps	Rationale	Special Considerations
12. With suction off, gently but quickly insert catheter with dominant hand into artificial airway during inspiration until resistance is met; then pull back 1 cm.	Catheter is now in tracheobronchial tree. Application of suction pressure upon insertion increases hypoxia and results in damage to the tracheal mucosa.	If secretions are thick and sticky, instill 3 ml of sterile saline lavage down the artificial airway.
13. Apply intermittent suction by placing and releasing nondominant thumb over the control vent of the catheter. Rotate the catheter between dominant thumb and forefinger as you slowly withdraw the catheter.	Intermittent suction and catheter rotation prevent tracheal mucosa injury.	Entire suction pass can be safely carried out for up to 15 seconds without incurring serious drops in oxygenation. Each intermittent valve occlusion should last no longer than 5 seconds.
14. Replace oxygen delivery device. Hyperoxygenate with three hyperinflations following suction procedures and between passes of the suction catheter. This can be done by manually "bagging" the patient or pressing the "manual sigh" on the ventilator.	Replenishes oxygen. Recovery to baseline PaO_2 takes 1 to 5 minutes. Reduces incidence of hypoxemia.	
15. Rinse catheter and connecting tubing with normal saline until clear.	Removes catheter secretions.	
16. Repeat steps 11 to 15 as often as necessary to clear secretions.	Repeated passes assist in clearing the airway of secretions.	
17. Monitor patient's cardiopulmonary status during and between suction passes.	Observe for signs of hypoxemia, e.g., dysrhythmias, cyanosis, anxiety, bronchospasms, and changes in mental status.	
18. Once the lower airway has been adequately cleared of secretions, perform nasal and oral pharyngeal or upper airway suctioning (see Skill 1–3).	Removes upper airway secretions.	The catheter is contaminated following nasal and oral pharyngeal suctioning and should not be reinserted into the endotracheal or tracheostomy tube.
19. Upon completion of upper airway suctioning, wrap catheter around dominant hand. Pull glove off inside out. Catheter will remain in glove. Pull off other glove in same fashion and discard. Turn off suction device.	Reduces transmission of microorganisms.	
20. Reposition patient.	Supports ventilatory efforts; promotes comfort; communicates caring attitude.	
21. Wash hands.	Reduces transmission of microorganisms.	
22. Reassess patient's respiratory status.	Indicates need for artificial airway or emergency intervention.	
23. Discard remainder of normal saline and solution container. If basin is nondisposable type, place in soiled utility room. If 1000 cc bottle used, dispose of every 24 hours.	Reduces transmission of microorganisms.	
24. Dispose of suction cannisters, saline, and connecting tubing every 24 hours and set up new system.	Decreases incidence of organism colonization and subsequent pulmonary contamination. Universal precautions.	Check individual institutional policies.

Evaluation

Compare patient's respiratory assessment before and after suctioning. **Rationale:** Identifies the effects of suctioning.

Expected Outcomes

1. Removal of obvious secretions in upper airway and visual secretions in the tube. **Rationale:** Upper and lower airways are cleared of secretions.
2. Absent or diminished inspiratory wheezes and expiratory crackles, absent or diminished breath sounds, increased depth of respiration, absence of cyanosis, normalization of respiratory rate, normalization of heart rate. **Rationale:** Reduces the work of breathing.

Unexpected Outcomes

1. Patient becomes cyanotic and more restless, develops dysrhythmias and decreased level of consciousness, suffers cardiac arrest. **Rationale:** Suctioning removes oxygen and results in hypoxia and cardiopulmonary compromise.
2. Bloody secretions. **Rationale:** Trauma to tracheobronchial tree and/or presence of infection can result in bloody secretions.
3. Pneumonia. **Rationale:** Multiple catheter passes increase the incidence of bacterial colonization.
4. Dysrhythmias. **Rationale:** Hypoxemia and vagal stimulation affect heart rate and rhythm.
5. Inability to pass catheter. **Rationale:** Mucosal edema, foreign objects, soft tissue, and encrusted secretions may present as a partial or complete obstruction.

Documentation

Documentation in the patient record should include respiratory, cardiac, and vital signs assessment before and after suctioning; act of suctioning; amount, color, consistency, and odor of secretions obtained; patient's response to suctioning and postsuctioning respiratory assessment; date, time, and frequency with which procedure is performed. **Rationale:** Documents nursing care given and serves as a legal document of the series of events.

Patient/Family Education

1. Assess ability and readiness of patient and family to demonstrate tracheostomy care while in hospital setting. **Rationale:** Psychomotor and/or cognitive impairments may necessitate delaying patient and family teaching.
2. Explain the need for suctioning. **Rationale:** Reduces patient anxiety and provides patient/family education and patient/family/nurse communication.
3. Discuss and demonstrate the steps for preparation and completion of tracheostomy tube suctioning. **Rationale:** Encourages cooperation and understanding. Facilitates visibility and promotes comfort. Enables patient and family to ask questions throughout skill.
4. Explain the signs and symptoms indicating need for tracheostomy tube suctioning and signs and symptoms of respiratory tract infection. **Rationale:** Enables the patient and family to recognize when suctioning is indicated and when to notify the physician.

Performance Checklist
Skill 1–6: Endotracheal or Tracheostomy Tube Suctioning

Critical Behaviors	Complies	
	yes	no
1. Wash hands.		
2. Don goggles or glasses, and mask.		
3. Turn on suction apparatus and set vacuum regulator to correct negative pressure.		
4. Secure connecting tube to suction machine.		
5. Open sterile catheter package on a clean surface.		
6. Set up sterile solution container on sterile field and fill with 100 ml of normal saline.		
7. Don sterile gloves.		
8. Secure suction catheter to connecting tubes.		
9. Ensure that equipment is functioning properly.		
10. Expose artificial airway.		
11. Hyperoxygenate patient with 100% O$_2$.		
12. Insert catheter into tracheobronchial tree without application of suction and using sterile technique.		
13. Apply intermittent suction while rotating and withdrawing the catheter.		

Table continues on following page

Critical Behaviors	Complies	
	yes	no
14. Replace oxygen device and hyperoxygenate.		
15. Rinse catheter and connecting tube.		
16. Repeat passes as needed.		
17. Monitor patient's cardiopulmonary status.		
18. Perform nasal and oral pharyngeal suctioning following lower airway suctioning.		
19. Discard gloves, remaining contaminated saline, and solution container.		
20. Reposition patient.		
21. Wash hands.		
22. Reassess patient's respiratory system for expected and unexpected outcomes.		
23. Document procedure in patient record.		
24. Discard remainder of normal saline and solution container, if appropriate.		
25. Dispose of suction cannisters and connecting tubing every 24 hours.		

SKILL 1–7

Tracheal Tube Cuff Care

The tracheal tube cuff is an inflatable "balloon" that surrounds the shaft of the tracheal tube *near* its distal end. When inflated, the cuff presses against the tracheal wall to prevent air leakage and pressure loss from the lungs as well as the aspiration of secretions into the lung. Although a variety of cuffs exist, the most desirable cuff provides a maximum airway seal with minimal tracheal wall pressure. Currently, the most widely used cuff is the *high-volume, low-pressure cuff* (soft cuff) (Fig. 1–16). This cuff has a relatively large inflation volume that requires less filling pressure to obtain a seal (less than 25 mmHg or 34 cmH$_2$O). High-volume, low-pressure cuffs allow a large surface area to come into contact with the tracheal wall, thus distributing the pressure over a much greater area. The older cuff design, low-volume, high-pressure, can require as much as 40 mmHg (54.4 cmH$_2$O) to obtain an effective seal and is therefore undesirable. Ideally, most tubes will seal at pressures between 14 and 20 mmHg (19 to 27 cmH$_2$O). This range usually prevents mucosal ischemia and aspiration.

The amount of pressure and volume necessary to obtain a seal and prevent mucosal damage depends on the tube size and design, cuff configuration, mode of ventilation, and the individual's arterial blood pressure. Although rare since the use of high-volume, low-pressure devices, the adverse effects of tracheal tube cuff inflation include tracheal stenosis, necrosis, tracheoesophageal fistulas, and tracheomalacia.

Purpose

The nurse maintains the tracheal tube cuff on adult patients to

1. Stabilize the tracheal tube.
2. Protect the airway from aspiration.
3. Maintain an adequate airway seal.

The nurse performs tracheal tube cuff care to

1. Assess the airway and tracheal tube for leaks.
2. Maintain intracuff pressure at a safe level.
3. Prevent major pulmonary aspirations.
4. Prepare for tracheal extubation.
5. Decrease the risk of inadvertent extubation.
6. Provide a patent airway for ventilation and removal of secretions.
7. Decrease the risk of iatrogenic infections.
8. Maintain adequate ventilation volume.

Prerequisite Knowledge and Skills

Prior to performing tracheal tube cuff care, the nurse should understand

1. Principles of aseptic technique.
2. Universal precautions (see Skill 35–1).
3. Anatomy and physiology of the respiratory system.
4. Principles of gas exchange.
5. Principles of airway resistance.
6. Principles of suctioning.
7. Principles of airway management.
8. Physiologic effects of intraarterial tracheal capillary occlusion.

The nurse should be able to perform

1. Proper handwashing technique (see Skill 35–5).
2. Vital signs assessment.
3. Respiratory assessment.

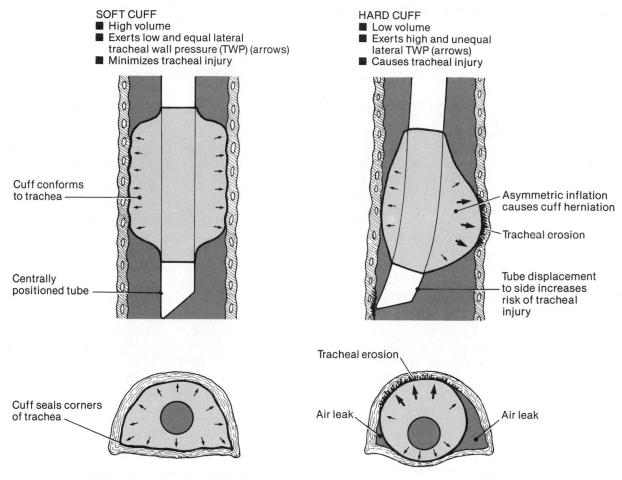

SOFT CUFF
■ High volume
■ Exerts low and equal lateral tracheal wall pressure (TWP) (arrows)
■ Minimizes tracheal injury

Cuff conforms to trachea

Centrally positioned tube

Cuff seals corners of trachea

HARD CUFF
■ Low volume
■ Exerts high and unequal lateral TWP (arrows)
■ Causes tracheal injury

Asymmetric inflation causes cuff herniation

Tracheal erosion

Tube displacement to side increases risk of tracheal injury

Tracheal erosion

Air leak   Air leak

FIGURE 1–16.   Cross-sectional view in D-shaped trachea. Effects of soft and hard cuff inflation on the tracheal wall. (Reprinted with permission from L. D. Kersten, *Comprehensive Respiratory Nursing: A Decision-Making Approach*. Philadelphia, Saunders, 1989, p. 648.)

4.   Oxygen administration techniques (see Skills 2–1 and 2–2).

5.   Tracheobronchial suction techniques (see Skills 1–4 and 1–6).

6.   Oropharyngeal and nasopharyngeal suctioning techniques (see Skill 1–3).

7.   Endotracheal and tracheostomy tube intubation (see Skill 1–5).

8.   Emergency advanced cardiac life support (ACLS) protocols.

Assessment

1.   Observe for signs and symptoms of inadequate ventilation, including rising arterial carbon dioxide tension, chest–abdominal dyssynchrony, patient–ventilator dyssynchrony, dyspnea, headache, restlessness, confusion, lethargy, and rising (early sign) or falling (late sign) arterial blood pressure and activation of expiratory/inspiratory volume alarms on the mechanical ventilator. **Rationale:** Inadequate ventilation results when cuff seal is improper or cuff leak is extensive.

2.   Assess signs and symptoms of cuff leakage, including audible or auscultated inspiratory leak over lar-

ynx, patient can audibly vocalize, pilot balloon deflation, and loss of inspiratory and expiratory volume on mechanically ventilated patients. **Rationale:** Adequate seal of cuff to tracheal wall will not permit air to flow past the cuff.

3.   Assess the need for monitoring cuff pressure, including transporting patient from one altitude to another (i.e., air transport) and hyperbaric therapy without environmental pressurization. **Rationale:** Boyle's law: At a constant temperature, the volume of a dry gas varies inversely with the pressure applied. Charles' law: If the pressure of a gas is held constant, the volume of a dry gas is directly proportional to the zero base temperature.

4.   Assess for signs of atelectasis, including localized dullness on percussion, decreased breath sounds on auscultation, increasing peak inspiratory pressure, decreased compliance, decreased PaO_2, and localized consolidation on chest radiograph. **Rationale:** Hypoventilation and conditions resulting in airway obstruction are amenable to nursing intervention (Goodnough et al., 1986).

5.   Assess the presence of a nasogastric tube. **Rationale:** The presence of a nasogastric tube displaces the posterior tracheal wall and indents the cuff. Elastic properties of the cuff are destroyed at the point of indentation

and allow full intracuff pressure to be transmitted to the tracheal mucosa (Kersten, 1989).

6. Assess conditions present that adversely affect tissue response to mucosal injury. **Rationale:** Poor perfusion and certain disease states allow mucosal ischemia to occur more easily, i.e., malnutrition, dehydration, infection, metastatic cancer, hypotensive states, and hypoxemia (MacKenzie, 1983).

7. Assess conditions present that may increase the incidence of inadvertent extubation. **Rationale:** Combative, thrashing conditions are not ideal for cuff and tube manipulation and may result in injury or tube dislodgment. Consider sedation or restraints when a safe airway cannot be ensured.

8. Assess the presence of anesthesia instillation through the tracheal tube. **Rationale:** Nitrous oxide tends to diffuse into thin cuffs and increase pressures (Kersten, 1989).

Nursing Diagnoses

1. **Impaired verbal communication related to presence of cuffed artificial airway. Rationale:** Sealed tracheal tube cuff prevents air from passing across vocal cords.

2. **Ineffective airway clearance related to retained secretions. Rationale:** Secretions, especially mucoid in nature, are sticky and tend to pool above the tracheal tube cuff.

3. **Altered tracheobronchial tissue perfusion related to reduced capillary flow. Rationale:** Mucosal ischemia occurs when lateral tracheal wall pressure exceeds capillary perfusion pressure, resulting in decreased mucosal blood flow. Arterial vessels occlude at 20 to 25 mmHg, venous vessels occlude at 18 to 20 mmHg, and lymphatic channels occlude at 5 to 8 mmHg. These values are based on normal arterial blood pressure readings.

Planning

1. Individualize the following goals for tracheal tube cuff care:
   a. Promote optimal ventilation. **Rationale:** Inadequate interface between tracheal cuff and tracheobronchial mucosa decreases inspiratory flow pressure to the acini.
   b. Promote optimal tracheobronchial tissue perfusion. **Rationale:** Excessive cuff pressure is cited as the most frequent problem of tracheal intubation and the best predictor of tracheolaryngeal injury (Rashkin and Davis, 1986).

c. Maintain tracheal tube cuff integrity. **Rationale:** Manipulation of the tracheal tube increases the likelihood of cuff disruption. Cuff leak or rupture is evident when the pressure on the manometer continues to fall despite inflation efforts, when air is audible through the patient's nose or mouth, when the low-pressure and/or low-volume alarm sounds on the mechanical ventilator, and if the patient can talk.

d. Mobilize secretions above the cuff. **Rationale:** Removal of secretions reduces the chance for partial or complete airway obstruction.

e. Maintain cuff inflation. **Rationale:** Hypoxemia, overinflation of the cuff upon reinflation, and pulmonary aspiration occur with periodic cuff deflations (Powaser et al., 1976). Cuff should be deflated only when problems arise or every 48 to 72 hours (Kersten, 1989).

2. Determine the best technique for cuff inflation, minimal leak volume (MLV) technique, minimal occlusion volume (MOV) technique. **Rationale:** Each technique has distinct advantages. MLV decreases mucosal injury and assists in mobilizing secretions forward into the pharynx. MOV decreases the incidence of aspirations and is most effective for patients who are changing position frequently and are at increased risk for tube movement.

3. Prepare all necessary equipment and supplies. **Rationale:** Assembly of equipment and supplies facilitates quick and efficient tracheal tube cuff care.
   a. Syringe, 10 cc.
   b. Pressure manometer with extension line.
   c. Three-way stopcock.
   For cuff inflation in the case of a faulty inflating line, gather in addition the following;
   d. Scissors.
   e. Short 18- to 23-gauge blunt needle.
   f. Tongue depressor.
   g. Tape, 1 in wide.
   h. Equipment necessary for reintubation (see Skill 1–5).
   i. Suction supplies (see Skill 1–3).

4. Prepare the patient and family.
   a. Explain the purpose and necessity of tracheal tube care. **Rationale:** Communication and explanation for therapy encourage cooperation, minimize risk and anxiety, and are important needs of patients and families (Parker et al., 1984; Viner, 1988).
   b. Place patient in semi-Fowler's position. **Rationale:** Promotes general relaxation, oxygenation, and ventilation. Reduces stimulation of gag reflex and risk of aspiration.

Implementation

Steps	Rationale	Special Considerations
Deflation/Inflation		
1. Wash hands.	Reduces transmission of microorganisms.	
2. Remove oxygen tubing attached to the endotracheal or tracheostomy tube.	Accesses tube opening.	
3. Suction the pharynx above the cuff prior to cuff deflation (see Skill 1–3).	Decreases incidence of aspiration into lower airway.	This catheter is considered contaminated and should not be used to suction the tracheobronchial tree.
4. Deflate cuff.	Prepares for measurement of cuff pressure.	When the inflating line becomes faulty and reintubation is undesirable, consider instituting an emergency cuff inflation technique (Fig. 1–17).
5. Stabilize the tube and instruct awake patient to cough.	Prevents unintentional extubation and assists in raising secretions to pharynx.	
6. Suction tracheobronchial tree (see Skill 1–4).	Clears secretions in the lower airway.	A fresh sterile catheter is necessary.
7. Insert air-filled 10-cc syringe tip into filling tube valve.	Provides a pathway between air source and cuff.	
For Minimal Occlusion Volume (MOV) Technique		
8. Place a stethoscope over larynx; have patient speak.	Indirectly assesses inflation of cuff.	
9. Slowly inject air until sounds cease over larynx.	Indicates that cuff is sealed against the tracheal mucosal wall.	Cuff hazards include: cuff overinflation, distension, and rupture.
10. Follow steps 14 to 18 to complete.		
For Minimal Leak Volume (MLV) Technique		
11. Follow steps 1 to 3.	Begins initial steps of procedure.	
12. Place a stethoscope over larynx.	Indirectly assesses inflation of cuff.	
13. Slowly withdraw air from the cuff until a small leak is heard.	Indicates air escaping through the larynx.	Cuff hazards include: cuff overinflation, distension, and rupture.
14. Remove syringe tip; check inflation of pilot balloon.	Indicates air placement into cuff.	
15. Replace any oxygen or humidity tubing and check and secure ventilator connections.	Allows for oxygen flow and prevents oxygen desaturation.	
16. Reassess patient's airway and respiratory status.	Identifies untoward results.	
17. Wash hands.	Reduces transmission of microorganisms.	
Cuff Measurement Technique: Aneroid Cuff Pressure Manometer (homemade pressure-monitoring device)		
1. Wash hands.	Reduces transmission of microorganisms.	
2. Connect the manometer line with a three-way stopcock (turn the position "off" to the patient) attached to the patient inflation system (Fig. 1–18).	Develops an intracuff pressure-monitoring device.	This device is easily made using parts of a blood pressure cuff (e.g., aneroid manometer device).

Table continues on following page

Table continues on following page

Steps	Rationale	Special Considerations
3. With your thumb, occlude the open port and with an air-filled syringe, inject air into the tubing leading to the manometer until the needle of the manometer reads between 14 and 20 mmHg (19 and 27 cmH$_2$O).	Measures the pressure of the air applied from the syringe.	Pressure should be kept at a level to maintain a seal between cuff and tracheal wall. The volume necessary to create the seal depends on tube size and cuff configuration.
4. Turn the "off" position of the stopcock to the open port (syringe). Read the cuff pressure now shown on the aneroid "face."	The connecting channel is now between the manometer and patient's inflation line.	
5. Turn the "off" position of the stopcock toward the inflating tube, and disconnect manometer line from the patient's inflation line.	The connecting channel to the inflating tube is now closed and thus maintaining air in the cuff.	
6. Detach the manometer line with three-way stopcock from the patient's inflation system.	Removes apparatus to monitor cuff pressure.	
7. Wash hands.	Reduces transmission of microorganisms.	

Troubleshooting of Tracheal Cuff Problems

Faulty Inflating Valve

1. Wash hands.	Reduces transmission of microorganisms.	
2. Identify faulty inflating valve.	Determines need for repair.	
3. Insert three-way stopcock into the distal opening of the inflating balloon.	Provides access to cuff.	
4. Inflate the cuff using MOV or MLV technique.	Allows for cuff inflation; restores tracheal wall/cuff seal.	
5. Clamp the inflating tube by applying a padded hemostat distal to the pilot balloon.	Maintains air in cuff; provides a quick occlusion of the inflating tube.	
6. Turn the stopcock to the "off" position toward the inflating tube; remove clamp.	Provides for temporary use of the tracheal tube while maintaining cuff pressure.	

Faulty Inflating Line

1. Wash hands.	Reduces transmission of microorganisms.	
2. Identify malfunctioning of inflating line.	Determines need for and method of repair.	
3. Cut off faulty end of inflation line with scissors (see Fig. 1–17).	Prepares inflation line for repair.	
4. Insert short 18- to 23-gauge blunt needle into inflation line.	Provides for inflation access.	Maintain care to avoid puncture or severing of inflation line. Use care not to puncture your skin.
5. Attach a three-way stopcock to a blunt needle.	Provides control of airflow in and out of inflating line.	
6. Using a 10-cc syringe inflate the cuff with air using MOV or MLV technique.	Allows cuff inflation; restores tracheal wall/cuff seal.	

Table continues on following page

Steps	Rationale	Special Considerations
7. Turn the stopcock to the "off" position toward the inflating tube.	Provides for temporary use of the tracheal tube while maintaining cuff pressure.	
8. Secure assembled device with tape to a tongue depressor.	Provides for stabilization and protection (Sills, 1986).	

Evaluation

Compare patient's respiratory status before and after tracheal tube cuff care. **Rationale:** Identifies the effects of tracheal tube cuff care.

Expected Outcomes

1. Tracheal tube remains in correct position. **Rationale:** Manipulation of the tube and cuff increases the incidence of inadvertent extubation.

2. Cuff pressure will be kept at a level to maintain a seal between cuff and tracheal wall (usually between 14 and 20 mmHg, or 19 and 27 cmH$_2$O) depending on tube size and cuff configuration. **Rationale:** Decreases the incidence of mucosal necrosis.

3. Cuff will remain intact. **Rationale:** Provides accurate pressure readings, maintains tube stability, prevents aspiration of secretions, and provides seal for mechanical ventilation efforts.

Unexpected Outcomes

1. Extubation or tube dislodgement. **Rationale:** Unintentional extubation and tube manipulation can occur with ineffective restraint, inadequate securing of the tube, inadequate sedation, incorrect tube size and length, improper support or respiratory underinflation of endotracheal cuff, and prolonged intubation (Pesiri et al., 1990).

2. Mucosal ischemia. **Rationale:** Cuff pressures greater than 25 mmHg exceed capillary perfusion pressure, resulting in decreased mucosal blood flow.

3. Faulty cuff and inflating line. **Rationale:** Manip-

ulation of the tube and cuff increases the incidence of tube and cuff damage.

4. Cuff overinflation and distension over the end of the tube. **Rationale:** Large air volume instillation creates a potential hazard and may result in tracheal stenosis, necrosis, and tracheoesophageal fistulas.

5. Cuff rupture. **Rationale:** Overinflation may cause rupture of cuff, allow foreign matter to enter lungs, and allow the escape of positive pressure.

Documentation

Documentation in the patient record should include respiratory and vital signs assessment before and after procedure; method of cuff inflation; nursing care given; use of medications; use of restraints; unexpected outcomes; cuff inflation volume and cuff pressure; date, time, and frequency with which procedure is performed. **Rationale:** Documents nursing actions and patient responses; serves as a legal document of the series of events.

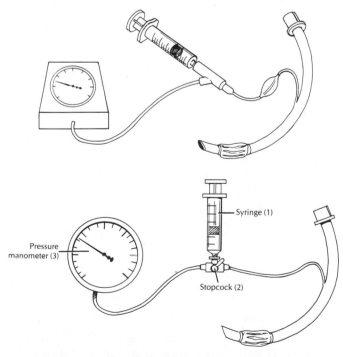

FIGURE 1–18. Measuring cuff pressure by way of homemade pressure monitor. (Reproduced with permission from D. H. Eubanks and R. C. Bone, *Comprehensive Respiratory Care: A Learning System*, 2d Ed. St. Louis, Mosby, 1990, p. 559.)

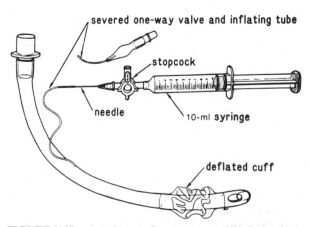

FIGURE 1–17. Attachments for emergency cuff inflation for faulty inflating line. (Reproduced with permission from J. Sills, An emergency cuff inflation technique. *Respir. Care* 31(3):200, 1986.)

Patient/Family Education

1. Assess level of understanding of patient and significant others regarding condition and rationale for tracheal cuff care. **Rationale:** Identifies misconceptions regarding patient's condition and the necessity for tube care. Identification of predicted outcomes and potential risks allows for additional communication and clarification.

2. Frequently communicate to patient and significant others the patient's inability to speak, condition, progress, prognosis, and expected outcomes. **Rationale:** Frequent updates regarding patient's condition, prognosis, progress, and expected outcomes are continually cited as important needs of patients and families (Hickey, 1990; Viner, 1988).

3. Explain how patient and significant others can best communicate. **Rationale:** Encourages an environment of caring and trust.

4. Instruct family on how to perform direct patient care activities such as pharyngeal suctioning and oral hygiene. **Rationale:** Significant others express the need to assist in patient care (O'Neill-Norris and Grove, 1986). Protective caregiving of the frail and elderly is a primary task of the nuclear family (Bowers, 1987).

Performance Checklist
Skill 1–7:   Tracheal Tube Cuff Care

Critical Behaviors	Complies yes	no
INFLATION TECHNIQUE 1. Wash hands.		
2. Remove oxygen tubing.		
3. Suction pharynx (see Skill 1–3).		
4. Deflate cuff.		
5. Instruct awake patient to cough.		
6. Suction tracheobronchial tree (see Skill 1–4).		
7. Attach syringe tip to filling tube valve.		
For Minimal Occlusion Volume (MOV) Technique 8. Place stethoscope over larynx; instruct patient to vocalize.		
9. Inject air until sounds cease.		
10. Follows steps 14 to 18 to complete.		
For Minimum Leak Volume (MLV) Technique 11. Follow steps 1 to 3.		
12. Place stethoscope over larynx.		
13. Inflate cuff until sound ceases.		
14. Slowly withdraw air from the cuff until a small leak is heard.		
15. Remove syringe tip; check pilot balloon.		
16. Replace oxygen and/or humidity tubing, check ventilator connection.		
17. Reassess patient's airway and respiratory status.		
18. Wash hands.		
19. Document procedure in patient record.		
CUFF MEASUREMENT TECHNIQUE 1. Wash hands.		
2. Connect manometer line and stopcock to patient inflation system.		
3. Occlude open port; inject air with syringe until manometer reads between 14 and 20 mmHg (19 and 27 cmH_2O).		
4. Turn "off" position of stopcock to the open port; read pressure.		

Table continues on following page

Critical Behaviors	Complies	
	yes	no
5. Turns "off" position of the stopcock toward inflating tube and disconnect manometer line.		
6. Detach manometer line and stopcock from the patient inflating system.		
7. Wash hands.		
8. Document procedure in patient record.		
TROUBLESHOOTING OF TRACHEAL CUFF *Faulty Inflating Valve* 1. Wash hands.		
2. Identify faulty inflating valve.		
3. Insert stopcock into distal opening of inflating balloon.		
4. Inflate cuff.		
5. Clamp inflating tube with padded hemostat.		
6. Turn stopcock "off" to inflating tube; remove clamp.		
7. Document procedure in patient record.		
Faulty Inflating Line 1. Wash hands.		
2. Identify malfunctioning of inflating line.		
3. Cut faulty end of inflation line.		
4. Insert blunt needle into inflation line.		
5. Attach stopcock.		
6. Inflate cuff.		
7. Turn stopcock "off" toward inflating tube.		
8. Secure assembled device.		
9. Document procedure in patient record.		

SKILL 1–8

Extubation and Decannulation

Extubation refers to removal of an endotracheal tube, whereas *decannulation* refers to removal of a tracheostomy tube. Most extubations or decannulations are planned. Planning allows for preparation of the patient, both physically and emotionally, and decreases the likelihood of reintubation and hypoxic sequelae. Unintentional (unplanned) extubation complicates a patient's overall recovery and has been the center of investigation (Pesiri et al., 1990). In this study, 60 percent of unintentional extubations occurred during the first 7 days following intubation, with more than half occurring during the daytime hours. Causative factors for unintentional extubation include improper patient sedation, ineffective patient restraint, inadequate securing of the endotracheal tube, underinflation of tracheal cuffs, and improper tubing support. These factors can be affected by a variety of nursing actions (see Table 1–7).

Extubation or decannulation is indicated when the needs for intubation are no longer present, the patient can clear his or her own secretions, and the patient can protect his or her own airway from aspirations.

Purpose

The nurse removes the artificial airway to

1. Allow the patient to breathe independently.
2. Allow the patient to remove secretions independently.

Prerequisite Knowledge and Skills

Prior to removing the artificial airway, the nurse should understand

1. Principles of aseptic technique.
2. Universal precautions.

3. Anatomy and physiology of the respiratory system.
4. Principles of suctioning.
5. Principles of airway management.
6. Contraindications of extubation.
7. Extubation and decannulation procedure.
8. Concepts of anxiety.

The nurse should be able to perform

1. Proper handwashing technique (see Skill 35–5).
2. Vital signs assessment.
3. Respiratory assessment.
4. Oxygen and humidification administration techniques (see Skills 2–1 and 2–2).
5. Oropharyngeal and nasopharyngeal suctioning techniques (see Skill 1–3).
6. Tracheobronchial suctioning techniques (see Skills 1–4 and 1–6).
7. Endotracheal tube insertion techniques (see Skill 1–5).
8. Emergency advanced cardiac life support (ACLS) protocols.
9. Universal precautions (Skill 35–1).

Assessment

1. Observe for signs and symptoms associated with independent breathing, including stable respiratory rate of 24 breaths per minute or less, even, deep, symmetrical chest expansion, PaO_2 of 70 to 90 mmHg on 5 cmH_2O of CPAP and an FIO_2 of 0.4 or less, pH of at least 7.35 on CPAP 30 minutes, Vd/Vt of 0.6, ability to lift head for 5 seconds, ability to grip hand appropriately on command, FVC of at least 15 ml/kg, PNP of at least -25 cmH_2O (Davis and Gammage, 1988), stable pulse and blood pressure, and absence of serious cardiac dysrhythmias. **Rationale:** Identifies that the need for intubation is no longer present.
2. Assess patient's ability to cough. **Rationale:** The ability to cough and clear secretions is important for successful extubation.

Nursing Diagnoses

1. Potential for aspiration related to pooled secretions. **Rationale:** Failure to suction or ineffective suctioning of the pharynx allows accumulated secretions to further advance into the trachea upon cuff deflation.

2. Activity intolerance related to deconditioning of muscles. **Rationale:** Patients on bed rest are subjected to limited mobilization.
3. Anxiety related to dependence on caregivers to meet basic human needs. **Rationale:** As a result of mobility and communication deficits, the patient relies on others to perform activities of daily living.
4. Fear-related uncertainty about prognosis and inadequate communication. **Rationale:** Insecurities surrounding discontinuing of mechanical ventilation are real to the patient.

Planning

1. Individualize the following goals for extubation:
   a. Promote optimal oxygenation. **Rationale:** Decreases the incidence of oxygen desaturation immediately following extubation.
   b. Encourage coughing and deep breathing. **Rationale:** Prevents atelectasis and secretion accumulation.
   c. Provide for resuscitation and emergency reintubation. **Rationale:** Premature extubation and patient fatigue can result in respiratory failure.
2. Prepare all necessary equipment and supplies. **Rationale:** Assembly of equipment and supplies facilitates quick and efficient extubation.
   a. Suctioning equipment.
   b. Scissors.
   c. Sterile gloves.
   d. Supplemental oxygen with aerosol setup (see Skill 2–2).
   e. Endotracheal intubation supplies (see Skill 1–5).
   f. Stethoscope.
   g. Syringe, 10 cc.
   h. Emergency cart.
   i. Yankauer suction catheter.
   j. Sterile dressing for tracheal stoma.
3. Prepare the patient and family.
   a. Explain the purpose and necessity of extubation. **Rationale:** Communication and explanation for therapy encourage cooperation, minimize risk and anxiety, and are important needs of patients and families (Parker et al., 1984; Viner, 1988).
   b. Place patient in semi-Fowler's position. **Rationale:** Respiratory muscles are more effective in an upright versus a prone position. This position facilitates cough and minimizes the risk of vomiting and consequent aspiration.

Implementation

Steps	Rationale	Special Considerations
1. Wash hands.	Reduces transmission of microorganisms.	
2. Don goggles, glasses, and mask.	Universal precautions.	

Table continues on following page

Steps	Rationale	Special Considerations
3. Cut twill tape or remove tape to free tube.	Removes outer means for securing the tube.	
4. Don gloves, and suction pharynx with Yankauer tonsil-tip catheter (see Skill 1–3).	Removes pooled secretions above the cuff.	
5. Hyperoxygenate and hyperinflate the patient with 3 breaths.	Prevents oxygen desaturation.	
6. Insert syringe into one-way valve in pilot balloon.	Prepares for cuff deflation.	
7. Instruct patient to deep breathe.	Promotes hyperinflation.	A manual resuscitator can assist in hyperinflation.
8. Insert sterile suction catheter 1 to 2 in (5 cms.) below distal end of tracheal tube.	Positions catheter correctly for removal of secretions.	
9. At the peak of a deep inspiration, deflate cuff and pull out the tube while applying suction to the catheter quickly in one motion on expiration.	Assists in a smooth, quick, less traumatic removal and prevents aspiration of mucus that may be in the tube.	Tracheostomy stoma closure usually occurs within a few days.
10. Encourage the patient to deep breathe and cough.	Promotes hyperinflation; helps remove secretions.	
11. Suction the pharynx.	Removes secretions.	
12. Apply supplemental oxygen and aerosol.	Promotes warmth and moisture and prevents oxygen desaturation.	
13. Assess patient's airway and respiratory status.	Identifies untoward effects.	Problems generally occur within the first hour of extubation.
14. Wash hands.	Reduces transmission of microorganisms.	
15. Discard tubes, supplies, catheter, and gloves in appropriate receptacle.	Reduces transmission of microorganisms. Universal precautions.	
16. Monitor the patient closely for signs of respiratory failure and/or until patient feels confident that he or she can breathe on his or her own without difficulty.	Assists with early identification of problems.	
17. Monitors arterial blood gases.	Provides for accurate assessment of patient's respiratory system.	Arterial blood gas analysis should be done initially following extubation, one hour following extubation, and if signs of respiratory compromise result.

Evaluation

Compare patient's respiratory status before and after tracheal extubation. **Rationale:** Identifies the effects of extubation.

Expected Outcomes

1. Smooth, atraumatic extubation. **Rationale:** Following protocol assists in reduction of mucosal and tissue trauma.
2. Stable respiratory status. **Rationale:** The decision for extubation is based on objective findings.

Unexpected Outcomes

1. Fatigue and respiratory failure. **Rationale:** Patients may be weak, fatigued, or malnourished and unable to maintain normal oxygenation and ventilation and be able to mobilize secretions.
2. Persistent hoarseness. **Rationale:** Indicates underlying problem (i.e., swelling, edema, laryngeal injury).
3. Tracheal stoma narrowing. **Rationale:** Stoma size often decreases to that of the tracheostomy tube, creating "drag" and difficulty in tube removal.

Documentation

Documentation in the patient record should include respiratory and vital signs assessment before and after procedure; nursing care given; unexpected outcomes; arterial blood gas results; patient response; date and time when procedure is performed. **Rationale:** Documents nursing actions and patient responses; serves as a legal document of the series of events.

Patient/Family Education

1. Discuss the rationale for removal of the artificial airway. Discuss the suctioning process and importance of coughing and deep breathing. **Rationale:** Encourages cooperation and trust and decreases fear and anxiety.

2. Frequently communicate to patient and significant others the patient's condition, progress, prognosis, and expected outcomes. **Rationale:** Frequent updates regarding patient's condition, prognosis, progress, and expected outcomes are continually cited as important needs of patients and families (Viner, 1988; Hickey, 1990).

Performance Checklist
Skill 1–8: Extubation and Decannulation

Critical Behaviors	Complies	
	yes	no
1. Wash hands.		
2. Remove tape securing tube.		
3. Suction pharynx.		
4. Hyperoxygenate patient.		
5. Insert syringe into one-way valve in pilot balloon.		
6. Instruct patient to deep breathe.		
7. Insert suction catheter into endotracheal or tracheostomy tube.		
8. Deflate cuff and remove tube while applying suction.		
9. Encourage deep breathing and coughing.		
10. Suction pharynx.		
11. Apply supplemental oxygen and aerosol.		
12. For tracheostomy tube, apply sterile occlusive dressing to stoma.		
13. Assess patient's airway and respiratory status.		
14. Wash hands.		
15. Discard supplies.		
16. Document procedure in patient record.		
17. Monitor patient.		
18. Monitor arterial blood gases.		

SKILL 1–9

Tracheotomy and Tracheostomy Tube Care

Tracheotomy refers to an incision made below the cricoid cartilage through the second to fourth tracheal rings (Fig. 1–19). *Tracheostomy* refers to the opening, or stoma, made by the incision. The tracheostomy tube is the artificial airway inserted into the trachea during tracheotomy (Fig. 1–20). A tracheotomy is performed either as an elective or an emergency procedure for a variety of reasons (Table 1–8).

More often, the procedure is elective and takes place in the operating room under sterile conditions. An emergency tracheotomy usually takes place at the bedside under aseptic technique. Protocols for emergency tracheotomy vary among institutions. Often nurses at the bedside take an active role in assisting with insertion; however, some institutions have surgical personnel go to

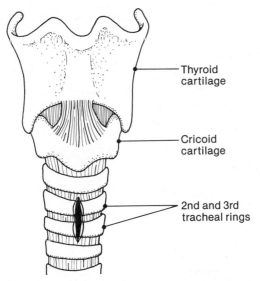

FIGURE 1–19. Vertical tracheal incision during a tracheotomy procedure. (Reproduced with permission from L. D. Kersten, *Comprehensive Respiratory Nursing: A Decision-Making Approach.* Philadelphia, Saunders, 1989, p. 654.)

TABLE 1–8 RATIONALE FOR TRACHEOTOMY

Bypass acute upper airway obstruction
Prolonged need for artificial airway
Prophylaxis for anticipated airway problems
Reduction of anatomic dead space
Prevention of pulmonary aspiration
Retained tracheobronchial secretions
Chronic upper airway obstruction

the bedside to help manage the care. During the initial 36 hours following tracheostomy tube insertion, the tube should not be removed. If the tube is removed too early, a newly created stoma may collapse, making reintubation difficult. During this immediate postintubation period, the head of the bed should be kept elevated at 30 degrees to assist in oropharyngeal and nasopharyngeal drainage.

Tracheostomy tubes are comprised of a variety of parts (Fig. 1–21) and come in various styles (Table 1–9). Al-

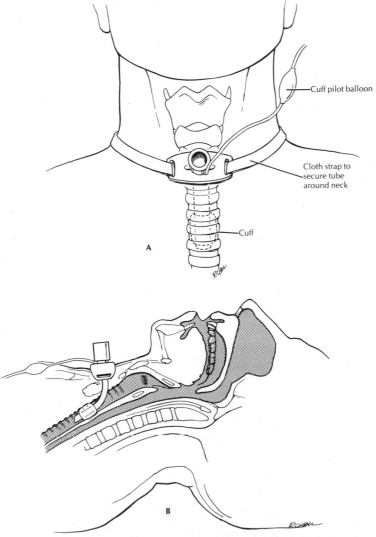

FIGURE 1–20. (*A*) Anterior view of a tracheostomy tube after insertion. (*B*) Lateral view of a tracheostomy tube after insertion. (Reproduced with permission from D. H. Eubanks and R. C. Bone, *Comprehensive Respiratory Care: A Learning System*, 2d Ed. St. Louis, Mosby, 1990, p. 554.)

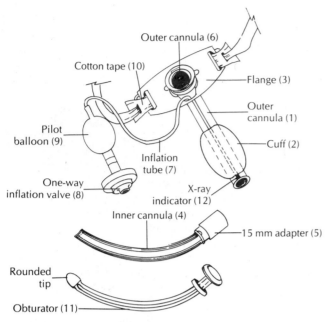

FIGURE 1–21. **Parts of a tracheostomy tube. (Reproduced with permission from D. H. Eubanks and R. C. Bone, *Comprehensive Respiratory Care: A Learning System*, 2d Ed. St. Louis, Mosby, 1990, p. 570.)**

though similar in diameter to an endotracheal tube, a tracheostomy tube is shorter and has a squared-off distal tip for maximizing airflow. The *outer cannula* forms the body of a tracheostomy tube with a cuff. In the event of expected mechanical ventilation a cuffed tube is necessary (see Fig. 1–21). The neck *flange* is attached to the outer cannula (see Fig. 1–21). It assists in stabilizing the tube in the trachea and provides the small holes necessary for proper securing of the tube around the neck.

Some tracheostomy setups have an *inner cannula* that is inserted into the outer cannula. The inner cannula is removable for easy cleaning without compromising the airway. The *cuff* consists of a balloon that is inflated with air to maintain a seal around the tube. Cuff inflation occurs when an air-filled syringe is inserted into the *inflation valve* and the syringe plunger is activated. As the air flows through the one-way inflation valve, the pilot

balloon inflates, indicating the volume of air present in the cuff. During insertion, the *obturator* replaces the inner cannula. Its smooth surface protrudes from the outer cannula and minimizes tracheal trauma. Once the tracheostomy tube is inserted, the obturator is pulled out and replaced with the inner cannula, which locks in place. The obturator is then placed in a plastic bag and kept at the bedside for emergency use.

Purpose

The nurse assists the physician in the placement of a tracheostomy tube to

1. Maintain airway patency.
2. Prevent further laryngeal injury from the translaryngeal tube.
3. Improve patient comfort.
4. Permit speech for the patient.
5. Facilitate nursing care (i.e., suctioning and mouth care).
6. Increase patient mobility.
7. Facilitate oral nourishment.
8. Facilitate transfer from the ICU.

Prerequisite Knowledge and Skills

Prior to a tracheostomy tube being placed, the nurse should understand

1. Principles of surgical technique.
2. Anatomy and physiology of the respiratory system.
3. Anatomy of the neck.
4. Indications for tracheostomy tube placement.
5. Contraindications for tracheostomy tube placement.
6. Principle of gas exchange.
7. Principles of airway resistance.
8. Principles of chest radiograph interpretation.

The nurse should be able to perform

1. Proper handwashing technique (see Skill 35–5).

TABLE 1–9   TRACHEOSTOMY TUBE STYLES AND DESCRIPTIONS

Style Name	Description
Shiley, Portex, National	A plastic tube usually comprised of three parts: a disposable inner cannula, an obturator, and a soft cuff. Some Portex brand tubes do not have inner cannulas.
Lanz	A plastic tube with a pressure-regulating valve, a soft cuff, and an external balloon.
Fenestrated	A tube with precut openings in the outer cannula, useful in weaning patients from mechanical ventilation or for long-term airway management.
Kamen-Wilkinson	A foam-filled plastic tube without an inner cannula that requires minimal air for inflation.
Jackson	A metal tube with an inner cannula and obturator. This tube is uncuffed and designed for long-term usage.
Kistner	Also referred to as a tracheostomy button, its one-way valve attached to the outer cannula permits airflow through the tube during inspiration and closes on expiration. This tube permits speaking and coughing.
Pitt Trach Speaking Tube	This tube permits speaking and coarse whispers in the presence of continuous air/oxygen ventilation.

2. Vital signs assessment.
3. Respiratory assessment (inspection, palpation, percussion, and auscultation).
4. Oxygen administration and ventilation via manual resuscitator bag (see Skill 4–2).
5. Basic cardiac life-support techniques.
6. Advanced cardiac life-support techniques.
7. Tracheal tube suctioning techniques (see Skill 1–4).
8. Nasopharyngeal and oropharyngeal suctioning techniques (see Skill 1–3).
9. Oral hygiene.
10. Universal precautions (see Skill 35–1).

Assessment

Tracheotomy with Tracheostomy Intubation

1. Observe for signs and symptoms requiring tracheostomy intubation, including patient's having translaryngeal intubation greater than 21 days, prolonged ventilator-dependent patients, airway suppuration with copious secretions or hemorrhage, acute upper airway obstruction (laryngeal and pharyngeal) where endotracheal intubation is undesirable or impossible, and chronic upper airway obstruction (i.e., obstructive sleep apnea). **Rationale:** Tracheostomy intubation bypasses upper airway structures to allow for air to flow from the stoma into the lower airways.
2. Observe for the presence of cervical vertebra damage or spinal cord injury. **Rationale:** Indicates injuries or dysfunctional problems prior to the procedure that may be mistaken for complications of the actual tracheotomy procedure.
3. Observe for anxiety and fear. **Rationale:** Tracheotomy is a surgical procedure that will require anesthetic and/or analgesics. Patients tend to be very apprehensive and fearful of choking or inability to breathe, or exhibit hypoxic episodes.
4. Identify signs and symptoms indicating the need for premedication, including combativeness, thrashing about, and uncooperative behavior. **Rationale:** Medications sedate agitated patients, provide temporary paralysis, and reduce salivation, bronchial secretions, and potential vagal-induced bradycardia.

Tracheostomy Tube Care

1. Observe for increased production of secretions. **Rationale:** Tube irritation to the mucosa results in an increased production of secretions.
2. Immediately after intubation, observe for swallowing ability. **Rationale:** Functional glottic incompetence diminishes swallowing as a result of muscular dysfunction. Swallowing is also diminished with anesthesia use.
3. Observe for excessive bleeding. **Rationale:** A small amount of bleeding is normal over 3 to 4 days following tracheotomy. A constant ooze may require blood vessel ligation. Stoma hemorrhage occurs in 36 percent of all tracheotomies (Stauffer et al., 1981).
Observe for signs and symptoms of stoma infection, including elevated temperature, purulent exudate at the site, increasing white blood cell count, cellulitis, and pain at the stoma site. **Rationale:** Infection at the stoma site occurs in 36 percent of all tracheotomies (Stauffer et al., 1981).

Nursing Diagnoses

Tracheotomy

1. Potential for suffocation related to upper airway obstruction and mechanical inability to ventilate. **Rationale:** Physical signs and symptoms result when gas flow is impeded.
2. Impaired tissue integrity of the tracheal mucosa and larynx. **Rationale:** Prolonged (greater than 21 days) translaryngeal intubation increases the risk of tissue necrosis and injury.
3. Potential for aspiration related to glottic dysfunction. **Rationale:** Glottic dysfunction results from trauma or cerebrovascular disease.
4. Altered nutrition, less than body requirements related to translaryngeal tube placement. **Rationale:** Translaryngeal intubation does not allow for eating, whereas a tracheotomy clears the pharynx, promoting oral nutrition and speech.

Tracheostomy Tube Care

1. Potential for infection related to impaired skin integrity. **Rationale:** Stoma site infection occurs in 36 percent of all tracheostomies (Stauffer et al., 1981). Colonization of the tracheobronchial tree with *Pseudomonas* or enteric gram-negative bacteria occurs in 60 to 100 percent of all long-term tracheostomy sites (Heffner et al., 1986). Inadequate stoma care and poor nutrition predispose patients to infection.
2. Decreased cardiac output related to loss of blood volume. **Rationale:** Initial stoma bleeding occurs in 36 percent of all tracheostomies.
3. Potential for trauma related to tracheal mucosa disruption. **Rationale:** Excessive cuff pressures alter capillary perfusion and lead to tissue necrosis.

Planning

1. Individualize the following goals for performing a tracheotomy.

TRACHEOTOMY
   a. Establish and maintain a patent airway. **Rationale:** Upper airway obstructions and technique used during endotracheal tube removal with simultaneous tracheostomy tube insertion can result in loss of airway patency.
   b. In collaboration with the physician, determine the optimal time for performing a tracheotomy (planned tracheotomy). **Rationale:** Tracheotomy is a surgical procedure not without risks and complications. Each case must be individually evaluated and the benefits and risks weighed.

TRACHEOSTOMY TUBE CARE

   a. Maintain mucosal tissue integrity. **Rationale:** Constant pressure and irritation of the mucosal tissue can result in blood vessel and cellular damage.

   b. Prevent stoma infection. **Rationale:** Inadequate tracheostomy care and prolonged tracheostomy are associated with a 60 to 100 percent colonization of the tracheobronchial tree (Heffner et al., 1986).

2. Prepare all necessary equipment and supplies. **Rationale:** Assembly of necessary equipment and supplies facilitates quick and efficient completion of a tracheotomy.

TRACHEOSTOMY

   Check institutional policies as surgical personnel may assist at the bedside.

   a. Remove headboard from the bed.

   b. Tracheotomy tray containing scalpel handle, no. 10 or no. 15 scalpel blade, needle holder, curved Kelly hemostats, two Allis clamps, two Army-Navy retractors, 1 small self-retaining retractor, 1 vein retractor, 1 package of 4-0 silk ties, 1 package of 4-0 silk sutures, straight surgical scissors, toothed forceps.

   c. Cuffed tracheostomy tube.

   d. Twill tape.

   e. Syringe, 10 cc.

   f. Sterile towels and sheet.

   g. Surgical masks and caps.

   h. Sterile 4 × 4 gauze sponges.

   i. Povidone-iodine solution.

   j. Xylocaine with epinephrine.

   k. 5-ml syringe with 23- or 25-gauge needle for anesthetic infiltration.

   l. Suction apparatus.

   m. Suction equipment and supplies (see Skill 1–6).

   n. Oxygen source and connecting tubes.

   o. Self-inflating resuscitation bag with mask connected to 100% oxygen (see Skill 4–2).

   p. Swivel adapter.

   q. Overhead light source.

   r. Emergency cardiac cart.

   s. ECG monitoring (see Skill 7–1).

TRACHEOSTOMY TUBE CARE

   Some institutions may use tracheostomy care kits, which include some or all of the following:

   a. Suction supplies.

   b. Two sterile gloves.

   c. Hydrogen peroxide.

   d. Normal saline.

   e. Twill tape or trach ties.

   f. Sterile cotton swabs.

   g. Sterile basin.

   h. Towel.

   i. Sterile 4 × 4 gauze.

   j. Sterile precut tracheostomy dressing.

   k. Small sterile brush.

   l. Scissors.

   m. Sterile tracheostomy care kit.

   n. Sterile disposable inner cannula (if disposable setup is used).

3. Secure additional personnel to assist with tracheotomy and tracheostomy tube care. **Rationale:** Prevents accidental extubation.

   a. Intubation: At least three persons are necessary: (1) a nurse, respiratory therapist, or physician to remove the endotracheal tube (if present), (2) an assistant for the procedure, and (3) a nurse or anesthesiologist to monitor the patient, administer medications, and document in patient record. All persons must don surgical attire including mask, cap, and gown.

   b. Tracheostomy tube care: At least two persons are necessary: (1) person to activate the self-inflating resuscitation bag, stabilize the inner cannula, and provide reassurance to the patient, and (2) nurse to remove and clean the inner cannula using sterile technique, or to insert sterile disposable cannula.

4. Prepare the patient and family.

   a. Prepare the patient for tracheotomy in a supine, head-extended position. **Rationale:** Allows for easy location of and access to the second, third, and fourth tracheal cartilaginous rings.

   b. Prepare the patient for tracheostomy tube care by assisting to a semi-Fowler's position. **Rationale:** Promotes comfort and provides easy access for the health care provider.

   c. Explain the purpose and necessity of tracheotomy and/or tracheostomy care. **Rationale:** Communication and explanation for therapy encourage cooperation, minimize risk and anxiety, and are a continually stated patient and family need (Parker et al., 1984; Viner, 1988).

   d. Premedicate patient as necessary for tracheotomy. **Rationale:** Medication administration allows for a more controlled intubation and reduces the likelihood of laryngospasms, insertion trauma, and improper tube placement.

Implementation

Steps	Rationale	Special Considerations
Assisting with Tracheotomy		
1. Wash hands.	Reduces transmission of microorganisms.	

Table continues on following page

Steps	Rationale	Special Considerations
2. Hyperoxygenate patient and hyperinflate lungs.	Protects against hypoxemia (Goodnough, 1985).	
3. Suction endotracheal tube and then oropharynx (see Skill 1–6).	Removes secretions and diminishes patient need to cough during the procedure.	
4. Monitor continuous ECG tracing (see Skill 7–1).	Allows for immediate visualization of cardiac electrical activity.	
5. Perform vital signs assessment (i.e., blood pressure, pulse, respiration).	Provides information regarding immediate patient status.	
6. Establish and/or ensure patency of intravenous catheter (see Skill 9–1).	Provides immediate "lifeline" access for emergency medication administration.	
7. Administer sedatives and/or analgesics as ordered.	Provides for muscle relaxation.	
8. Move oxygen tubes, ventilator tubes, etc., away from the tracheotomy site.	Promotes clear field and easy access.	
9. Prepare the surgical area, from the mandible to the clavicles, with povidone-iodine solution for 5 minutes and allow to dry.	Tracheotomy is performed under sterile technique.	
10. Don sterile gown, mask, cap, and gloves.	Tracheotomy is performed under sterile technique. Universal precautions maintained.	
11. Check tracheostomy cuff prior to insertion.	Validates cuff integrity.	
12. Assist the physician by holding retractors, suctioning, passing necessary equipment, and monitoring patient's status as requested.	Helps ensure that the procedure is carried out efficiently and safely.	
13. Secure trach ties and apply sterile dressing.	Keeps stoma site clean and decreases the risk of infection.	
14. Attach swivel adapter to the tracheostomy tube.	Allows for ease of patient movement while minimizing pulling or tugging of the tube.	
15. Replace oxygen source or connect to mechanical ventilation.	Reduces incidence of hypoxia.	
16. Reassess patient's vital signs and respiratory status.	Determines patient's response to procedure.	
17. Place obturator in a protective bag secured at the bedside. Keep an extra properly sized tracheostomy tube at the bedside.	Retained for emergency use.	
18. Measure cuff pressure (see Skill 1–7).	Minimizes mucosal necrosis.	
19. Obtain a chest radiograph.	Identifies actual tube placement.	
20. Obtain arterial blood gases.	Provides information regarding ventilation and perfusion.	
21. Discard supplies in appropriate receptacle.	Reduces transmission of microorganisms. Universal precautions (see Skill 35–1).	

Table continues on following page

Steps	Rationale	Special Considerations
22. Reposition patient.	Promotes comfort.	
23. Wash hands.	Reduces transmission of microorganisms.	

Tracheostomy Care

Steps	Rationale	Special Considerations
1. Wash hands.	Reduces transmission of microorganisms.	
2. Hyperoxygenate patient and hyperinflate lungs.	Protects against hypoxemia (Goodnough, 1985).	
3. Suction trachea and pharynx (see Skills 1–3 and 1–4); remove soiled dressing.	Removes secretions and diminishes patient's need to cough during the procedure.	
4. Set up sterile solution container or sterile field. Be careful not to touch the inside of the container. Fill with approximately 100 ml of normal sterile saline or water.		
5. Don sterile gloves.	Reduces transmission of microorganisms. Universal precautions.	
6. Remove oxygen source and remove inner cannula, placing it in 1:1 solution of H_2O_2 and normal saline.	Removes inner cannula for cleaning. Hydrogen peroxide loosens debris from inner cannula.	Disposable inner cannulas do not require this step.
7. Apply tracheostomy collar oxygen source over the outer cannula, or if ventilator assistance is needed, attach outer cannula to connector or ventilator.	Maintains oxygen supply.	
8. Clean inner cannula with pipe cleaners or small brush provided in the trach kit (see Fig. 1–21).	Assists in the removal of debris and thick secretions.	
9. Rinse inner cannula by pouring normal saline over the cannula.	Removes H_2O_2 and debris.	
10. Remove oxygen source from over outer cannula.	Allows access to opening of outer cannula.	
11. Insert inner cannula and lock into place.	Secures inner cannula.	
12. Reapply oxygen or ventilator oxygen source.	Reestablishes oxygen supply.	
13. Moisten swabs and 4 × 4 gauze pads with hydrogen peroxide. Clean stoma site and outer cannula surface by wiping with cotton-tipped swabs, and 4 × 4 gauze pads.	Removes debris and secretions from the stoma area.	
14. Rinse stoma site and outer cannula with normal saline–soaked cotton-tipped swabs and 4 × 4 gauze.	Rinses hydrogen peroxide and removes additional debris.	
15. Pat dry skin area surrounding stoma site.	Dry surface decreases likelihood of microorganism growth.	

Table continues on following page

Steps	Rationale	Special Considerations
16. To make new ties, cut twill tape at length that will wrap around the patient's neck two times.	Provides length for circumferential wrapping around the patient's neck.	
17. Have assistant hold neckplate securely.	Decreases the incidence of trach tube decannulation.	Assistant must maintain a hold while ties are not secure.
18. Cut and remove current twill tape.	Prepares for new twill tape.	
19. Insert one tie end through the faceplate and pull until one half of the tape is through the eyelet. (Tape will not be "doubled.") Slide the doubled tie around the back of neck, insert through the second eyelet, bring one tie around neck, pull snug, and tie in double square knot on the side of the neck (Fig. 1–22).	Reestablishes secure trach faceplate.	Allow one finger space between twill tape and neck to allow for venous outflow.
20. Apply clean pre-cut tracheostomy dressing under faceplate.	Promotes drainage absorption.	Never cut a 4 × 4 gauze pad because cut edges fray and provide a potential source for infection.
21. Remove gloves and discard in appropriate receptacle.	Prevents transmission of microorganisms. Universal precautions.	
22. Reassess patient's respiratory status.	Identifies effects of trach care.	
23. Discard supplies in appropriate receptacle.	Prevents transmission of microorganisms. Universal precautions.	
24. Wash hands.	Prevents transmission of microorganisms.	

Evaluation

Compare patient assessment before and after tracheotomy and with tracheostomy tube care. **Rationale:** Identifies patient responses.

Expected Outcomes

TRACHEOTOMY

1. Successful tracheotomy. **Rationale:** A successfully performed tracheotomy results in an artificial airway that is properly placed, patent, and secure.

2. Improvement in respiratory status, as evidenced by respiratory rate between 8 and 20 breaths per minute, even, deep, symmetrical chest expansion, PaO_2 between 80 and 100 mmHg, $PaCO_2$ between 35 and 45 mmHg, pH between 7.35 and 7.45, and O_2 saturation at 95 percent or greater. **Rationale:** Proper oxygenation and ventilation assists the lungs in meeting demands of the body.

3. Patent airway. **Rationale:** Facial trauma and a variety of diseases and congenital anomalies may make oral and/or nasal intubation less desirable and tracheotomy the choice for circumventing upper airway obstructions.

4. Removal of tracheobronchial secretions. **Rationale:** Definitive and direct lower airway channel allows for hypopharyngeal secretion removal.

TRACHEOSTOMY TUBE CARE

1. Secured and properly positioned tracheostomy tube. **Rationale:** Technique of procedure is successfully executed.

2. Decreased airway resistance. **Rationale:** Permits the passage of a larger-diameter, shorter-length tube, which in turn decreases turbulent airflow and airway resistance.

3. Improvement in condition of oral and nasal mucosa. **Rationale:** Prolonged use of artificial airways for greater than 3 weeks has been associated with upper airway complications (Kersten, 1989; Stauffer et al., 1981).

4. Improvement in comfort. **Rationale:** Eliminates tube in nose and mouth. Tracheostomy is associated with an improved sense of well-being, as well as a reduction in frustration.

Unexpected Outcomes

1. Prolonged apnea, increasing hypoxemia, and/or cardiopulmonary arrest. **Rationale:** Tracheotomy must be performed efficiently while maintaining a functional airway.

2. Hemorrhage, subcutaneous emphysema, pneumothorax, and thyroid gland injury. **Rationale:** Surgical

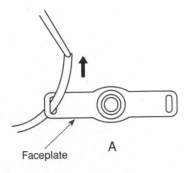

Faceplate

A

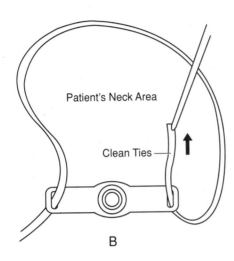

Patient's Neck Area

Clean Ties

B

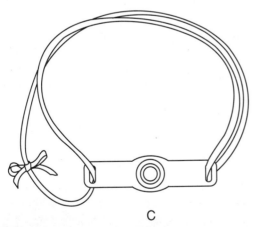

C

FIGURE 1–22. Placement of tracheostomy twill tape: (*A*) faceplate with threading of twill tape (to prevent decannulation, an additional person will need to stabilize the faceplate), (*B*) advancing the twill tape around the back of the neck and looping through the other side of faceplate, (*C*) doubling the twill tape and securing in a knot.

procedure increases the risk of potential injury to adjacent tissues and structures.

3. Cardiac dysrhythmias. **Rationale:** Hypoxemia and vagal stimulation affect heart rate and rhythm.

4. Tube-tip erosion into the tracheal innominate artery. **Rationale:** Stoma placement below the second and third cartilaginous ring results in an increased incidence. Palpation of the tube for pulsations is suggestive of impending erosion of major blood vessels (Kersten, 1989, p. 655).

5. Stoma infection. **Rationale:** Poor nutritional status, general debilitative condition, inadequate tracheostomy care, and constant stoma manipulation and/or irritation predispose patient to infection.

6. Excessive cuff pressure. **Rationale:** Failure to monitor proper cuff pressures can result in improper pressures. Excessive cuff pressures account for 23 percent of tracheostomy complications (Heffner et al., 1986).

7. Leaking airway cuff. **Rationale:** Defective cuff decreases the effectiveness for airway management and results in underinflation of the cuff and underventilation of the lungs.

8. Agitation. **Rationale:** Pain and discomfort increase the incidence of anxiety and disorientation.

9. Tracheal stenosis, malacia, and/or tracheoesophageal fistula. **Rationale:** Long-term use of tracheostomy predisposes the patient to potential complications.

Documentation

Documentation in the patient record should include respiratory and vital signs assessment before and after procedure; type and size of tube; persons assisting with the procedure; nursing care given; use of medications; measurement of cuff pressures and cuff volume; placement of inner cannula; expected and unexpected outcomes; patient response to procedure; date, time, and frequency with which procedure is performed. **Rationale:** Records nursing actions and patient responses; serves as a legal document of the series of events.

Patient/Family Education

1. Assess level of understanding of patient and significant others regarding condition and rationale for tracheotomy and tracheostomy tube care. **Rationale:** Identification of misconceptions regarding patient's condition, tracheotomy, and/or tracheostomy tube care, predicted outcome, and potential risks allows for additional communication and clarification.

2. Teach the patient and significant others how to perform direct-care activities. **Rationale:** The patient and significant other will have responsibilities for providing continuous care at home.

3. Maintain and encourage effective communication. **Rationale:** Communication assists caregiver in meeting needs. Communication can decrease isolation and feelings of anxiety, fear, and panic. Frequent communication of patient condition and progress is cited as an important patient (Viner, 1988) and family need (Hickey, 1990).

Performance Checklist
Skill 1–9: Tracheotomy and Tracheostomy Tube Care

Critical Behaviors	Complies	
	yes	no
TRACHEOTOMY		
1. Wash hands.		
2. Hyperoxygenate patient and hyperinflate lungs.		
3. Suction endotracheal tube and then oropharynx.		
4. Monitor ECG tracing.		
5. Assess vital signs.		
6. Establish patency of intravenous catheter.		
7. Administer sedation/analgesics as ordered.		
8. Establish clear site for tracheotomy.		
9. Prep the neck area.		
10. Don sterile attire.		
11. Check tracheotomy cuff.		
12. Assist the physician.		
13. Secure trach ties.		
14. Attach swivel adapter.		
15. Replace oxygen source and connect to ventilator as needed.		
16. Reassess respiratory and vital signs.		
17. Place obturator and correctly sized tracheostomy tube at the bedside.		
18. Measure cuff pressure.		
19. Obtain chest radiograph.		
20. Obtain arterial blood gases.		
21. Discard supplies.		
22. Reposition patient.		
23. Wash hands.		
24. Document procedure in patient record.		
TRACHEOSTOMY TUBE CARE		
1. Wash hands.		
2. Hyperoxygenate patient and hyperinflate lungs.		
3. Suction trachea and pharynx.		
4. Remove soiled dressing.		
5. Set up sterile solution container or field.		
6. Don sterile gloves.		
7. Remove oxygen source and inner cannula and place in 1:1 solution of H_2O_2 and normal saline.		
8. Apply tracheostomy collar and oxygen source.		

Table continues on following page

Critical Behaviors	Complies	
	yes	no
9. Clean inner cannula.		
10. Rinse inner cannula.		
11. Remove oxygen source from outer cannula.		
12. Replace inner cannula and lock into place.		
13. Reapply oxygen or ventilator source.		
14. Clean stoma site.		
15. Rinse stoma site.		
16. Pat skin dry surrounding stoma site.		
17. Prepare and cut twill tape.		
18. Cut and remove soiled twill tape.		
19. Insert twill tape to faceplate and secure.		
20. Apply clean tracheostomy dressing.		
21. Remove and discard gloves.		
22. Reassess patient's respiratory status.		
23. Discard supplies.		
24. Wash hands.		
25. Document care in patient record.		
26. Check to make sure that an extra obturator and correctly sized tracheostomy tube is placed at the bedside.		

REFERENCES

Baker, T., Taylor, M., Wilson, M., et al. (1989). Evaluation of a closed system endotracheal suction catheter. *Am. J. Infection Control* 17:97.

Berlauk, J. F. (1986). Prolonged endotracheal intubation vs. tracheotomy. *Crit. Care Med.* 14(8):742–745.

Bostick, J., and Wendelgass, St. T. (1987). Normal saline instillation as part of the suctioning procedure: Effects on PaO_2 and amount of secretions. *Heart Lung* 16(5):532–537.

Bowers, B. (1987). Intergenerational caregiving: Adult caregivers and their aging parents. *Adv. Nurs. Sci.* 9(2):20–31.

Chulay, M. (1988). Arterial blood gas changes with a hyperinflation and hyperoxygenation suctioning intervention in critically ill patients. *Heart Lung* 17(6):654–661.

Cunningham, C., and Sergent, J. (1983). A preliminary view of the contamination of suction apparatus. *Focus Crit. Care* 10(4):10–14.

Czarnik, R. E., Stone, K. S., Everhart, C. C., and Preusser, B. A. (1991). Differential effects of continuous versus intermittent suction on tracheal tissue. *Heart Lung* 20(2):144–151.

Davis, R. F., and Gammage, G. W. (1988). Postoperative Management of the Cardiac Surgery Patient. In J. M. Civetta, R. W. Taylor, and R. Kirby (Eds.), *Critical Care* (p. 557).

Estabrooks, C. A. (1989). Touch: A nursing strategy in the intensive care unit. *Heart Lung* 18(4):392–401.

Eubanks, D. H., and Bone, R. C. (1990). *Comprehensive Respiratory Care: A Learning System* (pp. 491–495). St. Louis: Mosby.

Flunk, R. R., Jr. (1985). Suctioning—intermittent or continuous? *Respir. Care* 30:837–838.

Goodnough, S. (1985). The effects of oxygen and hyperinflation on arterial oxygen tension after endotracheal suctioning. *Heart Lung* 14(1):11–17.

Goodnough, S., Bines, A., and Schneider, W. (1986). The effects of clinical nursing expertise on patient outcomes. *Crit. Care Med.* 14:358.

Gotta, A. (1988). Airway management for maxillofacial trauma. *Curr. Rev.* 114–119.

Habib, M. (1989). Physiologic implications of artificial airways. *Chest* 96(1):180–184.

Heffner, J., Miller, K., and Sahn, S. (1986). Tracheostomy in the intensive care unit: 2. Complications. *Chest* 90(3):430–436.

Herndon, D. N., Traber, D. L., Niehaus, G. D., et al. (1984). The pathophysiology of smoke inhalation injury in a sheep model. *J. Trauma* 24:1044–1051.

Hickey, M. (1990). What are the needs of families of critically ill patients? A review of the literature since 1976. *Heart Lung* 19(4):401–415.

Johnson, J., Rice, V., Fuller, S., and Endress, M. (1978). Sensory information, instruction in a coping strategy and recovery from surgery. *Res. Nurs. Health* 1:4–17.

Jung, R., and Gottlieb, L. (1976). Comparison of tracheobronchial suction catheters in humans. *Chest* 69(2):179–181.

Kacmarek, R., Mack, C., Dimas, S. (1990). *The Essentials of Respiratory Care* (p. 430). St. Louis, Mosby.

Kersten, L. D. (1989). *Comprehensive Respiratory Nursing: A Decision-Making Approach* (pp. 630–635). Philadelphia: Saunders.

Landa, J. F., Kwoka, M. A., Chapman, G. A., et al. (1980). Effects of suctioning on mucociliary transport. *Chest* 77:202–207.

MacKenzie, C. (1983). Compromises in the choice of orotracheal or nasotracheal intubation and tracheostomy. *Heart Lung* 12(5):485–492.

Miracle, V. A., and Allnutt, D. R. (1990). How to perform basic airway management. *Nursing* 90:55–60.

Moloney-Harmon, P. (1991). "Initial assessment and stabilization of the critically injured child," *Critical Care Nursing Clinics of North America*, Vol 3, no. 3, Philadelphia, Saunders, pp. 399–409.

Noll, M. L., Hix, C. D., Scott, G. (1990). Closed tracheal suction systems: effectiveness and nursing implications. *AACN Clinical Issues in Critical Care Nursing* 1:318–326.

O'Neill-Norris, L., and Grove, S. K. (1986). Investigation of selected psychosocial needs of family members of critically ill patients. *Heart Lung* 15:194–199.

Parker, M. M., Schubert, W., Shelhamer, J. H., and Parrillo, J. E. (1984). Perceptions of a critically ill patient experiencing therapeutic paralysis in an ICU. *Crit. Care Med.* 12:69.

Perry, A., and Potter, P. (1986). *Clinical Nursing Skills and Techniques: Basic, Intermediate, and Advanced* (pp. 452–455). St. Louis: Mosby.

Pesiri, A. J., Stewart, K., Kobe, E., and Stewart, W. (1990). Protocol for prevention of unintentional extubation. *Crit. Care Nurs. Q.* 87–90.

Plum, F., and Dunning, M. F. (1956). Techniques for minimizing trauma to the tracheobronchial tree after tracheotomy. *N. Engl. J. Med.* 254:193–200.

Powaser, M., et al. (1976). The effectiveness of hourly cuff deflation in minimizing tracheal damage. *Heart Lung* 5(5):734–741.

Rashkin, M., and Davis, T. (1986). Acute complications of endotracheal intubation; relationship to reintubation, route, urgency, and duration. *Chest* 89(2):165–167.

Rindfleisch, S., and Tyler, M. (1983). Points of view, duration of suctioning: An important variable. *Respir. Care* 28(4): 457–459.

Rosen, M., and Hillard, E. K. (1962). The effects of negative pressure during tracheal suction. *Anesth. Analg.* 41:50–57.

Sackner, M., Landa, J., Greeneltch, N., and Robinson, M. (1973). Pathogenesis and prevention of tracheobronchial damage with suction procedures. *Chest* 64(3):284–290.

Schumann, L., and Parsons, G. (1985). Tracheal suctioning and ventilator tubing changes in adult respiratory distress syndrome: Use of a positive end-expiratory pressure valve. *Heart Lung* 14(4):362–367.

Sills, J. (1986). An emergency cuff inflation technique. *Respir. Care* 31(3):199–201.

Stauffer, J. L., Olson, D. E., and Petty, T. L. (1981). Complications and consequences of endotracheal intubation and tracheotomy: A prospective study of 150 critically ill adult patients. *Am. J. Med.* 70:65.

Viner, E. (1988). *At the Other End of the Endotracheal Tube* (videotape). Washington: Foundation for Critical Care.

Weigelt, J. A., and McCormack, A. (1988). Mechanism of Injury. In V. Cardona, P. Hurn, P. Mason, et al. (Eds.), *Trauma Nursing from Resuscitation Through Rehabilitation* (p. 121). Philadelphia: Saunders.

BIBLIOGRAPHY

Block, A. J., and Cicale, M. J. (1988). Acute Respiratory Failure in Chronic Obstructive Pulmonary Disease. In J. Civetta, R. Taylor, and R. Kirby (Eds.), *Critical Care* (p. 1106). Philadelphia: Lippincott.

Chuley, M. (in press). Airway and Ventilatory Management. In B. Dossey, C. Guzzetta, and C. Kenner (Eds.), *Critical Care Nursing: Body-Mind-Spirit*, 3d Ed. Philadelphia: Lippincott.

Dail, D. H. (1982). Anatomy of Respiratory System. In K. M. Moser and R. G. Spragg (Eds.), *Respiratory Emergencies*, 2d Ed. St. Louis: Mosby.

Haberman, P., Green, H., et al. (1973). Determinants of successful selective tracheobronchial suctioning. *N. Engl. J. Med.* 289(20):1060–1063.

Heffner, J. E. (1989). Medical indications for tracheotomy. *Chest* 96(1):186–192.

2

OXYGEN THERAPY

BEHAVIORAL OBJECTIVES

After completing this chapter, the nurse will be able to

- Define the key terms.
- Indicate the purpose of oxygen therapy.
- State the indications for oxygen therapy.
- Identify oxygen delivery systems.
- Describe the hazards related to oxygen therapy.
- Identify conditions requiring special precautions related to oxygen administration.
- Demonstrate the skills used in oxygen therapy.

Oxygen is essential for cellular function. Without adequate oxygenation, cellular destruction and eventually death will occur. Organs most susceptible to oxygen deprivation include the brain, the adrenal glands, the heart, the kidneys, and the liver.

Oxygen concentrations within the body are measured by a variety of methods. The most common methods include arterial blood gas analysis, mixed venous oxygen saturation by pulmonary artery catheters, and transcutaneous oximetry.

There are three purposes for oxygen therapy: (1) to treat hypoxemia, (2) to decrease respiratory effort, and (3) to decrease the workload of the heart.

Like all drugs, oxygen has its indications, contraindications, side effects, and special administration techniques and precautions. The primary indication for oxygen therapy is a decreasing PaO_2 or clinical signs and symptoms of hypoxemia, including dyspnea, tachypnea, extreme paleness or cyanosis, disorientation, restlessness, impaired judgment, combativeness, hypotension with a decrease in heart rate, or acute hypertension with an increased heart rate. Clinical conditions that may indicate oxygen therapy include, but are not limited to, respiratory arrest, acute respiratory failure during anesthesia administration, congestive heart failure, acute myocardial infarction, shock, cardiac arrest, and noxious gas poisonings.

There are no absolute contraindications for oxygen therapy. However, there are several conditions that require special consideration regarding the administration of high oxygen concentrations. These conditions include, but are not limited to, prematurity, chronic obstructive pulmonary disease (COPD), and advanced age.

In healthy individuals, the normal stimulus to breathe is increased levels of carbon dioxide in the blood. This increased level of carbon dioxide stimulates the respiratory center of the brain, causing the individual to breathe more rapidly and deeply to thereby rid the body of the excess carbon dioxide. However, individuals with COPD naturally retain higher levels of carbon dioxide as a result of their alveolar destruction. Such individuals develop a tolerance to high carbon dioxide levels, and their stimulus to breathe becomes a decreased oxygen level. Administration of high concentrations of oxygen may seriously decrease their stimulus to breathe, particularly at night.

Premature infants cannot tolerate concentrations of oxygen that would increase their PaO_2 greater than 100 percent because of the possibility of retinal artery damage. This damage may result in retrolental fibroplasia. PaO_2 levels above 145 to 155 mmHg for as little as 4 to 5 hours may damage the retinal arteries enough to cause blindness.

In the elderly, there is a reduced ability of the lungs to expel carbon dioxide, therefore leading to increased carbon dioxide levels in the body. Administration of high concentrations of oxygen raises the blood oxygen level and stimulates the respiratory center of the brain to decrease the respiratory rate. This, in turn, further increases the carbon dioxide levels in the body and can lead to carbon dioxide narcosis and possibly death.

Oxygen therapy is administered by a variety of methods. These include, but are not limited to, nasal cannula, nasal catheter, simple mask, partial and nonrebreathing mask, Venturi mask, esophageal obturator airway, endotracheal tube, or tracheostomy tube. Regardless of the method of administration, oxygen therapy involves maintaining a patent airway and administering the oxygen in the appropriate quantity and quality for each individual.

The recommended acceptable PaO_2 is one that is greater than 60 mmHg. Therefore, use the lowest oxygen concentration and the best delivery system to achieve the desired PaO_2. This will decrease the risk for development of oxygen toxicity and other complications of oxygen therapy.

Complications of oxygen therapy include, but are not limited to, induced hypoventilation, microatelectasis, retrolental fibroplasia, oxygen toxicity, drying of the mucous membranes, and decreased mucociliary movement.

KEY TERMS

alveolar ventilation
artificial airway
atelectasis
carbon dioxide narcosis
carbon dioxide toxicity

cardiac output
chronic obstructive pulmonary
  disease (COPD)
endotracheal tube
entrain

esophageal obturator
  airway
FıO₂
high-flow oxygen delivery
  system
hyperinflated
hyperventilation
hypoventilation
hypoxemia
hypoxia
low-flow oxygen delivery
  system

microatelectasis
oronasal mask
oxygen toxicity
pulmonary congestion
respiratory failure
retrolental fibroplasia
supplemental oxygen
tidal volume
trachea
tracheal tube
transcutaneous ear
  oximetry

SKILLS

2–1 Nasal Cannula Application
2–2 Oxygen Mask Application
2–3 Portable Oxygen Tank Preparation and Setup
2–4 Incentive Spirometry
2–5 Intermittent Positive-Pressure Breathing Treatment

GUIDELINES

The following assessment guidelines assist the nurse in formulating a nursing diagnosis and an individualized plan of care for the patient to maintain an adequate arterial oxygen level:

1. Know the patient's baseline respiratory status.
2. Know the patient's baseline vital signs.
3. Know the patient's past medical history.
4. Know the patient's present treatment plan.
5. Perform a systematic assessment of the patient's status in a timely manner.

6. Determine appropriate interventions from the assessment data.
7. Become adept with equipment necessary to provide oxygen therapy.

SKILL 2–1

Nasal Cannula Application

The nasal cannula is a low-flow oxygen device that directs oxygen flow through two plastic prongs that have been inserted into the nares (Fig. 2–1). When the patient inspires through the mouth or nose, room air is drawn in to mix with the oxygen. The nasal cannula is available to all age groups and may be used for short- and long-term oxygen therapy.

Nasal cannulas provide an FıO₂ of 0.24 to 0.50 with a flow rate of 1 to 6 L/min. Flow rates in excess of 6 L/min may produce discomfort as a result of drying of the airway mucosa of the nares.

The concentration of oxygen increases by 4% for each 1-L/min increase in flow rate. Mean values of inspired oxygen concentration on a nasal cannula at various oxygen flow rates are shown in Table 2–1.

Purpose

The nurse administers oxygen by nasal cannula to

1. Correct or prevent hypoxemia, decrease the work of breathing, and decrease myocardial work.
2. Provide an oxygen device that allows the patient comfort in talking, eating, and coughing.
3. Deliver low oxygen concentrations.

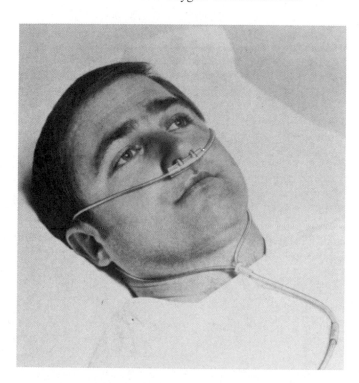

FIGURE 2–1. Standard nasal cannula: (*A*) nasal prongs, (*B*) slide, and (*C*) tubing. (From R. J. Craig, *Nursing Clinics of North America*, Vol. 16. Philadelphia: Saunders, 1981, with permission.)

TABLE 2–1 OXYGEN CONCENTRATIONS BY NASAL CANNULA AT VARIOUS FLOW RATES

Oxygen Flow Rate, L/min	Approximate FIO_2
1	0.24
2	0.28
3	0.32
4	0.36
5	0.40
6	0.44

Source: From Craig, R. J. *Nursing Clinics of North America*, Vol. 16. Philadelphia, Saunders, 1981, with permission.

Prerequisite Knowledge and Skills

Prior to applying a nasal cannula, the nurse should understand

1. Anatomy and physiology of the upper and lower respiratory system.
2. Principles of gas exchange.

The nurse should be able to perform

1. Respiratory system assessment.
2. Vital signs assessment.
3. Proper handwashing technique (see Skill 35–5).
4. Universal precautions (see Skill 35–1).

Assessment

1. Observe for signs and symptoms of hypoxemia requiring oxygen therapy, including increased respiratory rate, irregular/altered breathing patterns, restlessness, decreased level of consciousness, tachycardia or bradycardia, cyanosis (late), hypotension or hypertension, dizziness, fatigue, dyspnea, and dysrhythmias. **Rationale:** Physical signs and symptoms evidenced by hypoxemia may progress to dysrhythmias and death.
2. Assess and trend arterial blood gas (ABG) and/or pulse oximetry results. **Rationale:** The need for supplemental oxygen and the effects of oxygen therapy are objectively documented over time.
3. Assess patient for patent nasal passages and remove airway secretions (i.e., examine for deviated septum, mucosa edema, and polyps). **Rationale:** Oxygen is unable to enter the nares in the presence of obstructed passages.

Nursing Diagnoses

1. Activity intolerance related to insufficient oxygenation for activities of daily living. **Rationale:** Patient experiences a decreased exchange of gases (oxygen and carbon dioxide) between the alveoli of the lungs and the vascular system.
2. Potential for impaired skin integrity related to friction from the nasal cannula. **Rationale:** Irritation and ulceration on the tops of the ears can occur as a result of friction from the plastic cannula.

Planning

1. Individualize the following goals for low-flow oxygen administration via nasal cannula:
   a. Maintain normal PaO_2 and SaO_2 levels. **Rationale:** Demonstrates the effectiveness of oxygen therapy.
   b. Provides patient education. **Rationale:** Promotes compliance with oxygen therapy.
   c. Maintain skin integrity. **Rationale:** Impaired skin integrity causes discomfort for the patient and provides an entry route for microorganisms.
2. Prepare all necessary equipment and supplies. **Rationale:** Assembly of all equipment at the bedside ensures efficient and quick application of the nasal cannula.
   a. Flowmeter.
   b. Humidifier.
   c. Nasal cannula.
   d. Delivery tube, normally 3 to 5 ft in length, connecting nasal cannula to humidifier outlet. **Rationale:** Delivers humidified oxygen to nasal cannula while allowing patient movement.
3. Prepare the patient.
   a. Explain the procedure as appropriate to the patient's condition and familiarity with the procedure. **Rationale:** Patient has knowledge of procedure, which increases compliance and reduces anxiety.
   b. Communicate and enforce safety precautions. Fire hazards are involved with oxygen administration. **Rationale:** Although oxygen alone will not explode, it supports combustion and causes flammable substances to burn rapidly. Enforce the "No Smoking" rule for patients and anyone else in the area when oxygen is being administered.
4. Display "No Smoking" and "Oxygen in Use" signs in ready view. **Rationale:** Promotes safety to patient, visitors, and staff while oxygen is in use.

Implementation

Steps	Rationale	Special Considerations
1. Wash hands.	Reduces transmission of microorganisms (see Skill 35–1).	
2. Attach humidifier to flowmeter.	Oxygen is extremely dry as it comes from the wall outlet or cylinder.	
3. Connect flowmeter to oxygen source, and check operation of flowmeter and humidifier.	Ensures proper working condition of equipment.	
4. Open cannula package and attach to humidifier with care to avoid contamination of cannula nasal tips.	Prevents transmission of microorganisms (see Skill 35–1).	
5. Turn oxygen flowmeter on to prescribed liter flow/oxygen concentration prior to applying cannula (see Table 2–1). Observe that water in humidification container is bubbling.	Validates gas flow through the device.	
6. Insert the nasal tips into the nares. Direct prongs posteriorly.	Directs oxygen flow into nares.	For pediatric application (8 years and under), a lower flow rate of ¼ to ½ L/min, is recommended. Trim nasal tips with scissors. For long-term use, consider nasal cannula with soft, pliable prongs slightly flared at the ends to ensure smooth gas flow.
7. Loop the two plastic tubes of the cannula over the ears and under the chin, or place elastic band around the head.	Secures cannula comfortably in place.	Avoid ear soreness by padding the area behind the ear with a cotton ball or gauze pad.
8. Gently adjust the plastic slide until cannula is secure.	Ensures that nasal cannula will remain in secure position to deliver oxygen.	If the tube is too loose, the tips may fall out of the nares; if it is too tight, the tips will press against the surface of the nares causing irritation and misdirected gas flow.
9. Wash hands.	Reduces transmission of microorganisms.	

Evaluation

1. Compare the patient's PaO_2 and/or SaO_2 before and after oxygen administration. **Rationale:** Identifies the effectiveness of oxygen administration.

2. Reassess and compare the patient's respiratory status before and after application of nasal cannula. **Rationale:** Identifies the effects of oxygen administration on hypoxemia.

3. Assess placement and patency of the prongs entering the nares. **Rationale:** Prongs can be dislodged easily or may become plugged with nasal secretions.

4. Observe for skin breakdown of nares and skin above and behind ears. **Rationale:** Oxygen administration can cause drying to nares. Skin breakdown and irritation can occur from friction of the elastic band or plastic tubes.

Expected Outcomes

1. Improvement in PaO_2 or SaO_2, increased level of consciousness, normalization of respiratory and heart rate, and absence of cyanosis. **Rationale:** Improved arterial oxygenation.

2. Maintenance of skin integrity. **Rationale:** Skin breakdown and irritation are adverse effects of the nasal cannula.

Unexpected Outcomes

1. Persistent hypoxemia. **Rationale:** Respiratory failure can precipitate respiratory arrest, cardiac dysrhythmias, and death.

2. Decreased ventilatory drive in patients with COPD. **Rationale:** Excessive oxygen dulls the hypoxic drive, and the stimulus to breathe.

3. Skin breakdown. **Rationale:** Skin irritation from the plastic tubing or elastic strap over ears can cause skin breakdown.

4. Nasal trauma. **Rationale:** Tissue damage results from pressure of nasal prongs resting on the nares mucosa, or prolonged nasal cannula application.

Documentation

Documentation in the patient record should include respiratory assessment before and after oxygen administration, nasal cannula application, and oxygen flow (L/min); patient's response to oxygen administration; date and time of administration; and assessment of skin integrity and patient complaints of oxygen-related discomforts (e.g., substernal discomfort or drying of the nose, mouth, or throat). **Rationale:** Documents nursing care given, patient's respiratory status, and expected and unexpected outcomes.

Patient/Family Education

1. Assess ability and readiness of patient and family to apply nasal cannula. **Rationale:** Patient or family may not be emotionally or physically ready or able to apply device.

2. Discuss and demonstrate the steps for nasal cannula application and maintenance. **Rationale:** Encourages the patient and family to participate. Promotes comfort and encourages questions from patient and family.

3. Explain the signs and symptoms of hypoxemia, indicating need for oxygen therapy. **Rationale:** Enable patient and family to recognize the need for oxygen therapy.

4. Explain the possible complications and their preventive measures for nasal cannula therapy. **Rationale:** Patient and family will be able to recognize, prevent, and/or act upon complications.

Performance Checklist
Skill 2–1: Nasal Cannula Application

Critical Behaviors	Complies	
	yes	no
1. Wash hands.		
2. Attach humidifier to flowmeter.		
3. Connect flowmeter to oxygen, and check for proper operation.		
4. Open cannula package on a clean surface and attach cannula to humidifier, avoiding contamination of cannula tips.		
5. Turn on oxygen flowmeter to prescribed liter flow.		
6. Insert the nasal tips into the nares.		
7. Loop the two plastic tubes of the cannula over the ears and under the chin.		
8. Gently adjust the plastic slide until the cannula is secure.		
9. Wash hands.		
10. Document the application in patient record.		

SKILL 2–2

Oxygen Mask Application

Oxygen delivery systems are traditionally divided into low-flow and high-flow systems. The approach to oxygen therapy is usually dictated by the patient's condition.

The nasal cannula is used when lower concentrations of oxygen are indicated. For delivery of a specified oxygen concentration, the system used is the Venturi mask. For higher oxygen concentration delivery, the oronasal mask system is used. The lowest concentration is attained with the use of a simple mask, and the highest concentration by a nonrebreather mask.

When a patient's PaO_2 cannot be maintained with the nonrebreather mask, the need for intubation and mechanical ventilation is imminent.

The *simple face mask* is a low-flow system that uses the nose, nasopharynx, and oropharynx as an anatomic reservoir. The simple face mask is a dome-shaped, disposable, plastic apparatus that fits over the mouth and nose and is secured by a strap around the back of the head. It is adjusted to the patient's face by a malleable metal nose piece incorporated into the mask. It has a series of small holes, or ports, on each side that act as exhalation ports. Room air is also entrained through these ports, thus reducing the delivered oxygen concentrations (Fig. 2–2).

The simple face mask can deliver a moderate range of

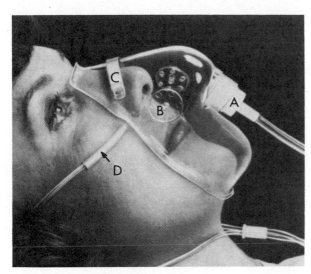

FIGURE 2–2. Simple face mask: (*A*) oxygen tubing, (*B*) exhalation ports, (*C*) malleable metal piece that conforms to shape of nose, and (*D*) restraining strap. (From R. J. Craig, *Nursing Clinics of North America*, Vol. 16. Philadelphia: Saunders, 1981, with permission.)

clinical advantage to the Venturi mask is that a predetermined oxygen percentage can be delivered to the patient regardless of wide deviations in the patient's respiratory rate. A Venturi mask reliably and predictably provides controlled low to moderate oxygen concentrations (Table 2–2).

The *partial rebreathing mask* is a simple face mask with an attached reservoir bag. It contains no valves and is generally used on acutely ill patients requiring an oxygen concentration between 40% to 60%. The use of a 500- to 1000-ml reservoir bag provides a range of oxygen concentrations from 35% to 60% at 6 to 10 L/min (Table 2–3). The reservoir allows reserve oxygen-rich air to be inhaled from the bag during inspiration. The first third of the patient's exhaled volume returns to the bag as the patient exhales, and the remaining two-thirds are exhaled through the mask's side ports (Fig. 2–4).

The *nonrebreathing face mask* is a simple mask with a reservoir bag that includes a one-way valve between the

oxygen concentrations (40% to 60% oxygen at 5 to 8 L/min). A minimum flow of 5 L/min is required to flush carbon dioxide from the mask.

A *Venturi mask* delivers a specified amount of oxygen through a restriction or jet (Fig. 2–3). Static room air is then drawn in through entrainment ports into the moving stream of oxygen. Varying concentrations of oxygen are delivered by changing the size of the jet. The major

TABLE 2–2   OXYGEN CONCENTRATIONS BY VENTURI MASK AT VARIOUS FLOW RATES

Oxygen Flow Rate, L/min	Approximate F_IO_2
4	0.24
4–6	0.28
6–8	0.31
8–10	0.35
8–12	0.40
12	0.50

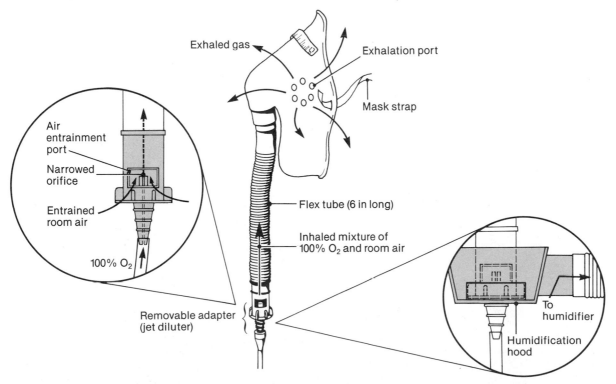

FIGURE 2–3.   Venturi mask. The arrows indicate the movement of gas during respiration. A humidification hood is added to protect air entrainment ports and to provide humidification. (From L. D. Kersten, *Comprehensive Respiratory Nursing*. Philadelphia: Saunders, 1989, with permission.)

TABLE 2–3   OXYGEN CONCENTRATIONS BY PARTIAL REBREATHING MASK AT VARIOUS FLOW RATES

Oxygen Flow Rate, L/min	Approximate FiO₂
6	0.35
7	0.40
8	0.45
9	0.50
10	0.60

TABLE 2–4   OXYGEN CONCENTRATIONS BY NONREBREATHING MASK AT VARIOUS FLOW RATES

Oxygen Flow Rate, L/min	Approximate FiO₂
6	0.55–0.60
8	0.60–0.80
10	0.80–0.90
12	0.90
15	0.90–1.00

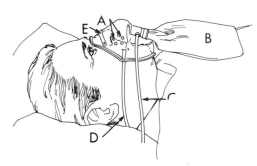

FIGURE 2–4.   Partial rebreathing mask: (*A*) exhalation ports, (*B*) reservoir bag, (*C*) oxygen tubing, (*D*) restraining strap, and (*E*) malleable metal piece that conforms to shape of nose. (From K. P. Rarey and J. W. Youtsey, *Respiratory Patient Care*. © 1981, pp. 23, 24. Reprinted by permission of Prentice-Hall, Inc., Englewood Cliffs, New Jersey.)

bag and the mask and two one-way valves on the mask's exhalation side ports (Fig. 2–5). These valves prevent the entrainment of room air through the exhalation ports and require that the patient receive pure oxygen from the reservoir bag and mask. Inhaled gas with a properly fitted mask comes only from the bag, and the exhaled gas goes only to the room. The gas concentration delivered depends on the concentration of the source gas (Table 2–4). The nonrebreathing mask delivers an FiO₂ of between 6 to 15 L/min and is indicated for short-term use in acutely ill patients.

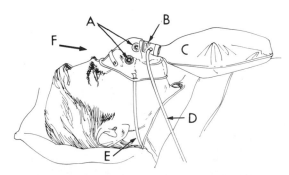

FIGURE 2–5.   Nonrebreathing mask: (*A*) one-way valve to exhalation, (*B*) one-way valve for inhalation from reservoir, (*C*) reservoir bag, (*D*) oxygen tubing, (*E*) restraining strap, and (*F*) malleable metal piece that conforms to shape of nose. (From K. P. Rarey and J. W. Youtsey, *Respiratory Patient Care*. Englewood Cliffs, N.J.: Prentice-Hall, 1981, pp. 23, 24. Reprinted by permission of Prentice-Hall, Inc.)

Purpose

The nurse administers oxygen via face mask to

1.   Correct or prevent hypoxemia, decrease the work of breathing, and decrease myocardial work.
2.   Deliver concentrations of oxygen ranging from 24 to 100 percent.
3.   Deliver constant humidification to the upper respiratory airway.

Prerequisite Knowledge and Skills

Prior to applying an oronasal face mask, the nurse should understand

1.   Anatomy and physiology of the upper and lower respiratory system.
2.   Principles of gas exchange.
3.   Arterial blood gas analysis.
4.   Conditions affecting oxygenation.

The nurse should be able to perform

1.   Respiratory system assessment.
2.   Vital signs assessment.
3.   Proper handwashing technique (see Skill 35–5).
4.   Universal precautions.

Assessment

1.   Observe for signs and symptoms of hypoxemia requiring oxygen therapy, including increased respiratory rate, increased work of breathing, restlessness, decreased level of consciousness, tachycardia or bradycardia, cyanosis, hypotension or hypertension, dyspnea, cardiac dysrhythmias, and dizziness. **Rationale:** Physical signs and symptoms of hypoxia may progress to cardiac dysrhythmias and death.
2.   Assess the patient for facial burns, nasogastric tubes, or where nursing care requires frequent access to the patient's face. **Rationale:** Alternate oxygen administration devices should be used to allow a proper fit of the mask and consistent delivery of oxygen.
3.   Observe for patent airway. **Rationale:** Additional tubes and secretions may occlude the airway.
4.   Assess and trend arterial blood gas (ABG) results. **Rationale:** The initiation and effect of supplemental oxygen objectively corrects hypoxemia.

Nursing Diagnoses

1. Activity intolerance related to insufficient oxygenation for activities of daily living. **Rationale:** Patient experiences a decreased exchange of gases (oxygen and carbon dioxide) between the alveoli of the lungs and the vascular system.
2. Ineffective airway clearance and potential for aspiration related to oronasal mask. **Rationale:** Face mask inhibits the clearance of vomitus from around the mask.
3. Potential for impaired skin integrity related to oxygen administration via face mask. **Rationale:** Irritation and ulceration of the skin can occur from friction of the plastic mask and the restraining strap. Oxygen administration can dry out and irritate oral and nasal mucous membranes.
4. Impaired verbal communication related to oronasal face mask. **Rationale:** Mask over the nose and mouth makes speech difficult to understand.

Planning

1. Individualize the following goals for oxygen therapy via face mask:
   a. Maintain SaO_2 greater than 85 mmHg or PaO_2 greater than 90 mmHg. **Rationale:** Corrects hypoxemia.
   b. Promote level of consciousness. **Rationale:** Increased oxygen in the blood improves the chances for cerebral perfusion.
   c. Maintain patent airway. **Rationale:** Patient should be closely observed for vomiting and for proper head position.
2. Prepare all necessary equipment and supplies. **Rationale:** Assembly of all equipment at the bedside ensures application of the face mask quickly and efficiently.
   a. Flowmeter.
   b. Humidifier (not used with a Venturi mask because water droplets will occlude the oxygen inlet to the mask and alter entrainment.
   c. Oxygen mask
      (1) Simple
      (2) Venturi mask: appropriate percentage jet adapters; oxygen connecting tubing
      (3) Partial rebreathing mask
      (4) Nonrebreathing mask
      (5) Nipple adapter/connector.
   d. Oxygen source.
   e. Sterile water.
3. Prepare the patient.
   a. Explain the procedure to patient. **Rationale:** Minimizes risks and reduces anxiety.
   b. Assist the patient to a position that promotes comfort and facilitates ease of respirations. **Rationale:** Promotes comfort and reduces respiratory work.
4. Display "No Smoking" and "Oxygen in Use" signs in ready view. **Rationale:** Promotes safety to patient, visitors, and staff while oxygen is in use.
5. Verify physician's order. **Rationale:** Ensures that procedure will be carried out efficiently.

Implementation

Steps	Rationale	Special Considerations
Simple and Partial Rebreathing Masks		
1. Wash hands.	Reduces transmission of microorganisms.	
2. Attach humidifier to flowmeter.	Oxygen is extremely dry as it comes from wall outlet or cylinder.	
3. Connect flowmeter to oxygen source, and check operation of flowmeter and humidifier. Set prescribed oxygen flow.	Ensures proper working condition of equipment.	
4. Attach oxygen mask connecting tubing to humidifier and flowmeter.	Delivers humidified oxygen to the mask.	Select a properly sized mask. Masks are often poorly tolerated by infants. The soft vinyl pediatric mask may be accepted by children.
5. Turn on oxygen.	Begins gas flow.	
6. Place mask on patient's mouth and nose. Adjust elastic or tubing for a snug fit.	Ensures precise oxygen concentration is delivered.	If using the partial rebreathing mask, cover your thumb or index finger with a clean tissue and occlude the reservoir bag opening, allowing the oxygen flow to fill the bag before placing it on the patient.

Table continues on following page

Steps	Rationale	Special Considerations
7. Check oxygen flow.	Validates prescribed oxygen concentration.	Adjust to ordered liter flow if simple mask or adjust to prevent bag deflation if partial rebreathing mask.
8. Stress fire hazards involved with oxygen administration.	Although oxygen alone will not explode, it will support combustion and cause flammable substances such as a face mask to burn rapidly.	Always enforce the "No Smoking" rule.
9. Wash hands.	Reduces transmission of microorganisms.	
Venturi Face Mask		
1. Wash hands.	Reduces transmission of microorganisms. (see Skill 35–5).	
2. Choose proper Venturi mask jet adapter for oxygen percentage.	Ensures proper oxygen percentage is delivered.	
3. Attach one end of connecting tube to Venturi mask jet adapter and the other end to nipple of flowmeter.	Delivers oxygen while allowing movement for the patient.	
4. Turn on oxygen to proper liter flow.	Ensures proper oxygen concentration is delivered.	Proper liter flow will be identified on the Venturi mask jet.
5. Listen for the "hiss" of the Venturi mask jet entraining room air.	Validates a proper connection with the jet and that oxygen is being mixed with room air.	Room air is necessary to control the concentration of oxygen being delivered to the patient.
6. Place the mask over the patient's nose and mouth. Adjust restraining straps and mold metal strip to fit the bridge of the nose.	Proper fit of the mask is required to ensure precise oxygen concentrations are delivered.	Adjust the restraining strap for a snug fit.
7. Stress fire hazards involved with oxygen administration.	Although oxygen alone will not explode, it will support combustion and cause flammable substances such as a face mask to burn rapidly.	Always enforce the "No Smoking" rule.
8. Wash hands.	Reduces transmission of microorganisms.	
Nonrebreathing Face Mask		
1. Wash hands.	Reduces transmission of microorganisms.	
2. Attach the oxygen connecting tubing to the oxygen flowmeter.	Delivers oxygen to the mask while allowing patient movement.	The tubing adaptor on the mask swivels for use on either side of the patient.
3. Set the oxygen to the prescribed flow, and check the gas flow through the device (see Table 2–4).	Ensures proper oxygen percentage will be delivered.	
4. Prior to placing the mask on the patient's face, check the reservoir bag to be sure it is inflated (distended).	Reservoir bag serves as an inlet for oxygen only. A one-way valve prevents backflow of exhaled gases into the bag.	
5. Place the mask over the patient's nose and mouth, expanding the sides of the mask to contour to the patient's cheek. Mold the metal strip to fit the bridge of the nose.	Proper positioning of the mask on the patient's face provides for a leakproof seal that will ensure exact oxygen concentrations will be delivered.	

Table continues on following page

Steps	Rationale	Special Considerations
6. Tighten the restraining strap to secure mask in place.	Proper fit of the mask is required to ensure precise oxygen concentrations are delivered.	
7. Check mask for leaks by feeling for gas escape and noting movement of the reservoir bag.	In a tight system, the bag will respond to the patient's slightest inspiratory efforts.	*Caution: Do not* use excessive gas flows into the mask. Once the reservoir is inflated, use only enough gas to keep it partially inflated.
8. Wash hands.	Reduces transmission of microorganisms.	

Evaluation

1. Compare the patient's respiratory assessment and arterial blood gases and/or pulse oximetry before and after face mask application. **Rationale:** Identifies the effects of oxygen administration via face mask.
2. Check the placement of a simple face mask and Venturi mask for restraining strap position and patient comfort and mask position.
3. Check the placement of the partial and nonrebreathing mask for mask and strap position and patient comfort and oxygen flow and the reservoir bag's ability to remain inflated during inspiration. **Rationale:** Proper fit of the oronasal face mask must be maintained for the delivery of accurate oxygen concentrations.
4. Observe the patient for any signs of nausea, and if possible, place the patient in a modified Fowler's position. **Rationale:** Decreases the risk of aspiration should vomiting occur.
5. Assist patient with alternate methods of communication. **Rationale:** Face mask over nose and mouth impairs patient's verbal communication.
6. Frequently inspect patient's skin and mucous membranes for signs of breakdown. **Rationale:** Use of a face mask and restraining strap creates friction to the patient's skin, and oxygen administration dries out mucous membrane.

Expected Outcomes

Improved arterial blood gases or pulse oximetry (SaO_2), absence of cyanosis, improved level of consciousness, normalization of respiratory rate, and normalization of heart rate. **Rationale:** Signs and symptoms of improved arterial oxygenation.

Unexpected Outcomes

1. Hypoxemia. **Rationale:** Hypoxemia can precipitate cardiac dysrhythmias, respiratory arrest, and death.
2. Aspiration. **Rationale:** Masks inhibit clearance of the vomitus from around the mouth especially in the unconscious and comatose patient.
3. Dehydration. **Rationale:** High oxygen flows (8 to 10 L/min) can result in dehydration of the airway mucosa and subsequent thickening of secretions.
4. Inaccurate oxygen concentrations. **Rationale:** Proper fitting mask and seals must be maintained with face masks to deliver accurate oxygen concentrations to the patient.
5. Suffocation. **Rationale:** If the oxygen flow from the oxygen flowmeter is obstructed with a non-rebreathing mask, the reservoir will be unable to fill with oxygen. When the patient inspires, no gas will be available for inhalation except that which can be entrained from around the edges of the mask. Two basic safety systems are used to prevent suffocation. In one device, one of the one-way valves is omitted from the exhalation ports, allowing the patient to inspire room air through this exhalation port. A second device is a spring valve mechanism located between the reservoir bag and the mask that can be pulled open when the patient inspires, creating a negative pressure and allowing the patient to inspire room air.
6. Skin/mucous membrane breakdown. **Rationale:** Skin irritation can occur from a snug face mask and from the contact of oxygen with the patient's skin.

Documentation

Documentation in the patient record should include respiratory assessment before and after face mask application; type of face mask applied; oxygen flow in L/min and percentage; patient's response to oxygen administration; date and time of administration; and routine observations for skin integrity and patient complaints of oxygen-related discomforts (e.g., drying of the nose, mouth, throat; thickening of secretions; and skin irritation). **Rationale:** Documents nursing care given, patient's respiratory status, and expected and unexpected outcomes.

Patient/Family Education

1. Discuss and demonstrate the steps for face mask application to the patient and family. **Rationale:** Promotes comfort and encourages questions from patient and family.
2. Explain the signs and symptoms of respiratory failure to the patient and family. **Rationale:** Enables the

patient and family to recognize when oxygen therapy is needed and when the physician needs to be notified.

3. Explain the possible complications and their pre-ventive measures for oronasal face mask therapy. **Rationale:** Patient and family will be able to prevent or recognize complications.

Performance Checklist
Skill 2–2: Oxygen Mask Application

Critical Behaviors	Complies yes	no
SIMPLE AND PARTIAL REBREATHING MASKS		
1. Wash hands.		
2. Attach humidifier to oxygen flowmeter.		
3. Connect flowmeter to oxygen source, and check proper operation of flowmeter and humidifier.		
4. Attach oxygen mask connecting tubing to humidifier and flowmeter. For partial rebreathing mask, occlude the reservoir bag opening, allowing oxygen to fill and inflate bag.		
5. Place mask on patient's mouth and nose. Mold metal strip to fit the bridge of the nose, and adjust restraining strap for a snug fit.		
6. Check oxygen flow.		
7. Stress fire hazards with oxygen.		
8. Wash hands.		
9. Document procedure in patient record.		
VENTURI FACE MASK		
1. Wash hands.		
2. Assemble equipment.		
3. Choose proper Venturi mask jet for appropriate oxygen percentage.		
4. Attach one end of connecting tube to Venturi mask jet adapter and other end to nipple of flowmeter.		
5. Turn on oxygen to proper liter flow.		
6. Check for proper connection with the jet to ensure that oxygen is being entrained with room air.		
7. Place mask over the patient's mouth and nose and secure a proper fit.		
8. Stress fire hazards with oxygen.		
9. Wash hands.		
10. Document procedure in patient record.		
NONREBREATHING FACE MASK		
1. Wash hands.		
2. Attach oxygen connecting tubing to the flowmeter.		
3. Set prescribed oxygen flow, and check gas flow through the device.		
4. Check the reservoir bag to be sure it is inflated (distended).		
5. Place the mask over the patient's mouth and nose. Mold the metal strip to fit the bridge of the nose.		
6. Tighten the restraining strap.		
7. Check mask for gas leaks.		
8. Wash hands.		
9. Document procedure in patient record.		

SKILL 2–3

Portable Oxygen Tank Preparation and Setup

Portable oxygen therapy may be required to maintain adequate oxygenation in certain patient situations. These situations include, but are not limited to, patient transportation and oxygen therapy in locations without accessible oxygen outlets. When using a portable oxygen tank, it is of utmost importance to follow some basic safety principles. Keep the oxygen tank away from open flames, fuel, an ignition source, or other gases. Oxygen tanks must be stored in an environment that is less than 126°F, and in an upright, anchored position. During use and/or transport, the tank should be secured in a portable carrier or skirt to prevent the tank from falling.

Administration of oxygen with a portable tank requires use of equipment that will allow safe access to the tank and provide for regulation of the flow rate.

Purpose

The nurse prepares and sets up portable oxygen tanks to

1. Maintain oxygen therapy in situations without accessible oxygen outlets (e.g., situations requiring patient transport).
2. Supply oxygen therapy during emergency situations.

Prerequisite Knowledge and Skills

Prior to preparing and setting up a portable oxygen tank, the nurse should understand

1. Anatomy and physiology of the upper and lower respiratory system.
2. Principles of oxygen therapy.
3. Principles of safety with portable tanks.

The nurse should be able to perform

1. Proper handwashing techniques (see Skill 35–5).
2. Vital signs assessment.
3. Respiratory system assessment.
4. Oxygen tank preparation.

Assessment

Observe for signs and symptoms of hypoxemia, including extreme paleness or cyanosis, hypotension with decreased heart rate, dyspnea, tachypnea, acute hypertension with increased heart rate, restlessness, disorientation, impaired judgment, and combativeness. **Rationale:** The body is able to store only a small amount of oxygen and must have a continual supply to maintain body functions.

Nursing Diagnosis

Impaired gas exchange related to altered oxygen supply. **Rationale:** A decrease in oxygen supply results in decreased oxygen delivery to arterial blood.

Planning

1. Individualize the following goals for accessing a portable oxygen tank and proper setup:
   a. Provide supplemental oxygen. **Rationale:** Oxygen is needed to maintain the metabolic needs of tissues and cells.
   b. Maintain patent airway. **Rationale:** Patent airways allow oxygen delivery to arterial blood (see Skills 1–1 through 1–9).
2. Prepare all necessary equipment and supplies. **Rationale:** Assembly of all equipment and supplies ensures quick and efficient availability of needed supplemental oxygen therapy.
   a. Portable oxygen tank.
   b. Portable carrier.
   c. Oxygen tubing.
   d. Regulator with flowmeter, cylinder pressure gauge.
   e. Nipple adapter.
   f. Some systems require a key, regulator knob, or slotted wrench.
3. Prepare the patient. **Rationale:** Encourages cooperation and reduces anxiety.
   a. Explain to the patient the need for supplemental oxygen. **Rationale:** Encourages cooperation and reduces anxiety.
   b. Assist in patient positioning. **Rationale:** Promotes comfort, reduces anxiety, and facilitates breathing.

Implementation

Steps	Rationale	Special Considerations
1. Bring oxygen tank to the patient bedside by portable carrier.	Prevents tank from being dragged, slid, or dropped.	Oxygen tanks have the potential of becoming dangerous or lethal missiles if dropped or mishandled.
2. Ensure that the environment is safe for portable oxygen use.	Oxygen supports and accelerates the combustion of other materials, making fire a potential hazard of gaseous oxygen.	Other gases, dirt, rust, oil, grease, hydrocarbons, and fuel or potential ignition sources must be kept away from oxygen regulator and cylinder valve.

Table continues on following page

Steps	Rationale	Special Considerations
3. Secure oxygen tank in an upright position.	Prevents tank from being dragged, slid, or dropped.	
4. Inspect tank and cylinder valve for damage. If damage is present, do not use.	Damaged cylinder valve may cause malfunction.	
5. Point the outlet valve away from any person, stand to one side, and open the valve slowly clockwise and then close. This is called *cracking* or *bleeding*. A "hissing" sound is generally present when this is done. Some cylinders may have a protective cap that will need to be removed. If necessary, a slotted wrench may be used, except on those valves equipped with a handwheel.	Cracking will blow the cylinder valve free of particulate matter.	Do not force valve. If unable to open, tag tank and return it to appropriate source.
6. If not currently in place, attach regulator and/or pressure-relief device to oxygen tank following manufacturer's instructions (Fig. 2–6). Ensure that only one O ring is present.	Monitor oxygen pressure and volume in the tank. Never use medical oxygen at full cylinder pressure. More than one O ring will cause oxygen leakage.	Identify and inspect the regulator for signs of damage. If damage is present, do not use. *Do not* attempt repairs yourself. Check with respiratory therapy department or appropriate hospital source handling oxygen supplies.
7. Attach all necessary tubing and other equipment if needed to the regulator. Slowly turn cylinder one full turn, then back a quarter turn, and then regulate flow.	Provides oxygen flow.	The dial indicating the amount of pressure should move.
8. Check the system for both visual and audible leaks.	Leaking system may be a hazard.	If cylinder is leaking, move to an isolated, well-ventilated area. Mark the cylinder and notify the respiratory therapy department.
9. To shut the cylinder down or to replace the cylinder, close the cylinder valve by turning counterclockwise until tightly sealed. Turn flowmeter to "off" and then back to "on" position. This will "bleed" the oxygen from the regulator. Then, turn the flowmeter off, disconnect the regulator from the cylinder, and replace with the cylinder valve cap.	Prevents pressure buildup.	Never use cylinder if less than 500 lb/in^2 or less than one-quarter full. Particles settle in the bottom of the cylinder and may be pulled into the patient's airway if such a cylinder is used. Tank reads 2200 lb/in.^{2} when full and 0 lb/in^2 when empty.
10. Place "Oxygen in Use" sign in immediate area.	Increases awareness and promotes use of oxygen safety rules.	

Evaluation

Compare the respiratory status before and after supplemental oxygen therapy setup. **Rationale:** Identifies the effectiveness of supplemental oxygen.

Expected Outcomes

1. Maintain a PaO_2 within normal range. **Rationale:**

Normal PaO_2 helps maintain adequate tissue oxygenation.

2. Respiratory rate remains within 5 breaths per minute of baseline. **Rationale:** Tachypnea or bradypnea will contribute to altered oxygen levels.

Unexpected Outcomes

1. Patient develops hypoxia or oxygen toxicity. **Ra-**

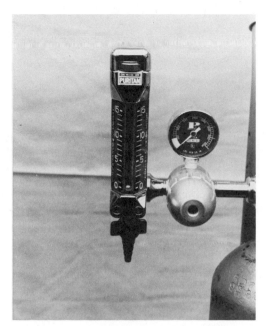

FIGURE 2–6. Oxygen regulator and flowmeter attached to portable oxygen tank.

tionale: Without proper flow-rate adjustment, too much or too little oxygen may be given.

2. Mechanical problem with tank or delivery system.

Rationale: All manufactured equipment is subject to malfunction.

Documentation

Documentation in the patient record should include flow rate of oxygen; delivery system used; patient's color, respiratory rate, depth, and rhythm; complaints of dyspnea, headache, and restlessness; nursing interventions and patient responses; date and time that the procedure is performed. **Rationale:** Documents nursing care given, patient's respiratory status, and expected and unexpected outcomes.

Patient/Family Education

1. Discuss signs and symptoms of respiratory distress and actions. **Rationale:** Increases patient and family awareness of signs and symptoms or change in conditions.

2. Should long-term oxygen therapy be needed, assess ability and readiness of patient and family to demonstrate oxygen tank care while in hospital setting. **Rationale:** Psychomotor and/or cognitive impairments may necessitate delaying patient and family teaching.

3. Discuss and demonstrate the steps for oxygen tank setup, maintenance, shutdown, and safety. **Rationale:** Encourages cooperation and understanding; allows for the correction of errors in technique; enables patient and family to ask questions.

Performance Checklist
Skill 2–3:   Portable Oxygen Tank Preparation and Setup

Critical Behaviors	Complies yes	no
1. Obtain oxygen tank.		
2. Ensure safe environment.		
3. Secure oxygen tank in upright position.		
4. Inspect cylinder valve and tank for damage.		
5. Open and "crack" tank.		
6. Attach regulator and/or pressure-relief device.		
7. Attach necessary tubing and other equipment.		
8. Check for leaks.		
9. Close and "bleed" tank.		
10. Place "Oxygen in Use" sign in immediate area.		
11. Document procedure in patient record.		

SKILL 2–4

Incentive Spirometry Treatments

Incentive spirometry treatments are used to increase the depth of inspiration in a patient who otherwise may not take adequate inspirations on his or her own. Patients who have had thoracic or abdominal surgery or have suffered trauma, restrictive pulmonary pathology, or obesity will often not inhale deep enough to maintain normal lung expansion and keep all alveoli open. Postoperative pain also results in a decreased inspiratory capacity.

Purpose

The nurse assists the patient with the use of incentive spirometry to

1. Prevent or assist with reversing atelectasis.
2. Promote normal lung expansion.
3. Improve oxygenation.
4. Provide an observable method for the patient to participate in his or her own care.

Prerequisite Knowledge and Skills

Prior to assisting with incentive spirometry, the nurse should understand

1. Anatomy and physiology of the upper and lower respiratory system.
2. Pathologic process of atelectasis.
3. Effects of surgery and immobilization on lung expansion and oxygenation.

The nurse should be able to perform

1. Proper handwashing technique (see Skill 35–5).
2. Vital signs assessment.
3. Patient teaching.
4. Respiratory assessment.
5. Coughing and deep breathing exercises.
6. Universal Precautions (see Skill 35–1).

Assessment

1. Observe for crackles, fever, increased respiratory rate, dyspnea, chest pain with deep inspiration, and development of sudden cough and/or production of sputum. **Rationale:** Physical signs and symptoms resulting from collapsed alveoli which indicate the need for incentive spirometry.
2. Identify patients who may benefit from the use of incentive spirometry, including preoperative patients scheduled for thoracic, abdominal, cardiac, or orthopedic surgery and patients with a history of smoking, recent colds, pneumonia, atelectasis, or immobility problems. **Rationale:** Allows for preoperative instruction and practice with incentive spirometry.

Nursing Diagnoses

1. Impaired gas exchange related to pain response from surgical incision or trauma; bedrest, immobility and decreased chest-wall movement. **Rationale:** Collapsed alveoli decrease surface area available for gas exchange. Decreased chest expansion reduces oxygen delivery to the lungs and arterial blood.
2. Ineffective airway clearance related to decreased chest-wall motion. **Rationale:** Failure to clear the airway may result in collapsed alveoli and accumulated secretions.
3. Impaired gas exchange related to accumulated secretions. **Rationale:** Presence of secretions will decrease gas exchange across the alveoli.

Planning

1. Individualize the following goals for incentive spirometry treatment: Maintain normal lung expansion. **Rationale:** Collapsed alveoli aggravate gas exchange.
2. Prepare all necessary equipment and supplies. **Rationale:** Assembly of all equipment ensures efficiency.
   a. Incentive spirometer
   b. Tissues
   c. Basin
3. Prepare the patient.
   a. Explain the procedure. **Rationale:** Minimizes anxiety and encourages patient.
   b. Assist patient to sitting position. Semi-Fowler's and high Fowler's are positions of choice to facilitate deep breathing. **Rationale:** Promotes lung expansion.
   c. Collaborate with patient in planning treatments. **Rationale:** Patients are more likely to participate if given an opportunity to assist with planning care.

Implementation

Steps	Rationale	Special Considerations
1. Wash hands.	Reduces transmission of microorganisms.	
2. Instruct patient to insert mouthpiece so that lips cover it completely, take a deep, slow, even breath and hold it for at least 3 seconds.	Breathing deeply and holding breath expand alveoli. Demonstration and instruction assist in teaching and promote an atmosphere conducive to further communication and learning.	Moist oral mucous membranes and lips will make holding of mouthpiece in mouth easier.

Table continues on following page

Steps	Rationale	Special Considerations
3. Instruct patient to exhale in a slow, passive manner. Encourage pursed-lip inhalation.	Pursed lips will keep the airway open longer.	
4. Instruct patient to breathe normally for a few minutes.	Prevents fatigue and hyperventilation.	
5. Instruct the patient to try and increase inspired volume by 100 to 250 ml per each successive deep breath. Once maximum volume is achieved, practice inspiring this volume 10 times.	Facilitates lung expansion.	Incentive spirometry will keep alveoli open for 1 hour after treatment. A realistic goal is to achieve an inspiratory capacity equal to the baseline pulmonary function test results.
6. Maintain cleanliness of spirometer by keeping mouthpiece covered when not in use and cleaning the mouthpiece with hydrogen peroxide.	Reduces transmission of microorganisms.	
7. Wash hands.	Reduces transmission of microorganisms.	

Evaluation

Compare patient's respiratory assessment before and after treatment to evaluate response to incentive spirometry.

Expected Outcomes

1. Absent or diminished crackles, fever, and chest pain with deep inspiration. **Rationale:** Optimal pulmonary function will be maintained or restored.
2. Reduction of atelectasis. **Rationale:** Deep inspiration will promote alveolar expansion.

Unexpected Outcome

Inability to achieve planned expansion due to pain. **Rationale:** Increased depth of inspiration may increase level of pain. Medicate as needed to promote patient cooperation. May need to consider intermittent positive-pressure breathing (IPPB) therapy to assist with lung expansion.

Documentation

Documentation in the patient record should include respiratory assessment; patient compliance; frequency and number of repetitions; cough and sputum production, color, and consistency; and date, time, and frequency with which the procedure is performed. **Rationale:** Documents patient's progress, facilitates communication of health care providers, and promotes continued patient care planning.

Patient/Family Education

1. Assess ability and readiness of patient to demonstrate incentive spirometry treatments. **Rationale:** Patient understanding promotes participation.
2. Reinforce proper technique. **Rationale:** Reinforcement and encouragement promote use of proper techniques.

Performance Checklist
Skill 2–4: Incentive Spirometry Treatments

Critical Behaviors	Complies	
	yes	no
1. Wash hands.		
2. Prepare and position patient.		
3. Give spirometer to patient.		
4. Instruct and encourage patient to take a deep breath.		
5. Assess patient during treatment.		
6. Place spirometer in clean place.		

Table continues on following page

Critical Behaviors	Complies	
	yes	no
7. Wash hands.		
8. Document procedure in patient record.		

SKILL 2–5

Intermittent Positive-Pressure Breathing Treatment

Intermittent positive-pressure breathing (IPPB) treatment is a therapy in which aerosol is delivered to the lungs or the lungs are hyperinflated during inspiration by applying positive pressure within the airways. Following inspiration, the IPPB machine cycles off, allowing the patient to passively exhale. Each inspiration will trigger the IPPB machine to provide the preset pressure within the airways. There are a number of clinical conditions in which IPPB is indicated. Clinical indications include, but are not limited to,

1. Hypoventilation due to pulmonary disease, muscle weakness, restrictive disease, obesity, or medication administration.
2. COPD (asthma, bronchitis, emphysema).
3. Chronic heart failure (CHF) and pulmonary edema.
4. Partial airway obstruction due to foreign body, stenosis, infection, or tumor.
5. Preoperatively to promote lung expansion and prepare the patient for postoperative treatments.
6. Pulmonary complications secondary to surgery.

There are some clinical conditions in which IPPB treatment is contraindicated. These include, but are not limited to,

1. Untreated tension pneumothorax.
2. Untreated tuberculosis.
3. Altered level of consciousness.
4. Increased intracranial pressure.
5. Subcutaneous emphysema.

When properly instituted, IPPB treatments can improve the uniformity and distribution of inhaled gases within the airways, increase effective alveolar ventilation, improve humidification of the airways, and also prevent atelectasis.

Purpose

The nurse administers an IPPB treatment to

1. Improve alveolar ventilation.
2. Expand airways.
3. Decrease the effort and work of breathing.
4. Improve and promote expectoration.
5. Prevent or correct atelectasis.
6. Deliver aerosolized medications.

Prerequisite Knowledge and Skills

Prior to administering an IPPB treatment, the nurse should understand

1. Anatomy and physiology of upper and lower respiratory system.
2. Principles of gas exchange.
3. Principles of aseptic technique.
4. Principles of medication administration.
5. Effects of surgery and immobilization on lung expansion and oxygenation.

The nurse should be able to perform

1. Proper handwashing technique (see Skill 35–5).
2. Vital signs assessment.
3. Respiratory system assessment.
4. Patient education.
5. Dosage calculations.
6. Safety precautions with O_2 therapy.
7. Coughing and deep breathing exercises.
8. Universal precautions (see Skill 35–1).

Assessment

1. Assess patient's vital signs. **Rationale:** Provides baseline values for comparison during and after treatment.
2. Assess patient's chest, including breathing pattern, equality of chest expansion, breath sounds, and use of any accessory muscles. **Rationale:** Provides baseline assessment and detection of any clinical conditions that would contraindicate treatment.
3. Assess patient's ability to cough. **Rationale:** Inability to cough may result in retained secretions and development or progression of atelectasis.
4. Assess patient's position and comfort level. **Rationale:** Proper positioning will enhance IPPB treatment outcomes.
5. Assess patient's knowledge base regarding IPPB treatment. **Rationale:** Patient understanding of procedure will decrease anxiety, promote participation, and enhance outcome.

Nursing Diagnoses

1. Impaired gas exchange related to excessive or thick secretions, infection, neuromuscular impairment, anesthesia, medications, bedrest, surgery, pain, or fatigue. **Rationale:** Presence of any of these conditions will decrease gas exchange at the alveolar level.

2. Ineffective airway clearance related to decreased chest-wall motion. **Rationale:** Failure to clear the airway results in airway obstruction and ineffective gas exchange.

3. Ineffective breathing pattern related to excessive or thick secretions, infection, neuromuscular impairment, anesthesia, medications, bedrest, surgery, pain, or fatigue. **Rationale:** Collapsed alveoli decrease surface area for gas exchange.

4. Potential for infection related to retained secretions. **Rationale:** Retained secretions provide a medium for bacterial growth.

Planning

1. Individualize the following goal for performing an IPPB treatment: Promote normal lung expansion. **Rationale:** Collapsed alveoli do not promote gas exchange.
2. Obtain all necessary equipment and supplies. **Rationale:** Having all necessary equipment and supplies ensures that the IPPB treatment can be completed in an efficient manner.
   a. IPPB machine (Bird, Bennett).
   b. Breathing circuit.
   c. Mouthpiece, lip seal, nose clips, mask, and endotracheal or tracheostomy adapter as indicated.
   d. Medications as prescribed (saline or prescribed inhalant).
   e. Tissues and emesis basin.
   f. Specimen cup if indicated.
   g. Suction equipment if needed.
   h. Stethoscope and blood pressure cuff.
3. Prepare the patient.
   a. Assess knowledge base of patient about procedure. State purpose and describe IPPB treatment to patient and family. **Rationale:** Patient and family understanding will decrease anxiety, promote participation, and enhance outcome.
   b. Assist patient to sitting position, high Fowler's if possible. **Rationale:** Sitting upright will maximize success of an IPPB treatment.
   c. Plan treatment times to avoid meal times. **Rationale:** IPPB treatments may cause gastric distension.
   d. Collaborate with patient in planning treatments. **Rationale:** Patients are more likely to participate in treatment when given an opportunity to assist in the planning aspects of their care.
   e. Instruct patient in correct breathing techniques: Relaxation and slow, deep breaths with machine during inspiration; pause at the end of inspiration; exhale slowly and passively. Promotes optimal lung expansion.

Implementation

Steps	Rationale	Special Considerations
1. Review physician's treatment order and medications to be administered. Note patient allergies.	Reduces risk of error.	Institutions vary as to who administers and assists with IPPB treatments. Check institutional policies and procedures for guidance.
2. Wash hands.	Reduces transmission of microorganisms.	
3. Secure patient breathing circuit to IPPB machine and attach mouthpiece, mask, or tracheostomy/endotracheal adapter to tubing.	Ensures airtight system.	Machines may vary. Check manufacturer's recommendations for further guidelines or information.
4. Add prescribed dosage of medication to medication cup attached to patient breathing circuit.	Ensures patient will receive medication ordered.	Make sure there is enough solution in medication cup to last entire treatment.
5. Have patient place mouthpiece in mouth and place lips firmly around entire mouthpiece.	Ensures airtight system.	
6. Adjust sensitivity dial appropriate for patient effort (Fig. 2–7). Start at most sensitive and progress to least sensitive.	Ensures that patient does not tire from too much effort to initiate treatment.	*Sensitivity* refers to the patient effort required to initiate inspiration. If effort is more than -2 cmH$_2$O pressure, sensitivity needs to be increased. Check with your hospital respiratory care department for further guidelines on setting sensitivity, pressure, and flow dials.

Table continues on following page

Steps	Rationale	Special Considerations
7. Pull air-mix knob to "out" position (Fig. 2–8).	Ensures that patient does not receive 100% O_2.	Some physicians may want to administer 100% O_2.
8. Set flow rate dial to start at 10 L/min for the average patient (see Fig. 2–8).	Ensures slow, deep inspiration.	Range is 0 to 40 L/min. Adjust flow to deliver slow, deep inspiration.
9. Set inspiratory pressure control to start at 10 cmH$_2$O for average patient (Fig. 2–9).	Ensures maximum effective inflation of airways.	Range is 0 to 40 cmH$_2$O. Adjust according to patient breath sounds, expansion of patient chest, or tidal volume.
10. Apply nose clips if patient is breathing by nose and mouth.	Helps ensure airtight system by sealing nose.	
11. Instruct patient to begin a deep breath to trigger machine, relax and let mist flow into lungs, pause 1 to 3 seconds before exhaling. Instruct patient to exhale slowly through mouthpiece without straining. Have patient pause a few seconds prior to taking the next breath and when coughing occurs.	Promotes optimal lung expansion and successful treatment.	Strive to make pressure indicator rise evenly with each breath. Diaphragmatic breathing will make treatment more effective. If patient becomes tachycardic or develops dysrhythmias; or if he or she develops dizziness, concentrate on breathing more slowly. Should problems persist, medication dosage may need to be adjusted. Notify the physician and stop treatment.
12. Observe patient during treatment for changes in heart rate, blood pressure, respiratory rate, and breathing pattern. Observe also for development of any signs and symptoms indicating complications.	Provides early detection of complications from IPPB treatment.	Complications may include, but are not limited to, hyperventilation, hypoventilation, decreased cardiac output, bloody sputum, gastric distension, infection, or barotrauma.
13. Assist patient to achieve a productive cough. Observe for change in color of sputum.	IPPB treatment helps loosen and mobilize secretions. Discoloration of sputum may indicate infection.	Patients with altered level of consciousness may require suctioning.
14. Perform respiratory and vital signs assessment and evaluate tolerance to treatment.	Identifies effectiveness of IPPB treatment.	
15. Clean medication cup and mouthpiece with water and hydrogen peroxide. Store equipment and supplies for future treatment.	Removes secretions and decreases chance of transmitting microorganisms.	
16. Wash hands.	Reduces transmission of microorganisms.	

Evaluation

Compare respiratory and vital signs assessment findings before and after an IPPB treatment. **Rationale:** Identifies effectiveness of an IPPB treatment.

Expected Outcomes

1. Productive cough. **Rationale:** IPPB treatment helps loosen and mobilize secretions.
2. Absence of adventitious breath sounds. **Rationale:** Airways are clear, and respiratory workload is decreased.
3. Reduction of atelectasis. **Rationale:** Normal expansion of the lungs will decrease potential for development or progression of atelectasis.
4. Patient and family demonstrate appropriate technique. **Rationale:** Demonstration of psychomotor skills allows for immediate feedback and evaluation of learning.

Unexpected Outcomes

1. Patient begins to hyperventilate (symptoms include dizziness, paresthesia, agitation, confusion, and increased respiratory rate). **Rationale:** IPPB treatment increases tidal volume and respiratory rate.

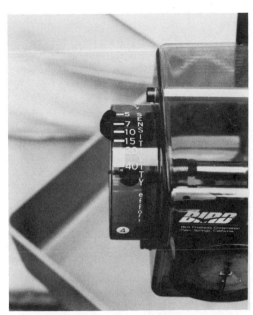

FIGURE 2–7. Sensitivity effort dial of Bird pressure ventilator.

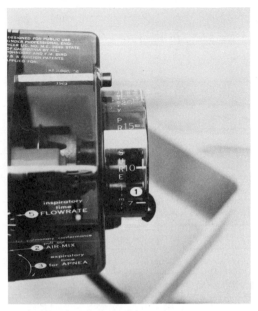

FIGURE 2–9. Inspiratory pressure control on pressure ventilator.

2. Patient develops symptoms of oxygen-induced hypoventilation (drowsiness, confusion, disorientation, and coma). **Rationale:** In COPD patients, low PaO_2 stimulates ventilation. Administration of high concentrations of oxygen may remove this stimulus to breathe.

3. Patient develops symptoms of decreased cardiac output (tachycardia, decreased blood pressure, confusion, and disorientation). **Rationale:** IPPB treatment replaces normal negative pressure with positive pressure as the drive for inspiration. High positive lung pressures can decrease the venous return to the heart, thus decreasing cardiac output.

4. Bloody sputum. **Rationale:** May be the result of bronchial irritation from improved cough.

5. Gastric distension. **Rationale:** Delivery of oxygen at a higher pressure or flow than needed forces air into stomach.

6. Infection. **Rationale:** Application of positive pressure within the airways provides a means for spreading bacterial infection.

7. Patient may develop symptoms of barotrauma or pneumothorax (sharp chest pain, tachycardia, acute shortness of breath, and decreased blood pressure). **Rationale:** COPD patients may have blebs or bullae that rupture during IPPB treatment.

8. Patient and family demonstrate unsafe techniques or use of equipment. **Rationale:** Demonstrates knowledge deficit.

Documentation

Documentation in the patient record should include vital signs and respiratory assessment before, during, and after treatment; length of treatment, pressures used, solutions and/or medications administered, and gas source; effectiveness of cough, and patient tolerance of procedure; side effects or complications of treatment; and date, time, and frequency with which the procedure is performed. **Rationale:** Documents care given, patient status, and expected or unexpected outcomes of procedure.

Patient/Family Education

1. Assess knowledge base of patient and family about purpose of IPPB treatment and actual steps in procedure. **Rationale:** Patient and family understanding of procedure will decrease anxiety, promote participation, and enhance outcome.

2. Support patient to achieve a productive cough. **Rationale:** Productive coughing helps mobilize and eliminate retained secretions.

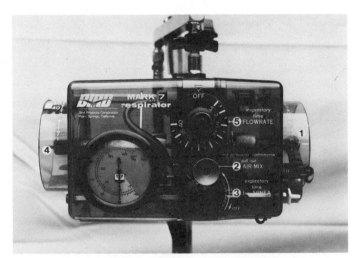

FIGURE 2–8. Pressure ventilator used for IPPB treatments: (1) inspiratory pressure control, (2) air-mix knob, (3) expiratory time for apnea, (4) sensitivity effort dial, and (5) inspiratory time flowrate.

Performance Checklist
Skill 2–5: Intermittent Positive-Pressure Breathing (IPPB) Treatment

Critical Behaviors	Complies yes	no
1. Review physician's orders for treatment and medication.		
2. Wash hands.		
3. Secure breathing circuit to IPPB machine.		
4. Attach mouthpiece, mask, or tracheal/endotracheal adapter to tubing.		
5. Add correct medication to medication cup.		
6. Position patient's mouthpiece correctly.		
7. Select sensitivity dial reading.		
8. Turn air-mix knob to "out" position.		
9. Select flow and pressure settings.		
10. Apply nose clips as necessary.		
11. Administer treatment.		
12. Observe patient during treatment for development of complications.		
13. Assist patient to achieve productive cough.		
14. Perform respiratory and vital signs assessment.		
15. Clean and store equipment.		
16. Wash hands.		
17. Document procedure in patient record.		

REFERENCES

Craig, R. J. (1981). *Nursing Clinics of North America*, Vol. 16. Philadelphia: Saunders.
Kersten, L. D. (1989). *Comprehensive Respiratory Nursing*. Philadelphia: Saunders.
Rarey, K. P., and Youtsey, J. W. (1981). *Respiratory Patient Care*. Englewood Cliffs, N.J.: Prentice-Hall.

BIBLIOGRAPHY

Alspach, J., and Williams, S. (1985). *Core Curriculum for Critical Care Nursing* 3d Ed. Philadelphia: Saunders.
Carpenito, L. (1990). *Handbook of Nursing Diagnosis*. Philadelphia: Lippincott.
Eliopoulos, C. (1987). *Gerontological Nursing Review: A Self-Instructional Text*. National Health Publishing.

3

CHEST PHYSIOTHERAPY

BEHAVIORAL OBJECTIVES

After completing this chapter, the nurse will be able to

- Define key terms.
- Describe the purpose of chest physiotherapy.
- Discuss the indications for chest physiotherapy.
- Demonstrate the skills used in chest physiotherapy.

Accumulation of secretions within the respiratory tract resulting from ineffective airway clearance is a common factor contributing to impaired gas exchange. Other factors, such as immobility, level of hydration, and underlying cardiopulmonary disease, create an increased risk to the patient in a critical care setting. Chest physiotherapy is aimed at supporting the patient's ability to mobilize secretions and assist in their removal.

KEY TERMS

percussion
vibration
postural drainage

SKILLS

3–1   Postural Drainage
3–2   Percussion and Vibration

GUIDELINES

The following assessment guidelines assist the nurse in formulating a nursing diagnosis and an individualized plan for a specific type of chest physiotherapy:

1.   Know the patient's baseline respiratory assessment.
2.   Know the patient's baseline vital signs.
3.   Know the patient's medical history.
4.   Know the patient's medical treatment, including current medications.
5.   Perform systematic respiratory assessments prior to and following the performance of chest physiotherapy.
6.   Assess scheduling of bronchodilator administration and meals.

SKILL 3–1

Postural Drainage

Postural drainage is performed by positioning the patient in a series of positions to facilitate gravitational drainage of smaller peripheral lung segments into larger, more central airways, where the secretions can be coughed or suctioned out. Systemic hydration and the use of bronchodilators assist in thinning secretions for easier mobilization. Figure 3–1 illustrates the positions employed for draining each segment of the lung.

Purpose

The nurse performs postural drainage to

1.   Maintain a patent airway by mobilizing secretions into larger airways, where they can be coughed or suctioned.
2.   Increase respiratory gas exchange by increasing the available surface area at the alveolar level.
3.   Decrease the incidence of respiratory infection.

Prerequisite Knowledge and Skills

Prior to performing postural drainage, the nurse should understand

1.   Anatomy and physiology of the tracheobronchial system.
2.   Principle of gas exchange.

The nurse should be able to perform

1.   Vital signs assessment.
2.   Respiratory system assessment.
3.   Proper positioning techniques.
4.   Proper body mechanics.
5.   Proper handwashing technique (see Skill 35–5).
6.   Universal precautions (see Skill 35–1).

Assessment

1.   Auscultate lungs to determine location and degree of retained secretions. **Rationale:** Bronchial, diminished, and absent breath sounds can indicate obstructed airways and reduced airflow.
2.   Verify assessment with recent chest radiographs. **Rationale:** Chest radiographs offer documentation of as well as indication for the need to perform postural drainage.
3.   Assess for symptoms of increased intracranial pressure or spinal fractures. **Rationale:** Head-down positions are contraindicated with these conditions.

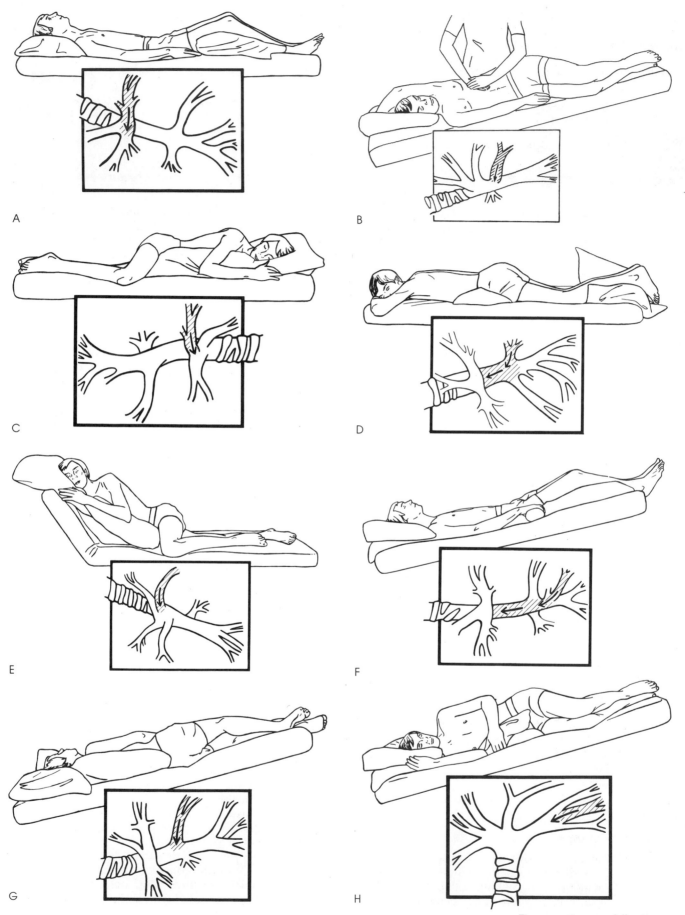

A

B

C

D

E

F

G

H

Figure continues on following page

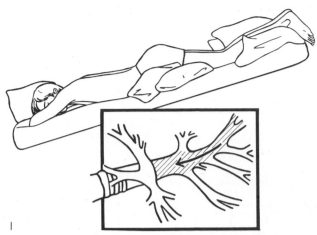

FIGURE 3–1. Positions for complete postural drainage (in sequence). (*A*) Upper lobes, anterior segments. (*B*) Upper lobe, posterior segment, right posterior bronchus. (*C*) Upper lobe, posterior segment, left posterior bronchus. (*D*) Right middle lobe. (*E*) Left lingula. (*F*) Lower lobes, apical segment. (*G*) Lower lobes, anterior basal segment. (*H*) Lower lobe, lateral basal segment. (*I*) Lower lobes, posterior basal bronchus. (Figure adapted from M. L. Morrison (Ed.), *Respiratory Intensive Care Nursing*, 2nd ed. Boston, Little, Brown and Co., 1979. Reproduced by permission.)

4.   Identify what time the patient consumed his or her last meal. **Rationale:** To avoid aspiration, postural drainage should be performed 1 to 2 hours following a meal. If patient is receiving continuous tube feedings, the feeding should be turned off and head-down positions should be avoided for 1 to 2 hours before postural drainage is initiated.

Nursing Diagnoses

1.   Impaired gas exchange related to accumulated secretions. **Rationale:** Secretions retained in lower airway decrease gas exchange at the alveolar level.

2.   Potential for infection related to retained secretions. **Rationale:** Accumulated secretions provide a medium for microorganisms.

3.   Ineffective airway clearance related to immobility. **Rationale:** Bedrest decreases the effectiveness of the airway's natural clearing defense mechanism.

4.   Potential for aspiration related to presence of gastric contents. **Rationale:** Head-dependent positioning can increase the risk of aspiration.

Planning

1.   Individualize the following goals for performing postural drainage:
    a.   Maintain a patent airway. **Rationale:** Retained secretions reduce the amount of alveolar surface available for gas exchange.
    b.   Mobilize secretions. **Rationale:** Mobilizing secretions from smaller peripheral lung segments to larger, more central airways will increase the flow of respiratory gases at the alveolar level.
    c.   Removal of secretions. **Rationale:** Removal of airway secretions decreases the favorable medium available to support microorganisms.
    d.   Prevention of aspiration. **Rationale:** Postural drainage should be scheduled 1 to 2 hours following a meal to allow for emptying of the stomach.

2.   Obtain all necessary equipment and supplies. **Rationale:** Assembly of all the necessary equipment and supplies at the bedside facilitates performing postural drainage with minimal fatigue and discomfort to the patient.
    a.   Pillows and positioning aids.
    b.   Facial tissues.
    c.   Emesis basin.
    d.   Suction equipment (if indicated).
    e.   Stethoscope.

3.   Prepare the patient.
    a.   Explain the procedure to the patient. **Rationale:** Minimizes risks and reduces anxiety.
    b.   Explain patient's participation and importance of coughing at the end of each position. **Rationale:** Encourages cooperation and facilitates secretion removal.

Implementation

Steps	Rationale	Special Considerations
1. Wash hands.	Reduces transmission of microorganisms.	
2. Position yourself close to bed, and adjust the height of the bed.	Promotes use of proper body mechanics.	
3. Assist the patient into first planned position.	Proper positioning is utilized to increase efficiency of gravity drainage.	Children may be positioned on parent's lap.
4. Ensure patient comfort and support.	Positioning will be maintained for 10 to 20 minutes.	

Table continues on following page

Steps	Rationale	Special Considerations
5. Monitor breathing pattern, heart rate and rhythm, and skin color.	Development of dyspnea, cyanosis, or dysrhythmia is an indication for stopping procedure.	
6. Maintain position for 10 to 20 minutes as tolerated.	Allows for adequate time to drain lung segment.	Length of time and head positioning should be altered based on patient's condition and tolerance.
7. Assist patient in coughing.	Controlled coughing will aid in removal of drained secretions (Hoffman et al., 1987; Potter, 1987).	
8. If patient is unable to produce effective cough, perform suctioning (see Skill 1–3).	Secretions not expelled will serve as medium for microorganisms.	
9. Allow patient to rest based on tolerance.	Decreases occurrence of hypoxia (Kersten, 1989).	
10. Reposition for next planned segment to be drained and repeat steps 3 to 8 until entire planned sequence is complete.	Allows for all areas to be drained.	Sequencing is top to bottom and altered based on patient's condition and tolerance.
11. Assist patient to a comfortable position (semi-Fowler's).	Facilitates respirations.	
12. Properly dispose of secretions.	Universal precautions.	
13. Wash hands.	Decreases transmission of microorganisms.	

Evaluation

Compare patient respiratory assessment pre and post postural drainage. **Rationale:** Identifies the effect of postural drainage.

Expected Outcomes

1. Sputum production from coughing or suctioning. **Rationale:** Effective movement of secretions from smaller, peripheral segments to larger, central segments.
2. Increased airflow and decreased respiratory rate. **Rationale:** Removal of secretions decreases the work of breathing.
3. Decreased or coarser adventitious breath sounds. **Rationale:** Increased flow of air into peripheral lung.

Unexpected Outcomes

1. Patient becomes cyanotic, dyspneic, or develops dysrhythmias. **Rationale:** Patient developing signs of hypoxia due to intolerance of positioning. Procedure should be stopped.
2. Patient becomes restless and diaphoretic, with gurgling sounds on auscultation and accompanied choking and pallor. **Rationale:** Patient exhibiting symptoms of aspiration. Place patient on left side, monitor vital signs, and seek medical assistance.
3. Patient does not bring up secretions. **Rationale:** Secretions may be too thick to mobilize or absent in the tracheobronchial tree.
4. Hemoptysis. **Rationale:** May result from infection, damaged blood vessel, or other pathophysiology.

Documentation

Documentation in the patient record should include respiratory assessment and vital signs before and after treatment; patient's tolerance of postural drainage; color, consistency, amount, and odor of secretions obtained; patient's level of cooperation with treatment; date, time, and frequency with which procedure is performed. **Rationale:** Documents nursing care given, patient's cardiopulmonary status, and expected and unexpected outcomes.

Patient/Family Education

1. Discuss needs and indications for postural drainage. **Rationale:** Encourages cooperation and understanding; facilitates continuance of therapy at home.
2. Demonstrate positioning techniques and allow for return demonstration. Provide pictorial handouts with step-by-step instructions. **Rationale:** Adult learners tend to be more visually oriented and benefit from a review tool.
3. Explain signs and symptoms that are indicators for stopping the procedure. Provide a handout with unexpected outcomes and what action to take in the event they occur. **Rationale:** Enables the patient and family to recognize the need for stopping the procedure.

Performance Checklist
Skill 3-1:   Postural Drainage

Critical Behaviors	Complies	
	yes	no
1. Wash hands.		
2. Position self close to bed and adjust bed.		
3. Assist patient into first planned position.		
4. Ensure patient comfort and support.		
5. Monitor breathing pattern, heart rate and rhythm, and color.		
6. Maintain position for 10 to 20 minutes.		
7. Assist patient with coughing.		
8. If cough is ineffective, perform suctioning.		
9. Allow patient to rest.		
10. Reposition to next planned segment, and repeat steps 3 to 8.		
11. Assist patient to comfortable position.		
12. Properly dispose of secretions.		
13. Wash hands.		
14. Assess patient's respiratory status following postural drainage.		
15. Document procedure in patient record.		

SKILL 3-2

Percussion and Vibration

Chest percussion and vibration are utilized as adjuncts to postural drainage in dislodging and mobilizing secretions from small, peripheral airways to larger, more central airways, where they can be removed by coughing or suctioning. When properly instituted, chest percussion and vibration can increase the effectiveness of postural drainage. Chest percussion involves lightly striking the chest wall over the affected areas of the lung with cupped hands, as illustrated in Figure 3-2. The air trapped in the cupped hands exerts pressure on the lung segment without causing trauma to the chest wall. This pressure acts as a mechanical aid in moving secretions.

Chest vibration is performed during expiration only. The vibrations are created using both hands, one on top of the other, as illustrated in Figure 3-3. The hands are placed on the chest wall directly over the segment of the lung that is affected, and a shaking movement is applied. This increases the velocity of air movement, which loosens secretions.

Chest percussion and vibration are indicated in conditions in which large amounts of sputum are produced (generally greater than 30 ml per day), such as cystic fibrosis, bronchiectasis, and retained secretions and lobar atelectasis not related to cardiac surgery. There is some controversy regarding their usefulness in atelectasis associated with cardiac surgery (Hoffman et al., 1987).

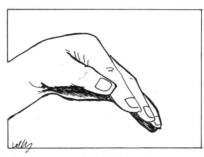

FIGURE 3-2.   Cupping of hands for performance of chest percussion. (Drawing by Bob Lilly.)

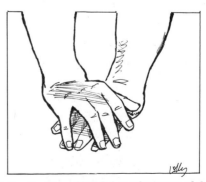

FIGURE 3-3.   Position of hands in performance of chest vibration. (Drawing by Bob Lilly.)

Contraindications for chest percussion and vibration include those conditions in which head-down positioning has a detrimental effect on patient status, such as acute myocardial infarction, increased intracranial pressure, eye surgery, or gastric reflux. Additionally, conditions in which the mechanical activity would adversely affect the medical surgical status, such as hemorrhage, bronchopulmonary fistula, acute chest trauma, lung abscess, or after surgical anastamoses of major blood vessels, provide a rationale for withholding therapy (Hoffman et al., 1987).

Purpose

The nurse performs chest percussion and vibration to

1. Enhance loosening of trapped secretions.
2. Increase the movement of secretions.
3. Decrease atelectasis.

Prerequisite Knowledge and Skills

Prior to performing chest percussion and vibration, the nurse should understand

1. Anatomy and physiology of the respiratory system.
2. Principles of gas exchange.
3. Proper positioning for postural drainage.

The nurse should be able to perform

1. Vital signs assessment.
2. Respiratory system assessment.
3. Postural drainage (see Skill 3–1).
4. Suctioning (see Skills 1–3, 1–4, and 1–9).
5. Cupping of hand for clapping.
6. Vibrating movement with one hand on top of the other.
7. Proper body mechanics.
8. Relaxation techniques.
9. Universal precautions (see Skill 35–1).

Assessment

1. Assess for the need to perform chest percussion and vibration, i.e., ineffective breathing patterns; ineffective airway clearance. **Rationale:** Bronchial, diminished, and absent breath sounds can indicate obstructed airways and reduced airflow.
2. Verify assessment with recent chest x-ray. **Rationale:** Aids in identifying location and degree of retained secretions.
3. Assess for contraindications to postural drainage positions. **Rationale:** Head-dependent positioning is not tolerated in conditions evidencing increased intracranial

pressure, in spinal fractures, and in patients with continuous gastric feedings.
4. Assess for symptoms of intrathoracic bleeding, lung abscess, or pleural effusion. **Rationale:** Chest percussion and vibration are contraindicated in the presence of these conditions.
5. Determine areas to be drained. (See Fig. 3–1 to determine positions and sequencing based on assessment.) Document plan to allow for continuity. **Rationale:** Performance of these procedures may be taxing to the patient's energy level, and focus should therefore be on affected areas.
6. Assess patient's understanding and cooperative ability. **Rationale:** Identifies potential knowledge and self-care deficits.

Nursing Diagnoses

1. Ineffective airway clearance related to accumulated secretions. **Rationale:** Presence of secretions in respiratory tract decreases gas exchange.
2. Potential for infection related to retained secretions. **Rationale:** Accumulation of secretions provides a favorable medium for the growth of microorganisms.

Planning

1. Individualize the following goals for performing chest percussion and vibration:
   a. Maintain patent airway. **Rationale:** Removal of secretions increases the number of alveoli available for gas exchange.
   b. Mobilize airway secretions. **Rationale:** Removal of secretions decreases the favorable environment for the growth of microorganisms.
2. Prepare all necessary equipment and supplies. **Rationale:** Assembly of all the necessary equipment and supplies ensures procedure can be performed more efficiently.
   a. Pillows and positioning aides.
   b. Stethoscope.
   c. Facial tissues.
   d. Emesis basin.
   e. Suctioning equipment.
   f. Light towel (optional).
3. Prepare the patient and family.
   a. Explain the procedure to the patient and family. **Rationale:** Encourages participation and reduces anxiety.
   b. Explain the importance of participation and relaxation. **Rationale:** Facilitates procedure and aids movement of secretions.
   c. Discuss the importance of coughing. **Rationale:** Encourages cooperation and facilitates removal of secretions.

Implementation

Steps	Rationale	Special Considerations
1. Wash hands.	Reduces transmission of microorganisms.	
2. Position yourself close to bed, and adjust height of the bed.	Promotes use of proper body mechanics.	
3. Assist patient into first planned position.	Increases efficiency of gravity drainage.	Refer to Figure 3–1 for proper positioning.
4. Ensure patient comfort and support.	Positioning to be maintained 10 to 20 minutes.	Relaxation and imaging techniques may assist in patient comfort and cooperation.
5. Cover chest area to be percussed and vibrated with a light towel.	Minimizes skin trauma.	Thoracotomy incision, chest-tube insertion sites, and female breasts are to be avoided.
6. Monitor breathing pattern, heart rate and rhythm, and skin color.	Development of dyspnea, cyanosis, or dysrhythmias are indications for stopping procedure.	
7. Begin percussion. Using cupped hands, alternately strike the chest over desired segment.	Provides mechanical loosening of secretions.	For infant or small child, a small padded face mask with the opening covered can be used for proportional cupping.
8. Continuously assess patient's response, including comfort, vital signs, and respiratory pattern.	Patient tolerance will determine altering length of procedure.	
9. Continue clapping for 2 to 3 minutes until entire segment is completed.	Allow time for loosening secretions.	Pressure of clapping must be adjusted for infants, children, and the elderly.
10. Position hands with one on top of the other, and apply to area just percussed.	Proper hand position for vibration.	
11. Instruct patient to breathe slowly and deeply through nose.	Air movement assists movement of secretions.	
12. Instruct patient to exhale with mouth open, avoiding straining.	Allows for easy air movement.	
13. Begin gentle vibration as the patient begins to exhale using the flat palm of the hand (see Fig. 3–3).	Loosens secretions.	Pressure of vibrations must be adjusted for infants, children, and the elderly.
14. Stop vibration when patient begins next inhalation cycle. Repeat vibrations through five exhalation cycles.	Perform only during exhalation.	Do not allow the patient to sit up between positions, since mucus will slide back down the airways.
15. Assist patient in controlled coughing by instructing patient to do small coughs until the end of breath.	Removes secretions.	
16. If cough ineffective, perform suctioning.	Removes secretions.	
17. Repeat steps 2 to 16 until entire planned sequence is completed.	Ensures that all segments are drained.	
18. Assist patient to semi-Fowler's position.	Aids in lung expansion.	
19. Dispose of secretions in appropriate receptacle.	Reduces transmission of microorganism.	

Table continues on following page

Steps	Rationale	Special Considerations
20. Wash hands.	Reduces transmission of microorganisms.	

Evaluation

Compare patient respiratory assessments before and after chest percussion and vibration. **Rationale:** Identifies the effects of percussion and vibration.

Expected Outcomes

1. Effective movement and removal of secretions in airways. **Rationale:** Upper and lower airways cleared of secretions.
2. Lungs sound clear with absent or more coarse adventitious breath sounds. **Rationale:** Increased airflow in lungs.

Unexpected Outcomes

1. Patient becomes cyanotic, dyspneic, or develops dysrhythmias. **Rationale:** Signs of hypoxia due to intolerance of positioning and/or procedure. Procedure should be stopped immediately.
2. Skin becomes reddened, traumatized. **Rationale:** Percussion and vibration have traumatized chest wall.
3. Patient does not bring up secretions. **Rationale:** Secretions may be too thick to mobilize or absent.
4. Hemoptysis. **Rationale:** May result from infection, damaged blood vessel, or other pathophysiology.

Documentation

Documentation in the patient record should include respiratory and vital signs assessment before and after treatment; implementation of postural drainage, chest percussion, and vibration; patient's response to and tolerance of procedure; patient's participation in procedure; color, consistency, odor, and amount of secretions obtained; date, time, and frequency with which procedure is performed. **Rationale:** Documents nursing care given, patient's cardiopulmonary status, and expected and unexpected outcomes.

Patient/Family Education

1. Discuss and demonstrate the steps for preparation and performance of chest percussion and vibration. Provide pictorial and written handouts. **Rationale:** Encourages understanding; enables family to ask questions throughout procedure.
2. Explain the expected and unexpected outcomes and indications for stopping procedure. **Rationale:** Provides feedback to family regarding results of treatment.

Performance Checklist
Skill 3–2:   Percussion and Vibration

Critical Behaviors	Complies	
	yes	no
1. Wash hands.		
2. Position patient to drain target area.		
3. Cup hand to produce hollow sound when percussing.		
4. Percuss area, alternating hands, for 2 to 3 minutes.		
5. Assess patient's comfort and tolerance.		
6. Position one hand on top of the other, and apply to target area on chest wall.		
7. Instruct patient to breathe slowly and deeply.		
8. Vibrate target area through expiration.		
9. Repeat vibrations through five cycles.		
10. Assist patient in coughing.		
11. Perform suctioning if cough is ineffective.		
12. Repeat steps 3 to 12 until all planned segments are completed.		
13. Assist patient to semi-Fowler's position.		

Critical Behaviors	Complies	
	yes	no
14. Properly dispose of secretions.		
15. Wash hands.		
16. Document procedure in patient record.		

REFERENCES

Hilman, E. (1978). *The "How" and "Why" of Bronchial Drainage-Guide for Your Home Care Program.* New York: Breon Labs (Winthrop-Breon Co.). Copyright Sterling Drug, pp. 546–550.

Hoffman, L., Mazzocco, M., and Roth, J. (1987). Fine tuning your chest PT. *Am. J. Nurs.* 12:1566–1570.

Kersten, L. D. (1989). *Comprehensive Respiratory Nursing* (pp. 534–554). Philadelphia: Saunders.

Potter, P. (1987). *Basic Nursing Theory and Practice* (pp. 781–799). St. Louis: Mosby.

BIBLIOGRAPHY

Brunner, L. S., and Suddarth, D. S. (1988). *Medical Surgical Nursing,* 6th Ed. (pp. 428–431). Philadelphia: Lippincott.

Kirilloff, L. et al. (1985). Does chest PT work? *Chest* 88:436–443.

McHugh, J. (1987). Perfecting the three steps of chest physiotherapy. *Nursing* 11:54–57.

Persons, C. B. (1987). *Critical Care Procedures and Protocol* (pp. 310–315). Philadelphia: Lippincott.

Smith, A. J., and Johnson, J. (1990). *Nurse's Guide to Clinical Procedures* (pp. 77–84). Philadelphia: Lippincott.

4

VENTILATORY MANAGEMENT

BEHAVIORAL OBJECTIVES

After completing this chapter, the nurse will be able to

- Define the key terms.
- Describe methods for initiating mechanical ventilatory support.
- Discuss methods for managing mechanical ventilatory support.
- Discuss techniques used to wean patients from mechanical ventilatory support.
- Demonstrate the skills involved in the use and management of mechanical ventilatory support.

Management of the patient receiving mechanical ventilatory assistance poses continual challenges to the nurse. The dynamic interactions between underlying disease processes, the effect of mechanical ventilation on organs other than the lungs, and the psychosocial dependence of the patient and family on trained professionals and life-support technology mandate that the nurse devote vigilance to the patient receiving mechanical ventilatory assistance. Collaboration with physicians, respiratory therapists, and other health care professionals is essential to initiate, manage, and terminate mechanical ventilatory assistance. However, the second-to-second monitoring and management of the patient–respiratory support system rests with the nurse.

This chapter discusses the skills necessary for instituting mechanical ventilatory assistance and for managing the patient from onset through weaning from mechanical ventilatory support.

Conventional mechanical ventilation relies on the application of positive or negative pressure to the pulmonary system. Although negative-pressure ventilation (e.g., the iron lung) was used extensively earlier in this century, introduction of the cuffed endotracheal tube has resulted in the dominance of positive-pressure ventilation in clinical practice during the second half of the twentieth century. There continues to be sporadic renewed interest in negative-pressure ventilation, but the ready access to the patient (and to the airway in particular) and the ability to alter the ventilatory parameters afforded by positive-pressure ventilation preclude a serious resurgence of negative-pressure ventilation in the foreseeable future.

Positive-pressure ventilators may be categorized into volume-preset and pressure-preset ventilators. Volume-preset ventilators are characterized by inspiratory cycles that terminate at preset inspiratory volumes. Pressure-preset ventilators are characterized by inspiratory cycles that terminate at preset peak inspiratory pressures. Because the delivered tidal volume may be quite variable with pressure-preset ventilators, these ventilators are not used for prolonged respiratory support and are not discussed in this chapter. The skills discussed in this chapter use volume-preset positive-pressure ventilators.

KEY TERMS

airway resistance (R_{aw})
alveolar-arterial oxygen gradient difference (A-aDO_2)
arterial oxygen tension to fraction of inspired oxygen ratio (respiratory index, PaO_2/FiO_2)
arterial-venous oxygen difference (a-$\bar{v}DO_2$)
assist-control (A-C)
auto-PEEP
barotrauma
chemical paralysis
content of oxygen in the arterial blood (CaO_2)
content of oxygen in the mixed venous blood ($C\bar{v}O_2$)
continuous positive airway pressure (CPAP)
controlled mandatory ventilation (CMV)
dead space (Vd/Vt)
frequency of respirations (f)
fraction of inspired oxygen (FiO_2)
high-frequency ventilation (HFV)
inspiratory-to-expiratory ratio (I:E ratio)
independent lung ventilation (ILV)
intermittent mandatory ventilation (IMV)
maximum voluntary ventilation (MVV)
mechanical sigh
minute ventilation ($\dot{V}_E$)
negative inspiratory pressure/force (NIP, NIF)
partial pressure of oxygen in arterial blood (PaO_2)
partial pressure of carbon dioxide in the arterial blood ($PaCO_2$)
partial pressure of oxygen in mixed venous blood ($P\bar{v}O_2$)
patient–ventilator synchrony
peak inspiratory flow (PIF)
peak (maximum) inspiratory pressure (PIP, MIP)
physiologic dynamic compliance (CMP_{dyn})
positive end-expiratory pressure (PEEP)
positive-pressure ventilation (PPV)
pressure support (PS)
saturation of hemoglobin with oxygen in arterial blood (SaO_2)
saturation of hemoglobin with oxygen in mixed venous blood ($S\bar{v}O_2$)
static (effective) compliance (CMP_{st})

synchronized intermittent mandatory ventilation (SIMV)
T-piece (T-bar, blow-by)
tidal volume (V_T)
work of breathing (inspiration) (WOB, WKIN)
venous admixture (percent shunt, $\dot{Q}s/\dot{Q}t$)
vital capacity (VC)

SKILLS

GUIDELINES

The following assessment guidelines assist the nurse in formulating nursing diagnoses and individualized care plans to initiate, manage, and terminate mechanical respiratory support:

1.   Know the patient's baseline respiratory assessment.

2.   Know the patient's baseline vital signs.

3.   Know the patient's baseline hemodynamic status.

4.   Know the patient's medical history.

5.   Know the patient's social history.

6.   Know the patient's current medical treatment.

7.   Know the therapeutic goals for the patient.

8.   Perform systematic respiratory assessments in a timely fashion.

9.   Perform frequent patient–ventilator "quick checks."

10. Become adept with equipment used for mechanical ventilatory support.

11. Determine appropriate intervention for assessed findings.

SKILL 4–1 _____

Initiation and Management of Positive-Pressure Ventilation (PPV)

Positive-pressure ventilation (PPV) is the traditional method of providing mechanical ventilatory assistance. PPV is delivered through an artificial airway—either an oral endotracheal tube, a nasotracheal tube, or a tracheostomy tube (see Chap. 1). PPV is indicated for the patient with respiratory or ventilatory failure, which may be caused by acute or chronic lung injury, neurologic disorders, multisystem failure, chemical respiratory depressants (e.g., anesthesia, sedation), or trauma. Hypoxemia, metabolic acidosis, respiratory acidosis, signs of inadequate tissue oxygenation, and respiratory muscle fatigue frequently indicate the need for PPV.

The ventilator delivers gas into the lungs, producing positive intrathoracic and airway pressures during inspiration. The rate and distribution of inspired gas are a function of the resistance and compliance of the lung. Increased airway resistance and/or decreased lung compliance secondary to disease necessitate high pressures to deliver the desired tidal volume at the desired rate. High inspiratory pressures put the patient at risk for cardiovascular depression and pulmonary barotrauma.

The extent of hemodynamic changes seen in a given patient depends on the level of positive pressure applied, the duration of positive pressure during different phases of the breathing cycle, the amount of pressure transmitted to the vascular structures, the patient's intravascular volume, and the adequacy of hemodynamic compensatory mechanisms. PPV can reduce venous return, shift the interventricular septum to the left, and increase right ventricular afterload as a result of increased pulmonary vascular resistance (Fig. 4–1). The hemodynamic effects of PPV may be prevented or corrected by optimizing filling pressures to accommodate the PPV-induced changes in intrathoracic pressures, by minimizing the peak inspiratory pressure (PIP), and by optimizing the inspiratory-to-expiratory (I:E) ratio.

Pulmonary barotrauma is damage to the lung from extrapulmonary air that may result from changes in intrapleural pressure during PPV. Barotrauma is manifested by pneumothorax, pneumomediastinum, pneumopericardium, pneumoperitoneum, or subcutaneous emphysema. The risk of barotrauma in the patient receiving positive-pressure ventilation is increased with preexisting lung lesions (e.g., localized infections, blebs), high inflation pressures (i.e., large tidal volumes, positive end-expiratory pressure, mainstem bronchus intubation, patient–ventilator asynchrony), and invasive thoracic procedures (e.g., subclavian catheter insertion, bronchoscopy, thoracentesis). Barotrauma from PPV may be prevented or corrected by decreasing PIP, decreasing positive end-expiratory pressure (PEEP), optimizing patient–ventilator synchrony, ensuring proper position of the tip of the artificial airway, and pleural or mediastinal decompression (Guthrie et al., 1983).

The overriding goal for every patient on PPV is timely and successful discontinuance of PPV. Timely discontinuance is defined differently for each patient but generally means the patient will not be on PPV longer than needed. Successful discontinuance of PPV also is defined differently for each patient but generally means that the patient will not require reinstitution of PPV within 24 to 48 hours following discontinuance.

Once the goals have been formulated, the roles and responsibilities of each provider, the patient, and the family are delineated. Clearly, the burden of managing the patient on PPV rests with the nurse. The nurse co-

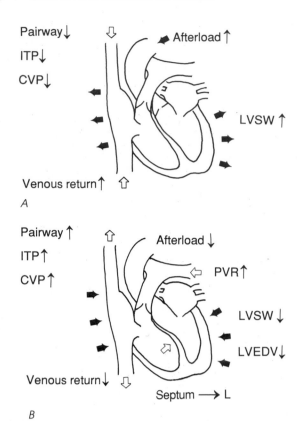

Pairway↓
ITP↓
CVP↓
Afterload↑
LVSW↑
Venous return↑

A

Pairway↑
ITP↑
CVP↑
Afterload↓
PVR↑
LVSW↓
LVEDV↓
Venous return↓
Septum → L

B

FIGURE 4–1. Effects of positive-pressure ventilation (PPV), positive end-expiratory pressure (PEEP), and continuous positive airway pressure (CPAP) on cardiac function. (*A*) Effects of reduced airway and intrathoracic pressures (ITP) on cardiac function. Central venous pressure (CVP) is decreased. Venous return, afterload, and left ventricular stroke work (LVSW) are increased. These are the typical effects of spontaneous ventilation. (*B*) Effects of increased airway and intrathoracic pressures on cardiac function. Venous return and afterload are decreased. Pulmonary vascular resistance (PVR) rises, the interventricular septum shifts into the left ventricle, and left ventricular end-diastolic volume (LVED) decreases along with left ventricular stroke work (LVSW). These are the typical effects of PPV, PEEP, and CPAP. (From C. W. Bryan-Brown. Ventilatory Management of Cardiovascular Disease. In L. C. Weeks (Ed.), *Advanced Cardiovascular Nursing*. Boston: Blackwell Scientific, 1986. Reproduced by permission from L. C. Weeks, Blackwell Scientific Publications; copyrighted by The C. V. Mosby Co., St. Louis.)

ordinates multiple efforts, teaches and supports the patient and family, monitors and intervenes in the patient–ventilator system, and ensures that the patient's complex needs are met during PPV.

When appropriately initiated and managed, PPV can provide adequate ventilation, promote adequate respiration, and provide rest for the patient until the need for mechanical ventilatory assistance is relieved.

Purpose

The nurse collaborates with the physician and respiratory therapist in the initiation and management of positive-pressure ventilation to

1. Maintain or improve ventilation.
2. Maintain or improve oxygenation levels in the arterial blood.

3. Decrease the work of breathing and improve patient comfort.

Prerequisite Knowledge and Skills

Prior to initiating positive-pressure ventilation, the nurse should understand

1. Principles of aseptic technique.
2. Anatomy and physiology of the upper and lower respiratory and cardiopulmonary systems.
3. Principles of airway management.
4. Principles of gas exchange.
5. Principles of airway resistance.
6. Principles of lung compliance.
7. Principles of arterial blood gas interpretation.
8. Principles of chest radiograph interpretation.
9. Principles of positive-pressure ventilation.
10. Mechanics of positive-pressure ventilation.
11. Verbal and nonverbal communication strategies.

The nurse should be able to perform

1. Proper handwashing technique (see Skill 35–5).
2. Vital signs assessment.
3. Ventilation via mouth-to-mouth, mouth-to-nose, or face mask–to–mouth and nose techniques.
4. Respiratory physical assessment (inspection, palpation, percussion, and auscultation).
5. Hemodynamic assessment.
6. Oral airway, nasal airway, or bite-block insertion (see Skills 1–1, 1–2).
7. Confirmation of endotracheal tube placement.
8. Endotracheal tube care (see Skill 1–5).
9. Tracheostomy tube care (see Skill 1–9).
10. Measurement of cuff pressures (see Skill 1–7).
11. Endotracheal suctioning (see Skill 1–6).
12. Nasal and oral pharyngeal suctioning (see Skill 1–3).
13. Sputum specimen collection from endotracheal or tracheostomy tube.
14. Extubation (see Skill 1–8).
15. Continuous oxygen saturation monitoring (arterial, mixed venous, and/or pulse oximetry (see Skills 6–1, 6–3).

Assessment

1. Observe for signs and symptoms of inadequate ventilation, including rising arterial carbon dioxide tension (definitive sign), chest–abdominal dyssynchrony, shallow respirations, irregular respirations, apnea, tachypnea, bradypnea, dyspnea, asterixis, headache, restlessness, confusion, lethargy, rising (early sign) or falling (late sign) arterial blood pressure, tachycardia, atrial and/or ventricular dysrhythmias, and depressed deep tendon reflexes. **Rationale:** Inadequate ventilation may indicate the need for initiation of PPV. While PPV is being considered and assembled, provide adequate ventilation via (1) a manual self-inflating resuscitation bag and face mask (see Skill 4–2), (2) mouth-to-mouth ventilation, or (3) coached breathing.

2. Assess arterial carbon dioxide tension and pH. Inadequate ventilation is confirmed by acute or chronic respiratory acidosis with a $PaCO_2$ greater than 45 mmHg. **Rationale:** Ventilatory failure is an indication for PPV.

3. Observe for signs and symptoms of inadequate oxygenation, including falling arterial oxygen tension (definitive sign), tachypnea, dyspnea, central cyanosis, restlessness, confusion, agitation, tachycardia (early sign), bradycardia (late sign), dysrhythmias, intercostal and suprasternal retractions, rising (early sign) or falling (late sign) arterial blood pressure, adventitious breath sounds, falling urine output, and metabolic acidosis. **Rationale:** Inadequate oxygenation may indicate the need for PPV. While PPV is being considered and assembled, provide 100% oxygen and humidity via face mask, T-tube, or trach collar. *Caution:* A self-inflating manual resuscitation bag and face mask should be on standby for emergency ventilation of the patient who has chronic carbon dioxide retention. High supplemental oxygen may depress ventilation significantly (Martin, 1987). Inadequate oxygenation can be addressed with changes in ventilator parameters and by treating the underlying pathophysiologic mechanism.

4. Assess arterial oxygen tension or saturation. Hypoxemia is confirmed by a falling PaO_2 and/or SaO_2 or an absolute PaO_2 of less than 60 mmHg and/or an absolute SaO_2 of less than 90 percent. **Rationale:** Hypoxemia may indicate the need for PPV. Hypoxemia is confirmed by a falling PaO_2 and/or SaO_2 or an absolute PaO_2 that exceeds the therapeutic guidelines for arterial oxygen level.

5. Observe for signs and symptoms of inadequate breathing pattern, including dyspnea, chest–abdominal dyssynchrony, shallow respirations, irregular respirations, intercostal retractions, suprasternal retractions, tracheal tug (upward and downward movement of larynx with inspiration and expiration), and dyspnea. **Rationale:** Respiratory distress is an indication for PPV. Comfortable breathing pattern is a goal of PPV. An inadequate breathing pattern can be corrected by changing the ventilator parameters or by finding and treating the underlying acute cause (e.g., malpositioned endotracheal tube, leak in the endotracheal tube cuff, improper assembly of ventilator component, etc.)

6. Assess for signs of atelectasis, including localized changes in auscultation (decreased or bronchial breath sound), localized dullness to percussion, increased breathing effort, tracheal deviation toward the side of abnormal findings, increased peak inspiratory pressure (PIP), decreased compliance, decreased PaO_2 or SaO_2 with constant ventilator parameters, and localized consolidation ("white out," opacity) on chest radiograph. **Rationale:** Early detection of atelectasis indicates the need for altering interventions to promote resolution (e.g., hyperinflation techniques, increased positioning, increased supplemental oxygen, etc.). Noncompression atelectasis caused by mucous plug or other peripheral airway obstruction and by hypoventilation is amenable to nursing interventions (Goodnough et al., 1986). Compression atelectasis caused by tumor, pleural effusion, or other pathology requires physician consultation.

7. Assess for signs and symptoms of pulmonary barotrauma, including acute, increasing, or severe dyspnea, restlessness, agitation, panic, localized changes in auscultation (decreased or absent breath sounds), localized hyperresonance or tympany to percussion, increased breathing effort, tracheal deviation away from the side of abnormal findings, increased PIP, decreased compliance, decreased PaO_2 or SaO_2 with constant ventilator parameters, subcutaneous emphysema, and localized intrapleural air ("black out," lucency) on chest radiograph. **Rationale:** Early detection of pneumothorax is essential to minimize progression and the adverse effects on the patient. Signs of barotrauma require physician collaboration. Tension pneumothorax requires emergency treatment by the most qualified person available.

8. Observe for signs of cardiovascular depression, particularly after an increase in tidal volume, PEEP, or CPAP or with hyperinflation. Signs include acute or gradual fall in arterial blood pressure, tachycardia (early sign), bradycardia (late sign), dysrhythmias, weak peripheral pulses, respiratory swing in arterial or pulmonary arterial waveforms (Fig. 4–2), decreased pulse pressure, acute or gradual increase in pulmonary capillary wedge pressure, and decreased mixed venous oxygen tension. **Rationale:** PPV can cause decreased venous return and afterload due to the increase in intrathoracic pressure (see Fig. 4–1). This mechanism often is manifested during the first 24 hours of PPV and following initiation of or increase in large tidal volumes, PEEP, CPAP, and other

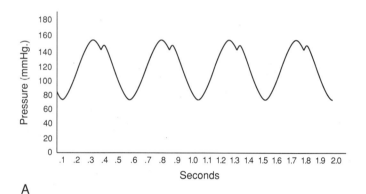

A

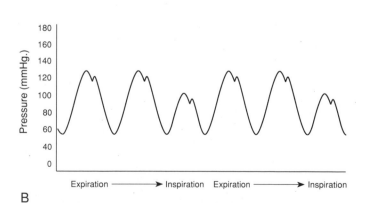

B

FIGURE 4–2. Comparison of normal arterial pressure pulse contour (*A*) with "respiratory swing" in arterial pressure waveform (*B*). (Courtesy of Sandra K. Goodnough-Hanneman.)

hyperinflation techniques (Goodnough, 1985). Cardiovascular depression associated with manual or periodic ventilator hyperinflations is immediately reversible with cessation of hyperinflation (Goodnough, 1985). Other interventions for cardiovascular depression require physician collaboration.

9. Continuously monitor for signs and symptoms of inadvertent extubation, including vocalization, activated low-pressure ventilator alarm, bilateral changes in anterior upper lobe auscultation (decreased or absent breath sounds), and gastric distension, and for signs and symptoms of inadequate ventilation, oxygenation, and breathing pattern in Assessment items 1 through 5. **Rationale:** Inadvertent extubation is defined as unplanned extubation (Goodnough et al., 1986, 1988). Inadvertent extubation is sometimes obvious (e.g., the endotracheal tube is in the patient's hand). Often, however, the tip of the endotracheal tube is in the hypopharynx or the esophagus, and inadvertent extubation is not immediately apparent. Reintubation is required. While awaiting reintubation, ventilation and oxygenation must be assisted with a self-inflating manual resuscitation bag and face mask (Fig. 4–3) or with mouth-to-mouth, mouth-to-nose, or face mask–to–mouth and nose technique.

10. Continuously monitor for signs and symptoms of malpositioned endotracheal tube, including dyspnea, restlessness, agitation, unilateral changes in auscultation (decreased or absent breath sounds), unilateral dullness to percussion, increased breathing effort, asymmetrical chest expansion, increased PIP, and radiographic evidence of the tip of the endotracheal tube less than 2 cm (.787 in) or more than 8 cm (3.15 in) above the carina (Goodnough et al., 1986, 1988). **Rationale:** Early detection and correction of a malpositioned endotracheal tube can prevent inadvertent extubation, atelectasis, barotrauma, and problems with gas exchange.

11. Observe for signs and symptoms of nosocomial lung infection, including purulent secretions, dyspnea, cough, increased breathing effort, localized changes in auscultation (decreased or bronchial breath sounds, coarse rales, wheezes), localized dullness to percussion, increased PIP, decreased compliance, tachycardia, de-

creased PaO_2 or SaO_2, positive sputum Gram stain, positive sputum and/or blood culture, decrease in respiratory mucus pH (Karnad et al., 1990), and localized or diffuse radiographic evidence of persistent or progressive infiltrates ("white-out," opacities, consolidation). **Rationale:** The prevalence of nosocomial pneumonia in patients on PPV ranges from 2 percent (Rutherford et al., 1990) to 59 percent (Goodnough et al., 1986; Pagliarello and Carter, 1990; Roberts et al., 1988; Sherry et al., 1990). *Caution*: Clinical, microbiologic, and radiologic indicators of pneumonia are not reliable (Karnad et al., 1990; Tobin and Grenvik, 1984). Physician consultation is required to make a differential diagnosis.

12. Observe for signs of nutritional deficiencies, including progressive weight loss, changes in anthropometric measurements, decreased urine creatinine, decreased skinfold measurement, decreased serum plasma proteins (e.g., albumin, prealbumin, transferrin, etc.), decreased lymphocyte count, deterioration in skin turgor, loss of hair, slow wound healing, and lethargy. **Rationale:** Because usual nutritional intake is prohibited by the endotracheal tube, extra attention is given to ensuring adequate nutrition in the patient on PPV. Adequate nutrition is defined relative to the patient's particular needs (e.g., tissue healing, increased work of breathing, etc.). Dietary consultation frequently is indicated to ensure adequate nutrition. The association between nutrition and pulmonary function is well established (Grant, 1988). Inadequate nutrition decreases diaphragmatic muscle mass, decreases pulmonary function performance, and increases mechanical ventilation requirements. *Caution*: Excessive carbohydrate loads may increase carbon dioxide production to the point of causing hypercapnia in patients on PPV (Grant, 1988).

Nursing Diagnoses

1. Impaired gas exchange related to hypercapnia and/or hypoxemia. **Rationale:** Hypercapnia associated with a pH less than 7.35 is acute respiratory acidosis, indicative of an inability to adequately eliminate carbon dioxide relative to its production. If the $PaCO_2$ continues to rise and the pH continues to fall despite alternative therapy, PPV will need to be initiated to mechanically assist with gas exchange. Hypoxemia that is unresponsive to high supplemental oxygen and other interventions indicates a need for PPV. Impaired gas exchange related to hypercapnia and/or hypoxemia is also a potential nursing diagnosis during and after initiation of PPV. Multiple pathophysiologic (e.g., atelectasis) and mechanical (e.g., tubing leak or disconnect) factors can result in impaired gas exchange while the patient is receiving PPV.

2. Potential for impaired breathing pattern related to hypoxemia, hypercapnia, atelectasis, barotrauma, nosocomial pneumonia, vigorous attempts to communicate, ventilator malfunction, patient–ventilator dyssynchrony, patient–ventilator system problems, malpositioned endotracheal tube, inadvertent extubation, decreased inspiratory muscle strength, decreased inspiratory muscle endurance, inappropriate ventilator settings, or leak in

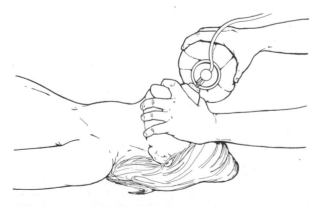

FIGURE 4–3. Proper technique for ventilation with manual self-inflating resuscitation bag and face mask. (Reproduced with permission from C. L. Scanlon, C. B. Spearman, and R. L. Sheldon, (Eds.), *Egan's Fundamentals of Respiratory Care*, 5th Ed. St. Louis: Mosby, 1990, p. 538.)

the endotracheal tube cuff. **Rationale:** As the list of etiologies suggests, many events in addition to the underlying disease process potentially can cause impaired breathing pattern.

3. Impaired airway clearance related to incomplete glottic closure, decreased mucociliary transport, hypersecretion of mucus, and abnormal viscosity of mucus. **Rationale:** The presence of an endotracheal tube prevents complete glottic closure, reducing the cough efficiency. The presence of an artificial airway and invasive procedures of the tracheobronchial tree (e.g., suctioning) irritate the mucosa, resulting in changes in secretion rate and viscosity of mucus and decreased mucociliary transport (Landa et al., 1980).

4. Potential for fluid volume deficit related to increased intrathoracic pressure. **Rationale:** PPV can cause transient or prolonged hypovolemia (relative) due to the increase in intrathoracic pressure from large tidal volumes, PEEP, auto-PEEP, or CPAP.

5. Potential for infection related to presence of artificial airway, contamination of equipment, breaks in aseptic technique, decreased mucociliary transport, ineffective airway clearance, and leak in the cuff of the artificial airway. **Rationale:** Within a few days, almost all intubated patients become colonized with pathogenic organisms (Hoyt, 1988; Jimenez et al., 1989). The oropharyngeal flora contain gram-negative organisms that may be aspirated around the endotracheal tube into the lower respiratory tract (Goodnough, 1988; Hoyt, 1988). Respiratory therapy equipment can be a source of both gram-negative and gram-positive hospital-acquired infections (Craven et al., 1984; Villers and Derriennic, 1983). The respiratory tract of the patient on PPV is at very high risk for contamination, colonization, and subsequent infection from suctioning, tracheal irrigation, condensed fluid in ventilator circuit, contaminated ventilators and other respiratory therapy equipment, and inhaled drugs (Pagliarello and Carter, 1990; Paluch, 1986; Powner et al., 1986; Roberts et al., 1988; Rutherford et al., 1990; Yannelli and Gurevich, 1988).

6. Potential for injury related to artificial airway and PPV. **Rationale:** The patient is at risk for injury to the trachea from the endotracheal or tracheostomy tube (Goodnough, 1988) and to the lung from PPV, particularly when large inflation pressures are required.

7. Potential for decreased cardiac output related to increased intrathoracic pressure. **Rationale:** PPV can cause a transient or prolonged decrease in cardiac output (see Figs. 4–1 and 4–2) as a result of decreased venous return and decreased afterload from increased intrathoracic pressure. The patient receiving large tidal volumes, PEEP, CPAP, and other hyperinflation techniques (Goodnough, 1985) is particularly at risk.

8. Potential for suffocation related to obstructed airway or improper ventilator assembly. **Rationale:** Many patients on PPV are dependent on a patent artificial airway that is properly positioned and a functioning ventilator that is set to meet their needs. Reversal of ventilator expiratory valve during assembly or complete herniation of the cuff over the tip of the endotracheal or tracheostomy tube can result in suffocation.

9. Potential for aspiration related to a leak in the cuff of the artificial airway. **Rationale:** Research suggests that the variables in cuff wall thickness and intracuff pressure interact to either prevent or facilitate aspiration of oropharyngeal and gastric contents (Bernhard et al., 1982; Elpern et al., 1987; Goodnough, 1988; Macrae and Wallace, 1981; Mehta, 1982).

10. Impaired verbal communication related to presence of artificial airway. **Rationale:** PPV requires that the cuff of the artificial airway be sealed, thereby preventing vocalization.

Planning

1. Individualize the following goals for initiating positive-pressure ventilation. See Table 4–1 for the various modes of mechanical ventilatory assistance and Figure 4–4 for how each mode affects airway pressure.

   a. Maintain or improve ventilation. Determine the desired $PaCO_2$ range. Consider modes of mechanical ventilatory assistance to best meet patient's needs. **Rationale:** Mechanical ventilatory assistance will be needed until the underlying problem causing inadequate ventilation is corrected. A-C mode is used to provide total ventilatory support while permitting the patient to use respiratory effort to initiate volume-preset breaths. *Caution:* $PaCO_2$ must be monitored for respiratory alkalosis. If the $PaCO_2$ falls below desired level, A-C frequency can be reduced or IMV/SIMV mode can be used. IMV mode is used to provide total or partial ventilatory support by adjusting the frequency of mandatory breaths per minute. With IMV, the patient can take spontaneous breaths that are not volume-preset between the set breaths. Synchronized intermittent mandatory ventilation (SIMV) synchronizes the patient's spontaneous breaths with the volume-preset breaths. Synchronization prevents "stacking" of spontaneous and ventilator tidal volumes, thereby theoretically preventing the auto-PEEP phenomenon (discussed under Unexpected Outcomes, Hemodynamic instability; see also Skill 4–7).

   b. Maintain or improve oxygenation. (Determine desired PaO_2 range.) Consider a ventilator with controlled mandatory ventilation (CMV), A-C, IMV/SIMV, pressure support, positive end-expiratory pressure (PEEP), and continuous positive airway pressure (CPAP) mode options. **Rationale:** Mechanical ventilatory assistance will be needed until the patient is able to maintain an adequate PaO_2 with spontaneous breathing and supplemental oxygen of less than 40%. The CMV mode is indicated only for the patient with severe hypoxemia who requires total ventilatory support to reduce oxygen consumption. Frequently, chemical paralysis is induced to aid this effort. *Caution:* When on CMV mode, the pa-

TABLE 4–1 MODES OF MECHANICAL VENTILATORY ASSISTANCE

Mode	Explanatory Note
Controlled mandatory ventilation (CMV)	The patient automatically receives breaths with controlled tidal volume and frequency.
Assist-Control (A-C)	The patient triggers breaths with controlled tidal volume. If the patient does not trigger a breath, controlled tidal volume is delivered automatically at the preset frequency.
Intermittent mandatory ventilation (IMV)	The patient breathes spontaneously through the ventilator between mandatory breaths with controlled tidal volume and frequency.
Synchronized intermittent mandatory ventilation (SIMV)	The patient breathes spontaneously through the ventilator between mandatory breaths with controlled tidal volume and frequency. The mandatory breaths are synchronized with the patient's spontaneous breathing.
Sigh	The patient automatically receives periodic deep breaths with controlled sigh (hyperinflation) volume and frequency.
Positive end-expiratory pressure (PEEP)	A ventilatory adjunct that can be used in combination with CMV, A-C, IMV, and SIMV. Prevents the lung pressure from decreasing to atmospheric pressure during expiration.
Pressure support (PS)	The patient breathes spontaneously with pressure assistance to each spontaneous inspiration.
Continuous positive airway pressure (CPAP)	A ventilatory adjunct that can be used with spontaneous ventilation and in combination with the spontaneous breaths with IMV and SIMV. The patient breathes spontaneously through the ventilator at an elevated baseline pressure throughout the breathing cycle.

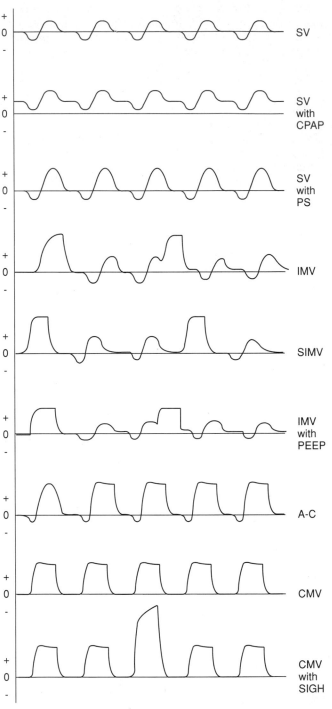

FIGURE 4–4. Airway pressure and mode of mechanical ventilatory assistance. A-C is assist-control, CMV is controlled mechanical ventilation, IMV is intermittent mandatory ventilation, PEEP is positive end-expiratory pressure, PS is pressure support, SIMV is synchronized intermittent mandatory ventilation, SV is spontaneous ventilation. (Courtesy of Sandra K. Goodnough-Hanneman.)

tient is totally dependent on the ventilatory support for gas exchange and must be continuously observed and monitored. The use of A-C or IMV/SIMV mode largely is based on preference, since the preset tidal volume and frequency of breaths per minute will affect oxygenation. To prevent oxygen toxicity from high fractions of inspired oxygen (FiO_2), large tidal volumes and PEEP may be used. Tidal volumes must be coordinated with frequency of breaths to maintain the minute ventilation within a range that produces desirable carbon dioxide levels. If the desired PaO_2 cannot be achieved without respiratory alkalosis, PEEP is indicated. *Caution*: PEEP can result in cardiovascular depression and pulmonary barotrauma. The patient on PEEP needs extensive and frequent cardiopulmonary assessment and monitoring.

IMV and SIMV modes increase the patient's work of breathing as a result of (1) resistance to inspired gas flow in the ventilator tubing and endotracheal tube, (2) patient effort required to open the ventilator demand valve, and (3) inadequate flow rates of many ventilators when the demand valve is open. When the patient triggers a spontaneous breath with IMV or SIMV, airway pressure is reduced. The reduction in airway pressure causes a demand valve in the ventilator to open, allowing gas flow for spontaneous breathing. The spontaneous tidal volume depends on maintaining a reduced airway pressure; when the airway pressure equalizes, the flow of gas is interrupted and the inspired volume ends.

Pressure support (PS) is a ventilatory adjunct that can be used with spontaneous, IMV, and SIMV modes of ventilation. PS provides sustained pressure throughout the spontaneous inspiratory phase, theoretically permitting more even distribution of inspired gas. With PS, the drop in airway pressure triggers a gas flow sufficient to increase the airway pressure to a preset level, which results in an increased tidal volume. The increased tidal volume is relative to the preset level of pressure support; the higher the pressure support, the larger is the tidal volume. Patients on IMV report greater comfort with PS. A decrease in the work of breathing in postoperative and critically ill patients has been shown with PS (Viale et al., 1988).

Like PS, continuous positive airway pressure (CPAP) permits more even distribution of inspired gas. CPAP, however, does this by maintaining airway pressure higher than atmospheric pressure during both inspiration and expiration. CPAP increases the functional residual capacity (FRC), permitting increased surface area for gas exchange. *Caution*: When CPAP is used with the patient breathing totally with the spontaneous mode of ventilation, the patient must be monitored for adequate spontaneous minute ventilation.

c. Maintain or improve breathing pattern (determine optimal breathing patterns). Consider desirable inspiratory-to-expiratory (I:E) ratio, and adjust peak inspiratory flow or inspiratory time accordingly. Provision must be made to ensure that the desired tidal volume is delivered within a comfortable time. With most volume-preset ventilators, a flow-rate control permits regulation of the length of the inspiratory phase. Peak

inspiratory flow (PIF) controls the peak flow rate of inspired gas from the ventilator during the CMV and A-C modes and the mandatory breaths during the IMV and SIMV modes. A formula can be used to determine the initial PIF setting (Dupuis, 1986). The formula and examples of applying the formula to different patients are demonstrated in Table 4–2. Low inspiratory flow rates result in a longer inspiratory phase; high inspiratory flow rates result in a shorter inspiratory phase and allow more time for expiration. The flow rate should be correlated with the respiratory rate to produce the desired I:E ratio. Increased peak flows are needed for fast respiratory rates or long expiratory phases; lower peak flows are indicated for slow respiratory rates. Inspiratory peak flows of 60 to 100 L/min have been shown to improve gas exchange by permitting better lung emptying in patients with COPD who are mechanically ventilated. *Caution*: The calculated flow is limited by increased airway pressures. Many patients who require initiation of positive-pressure ventilation will require higher peak inspiratory flow rates than those calculated using the formula in Table 4–2. Ventilators using flow rates to adjust I:E ratio have peak flow rates ranging from 10 to 200 L/min. Other ventilators have inspiratory and/or expiratory time controls. The desirable I:E ratio is determined (e.g., 1:2) for the patient. The total time for each breathing cycle is determined by dividing 60 (s/min) by the frequency (e.g., 60/12 breaths per minute = 5

TABLE 4–2 DETERMINATION OF INITIAL PEAK INSPIRATORY FLOW RATE

Formula for determining initial peak inspiratory flow setting:

$$\dot{V} = (V_T \times f) \times (I + E)$$

where $\dot{V}$ = flow rate (L/min)
V_T = tidal volume (liters)
f = frequency of breaths per minute
I = inspiratory portion of breathing cycle
E = expiratory portion of breathing cycle

Application of formula to two patients:

Patient A has normal lungs and neuromuscular disease.

Patient Parameters — *Initial PIF Setting*
$V_T = 0.5$ L
$f = 12$
I:E ratio = 1:3
$\dot{V} = (0.5 \times 12) \times (1 + 3)$
$= 24$ L/min ($= 0.4$ L/s)

Patient B has chronic obstructive pulmonary disease.
Patient Parameters — *Initial PIF Setting*
$V_T = 0.5$ L
$f = 12$
I:E ratio = 1:5
$\dot{V} = (0.5 \times 12) \times (1 + 5)$
$= 36$ L/min ($= 0.6$ L/s)

seconds per breath). With an I:E ratio of 1:2, the inspiratory time should be one-half the expiratory time. Multiply 5 (seconds per breath) by 34 percent (percentage of breathing cycle devoted to inspiration) to obtain an inspiratory time of 1.7 seconds. Some ventilators have I:E ratio controls with optional settings. Other ventilators have a fixed I:E ratio that cannot be altered.

d. Maintain a communication system. **Rationale:** Recognizing that the system may need to be altered periodically, the primary caregivers and the family need to be able to understand nonverbal communication from the patient.

2. Prepare all necessary equipment and supplies. **Rationale:** Equipment and supplies need to be readily available and functional to initiate PPV and to immediately troubleshoot problems that may occur during initiation. It is assumed that the patient is already on an ECG monitor.

   a. Manual self-inflating resuscitation bag capable of delivering 100% oxygen and large inflation volumes.
   b. PEEP valve (Fig. 4–5) on standby for the patient with severe hypoxemia.
   c. Appropriately sized resuscitation face mask.
   d. Multiple oxygen sources (at least two, one for the ventilator and one for the resuscitation bag)
   e. Ventilator.
   f. Spirometer for measuring exhaled tidal volume.
   g. Heated humidifier with filter and in-line thermometer.
   h. Oxygen analyzer.
   i. Rubber test lung.
   j. Oxygen blender and oxygen and air flow meters, if needed for ventilator.
   k. Distilled sterile water.
   l. Swivel adapter.
   m. Replacement artificial airway.
   n. Clean gloves.
   o. Suction equipment (see Skills 1–4, 1–9).
   p. Yaukauer suction catheter.
   q. Manometer for measuring cuff pressure (Figure 4–4) (see Skill 1–7).
   r. Rubber-tipped clamp or hemostat.
   s. 12 cc syringe for cuff inflation.
   t. Equipment for arterial blood gas (ABG) analysis (see Skill 9–2).
   u. Chest tube insertion tray or 14-gauge needle.
   v. Writing pad or other method for patient communication.
   w. Call bell within patient reach.
   x. Stethoscope.
   y. Backup ventilator alarm(s).
   z. Water-insoluble marker.
   aa. Sterile scissors.
   bb. Tincture of benzoin (or comparable preparation).
   cc. Container for draining condensate from ventilator tubing.
   dd. Bite block or nasal or oral airway

3. Prepare the patient.
   a. Explain the procedure and why PPV is being initiated. **Rationale:** Communication and explanation for therapy are cited as important needs of patients (Viner, 1988).
   b. Discuss the sensations the patient will experience, such as relief of dyspnea, big lung inflations, noise of ventilator operation, and alarm sounds. **Rationale:** Knowledge of anticipated sensory experiences reduces anxiety and distress (Viner, 1988).
   c. Encourage the patient to relax. **Rationale:** Promotes general relaxation, oxygenation, and ventilation.
   d. Explain that the patient will be unable to speak. Establish a method of communication in conjunction with the patient and family. **Rationale:** Information about the patient's condition and therapy is consistently cited as an important need of patients (Baier and Zimmeth, 1986; Foundation for Critical Care, 1988; Harvey et al., 1991; Viner, 1988) and family members (Hickey, 1990).

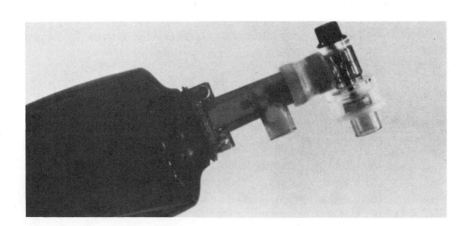

FIGURE 4–5. Manual self-inflating resuscitation bag with adjustable positive end-expiratory pressure (PEEP) valve. (Reproduced with permission from J. M. McHugh, Ventilatory Management. In S. Millar, L. K. Sampson, and S. M. Soukup (Eds.), *AACN Procedure Manual for Critical Care*, 2d Ed. Philadelphia: Saunders, 1985, p. 249.)

Implementation

Steps	Rationale	Special Considerations
Initiation		
1. Set tidal volume of 7 to 15 cc/kg as prescribed.	Conservative tidal volumes may be indicated in patients with chronic carbon dioxide retention or those with neuromuscular diseases who have normal lungs to prevent undesirable mechanical hyperventilation and associated alkalosis.	Use 7 to 10 cc/kg for patients with chronic CO_2 retention and patients with neuromuscular disease who have normal lungs.
	Patients with hypoxemia need large tidal volumes to optimize gas exchange.	Use 12 to 15 cc/kg for patients with hypoxemia.
2. Set respiratory rate between 8 and 20 breaths per minute, as prescribed.	Respiratory rate, like tidal volume, should be selected based on the patient's underlying disease process.	
	Normal respiratory rate is indicated for patients with neuromuscular disease and normal lungs.	Use 12 to 15 breaths per minute for patients with normal lungs.
	Faster respiratory rates are more comfortable for patients with hypoxemia and some neurologic disorders that result in rapid breathing patterns. Faster rates often permit patient–ventilator synchrony, thereby reducing the risk of pulmonary barotrauma.	Use 16 to 20 breaths per minute for patients with rapid spontaneous respiratory rates.
	Patients with chronic carbon dioxide retention often need slower rates to permit longer expiratory phase.	Use 8 to 12 breaths per minute for patients with chronic obstructive lung disease.
3. Set fraction of inspired oxygen (FiO_2) to 1.0 (100% oxygen concentration).	Initiating PPV with maximum oxygen concentration avoids hypoxemia while optimal ventilator settings are being determined and evaluated. Additionally, it permits measurement of the percentage of venous admixture (shunt), which provides an estimate of the severity of the gas-exchange abnormality.	Patients with chronic carbon dioxide retention on IMV or SIMV at low mandatory rates should have an FiO_2 of less than 0.40.
4. Set peak inspiratory flow of 20 to 100 L/min, as prescribed (see Table 4–2). Adjust as necessary.	*Inspiratory flow* refers to the speed with which a tidal volume is delivered during inspiration. Achieves the desired I:E ratio and comfortable breathing patterns.	Use 20 to 40 L/min for respiratory rates of 12 to 15 breaths per minute.
	Higher peak inspiratory flows may be needed in patients with poor lung compliance or high airway resistance to promote patient–ventilator synchrony and ensure adequate minute ventilation.	Use 40 to 60 L/min for respiratory rates of 16 to 20 breaths per minute. Use 80 to 100 L/min for patients with COPD who have respiratory rates of 8 to 12 breaths per minute.
5. Set the prescribed mode of ventilation (see Table 4–1).	Mode selection is often arbitrary and depends on the patient's clinical situation.	CMV is indicated for heavily sedated or paralyzed patients. CMV may be preferred in patients with respiratory muscle fatigue to prevent respiratory muscle exertion.
6. Set the sigh volume at 150 percent of the tidal volume and sigh rate at 4 to 6 breaths per minute.	Mechanical sighs replace the normal sigh mechanisms of cough, deep breath, yawn, etc. that occur every minute during the awake hours.	Patients with large tidal volumes, PEEP, or high peak inspiratory pressures should not have sighs set. Mechanical sighs may increase their

Table continues on following page

Steps	Rationale	Special Considerations
	Studies have shown that monotonous tidal volumes can cause progressively decreasing pulmonary compliance and resting lung volumes.	PIP to dangerously high levels, increasing the risk of barotrauma. Ventilator sighs are indicated in patients who have normal lungs (e.g., neuromuscular disorders, drug overdose) to prevent the complications of monotonous tidal volumes (Eubanks and Bone, 1990) and in patients with noncompression atelectasis.
7. Fill (or check) the humidifier with sterile distilled water and adjust the thermostat setting according to manufacturer's recommendation or unit protocol.	Since the inspired gas will bypass the patient's normal humidification mechanism in the upper airway, the gas must be humidified at 37°C (98.6°F) prior to entering the artificial airway.	
8. Plug the power cord into a grounded 110-volt ac outlet.	Most ventilators are electrically operated.	Audible or visual alarm should activate, indicating loss of oxygen source.
9. Attach high-pressure oxygen hose to a 50-lb/in² oxygen source and high-pressure air hose to 50-lb/in² compressed-air source.	Ventilators operate on a pneumatic source of wall oxygen (and air) under pressure.	Most ventilators have an internal compressor that allows the ventilator to generate its own air supply should the wall air source fail. Audible or visual alarm indicating loss of oxygen should turn off when attachment is completed.
10. Attach an oxygen analyzer to the inspiratory circuit. Attach rubber test lung to the analyzer. Ventilate test lung for 2 minutes. Check oxygen analyzer. The reading should be within 5 percent of the oxygen setting.	Validates percentage of oxygen to be administered.	Oxygen wash-in time is variable, depending on ventilator and minute volume ($V_T \times f$).
11. Replace oxygen analyzer with a portable respirometer (e.g., Wright).	Ensures that delivered V_T is the same as set V_T.	Variance between delivered and set V_T may require calibration, adjustment, or repair of ventilator.
12. Set high-pressure limit to 20 cmH$_2$O higher than PIP. Squeeze the test lung for three breaths.	Prevents the delivery of oxygen at high peak pressures, thus decreasing the risk of barotrauma.	Audible or visual high-pressure alarm should activate, indicating PIP has exceeded high-pressure limit.
13. Remove respirometer and test lung. Attach swivel adapter. Connect swivel adapter to artificial airway.	Initiates mechanical ventilation.	Ventilator is checked and ready to attach to the patient's airway.
14. Observe patient's breathing pattern. Count respiratory rate, (f), and note the I:E ratio.	Ascertains adequate breathing pattern.	With inadequate breathing patterns, disconnect the ventilator and manually bag the patient.
15. Note PIP and adjust high-pressure limit, if necessary, to 20 cmH$_2$O higher than PIP.	High-pressure limit shunts remaining tidal volume to the atmosphere, limiting high pressure to that set and reducing the risk of barotrauma.	
16. Measure exhaled tidal volume with respirometer. Adjust set tidal volume, if necessary, to achieve desired delivered tidal volume.	Several variables can result in a discrepancy between set and delivered tidal volume, such as leak in endotracheal tube cuff, leak in ventilator connection sites, etc.	
17. Measure dynamic compliance (see Skill 4–4).	Serves as an indicator of airway resistance.	

Table continues on following page

Steps	Rationale	Special Considerations
18. Measure static compliance (see Skill 4–4).	Serves as an indicator of lung compliance.	
19. *Activate all alarms*—ventilator and cardiac.	Alerts the nurse to actual or potential life-threatening problems.	
20. Place the call bell within the reach of patients who are able to use it.	Reduces fear, anxiety, and panic associated with dependence on life-support technology (Bergbom-Engberg and Haljamae, 1989).	
21. Place manual self-inflating resuscitation bag with face mask attached to an oxygen flowmeter which is turned on at the head of the bed.	Safety precaution to provide ventilatory support should the patient become extubated, experience cardiopulmonary arrest or with ventilator malfunction.	

Management

Steps	Rationale	Special Considerations
1. Check that ventilator and cardiac monitor alarm systems are functional and appropriately set.	Ensures monitoring and warning of potential major problems when nurse is away from the bedside. Enhances feeling of security in patient when nurse leaves the bedside.	Cardiac alarm upper and lower limits should be set within 20 percent of patient's heart rate. High-pressure ventilator alarm should be set 15 cmH$_2$O higher than peak inspiratory pressure. Low-volume ventilator alarm should be set within 10 percent of delivered tidal volume.
2. Check for secure stabilization of the artificial airway.	Reduces the risk of inadvertent extubation.	Stabilization can be ascertained by lifting the patient's head slightly off the pillow by pulling on the endotracheal tube. If any movement of the tube is noted, resecure. An example of one method of securing the artificial airway is shown in Figure 4–6.
3. Check that replacement artificial airway is readily available at the head of the patient's bed. Ensure that type and size of replacement tube match the indwelling tube.	Ensures quick reestablishment of artificial airway in the event of inadvertent extubation.	
4. Check that appropriately sized face mask is at the bedside.	Ensures capability of providing immediate ventilation and oxygenation with a manual self-inflating resuscitation bag in the event of inadvertent extubation (see Fig. 4–3).	
5. Check tracheal tube size and date of insertion in patient record.	Provides data for decision-making about the appropriateness of a tracheostomy in the patient who has been intubated for a long time and is expected to require prolonged PPV.	
6. Auscultate and observe expansion of anterior chest at least hourly and immediately after manipulation of artificial airway, patient position change, chest physical therapy, and suctioning.	Increases the likelihood of detecting malpositioned endotracheal tube or inadvertent extubation.	
7. Request verification from radiology, or verify directly, that endotracheal tube tip is positioned properly as soon as possible after every chest radiograph.	Increases likelihood of early detection and correction of malpositioned endotracheal tube.	A ruler that measures in centimeters should be available at the view box for measuring distance between the tip of the endotracheal tube and the carina on chest films.
8. Use minimal occlusion volume (MOV) cuff inflation technique (Goodnough, 1988) (see Skill 1–6).	Reduces risk of bronchospasm and aspiration pneumonia due to leak in the artificial airway cuff.	Minimal leak cuff inflation technique may be indicated in the patient with suspected or documented tracheal injury.

Table continues on following page

Steps	Rationale	Special Considerations
		The risks (aspiration) versus benefits (reduced cuff contact with tracheal wall) of using minimal leak technique instead of MOV should be documented.
9. Continuously assess for gurgling sounds, vocalization, air leak around nose and mouth, loss of tidal volume, and decrease in peak inspiratory pressure.	Enhances early detection and correction of leak in the artificial airway cuff.	
10. Evaluate the need for a nasogastric tube to decompress stomach.	Reduces risk of aspiration pneumonia.	
11. Maintain semiprone position (Fig. 4–7) and/or elevate head of bed during enteral feedings unless contraindicated.	Reduces risk of aspiration.	
12. Suction oropharynx or nasopharynx after endotracheal suctioning and before any manipulation of the artificial airway cuff.	Decreases accumulation of secretions in the hypopharynx, thereby reducing risk of aspiration.	
13. Before repositioning artificial airway, hyperinflate the patient with sustained inspiratory pause *just before* deflating artificial airway cuff. (This maneuver requires two people, one to hyperinflate and one to manipulate tube.)	Forces exhalation, theoretically causing secretions on top of the cuff to be expelled out of the trachea, during cuff deflation. Although no research exists to document this phenomenon, it is logically a useful procedure to reduce the risk of aspiration. Suctioning the hypopharynx does not remove tracheal secretions on top of the cuff.	
14. Monitor artificial airway cuff pressure continuously if technology permits. Otherwise, monitor every 2 to 4 hours and record the measurement (Goodnough, 1988).	Decreases the risks of tracheoesophageal fistula, tracheomalacia, cuff rupture or herniation, and tracheal wall necrosis due to high cuff pressure.	If cuff pressure is greater than 25 mmHg (34 cmH$_2$O), deflate and reinflate cuff with MOV technique. If pressure is still greater than 25 mmHg, notify physician; a larger artificial airway may be needed. Document risk-benefit rationale for decision to tolerate cuff pressure greater than 25 mmHg (34 cmH$_2$O).

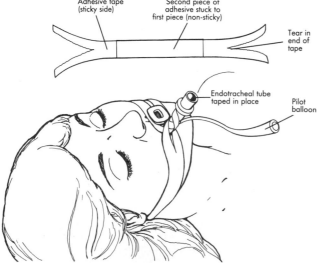

FIGURE 4–6.   One method of securing the endotracheal tube. (Reproduced with permission from C. L. Scanlon, C. B. Spearman, and R. L. Sheldon, (Eds.), *Egan's Fundamentals of Respiratory Care*, 5th Ed. St. Louis: Mosby, 1990, p. 495.)

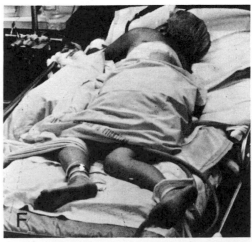

FIGURE 4–7.   Right semiprone position. (Reproduced with permission from C. F. Mackenzie, P. C. Imle, and N. Ciesla, *Chest Physiotherapy in the Intensive Care Unit*, 2d Ed. Baltimore: Williams & Wilkins, 1989, p. 97.)

Table continues on following page

Steps	Rationale	Special Considerations
15. Avoid tension on the endotracheal tube by cutting excess length of tube to 1 to 1½ in (2.54 to 3.81 cm) of the fixation point.	Reduces risk of necrosis of the nose, mouth, and oropharynx from pressure and movement of the endotracheal tube. Additionally, shortening the tube decreases resistance to breathing from the tube, thereby decreasing the work of breathing.	Verify proper position of the tip of the endotracheal tube from chest radiograph and clinical assessment prior to cutting excess tube. Document the length of tubing cut.
16. Use swivel adapter between artificial airway and ventilator.	Reduces risk of necrosis of the nose, mouth, and pharynx from pressure and movement of the endotracheal tube. Reduces risk of inadvertent extubation and malpositioned endotracheal tube.	
17. Stabilize endotracheal tube securely with tincture of benzoin (or comparable preparation) on face (see Skill 1–5 or Fig. 4–6).	Reduces risk of necrosis of the nose, mouth, and pharynx from pressure and movement of the endotracheal tube. Reduces risk of inadvertent extubation and malpositioned endotracheal tube.	Consider using double tape on hair and neck to promote comfort during removal of the tape. (An example of one method for securing the endotracheal tube is shown in Figure 4–6.)
18. Rotate endotracheal tube from one corner of the mouth to the other at least every 24 hours (see Skill 1–5).	Reduces risk of necrosis of the nose, mouth, and pharynx.	
19. Suction with low-trauma suction catheters (see Skills 1–3, 1–4, and 1–6).	Reduces risk of tracheobronchial mucosal trauma and subsequent risk of respiratory infection.	
20. Suction only when necessary. Attempt other secretion removal techniques when appropriate.	Reduces risk of tracheobronchial mucosal trauma and subsequent risk of respiratory infection. Reduces patient discomfort (Bergbom-Engberg and Haljamae, 1989) and risks of barotrauma and cardiovascular depression from subsequent patient–ventilator dyssynchrony.	
21. Continuously monitor in-line thermometer to maintain inspired gas temperature range of 36 to 38°C (96.8°F to 100.4°F) (15.24 cm) from the proximal airway.	Reduces risk of thermal injury from overheated inspired gas and risk of poor humidity from underheated inspired gas.	
22. Keep ventilator tubing clear of condensation (drain tubing from clean to dirty).	Reduces risk of respiratory infection by decreasing inhalation of contaminated water droplets.	
23. Keep manual self-inflating resuscitation bag with supplemental oxygen continuously on at 15 L/min to "flush" at the head of the bed.	Provides capability for immediately delivering ventilation and oxygenation to relieve acute respiratory distress due to hypoxemia and/or acidosis.	Attach a PEEP valve if the patient is on therapeutic PEEP (>5 cmH$_2$O).
24. Check ventilator for baseline FIO$_2$, PIP, and alarm activation after removal of ventilator from patient for suctioning, cough, bagging, draining ventilator tubing, etc.	Ensures that ordered ventilator parameters are used (i.e., 100% oxygen used for suctioning is not delivered after suctioning procedure), provides diagnostic data to evaluate intervention (e.g., PIP is reduced after suctioning, cough, or bagging), and ensures that the monitoring/warning function of the ventilator is functional (i.e., alarms).	
25. Explore any changes in peak inspiratory pressure greater than 2 to 4 cmH$_2$O.	Acute changes in PIP may indicate mechanical malfunction such as tubing disconnect; tubing, cuff, or connector leaks; tubing or airway kinks; and worn or improperly assembled parts.	

Table continues on following page

Steps	Rationale	Special Considerations
26. Assess at least hourly and after position change, suctioning, chest physical therapy, and visits to the bedside by others: anterior chest expansion and breath sounds, patient–ventilator synchrony, vital signs, ventilator sounds, all connections and alarm settings, PIP, frequency, I:E ratio, PEEP, V_T, and FiO_2.	The nurse bears continuous and ultimate accountability for monitoring the patient–ventilator interaction and the development of complications.	
27. Place bite block between the teeth if the patient is biting on the oral endotracheal tube.	Eliminates the effective airway obstruction and consequent high PIPs from narrowing of the tube lumen.	An oral airway serves the same purpose but may not be tolerated as well as the bite block.
28. Change the patient's body position as often as possible, but at least every 2 hours.	Frequent position changes are indicated to reduce the risks of noncompression atelectasis and pneumonia due to secretion stasis as well as the risk of microatelectasis due to loss of normal sigh maneuvers.	Place patient in semiprone position when possible (see Fig. 4–7) for optimal matching of ventilation and perfusion (Mackenzie et al., 1989) and to promote drainage of secretions. Schmitz (1988) demonstrated that the semiprone position can be used safely and comfortably in critically ill patients with multiple tubes and lines and that the semiprone position resulted in improved oxygenation in patients with adult respiratory distress syndrome (ARDS). *Caution:* Monitor patients with lung disease closely while turning. A marked deterioration in oxygenation and hemodynamics may occur.
29. If the patient is receiving a monotonous tidal volume (i.e., on CMV or A-C), alter pattern and depth of ventilation at least hourly for three consecutive breaths.	Reduces risk of noncompression atelectasis due to loss of normal sigh maneuvers and normal mobility. Reduces noncompression atelectasis by increasing collateral ventilation (Mackenzie et al., 1989).	
30. Sit the patient in a chair or ambulate at least three times daily, unless contraindicated.	Reduces risk of noncompression atelectasis due to loss of normal sigh maneuvers and impaired mobility. Conditions respiratory muscles as well as other body muscles.	Patients on PPV can be ambulated with portable oxygen and a manual self-inflating resuscitation bag as long as the bag and the "bagger" are capable of replicating the ventilator parameters. If the patient does not tolerate ambulation, walking in place at the bedside can be tried.
31. Explore the cause of high-pressure alarm activation within 15 seconds of detection.	Reduces the risk of barotrauma due to high airway pressures or detects barotrauma for early intervention.	
32. Explore patient–ventilator dyssynchrony by manually ventilating the patient with a self-inflating resuscitation bag (see Skill 4–2).	Reduces risks of barotrauma and cardiovascular depression or detects barotrauma for early intervention.	If patient breathes in synchrony with bagging, consider changes in ventilatory pattern or parameters of PPV. If patient does not breathe synchronously with bagging, explore differential diagnoses of problems distal to the airway. Physician consultation may be required.
33. Determine and maintain high-pressure limit setting 15 to 20 cmH_2O higher than PIP.	Reduces risk of barotrauma from high airway pressures.	
34. Explore any sudden increase in PIP of greater than 6 cmH_2O.	A sudden rise in peak inspiratory pressure indicates a rise in intrathoracic pressure. Reduces risk of barotrauma or	

Table continues on following page

Steps	Rationale	Special Considerations
	detects barotrauma for early intervention.	
35. For a combination of any two of the following signs: unilateral decreased breath sounds, unilateral hyperresonance, tracheal deviation away from the hyperresonant side, increased pulse and blood pressure followed by decreased pulse and blood pressure, acute increased PIP, severe respiratory distress, and subcutaneous emphysema: a. Turn FiO₂ on ventilator to 1.0. b. Remove the patient from the ventilator and manually ventilate. c. Have someone else call the physician immediately, and remain with the patient.	A combination of the signs listed indicates tension pneumothorax. Early nursing interventions may save the patient's life.	Frequently assess patients with PIPs greater than 40 cmH₂O for signs listed in step 35. Assess all patients after intubation and central line insertion for signs listed in step 35.
36. Keep chest tube insertion equipment and/or 14- to 16-gauge needles in the unit.	Provides capability for treating pneumothorax and for immediate decompression of tension pneumothorax.	
37. Weigh the patient daily, unless contraindicated.	Provides trend data to interpret weight gain or loss.	A daily weight change of greater than 0.5 kg and/or a respiratory swing of more than 10 mmHg may indicate an inadequate circulating volume secondary to positive intrathoracic pressure.
38. Observe arterial waveform with manual hyperinflation. If mean arterial pressure decreases more than 30 mmHg, abort hyperinflation, document, and notify physician.	Indicates relative functional changes in circulating volume due to positive intrathoracic pressure.	
39. Observe, document, and report to the physician any of the following hemodynamic changes associated with increased tidal volume or PEEP: decreased blood pressure, heart rate increase or decrease of more than 10 percent, arterial or venous respiratory swing, decreased cardiac output, decreased mixed venous oxygen tension, and increased arterial-venous oxygen difference (a-v̄DO₂; see Skill 4–5).	Indicates relative functional changes in circulating volume due to positive intrathoracic pressure.	
40. Discuss the patient's nutritional status with the physician daily.	Because the patient's usual nutritional intake is prohibited by the artificial airway, extra attention is given to ensuring adequate nutrition in the patient on PPV. Inadequate nutrition decreases diaphragmatic muscle mass, decreases pulmonary function performance, and increases mechanical ventilation requirements (Grant, 1988). Malnutrition (serum albumin less than 30 g/L) has been associated with an increased predisposition to pulmonary infection (Garibaldi et al., 1981).	Excessive carbohydrate loads may increase carbon dioxide production to the point of causing hypercapnia in patients on PPV (Askanazi et al., 1980; Grant, 1988).

Table continues on following page

Steps	Rationale	Special Considerations
41. Obtain coverage for meals, breaks, and other nurse absences from the bedside. Tell the patient that you are leaving but that nurse _____will be watching them during your absence.	Ensures that the patient will not be left unmonitored while on acute life-support equipment and that alarms will be responded to within 15 seconds. Reduces fear, anxiety, and panic associated with dependence on life-support technology (Bergbom-Engberg and Haljamae, 1989).	
42. Always leave the call bell within reach of patients who are able to use it.	Reduces fear, anxiety, and panic associated with dependence on life-support technology (Bergbom-Engberg and Haljamae, 1989).	
43. Discuss the goals of PPV with the physician, respiratory therapist, patient, and family daily, and communicate the progress toward the goals.	Clarity of the goals of PPV helps all concerned focus on achieving the goals (Goodnough-Hanneman, 1990). Promotes timely and successful discontinuance of PPV.	
44. Monitor gastric pH continuously, if technology permits, or periodically.	Studies have demonstrated a greater incidence of pneumonia in patients who have increased gastric pH (Craven et al., 1986).	The incidence of pneumonia in patients on PPV is higher in patients given antacids or histamine type 2 (H2) blockers for stress ulcer prophylaxis (Craven et al., 1986) compared with sucralfate (Driks et al., 1987). Driks and colleagues (1987) suggested that sucralfate preserves the natural gastric acid barrier against bacterial overgrowth and prevents gastric colonization of the airway, thereby reducing the risk of nosocomial pneumonia in patients on PPV.
45. Wash hands.	Reduces transmission of microorganisms.	

Evaluation

1. Observe for signs and symptoms of adequate ventilation, including $PaCO_2$ within desired range (definitive criterion), bilateral anterior chest expansion, breath sounds present and equal bilaterally, chest–abdominal synchrony, comfortable appearance, stable blood pressure and heart rate, and absence of the following: headache, visual disturbances, dyspnea, asterixis, somnolence, and confusion. **Rationale:** These criteria indicate adequate ventilation. If any of the criteria are not met, assess patient–ventilator system and intervene appropriately.

2. Observe for signs and symptoms of adequate oxygenation, including PaO_2/SaO_2 within desired range (definitive criterion), chest–abdominal synchrony, regular respirations, adequate urine output, stable hemodynamic status, and absence of the following: dyspnea, central cyanosis, and accessory muscle use. **Rationale:** These criteria indicate adequate oxygenation. If any of the criteria are not met, assess the patient–ventilator system and intervene appropriately.

3. Observe for signs and symptoms of adequate breathing pattern, including adequate depth, timing, and rhythm of respirations, chest–abdominal synchrony, symmetrical anterior chest expansion, comfortable appearance, patient indicates satisfactory breathing, and absence of the following: nasal flaring, retractions, and accessory muscle use. **Rationale:** These criteria indicate absence of respiratory distress. If any of the criteria are not met, assess the patient–ventilator system and intervene appropriately.

4. Evaluate progress toward discontinuance of positive-pressure ventilation and on a daily basis. Indicators of progress toward this goal include decreasing levels of PEEP, CPAP, and FiO_2 with corresponding stability or improvement in arterial blood gases, improvement of underlying pathology for which PPV was initiated and maintained, stability or improvement in hemodynamic parameters, and patient's ability to assume a greater proportion of the minute volume. Caution must be exercised when evaluating the last indicator. Rapid, shallow breathing does not indicate patient capacity for spontaneous breathing. Low tidal volumes and frequencies greater than 30 breaths per minute correlate with the reinstitution of PPV (Tobin et al., 1986). Therefore, effective spontaneous breathing contribution to minute volume is interpreted as a tidal volume greater than 300 ml and a frequency of less than 20 breaths per minute. **Rationale:** Achieving the overriding goal of timely and successful discontinuance of PPV requires daily assess-

ment of progress. If progress is not evident, reassessment and revision of interventions are warranted.

5. Evaluate progress toward achievement of the individual goals of PPV formulated for the patient daily in collaboration with the physician, respiratory therapist, patient, and family as appropriate. **Rationale:** Achievement of the individual goals requires daily assessment of progress. If progress is not evident, reassessment and revision of interventions are warranted. Although generic standards of care for the patient receiving PPV guide the plan of care, goals are individualized to each patient.

6. Observe for signs and symptoms of the iatrogenic complications of inadequate ventilation, inadequate oxygenation, inadequate breathing pattern, noncompression atelectasis (Goodnough et al., 1986), barotrauma, cardiovascular depression, inadvertent extubation, malpositioned endotracheal tube, nosocomial lung infection, nutritional deficiencies, and tracheal injury. Specific signs and symptoms are discussed under Assessment. **Rationale:** It is desirable to prevent the development of iatrogenic complications. In the event that an iatrogenic complication is not (or cannot be) prevented, early detection and intervention are necessary.

Expected Outcomes

1. Maintenance of adequate $PaCO_2$. **Rationale:** Adequate ventilation is one purpose of initiating PPV. Except in rare circumstances, such as the patient with terminal respiratory distress syndrome, this outcome is achievable with vigilant assessment and intervention.

2. Maintenance of adequate PaO_2. **Rationale:** Adequate oxygenation is one purpose of initiating PPV. With the exception of the patient with severe hypoxemia, in whom a less than adequate PaO_2 may be tolerated in lieu of severe barotrauma or cardiovascular depression, this outcome is achievable with vigilant assessment and intervention.

3. Maintenance of adequate breathing pattern. **Rationale:** Adequate breathing pattern is one purpose of initiating PPV. This outcome is achievable with vigilant assessment and intervention when expected outcomes 1 and 2 are achieved.

4. Timely and planned discontinuation of PPV. **Rationale:** Premature discontinuation will result in the need for reestablishment of PPV (and perhaps reintubation) with consequent deterioration in physical and psychological state of the patient. Maintaining PPV beyond need puts the patient at risk for preventable, iatrogenic complications (e.g., tracheal injury, barotrauma, infection, etc.).

Unexpected Outcomes

1. Hemodynamic instability. **Rationale:** High mean airway pressure (caused by poor lung compliance, high airway resistance, large tidal volumes, PEEP, I:E ratio approaching or greater than 1, and patient–ventilator dyssynchrony) can depress cardiac output. Acute respiratory alkalosis can depress cardiac output by shifting the oxyhemoglobin dissociation curve. *Auto-PEEP phenom-*

enon (intrinsic PEEP) can depress hemodynamic function (Pepe and Marini, 1982), particularly in patients with chronic obstructive pulmonary disease (COPD). With CMV, A-C, and IMV modes, the ventilator may initiate the inspiratory cycle before the patient has completed the expiratory cycle. Alveolar pressure remains elevated, thus creating a PEEP effect (see Skill 4–7).

2. Pulmonary barotrauma. **Rationale:** High intrapleural pressures from high inflation pressures (caused by poor lung compliance, high airway resistance, large tidal volume, PEEP, patient–ventilator dyssynchrony, and malpositioned endotracheal tube) can cause pneumothorax, pneumomediastinum, pneumopericardium, pneumoperitoneum, and/or subcutaneous emphysema. A pneumothorax during PPV constitutes a potential emergency because it may become a tension pneumothorax with subsequent tracheal deviation, displaced mediastinum, and cardiopulmonary collapse. Following alveolar rupture, air may escape into the interstitium, producing subcutaneous emphysema.

3. Noncompression atelectasis. **Rationale:** Noncompression atelectasis, caused by mucous plug or other peripheral airway obstruction and by hypoventilation, is amenable to nursing interventions (Goodnough et al., 1986). Compression atelectasis, caused by tumor, pleural effusion, or other pathology, is not amenable to independent nursing interventions.

4. Inadvertent extubation. **Rationale:** Inadvertent extubation is defined as unplanned extubation (Goodnough et al., 1986, 1988) and may result in impaired gas exchange and cardiopulmonary arrest.

5. Malpositioned endotracheal tube. **Rationale:** Malpositioned endotracheal tube is defined as the tip of the tube being less than 2 cm or more than 8 cm (3.15 in) above the carina (Goodnough et al., 1986, 1988). This complication may result in inadvertent extubation, atelectasis, barotrauma, and impaired gas exchange.

6. Nosocomial lung infection. **Rationale:** The prevalence of nosocomial pneumonia in patients on PPV ranges from 2 percent (Rutherford et al., 1990) to 59 percent (Goodnough et al., 1986; Pagliarello and Carter, 1990; Roberts et al., 1988; Sherry et al., 1990; Tobin and Grenvik, 1984).

7. Acid–base disturbance. **Rationale:** Inappropriate ventilator settings may result in respiratory alkalosis or respiratory acidosis. Patients with chronic carbon dioxide retention ventilated with inappropriately large tidal volumes will develop an acute respiratory alkalosis with a concomitant shift to the left in the oxyhemoglobin dissociation curve and decreased cerebral blood flow.

8. Fluid retention. **Rationale:** Fluid retention occurs in 20 percent of patients requiring PPV, without evidence of heart failure (Montenegro, 1987). Theoretical mechanisms of fluid retention include release of antidiuretic hormone and changes in renal perfusion.

9. Gastrointestinal (GI) bleeding. **Rationale:** GI bleeding occurs in up to 20 percent of patients with PPV (Montenegro, 1987). Theoretical mechanisms of GI bleeding include gastric mucosal ischemia due to impaired gas exchange, underlying disease processes, and the hemodynamic alterations seen upon initiation of PPV

and abnormal quantity and quality of gastric secretions associated with hypoxemia and hypercapnia.

10. Jaundice. **Rationale:** Elevation of serum bilirubin levels has been reported in up to a third of patients in surgical critical care units who are receiving PPV. While this may be related to episodes of hypotension or sepsis, it is hypothesized that the hemodynamic changes seen with initiation of PPV affect portal circulation, inducing liver dysfunction (Montenegro, 1987).

11. Nutritional deficiencies. **Rationale:** The association between nutrition and pulmonary function is well established (Grant, 1988). Inadequate nutrition decreases diaphragmatic muscle mass, decreases overall pulmonary function performance, and increases mechanical ventilation requirements. Excessive carbohydrate loads can increase carbon dioxide production to the point of causing hypercapnia in patients on PPV, particularly in patients with chronic lung disease and those who are subjected to vigorous refeeding after a period of malnutrition (Grant, 1988).

12. Tracheal injury. **Rationale:** Dynamic interplay of physiologic, clinical, and mechanical factors causes tracheal injury (Goodnough, 1988), and these factors are exacerbated with PPV.

13. Constraint of patient's nonverbal communication. **Rationale:** Obstacles to communication cause frustration, anxiety, panic, and fear (Bergbom-Engberg and Haljamae, 1989). Unsuccessful and vigorous attempts at communication affect pulmonary function and patient–ventilator synchrony.

Documentation

Documentation in the patient record should include date and time ventilatory assistance was instituted, ventilator settings and patient mechanics, including: FIO_2, delivered/exhaled V_T, mode of ventilation, frequency of breaths per minute, (mandatory/spontaneous or mandatory/total), PEEP, I:E ratio or inspiratory time, PIP, CMP_{dyn} and CMP_{st}, date and time for changes in ventilator parameters and patient position (e.g., left side) when arterial blood gas (ABG) sampling and SaO_2 reading are performed and the need for initiating PPV, patient responses to initiation of PPV, including the patient's indication of level of comfort and respiratory complaints, hemodynamic and vital signs responses, and respiratory assessment findings, date and times of cuff pressure measurements, daily weight changes greater than 0.5 kg, respiratory swings greater than 10 mmHg (see Fig. 4–10) on arterial or venous waveforms, decreased cardiac output, and/or widened a-$\bar{v}DO_2$. **Rationale:** Provides data to evaluate therapeutic efficacy of PPV and provides historical data for decision-making regarding discontinuance of PPV.

Patient/Family Education

1. Explain to the patient and family why PPV is being initiated and what the goals are for the patient during PPV. Discuss how the patient and family can help promote the patient's recovery (and/or comfortable breathing) during PPV, such as encouraging the patient to relax and allow the ventilator to inflate the lungs and using alternative communication methods to mouthing and trying to talk. **Rationale:** Information about the patient's condition and therapy, including the rationale for therapy, are consistently cited as an important need of patients (Foundation for Critical Care, 1988; Parker et al., 1984; Viner, 1988) and family members (Dunbar et al., 1990; Hickey, 1990).

2. Discuss the sensory experiences associated with PPV, such as relief of dyspnea, big lung inflations, sounds of ventilator operation, and alarm sounds. Explain that the high-pressure alarm may be activated with coughing, repositioning, and physical effort. **Rationale:** Knowledge of anticipated sensory experiences decreases anxiety and distress (CURN Project, 1981; Johnson, 1972; Johnson and Rice, 1974; Johnson et al., 1975, 1978; Viner, 1988).

3. Teach the family how to perform desired and appropriate activities of direct patient care, such as pharyngeal suction with the tonsil sucker, range-of-motion exercises, and hygiene tasks. **Rationale:** Family members have identified the need to help in the patient's care (Daley, 1984; Dunbar et al., 1990; Harvey et al., 1991; O'Neill-Norris and Grove, 1986).

4. Instruct and encourage the patient to communicate anxiety, fear, panic, and concerns about security with the established communication method. **Rationale:** Inability to communicate has been implicated as the dominant reason for severe emotional reactions in patients who experience PPV. The isolation due to communication difficulties was seen as a greater problem than direct airway and ventilator-related activities (Bergbom-Engberg and Haljamae, 1989).

5. Evaluate the patient's need for long-term mechanical ventilation. **Rationale:** Allows nurse to anticipate patient and family needs for the patient's discharge home on PPV.

6. Show the patient (if appropriate) and family how to reconnect the ventilator to the artificial airway, and perform demonstration and return demonstration of the use of the call bell. **Rationale:** Minimizes disconnect time and subsequent physiologic instability and ensures that the patient and family can summon the nurse when needed. Further, family members have identified the need to help in the patient's care (Daley, 1984; Harvey et al., 1991; O'Neill-Norris and Grove, 1986).

7. Instruct the patient to communicate discomfort with breathing to the nurse via the call bell, or establish a communication method. **Rationale:** The patient should feel secure that the nurse will respond promptly to complaints of respiratory distress.

8. Provide the patient and family with information on the critical nature of the patient's dependence on PPV. **Rationale:** Knowing the prognosis, probable outcome, or chance for recovery is cited as an important need of patients and families (Dunbar et al., 1990; Hickey, 1990; Viner, 1988).

9. Offer the opportunity for both patient and family to ask questions about PPV. **Rationale:** Asking questions

and having questions answered honestly are cited consistently as the most important need of patients (Dunbar et al., 1990) and families (Hickey, 1990).

10. Evaluate patient's need for long-term mechanical ventilatory assistance. **Rationale:** Allows nurse to anticipate patient and family needs for the patient's discharge home with a mechanical ventilator.

Performance Checklist
Skill 4–1: Initiation and Management of Positive-Pressure Ventilation (PPV)

Critical Behaviors	Complies yes	no
INITIATION		
1. Set selected V_T.		
2. Set selected respiratory rate.		
3. Set FiO_2.		
4. Set selected PIF (or inspiratory time, I:E ratio, as appropriate).		
5. Set selected mode of ventilation.		
6. Set selected sigh volume and rate.		
7. Fill humidifier and adjust humidifier thermostat setting.		
8. Plug in power cord into grounded 110-volt ac outlet.		
9. Attach high-pressure hose(s) to 50-lb/in² source(s).		
10. Attach oxygen analyzer and test lung to patient ventilator circuit and ventilate test lung for 2 minutes.		
11. Measure FiO_2 and replace oxygen analyzer with portable respirometer.		
12. Measure exhaled V_T from test lung with portable respirometer.		
13. Set high-pressure limit to 20 cmH₂O higher than PIP with test lung.		
14. Replace respirometer and test lung with swivel adapter, and connect swivel adapter to artificial airway.		
15. Observe patient's breathing pattern.		
16. Count mandatory respiration rate, total respiration rate, and I:E ratio.		
17. Check PIP, and adjust high-pressure limit to 20 cmH₂O higher than PIP.		
18. Measure exhaled V_T with respirometer and compare with set V_T, and adjust set V_T if necessary.		
19. Measure dynamic compliance.		
20. Measure static compliance.		
21. Activate all ventilator alarms.		
22. Place call bell within patient reach.		
23. Document procedure and patient response in patient record.		
MANAGEMENT		
1. Check that ventilator and cardiac monitor alarm systems are functional and appropriately set.		
2. Check for secure stabilization of the artificial airway. Resecure if not stable.		
3. Assure availability of replacement artificial airway.		
4. Check that appropriately sized face mask is at the bedside.		
5. Check that tracheal tube size and date of insertion are recorded in patient record.		

Table continues on following page

Critical Behaviors	Complies	
	yes	no
6. Auscultate and observe expansion of anterior chest at least hourly and after patient or airway manipulated.		
7. Verify tracheal tube tip position.		
8. Inflate cuff using MOV or MLC technique as appropriate.		
9. Assess for cuff leak.		
10. Evaluate the need for a nasogastric tube.		
11. Maintain semiprone position or elevate the head of the bed as appropriate.		
12. Suction oropharynx or nasopharynx as indicated.		
13. Hyperinflate the patient with sustained inspiratory pause *just before* deflating artificial airway cuff.		
14. Monitor artificial airway cuff pressure.		
15. Cut excess length of endotracheal tube if necessary.		
16. Use swivel adapter between artificial airway and ventilator.		
17. Stabilize endotracheal tube securely with tincture of benzoin (or comparable preparation) on face.		
18. Rotate endotracheal tube from one corner of the mouth to the other at least every 24 hours.		
19. Suction with low-trauma suction catheters as needed to maintain patent airway.		
20. Continuously monitor in-line thermometer.		
21. Drain condensate from ventilator tubing from clean to dirty.		
22. Keep manual self-inflating resuscitation bag with supplemental oxygen continuously on at 15 L/min to "flush" at the head of the patient's bed.		
23. Check ventilator for baseline settings (FiO$_2$, tidal volume, frequency, PIP, and alarm activation) after removal of the ventilator from the patient.		
24. Explore changes in peak inspiratory pressure.		
25. Assess anterior chest expansion, anterior breath sounds, patient–ventilator synchrony, vital signs, ventilator sounds, all ventilator connections and alarm settings, and all ventilator settings.		
26. Place bite block (or oral airway) between the teeth if the patient is biting on the oral endotracheal tube.		
27. Change the patient's body position as appropriate.		
28. Alter pattern and depth of ventilation.		
29. Sit the patient in a chair, ambulate, or have the patient walk in place at least three times daily, unless contraindicated.		
30. Explore the cause of high-pressure alarm activation.		
31. Explore patient–ventilator dyssynchrony.		
32. Determine and maintain high-pressure limit setting.		
33. Explore sudden increase in PIP.		
34. Assess for tension pneumothorax and respond appropriately.		
35. Weigh the patient daily, unless contraindicated.		
36. Observe arterial pressure waveform with manual hyperinflation.		
37. Observe and document hemodynamic changes associated with increased tidal volume or PEEP.		
38. Discuss the patient's nutritional status with the physician daily.		

Table continues on following page

Critical Behaviors	Complies	
	yes	**no**
39. Obtain coverage for absences from the bedside.		
40. Place the call bell within reach of the patient who is able to use it.		
41. Discuss the goals of PPV with the physician, respiratory therapist, patient, and family daily.		
42. Monitor gastric pH continuously.		
43. Wash hands.		
44. Document procedure in patient record.		

SKILL 4–2

Ventilation with Manual Self-Inflating Resuscitation Bag

There are multiple diagnostic and therapeutic uses of the manual self-inflating resuscitation bag. Skill with bagging techniques is essential for the nurse working with patients on mechanical ventilators. A manual self-inflating resuscitation bag (bag) and anesthesia face mask must be at the bedside of every patient who is receiving mechanical ventilatory assistance, has an artificial airway, or is at high risk for or exhibiting signs and symptoms of cardiopulmonary deterioration. The Society of Critical Care Medicine (SCCM) recently formalized this guideline as a minimum standard in the care of the critically ill patient on PPV (SCCM, 1991). The bag is attached to oxygen with the capability of delivering 100% oxygen. Adjunctive equipment needs (e.g., PEEP valve, reservoir tubing) are determined by the patient's physiologic condition.

The bag is used for diagnostic, therapeutic, and emergency purposes in the patient receiving mechanical ventilatory assistance (Table 4–3). The patient is ventilated with the manual self-inflating resuscitation bag—hereafter referred to as *bagging*—as part of the respiratory assessment to collect diagnostic data about lung compliance, breath sounds, position of the endotracheal tube, inflation of the artificial airway cuff, and lung pathology.

Bagging the patient provides the nurse with qualitative information about lung compliance. An increase in difficulty deflating the bag may indicate a decrease in lung compliance; conversely, a decrease in difficulty deflating the bag may indicate an increase in lung compliance. Assessing lung compliance with bagging is subjective; bag volumes and flows vary breath to breath and nurse to nurse. Although bagging is far less accurate than calculating compliance (see Skill 4–4), it provides quick, easy, and useful qualitative information about lung compliance.

Eliciting the help of another clinician to bag the patient permits the nurse to auscultate breath sounds and assess the position of the endotracheal tube and the presence of a leak in the cuff of the artificial airway without the interference of adventitious sounds produced by the ventilator. The flow characteristics of inspired gas are more easily altered with the resuscitation bag than with the ventilator, allowing detection of subtle changes in adventitious breath sounds.

Elevation of peak inspiratory pressure (PIP) in the absence of audible secretions may indicate the need for endotracheal suctioning (see Skill 1–6). Bagging the patient for several breaths aids in diagnosing the presence

TABLE 4–3   USES OF MANUAL SELF-INFLATING RESUSCITATION BAG

Diagnostic	Therapeutic	Emergency
Assess lung compliance	Provide hyperinflation	Provide ventilation for CPR, inadvertent extubation, ventilator malfunction, and severe respiratory distress
Determine need for suctioning	Provide supplemental oxygenation	
Assess breath sounds	Promote patient–ventilator synchrony	
Assess position of endotracheal tube	Alter ventilatory pattern	
Assess artificial airway cuff inflation	Provide ventilation during transport, ambulation, ventilator maintenance, and other needs for ventilator disconnection	
Assess cause of patient–ventilator dyssynchrony		
Assess cause of patient–ventilator problems		
Assess lung pathology		

of secretions in the large airways. Most important, bagging the patient is indicated for assessing the cause of patient–ventilator dyssynchrony or patient–ventilator problems. Prior to checking the ventilator, the patient is bagged manually to rule out problems distal to the artificial airway.

Therapeutically, the bag often is used in lieu of the ventilator to provide hyperinflation and/or supplemental oxygenation before and after endotracheal suctioning (Bostick and Wendelgass, 1987; Chulay, 1988; Goodnough, 1985; Preusser et al., 1988; Rogge et al., 1989; Schumann and Parsons, 1985), intubation or repositioning of the endotracheal tube, and bronchoscopy. Manual hyperinflation and oxygenation have the advantages of being quick and easy, permitting the delivery of variable rates and volumes, and avoiding resetting of the ventilator. The disadvantages include the need for an assistant to bag and the inability of many bags to deliver more than a liter of volume unless completely compressed. Caution should be exercised with large hyperinflation volumes, particularly in patients with hemodynamic instability. Clinically significant drops in blood pressure and heart rate with hyperinflation at 150 percent of the patient's baseline tidal volume have been reported (Goodnough, 1985). The arterial pressure waveform and

cardiac monitor should be observed during hyperinflation, and hyperinflation should be discontinued immediately when a significant decrease is observed.

The bag oxygen delivery system should be analyzed for FIO_2 with various hyperinflation volumes. The design of the bag, the flow rate of oxygen, and the volume delivered interact to produce varying oxygen concentrations (Preusser, 1985). Reservoir tubing or a reservoir bag (Fig. 4–8) may need to be added to the bag oxygen delivery system to reduce room air entrainment, thus permitting oxygen concentrations approaching 100%.

The patient who is breathing dyssynchronously with the ventilator—sometimes referred to as "out of phase" (Martz et al., 1984)—may be trying to communicate dyspnea for any number of reasons. Prior to making adjustments in ventilator settings or obtaining diagnostic tests, bagging the patient should be attempted. The manual ventilation and oxygenation may reduce carbon dioxide, dislodge a mucous plug, reduce anxiety, or otherwise alleviate the dyspnea. At first, the nurse manually ventilates at the patient's rate but with deeper breaths. Gradually, both the volume and rate should approximate that of the ventilator. When the patient is breathing comfortably with the bag, the ventilator can be reconnected.

Research indicates that monotonous tidal volumes of

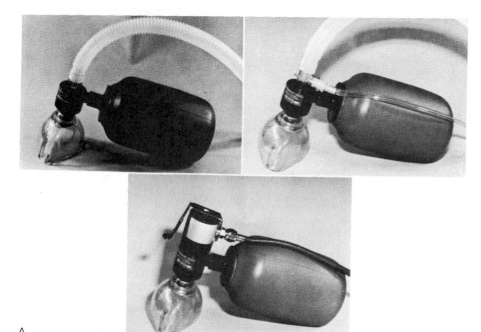

A

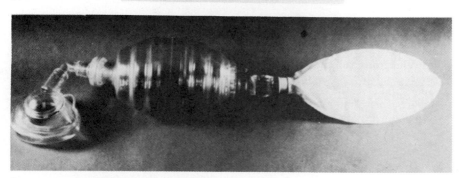

B

FIGURE 4–8. Manual self-inflating resuscitation bags with (A) reservoir tubing and (B) reservoir bag to increase the concentration of oxygen delivered to the patient. (Modified with permission from S. P. McPherson, *Respiratory Therapy Equipment*, 4th Ed. St. Louis: Mosby, 1990, pp. 127, 134.)

fixed amounts delivered with mechanical ventilators produce atelectasis (Zimmerman, 1989). The implied mechanism is that elimination of the normal sigh maneuvers (e.g., yawn, cough) and the absence of normal variability in tidal volume from speech and body movement alter surfactant production or function. The use of IMV/SIMV mediates this concern if the patient is breathing spontaneously between mandatory breaths. However, if the patient is receiving total mechanical ventilatory support, bagging is indicated frequently (every 5 to 10 minutes is ideal, but at least once an hour) to alter the pattern of ventilation. Three to four consecutive breaths with the bag are sufficient for this purpose. Alternatively, the sigh mechanism on the ventilator can be used in patients who have tidal volumes less than 10 ml/kg.

Therapeutically, bagging is also used to provide ventilation whenever the ventilator is disconnected, such as for patient transport, ambulation, power failure, and ventilator maintenance or troubleshooting. In these situations, the bagging technique simulates the ventilator breaths as closely as possible in volume, rate, FIO_2, and I:E ratio.

The patient on a mechanical ventilator is at risk for such respiratory emergencies as inadvertent extubation and ventilator malfunction. Most patients on ventilators are critically ill and therefore are at risk for nonrespiratory emergencies as well. The bagging technique used depends on the nature of the emergency. For instance, during cardiopulmonary resuscitation, 100% oxygen is delivered with large tidal volume and the rate of one breath every 5 seconds, coordinated with chest compressions. If ventilator malfunction is detected prior to the patient developing respiratory distress, manual breaths that simulate ventilator breaths are delivered. If respiratory distress is present, rapid, deep breaths are indicated until the distress is relieved. In the event of inadvertent extubation, the face mask is attached to the bag, and the bagging technique is dictated by the absence or presence of respiratory distress.

Purpose

The nurse uses the manual self-inflating resuscitation bag to

1. Provide ventilation.
2. Assess respiratory status.
3. Assess placement and function of the artificial airway.
4. Determine the need for therapeutic intervention.
5. Diagnose patient–ventilator problems.
6. Provide hyperinflation and supplemental oxygenation before and after interventions.
7. Alter ventilatory pattern.

Prerequisite Knowledge and Skills

Prior to using the manual self-inflating resuscitation bag, the nurse should understand

1. Anatomy and physiology of the upper and lower respiratory and cardiac systems.
2. Principles of airway resistance.
3. Principles of lung compliance.
4. Principles of positive-pressure ventilation.
5. Principles of gas flow.

The nurse should be able to perform

1. Ventilation via mouth-to-mouth, mouth-to-nose, or face mask-to-mouth and nose techniques.
2. Respiratory physical assessment (inspection, palpation, percussion, and auscultation).
3. Hemodynamic vital signs assessment.
4. Confirmation of endotracheal tube placement.
5. Securing of endotracheal tracheostomy tube (see Skills 1–5, 1–9).
6. Measurement of cuff pressure (see Skill 1–7).
7. Endotracheal suctioning (see Skill 1–6).
8. Detection of tension pneumothorax.

Assessment

1. Assess lung compliance by bagging the patient with breaths that are as consistent in volume and rate as possible. Compliance represents the forces resisting expansion of the lung and is expressed as the relationship between pressure and volume (see Skill 4–4). The resistance to bag deflation will be altered with different volumes and rates. Focus on the degree of ease (or difficulty) with which the bag is deflated during inspiration. If both hands and a lot of pressure are required to deflate the bag, the dynamic compliance is decreased. Look for causes of high airway resistance (e.g., obstructed airway, bronchospasm) and/or low lung compliance (e.g., pulmonary edema, pneumonia, pleural effusion). Monitor the trend in dynamic compliance by assessing the degree of difficulty in bagging daily and after therapeutic interventions. **Rationale:** Gross improvement or deterioration in lung function can be followed with this diagnostic technique.
2. Assess placement and function of the artificial airway (see Skills 1–1, 1–2, 1–5, and 1–9). **Rationale:** Ensures the positioning and patency of the airway.
3. Assess the need for therapeutic intervention by observing for signs and symptoms of upper and lower airway obstruction, including audible rhonchi, wheezes, or gurgling, restlessness, dyspnea, altered level of consciousness, patient–ventilator dyssynchrony, decreased or unequal breath sounds, adventitious breath sounds, inspiratory or expiratory wheezes, tachycardia or bradycardia, dysrhythmias, cyanosis, hypertension, or hypotension. **Rationale:** Bagging can aid in the diagnosis of airway obstruction and may alleviate the cause. If signs and symptoms persist despite bagging, other therapeutic interventions (suctioning, endotracheal tube repositioning, bronchodilators, bronchoscopy, etc.) need to be considered.
4. Assess for patient–ventilator problems (see Skill 4–1). **Rationale:** Allows for quick response.
5. Monitor the peak inspiratory pressure (PIP) on

the ventilator. An acute increase in PIP indicates accumulation of secretions, presence of mucous plug, obstruction of the endotracheal tube, malpositioned endotracheal tube, bronchospasm, or pneumothorax. A gradual increase in PIP when tidal volume and PEEP are constant indicates the advent or progression of lung pathology (atelectasis, pneumonia, pleural effusion, pulmonary edema, ARDS, etc.). **Rationale:** Bagging the patient will help diagnose the cause of a sudden or gradual increase in PIP.

Nursing Diagnoses

1. Impaired gas exchange related to hypercapnia and/or hypoxemia. **Rationale:** Multiple pathophysiologic and mechanical factors can result in impaired gas exchange.
2. Ineffective breathing pattern related to pathophysiologic and mechanical factors. **Rationale:** Ventilating the patient with the manual self-inflating resuscitation bag may provide diagnostic data as well as immediate improvement in breathing pattern.
3. Ineffective airway clearance related to secretions or aspiration. **Rationale:** Use of the manual self-inflating resuscitation bag determines or confirms the need for secretion mobilization and removal. Bagging is an excellent technique for mobilizing secretions.
4. Potential for anxiety and fear related to dyspnea. **Rationale:** Dyspnea causes anxiety and fear (Bergbom-Engberg and Haljamae, 1989; DeVito, 1990; Lush et al., 1988).
5. Potential for sensory/perceptual alterations in vision and reality interpretation related to hypercapnia and/or hypoxemia. **Rationale:** Confusion, delusions, and hallucinations can result from carbon dioxide retention and/or hypoxemia. Bagging may improve gas exchange.

Planning

1. Individualize the following goals for bagging based on the critical nature of the situation and patient need.
   a. Relieve respiratory distress within 2 minutes of onset. **Rationale:** Dyspnea is uncomfortable and frightening. It leads to anxiety, fear, and distrust of the nurse (Bergbom-Engberg and Haljamae, 1989; DeVito, 1990). Failure to promptly diagnose and alleviate the cause of respiratory distress puts the patient at risk for impaired gas exchange.
   b. Prevent or resolve noncompression atelectasis. **Rationale:** Atelectasis can cause hypoxemia. Atelectasis due to low alveolar volume or secretion stasis can be prevented or resolved with frequent alterations in tidal volume, periodic hyperinflations, and secretion mobilization.
   c. Maintain effective ventilation during periods of ventilator disconnection. **Rationale:** Maintain ventilation and oxygenation in order to prevent hypercapnia, hypoxemia, and dyspnea.
2. Prepare all necessary equipment and supplies. **Rationale:** Assists in a manual self-inflating resuscitation bag being used quickly and efficiently.
   a. Manual self-inflating resuscitation bag, with universal adapter, capable of delivering adequate volume, oxygen concentration, and PEEP. Desirable characteristics of the bag include the following: It refills quickly to permit rapid rates with large volumes, it is usable by persons with small hands, it is equipped with fittings to accept small-bore and wide-bore tubing, it is adaptable for delivery of 100 percent oxygen, and it can be sterilized (or is disposable). Since the patient's condition may change at any time, the bag should be capable of delivering at least a 1000-ml tidal volume, oxygen concentration of 100%, and PEEP of 20 cmH$_2$O.
   b. Appropriately sized face mask.
   c. Oxygen flowmeter. The bag should be attached to an oxygen flowmeter that is turned on at all times.
   d. Small-bore oxygen tubing.
   e. Wide-bore reservoir tubing, as appropriate. The longer the reservoir tubing, the higher is the delivered oxygen concentration.
   f. PEEP valve (see Fig. 4–5), as appropriate.
   g. Portable respirometer.
3. Prepare the patient and family generally for the indications and frequent use of the bag. **Rationale:** Information about the patient's therapy is cited consistently as an important need of patients (Foundation for Critical Care, 1988; Parker et al., 1984; Viner, 1988) and family members (Dunbar et al., 1990; Foundation for Critical Care, 1988; Hickey, 1990).

Implementation

Steps	Rationale	Special Considerations
Respiratory Distress		
1. Check that bag is attached to oxygen source which is turned on.	Safety precaution. Allows oxygen to flow to the bag.	
2. Disconnect patient from ventilator and connect (bag) to artificial airway.	Allows for manual ventilation.	

Table continues on following page

Steps	Rationale	Special Considerations
3. Observe patient's breathing pattern and rate. Bag patient at the same rate but with deeper breaths.	Helps patient gain control over breathing by ensuring hyperventilation and adequate oxygenation.	
4. Encourage patient to let you give him or her deep breaths.	Promotes synchrony between patient breathing and manual breaths.	
5. Gradually slow the rate of manual breaths to approximate the frequency (f) that is set on the ventilator.	Reestablishes synchrony with ventilator.	If respiratory distress can be relieved with same f and volume as that delivered by the ventilator, patient can be reconnected to the ventilator.
6. Ascertain whether patient is comfortable with the breaths.	Promotes comfort.	
a. If patient indicates yes, gradually decrease depth of breaths to approximate V_T set on ventilator (for modes of CMV, A-C, IMV/SIMV) or 400 to 500 ml.	Indicates that respiratory distress is relieved and patient can be reconnected to ventilator.	
b. If patient indicates no, continue bagging at faster rate with deeper breaths and call for assistance.	Indicates that respiratory distress cannot be relieved with bagging. Further assessment is required.	
7. Return patient to ventilator when respiratory distress is relieved. Reactivate and check ventilator alarm(s) and settings and observe breathing pattern, patient–ventilator synchrony, and PIP. Check that call bell is within patient reach, if appropriate.	Safety precaution. Ensures nurse is alerted to actual or potential life-threatening problems.	

Respiratory Status Assessment

Steps	Rationale	Special Considerations
1. Check that bag is attached to oxygen source which is turned on.	Safety precaution. Provides direct route for oxygen to flow into the bag.	
2. Disconnect patient from ventilator. Deactivate/silence ventilator alarm(s).	Because the nurse is at the bedside and there is no problem with the ventilator or patient, there is no reason for the alarm(s) to summon help or to disturb other patients.	
3. Insert portable respirometer between bag and artificial airway.	Helps the nurse deliver a relatively constant volume.	
4. Connect bag to patient.	Allows bagging to be initiated.	
5. Compress bag to predetermined volume (e.g., tidal volume). Repeat until approximate volume is reproducible.	Provides ventilation.	Tidal volume or hyperinflation volume can be used. A consistent volume and frequency are required to make comparisons in the ease of bag deflation from one assessment to the next.
6. Assess the ease (or difficulty) with which the bag can be deflated. Observe whether one or two hands are needed to provide the predetermined volume and the degree to which the bag must be deflated to achieve this volume.	The change in these qualitative distinctions provides gross trend data about increasing (improved) or decreasing (deteriorating) lung compliance.	

Table continues on following page

Steps	Rationale	Special Considerations
7. Reconnect patient to ventilator. Reactivate all ventilator alarms. Ensure that call bell is within reach of the patient.	Safety precautions. Ensure that nurse is alerted to actual or potential life-threatening events.	

Hyperinflation/Alternative Ventilatory Pattern

1. Check that bag is attached to oxygen source which is turned on.	Safety precaution. Provides direct route for oxygen to flow into the bag.	
2. Disconnect patient from ventilator. Deactivate/silence ventilator alarm(s).	Because the nurse is at the bedside and there is no problem with the patient or ventilator, there is no reason for the alarm(s) to summon help or to disturb other patients.	
3. Insert portable respirometer between bag and artificial airway.	Helps the nurse deliver a relatively constant flow.	
4. a. Hyperinflation: Provide hyperinflation breaths at 150 percent of tidal volume. Adjust bag compressions as necessary to achieve desired hyperinflation volume. Repeat until approximate hyperinflation volume is reproducible.	By definition, hyperinflation volume must exceed tidal volume, and 150 percent of tidal volume is used in experimental hyperinflation (Chulay, 1988; Goodnough, 1985).	If 150 percent of tidal volume produces excessively high PIP, hyperinflation volume should be scaled down to less than 150 percent of tidal volume to decrease risk of barotrauma.
b. Alternative ventilatory pattern: Bag patient with three to four breaths at variable tidal or hyperinflation volumes.	Mimics the physiologic sigh mechanisms of the healthy person.	
5. Monitor cardiac rhythm and rate and arterial pressure waveform during hyperinflation. Immediately discontinue hyperinflation for clinically significant change in hemodynamic parameters.	Hyperinflation volumes at 150 percent of tidal volume have been found to produce a clinically significant decrease in blood pressure and heart rate in some patients (Goodnough, 1985).	
6. Reconnect patient to ventilator. Reactivate ventilator alarm(s). Ensure that call bell is within patient reach.	Ventilator alarms ensure that the nurse will be alerted to actual or potential life-threatening problems.	

Maintenance Ventilation

1. Check that bag is attached to oxygen source which is turned on.	Safety precaution. Provides direct route for oxygen to flow into the bag.	
2. Disconnect patient from ventilator. Deactivate/silence ventilator alarm(s).	Because the nurse is at the bedside and there is no problem with the patient or ventilator, there is no reason for the alarm(s) to summon help or disturb other patients.	
3. Insert portable respirometer between bag and artificial airway.	Ensures same tidal volume delivery as ventilator provides.	
4. Bag patient at approximate rate, depth, and pattern as ventilator breaths.	Maintains the same ventilation as patient receives with ventilator.	

Table continues on following page

Steps	Rationale	Special Considerations
5. Analyze average V_T delivered manually. Adjust bag compressions as necessary to produce V_T that approximates ventilator V_T. Repeat until approximate V_T is reproducible.	Achieves reproducible manual breaths.	
6. Remove portable respirometer and insert portable oxygen analyzer between bag and artificial airway.	Allows for FIO_2 to be analyzed.	
7. Analyze FIO_2 delivered. Adjust liter flow of oxygen to produce same FIO_2 as ventilator breaths.	Prevents hypoxia and maintains prescribed FIO_2.	FIO_2 delivered with bag depends on oxygen liter flow and minute volume delivered (Preusser, 1985). Add/extend reservoir tubing if unable to achieve desired FIO_2.
8. Remove oxygen analyzer and manually ventilate patient at V_T, f, and FIO_2 that approximate ventilator settings.	Approximates baseline ventilation and oxygenation.	
9. Periodically ascertain that the patient is comfortable with the bagging technique. Adjustments may be needed to maintain patient comfort with manual ventilation.	Promotes patient comfort.	The patient who is being ambulated may require a larger minute ventilation than usual to match increased CO_2 production and oxygen consumption from activity.
10. Reconnect patient to ventilator. Reactivate ventilator alarm(s). Ensure that call bell is within patient reach.	Safety precaution. Ensures that the nurse will be alerted to actual or potential life-threatening problems.	

Evaluation

1. Evaluate trends or sudden changes in lung compliance. **Rationale:** Improvement or deterioration in lung function can be approximated by daily evaluation of patient's response to bagging.

2. Observe for signs and symptoms of patent upper and lower airways, including comfortable appearance, stable or improved level of consciousness, patient–ventilator synchrony, equal breath sounds, stable heart rate, rhythm, and blood pressure, and absence of rhonchi, wheezes, and dyspnea. **Rationale:** Successful intervention(s) will alleviate upper and lower airway obstruction.

3. Observe the patient during bagging. The patient should look comfortable. The chest should rise and fall evenly with bag deflations and inflations. **Rationale:** Proper technique will result in a comfortable, synchronous breathing pattern.

4. Monitor clinical assessment findings and chest x-rays for noncompression atelectasis. **Rationale:** Frequent alteration of ventilatory pattern helps prevent noncompression atelectasis.

5. Monitor SaO_2, if oximetry used, for maintenance of adequate oxygenation during bagging. **Rationale:** If adequate oxygen is being delivered with the bag, SaO_2 should be unchanged or increase with bagging techniques.

Expected Outcomes

1. Maintenance of adequate ventilation. **Rationale:** One purpose of bagging is specifically to provide ventilation. Regardless of bagging technique or purpose for bagging, adequate ventilation must be provided during this procedure.

2. Maintenance of adequate oxygenation. **Rationale:** The bag must provide adequate oxygen to meet the needs of the patient during basal metabolism and periods of high oxygen consumption.

3. Absence, or resolution, of noncompression atelectasis. **Rationale:** Frequent alteration of ventilatory pattern is hypothesized to help prevent atelectasis due to monotonous tidal volume. Proper diagnostic use of the bag will ensure that the patient undergoes adequate secretion mobilization and removal.

4. Acute respiratory distress will be alleviated within 2 minutes or less. **Rationale:** Most episodes of acute respiratory distress, including those due to inadvertent extubation, can be reversed with adequate ventilation and oxygenation provided by the bag within 2 minutes. If the distress cannot be relieved within 2 minutes, immediate

consultation is needed to assist with diagnosis and treatment.

Unexpected Outcomes

1. Hemodynamic instability. **Rationale:** Large hyperinflation volumes have been found to significantly decrease blood pressure and heart rate in some patients (Goodnough, 1985).

2. Pulmonary barotrauma. **Rationale:** Increased intrathoracic pressure from high inflation pressures can cause pneumothorax, pneumomediastinum, pneumopericardium, pneumoperitoneum, and/or subcutaneous emphysema.

3. Acid–base disturbance. **Rationale:** Delivery of excessive minute volumes with the bag will result in acute respiratory alkalosis. Conversely, delivery of too small a minute volume will result in acute respiratory acidosis.

4. Inadvertent extubation. **Rationale:** Excessive torque on the artificial airway during bagging can result in dislodgement.

5. Asphyxiation. **Rationale:** Improper assembly or malfunction of the bag can result in failure to ventilate.

6. Pulmonary infection. **Rationale:** Bedside resuscitation bags have been found to be a source of both gram-positive and gram-negative bacterial contamination (Hoyt, 1988; Thompson et al., 1985).

Documentation

Documentation in the patient record should include initial and periodic determinations of approximate FIO_2 delivered with the bag; purpose of and patient response to bagging; and dates on which the manual self-inflating resuscitation bag system was changed. **Rationale:** Provides diagnostic and trend data to evaluate patient improvement or deterioration.

Patient/Family Education

1. Explain to the patient and family why bagging is performed. Discuss how the patient and family can help to promote a comfortable and effective breathing pattern during bagging. **Rationale:** Information about the patient's therapy, including rationale, is cited consistently as an important need of patients (Foundation for Critical Care, 1988; Parker et al., 1984; Viner, 1988) and family members (Dunbar et al., 1990; Hickey, 1990).

2. Discuss the sensory experiences associated with bagging. **Rationale:** Knowledge of anticipated sensory experiences decreases anxiety and distress (CURN Project, 1981; Johnson, 1972; Johnson and Rice, 1974; Johnson et al., 1975; Johnson et al., 1978; Viner, 1988).

3. Instruct the patient to communicate discomfort with breathing during bagging to the nurse. **Rationale:** The bagging technique can be altered to produce a comfortable breathing pattern.

4. Offer the opportunity for both patient and family to ask questions about bagging. **Rationale:** Asking questions and having questions answered honestly are cited consistently as the most important needs of patients and families (Dunbar et al., 1990; Hickey, 1990).

5. Evaluate the patient's need for long-term use of an artificial airway. **Rationale:** Allows nurse to anticipate the family's need to learn how to use bagging techniques for the patient's long-term care.

Performance Checklist
Skill 4–2: Ventilation with Manual Self-Inflating Resuscitation Bag

Critical Behaviors	Complies yes	no
RESPIRATORY DISTRESS		
1. Turn on oxygen source and check that bag is attached.		
2. Disconnect patient from ventilator and connect (bag) to artificial airway.		
3. Observe patient's breathing and bag at the same rate with deeper breaths.		
4. Encourage patient to relax.		
5. Gradually slow manual breathing rate to approximate ventilator frequency.		
6. Monitor comfort of patient.		
7. Reconnect patient to ventilator once respiratory distress relieved.		
RESPIRATORY STATUS ASSESSMENT		
1. Turn on oxygen source and check that bag is attached.		
2. Disconnect patient from ventilator.		
3. Attain portable respirometer between bag and artificial airway.		
4. Connect bag to patient.		
5. Compress bag to predetermined volume; repeat until approximate volume is reproducible.		

Table continues on following page

Critical Behaviors	Complies	
	yes	no
6. Assess the ease or difficulty with which the bag is deflated.		
7. Reconnect patient to ventilator, reactivate ventilator alarms, and ensure call bell is within reach.		
HYPERINFLATION/ALTERNATIVE VENTILATORY PATTERN 1. Turn on oxygen source and check that bag is attached.		
2. Disconnect patient from ventilator, silence alarms.		
3. Attach portable respirometer between bag and artificial airway.		
4. a. Provide hyperinflation breaths at 150% of tidal volume. b. Provide alternative ventilatory pattern.		
5. Monitor cardiac rhythm, rate, and arterial pressure during hyperinflation. Discontinue hyperinflation with significant change in hemodynamic status.		
6. Reconnect patient to ventilator, reactivate ventilator alarms, and ensure call bell is within reach.		
MAINTENANCE VENTILATION 1. Turn on oxygen source and check that bag is atached.		
2. Disconnect patient from ventilator, silence alarms.		
3. Attach portable respirometer between bag and artificial airway.		
4. Bag patient to match rate and depth of ventilator breaths.		
5. Analyze V_T manually delivered and adjust bag compressions to match V_T on ventilator.		
6. Remove portable respirometer and insert portable oxygen analyzer between bag and artificial airway.		
7. Analyze FIO_2 delivered and adjust liter flow of oxygen to produce same FIO_2 as ventilator breaths.		
8. Remove oxygen analyzer and manually ventilate patient at V_T, f, and FIO_2 approximate to ventilator settings.		
9. Monitor comfort of patient.		
10. Reconnect patient to ventilator, reactivate ventilator alarms, and ensure call bell is within reach.		

SKILL 4–3

Alveolar-Arterial Oxygen Difference (A-aDO₂) Calculation

Calculation of A-aDO₂ is helpful in diagnosing the primary mechanism of hypoxemia (e.g., intrapulmonary shunting) and, subsequently, in determining the appropriate therapy. The oxygen that comes to the lungs in mixed venous blood for gas exchange equilibrates with the alveolar gas and leaves the lungs with an alveolar oxygen tension (P_AO_2) of approximately 100 mmHg. The bronchial veins bring desaturated blood to the left atrium, bypassing the pulmonary circulation. Thus a small amount of blood is shunted past the lungs and mixes with oxygenated blood in the left ventricle, resulting in an arterial oxygen tension (PaO_2) of 80 to 90 mmHg. This physiologic phenomenon is called the *alveolar-to-arterial oxygen difference* (A-aDO₂) or the *alveolar-to-arterial oxygen gradient* [$P(A-a)O_2$].

The normal A-aDO₂ is 10 to 35 mmHg (Nunn, 1989) and less than 50 mmHg for the patient being mechanically ventilated. If the difference is wider than 50 mmHg in the mechanically ventilated patient, hypoxemia is caused by right-to-left intrapulmonary shunting or low ventilation-to-perfusion mismatching ($\dot{V}/\dot{Q}$ mismatch). Calculation of A-aDO₂ with the patient breathing 100% oxygen further delimits the mechanism of hypoxemia. An increased A-aDO₂ due to shunt will not respond significantly to increased inspired oxygen, whereas an increased A-aDO₂ related to $\dot{V}/\dot{Q}$ mismatch will be decreased with an FIO_2 of 1.0. As a rule of thumb, every 100 mmHg of A-aDO₂ is equivalent to a 5 percent intrapulmonary shunt when breathing 100% oxygen (Williams-Colon and Thalken, 1990).

A-aDO₂ provides useful trend data about oxygenation as long as the calculations are based on the patient breathing 100% oxygen. The relationship between A-aDO₂ and FIO_2 is linear. The alveolar oxygen tension is influenced by alveolar carbon dioxide tension and venous oxygen content. Further, when $\dot{V}/\dot{Q}$ mismatch is severe, the alveolar oxygen tension may change very little until very high concentrations of oxygen are administered.

Monitoring the trends in A-aDO$_2$ can evaluate an increase or decrease in shunt and permit timely and safe decreases in hyperinflation and supplemental oxygen.

The a:A ratio (PaO$_2$/PAO$_2$), respiratory index (RI), and P:F ratio are calculations that combine alveolar and arterial oxygen tension to assess oxygenation with changing FIO$_2$ values. These ratios give a constant value for a given degree of shunt regardless of FIO$_2$ and are compared with A-aDO$_2$ in Table 4–4. Calculation of A-aDO$_2$ is emphasized here as a skill because it is also used to calculate the respiratory index.

Purpose

The nurse calculates A-aDO$_2$ in the mechanically ventilated patient to

1. Diagnose shunt as the primary mechanism of hypoxemia.
2. Assess trends in respiratory status.
3. Determine effectiveness and titration of therapy.

Prerequisite Knowledge and Skills

Prior to calculating A-aDO$_2$, the nurse should understand

1. Physiologic mechanisms of hypoxemia.
2. Principles of lung compliance.
3. Principles of positive-pressure ventilation.
4. Principles of gas exchange.

The nurse should be able to perform

1. Simple mathematical calculations.
2. Ventilator adjustments of inspired oxygen.
3. Ventilator adjustments of tidal volume.
4. Ventilator adjustments of PEEP.
5. Hemodynamic assessment.
6. Respiratory physical assessment (inspection, palpation, percussion, and auscultation).
7. Interpretation of arterial blood gas analysis.

Assessment

1. Observe for signs and symptoms of inadequate oxygenation, including falling arterial oxygen tension (definitive sign), tachypnea, dyspnea, central cyanosis, restlessness, confusion, agitation, tachycardia (early sign), bradycardia (late sign), dysrhythmias, intercostal and suprasternal retractions, rising (early sign) or falling (late sign) arterial blood pressure, adventitious breath sounds, falling urine output, and metabolic acidosis. **Rationale:** Calculation of A-aDO$_2$ is indicated only for differentiating the mechanisms of hypoxemia.

2. Assess arterial oxygen tension or saturation. Hypoxemia is confirmed by a falling PaO$_2$ and/or SaO$_2$ or an absolute PaO$_2$ of less than 60 mmHg and/or an absolute SaO$_2$ of less than 90 percent. **Rationale:** Calculation of A-aDO$_2$ is indicated only for differentiating the mechanisms of hypoxemia.

3. Monitor trend of A-aDO$_2$ on 100% oxygen. **Rationale:** An increase in A-aDO$_2$ indicates an increase in

TABLE 4–4 OPTIONS FOR CLINICAL DETERMINATION OF OXYGENATION

	A-aDO$_2$	a:A Ratio	RI	P:F Ratio
Definition	Difference between alveolar and arterial oxygen tension	Arterial oxygen tension divided by alveolar oxygen tension	Difference between alveolar and arterial oxygen tension divided by arterial oxygen tension	Arterial oxygen tension divided by fraction of inspired oxygen
FIO$_2$ Recommended for Calculation	1.0	0.21–1.0	0.21–1.0	0.21–1.0
Normal Value(s)	10–35 (spontaneous breathing) <50 (mechanical ventilation) <100 (FIO$_2$ of 1.0)	0.74 (elderly)–0.90	0.07–1.0	>200
Value(s) Indicating V̇/Q̇ Mismatch	>100	<0.6	1.0–5.0	<200
Value(s) Indicating Intrapulmonary Shunting	>350	<0.15	>5.0	<150

FIO$_2$ = fraction of inspired oxygen; V̇/Q̇ = ratio of ventilation to perfusion.

shunting; a decrease in A-aDO$_2$ indicates a decrease in shunting.

Nursing Diagnoses

1. Impaired gas exchange related to hypoxemia caused by shunting. **Rationale:** An intrapulmonary shunt results in unoxygenated blood bypassing alveoli. The shunted blood remains poorly oxygenated. Mixing of poorly oxygenated blood with blood that does pass functional alveoli decreases the arterial oxygen tension in proportion to the percent of cardiac output shunted, resulting in hypoxemia.
2. Potential for impaired gas exchange related to hypoxemia caused by barotrauma. **Rationale:** Hyperinflation treatment modalities for hypoxemia (e.g., large tidal volume, PEEP) put the patient at risk for barotrauma. Barotrauma causes hypoxemia and, if untreated, hypercapnia.
3. Potential for impaired gas exchange related to hypoxemia caused by oxygen toxicity. **Rationale:** Oxygen toxicity causes parenchymal lung damage, mimicking adult respiratory distress syndrome (ARDS). The risk of oxygen toxicity increases with FIO_2 levels greater than 0.50. Hypoxemia (and hypercapnia in advanced stages of lung injury) results from the parenchymal damage.

Planning

1. Individualize the following goals based upon the patient's critical nature.
    a. Improve oxygenation. **Rationale:** Calculation of A-aDO$_2$ provides objective data useful in diagnosing the mechanisms of hypoxemia.
    b. Improve ventilation. **Rationale:** Calculation of A-aDO$_2$ provides information regarding effectiveness of therapies used to improve hypoxemia.
2. Gather all necessary data and equipment. **Rationale:** Assists in the procedure being completed efficiently and quickly.
    a. Results of arterial blood gas analysis after breathing 100% oxygen for 15 minutes (Marini and Wheeler, 1989) or more.
    b. Calculator.

Implementation

Steps	Rationale	Special Considerations
1. The following equation is used for clinical purposes: $P_{AO_2} = P_{IO_2} - (1.25 \times PaCO_2)$ Subtract PaO$_2$ from P$_{AO_2}$. [A-aDO$_2$ $= P_{AO_2} - PaO_2$.]	Only approximation is needed for clinical purposes.	For research purposes, use the following formula: $P_{AO_2} = P_{IO_2} - PaCO_2/R + [PaCO_2 \times F_{IO_2} \times (1 - R)/R]$
2. Document A-aDO$_2$ in patient record with the following data:	All the data viewed together are needed for decision-making regarding changes in therapy.	
a. Arterial blood gas (ABG) results.		
b. Ventilator parameters, including FIO_2, at the time ABGs drawn.		
c. Position of patient at the time the blood was drawn.		
d. Date and time ABGs drawn.		
e. Changes in therapy, if any, based on A-aDO$_2$.		

Evaluation

1. Observe trend in A-aDO$_2$. An increasing difference indicates worsening of disease process or ineffective therapy. A decreasing difference indicates improving disease process or effective therapy. **Rationale:** A-aDO$_2$ reflects the approximate degree of shunting as a mechanism of hypoxemia.
2. Observe for increasing PaO$_2$ and/or SaO$_2$. When PaO$_2$ > 60 mmHg and/or SaO$_2$ > 90 percent on an FIO_2 of less than 0.40, monitoring of A-aDO$_2$ is no longer needed. **Rationale:** Shunting, as a mechanism of hypoxemia, requires high oxygen concentrations to maintain marginal oxygenation. Shunting is not contributing significantly to hypoxemia if the patient has an adequate arterial oxygen tension on an FIO_2 of less than 0.40.

Expected Outcomes

1. Maintenance of adequate PaO$_2$. **Rationale:** A-aDO$_2$ provides data delineating the mechanism of hy-

poxemia as shunting and directs therapy toward both minimizing the effects of shunting and resolving the underlying disease process.

2. Timely titration of alveolar hyperinflation and supplemental oxygen therapy. **Rationale:** As A-aDO₂ decreases, the therapies for treating shunting are scaled downward. That is, PEEP, FiO₂, and tidal volume are progressively decreased.

Unexpected Outcomes

1. Hemodynamic instability. **Rationale:** High mean airway pressure caused by PEEP and large tidal volumes can decrease cardiac output.

2. Pulmonary barotrauma. **Rationale:** High intrapleural pressures caused by PEEP and large tidal volumes can cause pneumothorax, pneumomediastinum, pneumopericardium, and subcutaneous emphysema.

3. Oxygen toxicity. **Rationale:** There is no consensus on exactly how much oxygen for exactly how long results in toxic effects on the lungs. In general, some degree of oxygen toxicity is believed to occur within 24 to 48 hours with an FiO₂ greater than 0.50; the higher the FiO₂, the greater is the degree and likelihood of oxygen toxicity. Therefore, it is desirable to maintain an FiO₂ that is less than 0.40 to 0.50 (Daly and Allen, 1987).

Documentation

Documentation in the patient record should include the A-aDO₂; ABG results and FiO₂ with which it was calculated; the time, date, position of patient (e.g., supine, left lateral, etc.), and ventilator parameters at the time the blood was drawn; changes in therapy based on the A-aDO₂; and patient response to the intervention(s). **Rationale:** Provides integrated trend data to evaluate recovery or deterioration and permits calculations to be rechecked and demonstrates appropriate use of diagnostic tests to evaluate, and alter if needed, therapy. The PaO₂ (and therefore A-aDO₂) is affected by ventilator parameters and patient position.

Patient/Family Education

Inform the patient and family about the patient's oxygenation status and the rationale and implications for changes in therapy. If the patient or family requests specific information about alveolar-arterial oxygen differences, explain the general relationship between A-aDO₂ and hypoxemia. **Rationale:** Most patients and families are less concerned with the diagnostic and therapeutic details and more concerned with how the patient is progressing overall or in relation to a specific physiologic function (Dunbar et al., 1990).

Performance Checklist
Skill 4–3: Alveolar-Arterial Oxygen Difference (A-aDO₂) Calculation

Critical Behaviors	Complies yes	no
1. Adjust FiO₂ to 1.0, as appropriate, for 15 minutes before sampling for ABG analysis, obtain ABG sample, and send for analysis. Return FiO₂ to baseline setting.		
2. Calculate PaO₂ using modified alveolar gas equation or simplified formula for clinical use.		
3. Subtract PaO₂ from PaO₂.		
4. Document A-aDO₂ in patient record with the following additional data: ABG results; ventilator parameters at the time ABGs were drawn; position of patient at the time ABGs were drawn; date and time ABGs were drawn; and changes in therapy, if any, based on A-aDO₂.		

SKILL 4–4

Compliance Measurement

Although spirometry or plethysmography is required to measure lung compliance accurately, the bedside method of measuring compliance of a patient receiving mechanical ventilation can produce approximate compliance data. Measurements of dynamic compliance (CMP_dyn) and static compliance (CMP_st) are useful in assessing trends in respiratory status.

Compliance is a measure of the distensibility of the lungs and thorax, that is, the ease with which the lungs can be inflated. Compliance is the inverse of elasticity—the property that causes the lungs to recoil to their resting state. Compliance is expressed in milliliters per centi-

meter of water (ml/cmH₂O) and is defined as the unit change in volume per unit change in pressure.

Technically, the term *dynamic compliance* is misleading. Measurements of CMP_dyn are made during the breathing cycle when flow, albeit variable, is present. Measurement during a flow state captures both the compliance and the resistance components of lung mechanics. Dynamic compliance is quickly, easily, and safely determined in the mechanically ventilated patient and is helpful in the assessment of respiratory status.

A CMP_dyn of 35 to 50 ml/cmH₂O is considered normal (Scanlon et al., 1990). Because CMP_dyn does not separate the resistance forces from compliance forces, conditions that increase airway resistance can significantly alter the value obtained. The presence of bronchospasm, secretions, a small endotracheal tube relative to the size of the trachea, and other conditions that narrow the effective airway will result in a low value for CMP_{dyn} and yet not necessarily reflect a decrease in lung compliance.

In contrast, the measurement of *static*, or *effective*, *compliance* separates the compliance and resistance forces by imposing an end-inspiratory pause maneuver. The pause at end-inspiration holds the delivered tidal volume in the lungs under no-flow conditions. Resistance is eliminated; the unit change in volume per unit change in pressure reflects lung compliance.

A CMP_{st} of 60 to 100 ml/cmH$_2$O is considered normal. Values less than 25 ml/cmH$_2$O indicate that excessive work of breathing is required to inflate the lungs (Scanlon et al., 1990). Any condition that makes it more difficult to distend the lungs will decrease compliance and produce a low CMP_{st}. Such conditions include obesity, pregnancy, kyphoscoliosis, pulmonary fibrosis, ascites, respiratory distress syndrome, atelectasis, pneumonia, pulmonary edema, pneumothorax, pleural effusion, sarcoidosis, and pneumoconiosis. Increased compliance is caused primarily by emphysema, in which the elastic properties of the lung have been damaged, causing lung inflation to be largely unopposed by the usual mechanical properties of the lung.

A baseline value of dynamic compliance should be obtained after every tidal volume change. Thereafter, CMP_{dyn} should be monitored at least once a shift. If the value increases acutely and no obvious signs of airway resistance are apparent, static compliance should be measured. Caution must be exercised when measuring plateau pressure. Stopping expiration, thereby holding the lungs in an inflated state, can cause pneumothorax and cardiovascular depression (Levitzky et al., 1990). The longer the inspiratory hold, the greater is the risk of barotrauma and cardiovascular depression; therefore, inspiration should be held just long enough for the PIP needle to drop to a lower level (usually less than 2 seconds).

A decrease in static compliance has several implications for diagnostic and therapeutic interventions. First, the development or progression of an acute event (e.g., ascites, lobar atelectasis, pneumothorax, etc.) should be assessed. If a short-term, reversible event is not diagnosed, interventions should be directed toward assisting the patient with lung inflations. The patient being ventilated with low-frequency IMV/SIMV may benefit from increased frequency of mandatory breaths. Tidal volumes may need to be increased or PEEP may need to be added. And, of course, the underlying pathology causing low compliance should be treated.

Please note that the measurements of compliance discussed here do not take into account the compliance of the ventilator tubing. In mechanically ventilated patients, the respiratory system, in effect, includes the ventilator and ventilator circuitry as well as the patient's lungs and chest wall. The ventilator and the ventilator circuitry have a compliance of their own that interacts with the compliance of the patient's lungs and chest wall. Ventilator compliance results from the elastic properties of the materials and the compressibility of the gas volume

in the circuitry. This mechanical compliance is usually in the range of 3 to 5 ml/cmH$_2$O for nondisposable circuits (Dupuis, 1986) and in the range of 1 to 3 ml/cmH$_2$O for disposable circuits. Determination of tubing and ventilator compliance requires removing the patient from the ventilator. The intent of this skill is to provide quick and easy data to assess trends in respiratory status that can guide interventions. Therefore, measuring ventilator circuitry compliance is purposefully eliminated.

Purpose

The nurse measures compliance in the mechanically ventilated patient to

1. Assess trends in respiratory status.
2. Determine the effectiveness and titration of therapy.

Prerequisite Knowledge and Skills

Prior to measuring compliance, the nurse should understand

1. Principles of lung compliance.
2. Principles of airway resistance.
3. Principles of positive-pressure ventilation.

The nurse should be able to perform

1. Simple mathematical calculations.
2. Ventilator adjustments of tidal volume (see Skill 4–1).
3. Ventilator adjustments of PEEP.
4. Ventilator adjustments of mandatory respiration rates (see Skill 4–1).
5. Determination of auto-PEEP (see Skill 4–7).
6. Measurement of plateau pressure.
7. Hemodynamic assessment.
8. Respiratory assessment.
9. Endotracheal suctioning (see Skill 1–6).

Assessment

1. Observe PIP for gradual or acute changes. **Rationale:** Given a constant tidal volume, a change in PIP indicates a change in airway resistance or lung compliance.
2. Note any changes in ease, or difficulty, in compressing the manual self-inflating resuscitation bag. **Rationale:** Compliance is change in volume for a change in pressure. If more pressure is required to inflate the lungs, volume delivery will be affected.

Nursing Diagnoses

1. Potential for impaired gas exchange related to hypoxemia. **Rationale:** Barotrauma is a potential risk when measuring static compliance. Barotrauma can cause hypoxemia or seriously augment existing hypoxemia, causing increased work of breathing.

2. Potential for ineffective breathing pattern related to insufficient lung inflation and increased work of breathing. **Rationale:** The patient may demonstrate an ineffective breathing pattern in the attempt to improve gas exchange.

Planning

1. Individualize therapeutic guidelines for management of PPV when compliance is changed. **Rationale:** Hyperinflation therapies may need to be altered and, in the presence of increased airway resistance, suctioning or bronchodilator therapies may need to be reevaluated.

2. Prepare all the necessary equipment and data: calculator, PIP reading, tidal volume reading, PEEP or auto-PEEP reading, and plateau pressure reading. **Rationale:** Assists in data being collected efficiently and accurately.

Implementation

Steps	Rationale	Special Considerations
Dynamic Compliance		
1. Identify the peak inspiratory pressure (PIP).	PIP is used as a rough estimate of the mechanical properties of the lung and chest wall.	
2. Identify the delivered tidal volume (V_T).	Datum collection for calculation.	Air leaks around the artificial airway or through chest tubes will prevent an accurate measurement of dynamic compliance (Martz et al., 1984).
3. Identify the amount of PEEP and/or auto-PEEP.	Datum collection for calculation.	
4. Record the PIP, V_T, and PEEP.	Data collection for calculation.	
5. Subtract PEEP/auto-PEEP from PIP.	Reflects PIP without PEEP.	
6. Divide V_T by the number obtained in step 5. The result equals the CMP_{dyn}.	Compliance is defined as the unit change in volume per unit change in pressure.	
7. Record CMP_{dyn} in ml/cmH_2O.	Communicates datum.	
8. If this is the first value obtained for the given V_T, or if the CMP_{dyn} value is decreased from the previous value, measure CMP_{st}.	Separates airway resistance factor from the compliance factor (Martz et al., 1984).	
Static Compliance		
1. Perform steps 1 through 4 under Dynamic Compliance.		
2. Observe several ventilator respiratory cycles.	Determines timing of the end of inspiration.	
3. Identify the initiation of the ventilator inspiratory cycle.	Determines timing of the beginning of inspiration.	
4. At the end of inspiration, activate the inspiratory pause (inflation hold), while watching on pressure gauge. Note the slight drop in the PIP needle (plateau pressure) and immediately deactivate the inspiratory pause, allowing exhalation.	At this point, the flow of gas through the airway stops, causing inspiratory pressure to drop slightly.	This maneuver requires hand–eye coordination to ensure an inspiratory pause of less than 2 seconds.
5. Record the plateau pressure.	Datum collection for calculation.	
6. Subtract PEEP/auto-PEEP from plateau pressure.	Reflects PIP without PEEP.	

Table continues on following page

Steps	Rationale	Special Considerations
7. Divide V_T by the number obtained in step 6.	CMP_{st} is the relationship of the tidal volume to the plateau pressure.	Air leaks around the artificial airway or through chest tubes will prevent an accurate measurement of static compliance (Martz et al., 1984).
8. Record CMP_{st} in ml/cmH$_2$O.	Communicates datum.	
9. Perform physical assessment to monitor for barotrauma.	Barotrauma is a potential risk of measuring static compliance.	

Evaluation

Observe trends in CMP_{dyn} and/or CMP_{st}. **Rationale:** Increasing compliance values, with a constant tidal volume, indicate improvement in underlying disease process and effectiveness of interventions. Decreasing compliance values, with constant tidal volume, indicate increased airway resistance (CMP_{dyn}) or progression of underlying disease process and ineffective interventions (CMP_{dyn} and CMP_{st}).

Expected Outcome

Therapy titrated to patient response. **Rationale:** Bedside compliance values provide additional respiratory assessment data to determine appropriate interventions, such as suctioning, change of artificial airway, drug therapy, changes in ventilator parameters, etc.

Unexpected Outcomes

1. Pulmonary barotrauma. **Rationale:** Holding the lungs in an inflated state to obtain the plateau pressure for calculation of CMP_{st} can' cause pneumothorax (Levitsky et al., 1990).
2. Cardiovascular depression. **Rationale:** Holding the lungs in an inflated state to obtain the plateau pressure for calculation of CMP_{st} can cause a decrease in cardiac output (Levitsky et al., 1990).

Documentation

Documentation in the patient record should include both CMP_{dyn} and CMP_{st} values measured after any change in tidal volume. **Rationale:** Compliance is the relationship between pressure and volume. Changes in tidal volume are expected to produce changes in PIP and plateau pressure.

Patient/Family Education

Inform the patient and family about the patient's respiratory status, changes in therapy, and how to interpret the changes. If the patient or family requests specific information about compliance measurements, explain the general relationship between pressure and volume. **Rationale:** Most patients and families are less concerned with the diagnostic and therapeutic details and more concerned with how the patient is progressing overall or in relation to a specific physiologic function (Dunbar et al., 1990).

Performance Checklist
Skill 4–4:   Compliance Measurement

Critical Behaviors	Complies	
	yes	no
DYNAMIC COMPLIANCE		
1. Identify the peak inspiratory pressure (PIP).		
2. Identify the delivered tidal volume (V_T).		
3. Identify the amount of PEEP and/or auto-PEEP.		
4. Record PIP, V_T, and PEEP.		
5. Subtract PEEP/auto-PEEP from PIP.		
6. Divide V_T by the number obtained in step 5.		
7. Record the CMP_{dyn} in ml/cmH$_2$O in patient record.		
8. Calculate static compliance if appropriate.		
9. Document procedure in patient record.		

Table continues on following page

Critical Behaviors	Complies	
	yes	no
STATIC COMPLIANCE 1. Repeat steps 1 through 4 under Dynamic Compliance.		
2. Observe several ventilator respiratory cycles.		
3. Identify the initiation of the ventilator inspiratory cycle.		
4. Determine and record the plateau pressure. At the end of inspiration, activate the inspiratory pause (or inflation hold), keeping eye on the pressure gauge.		
5. Subtract PEEP/auto-PEEP from the plateau pressure.		
6. Divide V_T by the number obtained in Step 5.		
7. Record CMP_{st} in ml/cmH$_2$O in patient record.		
8. Perform physical assessment to monitor for barotrauma.		

SKILL 4–5

Arterial-Venous Oxygen Difference (a-v̄DO$_2$) Calculation

Despite increasing research, there remains no satisfactory method for assessing the adequacy of tissue oxygenation. The measurement of oxygen delivery tells us little about peripheral tissue utilization of oxygen. Lactic acidosis has been proposed as an indicator of inadequate tissue oxygenation, but it often occurs as a late manifestation when the clinical condition is irreversible. Mixed venous oxygen tension (Pv̄O$_2$) and mixed venous oxygen saturation (Sv̄O$_2$) also have been proposed as indicators of tissue oxygenation. However, mixed venous blood represents a weighted mean tissue oxygen tension from all body tissues (Bone, 1985). Each tissue differs greatly in total blood flow, metabolic rate, and thus oxygen extraction ratios. A normal or high Pv̄O$_2$ can be maintained in the face of insufficient tissue oxygenation if tissues with low oxygen extraction ratios receive a disproportionate share of blood flow. While it may be assumed that a very low Pv̄O$_2$ (e.g., <30 mmHg) indicates tissue hypoxia, a normal Pv̄O$_2$ should not be assumed to reflect adequate tissue oxygenation. Pv̄O$_2$ provides an accurate assessment of tissue oxygenation in patients with hemorrhagic and hypoxic shock but is falsely high in patients with endotoxin shock due to peripheral arteriovenous shunting. Pv̄O$_2$ is not a useful indicator of tissue oxygenation in patients with anemic shock or in patients receiving positive end-expiratory pressure (Bone, 1985).

The product of cardiac output and arterial content of oxygen defines the overall rate of oxygen delivery (Marini and Wheeler, 1989). The product of cardiac output (CO) and the oxygen content difference between arterial and mixed venous blood defines oxygen consumption. Pv̄O$_2$ and Sv̄O$_2$ reflect tissue oxygenation under most conditions. When blood flow does not increase to meet higher tissue oxygen demands (hypodynamic flow), more oxygen is extracted from the arterial blood, and the Pv̄O$_2$ and Sv̄O$_2$ fall. The difference between arterial oxygen content (CaO$_2$) and mixed venous oxygen content (Cv̄O$_2$) widens. Conversely, when blood flow is increased beyond tissue oxygen demand (hyperdynamic flow), less oxygen is extracted from the arterial blood, and Pv̄O$_2$ and Sv̄O$_2$ increase. The difference between arterial oxygen content and mixed venous oxygen content (a-v̄DO$_2$) decreases.

Reduced flow (CO) or reduced supply (CaO$_2$) depresses oxygen transport, resulting in lower values for Pv̄O$_2$ and Sv̄O$_2$. Since CaO$_2$ depends on hemoglobin and arterial saturation levels, Sv̄O$_2$ is determined by four dynamic and interacting variables: SaO$_2$, CO, hemoglobin, and oxygen consumption. A decrease in Sv̄O$_2$ can be caused by reductions in SaO$_2$, cardiac output, and hemoglobin or by an increase in oxygen consumption. A change in Sv̄O$_2$ does not indicate which of these variables is responsible for the change.

Arterial oxygen content is used to calculate oxygen transport, or delivery, and a-v̄DO$_2$ is used to calculate oxygen consumption, or utilization. Because lung function and hemodynamic function both are directly affected by mechanical ventilation, and because both are components of a-v̄DO$_2$, the arterial–mixed venous oxygen content difference is a useful datum in ventilatory management. The normal a-v̄DO$_2$ is 5 vol% (range is 4 to 6 vol%).

Table 4–5 demonstrates how to calculate a-v̄DO$_2$ under normal and pathologic conditions. Technically, the dissolved oxygen (0.003 × PaO$_2$) is added to the equation. However, the clinical utility of this step does not compensate for the extra calculation time. The addition of dissolved oxygen is eliminated from the a-v̄DO$_2$ calculations in this skill. A narrowed a-v̄DO$_2$ (less than 4 vol%) reflects a hyperdynamic flow. A widened a-v̄DO$_2$ (greater than 6 vol%) reflects a hypodynamic flow. Note that hemoglobin, arterial oxygen saturation, and mixed venous oxygen saturation are needed to calculate the a-v̄DO$_2$. Blood drawn from a central venous catheter is not a mixed venous specimen. Mixed venous oxygen saturation must be obtained from the proximal pulmonary artery, necessitating a functional pulmonary artery catheter. Caution must be exercised to prevent contamination of the pulmonary artery blood sample with oxygenated

TABLE 4–5 CALCULATION OF A-$\overline{v}DO_2$

To calculate oxygen content, multiply the oxygen-carrying capacity (1.39)* times the hemoglobin (g% or grams per 100 ml blood) times the percentage of saturation (%sat).

	O₂-Carrying Capacity	×	Hemoglobin (g%)	×	%Sat	= O₂ Content
CaO_2	1.39	×	15	×	100% =	20.8
$C\overline{v}O_2$	1.39	×	15	×	75% =	15.6

$$a\text{-}\overline{v}DO_2 = CaO_2 - C\overline{v}O_2$$
$$a\text{-}\overline{v}DO_2 = 20.8 - 15.6 = 5.2$$

a. Effect of reduced hemoglobin (e.g., anemia):

CaO_2	1.39	×	10	×	100% =	13.9
$C\overline{v}O_2$	1.39	×	10	×	75% =	10.4

$$a\text{-}\overline{v}DO_2 = 13.9 - 10.4 = 3.5$$

b. Effect of reduced lung function (e.g., hypoxemia):

CaO_2	1.39	×	15	×	90% =	18.76
$C\overline{v}O_2$	1.39	×	15	×	75% =	15.6

$$a\text{-}\overline{v}DO_2 = 18.76 - 15.6 = 3.16$$

c. Effect of reduced perfusion (e.g., low cardiac output):

CaO_2	1.39	×	15	×	100% =	20.8
$C\overline{v}O_2$	1.39	×	15	×	65% =	13.55

$$a\text{-}\overline{v}DO_2 = 20.8 - 13.55 = 7.25$$

*From Bone et al., 1990; others use 1.34.

capillary blood. The blood sample must be withdrawn from the proximal pulmonary artery slowly, with the catheter balloon deflated and the catheter tip positioned in a major pulmonary arterial vessel (see Skill 10–9).

Purpose

The nurse calculates a-$\overline{v}DO_2$ in the mechanically ventilated patient to

1. Provide an indication of the adequacy of tissue oxygenation.
2. Provide an indication of blood flow, or perfusion.
3. Provide an indication of oxygen delivery.
4. Provide an indication of oxygen consumption.

Prerequisite Knowledge and Skills

Prior to calculating a-$\overline{v}DO_2$, the nurse should understand

1. Principles of oxygenation.
2. Principles of perfusion.
3. Principles of oxygen delivery.
4. Principles of oxygen utilization.

The nurse should be able to perform

1. Simple mathematical calculations.
2. Measurement of cardiac output (see Skills 10–9)

for oxygen delivery and oxygen consumption calculations only.

3. Confirmation of pulmonary artery catheter placement.

4. Sampling of arterial blood from indwelling catheter or arterial puncture (see Skills 9–2 and 10–7).

5. Sampling of mixed venous blood from pulmonary artery catheter (see Skill 9–2).

6. Interpretation of arterial blood gas analysis.

7. Interpretation of hemoglobin analysis.

Assessment

Observe for signs and symptoms of inadequate tissue oxygenation, including thirst, nausea, anxiety, apprehension (Whitman, 1988), skin warmth, bounding pulse, tachycardia, high cardiac output, and low systemic vascular resistance are signs of hyperdynamic flow, and cool skin, weak pulse, tachycardia, low cardiac output, hypotension, decreased mentation, lactic acidosis (late sign), metabolic acidosis, decreased pulse pressure, increased systemic vascular resistance, tachypnea, and decreased urine output are signs of hypodynamic flow. **Rationale:** Calculation of a-$\overline{v}DO_2$ is indicated to provide a rough quantitative estimate of tissue perfusion and oxygenation.

Nursing Diagnoses

1. Altered tissue perfusion related to hyperdynamic or hypodynamic blood flow states. **Rationale:** Patients on PPV are at risk for various types of shock (e.g., anemic, endotoxic, hemorrhagic, etc.) that can manifest altered perfusion. a-$\overline{v}DO_2$ measurement provides an indirect method of assessing tissue perfusion.

2. Potential for decreased cardiac output related to positive-pressure ventilation therapy. **Rationale:** High mean airway pressure from PPV, PEEP, and large tidal volumes can depress cardiac output.

Planning

1. Individualize the following goal for managing PPV in impaired tissue oxygenation states: Improve oxygenation. **Rationale:** Indicates prescribed therapies are working and decreasing lactic acidosis states.
2. Gather all necessary data and equipment. **Rationale:** Ensures a-$\overline{v}DO_2$ values are calculated accurately and efficently.
   a. Results of arterial blood gas analysis.
   b. Results of mixed venous blood gas analysis.
   c. Results of serum hemoglobin analysis.
   d. Calculator.

Implementation

Steps	Rationale	Special Considerations
1. Determine and record the value to be used for oxygen-carrying capacity. Either 1.39 or 1.34.	Consistently use the same oxygen-carrying capacity value for all a-$\overline{v}DO_2$ calculations per patient. Prevents erroneous results.	
2. Calculate CaO_2 using the modified Fick equation: $CaO_2 = 1.39 \text{ (or 1.34)} \times Hgb \times \%SaO_2$	Only approximation is needed for clinical purposes.	If using dissolved oxygen, add $(0.003 \times PaO_2)$.
3. Calculate $C\overline{v}O_2$ using the modified Fick equation: $C\overline{v}O_2 = 1.39 \text{ (or 1.34)} \times Hgb \times \%S\overline{v}O_2$	An approximation is useful for clinical purposes.	If using dissolved oxygen in the equation, add $(0.003 \times PaO_2)$.
4. Subtract $C\overline{v}O_2$ from CaO_2.	Results in a-$\overline{v}DO_2$ value.	
5. Consult with physician if needed changes in therapy exceed the therapeutic guidelines.	Large changes in a-$\overline{v}DO_2$ may indicate the need for either revising the therapeutic guidelines or, temporarily at least, discarding them.	

Evaluation

Observe trend in a-$\overline{v}DO_2$. A narrowing difference indicates hyperdynamic perfusion. A widening difference indicates hypodynamic perfusion. The effect of positive-pressure ventilation (PPV) therapy on perfusion needs to be explored. **Rationale:** PPV, particularly with a large tidal volume and PEEP, can compromise hemodynamics from increased intrathoracic pressure.

Expected Outcome

Titration of PPV parameters (e.g., tidal volume, PEEP, I:E ratio) to maintain adequate perfusion and tissue oxygenation. **Rationale:** A widened a-$\overline{v}DO_2$ indicates decreased perfusion and impaired tissue oxygenation and directs therapy toward alleviating or minimizing adverse effects of PPV on perfusion.

Unexpected Outcome

Hemodynamic instability. **Rationale:** High mean airway pressure from PPV, PEEP, and large tidal volumes can depress cardiac output.

Documentation

Documentation in the patient record should include the a-$\overline{v}DO_2$; the ABG and hemoglobin results with which it was calculated; the time, date, position of patient (e.g., supine, left semiprone, etc.), and ventilator parameters at the time the blood gas samples were drawn; changes in therapy based on the a-$\overline{v}DO_2$; and patient response to the intervention(s). **Rationale:** Provides integrated trend data to evaluate tissue oxygenation in light of the pulmonary function and ventilator parameters and demonstrates appropriate use of diagnostic and monitoring tests to evaluate therapy and alter therapy if needed.

Patient/Family Education

Inform the patient and family of the patient's perfusion status, changes in therapy, and how to interpret the changes. If the patient or family requests specific information about arterial-venous oxygen content differences, explain the general relationship between a-$\overline{v}DO_2$ and perfusion. **Rationale:** Most patients and families are less concerned with the diagnostic and therapeutic details and more concerned with how the patient is progressing overall or in relation to a specific physiologic function (Dunbar et al., 1990).

Performance Checklist
Skill 4–5: Arterial-Venous Oxygen Difference (a-$\overline{v}DO_2$) Calculation

Critical Behaviors	Complies	
	yes	no
1. Obtain arterial blood gas results, and note SaO_2.		
2. Obtain mixed venous blood gas, results, and note $S\overline{v}O_2$.		

Table continues on following page

Critical Behaviors	Complies	
	yes	no
3. Obtain hemoglobin results.		
4. Determine value to be used for oxygen-carrying capacity (either 1.39 or 1.34).		
5. Calculate CaO_2 using the modified Fick equation.		
6. Calculate $C\bar{v}O_2$ using the modified Fick equation.		
7. Subtract $C\bar{v}O_2$ from CaO_2.		
8. Document a-vDO$_2$ in patient record with the following additional data: arterial blood gas results; mixed venous blood gas results; hemoglobin results; ventilator parameters at time blood was drawn; position of patient at time blood was drawn; time blood was drawn; changes in therapy, if any, based on a-vDO$_2$.		
9. Consult with physician as necessary.		

SKILL 4–6

Shunt Calculation ($\dot{Q}s/\dot{Q}t$)

Right-to-left intrapulmonary shunting (variously called *physiologic shunting, wasted blood flow,* and *venous admixture*) is the pathologic phenomenon whereby venous blood is shunted past the alveoli without taking up oxygen. It therefore returns to the left side of the heart as venous blood with a low oxygen tension. There it mixes with arterialized blood with a high oxygen tension before circulating throughout the body.

Right-to-left intrapulmonary shunting is expressed as a fraction or percentage of shunted blood flow to total blood flow ($\dot{Q}s/\dot{Q}t$). The normal physiologic shunt is less than 5 percent and is due to venous blood from the bronchial and coronary veins returning to the left side of the heart as desaturated blood. Shunting of blood flow past the alveoli does not mean that a certain percentage of the blood does not course through the pulmonary vasculature, but that it courses through an area of lung that receives no ventilation. Nonventilated areas of the lung can be caused by conditions such as atelectasis, pneumonia, pulmonary edema with fluid-filled alveoli, and total bronchial obstruction. As the percentage of the shunted cardiac output increases, the mixture of venous shunted blood with arterial blood increases and there is a concomitant fall in the arterial oxygen tension. The extent of the hypoxemia depends on the amount of the lung parenchyma that is not ventilated.

The hallmark of right-to-left intrapulmonary shunting is that the hypoxemia cannot be totally corrected by high concentrations of inspired oxygen. Treating this mechanism of hypoxemia is difficult and complex. With a significantly large shunt (e.g., greater than 50 percent), the patient will still be hypoxemic while breathing 100% oxygen. Even though the oxygen tension of the well-oxygenated blood may exceed 600 mmHg, it is continually being diluted by the shunted blood with a low oxygen tension (Fig. 4–9).

The response of an increasing shunt in the lung, with a constant minute ventilation and cardiac output, to higher levels of oxygen is demonstrated in Figure 4–10.

The most striking feature is the muted response to increased oxygen concentrations. At low levels of shunting, there is a rise in PaO$_2$ as FiO$_2$ is increased as a result of the ability to increase the oxygen in the blood exposed to ventilated alveoli. At progressively higher levels of shunt, the blood exposed to ventilated alveoli is oxygenated maximally, but lesser percentages of the total blood flow are exposed to ventilated alveoli.

The muted response to increasing FiO$_2$ does not mitigate the need for high FiO$_2$ values in patients with severe shunting. Even though there is little increase in PaO$_2$ with the administration of 100% oxygen, the changes effected are at the knee (i.e., acute slope) of the oxyhemoglobin dissociation curve. With severe hypoxemia, even small increases in PaO$_2$ can increase oxygen content

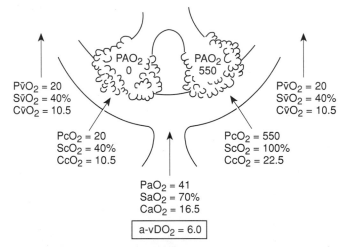

FIGURE 4–9. Schematic representation showing dilution of oxygenated blood with unoxygenated blood in a 50 percent right-to-left intrapulmonary shunt. P$_A$O$_2$ = alveolar oxygen tension, P$\bar{v}$O$_2$ = mixed venous oxygen tension, S$\bar{v}$O$_2$ = mixed venous oxygen saturation, C$\bar{v}$O$_2$ = mixed venous oxygen content, PcO$_2$ = capillary oxygen tension, ScO$_2$ = capillary oxygen saturation, CcO$_2$ = capillary oxygen content, PaO$_2$ = arterial oxygen tension, SaO$_2$ = arterial oxygen saturation, CaO$_2$ = arterial oxygen content, a-vDO$_2$ = difference between arterial and mixed venous oxygen content. (Reproduced with permission from S. K. Goodnough, *Advanced Pulmonary Critical Care Course*, Vol. 1. Houston: Hermann Hospital, 1983.)

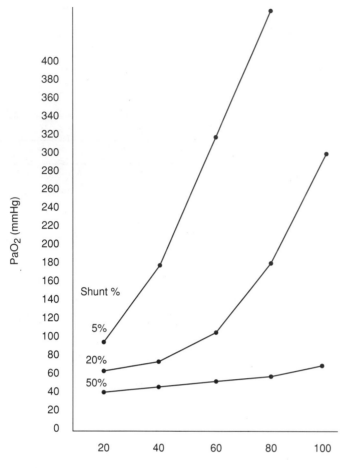

FIGURE 4–10. The response of PaO_2 to higher concentrations of inspired oxygen with increasing levels of right-to-left intrapulmonary shunting. Assumes a constant minute ventilation and a-$\bar{v}DO_2$ of 5 vol%, Hgb > 10 g%, and $PaCO_2$ of 25 to 40 mmHg. (Courtesy of Sandra K. Goodnough-Hanneman.)

and, therefore, oxygen delivery to the tissues significantly. The therapeutic emphasis, however, must be on reversing the underlying cause of the shunt. Table 4–6 demonstrates the percentage of shunt ($\dot{Q}s/\dot{Q}t$).

Purpose

The nurse calculates $\dot{Q}s/\dot{Q}t$ in the mechanically ventilated patient to

1. Differentiate shunting from other mechanisms of hypoxemia.
2. Quantify the shunt.
3. Assess trends in progression or improvement of shunting.
4. Determine effectiveness and titration of therapy.

Prerequisite Knowledge and Skills

Prior to calculating $\dot{Q}s/\dot{Q}t$, the nurse should understand

1. Physiologic mechanisms of hypoxemia.
2. Principles of lung compliance.
3. Principles of positive-pressure ventilation.
4. Principles of gas exchange.
5. Principles of oxygen therapy.
6. Principles of the oxyhemoglobin dissociation curve.
7. Principles of blood flow.

The nurse should be able to perform

1. Simple mathematical calculations.
2. Ventilator adjustments of inspired oxygen.
3. Ventilator adjustments of tidal volume (see Skill 4–1).
4. Ventilator adjustments of PEEP.
5. Hyperinflation maneuvers.
6. Hemodynamic assessment.
7. Respiratory assessment.
8. Interpretation of arterial blood gas analysis.

Assessment

1. Observe for signs and symptoms of inadequate oxygenation, including falling arterial oxygen tension (definitive sign), tachypnea, dyspnea, central cyanosis, restlessness, confusion, agitation, tachycardia (early sign), bradycardia (late sign), dysrhythmias, intercostal

TABLE 4–6 CALCULATION OF $\dot{Q}s/\dot{Q}t$

$$\dot{Q}s/\dot{Q}t = \frac{CAO_2 - CaO_2}{CAO_2 - C\bar{v}O_2}$$

where $\dot{Q}s$ = intrapulmonary shunt

$\dot{Q}t$ = total lung blood flow

CAO_2 = alveolar oxygen content

Hgb = hemoglobin in g%

CaO_2 = arterial oxygen content in ml/100 ml of blood equals
the product $0.003 \times PaO_2 + 0.0134 \times (SaO_2 \times Hgb)$

$C\bar{v}O_2$ = mixed venous oxygen content in ml/100 ml of
blood equals the product $0.003 \times P\bar{v}O_2 + 0.0134 \times (S\bar{v}O_2 \times Hgb)$

Shunt must be calculated with arterial blood gas values on an FO_2 of 1.0 to eliminate the contribution of $\dot{V}/\dot{Q}$ inequalities.

and suprasternal retractions, rising (early sign) or falling (late sign) arterial blood pressure, adventitious breath sounds, falling urine output, and metabolic acidosis. **Rationale:** Calculation of $\dot{Q}s/\dot{Q}t$ is indicated to help differentiate mechanisms of hypoxemia.

2. Monitor arterial oxygen tension or saturation. Hypoxemia due to right-to-left intrapulmonary shunting is confirmed by a low PaO_2 and low SaO_2 with increasing supplemental oxygen. **Rationale:** Calculation of $\dot{Q}s/\dot{Q}t$ is indicated to help differentiate mechanisms of hypoxemia and to provide interventions appropriate to the mechanism of hypoxemia.

3. Monitor trend of $\dot{Q}s/\dot{Q}t$ on 100% oxygen. **Rationale:** "True" shunt (as opposed to ventilation-perfusion inequality) is determined during administration of 100% inspired oxygen (Bone et al., 1990).

Nursing Diagnoses

1. Impaired gas exchange related to hypoxemia caused by right-to-left intrapulmonary shunt. **Rationale:** Right-to-left intrapulmonary shunting of blood causes hypoxemia that is often refractory to high levels of oxygen.

2. Potential for impaired gas exchange related to hypoxemia caused by pulmonary barotrauma. **Rationale:** The hyperinflation modalities used to treat shunt put the patient at risk for barotrauma. Even when the shunt is resolved, the patient may experience hypoxemia from barotrauma.

3. Potential for impaired gas exchange related to hypoxemia caused by oxygen toxicity. **Rationale:** The high FiO_2 (>0.50) used to maximize oxygenation during shunting puts the patient at risk for oxygen toxicity. Even when the original cause of the shunt has been treated successfully, the patient may experience hypoxemia from parenchymal lung damage caused by oxygen toxicity.

Planning

1. Individualize the following goals for treating shunt.
   a. Correct hypoxemia. **Rationale:** Reduces the amount of desaturated blood returning to the tissues.
   b. Prevents barotrauma. **Rationale:** Hyperinflation modalities increase the incidence.
   c. Decreasing shunt. **Rationale:** Indicates improving condition and or effective therapy.

2. Prepare necessary equipment and data. **Rationale:** Ensures calculation of $\dot{Q}s/\dot{Q}t$ will be performed quickly and accurately.
   a. Results of arterial blood gas analysis after breathing 100% oxygen for 15 minutes (Marini and Wheeler, 1989) or more.
   b. Results of mixed venous blood gas analysis.
   c. Calculator.

Implementation

Steps	Rationale	Special Considerations
1. Obtain $\dot{Q}s/\dot{Q}t$ by using the equation in Table 4–6 (Bone, 1988; Marini and Wheeler, 1989).	Provides data to determine appropriate interventions or changes in therapy.	The $a-\bar{v}DO_2$ and $A-aDO_2$ are easier to calculate, since the step of alveolar oxygen content is omitted.
2. Record $\dot{Q}s/\dot{Q}t$.	Provides data for evaluation.	

Evaluation

1. Observe trend in $\dot{Q}s/\dot{Q}t$. An increasing shunt indicates worsening of the disease process or ineffective therapy. A decreasing shunt indicates improving disease process or effective therapy. **Rationale:** The greater the blood flow past unoxygenated alveoli, the greater the shunt and the greater the hypoxemia.

2. Observe for increasing PaO_2 and/or SaO_2. When $PaO_2 > 60$ mmHg and/or $SaO_2 > 90$ percent on an FiO_2 of 0.40 or less, monitoring of $\dot{Q}s/\dot{Q}t$ is no longer necessary. **Rationale:** Shunt, as a mechanism of hypoxemia, requires high oxygen concentrations to maintain marginal oxygenation. Shunting is not contributing significantly to hypoxemia if the patient has adequate arterial oxygen tension on an FiO_2 of 0.40 or less.

3. Gather all necessary data and equipment. **Rationale:** Facilitates quick and accurate values.

Expected Outcomes

1. Maintenance of adequate PaO_2. **Rationale:** $\dot{Q}s/\dot{Q}t$ provides data delineating the mechanism of hypoxemia as shunting and directs therapy toward both minimizing the effects of shunting and resolving the underlying disease process.

2. Timely titration of alveolar hyperinflation and supplemental oxygen therapy. **Rationale:** As $\dot{Q}s/\dot{Q}t$ decreases PEEP, FiO_2, and V_T are progressively decreased.

Unexpected Outcomes

1. Hemodynamic instability. **Rationale:** High intrathoracic pressures caused by the interventions to maintain adequate oxygenation in the presence of shunting (e.g., PEEP and large tidal volume) can depress cardiac output.

2. Pulmonary barotrauma. **Rationale:** High intra-

pleural pressures caused by the interventions to maintain adequate oxygenation in the presence of shunting (e.g., PEEP and large tidal volumes) can cause pneumothorax, pneumomediastinum, pneumopericardium, pneumoperitoneum, and subcutaneous emphysema.

3. Oxygen toxicity. **Rationale:** There is not consensus on exactly how much oxygen for exactly how long results in toxic effects on the lungs. In general, however, it is desirable to maintain the FIO_2 at 0.40 to 0.50 or less (Daly and Allen, 1987) to avoid oxygen toxicity.

Documentation

Documentation in the patient record should include date and time the $\dot{Q}s/\dot{Q}t$ was performed; the arterial and mixed venous blood gas results and FIO_2 with which it was calculated; the time, date, position of patient (e.g., supine, left lateral, etc.), and ventilator parameters at the time the blood gases were drawn; changes in therapy based on the calculated $\dot{Q}s/\dot{Q}t$; and patient response to

the intervention(s). **Rationale:** Provides integrated trend data to evaluate recovery or deterioration and permits calculations to be rechecked. PaO_2 and $P\bar{v}O_2$ (and therefore $\dot{Q}s/\dot{Q}t$) are affected by ventilator parameters and patient position. Demonstrates appropriate use of diagnostic tests to evaluate, and alter if needed, therapy.

Patient/Family Education

Keep the patient and family informed about the patient's oxygenation status in general. Inform them of changes in therapy and how to interpret the changes. If the patient or family requests specific information about intrapulmonary shunting, explain the general relationship between $\dot{Q}s/\dot{Q}t$ and hypoxemia. **Rationale:** Most patients and families are less concerned with the diagnostic and therapeutic details and more concerned with how the patient is progressing overall or in relation to a specific physiological function (Dunbar et al., 1990).

Performance Checklist
Skill 4–6: Shunt Calculation ($\dot{Q}s/\dot{Q}t$)

Critical Behaviors	Complies	
	yes	no
1. Wash hands.		
2. Obtain arterial and mixed venous blood gas samples and send for analysis.		
3. Calculate $\dot{Q}s/\dot{Q}t$.		
4. Document $\dot{Q}s/\dot{Q}t$ in patient record.		

SKILL 4–7

Determination of Auto-PEEP

Auto-PEEP is the phenomenon whereby alveolar pressure inadvertently remains above atmospheric pressure at end-expiration. Insufficient time exists between respiratory cycles to permit complete emptying of the lungs and to reestablish the resting position of the respiratory system. Mechanically ventilated patients with increased airway resistance, patients with severe airway disease who are ventilated with fast respiratory frequencies or shorter expiratory times than needed, and patients with high minute ventilations (Marini and Wheeler, 1989) are exposed to initiation of the next inspiratory breath before the previous expiration is completed. Alveolar pressure remains positive throughout both phases of the respiratory cycle, thus generating continuous lung distension (Fig. 4–11). Intentional creation of this phenomenon is done with the application of PEEP or CPAP in patients with refractory hypoxemia. The inadvertent presence of continuous lung distension due to PPV is auto-PEEP (variously called *intrinsic PEEP* or *inadvertent PEEP*).

The incidence of auto-PEEP has been reported to be

as high as 47 percent in patients receiving positive-pressure ventilation (Wright and Gong, 1990). The incidence increases with minute ventilations greater than 18 L/min, respiratory frequencies greater than 27 breaths per minute, and therapeutic PEEP greater than 10 cmH_2O. Auto-PEEP appears to be present more frequently, and to a greater degree, in patients in medical critical care units, although an incidence rate of 29 percent has been found in surgical critical care unit patients (Wright and Gong, 1990).

As with intentional PEEP applied for therapeutic purposes, auto-PEEP subjects the patient to high risk for hemodynamic compromise and barotrauma. Additionally, auto-PEEP increases the work of breathing by increasing the threshold load to triggering inspiration with A-C, IMV, and SIMV modes of ventilation. Often auto-PEEP can be eliminated by resetting the ventilator parameters (e.g., frequency and I:E ratio) to permit longer exhalation time. Auto-PEEP must be assessed and quantified to determine dynamic and static compliance (see Skill 4–4).

The phenomenon of auto-PEEP cannot be detected by observing the ventilator pressure gauge, since most ventilators are exposed to atmospheric pressure during

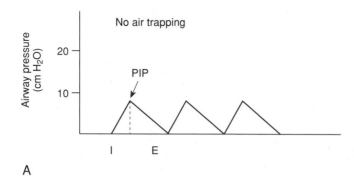

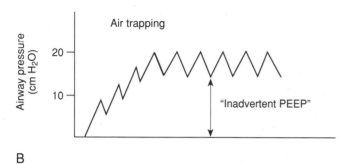

FIGURE 4–11. Auto-PEEP ("inadvertent PEEP") may result from insufficient expiratory time. (*A*) Complete exhalation of gas before subsequent ventilator breaths. (*B*) Incomplete exhalation of gas before subsequent ventilator breaths, causing trapping of gas, overexpansion of the lungs, and auto-PEEP. PIP is peak inspiratory pressure. (Modified with permission from M. J. Banner. Technical aspects of high frequency ventilation. *Curr. Rev. Respir. Ther.* 7:89, 1985.)

expiration, resulting in the return of the peak inspiratory pressure (PIP) needle to zero pressure at the end of expiration. To detect auto-PEEP, the expiratory port of the ventilator must be occluded at the end of expiration. Occlusion must be done just before the subsequent breath is delivered by the ventilator.

Purpose

The nurse measures auto-PEEP in the mechanically ventilated patient to

1. Identify its presence.
2. Quantify the level for assessing patient risk and possible subsequent changes in ventilator therapy.
3. Quantify the level for calculating dynamic and static compliance.

Prerequisite Knowledge and Skills

Prior to measuring auto-PEEP, the nurse should understand

1. Principles of lung compliance.
2. Principles of airway resistance.
3. Principles of positive-pressure ventilation.
4. Mechanics of positive-pressure ventilation.
5. Principles of hemodynamics (particularly hemodynamic response to increased intrathoracic pressure).

The nurse should be able to perform

1. Ventilator adjustments of tidal volume (see Skill 4–1).
2. Ventilator adjustments of respiratory frequency (see Skill 4–1).
3. Ventilator adjustments of I:E ratio (see Skill 4–1).
4. Hemodynamic assessment.
5. Respiratory assessment (including inspection, palpation, percussion, and auscultation).

Assessment

Observe PIP for gradual or acute changes. **Rationale:** Given a constant tidal volume, a change in PIP indicates a change in airway resistance or lung compliance.

Nursing Diagnoses

1. Potential for ineffective breathing pattern related to incomplete lung deflation and increased work of breathing (Marini and Wheeler, 1989). **Rationale:** Auto-PEEP increases the work of breathing by increasing the threshold load to trigger inspiration. Increased work of breathing may cause fatigue and accessory muscle use.
2. Potential for impaired gas exchange related to hypoxemia from barotrauma. **Rationale:** Auto-PEEP, like intentional PEEP, puts the patient at risk for barotrauma because of increased airway and intraalveolar pressures.
3. Potential for altered tissue perfusion related to hemodynamic compromise. **Rationale:** Auto-PEEP, like intentional PEEP, puts the patient at risk for hemodynamic compromise because of increased airway and intraalveolar pressures.

Planning

1. Individualize the following goals for determining the presence of degree of auto-PEEP.
   a. Positive alveolar pressure. **Rationale:** Generates continuous lung distension.
   b. Improved oxygenation. **Rationale:** Usage of auto-PEEP decreases the incidence of refractory hypoxemia.
2. Gather all necessary equipment, supplies, and data. **Rationale:** Ensures the skill is performed quickly and efficiently.
   a. Palm of hand.
   b. Ventilator with exhalation port.

Implementation

Steps	Rationale	Special Considerations
1. Wash hands.	Reduces transmission of microorganisms.	
2. Check the ventilator exhalation port with the hand to determine if airflow ceases during the expiratory phase.	If gas flow ceases, the patient does not have auto-PEEP. If gas flow cessation cannot be detected, measure auto-PEEP.	
3. Observe the pattern and timing of the phases of the respiratory cycle prior to occluding exhalation port.	Diminishes the risk of barotrauma from holding the lungs in a distended state.	
4. Occlude the expiratory port of the ventilator at end-expiration just before initiation of the subsequent mechanical breath. While watching the PIP gauge during this maneuver, note where the needle rests, and immediately release the expiratory port.	Determines the presence and degree of auto-PEEP.	This maneuver must be accomplished as quickly as possible to avoid barotrauma from holding the lungs in a distended state.

Evaluation

Assess patient for signs and symptoms of barotrauma following determination of auto-PEEP. **Rationale:** Barotrauma is a risk from holding the lungs in a distended state.

Expected Outcomes

1. Auto-PEEP will be eliminated, if present, or monitored. **Rationale:** Auto-PEEP is unintentional PEEP with attendant risks for barotrauma and hemodynamic compromise.
2. Therapy will be titrated, if possible, to minimize or eliminate auto-PEEP. **Rationale:** Auto-PEEP can be eliminated by adjusting ventilator parameters to permit complete exhalation.

Unexpected Outcomes

1. Pulmonary barotrauma. **Rationale:** Auto-PEEP puts the patient at risk for barotrauma by maintaining alveolar pressure above atmospheric pressure throughout the respiratory cycle. Quantifying auto-PEEP by occluding the ventilator expiratory port may cause the lungs to be held in various states of inflation.
2. Cardiovascular depression. **Rationale:** Lung distension can cause a decrease in cardiac output. Patients at risk for auto-PEEP who have normal or increased lung compliance will have normal transmission of alveolar pressure to the pleural space (Marini and Wheeler, 1989).

Thus the cardiovascular consequences of auto-PEEP may be more severe than those resulting from therapeutic PEEP used in patients with decreased lung compliance, in whom alveolar pressure is not as readily transmitted to the pleural space.

Documentation

Documentation in the patient record should include the presence and degree of auto-PEEP and any changes in the ventilator parameters. **Rationale:** Demonstrates appropriate use of diagnostic and monitoring data to evaluate therapy and to alter therapy when indicated.

Patient/Family Education

Inform the patient and family about the patient's respiratory status changes in therapy and how to interpret the changes. If the patient or family requests specific information about auto-PEEP measurements, explain the general relationship between auto-PEEP and work of breathing and risk of complications. **Rationale:** Most patients and families are less concerned with the diagnostic and therapeutic details and more concerned with how the patient is progressing overall or in relation to a specific physiologic function (Dunbar et al., 1990).

Performance Checklist
Skill 4–7: Determination of Auto-PEEP

Critical Behaviors	Complies	
	yes	no
1. Wash hands.		

Table continues on following page

Critical Behaviors	Complies	
	yes	no
2. Check the ventilator exhalation port with the hand to determine if airflow ceases during the expiratory phase.		
3. Occlude the expiratory port of the ventilator at end expiration just before initiation of the subsequent mechanical breath. Observe the PIP gauge during occlusion of the expiratory port, note where the needle comes to rest, and immediately release the expiratory port occlusion.		
4. Assess patient for signs and symptoms of barotrauma following determination of auto-PEEP.		
5. Wash hands.		
6. Document the presence and degree of auto-PEEP in patient record.		
7. Consult therapeutic guidelines, if appropriate, or notify physician to make changes in ventilator parameters.		

SKILL 4–8

Vital Capacity (VC) and Negative Inspiratory Pressure (NIP) Measurement

Vital capacity and negative inspiratory pressure—variously called *negative inspiratory force* (Allard, 1991), *peak negative pressure* (MacIntyre and Stock, 1990), *maximal inspiratory pressure* (Marini and Wheeler, 1989), or *maximal inspiratory force* (Luce, 1988)—evaluate the patient's respiratory muscle strength. Muscle strength is one criterion used to assess a patient's ability to breathe spontaneously. The generation of both vital capacity (VC) and negative inspiratory pressure (NIP) occurs against an occluded airway and requires voluntary patient effort. Full activation of the respiratory muscles to produce VC and NIP measurements that are useful for clinical decision-making requires patient cooperation with the procedures.

VC and NIP are used to determine whether a patient requires intubation and/or mechanical ventilatory assistance and therefore are used in the decision-making for both initiation and discontinuance of artificial airway and positive-pressure ventilation. Values that indicate the need for intubation or mechanical ventilation are a VC of less than 15 ml/kg (Montenegro, 1987) and a NIP of less than -20 cmH$_2$O (Luce, 1988; Montenegro, 1987) to less than -30 cmH$_2$O (MacIntyre and Stock, 1990). Conversely, values that indicate the discontinuance of positive-pressure ventilation or extubation are a VC of greater than 15 ml/kg (Montenegro, 1987) and a NIP of greater than -20 cmH$_2$O (Luce, 1988; Montenegro, 1987) to greater than -30 cmH$_2$O (MacIntyre and Stock, 1990).

Purpose

The nurse measures vital capacity and negative inspiratory pressure to evaluate the patient's respiratory muscle strength. **Rationale:** Determines the need for intubation or extubation and the initiation or discontinuance of positive-pressure ventilation.

Prerequisite Knowledge and Skills

Prior to measuring VC or NIP, the nurse should understand

1. Principles of pulmonary mechanics.
2. Principles of airway clearance.

The nurse should be able to

1. Utilize an aneroid manometer (Fig. 4–12).
2. Perform universal precautions (see Skill 35–1).

Assessment

Observe for signs and symptoms of inadequate ventilation, including rising arterial carbon dioxide tension (definitive sign), chest–abdominal dyssynchrony, shallow respirations, irregular respirations, apnea, tachypnea, bradypnea, dyspnea, asterixis, headache, restlessness, confusion, lethargy, rising (early sign) or falling (late sign) arterial blood pressure, tachycardia, atrial and/or ventricular dysrhythmias, depressed deep tendon reflexes. **Rationale:** Inadequate ventilation may indicate the need for positive-pressure ventilation. If signs and symptoms suggest inadequate ventilation, measurement

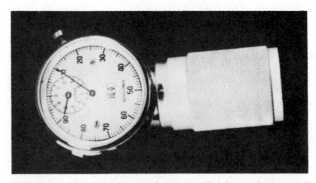

FIGURE 4–12. Portable respirometer (Wright respirometer, Harris Calorific, Cleveland, Ohio). (Reproduced with permission from S. P. McPherson, *Respiratory Therapy Equipment*, 4th Ed. St. Louis: Mosby, 1990, p. 150.)

of VC and NIP will provide data on respiratory muscle strength to use in the decision as to whether to initiate positive-pressure ventilation. Conversely, if no signs and symptoms of inadequate ventilation are present in the patient on positive-pressure ventilation, VC and NIP measurements provide data to determine discontinuance of PPV.

Nursing Diagnoses

1. Potential for impaired gas exchange related to hypercapnia due to poor respiratory muscle strength. **Rationale:** A low VC and NIP reflect the inability to spontaneously hyperinflate the lungs.
2. Potential for ineffective airway clearance related to respiratory muscle weakness. **Rationale:** Low VC and NIP reflect the inability to spontaneously hyperinflate the lungs. Lung hyperinflations are required for spontaneous airway clearance.

Planning

1. Individualize the following goals for measuring vital capacity and negative inspiratory pressure.
   a. Measurements will be true and accurate. **Rationale:** Measurements determine the type of therapy to be initiated or discontinued.

b. Discontinuation from mechanical ventilation. **Rationale:** Provides indirect assessment of respiratory muscle strength.
2. Prepare all necessary equipment and supplies. **Rationale:** Ensures VC and NIP are measured efficiently and correctly.
   a. Portable respirometer.
   b. Portable aneroid manometer.
   c. Clean gloves.
3. Prepare the patient.
   a. Explain the procedures and why they are being done. **Rationale:** Communication and explanation for therapy are cited as an important need of patients (Viner, 1988).
   b. Discuss the sensations the patient may experience, such as transient shortness of breath and fatigue. **Rationale:** Knowledge of anticipated sensory experiences reduces anxiety and distress (Viner, 1988).
   c. Explain to the patient the importance of cooperation and maximal effort to achieve valid and reliable measurements. **Rationale:** Information about the patient's therapy, including rationale, is cited consistently as an important need of patients (Foundation for Critical Care, 1988; Parker et al., 1984; Viner, 1988) and family members (Dunbar et al., 1990; Hickey, 1990).

Implementation

Steps	Rationale	Special Considerations
1. Wash hands.	Reduces transmission of microorganisms.	
2. Don exam gloves.	Universal precautions.	
3. Attach portable respirometer to airway.	Respirometer is used to measure VC.	
4. Instruct patient to inhale as deeply as possible, zero respirometer, and instruct patient to exhale as completely as possible.	A good VC effort mandates a maximum inspiration followed by a maximum expiration.	
5. If patient is on PPV, place back on ventilator to rest for a few minutes. Note the respirometer reading, and communicate the reading to the patient.	Provides an incentive to the patient to exceed effort.	
6. Repeat steps 3 to 5 two more times, coaching the patient to try to improve on previous reading.	The goal is to obtain the best effort the patient can make.	
7. Advise the patient that you will measure NIP four times.	Ensures best effort and evaluates reproducibility.	
8. Attach negative-pressure manometer to airway.	Negative-pressure manometer is used to measure NIP.	
9. Instruct the patient to inhale as deeply as possible. Observe the manometer needle during inspiration. Remove manometer for expiration.	The goal is to obtain the patient's best effort. One-way valve prevents exhalation through the manometer.	

Table continues on following page

Steps	Rationale	Special Considerations
10. Repeat the measurement 3 more times and place the patient back on the ventilator, if appropriate, to rest for a few minutes between each try.	Obtains patient's best effort.	
11. Tell patient what the readings were.	Provides incentive for patient to exceed effort.	
12. Wash hands.	Reduces transmission of microorganisms.	

Evaluation

Compare the VC and NIP measurements to the goals for the patient's parameters. **Rationale:** If the measurements are less than the goals, the patient may need either initiation of positive-pressure ventilation or continuance of mechanical ventilation. If the measurements equal or exceed the goals, the patient may remain breathing spontaneously or begin weaning from mechanical ventilation.

Expected Outcome

Valid and reliable measurements. **Rationale:** Decisions to intubate or extubate and to initiate or discontinue PPV are made, in part, on the results of these procedures.

Unexpected Outcome

Invalid and unreliable measurements. **Rationale:** These procedures are dependent on the patient's cooperative voluntary effort and the nurse's hand–eye coordination to zero the respirometer just prior to exhalation for VC.

Documentation

Documentation in the patient record should include the highest of consecutive VC measurements and the most negative of consecutive NIP measurements and patient responses, particularly adverse ones, to the procedures. **Rationale:** Serial measurements are taken for each procedure to ensure obtaining the results of the patient's maximal "best" effort. Patients with obstructive airway disease may manifest intense bronchospasm from the forced exhalation of VC and forced inspiration of NIP. This reaction suggests the potential for the development of complications such as atelectasis and nosocomial pneumonia, if untreated. Bronchodilators may be indicated to relieve the bronchospasm. VC less than 10 to 15 ml/kg predicts that the patient will be unable to effectively deep breathe and clear airway without assistance. NIP less than -20 to -30 cmH$_2$O predicts that the patient will be unable to sustain the ability to take deep breaths and cough.

Patient/Family Education

1. Inform the patient and family about the patient's respiratory status, changes in therapy, and how to interpret the changes. If the patient or family requests specific information about VC or NIP, explain the relationship between these measurements and respiratory muscle strength. **Rationale:** Most patients and families are less concerned with the diagnostic and therapeutic details and more concerned with how the patient is progressing overall (Dunbar et al., 1990). However, the concepts of VC and NIP are readily grasped by patients and families. They may wish to follow the patient's progress regarding mechanical respiratory assistance with these quantitative measurements. If so, the family can be recruited to help the patient provide a maximal effort during measurements.

2. Evaluate the patient's need for a long-term artificial airway and mechanical ventilatory assistance. **Rationale:** Consistently low measurements of VC and NIP may indicate the need for home ventilator therapy.

3. Evaluate the patient's need for modified airway clearance techniques. **Rationale:** The patient who cannot clear the airway with hyperinflation and cough techniques will need alternative techniques (e.g., postural drainage, percussion, vibration) to ensure the maintenance of a patent airway.

Performance Checklist
Skill 4–8: Vital Capacity (VC) and Negative Inspiratory Pressure (NIP) Measurement

Critical Behaviors	Complies yes	no
1. Wash hands.		
2. Don exam gloves.		

		Complies	
Critical Behaviors		yes	no
3. Attach portable respirometer to airway.			
4. Instruct patient to inhale as deeply as possible, zero respirometer, and instruct patient to exhale as completely as possible.			
5. Remove respirometer, put patient back on ventilator or oxygen support, if appropriate, and allow patient to rest for a few minutes.			
6. Note the respirometer reading and communicate the reading to the patient.			
7. Document highest VC reading in patient record.			
8. Advise patient that NIP will be measured four times.			
9. Attach negative-pressure manometer to airway.			
10. Instruct the patient to inhale as deeply as possible, observe the manometer needle during inspiration, and remove manometer for expiration.			
11. Repeat the measurement 4 times and place patient back on ventilator or oxygen support, as appropriate, to rest for a few minutes.			
12. Note the manometer readings and communicate both readings to patient.			
13. Wash hands.			
14. Document the most negative reading in the patient record.			

SKILL 4–9

Weaning from Positive Pressure Ventilation

Weaning is the process of withdrawing a patient from mechanical ventilation. Most patients who are placed on positive-pressure ventilation (PPV) for short-term purposes (e.g., to support respiration during anesthesia for surgery) do not require weaning. PPV is simply discontinued when the purpose for which it was instituted has been accomplished. The underlying disease process or the development of complications dictates that some patients, however, require PPV for longer periods of time. The patient becomes accustomed to mechanical ventilation and must be weaned from it. Generally, there is a linear relationship between the length of time on PPV and the time needed to wean from PPV (Schuster, 1990; Shekleton et al., 1984).

The overriding goal for the patient on PPV is timely and appropriate withdrawal of mechanical ventilation and the artificial airway to avoid the iatrogenic complications inherent in these therapies. Prolonged use of PPV and the concomitant need for an artificial airway put the patient at increased risk for the complications of tracheal injury (Goodnough, 1988), barotrauma (Guthrie et al., 1983; Sottile, 1988); cardiovascular depression (Goodnough, 1985; Montenegro, 1987), and nosocomial pneumonia (Hoyt, 1988; Pagliarello and Carter, 1990; Rutherford et al., 1990; Sherry et al., 1990; Yannelli and Gurevich, 1988). These complications are common, serious, and costly (Meijer et al., 1990; Rutherford et al., 1990).

The traditional weaning method is a trial-and-error approach. Sometimes the weaning is premature, and complications result from withdrawing support too soon. Other times the decision to wean is delayed, and complications result from continuing support too long. Studies have shown that using predetermined objective criteria for judging a patient's readiness to be weaned, in contrast to simply deciding to proceed on clinical grounds, improves success rates (Foster et al., 1984; Hilberman et al., 1976; Quasha et al., 1980; Shekleton et al., 1984; Shikora et al., 1990; Tobin et al., 1986). Conventional criteria for predicting successful weaning from mechanical ventilation are not always valid (Milic-Emili, 1986; Schuster, 1990; Shikora et al., 1990). Current weaning practice continues to reflect the quandary over which criteria are most helpful in predicting successful weaning from mechanical ventilation. This quandary is substantiated in the literature with reports and recommendations of multiple and variable subjective and objective criteria.

The two procedures in this skill are recommended as guidelines until more research-based directions become available.

Purpose

The nurse weans the patient from (PPV) support to

1. Discontinue positive-pressure ventilation (PPV) and artificial airway.
2. Reduce patient risk for iatrogenic complications from PPV.

Prerequisite Knowledge and Skills

Prior to weaning the patient from PPV support, the nurse should understand

1. Anatomy and physiology of the respiratory systems.
2. Principles of airway management (see Chap. 1).
3. Principles of gas exchange.
4. Principles of airway resistance.
5. Principles of lung compliance (see Skill 4–4).
6. Principles of blood gas interpretation.
7. Principles of positive-pressure ventilation.
8. Mechanics of positive-pressure ventilation.
9. Principles of work of breathing.
10. Stress and coping theory.
11. Concept of anxiety.
12. Principles of nutrition.
13. Verbal and nonverbal communication strategies.
14. Principles of pharmacology.
15. Principles of aseptic technique.

The nurse should be able to perform

1. Proper handwashing technique (see Skill 35–5).
2. Vital signs assessment.
3. Oxygen administration and ventilation via manual self-inflating resuscitation bag (see Skill 4–2).
4. Ventilation via mouth-to-mouth, mouth-to-nose, or face mask–to–mouth and nose techniques (see Fig. 4–3).
5. Respiratory physical assessment (inspection, palpation, percussion, and auscultation).
6. Hemodynamic assessment.
7. Level of consciousness assessment.
8. Confirmation of endotracheal tube placement.
9. Endotracheal suctioning (see Skill 1–6).
10. Nasopharyngeal and oropharyngeal suctioning (see Skill 1–3).
11. Extubation (see Skill 1–8).
12. Oxygen administration via face mask, hood, or nasal cannula (see Skills 2–1 and 2–2).
13. Measurement of vital capacity (see Skill 4–8).
14. Measurement of negative inspiratory pressure (see Skill 4–8).
15. Oxygen saturation monitoring by pulse oximetry (see Skill 6–1).

Assessment

1. Observe for signs and symptoms of adequate ventilation within desired limits for the patient, including stable arterial carbon dioxide tension (definitive sign), chest–abdominal synchrony, patient–ventilator synchrony, absence of dyspnea, absence of headache, level of consciousness and orientation, stable blood pressure, and cardiac rate and rhythm. **Rationale:** Adequate ventilation is a criterion for weaning from mechanical ventilation.
2. Observe for signs and symptoms of adequate oxygenation, within desired limits for the patient, including stable arterial oxygen tension (definitive sign), respira-

tory frequency within the therapeutic guidelines (generally less than 24 breaths per minute; Tobin et al., 1986), absence of dyspnea, absence of central cyanosis, level of consciousness and orientation, stable blood pressure, and cardiac rate and rhythm. **Rationale:** Adequate oxygenation is a criterion for weaning from PPV.
3. Evaluate the patient's breathing pattern for absence of accessory muscle use, retractions, tracheal tug, respiratory alternans, and respiratory muscle paradox. **Rationale:** An abnormal breathing pattern may indicate that the patient is not ready to be weaned from PPV.
4. Evaluate arterial blood gases on an FIO_2 of less than 0.40 for a pH of greater than 7.30 and less than 7.50, PaO_2 greater than 60 mmHg, and $PaCO_2$ greater than 30 mmHg and less than 50 mmHg. **Rationale:** Abnormal arterial blood gases indicate that the patient is not ready to be weaned from PPV.

Nursing Diagnoses

1. Potential for impaired breathing pattern related to hypoxemia and/or hypercapnia due to decreased inspiratory muscle strength and decreased inspiratory muscle endurance. **Rationale:** A high level of respiratory work (greater than 15 percent; Shikora et al., 1990) to maintain adequate gas exchange is needed in patients with decreased inspiratory muscle strength and endurance. Fatigue from the respiratory work of breathing is manifested by an impaired breathing pattern. Additionally, some weakening and discoordination of respiratory muscles occurs with prolonged PPV (Marini and Wheeler, 1989).
2. Ineffective breathing patterns related to hypoxemia, hypercapnia, and increased work of breathing. **Rationale:** Hypoxemia, hypercapnia, and increased work of breathing are associated with the recruitment of accessory respiratory muscle function during spontaneous breathing. Recruitment of accessory respiratory muscles during inspiration increases dyspnea (Breslin et al., 1990).
3. Fatigue related to alveolar hypoventilation. **Rationale:** Alveolar hypoventilation can be caused by respiratory muscle fatigue, inefficient gas exchange, and excessive ventilatory requirements (Tobin et al., 1986). With some systems, the FIO_2 delivered with spontaneous T-tube breathing is dependent on the minute volume, flow rate, set oxygen concentration, and the patient's breathing pattern (e.g., tidal volume). The interaction of these factors can result in a lower inspired oxygen concentration with the T-tube than on the ventilator. High-flow oxygen systems (e.g., continuous aerosol nebulizers, Venturi) provide all the inspired gas source. FIO_2 with these systems is independent of minute volume.
4. Impaired gas exchange related to alveolar hypoventilation due to increased work of breathing and resultant fatigue. **Rationale:** Alveolar hypoventilation can be caused by respiratory muscle fatigue, impaired gas exchange, and excessive ventilatory requirements (Tobin et al., 1986). Hypercapnia will result if clinical signs of increased work of breathing and fatigue (e.g., tachypnea,

respiratory alternans, and paradoxical breathing) go un-detected or untreated. Note that hyperalimentation may produce excessive carbohydrate loads with an increase in carbon dioxide production, which can lead to hyper-capnia in patients with lung disease (Askanazi et al., 1980; Dark et al., 1985; Herve et al., 1985).

5. Fatigue related to increased work of breathing and increased oxygen consumption. **Rationale:** The work of spontaneous breathing through demand valves, PEEP valves (Schuster, 1990), and narrowed endotracheal tube lumens can cause fatigue (Schuster, 1990; Shapiro et al., 1986). Clinical signs of fatigue, such as tachypnea, respiratory alternans, or paradoxical abdominal motion, indicate the need to increase ventilatory support.

Planning

1. Individualize the following goals for weaning the patient from PPV in collaboration with the physician, respiratory therapist, the patient, and family.
    a. Maintain alveolar ventilation. **Rationale:** Promotes gas exchange, thus decreasing the incidence of hypercapnia.
    b. Prevent fatigue. **Rationale:** Promotes "easy" breathing patterns and maintains normal oxygen consumption.
    c. Determine therapeutic guidelines for PaO_2 and $PaCO_2$ ranges in collaboration with the physician and respiratory therapist. **Rationale:** A desired range, as opposed to absolute numbers, permits titration of ventilator parameters (e.g., tidal volume, frequency, IMV, SIMV, pressure support, CPAP, FiO_2) to meet the patient response to weaning more quickly.

2. Gather and check all necessary equipment and supplies. **Rationale:** Listed equipment and supplies are necessary to wean the patient as efficaciously as possible.
    a. Manual self-inflating resuscitation bag capable of delivering 100% oxygen and large inflation volumes.
    b. Appropriately sized resuscitation face mask.
    c. Multiple oxygen sources and flowmeters (at least three, one for the ventilator, one for the resuscitation bag, and one for the T-tube [T-bar; T-piece]).
    d. Functional portable respirometer (see Fig. 4–12) for measuring vital capacity (see Skill 4–8), spontaneous tidal volume, and spontaneous minute volume.
    e. Functional heated aerosol for T-tube oxygen (Fig. 4–13). For weaning on the ventilator (IMV/SIMV, flowby, decreasing A-C support), ensure functional in-line thermometer for measuring inspired gas temperature.
    f. Portable oxygen analyzer.
    g. Distilled sterile water.
    h. Exam gloves.
    i. Suction equipment (see Chap. 1).
    j. Tonsil sucker suction catheter.
    k. Arterial blood gas testing equipment.

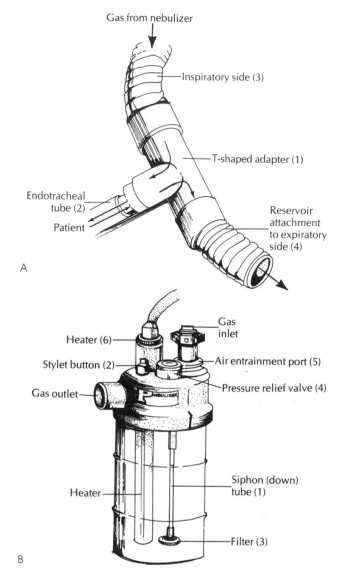

A

B

FIGURE 4–13. (*A*) Aerosol T-adapter for attachment to endotracheal or tracheostomy tube. (*B*) Mechanical jet nebulizer (Puritan-Bennett Corporation, Overland Park, Kansas). (Reproduced with permission from D. H. Eubanks and R. C. Bone, *Comprehensive Respiratory Care*, 2d Ed. St. Louis: Mosby, 1990, pp. 350, 352.)

    l. Portable aneroid manometer (see Skill 4–8).
    m. Implements for patient communication.
    n. Call bell.
    o. Stethoscope.
    p. Stop watch.
    q. T-tube, 3-in (7.62 cm) extension tubing, and large-bore tubing (see Fig. 4–13).

3. Prepare the patient and family.
    a. Explain the procedure(s) and why weaning is being initiated. **Rationale:** Anxiety is reduced when patients are prepared for the sensations they may experience during procedures (CURN Project, 1981; Johnson, 1972; Johnson et al., 1978).
    b. Take VC measurement. **Rationale:** Vital capacity evaluates the patient's ability to take deep breaths and cough. Taking the measurement

three times ensures best effort and evaluates re-producibility.
  c. Discuss the sensations the patient may experience, such as smaller lung inflations, dyspnea, change or absence of ventilator sounds, etc. **Rationale:** Patients (in particular those who have been on prolonged PPV support) report discomfort with resumption of spontaneous breathing (Bergbom-Engberg and Haljamae, 1989).

  d. Reassure the patient of the nurse's continuous presence during initiation of weaning. **Rationale:** Dependence on the nurse's support and monitoring makes it easier for the patient to accept relinquishing dependence on PPV support.
  e. Encourage the patient to relax and breathe comfortably. **Rationale:** Relaxation decreases muscle tension (Acosta, 1988).

Implementation

Steps	Rationale	Special Considerations
Weaning Trial from PPV		
1. Wash hands.	Reduces transmission of microorganisms.	
2. Don sterile gloves.	Maintain universal precautions.	
3. Remove ventilator circuit from artificial airway, and measure vital capacity three times (see Skill 4–8).	VC evaluates the patient's ability to take deep breaths and cough. Multiple measurements ensure best effort and evaluate reproducibility.	
4. Document highest VC reading. If reading is less than 10 ml/kg body weight, abort the procedure.	A VC of less than 10 to 15 ml/kg predicts that the patient will be unable to effectively deep breathe and clear secretions.	
5. Explain the purpose and procedure of negative inspiratory pressure measurement to the patient, explain that the measurement may stimulate transient dyspnea and coughing, and advise that you will measure negative inspiratory pressure four times.	Negative inspiratory pressure (NIP) evaluates the patient's ability to generate sufficient intrathoracic pressures for deep breathing and airway clearance.	
6. Remove ventilator circuit and measure NIP four times (see Skill 4–8).		
7. Document most negative reading. If reading is less than -20 cmH$_2$O, abort procedure.	Less negative inspiratory pressure indicates the patient will be unable to sustain the ability to take deep breaths and cough.	
8. Explain purpose and procedure of minute volume ($\dot{V}_E$) measurement, and advise patient that the measurement should not produce any discomfort and that you will perform it just once.	$\dot{V}_E$ is a good proxy indicator of work of breathing. If minute volume is high, the work of breathing is excessive and the patient will fatigue with spontaneous breathing.	
9. Remove ventilator circuit from artificial airway, attach portable respirometer (see Fig. 4–12), zero respirometer and stopwatch simultaneously, instruct patient to breathe normally, and count the frequency of respirations for 1 full minute. Remove respirometer at the end of 1 minute and place the patient back on the ventilator. **Rationale:** Promotes accurate measurement.		

Table continues on following page

Steps	Rationale	Special Considerations
10. Divide the frequency f into the minute volume to determine the average spontaneous tidal volume. Document the $\dot{V}_E$, f, and tidal volume (V_T). If $\dot{V}_E$ is greater than 10 L/min, abort procedure.	Minute volume greater than 10 L/min indicates that the patient is not ready to wean.	
11. Explain purpose and procedure of T-tube to patients, and place patient on T-tube with heated aerosol. Instruct patient to breathe normally, and monitor frequency, breathing pattern, heart rate, cardiac rhythm, and general appearance of patient.	Heated aerosol enhances secretion clearance by changing the nature of tracheobronchial mucus and replaces water that normally would be added by the upper airway if it were not bypassed by the endotracheal or tracheostomy tube.	Abort weaning for any of the following, and place patient back on PPV support: frequency greater than 24 breaths per minute, subjective complaint of dyspnea and/or fatigue, abnormal breathing pattern, heart rate greater than 10 percent of baseline, dysrhythmias, diaphoresis, pallor or cyanosis, confusion, restlessness, or agitation.
12. After 30 minutes of spontaneous breathing on the T-tube, obtain arterial blood gases, and place patient back on the ventilator.	Arterial blood gas values are objective data to assess patient response to weaning. The patient is placed back on the ventilator to rest until all data regarding weaning response can be assessed.	
13. Notify physician of patient response to weaning trial, including the arterial blood gas (ABG) results, and consult with physician regarding extubation.	Data assessment and consultation lead to a decision regarding extubation.	
Weaning Ventilator-Dependent Patients 1. Wash hands.	Reduces transmission of microorganisms.	
2. Proceed to steps in the decision tree algorithm for ventilator-dependent patients (Fig. 4-14).	If patient meets criteria for a weaning program determine weaning method to be used in collaboration with the physician, respiratory therapist, and patient.	
A. T-Tube (T-piece, T-bar) Weaning Method 1. Devise weaning schedule.	This method alternates periods of total spontaneous breathing with full PPV support until the patient can sustain comfortable and effective spontaneous breathing throughout wake and sleep cycles. A schedule is devised whereby the patient undergoes progressively longer periods on the T-tube during the day. Initially, the T-tube periods are short, lasting 5 to 10 minutes, and are followed by 2 hours of full PPV support. The patient remains on full PPV support at night to promote adequate rest. The intervals on the T-tube are progressively increased according to patient tolerance and response, and the intervals on full PPV support are progressively decreased. Generally, weaning is considered successful when the patient can breathe spontaneously for a continuous 24-hour period.	High-flow continuous positive airway pressure (CPAP) may be used during T-tube weaning in those patients who have borderline arterial oxygen tension levels. Demand-valve CPAP should not be used as it increases the work of breathing, causing fatigue and weaning setbacks. Due to the increased work of breathing with spontaneous ventilation through an endotracheal tube, the patient with borderline arterial oxygen tension may need a higher FIO_2 (e.g., $5 - 10\%$ higher) on the T-tube than on the ventilator.

Table continues on following page

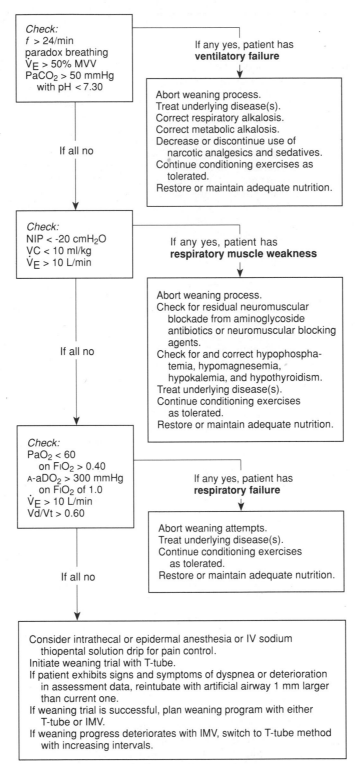

Check:
$f > 24/min$
paradox breathing
$\dot{V}_E > 50\%$ MVV
$PaCO_2 > 50$ mmHg
    with pH < 7.30

If any yes, patient has
ventilatory failure

Abort weaning process.
Treat underlying disease(s).
Correct respiratory alkalosis.
Correct metabolic alkalosis.
Decrease or discontinue use of
    narcotic analgesics and sedatives.
Continue conditioning exercises as
    tolerated.
Restore or maintain adequate nutrition.

If all no

Check:
NIP < -20 cmH$_2$O
$\dot{V}C < 10$ ml/kg
$\dot{V}_E > 10$ L/min

If any yes, patient has
respiratory muscle weakness

Abort weaning process.
Check for residual neuromuscular
    blockade from aminoglycoside
    antibiotics or neuromuscular blocking
    agents.
Check for and correct hypophospha-
    temia, hypomagnesemia,
    hypokalemia, and hypothyroidism.
Treat underlying disease(s).
Continue conditioning exercises
    as tolerated.
Restore or maintain adequate nutrition.

If all no

Check:
PaO$_2$ < 60
    on FiO$_2$ > 0.40
A-aDO$_2$ > 300 mmHg
    on FiO$_2$ of 1.0
$\dot{V}_E > 10$ L/min
Vd/Vt > 0.60

If any yes, patient has
respiratory failure

Abort weaning attempts.
Treat underlying disease(s).
Continue conditioning exercises
    as tolerated.
Restore or maintain adequate nutrition.

If all no

Consider intrathecal or epidermal anesthesia or IV sodium
    thiopental solution drip for pain control.
Initiate weaning trial with T-tube.
If patient exhibits signs and symptoms of dyspnea or deterioration
    in assessment data, reintubate with artificial airway 1 mm larger
    than current one.
If weaning trial is successful, plan weaning program with either
    T-tube or IMV.
If weaning progress deteriorates with IMV, switch to T-tube method
    with increasing intervals.

**FIGURE 4–14. Decision tree algorithm for ventilator-dependent
patients.**

Steps	Rationale	Special Considerations
2. Assess for signs and symptoms of fatigue, inadequate gas exchange, and impaired breathing pattern.	Provides data regarding patient's response to weaning.	
3. Communicate with patient throughout periods on the T-tube.	Attention is given to the patient's psychologic response to weaning. The nurse remains with the patient during the initial T-tube trials, coaches the patient with relaxation and breathing techniques, reinforces the goals and desired outcomes, reminds the patient that talking, eating, self-care activities, and mobilization will be facilitated by successful weaning and extubation, and celebrates progress with weaning with the patient.	
B. IMV/SIMV Weaning Method		
1. Gradually and progressively decrease IMV/SIMV breaths.	This method of weaning provides gradual decrements in full PPV support by permitting spontaneous breathing and periodic preset ventilator breaths. The preset breaths are progressively decreased as the patient assumes a greater proportion of the minute volume with spontaneous breathing. In the early stages of weaning, the patient is placed on full PPV support at night to promote adequate rest. Generally, weaning is considered successful when the patient can breathe spontaneously for a continuous 24-hour period with an IMV/SIMV rate of 2 breaths per minute or less.	IMV/SIMV demand valves offer high resistance to breathing and produce a lag between the patient's initiation of a breath and delivery of the inspired gas during spontaneous breathing (MacIntyre and Stock, 1990). These factors increase the work of breathing and subsequent fatigue with the IMV/SIMV method. To avoid this disadvantage, the system should be adapted to provide a high continuous flow of at least 40 L/min with a low-compliance reservoir bag in the inspiratory limb. High-flow continuous CPAP may be used during IMV/SIMV weaning in those patients who have borderline arterial oxygen tension levels. Demand-valve CPAP should not be used because it increases the work of breathing, causing fatigue and weaning setbacks.
2. Assess the patient for signs and symptoms of fatigue, inadequate gas exchange, and impaired breathing pattern with each decrement in IMV/SIMV support.	Determines patient response to weaning.	
3. Communicate with patient each time the IMV/SIMV rate is decreased.	Attention is given to the patient's psychological response to weaning. The nurse remains with the patient for the first 30 minutes after a decrease in IMV/SIMV rate, coaches the patient with relaxation and breathing techniques, reinforces the goals and desired outcomes, reminds the patient that talking, eating, self-care activities, and mobilization will be facilitated by successful weaning and extubation, and celebrates progress with weaning with the patient.	
C. Pressure-Support Weaning Method		
1. Set level of pressure support as determined in collaboration with	This weaning method provides a preset level of inspiratory pressure	PSV is a relatively new method and is not available on all ventilators.

Table continues on following page

Steps	Rationale	Special Considerations
the physician and respiratory therapist.	assist with each spontaneous breath. The patient initiates the breath, and the ventilator responds by supplying a rapid flow of gas, providing a constant pressure throughout the inspiratory cycle (Burns, 1990; MacIntyre and Stock, 1990). The patient determines the respiratory frequency and duration of inspiration. Initially, pressure-support ventilation (PSV) is set at a level to produce a tidal volume of the same size the patient is receiving on full PPV support. PSV is reduced gradually according to patient tolerance and response. Generally, weaning is considered successful when the patient can breathe spontaneously with PSV of 5 cmH$_2$O (MacIntyre and Stock, 1990) for a continuous 24-hour period.	
2. Monitor patient responses to weaning.	PSV reduces the work of breathing (Viale et al., 1988) and therefore should prevent fatigue. If the patient becomes fatigued, the level of PSV should be reevaluated.	An incompletely inflated artificial airway cuff can create a leak that prevents the PSV level from being reached during inspiration, thereby preventing the ventilator from cycling off (Burns, 1990). The patient is closely monitored for signs and symptoms of inadequate gas exchange and impaired breathing pattern.
3. Communicate with the patient throughout the weaning process.	Attention is given to the patient's psychologic response to weaning. The nurse remains with the patient for 15 to 30 minutes after each decrement in PSV level, coaches the patient with relaxation and breathing techniques, reinforces the goals and desired outcomes, reminds the patient that talking, eating, self-care activities, and mobilization will be facilitated by successful weaning and extubation, and celebrates progress with weaning with the patient.	

Evaluation

1. Evaluate progress toward achievement of the individual short-term goals every 5 to 30 minutes, as appropriate, in patients who are anticipated to be successful with weaning trial from PPV. **Rationale:** Successful weaning may be achieved within several hours in these patients if patient response is monitored closely and interventions are applied in tandem with patient response.

2. Evaluate progress toward achievement of the individual long-term goals daily in patients who are ventilator-dependent in collaboration with the physician, respiratory therapist, patient, and family as appropriate. **Rationale:** Successful weaning may be achieved within days to weeks in these patients if patient response is

methodically evaluated and interventions are applied in tandem with patient response.

3. Observe breathing pattern in response to decrements in PPV support in all patients being weaned. Note presence of accessory muscle use, retractions, tracheal tug, respiratory alternans, respiratory muscle paradox, and I:E ratio. **Rationale:** Abnormal breathing pattern may indicate either that the patient is not ready to wean or that the decrements in mechanical ventilatory support are inappropriate in magnitude or speed.

4. Evaluate changes in level of consciousness, nonverbal behavior, and patient complaints of dyspnea and/or fatigue. **Rationale:** Work of breathing may be such that the patient is maintaining adequate breathing pattern and gas exchange at the moment but does not have

sufficient reserves to continue expending energy to breathe. Patient exhaustion during weaning results in psychological and physiologic delays in the weaning progress.

5. Monitor spontaneous respiratory frequency. **Rationale:** The optimal rate and depth of breathing are those which produce adequate alveolar ventilation. Adequate alveolar ventilation can be achieved by rapid, shallow breathing or slow, deep breathing. However, when ventilation becomes rapid, the dead space ventilation per minute increases. The airflow increases, and added to the turbulence produced by the irregularity of bronchi, there is a significant impedance to ventilation. To overcome the increased airway resistance with rapid breathing, an increase in work of breathing is necessary. A spontaneous frequency of greater than 24 breaths per minute is associated with failure to wean (Shekleton et al., 1984; Tobin et al., 1986).

6. Evaluate vital capacity (see Skill 4–8). **Rationale:** Vital capacity evaluates the patient's ability to take deep breaths and cough. Generally, a vital capacity of 15 ml/kg or greater is predictive of successful weaning (Hilberman et al., 1976; Tobin et al., 1986).

7. Evaluate negative inspiratory pressure (see Skill 4–8). **Rationale:** Negative inspiratory pressure evaluates the patient's ability to generate sufficient intrathoracic pressure for deep breathing and airway clearance. Generally, a negative inspiratory pressure of -20 cmH$_2$O or greater is predictive of successful weaning (Hilberman et al., 1976; Tobin et al., 1986).

8. Evaluate spontaneous minute volume. **Rationale:** Minute volume is a proxy indicator of work of breathing. Generally, a minute volume ($\dot{V}_E$) of greater than 10 L/min indicates excessive work of breathing and that the patient will fatigue with continued spontaneous breathing (Marini and Wheeler, 1989).

9. Evaluate arterial carbon dioxide tension with spontaneous breathing. **Rationale:** PaCO$_2$ is the definitive indicator of the adequacy of ventilation. A PaCO$_2$ within the patient's normal physiologic range indicates that the patient's ventilation is adequate with spontaneous breathing. Note that if the arterial pH is less than 7.35 or greater than 7.45, the problem causing the acid–base disturbance needs to be corrected.

10. Evaluate arterial oxygen tension with spontaneous breathing. **Rationale:** PaO$_2$ is the definitive indicator of the adequacy of oxygenation. A PaO$_2$ within the patient's normal physiologic range indicates that the patient's oxygenation is adequate with spontaneous breathing. Generally, if the PaO$_2$ is greater than 60 mmHg on an FIO$_2$ of 0.4 or less, the patient can be weaned and given supplemental oxygen. It is difficult to ensure an FIO$_2$ greater than 0.4 to 0.5 with available supplementary oxygen devices. If the patient needs an FIO$_2$ greater than 0.4 to maintain adequate oxygenation, weaning should be postponed, and the patient should be placed back on PPV support until gas exchange improves.

11. Evaluate intrapulmonary shunting (see Skill 4–6). **Rationale:** In general, a shunt of less than 20 percent is one predictive criterion of successful weaning (Montenegro, 1987).

12. Monitor patient anxiety level. **Rationale:** Resumption of spontaneous breathing may cause anxiety, particularly in patients who have been on prolonged PPV support (Acosta, 1988; Bergbom-Engberg and Haljamae, 1989).

Expected Outcomes

1. Timely and successful discontinuance of PPV. **Rationale:** Appropriate discontinuance of PPV is the major purpose of weaning from PPV support. The patient is at risk for iatrogenic complications from withdrawing support too soon or continuing support too long.

2. Comfortable and adequate breathing pattern during the weaning process. **Rationale:** Weaning should progress in tandem with patient response. An uncomfortable and inadequate breathing pattern (e.g., tachypnea, respiratory alternans, accessory muscle use, abdominal paradoxical breathing) suggests that weaning attempts need to be postponed or the procedures altered (Milic-Emili, 1986; Schuster, 1990).

Unexpected Outcomes

1. Tracheal injury. **Rationale:** Prolonged PPV and an artificial airway place the patient at increased risk for acute and chronic tracheal injury (Goodnough, 1988).

2. Pulmonary barotrauma. **Rationale:** Patient–ventilator dyssynchrony during weaning with IMV or A-C modes of PPV support puts the patient at increased risk for pneumothorax, pneumomediastinum, pneumopericardium, pneumoperitoneum, and/or subcutaneous emphysema (Guthrie et al., 1983).

3. Cardiovascular depression. **Rationale:** Patient–ventilator dyssynchrony during weaning with IMV or A-C modes of PPV support puts the patient at increased risk for cardiovascular depression (Montenegro, 1987). Hyperinflation breaths used to relieve dyspnea during weaning may cause cardiovascular depression (Goodnough, 1985).

4. Fatigue. **Rationale:** Weaning that does not progress according to patient response can result in excessive work of breathing and subsequent fatigue (Breslin et al., 1990; Schuster, 1990; Shapiro et al., 1986).

5. Hypoxemia. **Rationale:** Hypoxemia during weaning indicates respiratory muscle fatigue, inefficient gas exchange, and/or excessive ventilatory requirements (Tobin et al., 1986). Weaning attempts need to be postponed or the procedures altered.

6. Hypercapnia. **Rationale:** Hypercapnia during weaning indicates respiratory muscle fatigue, inefficient gas exchange, and/or excessive ventilatory requirements (Tobin et al., 1986). Weaning attempts need to be postponed or the procedures altered.

7. Dyspnea. **Rationale:** While transient dyspnea when weaning is first initiated may be expected and tolerated, continued or escalating dyspnea means the patient is not ready to wean or that the weaning procedures need to be altered.

Documentation

Documentation in the patient record should include the individualized goals for weaning; the procedure used for weaning (e.g., T-piece, decreasing IMV/SIMV support, pressure support, PEEP, or CPAP); any of the following parameters, used to assess patient readiness to wean or tolerance of weaning: arterial blood gases, oximetry readings, vital capacity (Hilberman et al., 1976; Tobin et al., 1986), negative inspiratory pressure (Luce, 1988; MacIntyre and Stock, 1990; Marini and Wheeler, 1989; Schuster, 1990), spontaneous respiratory frequency (Shekleton et al., 1984; Tobin et al., 1986), spontaneous minute volume (Marini and Wheeler, 1989; Schuster, 1990), spontaneous maximal minute ventilation (MacIntyre and Stock, 1990), spontaneous tidal volume (Shekleton et al., 1984; Tobin et al., 1986), intrapulmonary shunt ($\dot{Q}s/\dot{Q}t$) percentage (Montenegro, 1987), work of breathing indices and measurements (Marini and Wheeler, 1989; Schuster, 1990; Shapiro et al., 1986; Shikora et al., 1990), dynamic and/or static (MacIntyre and Stock, 1990) compliance measurements, airway resistance (MacIntyre and Stock, 1990) measurement, and accessory muscle use (Breslin et al., 1990; Marini and Wheeler, 1989); and the patient response to decrements in mechanical ventilatory support. Document the time spent on T-tube, changes in IMV/SIMV rate, and patient response. Document each level of PSV and the patient's response. **Rationale:** Provides data to evaluate patient recovery and progress.

Patient/Family Education

1. Frequently provide information to the patient and family on progress with weaning. Discuss how the patient and family can help promote comfortable breathing during weaning, such as encouraging the patient to relax, using biofeedback and progressive relaxation techniques (Acosta, 1988), using the established communication methods, and promoting adequate rest. **Rationale:** Information about the patient's therapy, progress, and probable outcome is consistently cited as an important need of patients (Baier and Zimmeth, 1986; Foundation for Critical Care, 1988; Harvey et al., 1991; Viner, 1988) and families (Dunbar et al., 1990; Hickey, 1990).

2. Instruct and encourage the patient to communicate anxiety, fear, panic, and concerns about the ability to breathe with the established communication method. **Rationale:** Inability to communicate has been implicated as the dominant reason for severe emotional reactions in patients who are being weaned (Bergbom-Engberg and Haljamae, 1989). Concerns about the ability to breathe without mechanical ventilatory support are a particular problem in patients who have received prolonged PPV (Acosta, 1988; Henneman, 1989).

3. Frequently offer the opportunity for both patient and family to ask questions about the weaning procedure and progress. **Rationale:** Asking questions and having them answered honestly are cited consistently as important needs of patients (Foundation for Critical Care, 1988; Harvey et al., 1991, Viner, 1988) and families (Dunbar et al., 1990; Hickey, 1990).

4. Evaluate the patient's need for long-term mechanical ventilatory support. **Rationale:** Allows nurse to anticipate patient and family needs for the patient's discharge home on PPV.

Performance Checklist
Skill 4–9: Weaning from Positive Pressure Ventilation

Critical Behaviors	Complies	
	yes	no
WEANING TRIAL FROM **PPV**		
1. Wash hands.		
2. Don sterile gloves.		
3. Measure VC three times.		
4. Document highest VC reading.		
5. Explain the purpose and procedure of negative inspiratory pressure (NIP) to the patient.		
6. Measure NIP.		
7. Document most negative reading.		
8. Explain purpose and procedure of minute volume ($\dot{V}_E$) measurement to patient.		
9. Measure $\dot{V}_E$.		
10. Record the minute volume.		
11. Explain the purpose and procedure of T-tube to patient.		

Table continues on following page

Critical Behaviors	Complies	
	yes	no
12. Place patient on T-tube with heated aerosol.		
13. Monitor frequency, breathing pattern, heart rate, cardiac rhythm, and general appearance of the patient.		
14. Weaning as indicated.		
15. Obtain arterial blood gases (ABGs) after 30 minutes of spontaneous breathing on the T-tube.		
16. Place patient back on ventilator.		
17. Notify physician of patient response to weaning trial, including ABG results, and consult with physician regarding extubation.		
18. Document weaning data and subjective patient response to weaning trial in the patient record.		
WEANING VENTILATOR-DEPENDENT PATIENTS 1. Wash hands.		
2. Proceed with steps in the decision tree algorithm for ventilator-dependent patients (Fig. 4–14).		
3. Devise weaning plan and schedule (if appropriate).		
4. Remain with the patient for 15 to 30 minutes after decrement in PPV support.		
5. Monitor patient response to weaning.		
6. Communicate with patient throughout the weaning process.		
7. Document decrements in PPV support and patient responses to weaning in the patient record.		

SKILL 4–10

Management of High-Frequency Ventilation (HFV)

Positive-pressure ventilation (PPV) provides tidal volumes in excess of dead space volume by providing bulk gas flow into the lung. Oxygen and carbon dioxide diffusion occur at a rate determined by their respective alveolar-arterial gradients. The rate and distribution of the bulk gas flow are a function of airway resistance and lung compliance. High airway resistance and low lung compliance necessitate that bulk gas flow be delivered to the lung at high pressures. The high pressures put the patient at increased risk for pulmonary barotrauma and cardiovascular depression.

High-frequency ventilation (HFV) is a method of mechanical ventilatory support that uses faster respiratory rates (60 to 3000 oscillations per minute) and lower tidal volumes than PPV (Table 4–7). The tidal volumes used may be less than dead space volume. The rate and distribution of gas to the lung with HFV effect acceptable gas exchange, but the physiologic mechanisms differ from those with PPV. The physiologic mechanisms to explain gas exchange with HFV are hypothetical and multiple. The reader is referred to other texts for an indepth discussion of the postulated theories of axial transport of gas with radial mixing, convective exchange at the bifurcations, asynchronous alveolar ventilation, and regional variations in dead space volume (Supinski and Silverman, 1987, pp. 49–83). The theoretical advantage of HFV is that the small tidal volumes used result in lower peak inspiratory pressures than with PPV, thus reducing the incidences of barotrauma and cardiovascular depression. However, studies have suggested that the incidences of these iatrogenic complications are not reduced markedly with HFV as compared with PPV (Carlon and Howland, 1985; Carlon et al., 1983; Nochomovitz and Montenegro, 1987; Pilbeam, 1986).

Different modes of HFV are compared in Table 4–8. High-frequency positive-pressure ventilation (HFPPV) is analogous to PPV but with faster rates. Each breath is pushed into the lungs through a pneumatic or solenoid valve instead of being pumped into the lungs with a mechanical on–off valve. HFPPV is delivered through an

TABLE 4–7 COMPARISON OF POSITIVE-PRESSURE VENTILATION (PPV) WITH HIGH-FREQUENCY VENTILATION (HFV)

Parameter	PPV	HFV
Tidal volume	Greater than dead space, 10–15 ml/kg	Greater than or equal to dead space, <5 ml/kg
Frequency	<30 breaths per minute	>60–3000 breaths per minute
Inspiratory time	0.8–1.2 seconds	<0.3 seconds

TABLE 4–8 COMPARISON OF DIFFERENT MODES OF HIGH-FREQUENCY VENTILATION (HFV)

Parameter	HFPPV*	HFJV	HFO
Tidal volume	3–5 ml/kg	2–5 ml/kg	1–3 ml/kg (50–100 ml)
Frequency	60–150 breaths per min	100–300 breaths per min	900–30000 oscillations per min
Inspiratory time	<0.3 seconds	<0.2 seconds	Not applicable

*HFPPV = high-frequency positive-pressure ventilation; HFJV = high-frequency jet ventilation; HFO = high-frequency oscillation.

endotracheal or tracheostomy tube in the conventional manner. The frequency used varies from 60 breaths per minute to 150 breaths per minute, or 1 to 2.5 hertz (Hz).* HFPPV requires a ventilator with negligible compressible volume. Tidal volume is usually 3 to 4 ml/kg. The I:E ratio varies from 1:2 to 1:5. Peak inspiratory pressure (PIP) is low, proportional to the tidal volume. Airway pressure exceeds atmospheric pressure throughout inspiration and expiration. HFPPV has been used during bronchosurgery and laryngoscopy and for surgical anesthesia when the need exists for eliminating respiratory movements during thoracic surgery. HFPPV also has been used in combination with PEEP and in preterm infants with hyaline membrane disease (Supinski and Silverman, 1987).

High-frequency jet ventilation (HFJV) is based on the physical principles of the jet injector. A high-pressure source is used to deliver short bursts of gas into the airway. A fluid, pneumatic, or solenoid mechanism controls gas flow from the pressure source to the patient. HFJV is delivered through a small-bore cannula placed in the airway (Fig. 4–15) or through a 14-gauge needle placed at the elbow connector of an IMV ventilator circuit (Allen, 1989). HFJV requires a jet ventilator. Air from a second gas source (usually a backup positive-pressure ventilator) can be entrained by the jet stream (Pilbeam, 1986). The frequency used varies from 100 to 300 oscillations per minute (1.7 to 5 Hz). Tidal volume is usually 3 to 4 ml/kg. The I:E ratio varies from 1:2 to 1:5. PIP is a function of flow rate but is generally low. With HFJV, approximately three times the minute ventilation used with PPV is required to produce the same amount of alveolar ventilation (Supinski and Silverman, 1987).

High-frequency oscillation (HFO) produces oscillation of the column of gas present in the airway. A piston pump or radio loudspeaker is used to cause the vibrations, or oscillations. Fresh gas is provided through a side intake port, and old gas is vented through a side exit port placed at right angles to the piston. The cycles used vary from 900 to 3000 oscillations per minute (15 to 50 Hz). Tidal volume is usually 50 to 100 ml, less than the anatomic dead space volume (144 to 150 ml in the adult). The I:E ratio is 1:1. PIP is low. Airway pressures swing to negative values during the piston backstroke (Supinski and Silverman, 1987). HFO has been used in patients with ventilatory failure and in neonates with hyaline membrane disease.

HFV is not routinely used in practice. Clinical experience with HFV remains limited to procedures that are short term (e.g., laryngoscopy and bronchoscopy) and that require an immobilized surgical field (e.g., tracheal reconstruction) and in patients with bronchopleural or tracheoesophageal fistulas in whom adequate ventilation cannot be achieved with PPV. HFV has not been shown to offer any significant advantage over PPV to date (Allen, 1989; Burns, 1990; Hamilton et al., 1986; Martin, 1987; Pittet et al., 1990; Supinski and Silverman, 1987). Prospective studies with random assignment to PPV and HFV have shown the treatment modalities to be equivalent. No difference was found between groups in survival (Carlon et al., 1983), duration of respiratory support (Carlon et al., 1983), barotrauma (Carlon et al., 1983), cardiovascular depression (Sladen et al., 1984a, 1984b), intracranial pressure (Pittet et al., 1990), and cerebral blood flow (Pittet et al., 1990). The Food and Drug Administration has approved HFJV and HFPPV devices, up to rates of 150 breaths per minute, for treatment of bronchopleural fistulas, laryngoscopy, and bronchoscopy. Investigational approval and patient informed consent should be obtained for all other uses of HFV.

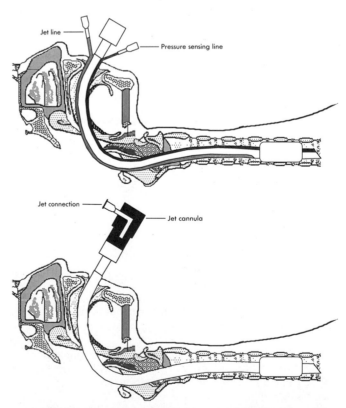

FIGURE 4–15. Diagram of high-frequency jet tube and cannula. (Reproduced with permission from S. P. McPherson, *Respiratory Therapy Equipment*, 4th Ed. St. Louis: Mosby, 1990, p. 177.)

*Note: 1 hertz (Hz) = 60 cycles per minute.

As with other methods of mechanical ventilatory support, iatrogenic complications are associated with the use of HFV modes. Potential complications from HFV therapy in general include airway obstruction from inadequate humidification of inspired gas, lung and airway damage from high-velocity streams of inspired gas, cardiac depression from the development of auto-PEEP, weaning failures, inadequate gas exchange from difficulty with monitoring airway pressures and ventilation volumes, mechanical failure of HFV ventilators, and inadvertent asymmetrical ventilation.

Purpose

The nurse manages high-frequency ventilation to

1. Achieve the goal of timely and successful discontinuance of mechanical ventilatory support and artificial airway.
2. Maximize oxygen delivery.
3. Maintain adequate ventilation.
4. Minimize the side effects of HFV.

Prerequisite Knowledge and Skills

Prior to managing the patient with high-frequency ventilation, the nurse should understand

1. Anatomy and physiology of the upper and lower respiratory systems.
2. Principles of airway management.
3. Principles of gas exchange.
4. Principles of airway resistance.
5. Principles of lung compliance (see Skill 4–4).
6. Principles of mucociliary transport.
7. Principles of high-frequency ventilation.
8. Mechanics of the HFV mode to be used.
9. Verbal and nonverbal communication strategies.
10. Principles of metal fatigue.
11. Principles of humidification.
12. Principles of airway pressure.
13. Principles of informed consent.
14. Principles of auto-PEEP (see Skill 4–7).
15. Principles of aseptic technique.
16. Stress and coping theory.
17. Principles of nutrition.

The nurse should be able to perform

1. Proper handwashing technique (see Skill 35–5).
2. Vital signs assessment.
3. Oxygen administration and ventilation via manual self-inflating resuscitation bag (see Skill 4–2).
4. Respiratory assessment (inspection, palpation, percussion, and auscultation).
5. Hemodynamic assessment.
6. Confirmation of endotracheal tube placement.
7. Endotracheal suctioning (see Skill 1–6).
8. Nasopharyngeal and oropharyngeal suctioning (see Skill 1–2).
9. Determination of auto-PEEP (see Skill 4–7).
10. Integrated assessment of psychosocial and physiologic needs.

11. Communication with an intubated patient.
12. Decompression of a tension pneumothorax.

Assessment

1. Observe for signs and symptoms of inadequate ventilation, including rising arterial carbon dioxide tension (definitive sign), dyspnea, headache, restlessness, tachypnea, confusion, lethargy, rising (early sign) or falling (late sign) arterial blood pressure, tachycardia, and atrial and/or ventricular dysrhythmias. **Rationale:** Assess success of ventilation.
2. Monitor arterial carbon dioxide tension and pH. **Rationale:** Inadequate ventilation is confirmed by acute or chronic respiratory acidosis with a $PaCO_2$ greater than 45 mmHg or an absolute $PaCO_2$ that exceeds the therapeutic guidelines for arterial carbon dioxide level.
3. Observe for signs and symptoms of inadequate oxygenation, including falling arterial oxygen tension (definitive sign), tachypnea, dyspnea, central cyanosis, restlessness, confusion, agitation, tachycardia (early sign), bradycardia (late sign), dysrhythmias, rising (early sign) or falling (late sign) arterial blood pressure, falling urine output, and metabolic acidosis. **Rationale:** Adequate oxygenation is a goal of mechanical ventilatory support. If adequate oxygenation cannot be maintained with PPV, a trial of HFV may be indicated.
4. Monitor arterial oxygen tension or saturation. **Rationale:** Hypoxemia is confirmed by a falling PaO_2 and/or SaO_2 or an absolute PaO_2 that exceeds the therapeutic guidelines for arterial oxygen level.
5. Assess for signs and symptoms of pulmonary barotrauma, including acute, increasing, or severe dyspnea, restlessness, agitation, and panic, localized changes in auscultation, localized hyperresonance or tympany to percussion, increased breathing effort, tracheal deviation away from the side of abnormal findings, increased PIP, decreased compliance, decreased PaO_2 or SaO_2 with constant ventilator parameters, subcutaneous emphysema, and localized intrapleural air ("black out," lucency) on chest radiograph. **Rationale:** Early detection minimizes progression and the adverse effects on the patient.
6. Observe for signs of cardiovascular depression, including an acute or gradual fall in arterial blood pressure, tachycardia (early sign), bradycardia (late sign), dysrhythmias, weak peripheral pulses, decreased pulse pressure, acute or gradual increase in pulmonary capillary wedge pressure, decreased mixed venous oxygen tension, and a widened $a-\bar{v}DO_2$. **Rationale:** HFV provides alveolar ventilation at lower peak inspiratory pressures, and should have less adverse effects on the cardiovascular system than PPV.

Nursing Diagnoses

1. Impaired verbal communication related to presence of artificial airway. **Rationale:** HFV may be administered with the cuff inflated or deflated. A deflated cuff impairs vocalization, and an inflated cuff prevents vocalization.

2. Impaired coping of the family related to the critical care experience and HFV. **Rationale:** The critical care experience disrupts the usual routines, roles, and relationships of the family (Halm, 1990; LaMontagne and Pawlak, 1990). In addition, limited access to the patient because of restricted visiting hours and the uncertainty about the patient's welfare cause stress for the family members (Dunbar et al., 1990; Foundation for Critical Care, 1988; Jacono et al., 1990; LaMontagne and Pawlak, 1990; Mishel, 1988; Riegel and Ehrenrich, 1989).

3. Fear related to uncertainty about prognosis and inadequate information or understanding of the critical care experience. **Rationale:** While the causes may be diverse and variable for a given patient, the transient or prolonged feeling of fear is common in patients on mechanical ventilatory support (Bergbom-Engberg and Haljamae, 1989).

4. Impaired airway clearance related to decreased mucociliary transport and abnormal viscosity of mucus. **Rationale:** HFV poses problems with the humidification of inspired gas, resulting in viscid secretions that can cause airway obstruction (Kan et al., 1990; Supinski and Silverman, 1987). Conventional humidifiers cannot operate at the high pressures used with HFV; therefore, special attention must be devoted to providing heated humidification of jet-stream gas and entrained air. The mucous plugging seen with HFV modes may be due to inadequate humidification (Kan et al., 1990), disruption of mucociliary transport, or other unknown mechanisms. In contrast, some reports have suggested that HFO actually facilitates airway clearance by vibrating secretions off the mucosa so that they can be effectively cleared by coughing and suctioning.

5. Potential for suffocation related to obstructed airway or mechanical failure. **Rationale:** Clinical experience with HFV has demonstrated significant problems with bronchial mucous plugging and inspissated secretions. The mucous plugging may be due to inadequate humidification, disruption of mucociliary transport, or unknown mechanisms. Although strides have been made in humidification techniques recently, the patient on HFV is at risk for obstructed airway. Life expectancies of the solenoid valve differ, depending on the device and manufacturer. Given the wear and tear on a mechanical component that must open and close up to 435,000 times a day, mechanical failure is a potential problem. Spare parts and personnel trained in replacing them should be available when HFV is used.

Planning

1. Individualize the following goals for managing the patient on high-frequency ventilation.
   a. Maintain or improve ventilation. **Rationale:** High-frequency ventilation will be needed until the underlying problem causing inadequate ventilation is corrected. The guidelines may be more strict with HFV owing to the experimental nature of this therapy as compared with PPV.
   b. Maintain or improve oxygenation. **Rationale:** HFV will be needed until the patient is able to maintain an adequate PaO_2.
   c. Initiate effective HFV. **Rationale:** The circuits, valves, injector, and other components of HFV ventilators determine the optimal functioning of the equipment and are unique to each ventilator. The ventilator should be tested clinically with the physician and respiratory therapist present at the bedside prior to developing guidelines for use in patient populations.
   d. Improve patient's nutritional needs. Consult with a registered dietician if indicated. **Rationale:** HFV interrupts normal gastrointestinal tract function. Caloric and nitrogen needs for a normal, hypocatabolic, or hypercatabolic state can be met with total parenteral nutrition or enteral feeding.

2. Assemble and check all necessary supplies and equipment. **Rationale:** Equipment and supplies need to be readily available and functional to initiate HFV and to immediately troubleshoot problems that may occur during initiation.
   a. Manual self-inflating resuscitation bag capable of delivering 100% oxygen and large inflation volumes.
   b. Appropriately sized resuscitation face mask that will attach to the manual resuscitation bag.
   c. Multiple oxygen sources (e.g., for high-frequency ventilator, backup ventilator, HFV humidifier, resuscitation bag, etc.).
   d. Functional humidifier with in-line thermometer for measuring inspired gas temperature of backup ventilator.
   e. Functional humidification system for high-frequency ventilator.
   f. Oxygen analyzer.
   g. Distilled sterile water.
   h. Swivel adapter.
   i. Replacement artificial airway.
   j. Replacement high-frequency jet tube, small-bore cannula (see Fig. 4-15), or 14-gauge needle for HFV.
   k. Exam gloves.
   l. Sterile gloves.
   m. Suction equipment (see Skills 1–4, 1–6).
   n. Tonsil sucker.
   o. Manometer for measuring cuff pressure (see Skill 1–7).
   p. Rubber-tipped clamp or hemostat.
   q. Syringe appropriate for cuff size.
   r. Chest tube insertion tray.
   s. Extra 14-gauge needles at the bedside for emergency tension pneumothorax decompression.
   t. Writing pad or other implement for patient communication.
   u. Call bell within patient reach.
   v. Functional ventilator alarms for backup ventilator and high-frequency ventilator.
   w. Stethoscope.
   x. Chest x-ray viewing capability.
   y. Sterile scissors.

z. Water-insoluble marker.

aa. Tincture of benzoin (or comparable preparation).

bb. Low-trauma suction catheters (see Skills 1–4 and 1–6).

cc. Container for draining condensate from ventilator tubing.

dd. PEEP valve or other apparatus if patient is on therapeutic PEEP.

ee. Second hand on watch, clock, or chronometer.

ff. Bite block or nasal or oral airway.

3. Prepare patient and family.

a. Explain the procedure(s) and why HFV is being initiated. **Rationale:** Anxiety is reduced when patients are prepared for the sensations they may experience during procedures (CURN Project, 1981; Johnson, 1972; Johnson et al., 1978).

b. Ensure that informed consent and/or investigational approval has been obtained. **Rationale:** The FDA has approved HFJV and HFPPV for the treatment of bronchopleural fistulas, laryngoscopy, and bronchoscopy. All other uses should have patient informed consent.

c. Perform frequent respiratory assessments. **Rationale:** Changes in respiratory assessment may indicate pulmonary complication or deteriorating respiratory status. Auscultatory changes in distribution of HFV flow or adventitious breath sounds should be explored. The inability to accurately measure distal airway pressure and delivered volume mandates vigilant attention to respiratory rate and pattern as proxy indicators of effective ventilation. A change in the presence or character of spontaneous ventilation should be explored. Auscultation should be done with the patient on HFV and with bagging. The turbulent flow generated with HFV requires a sensitive ear and practice with listening skills to differentiate interpretable changes. Spontaneous ventilation is suppressed in many patients receiving HFV. Tachypnea, in particular, may indicate the development of complications.

d. Check for secure stabilization of the artificial airway. **Rationale:** Reduces the risk of inadvertent extubation.

e. Check that replacement artificial airway and jet cannula or catheter, if appropriate, are readily available at the head of the patient's bed. **Rationale:** Ensures quick reestablishment of patent airway in the event of inadvertent extubation. Ensures that the type and size of replacements match the indwelling ones.

f. Place manual self-inflating resuscitation bag with supplemental oxygen continuously on at 15 L/min to "flush" and appropriately sized face masks at head of the bed. **Rationale:** Provides capability for immediately delivering ventilation and oxygenation to relieve acute respiratory distress due to hypoxemia, acidosis, or ventilator failure. Attach a PEEP valve if the patient is on PEEP.

Implementation

Steps	Rationale	Special Considerations
1. Wash hands.	Reduces transmission of microorganisms.	
2. Check ventilators for baseline parameters.	Ensures that ordered ventilator parameters are used.	
3. Check FiO_2 of both HFV flow and entrained gas.	Ensures actual oxygen concentration delivered is correct and duplicated in both gas sources.	
4. Frequently perform visual monitoring checks of airway pressure, cycles or hertz, amplitude, and PEEP or CPAP when used.	Ensures that any changes will be detected and explored quickly.	
5. Monitor patient response to changes in ventilator parameters.	Changes in driving pressure, inspiratory time, and/or cycles directly affect tidal volume and $PaCO_2$ and indirectly affect PaO_2. Changes in PEEP or CPAP directly affect PaO_2.	Higher frequencies (cycles, hertz) will result in lower delivered volume if inspiratory time remains constant. Expiration requires adequate time to prevent air trapping (auto-PEEP), which will increase mean airway pressure, increase the risk of barotrauma and cardiovascular depression, and increase dead space–to–tidal volume ratio. High PEEP or

Table continues on following page

Steps	Rationale	Special Considerations
		CPAP levels may alter the performance of the ventilator with a built-in demand valve (Gallagher, 1985). Modifications of the controls may be needed to maintain arterial blood gases within the therapeutic guidelines.
6. Frequently assess patency of the airway.	HFV poses particular problems with the humidification of inspired gas, resulting in mucous plugging and inspissated secretions that can cause airway obstruction.	Depending on the HFV setup, caution must be exercised when the driving pressure is changed. The humidification infusion rates must be altered to prevent excessive amounts of water from entering the airway (Kan et al., 1990).
7. Monitor tidal volume directly, if possible, or with the use of proxy measures such as verification of chest movements or recording of amplitude displacement.	Verification of chest movements or vibrations is recommended as an indicator of adequate tidal volume (Gallagher, 1985). Amplitude displacement can be used to display changes in airway pressure from baseline with each breath.	Airway pressures must be measured distal to the injector cannula with HFJV. Ensure that the tubing used for pressure monitoring remains patent. Frequent flushing of this line with normal saline is necessary to prevent clogging (Supinski and Silverman, 1987).
8. Frequently assess the patient for signs and symptoms of atelectasis, pulmonary barotrauma, cardiovascular depression, and nosocomial lung infection.	Early detection of pulmonary complications during HFV ensures appropriate treatment to promote resolution and prevent further complication(s).	
9. Evaluate the need for a nasogastric tube.	Reduces risk of aspiration and decompresses to stomach.	
10. Perform "quick check" evaluations at least hourly and after position change, suctioning, chest physiotherapy, and visits to the bedside by others of chest movement, breath sounds, vital signs, ventilator sounds, all connections and alarm settings, airway pressure, driving pressure, cycles, I:E ratio, PEEP or CPAP, and FiO_2.	The critical care nurse bears continuous and ultimate accountability for monitoring the patient–ventilator interaction and the development of complications.	

Evaluation

1. Evaluate progress toward discontinuance of high-frequency ventilation daily. Indicators of progress toward this goal include: decreasing levels of PEEP, supplemental oxygen, and driving pressure with corresponding stability or improvement in arterial blood gases; improvement of underlying pathology for which HFV was initiated and maintained; stability or improvement in hemodynamic parameters; and patient's ability to assume increasing proportions of minute ventilation. **Rationale:** Achieving the overriding goal of timely and successful discontinuance of HFV requires daily assessment of progress.

2. Monitor for adequacy of ventilation. **Rationale:** Adequate ventilation is a goal of HFV. Inadequate ventilation can be corrected by increasing the driving pressure or changing the inspiratory time (Carlon and Howland, 1985; Supinski and Silverman, 1987).

3. Monitor for adequacy of oxygenation. **Rationale:** Adequate oxygenation is a goal of HFV. Inadequate oxygenation may be addressed by changes in ventilatory parameters or by switching the patient to positive-pressure ventilation (PPV).

4. Monitor arterial blood gases. **Rationale:** Rapid changes in PaO_2 and $PaCO_2$ may occur with a change in one or more HFV ventilator parameters.

5. Monitor patient response to changes in driving pressure. **Rationale:** Driving pressure affects tidal volume and $PaCO_2$ directly and PaO_2 indirectly. Driving pressure is linearly correlated to flow rate (Gallagher, 1985) and therefore tidal volume, which is a function of flow rate and inspiratory time.

6. Monitor inspiratory time or I:E ratio for any

change in frequency. **Rationale:** Higher frequencies will result in lower delivered volume if inspiratory time remains constant. Expiration requires adequate time to prevent air trapping (auto-PEEP), which will increase mean airway pressure, increase the risk of barotrauma, and increase dead space–to–tidal volume ratio (VD/VT).

7. Monitor tidal volume directly, if possible, or by the use of proxy measures. **Rationale:** Accurate, direct measurement of tidal volume is very difficult with HFV. The techniques used to monitor volume and airway pressure with PPV cannot be applied to HFV because of the rapid changes in flow waveforms. The dead space of spirometers generally used for PPV is too large for the small volumes delivered with HFV. Pneumotachographs have inadequate response time to the high frequencies used with HFV. Experts recommend verifying the presence of chest movements as an indicator of adequate tidal volume (Gallagher, 1985). Although this is possible with HFPPV and HFJV, it is extremely difficult with HFO. Amplitude displacement can be used to display changes in airway pressure from the baseline with each breath. *Caution:* Airway pressures must be measured distal to the injector cannula with HFJV. Ensure that the tubing used for pressure monitoring remains patent. Frequent flushing of this line with normal saline is necessary to prevent clogging from airway secretions (Supinski and Silverman, 1987).

8. Monitor patient response to the addition of or change in PEEP or CPAP. **Rationale:** High PEEP or CPAP levels may alter the performance of the ventilator with a built-in demand valve (Gallagher, 1985). Modifications of the controls may be necessary to restore original arterial blood gas levels.

9. Continuously monitor or periodically check mean airway pressure and PEEP or CPAP with a strip-chart recorder, if appropriate. **Rationale:** The manometer pressure gauge on the HFV ventilator may be damped to prevent uncontrolled oscillation. The gauge will reflect an approximation of pressure only. A rapidly responding strip-chart recorder will give accurate measurements. Newer machines have an oscilloscopic display; when properly calibrated, the measurements are accurate and a recording is unnecessary. The level of PEEP or CPAP is read as the lowest pressure recorded or displayed during mechanical breathing (Gallagher, 1985).

10. Monitor the oxygen concentration of entrained gas and jet gas. **Rationale:** Accurate FIO_2 depends on the entrained gas being kept at the same concentration as the jet flow. Generally, this is achieved by using the same oxygen blender for both gas sources.

11. Constantly evaluate the interaction between the control settings of HFV and patient response. **Rationale:** Inadequate oxygenation can be corrected by higher PEEP/CPAP, increasing inspiratory time, increasing driving pressure, and increasing frequency. Each strategy for improving oxygenation is subject to potential adverse effects. Higher PEEP/CPAP will increase mean airway pressure, which may decrease venous return and depress cardiovascular function. Prolonging inspiratory time may have the same result. Increasing driving pressure will improve oxygenation if the I:E ratio is adjusted appro-

priately. If the expiratory phase is too short, auto-PEEP will develop with the attendant risk of barotrauma and possible cardiovascular depression. Increasing frequency may have the same result as increasing driving pressure. *Caution* must be exercised whenever the driving pressure is changed. The humidification infusion rates must be altered to prevent excessive amounts of water from entering the airway (Kan et al., 1990; Pilbeam, 1986). Excessive water can lead to fluid overload, particularly in infants and children, and can alter the function of the mucociliary system.

12. Continuously monitor patient response to HFV, particularly during the first 2 hours the patient is placed on HFV. **Rationale:** Our understanding of the mechanisms of respiratory failure and HFV is incomplete. HFV remains experimental despite its introduction in 1915 (Carlon and Howland, 1985) and both clinical and experimental use over the past 20 years. Patients sometimes deteriorate when placed on HFV and must be converted to PPV. At other times, HFV fails to improve gas exchange compared with PPV, and the benefit of using experimental technology is questionable.

13. Monitor carbon dioxide levels with transcutaneous PCO_2 analyzers. **Rationale:** Breath-to-breath measurements with carbon dioxide monitors cannot be used because of the slow response time of infrared analyzers. Additionally, gases sampled at the expiratory port do not represent alveolar gas during HFV and therefore cannot be used as a reliable indicator of arterial carbon dioxide values (Supinski and Silverman, 1987).

14. Ensure that the expiratory limb of the HFV circuit is open. **Rationale:** Occlusion can cause a rapid rise in airway pressure to dangerous levels. Airway pressure monitors and alarms are essential with HFV. A mechanism must exist to interrupt the solenoid valve to prevent jetting of gas, and the development of higher pressures, in the event of impediment to full expiration.

Expected Outcomes

1. Timely and successful discontinuance of HFV. **Rationale:** Appropriate discontinuance of all mechanical ventilatory support is the major purpose of any mode of mechanical ventilation, including HFV.

2. Maintenance of adequate $PaCO_2$ and PaO_2. **Rationale:** Adequate ventilation and oxygenation is a major purpose for initiation of HFV. If this outcome cannot be achieved within 1 to 2 hours of initiating HFV or making adjustments in HFV parameters, the patient should be switched to a nonexperimental mode of mechanical ventilation.

Unexpected Outcomes

1. Pulmonary barotrauma. **Rationale:** HFV increases mean airway pressure and alveolar pressure progressively with increasing frequency and driving pressure (Carlon and Howland, 1985).

2. Cardiovascular depression. **Rationale:** Although theoretically HFV should produce fewer adverse effects on the cardiovascular system than PPV, investigators have reported mixed effects of HFV on cardiovascular function (Carlon and Howland, 1985; Supinski and Sil-

verman, 1987). Like barotrauma, cardiovascular effects appear to be a function of mean airway pressure rather than peak airway pressure.

3. Tracheal injury. **Rationale:** Inadequate humidification and the high-velocity gas streams with HFV damage the tracheobronchial mucosa.

4. Severe emotional reactions during HFV. **Rationale:** Patients generally report greater comfort with HFV than with PPV. This comfort, as well as the apnea usually experienced, should decrease anxiety, fear, agony, panic, and insecurity reported retrospectively by patients who have been on PPV (Bergbom-Engberg and Haljamae, 1989). However, if barriers to communication produce the psychosocial stresses (Bergbom-Engberg and Haljamae, 1989), the patient on HFV may experience anxiety, fear, agony, and panic.

Documentation

Documentation in the patient record should include date and time patient is placed on HFV and when discontinued; mode of HFV, type of HFV ventilator and set parameters, type of backup ventilator and set parameters, other pertinent parameters specific to the ventilator(s) being used; FiO_2, I:E ratio, PEEP/CPAP; patient's indication of level of comfort and respiratory complaints, hemodynamic and vital signs responses, respiratory assessment findings, neurologic responses, arterial blood gas results following a change in parameters; adjuncts for delivering HFV (e.g., no. 8.5 NCC Hi-Lo endotracheal tube inserted 01/09/91 and 14 gauge jet cannula inserted 01/10/91), cuff pressure measurements with dates and times taken, and signs and symptoms indicating an iatrogenic complication and subsequent interventions. **Rationale:** Provides data to evaluate effectiveness of therapy and demonstrates appropriate linkages between assessment, monitoring, and intervention.

Patient/Family Education

1. Frequently provide information to the patient and family on progress toward the individualized goals of HFV. Discuss how the patient and family can help promote the patient's recovery during HFV. **Rationale:** Information about the patient's condition and therapy, prognosis, progress, and probable outcome is consistently cited as an important need of patients (Baier and Zimmeth, 1986; Foundation for Critical Care, 1988; Harvey, et al., 1991; Viner, 1988) and families (Hickey, 1990).

2. Teach the family how to perform desired and appropriate activities of direct patient care, such as pharyngeal suction with the tonsil sucker, range-of-motion exercises, hygiene tasks. **Rationale:** Family members have identified the need to help in the patient's care (Daley, 1984; Dunbar et al., 1990; Harvey et al., 1991; O'Neill-Norris and Grove, 1986).

3. Instruct and encourage the patient to communicate anxiety, fear, panic, concerns about security, and needs with the established communication method. **Rationale:** Inability to communicate has been implicated as the dominant reason for severe emotional reactions in patients who experienced mechanical ventilation. The isolation due to communication difficulties was seen as a greater problem than activities related to the direct airway and ventilator (Baier and Zimmeth, 1986; Bergbom-Engberg and Haljamae, 1989; Harvey et al.)

4. Frequently offer the opportunity for both patient and family to ask questions about the management of HFV. **Rationale:** In many situations, HFV is experimental therapy. Asking questions and having them answered honestly are cited consistently as the most important needs of patients (Bergbom-Engberg and Haljamae, 1989; Foundation for Critical Care, 1988; Harvey et al.; Viner, 1988) and families (Hickey, 1990).

5. Evaluate the patient's need for long-term mechanical ventilation. **Rationale:** At this point in time, the patient will not leave the critical care unit on HFV. However, the patient may be discharged with PPV. Anticipating the need for long-term PPV allows the nurse to begin patient and family preparation.

Performance Checklist
Skill 4–10: Management of High-Frequency Ventilation (HFV)

Critical Behaviors	Complies	
	yes	no
1. Wash hands.		
2. Check ventilators for baseline parameters.		
3. Check FiO_2 of both HFV flow and entrained gas.		
4. Frequently perform visual monitoring checks of airway pressure, cycles or hertz, amplitude, and PEEP/CPAP when used.		
5. Monitor patient response to changes in ventilator parameters.		
6. Frequently assess patency of the airway.		
7. Monitor tidal volume.		

Table continues on following page

Critical Behaviors	Complies	
	yes	no
8. Frequently assess the patient for signs and symptoms of atelectasis, pulmonary barotrauma, cardiovascular depression, and nosocomial lung infection.		
9. Evaluate the need for a nasogastric tube.		
10. Perform "quick check" evaluations at least hourly and after position change, suctioning, chest physiotherapy, and visits to the bedside by others of chest movement, breath sounds, vital signs, ventilator sounds, all connections and alarm settings, airway pressure, driving pressure, cycles, I:E ratio, PEEP or CPAP, and FiO_2.		
11. Document the following in the patient record: date and time HFV initiated; mode of HFV, type of HFV ventilator and set parameters, type of backup ventilator and set parameters, and other pertinent parameters specific to the ventilator(s) being used; patient responses to HFV and to changes in ventilatory parameters; and signs and symptoms indicating an iatrogenic complication and subsequent interventions.		

REFERENCES

Acosta, F. (1988). Biofeedback and progressive relaxation in weaning the anxious patient from the ventilator: A brief report. *Heart Lung* 17(3): 299–301.

Allard, K. S. (1991). Mechanical Ventilation. In *Cardiopulmonary Emergencies* (pp. 287–322). Springhouse, Pa.: Springhouse Corporation.

Allen, S. J. (1989). HFJV, PS, IRV, MMV, APRV: "New" Ventilatory Modes. In T. H. Stanley and R. J. Sperry (Eds.), *Anesthesia and the Lung* (pp. 215–219). Boston: Kluwer Academic Publishers.

AACN (1990). *Outcome Standards for Nursing Care of the Critically Ill.* Laguna Niguel, Calif.: American Association of Critical Care Nurses.

Askanazi, J., Elwyn, D. H., Silverberg, P. A., et al. (1980). Respiratory distress secondary to a high carbohydrate load: A case report. *Surgery* 87: 596.

Baier, S., and Zimmeth, M. (1986). *Bed Number Ten.* New York: CRC Press.

Banner, M. J. (1985). Technical aspects of high frequency ventilation. *Curr. Rev. Respir. Ther.* 7: 89.

Bergbom-Engberg, I., and Haljamae, H. (1989). Assessment of patients' experience of discomforts during respirator therapy. *Crit. Care Med.* 17(10): 1068–1072.

Bernhard, W. N., Yost, L., Joynes, D., et al. (1982). Just seal intracuff pressures during mechanical ventilation. *Anesthesiology* 57: A145.

Bone, R. C. (1985). Monitoring Respiratory and Hemodynamic Function in the Patient with Respiratory Failure. In R. R. Kirby, R. A. Smith, and D. A. Desautels (Eds.), *Mechanical Ventilation* (pp. 137–170). New York: Churchill-Livingstone.

Bone, R. C. (1988). Respiratory Monitoring. In R. J. Fallat and J. M. Luce (Eds.), *Cardiopulmonary Critical Care Management* (pp. 89–111). New York: Churchill-Livingstone.

Bone, R. C., Gravenstein, N., and Kirby, R. R. (1990). Monitoring Respiratory and Hemodynamic Function in the Patient with Respiratory Failure. In R. R. Kirby, M. J. Banner, and J. B. Downs (Eds.), *Clinical Applications of Ventilatory Support* (pp. 301–336). New York: Churchill-Livingstone.

Bostick, J., and Wendelgass, S. T. (1987). Normal saline instillation as part of the suctioning procedure: Effects on PaO_2 and amount of secretions. *Heart Lung* 16(5): 532–537.

Breslin, E. H., Garoutte, B. C., Kohlman-Carrieri, V., and Celli, B. R. (1990). Correlations between dyspnea, diaphragm and sternomastoid recruitment during inspiratory resistance breathing in normal subjects. *Chest* 98(2): 298–302.

Bryan-Brown, C. W. (1986). Ventilatory Management of Cardiovascular Disease. In L. C. Weeks (Ed.), *Advanced Cardiovascular Nursing* (pp. 705–725). Boston: Blackwell Scientific.

Burns, S. M. (1990). Advances in ventilator therapy. *Focus Crit. Care* 17(3): 227–237.

Carlon, G. C., Howland, W. S., and Ray, C. (1983). High frequency jet ventilation: A prospective randomized evaluation. *Chest* 84: 551.

Carlon, G. C., and Howland, W. S. (Eds.) (1985). *High-Frequency Ventilation in Intensive Care and During Surgery.* New York: Marcel Dekker.

Chulay, M. (1988). Arterial blood gas changes with a hyperinflation and hyperoxygenation suctioning intervention in critically ill patients. *Heart Lung* 17(6): 654–661.

Chulay, M., Brown, J., and Summer, W. (1982). Effect of postoperative immobilization after coronary artery bypass. *Crit. Care Med.* 10(3): 176–179.

Craig, C. P., and Connelly, S. (1984). Effect of intensive care unit nosocomial pneumonia on duration of stay and mortality. *Am. J. Infect. Control* 12: 233–238.

Craven, D. E., Lichtenberg, D. A., and Goularte, T. A. (1984). Contaminated medication nebulizers in mechanical ventilator circuits. *Am. J. Med.* 77: 834.

Craven, D. E., Kunches, L. M., Kilinsky, V., et al. (1986). Risk factors for pneumonia and fatality in patients receiving continuous mechanical ventilation. *Am. Rev. Respir. Dis.* 133: 792–796.

CURN Project (1981). *Distress Reduction Through Sensory Preparation.* New York: Grune & Stratton.

Daley, L. (1984). The perceived immediate needs of families with relatives in the intensive care setting. *Heart Lung* 13: 231–237.

Daly, B. J., and Allen, M. L. (1987). Nursing Care of the Mechanically Ventilated Patient. In M. L. Nochomovitz and H. D. Montenegro (Eds.), *Ventilatory Support in Respiratory Failure* (pp. 159–210). Mount Kisco, N.Y.: Futura.

Dark, D. S., Pingleton, S. K., and Kirby, G. R. (1985). Hypercapnia during weaning: A complication of nutritional support. *Chest* 88: 141.

DeVito, A. J. (1990). Dyspnea during hospitalizations for acute phase of illness as recalled by patients with chronic obstructive pulmonary disease. *Heart Lung* 19(2): 186–191.

Driks, M. R., Craven, D. E., Celli, B. R., et al. (1987). Nosocomial pneumonia in intubated patients given Sucralfate as compared with antacids or histamine type 2 blockers. *N. Engl. J. Med.* 317: 1376–1382.

Dunbar, S., Dugas, L., Birge, J. B., and Trinclisti, B. (1990). Family Panel: Working with Families in Critical Care. In *Proceedings Book of the 1990 National Teaching Institute* (p. 419). Newport Beach, Calif.: American Association of Critical-Care Nurses.

Dupuis, Y. G. (1986). *Ventilators.* St. Louis: Mosby.

Elpern, E. H., Jacobs, E. R., and Bone, R. C. (1987). Incidence of aspiration in tracheally intubated patients. *Heart Lung* 16(5): 527–531.

Eubanks, D. H., and Bone, R. C. (1990). *Comprehensive Respiratory Care*, 2d Ed. St. Louis: Mosby.

Flick, G. R., and Berger, M. B. (1990). Pulmonary Function Testing in the Critical Care Unit. In R. W. Taylor, J. M. Civetta, and R. R. Kirby (Eds.), *Techniques and Procedures in Critical Care* (pp. 105–119). Philadelphia: Lippincott.

Foster, G. H., Conway, W. A., Pamulkov, N., et al. (1984). Early extubation after coronary artery bypass: Brief report. *Crit. Care Med.* 12(11): 994–996.

Foundation for Critical Care (1988). *In Skilled and Caring Hands* (videotape). Washington: Foundation for Critical Care.

Gallagher, T. J. (1985). Clinical Use of High-Frequency Jet Ventilation in Intensive Care. In G. C. Carlon and W. S. Howland (Eds.), *High-Frequency Ventilation in Intensive Care and During Surgery* (pp. 159–174). New York: Marcel Dekker.

Garibaldi, R. A., Britt, M. R., Coleman, M. L., et al. (1981). Risk factors for postoperative pneumonia. *Am. J. Med.* 70: 677–680.

Goodnough, S. K. (1983). *Advanced Pulmonary Critical Care Course Syllabus*, Vol. 1. Houston: Hermann Hospital.

Goodnough, S. K. (1985). The effects of oxygen and hyperinflation on arterial oxygen tension after endotracheal suctioning. *Heart Lung* 14(1): 11–17.

Goodnough, S. K. (1988). Reducing tracheal injury and aspiration. *Dimens. Crit. Care Nurs.* 7(6): 324–332.

Goodnough, S. K., Bines, A., and Schneider, W. (1986). The effect of clinical nursing expertise on patient outcomes. *Crit. Care Med.* 14: 358.

Goodnough, S. K., Bines, A., and Schneider, W. (1988). The Effect of Clinical Nursing Expertise on Patient Outcomes. In *Proceedings of the Third International Intensive Care Nursing Conference* (p. 192). Newport Beach, Calif.: American Association of Critical-Care Nurses.

Goodnough-Hanneman, S. K. (1990). Relationships and Patterns Between Expert and Nonexpert Critical Care Nursing Practice and Patient Outcomes. Doctoral dissertation, Texas Woman's University. *Dissertation Abstracts International*, 51 (06B), 33273.

Goodnough-Hanneman, S. K. (1991). Physiologic predictors of successful early weaning from mechanical ventilation after cardiac surgery. (Submitted to Nursing Research).

Grant, J. P. (1988). Nutrition-Related Complications in Critically Ill Patients. In P. D. Lumb and C. W. Bryan-Brown (Eds.), *Complications in Critical Care Medicine* (pp. 220–246). Chicago: Year Book Medical Publishers.

Guthrie, A., Starck, P., Goodnough, S. K., et al. (1983). Barotrauma in the mechanically ventilated patient: A new look. *Radiology* 149(P): 23.

Halm, M. A. (1990). Effects of support groups on anxiety of family members during critical illness. *Heart Lung* 19(1): 62–71.

Hamilton, L. H., Neu, J., and Calkins, J. M. (1986). *High Frequency Ventilation*. Boca Raton, Fla.: CRC Press.

Harvey, M. A., Ninos, N. P., Adler, D., et al. (1991). Consensus Conference on Fostering More Humane Care: Creating a Healing Environment. In R. W. Taylor and W. C. Shoemaker (Eds.), *Critical Care: State of the Art*, Vol. 12. Fullerton, Calif.: Society of Critical Care Medicine.

Henneman, E. A. (1989). Effect of nursing contact on the stress response of patients being weaned from mechanical ventilation. *Heart Lung* 18(5): 483–489.

Herve, P., Simmonneau, G., Girard, P., et al. (1985). Hypercapnic acidosis induced by nutrition in mechanically ventilated patients: Glucose versus fat. *Crit. Care Med.* 13: 537.

Hickey, M. (1990). What are the needs of families of critically ill patients? A review of the literature since 1976. *Heart Lung* 19(4): 401–415.

Hilberman, M., Kamm, B., Lamy, M., et al. (1976). An analysis of potential physiologic predictors of respiratory adequacy following cardiac surgery. *J. Thorac. Cardiovasc. Surg.* 71(5): 711–720.

Hoyt, J. W. (1988). Complications of Infection in the Critically Ill Patient. In P. D. Lumb and C. W. Bryan-Brown (Eds.), *Complications in Critical Care Medicine* (pp. 205–219). Chicago: Year Book Medical Publishers.

Jacono, J., Hicks, G., Antonioni, C., et al. (1990). Comparison of perceived needs of family members between registered nurses and family members of critically ill patients in intensive care and neonatal intensive care units. *Heart Lung* 19(1): 72–78.

Jimenez, P., Torres, A., Rodriguez-Roisin, R., et al. (1989). Incidence and etiology of pneumonia acquired during mechanical ventilation. *Crit. Care Med.* 17(9): 882–885.

Johnson, J. E. (1972). Effects of structuring patients' expectations on their reactions to threatening events. *Nurs. Res.* 21: 499–504.

Johnson, J. E., and Rice, V. H. (1974). Sensory and distress components of pain: Implications for the study of clinical pain. *Nurs. Res.* 23: 203–209.

Johnson, J. E., Kirchhoff, K. T., and Endress, M. P. (1975). Altering children's distress behavior during orthopedic cast removal. *Nurs. Res.* 24: 404–410.

Johnson, J., Rice, V., Fuller, S., and Endress, M. (1978). Sensory information, instruction in a coping strategy, and recovery from surgery. *Res. Nurs. Health* 1: 4–17.

Kan, A. F., Gin, T., Lin, E. S., and Oh, T. E. (1990). Factors influencing humidification in high-frequency jet ventilation. *Crit. Care Med.* 18(5): 537–539.

Karnad, D. R., Mhaisekar, D. G., and Moralwar, K. V. (1990). Respiratory mucus pH in tracheostomized intensive care unit patients: Effects of colonization and pneumonia. *Crit. Care Med.* 18(7): 699–701.

Keszler, H. (1985). High-Frequency Jet Ventilation: Miscellaneous Uses. In G. C. Carlon and W. S. Howland (Eds.), *High-Frequency Ventilation in Intensive Care and During Surgery* (pp. 175–185). New York: Marcel Dekker.

LaMontagne, L. L., and Pawlak, R. (1990). Stress and coping of parents of children in a pediatric intensive care unit. *Heart Lung* 19(4): 416–421.

Landa, J. F., Kwoka, M. A., Chapman, G. A., et al. (1980). Effects of suctioning on mucociliary transport. *Chest* 77: 202–207.

Levitzky, M. G., Cairo, J. M., and Hall, S. M. (1990). *Introduction to Respiratory Care*. Philadelphia: Saunders.

Lewandowski, L., and Kositsky, A. (1983). Research priorities for critical care nursing: A study by the American Association of Critical-Care Nurses. *Heart Lung* 12: 35–44.

Loder, B. J., Guy, Y., and Carlon, G. C. (1984). Critical care nurse and high-frequency ventilation. *Crit. Care Med.* 12(9): 798–799.

Luce, J. M. (1988). Pathophysiology and Management of Ventilatory Failure. In R. J. Fallat and J. M. Luce (Eds.), *Cardiopulmonary Critical Care Management* (pp. 11–35). New York: Churchill-Livingstone.

Luce, J. M., and Culver, B. H. (1982). Respiratory muscle function in health and disease. *Chest* 81(1): 82–90.

Lush, M. T., Janson-Bjerklie, S., Carrieri, V. K., and Lovejoy, N. (1988). Dyspnea in the ventilator-assisted patient. *Heart Lung* 17(5): 528–535.

MacIntyre, N. R., and Stock, M. C. (1990). Weaning Mechanical Ventilatory Support. In R. R. Kirby, M. J. Banner, and J. B. Downs (Eds.), *Clinical Applications of Ventilatory Support* (pp. 263–276). New York: Churchill-Livingstone.

Mackenzie, C. F., Imle, P. C., and Ciesla, N. (1989). *Chest Physiotherapy in the Intensive Care Unit*, 2d Ed. Baltimore: Williams & Wilkins.

Macrae, W., and Wallace, P. (1981). Aspiration around high-volume, low-pressure endotracheal cuff. *Br. Med. J.* 283: 1220.

Marini, J. J., and Wheeler, A. P. (1989). *Critical Care Medicine: The Essentials*. Baltimore: Williams & Wilkins.

Martin, L. (1987). *Pulmonary Physiology in Clinical Practice: The Essentials for Patient Care and Evaluation*. St. Louis: Mosby.

Martz, K. V., Joiner, J. W., and Shepherd, R. M. (1984). *Management of the Patient-Ventilator System*, 2d Ed. St. Louis: Mosby.

McHugh, J. M. (1985). Ventilatory Management. In S. Millar, L. K. Sampson, and S. M. Soukup (Eds.), *AACN Procedure Manual for Critical Care*, 2d Ed. (pp. 240–254). Philadelphia: Saunders.

McPherson, S. P. (1990). *Respiratory Therapy Equipment*, 4th Ed. St. Louis: Mosby.

Mehta, S. (1982). Aspiration around high-volume, low-pressure endotracheal tube cuff. *Br. Med. J.* 284: 115–116.

Meijer, K., van Saene, H. K. F., and Hill, J. C. (1990). Infection control in patients undergoing mechanical ventilation: Traditional approach versus a new development—Selective decontamination of the digestive tract. *Heart Lung* 19(1): 11–20.

Mickschl, D. B., Davidson, L. J., Flournoy, D. J., and Parker, D. E. (1990). Contamination of enteral feedings and diarrhea in patients in intensive care units. *Heart Lung* 19(4): 362–370.

Milic-Emili, J. (1986). Is weaning an art or a science? *Am. Rev. Respir. Dis.* 143(6): 1107–1108.

Mishel, M. H. (1988). Uncertainty in illness. *Image* 20(4): 225–232.

Montenegro, H. D. (1987). Positive-Pressure Ventilation. In M. L. Nochomovitz and H. D. Montenegro (Eds.), *Ventilatory Support in Respiratory Failure* (pp. 1–25). Mount Kisco, N.Y.: Futura.

Nochomovitz, M. L., and Montenegro, H. D. (Eds.) (1987). *Ventilatory Support in Respiratory Failure*. Mount Kisco, N.Y.: Futura.

Nunn, J. F. (1989). What Is the Required Inspired Oxygen Consumption During Anesthesia? In T. H. Stanley and R. J. Sperry (Eds.), *Anesthesia and the Lung* (pp. 99–105). Boston: Kluwer Academic Publishers.

O'Neill-Norris, L., and Grove, S. K. (1986). Investigation of selected psychosocial needs of family members of critically ill patients. *Heart Lung* 15: 194–199.

Pagliarello, G., and Carter, J. A. (1990). A comparison of rates of nosocomial pneumonia in trauma vs. nontrauma intensive care unit patients. *Crit. Care Med.* 18(4): S201.

Paluch, B. R. (1986). Bacteriologic evaluation of the Servo 150 hygroscopic condenser-humidifier. *Crit. Care Med.* 14: 914.

Parker, M. M., Schubert, W., Shelhamer, J. H., and Parrillo, J. E. (1984). Perceptions of a critically ill patient experiencing therapeutic paralysis in an ICU. *Crit. Care Med.* 12: 69.

Pepe, P. E., and Marini, J. J. (1982). Occult positive end-expiratory pressure in mechanically ventilated patients with air flow obstruction: The auto-PEEP effect. *Am. Rev. Respir. Dis.* 126: 166.

Pilbeam, S. P. (1986). *Mechanical Ventilation: Physiologic and Clinical Applications.* St. Louis: Multi-Media Publishing.

Pittet, J., Forster, A., and Suter, P. M. (1990). High-frequency jet ventilation and intermittent positive-pressure ventilation: Effect of cerebral blood flow in patients after open heart surgery. *Chest* 97(2): 420–424.

Powner, D. J., Sanders, C. S., and Bailey, B. J. (1986). Bacteriologic evaluation of the Servo 150 hygroscopic condenser-humidifier. *Crit. Care Med.* 14: 135.

Preusser, B. A. (1985). The efficiency of commercially available manual resuscitation bags. *Focus Crit. Care* 12(3): 59–61.

Preusser, B. A., Stone, K. S., Gonyon, D. S., et al. (1988). Effects of two methods of preoxygenation on mean arterial pressure, cardiac output, peak airway pressure, and postsuctioning hypoxemia. *Heart Lung* 17(3): 290–299.

Quasha, A. L., Loeber, N., Feeley, T. W., et al. (1980). Postoperative respiratory care: A controlled trial of early and late extubation following coronary-artery bypass grafting. *Anesthesiology* 52(2): 135–141.

Riegel, B. E., and Ehrenrich, D. (1989). *Psychologic Aspects of Critical Care Nursing.* Rockville, Md.: Aspen.

Roberts, J., Barnes, W., Pennock, M., and Browne, G. (1988). Diagnostic accuracy of fever as a measure of postoperative pulmonary complications. *Heart Lung* 17(2): 166–170.

Rogge, J. A., Bunde, L., and Baun, M. M. (1989). Effectiveness of oxygen concentrations of less than 100% before and after endotracheal suction in patients with chronic obstructive pulmonary disease. *Heart Lung* 18(1): 64–71.

Rutherford, E., Rutledge, R., Fakhry, S., et al. (1990). The impact of complications on the resource utilization, hospital charges, and outcome in the surgical intensive care unit (SICU): A study in 1438 patients. *Crit. Care Med.* 18(4): S196.

Sackner, M. A., Hirsch, J., and Epstein, S. (1975). Effect of cuffed endotracheal tubes on tracheal mucous velocity. *Chest* 68: 774–777.

Sandowski, C. L. (1989). *Sexual Concerns When Illness or Disability Strikes.* Springfield, Ill.: Charles C. Thomas.

Scanlon, C. L., Spearman, C. B., and Sheldon, R. L. (Eds.) (1990). *Egan's Fundamentals of Respiratory Care,* 5th Ed. St. Louis: Mosby.

Schmitz, T. M. (1988). Effect of the Semiprone Body Position on Oxygenation. Masters thesis, University of Texas Health Sciences Center.

Schmitz, T. M. (1991). Fact or myth? Patients with pulmonary disease should be placed in the semi-Fowler's position. *Focus Crit. Care* 18(1): 58–64.

Schumann, L., and Parsons, G. (1985). Tracheal suctioning and ventilator tubing changes in adult respiratory distress syndrome: Use of a positive end-expiratory pressure valve. *Heart Lung* 14(4): 362–367.

Schuster, D. P. (1990). A physiologic approach to initiating, maintaining, and withdrawing mechanical ventilatory support during acute respiratory failure. *Am. J. Med.* 88(3): 268–278.

Shapiro, M., Wilson, K., Casar, G., et al. (1986). Work of breathing through different sized endotracheal tubes. *Crit. Care Med.* 14: 1028–1031.

Shekleton, M. E., Balk, R. A., Catrambone, C., et al. (1984). Contrasting ventilatory parameters in patients who succeed and fail weaning trials. *Am. Rev. Respir. Dis.* 132: A439.

Sherry, T. M., Morgan, A. S., and Hirvela, E. R. (1990). Pneumonia in the surgical ICU: Trauma vs. nontrauma patients. *Crit. Care Med.* 18(4): S189.

Shikora, S. A., Bistrian, B. R., Borlase, B. C., et al. (1990). Work of breathing: Reliable predictor of weaning and extubation. *Crit. Care Med.* 18(2): 157–162.

Shneerson, J. (1988). *Disorders of Ventilation.* Boston: Blackwell Scientific.

Sladen, A., Guntupalli, K., and Klain, M. (1984a). High-frequency jet ventilation versus intermittent positive-pressure ventilation. *Crit. Care Med.* 12(9): 788–792.

Sladen, A., Guntupalli, K., Marquez, J., and Klain, M. (1984b). High-frequency jet ventilation in the postoperative period: A review of 100 patients. *Crit. Care Med.* 12(9): 782–787.

Smith, R. N., and de Asla, R. A. (1988). Instrumentation. In M. R. Kinney, D. R. Packa, and S. B. Dunbar (Eds.), *AACN Clinical Reference for Critical-Care Nursing,* 2d Ed. (pp. 33–82). New York: McGraw-Hill.

Society of Critical Care Medicine (1991). Guidelines for standards of care for patients with acute respiratory failure on mechanical ventilatory support. *Crit. Care Med.* 19(2): 275–278.

Sottile, F. D. (1988). Complications of Mechanical Ventilation. In P. D. Lumb and C. W. Bryan-Brown (Eds.), *Complications in Critical Care Medicine* (pp. 12–44). Chicago: Year Book Medical Publishers.

Supinski, G. S., and Silverman, M. (1987). High-Frequency Ventilation. In M. L. Nochomovitz and H. D. Montenegro (Eds.), *Ventilatory Support in Respiratory Failure* (pp. 49–83). Mount Kisco, N.Y.: Futura.

Thompson, A. C., Wilder, B. H., and Powner, D. J. (1985). Bedside resuscitation bags: A source of bacterial contamination. *Infect. Control* 6: 231–232.

Tobin, M. J., and Grenvik, A. (1984). Nosocomial lung infection and its diagnosis. *Crit. Care Med.* 12(3): 191–199.

Tobin, M. J., Perez, W., Guenther, S. M., et al. (1986). The pattern of breathing during successful and unsuccessful trials of weaning from mechanical ventilation. *Am. Rev. Respir. Dis.* 134(6): 1111–1118.

Townsend, D. D. (1990). Between the Bedrails . . . Beyond the Door: The Critical Care Nurse as a Patient. In *Proceedings of the 1990 National Teaching Institute* (p. 414). Newport Beach, Calif.: American Association of Critical-Care Nurses.

Viale, J. P., Annat, G. J., Bouffard, Y. M., et al. (1988). Oxygen cost of breathing in postoperative patients: Pressure support ventilation vs continuous positive airway pressure. *Chest* 93: 506–509.

Villers, D., and Derriennic, M. (1983). Reliability of the bronchoscopic protected catheter brush in intubated and ventilated patients. *Chest* 88: 527–530.

Viner, E. (1988). *Life at the Other End of the Endotracheal Tube* (videotape). Washington: Foundation for Critical Care.

Whitman, G. R. (1988). Tissue Perfusion. In M. R. Kinney, D. R. Packa, and S. B. Dunbar (Eds.), *AACN Clinical Reference for Critical-Care Nursing,* 2d Ed. (pp. 115–159). New York: McGraw-Hill.

Williams-Colon, S., and Thalken, F. R. (1990). Management and Monitoring of the Patient in Respiratory Failure. In C. L. Scanlan, C. B. Spearman, and R. L. Sheldon (Eds.), *Egan's Fundamentals of Respiratory Care,* 5th Ed. (pp. 780–835). St. Louis: Mosby.

Wright, J., and Gong, H., Jr. (1990). "Auto-PEEP": Incidence, magnitude, and contributing factors. *Heart Lung* 19(4): 352–357.

Yannelli, B., and Gurevich, I. (1988). Infection control in critical care. *Heart Lung* 17(6): 596.

Zimmerman, G. A. (1989). Pulmonary Surfactant: An Endogenous Mediator of Alveolar Stability and a Therapeutic Agent. In T. H. Stanley and R. J. Sperry (Eds.), *Anesthesia and the Lung* (pp. 47–53). Boston: Kluwer Academic Publishers.

THORACIC CAVITY MANAGEMENT

BEHAVIORAL OBJECTIVES

After completing this chapter, the nurse will be able to

- Define the key terms.
- Identify the clinical indications for which management of the thoracic cavity is needed.
- List nursing diagnoses appropriate for patients undergoing procedures involving the thoracic cavity.
- Develop teaching plans for patients and families of patients undergoing procedures involving the thoracic cavity.
- Demonstrate proper procedure for the skills involved in thoracic cavity management.
- Evaluate patients for expected and unexpected outcomes following procedures involving the thoracic cavity.

The thoracic cavity is divided into three compartments: one compartment for each of the lungs and the mediastinum that lies between the lungs (Fig. 5–1). These structures are protected by the ribs, sternum, and intercostal muscles. The thoracic cavity is lined with a thin membrane called the *parietal pleura*. The lungs are similarly covered with a membrane, the *visceral* (or *pulmonary*) *pleura*. Between these two membranes is the pleural "space" (or cavity), which is not a true space at all but rather contains a thin layer (5 to 15 ml) of serous fluid. This fluid acts as a lubricant to keep the parietal and visceral membranes in contact with each other during respiration, allowing them to slide smoothly over one another. The potential exists for a space between these two membranes; hence it is called the *pleural space*.

The lungs and chest wall contain elastic tissue that tends to pull in opposite directions, the lungs pulling inward and the chest wall tending to pull outward. As these opposing forces try to pull the parietal and visceral pleura apart, a negative pressure is created within the pleural space. This negative intrapleural pressure keeps the pleural surfaces in contact, holding the lung against the chest wall and expanding the lungs to fill the pleural compartment completely. The intrapleural pressure must remain negative at all times in order to keep the lungs fully expanded. The extent of negative intrapleural pressure depends on the phase of respiration. At rest, the intrapleural pressure is -5 cmH$_2$O and the intrapulmonary pressure (pressure within the alveoli) equals atmospheric pressure. During inspiration, the thoracic cavity enlarges, decreasing intrapleural pressure to -6 to -12 cmH$_2$O and lowering intrapulmonary pressure 2 to 3 cmH$_2$O less than the atmosphere, causing air to be drawn into the lungs.

During expiration, the intrapleural pressure "increases" to -4 to -8 cmH$_2$O and intrapulmonary pressure increases 2 to 3 cmH$_2$O greater than the atmosphere, causing air to be passively forced out of the lungs.

Under normal conditions, the thoracic cavity is a closed, airtight space. Any disruption will result in a loss of negative pressure within the intrapleural space. Air and/or fluid collects, taking up the space within the pleural cavity that the lungs need in order to expand. The result is partial or total collapse of the lung.

KEY TERMS

atmospheric pressure	midaxillary
chemical pleurodesis	midclavicular
chest drainage system	negative pressure
chest tube	parietal pleura
cholothorax	pleural effusion
chyle	pleural space
chylothorax	positive pressure
empyema	pneumothorax
fluctuation	pyothorax
Heimlich valve	subcutaneous emphysema
hemopneumothorax	tension pneumothorax
hemothorax	thoracentesis
hydrothorax	thoracostomy
intercostal	thoracotomy
intrapleural	thorax
intrapulmonary pressure	vacuum
mediastinal tube	visceral pleura
mediastinum	water seal

SKILLS

5–1 Assisting with Chest Tube Placement
5–2 Closed Chest Drainage System (Bottle and Disposable Units)
5–3 Chest Tube Removal
5–4 Assisting with Open Chest Thoracotomy

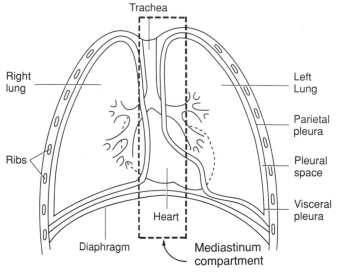

Trachea

Right lung

Left Lung

Parietal pleura

Pleural space

Ribs

Visceral pleura

Heart

Diaphragm

Mediastinum compartment

FIGURE 5–1. Thoracic cavity.

GUIDELINES

The following assessment guidelines assist the nurse to formulate nursing diagnoses and an individualized plan of care to manage patients undergoing procedures involving the thoracic cavity:

1. Know the patient's baseline respiratory/thoracic assessment.
2. Know the patient's baseline vital signs.
3. Know the patient's medical/surgical history and allergies.
4. Know the patient's presenting problem and mechanism of injury (if applicable).
5. Know the results of the radiologic and laboratory diagnostic tests (i.e., chest x-ray and arterial blood gas analysis).
6. Know the patient's current medical/surgical treatment.
7. Know appropriate interventions for the assessed findings.
8. Reassess respiratory/thoracic systems and vital signs in a timely manner.
9. Become adept with the equipment used for procedures involving the thoracic cavity.

SKILL 5–1

Assisting with Chest Tube Placement

Conditions that disrupt the normally negative pressure within the pleural space, either because of disease, injury, surgery, or iatrogenic causes, will result in a loss of negative pressure within the intrapleural space. Air, fluid, and/or blood collect, taking up the space within the pleural cavity that the lungs need in order to expand; the result is a partial or total collapse of the lung. The insertion of a chest tube (also known as a *thoracostomy tube* or *thoracic catheter*) assists with the removal of air, fluid, and blood from the intrapleural space. Negative

pressure is thus reestablished, allowing the collapsed lung to reexpand.

A mediastinal tube also may be indicated after heart surgery to drain fluid and blood from around the heart. While the pleurae usually remain intact and there is no pneumothorax, the blood and fluid, if allowed to accumulate in the mediastinum postoperatively, would create enough pressure to compress the heart, causing cardiac tamponade.

While a *pneumothorax* (the collection of air in the pleural space) is the most common condition requiring insertion of a chest tube, a *hemothorax* (the collection of blood) and a *hemopneumothorax* (the accumulation of air and blood in the pleural space) also may necessitate insertion of a chest tube. Less common indications for a chest tube are a *pyothorax* or *empyema* (the collection of pus), *chylothorax* (the collection of chyle from the thoracic duct), *cholothorax* (the collection of fluid containing bile), *hydrothorax* (the collection of noninflammatory serous fluid), and pleural effusions.

A pneumothorax may be open or closed. An *open pneumothorax* occurs with penetrating injury, due either to trauma (i.e., gunshot wounds, stab wounds, crushing chest injuries) or to a surgical incision in the thoracic cavity. With an open pneumothorax, there is a communication into the pleural space from the chest wall that allows air to enter from the atmosphere, collapsing the lung.

A *closed pneumothorax* is one in which the outer chest wall and parietal pleura remain intact, but injury to the visceral pleura on the surface of the lung allows air to enter the pleural space from within the lung. A closed pneumothorax may occur spontaneously following blunt traumatic injury or iatrogenically. A spontaneous pneumothorax occurs without apparent injury and is often seen in individuals with chronic lung disorders such as emphysema, cystic fibrosis, tuberculosis, and necrotizing pneumonia. A cyst, bulla, or bleb on the surface of the lung ruptures, causing air to enter into the pleural space. A spontaneous pneumothorax is more commonly seen in young, tall males who have a greater than normal height-to-chest width ratio. Subpleural blebs occur at the top of the long, upright lung because of mechanical stressors placed on the pleura by the increased lung height, predisposing the blebs to rupture. A closed pneumothorax may occur following blunt chest trauma if a fractured rib punctures the lung, allowing air to enter from the lung into the pleural space.

Iatrogenic pneumothorax occurs as a complication of medical treatment or surgical procedures. The use of intermittent positive-pressure breathing (IPPB) in individuals with weak lung tissue can overstretch the fragile lung, causing it to rupture. Mechanical ventilation with positive end-expiratory pressure (PEEP), used to prevent alveolar collapse in respiratory failure and adult respiratory distress syndrome (ARDS), may actually cause alveolar rupture with the resultant escape of air into the pleural space. Additionally, a lung may be unintentionally punctured during invasive procedures such as thoracentesis and central venous catheter insertion (particularly when a subclavian approach is used). A hydrothorax is a type of iatrogenically induced pleural effusion that may occur when a displaced central venous catheter allows IV fluids, serum, or total parenteral nutrition to be infused into the pleural space.

A *tension pneumothorax* may develop from either a closed pneumothorax or an open pneumothorax that has an occlusive dressing applied. This is a serious and life-threatening event that occurs when air leaks into the pleural space through a tear in the lung but has no means to escape, creating a one-way valve effect. With each breath the patient takes, air accumulates, intrapleural pressure increases, and the lung collapses. This causes the mediastinal structures, the heart, great vessels, and trachea, to shift to the opposite or unaffected side of the chest. Venous return and cardiac output are impeded, along with the possibility of collapse of the unaffected lung. This is a life-threatening emergency that requires prompt recognition and intervention.

The chest tube is a sterile, flexible, vinyl, silicone, or latex nonthrombogenic catheter that is approximately 20 in (51 cm) long and varies in size (Fig. 5–2). Adults usually require a 16- to 24-gauge chest tube for a simple pneumothorax, whereas a 28- to 36-gauge tube is used to drain liquid accumulations. Smaller chest tubes are available for children. The end of the chest tube that rests in the patient's pleural space has a number of drainage holes to prevent tip occlusion from clots or tissue, and the distal end connects to a chest drainage system.

One of two methods may be used by the physician to insert a chest tube after the insertion site is locally anesthetized and a small incision is made. The *trocar method* uses a pointed metal trocar to penetrate the thoracic cavity. The chest tube is passed through the hollow trocar, which is then removed, and the chest tube left in place (Fig. 5–3). The *blunt-dissection method* uses a forceps passed through a skin incision to penetrate the pleural space (Fig. 5–4). A finger is used to create the tract for the chest tube, lyse adhesions, and ensure intrapleural placement of the chest tube. The chest tube, clamped to the forceps, is then advanced into the pleural space. Once in place, the tube is sutured to the skin to prevent its displacement and is taped to prevent side-to-side movement; then an occlusive dressing is applied (Fig. 5–5).

The need for insertion of a chest tube is dependent on the size and severity of the pneumothorax. A small pneumothorax occupies less than 15 percent of the pleural space and may not require insertion of a chest tube. A moderate pneumothorax occupying 15 to 60 percent of the pleural space and a large pneumothorax occupying greater than 60 percent of the pleural space require placement of a chest tube.

The insertion site selected for the chest tube depends on the type of drainage. A chest tube inserted to drain air is placed near the apex of the lung (because air will rise) at the second intercostal space in the midclavicular line (Fig. 5–6A). If the tube is inserted to drain fluid (i.e., hemothorax, pleural effusions), it will be placed near the bottom of the lung (because gravity will pull fluid to the base of the lung) at the fourth to sixth intercostal space midaxillary line (Fig. 5–6B). In the event of a hemopneumothorax, two chest tubes may be inserted, one anteriorly in the apex to remove air and one laterally at the base of the lung to drain fluid. When two chest tubes are used, they are frequently attached to a single chest drainage system by a Y connector (Fig. 5–7). After heart surgery, one or two mediastinal tubes may be placed in the mediastinum to drain blood from in front of and behind the heart.

Following insertion, the chest tube is connected to a chest drainage system that removes air and/or fluid from the pleural space and prevents backflow into the pleural space. This facilitates reexpansion of the collapsed lung. All connection points are secured with tape or Parham bands to ensure that the system remains airtight (Fig. 5–8).

If the drainage from the chest tube is bloody or thick, the chest tube may need to be milked or stripped to keep it patent. Milking is a safer and gentler technique than stripping and can be done manually by squeezing and releasing the chest tubing between the fingers. Stripping the tube is controversial and should be done only when it is absolutely necessary to remove clots. Research has shown that stripping creates a transient, but high pulse of negative pressure (-200 to -400 cmH$_2$O) as compressed tubing is released and reexpands (Duncan and Erickson, 1982). This causes patient discomfort, and the excessive pressure may inflict lung tissue trauma and cause bleeding. A mechanical stripper may be used (Fig. 5–9), or it can be done manually (Fig. 5–10). Using the

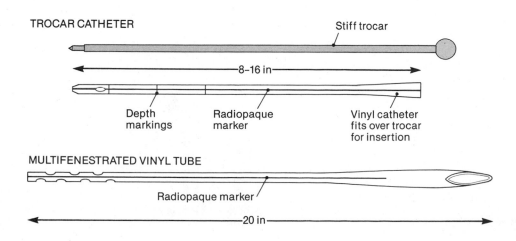

TROCAR CATHETER
Stiff trocar
8–16 in
Depth markings
Radiopaque marker
Vinyl catheter fits over trocar for insertion

MULTIFENESTRATED VINYL TUBE
Radiopaque marker
20 in

FIGURE 5–2. Straight chest tubes. (Used with permission from L. D. Kerston, *Comprehensive Respiratory Nursing: A Decision-Making Approach.* Philadelphia: Saunders, 1989, p. 771.)

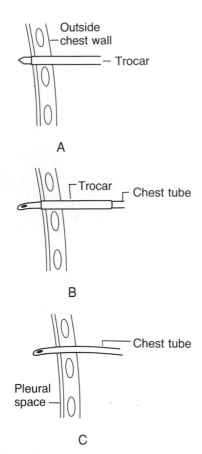

A

B

Pleural space

C

FIGURE 5–3. Trocar method of chest tube insertion. (*A*) Chest wall is pierced with trocar. (*B*) Chest tube is passed through the trocar. (*C*) Trocar is removed and chest tube remains resting in the pleural space.

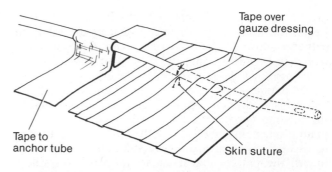

FIGURE 5–5. Occlusive chest tube dressing. (Used with permission from L. D. Kerston, *Comprehensive Respiratory Nursing: A Decision-Making Approach.* Philadelphia: Saunders, 1989, p. 772.)

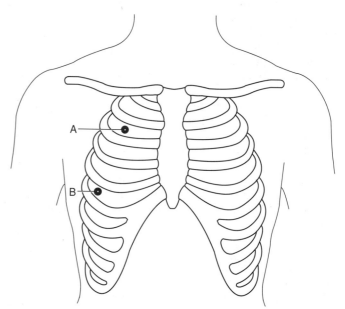

FIGURE 5–6. Standard sites for chest tube placement. (*A*) Second intercostal space, midclavicular line, for air. (*B*) Fifth intercostal space, midaxillary line, for fluid.

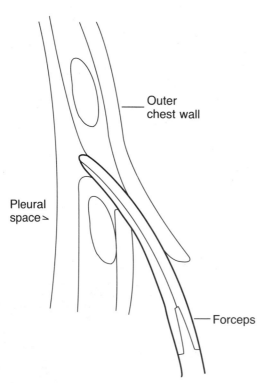

FIGURE 5–4. Blunt dissection method of chest tube insertion.

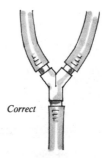

Correct

FIGURE 5–7. Y connector joining two chest tubes. (Courtesy of Atrium Medical Corporation, Hollis, N.H.)

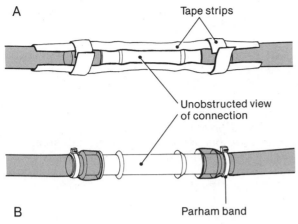

FIGURE 5–8. The securing of connection points: (*A*) tape, (*B*) Parham bands. (Used with permission from L. D. Kerston, *Comprehensive Respiratory Nursing: A Decision-Making Approach.* Philadelphia: Saunders, 1989, p. 783.)

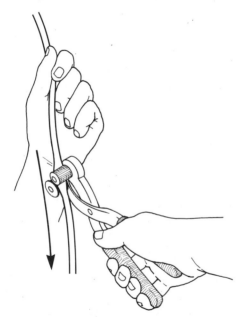

FIGURE 5–9. Hand stripper. (Used with permission from L. D. Kerston, *Comprehensive Respiratory Nursing: A Decision-Making Approach.* Philadelphia: Saunders, 1989, p. 782.)

thumb and index finger of the nondominant hand, stabilize the chest tube about 2 in. (approximately 5 cm) from the insertion site to prevent tension and possible dislodgment. Using the thumb and index finger of the dominant hand, compress the tubing as the fingers slide down the tube toward the drainage collection system. A lubricant such as lotion or KY Jelly may be used to make the stripping easier.

Clamping of chest tubes is generally not indicated, but it may be ordered prior to removing the chest tube (see Skill 5–3) or to locate the source of an air leak (indicated by continuous bubbling in the water-seal chamber). To clamp a chest tube, two covered or rubber-tipped Kelly clamps are attached to the tube in opposite directions near the insertion site (Fig. 5–11). Once clamped, air and fluid will accumulate in the pleural space, and with no method to escape, a tension pneumothorax may result. Therefore, clamps should only be left on less than a minute. To locate a leak, clamp the tubing at various points along its length. Once a clamp is located between the air leak and the water seal, the bubbling will stop. If the bubbling stops when the clamp is placed close to the chest, air may be escaping from the pleural space or from around the insertion site, and this should be reported. If the bubbling stops as the tubing is clamped along its length, check the connections to make sure they are airtight. If the bubbling does not stop, the chest drainage unit may be defective and may need to be replaced. The chest tube may be clamped to keep air from entering the pleural space while the collection unit is being replaced, but it is safer to immerse the distal end of the tubing into a container of sterile water or normal saline to create a temporary water seal during replacement.

Purpose

The nurse assists with placement of a chest tube to

1. Facilitate the removal of fluid, blood, and/or air from the pleural space or the mediastinum.
2. Assess the type and amount of drainage from the pleural space.
3. Restore negative pressure to the pleural space.
4. Promote reexpansion of a collapsed lung.
5. Relieve respiratory distress associated with a collapsed lung.
6. Improve ventilation and perfusion of the lung.

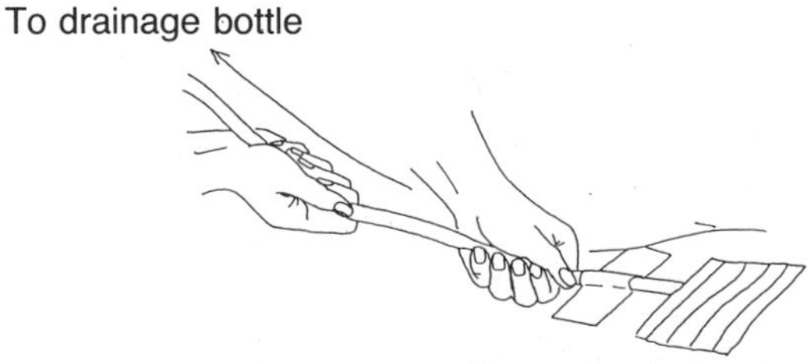

FIGURE 5–10. Manually stripping the chest tube.

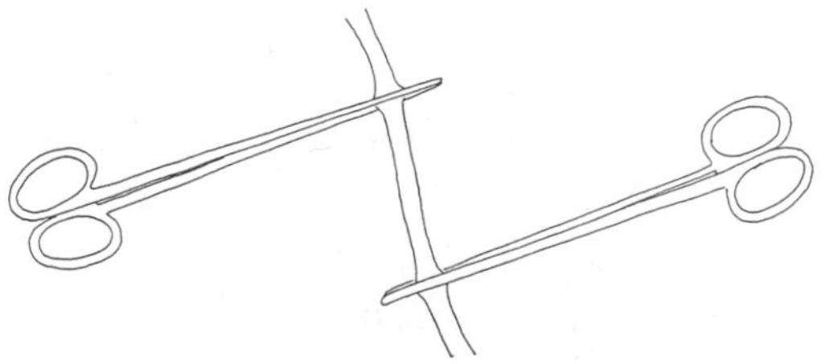

FIGURE 5–11. Clamping the chest tube.

Prerequisite Knowledge and Skills

Prior to assisting with insertion of a chest tube, the nurse should understand

1. Principles of aseptic technique.
2. Principles of universal precautions.
3. Anatomy and physiology of the thoracic cavity and respiratory systems.
4. Principles of closed chest drainage systems.

The nurse should be able to

1. Perform proper handwashing technique (see Skill 35–5).
2. Comply with universal precautions (see Skill 35–1).
3. Assess vital signs.
3. Perform respiratory/thoracic assessment.
4. Set up and manage chest drainage system (see Skill 5–2).

Assessment

1. Assess for significant medical history or injury, including chronic lung disease, spontaneous pneumothorax, pulmonary disease, therapeutic procedures associated with risk of pneumothorax/hemothorax, and mechanism of injury. **Rationale:** Medical history or injury may provide the etiologic basis for the occurrence of the pneumothorax or hemothorax.
2. Assess respiratory system for tachypnea, decreased or absent breath sounds on the affected side, crackles adjacent to the affected area, shortness of breath (dyspnea), asymmetrical chest excursion with respirations, cyanosis, hyperresonance in the affected side (pneumothorax), subcutaneous emphysema (pneumothorax), dullness/flatness in the affected side (hemothorax, pleural effusion), sudden sharp chest pain, anxiety, restlessness, or apprehension, tachycardia, hypotension, dysrhythmias, tracheal deviation to the unaffected side, and neck vein distension. **Rationale:** Physical signs and symptoms that result from a pneumothorax, hemothorax, or tension pneumothorax.
3. Assess results of chest x-ray and arterial blood gases (if patient's condition does not necessitate immediate intervention). **Rationale:** Diagnostic testing confirms the presence of air and/or fluid in the pleural space, a collapsed lung, hypoxemia, and respiratory compromise.

Nursing Diagnoses

1. Ineffective breathing pattern related to partial or total collapse of the lung. **Rationale:** Respiratory distress occurs as a result of decreased respiratory gas exchange and subsequent hypoxia.
2. Impaired gas exchange related to partial or total collapse of the lung. **Rationale:** Respiratory gas exchange is decreased or absent in collapsed lung tissue.
3. Alteration in skin integrity related to insertion of a chest tube. **Rationale:** A small incision is made into the chest wall to facilitate insertion of the chest tube.
4. Ineffective breathing pattern related to pain. **Rationale:** Pain at the site of chest tube insertion interferes with deep breathing and coughing exercises that facilitate drainage from the pleural space, promote lung expansion, and prevent respiratory complications.
5. Potential for injury: tension pneumothorax related to unrelieved pressure within the pleural space. **Rationale:** Tension pneumothorax is a life-threatening complication that can occur when air accumulates in the pleural space resulting in increased intrapleural pressure and collapse of the lung.

Planning

1. Individualize the following goals for assisting with insertion of a chest tube.
   a. Maintain effective breathing pattern. **Rationale:** Effective respirations are necessary for the exchange of oxygen and carbon dioxide.
   b. Improve gas exchange. **Rationale:** As gas exchange is improved, symptoms of respiratory distress are relieved.
   c. Promote the drainage of air, fluid, and/or blood from the intrapleural space. **Rationale:** As drainage from the intrapleural space occurs, negative intrapleural pressure will be reestablished with subsequent expansion of the lung.
   d. Absence of complications associated with a pneumothorax or hemothorax and chest tube insertion. **Rationale:** Tension pneumothorax, hemorrhage, and infection complicate the patient's recovery.
2. Prepare all necessary equipment and supplies. **Rationale:** Assembly of all the equipment and supplies facilitates the quick and efficient insertion of a chest tube.
   a. Sterile gown, gloves, and mask.
   b. Sterile drape(s) and bed protector.
   c. Antiseptic skin prep and swabs (usually povidone iodine).
   d. Local anesthetic (usually 1% lidocaine).
   e. 1¼-in 18- to 20-gauge needle (to draw up the anesthetic).
   f. ⅝-in 25- to 27-gauge needle (to administer the anesthetic).
   g. 10-ml syringe.
   h. Alcohol wipes.
   i. Scalpel with blade (usually no. 11).
   j. Hemostat.
   k. Trocar.
   l. Chest tube (nos. 16 to 24 for adult pneumothorax; nos. 28 to 36 for adult hemothorax) with connector.
   m. Suture material (usually 2-0 to 3-0 silk) with a cutting needle.
   n. Dressing materials (4 × 4 gauze pads, split drain sponges, petrolatum gauze, tape).
   o. Kelly clamps (two per chest tube).

p. Sterile connecting tube (6 ft).

q. Y connector (if two chest tubes).

r. Chest drainage system.

s. Suction source (a standard chest tube tray generally contains these items).

t. 1 in adhesive tape (1 roll).

3. Prepare the patient and family.

   a. Explain the procedure. **Rationale:** Explanations decrease patient and family anxiety and enhance cooperation.

   b. Explain the patient's participation. **Rationale:** The patient should remain as immobile as possible and do relaxed breathing.

   c. Follow hospital policy to obtain the consent of the patient (if able) or significant other. **Rationale:** Invasive procedures, unless performed under implied consent in a life-threatening situation, require the written consent of the patient or significant other.

   d. Assist the patient to the position the physician prefers. **Rationale:** The lateral position with the affected side upward, the supine position for a pneumothorax, or the semi-Fowler's position for a hemothorax.

   e. Administer prescribed pain medication as needed. **Rationale:** Pain medication reduces the discomfort and anxiety experienced, facilitating patient cooperation.

4. Set up chest drainage system (see Skill 5–2). **Rationale:** Once the chest tube is inserted, it needs to be immediately attached to a closed chest drainage system.

Implementation

Steps	Rationale	Special Considerations
1. Wash hands.	Reduces transmission of microorganisms.	
2. Open the chest tube tray using sterile technique.	Reduces transmission of microorganisms.	
3. Assist the physician with preparation of the insertion site.	Inhibits the growth of bacteria at the insertion site.	
a. Pour antiseptic solution into the basin using aseptic technique.	Used to saturate gauze pads for cleansing.	Determine that the patient has no allergies to the antiseptic solution.
b. Wipe the top of the vial of local anesthetic with an alcohol swab.	Disinfects the surface of the vial.	
c. Invert the vial so that the physician can withdraw the anesthetic solution into the syringe.	Maintains sterility.	
4. Assist the physician with insertion of the chest tube.		Sterile procedure performed by the physician; the nurse monitors and reassures the patient.
a. The physician infiltrates the insertion site with the anesthetic agent.	Results in loss of sensation and reduction of pain during insertion of the chest tube.	
b. The physician makes a small incision at the insertion site, using a "tunnel" approach to dissect the subcutaneous tissue and intercostal muscle.	Admits the diameter of the chest tube.	
c. The physician perforates the pleura using a trocar (see Fig. 5–3) or forceps (see Fig. 5–4).	Ensures that the opening is large enough for the chest tube and decreases the incidence of extrapleural positioning. Relieves air and/or fluid.	
d. The physician advances the chest tube through the incision and into the pleural space.	Places chest tube in correct position.	A trocar or hemostat may be used to facilitate insertion of the chest tube; listen for the return of a rush of air as it escapes and observe an initial fogging of the chest tube upon normal exhalation, which indicate proper placement.

Table continues on following page

Steps	Rationale	Special Considerations
5. Remove the adapter from the end of the 6-ft length of latex connecting tube, keeping the exposed end of the tube sterile and connected to the chest tube.	Maintains sterility and creates a closed system.	Length of connecting tube must be sufficient to allow patient movement and to decrease the chance that a deep breath by the patient will draw chest drainage back into the pleural space. The chest drainage system should be placed below the level of the patient's chest to promote gravity drainage and to prevent backflow; if two chest tubes are placed, a Y connector may be used to join them to a single drainage system (see Fig. 5–7).
6. Tape all connection points in the chest drainage system (see Fig. 5–8A).	Airtight connections keep the tubes together and prevent air leaks into the pleural space.	Parham bands may be used to secure connections instead of tape (see Fig. 5–8B).
a. One-inch tape is placed horizontally extending over connections (a portion of the connector may be left unobstructed by the tape).	Secures connections but allows visualization of drainage.	
b. Reinforce the horizontal tape with tape placed vertically so that it encircles both ends of the connector.	Secures connections.	
7. Instruct the patient to take a deep breath and exhale slowly.	Facilitates drainage and reexpansion of the lung.	
8. Assist the physician with suturing the chest tube to the skin.	Prevents displacement of the chest tube, the skin next to the tube is sutured and the ends of the suture are wrapped around the tube, anchoring the tube to the chest wall.	
9. Apply occlusive dressing (see Fig. 5–5).	Provides for an airtight seal around the insertion site.	
a. Apply split drain sponges around the chest tube, one over the top and one from underneath the tube.	Creates an airtight system.	A petrolatum gauze may be wrapped around the tube close to the insertion site if the air leak is large; however, this may cause maceration of the skin.
b. Apply 2 to 3 gauze pads (4 × 4) on top of the split drain sponges.	Creates an airtight system.	Determine that the patient is not allergic to the tape.
c. Tape the dressing to the skin.	Secures the dressing.	
10. Tape the chest tube to the skin.	Prevents side-to-side movement and accidental dislodgment of the chest tube.	
11. If prescribed, turn on suction source. (Physician will determine the amount of suction necessary.)	Assists in pulling drainage from the pleural cavity.	
12. Coil latex connecting tube and secure to sheet.	Drainage accumulating in dependent loops obstructs chest drainage into the collecting system.	Allow enough length for patient movement.
13. Order a stat portable chest x-ray per physician instruction/protocol.	Verifies correct placement and position of the chest tube.	
14. Dispose of equipment in appropriate receptacle.	Universal precautions.	
15. Wash hands.	Reduces transmission of microorganisms.	

Evaluation

1. Compare patient's vital signs and respiratory assessment after insertion of the chest tube with the baseline assessments done prior to the procedure. **Rationale:** Identifies the effects of chest tube insertion on the patient and the occurrence of developing complications.

2. Evaluate the insertion site for the presence of subcutaneous emphysema. **Rationale:** Subcutaneous emphysema, indicating an air leak, may have been present prior to insertion of the chest tube, and this should be monitored and reported to the physician if there is an increase. Subcutaneous emphysema present after the chest tube has been inserted needs to be reported immediately as it may indicate an air leak.

3. Evaluate the chest drainage system for the type and amount of drainage. **Rationale:** Immediately after the chest tube is inserted, the sound of air escaping should be heard. Depending on the reason the chest tube was inserted, drainage may be air, fluid, blood, or a combination of these. Rapid drainage of excessive amounts (200 cc per hour) of fluid or blood may result in shock, which should be reported to the physician immediately.

4. Evaluate the chest drainage system for bubbling and fluctuation in the water-seal chamber. **Rationale:** The water level in the water-seal chamber should rise and fall with the patient's respirations until the lung is fully expanded. The absence of fluctuation immediately after insertion needs to be identified and corrected. A chest x-ray will determine whether incorrect tube placement or dislodgment of the tube is the source of this problem. The chest drainage system should be checked for possible malfunction due to incorrect setup, obstruction in the tubing from kinks, the patient lying on the tubing, or the presence of fluid-filled loops that should be emptied into the chest drainage collection system. Bubbling in the water-seal chamber immediately after insertion of the chest tube and with exhalation and coughing is expected, but continued bubbling indicates an air leak that needs to be corrected, usually by increasing the amount of suction. Additionally, connection points should be checked and secured to ensure an airtight system.

Expected Outcomes

1. Removal of air, fluid, or blood from the pleural space. **Rationale:** Reduces the space-occupying accumulations that interfere with full lung expansion.

2. Fluctuations noted in the water-seal chamber. **Rationale:** The water level in the water-seal chamber should rise and fall with the patient's respirations until the lung is fully expanded.

3. Relief of respiratory distress. **Rationale:** As the lung reexpands, pulmonary exchange of gases occurs, hypoxia is relieved, and arterial blood gas results indicate improvement.

4. Reexpansion of the collapsed lung validated by chest x-ray. **Rationale:** As negative pressure is restored to the intrapleural space, the lung reexpands and bilateral breath sounds are heard in all lung fields.

Unexpected Outcomes

1. Tension pneumothorax. Increasing respiratory distress, dysrhythmias, tachycardia, hypotension, and tracheal deviation. **Rationale:** Occlusion of chest drainage system has occurred, creating intrapleural pressure and imminent life-threatening conditions.

2. Hemorrhagic shock. Continuous bloody drainage of 200 cc/hr must be reported to the physician immediately. **Rationale:** Vessel or mediastinal disruption is suspected.

3. Absence of drainage and fluctuations and/or continuous bubbling in the water-seal chamber with continued respiratory distress; lung does not show evidence of reexpansion. **Rationale:** Possible equipment malfunction, incorrect tube placement, dislodgment of tube, or air leak.

4. Fever, purulent drainage and redness around the insertion site, or purulent drainage in the chest tube. **Rationale:** Evidence of an infection in process.

Documentation

Documentation in the patient record should include respiratory/thoracic and vital signs assessment before and after the procedure; date and time the procedure was performed; procedure performed by whom, size of the chest tube, and insertion site; connection to either a bottle or disposable chest drainage system, amount of suction, fluctuations, and the type and amount of drainage; patient's tolerance of the procedure; and completion and results of the postinsertion chest x-ray and any other diagnostic tests ordered. **Rationale:** Documents interventions, nursing care given, and expected and unexpected outcomes and serves as a medical-legal record of the events.

Patient/Family Education

1. Assess the patient and family's understanding of the patient's condition, the rationale for chest tube insertion, and how the closed chest drainage system works. **Rationale:** Identifies patient and family knowledge deficits concerning the patient's condition, the procedure, expected benefits, and potential risks and allows time for questions to clarify information.

2. Instruct the patient to sit in a semi-Fowler's position (unless contraindicated). **Rationale:** Facilitates drainage from the lung by allowing air to rise and fluid to settle in order to be removed via the chest tube. This position also makes breathing easier.

3. Instruct the patient to turn and position every 2 hours. **Rationale:** Turning and repositioning prevent complications related to immobility and retained secretions.

4. Instruct the patient to cough and deep breathe, splinting the affected side. **Rationale:** Coughing and deep breathing raise intrapleural pressure, thus facilitating drainage, promoting lung reexpansion, and preventing respiratory complications associated with retained secre-

tions. The application of firm pressure over the chest tube insertion site (i.e., splinting) decreases pain and discomfort.

5. Instruct the patient not to lie on the tubing and to keep it free from kinks. **Rationale:** Maintains patency of tube, facilitates drainage, and prevents the accumulation of pressure within the intrapleural space that interferes with lung reexpansion.

6. Encourage active or passive range-of-motion exercises of the arm on the affected side. **Rationale:** The patient may splint the arm on the affected side to decrease discomfort at the insertion site.

7. Instruct the patient and family about activity as prescribed while maintaining the drainage system below the level of the chest. **Rationale:** Facilitates gravity drainage and prevents backflow into the pleural space.

8. Instruct the patient about the availability of prescribed analgesic medication. **Rationale:** Alleviates pain and facilitates coughing, deep breathing, positioning, and range-of-motion exercises.

Performance Checklist
Skill 5–1: Assisting with Chest Tube Placement

Critical Behaviors	Complies yes	no
1. Wash hands.		
2. Use aseptic technique to open chest tube tray.		
3. Assist physician with preparation of the insertion site.		
a. Pour antiseptic solution into the basin using aseptic technique.		
b. Cleanse the top of the vial of local anesthetic.		
c. Invert the vial for withdrawal of anesthetic solution.		
4. Assist physician during insertion of the chest tube.		
5. Connect the chest tube to the chest drainage system.		
6. Secure connections between chest tube and chest drainage system.		
7. Instruct patient to take a deep breath and to exhale slowly.		
8. Assist physician with suturing the chest tube to the skin.		
9. Apply an occlusive dressing.		
10. Tape chest tube to skin.		
11. Turn on suction source as prescribed.		
12. Coil latex connecting tube and secure.		
13. Order stat portable chest x-ray per physician instruction/protocol.		
14. Dispose of equipment.		
15. Wash hands.		
16. Document procedure in patient record.		

SKILL 5–2

Closed Chest Drainage System (Bottle and Disposable Units)

Closed chest drainage systems (single-, double-, triple-, and four-bottle setups, as well as disposable units) use gravity and/or suction to restore negative pressure and remove air, fluid, and/or blood from the pleural space so that the collapsed lung(s) can reexpand. Whenever a chest tube is inserted, it must be connected to a one-way mechanism that allows air to escape from the pleural space while preventing air to enter from the atmosphere. This can be accomplished by using an underwater seal mechanism. Drainage tubing from the chest tube (or connecting tubing between a multiple-bottle system) is attached to a strawlike tube immersed 2 cm ($\frac{3}{4}$ in) beneath the surface of a solution of sterile water or saline contained in a bottle. (Immersing the straw more than 2 cm beneath the surface of a solution increases the work of respiration.) Air or fluid can exit the pleural space as a result of gravity, but the water seal prevents it from being drawn back into the cavity.

Bubbling in the water-seal bottle is normal immediately after connecting the chest tube, during expiration, and with coughing, but continuous bubbling in the water seal indicates an air leak in the system. Fluctuations of 5 to 10 cm (2–5 in) of the water level in the straw of the water-seal bottle (rising with spontaneous inhalation and falling with exhalation) reflect pressure changes in the pleural space with respirations. If the patient is receiving mechanical ventilation, fluctuation patterns will be reversed, falling with inhalation and rising with exhalation. The fluctuations may be more if the patient exerts increased respiratory effort or less if the respirations are shallow.

Closed chest drainage systems require that the pressure within the chest be greater than that in the bottles to drain air and fluid. This is accomplished by keeping the drainage bottles below the level of the chest. However, drainage by gravity alone may not be sufficient when large volumes of air and/or fluid must be evacuated from the pleural space. The addition of a suction source, either from an Emerson pump or a wall unit, can enhance drainage while maintaining a low negative pressure. Suction pulls air from the bottles, causing the pressure within them to drop. This increases the pressure differences between the pleural space and the bottles, thus enhancing drainage from the pleural space.

The single-bottle system is used to drain air or small amounts of fluid from the pleural space (Fig. 5–12). A 2-L bottle serves as both the water-seal and drainage-collection bottle. An airtight seal is created by using a rubber stopper with two openings through which a strawlike tube is placed. With this arrangement, the drainage tube from the chest tube is attached to a long straw inserted through the rubber stopper and immersed 2 cm (1 in) beneath the surface of the solution, creating the water-seal bottle. A second short straw serves as an air vent to allow for the escape of air as it accumulates in the bottle from the pleural space. Without this air vent, pressure would increase in the bottle, interfering with air and fluid drainage.

There are two disadvantages to the single-bottle setup. First, as drainage continues to fill the bottle, resistance increases and more respiratory effort is needed for drainage to continue. Second, drainage from patients who have a hemopneumothorax in which air and fluid mixes causes a foamy solution that is difficult to measure. Both these drawbacks can be resolved by using a double-bottle system.

One of two double-bottle setups may be used (Fig. 5–13). With the first setup, one bottle serves as the drainage-collection bottle and the second is the water-seal bottle (Fig. 5–13A). The distal end of the patient's drainage tube connects to one of two short strawlike tubes inserted through the airtight rubber stopper in the drainage-collection bottle. The second short straw is connected by tubing to the long straw of the water-seal bottle. The air-vent tube in the water-seal bottle may be left open or may be connected to a suction source. The suc-

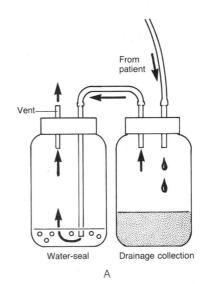

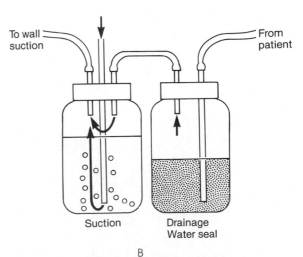

FIGURE 5–13. Double-bottle chest drainage system. (*A*) Drainage-collection and water-seal bottles. (Used with permission from J. M. Luce, M. L. Tyler, and D. J. Pierson, *Intensive Respiratory Care.* Philadelphia: Saunders, 1984, p. 164.) (*B*) Drainage-collection/water-seal and vacuum-control bottles. (Used with permission from L. D. Kerston, *Comprehensive Respiratory Nursing: A Decision-Making Approach.* Philadelphia: Saunders, 1989.)

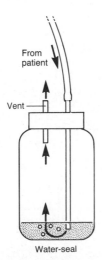

FIGURE 5–12. Single-bottle chest drainage system. (Used with permission from J. M. Luce, M. L. Tyler, and D. J. Pierson, *Intensive Respiratory Care.* Philadelphia: Saunders, 1984, p. 164.)

tion source is attached directly to the air vent on the water-seal bottle and generally set at a suction level of −20 cmH₂O. Drainage collects in the first bottle, and air escaping from the pleural space flows through the water-seal bottle to exit via the air vent. This setup keeps the water seal at a fixed level and allows for more accurate assessment of the amount and type of drainage. Bubbling and fluctuations in the water-seal chamber will occur as for the single-bottle system. The disadvantage to this system is that addition of the second bottle adds dead air space to the drainage system, which can be drawn back into the pleural cavity.

A second type of double-bottle setup uses one bottle as a combination water-seal/drainage-collection bottle (similar to the single-bottle system) and a second bottle as a vacuum-control bottle (see Fig. 5–13B). With this arrangement, the drainage tube from the chest tube is connected to the long straw of the water-seal/drainage bottle that is immersed 2 cm (1 in) beneath the surface of the water. The air vent of the water-seal/drainage bottle is connected by tubing to the vacuum-control bottle. The vacuum-control bottle has an airtight rubber stopper with three holes. A long straw is inserted through the center opening and immersed beneath the surface of a sterile water or normal saline solution, usually 20 cm (1 in). The other end of this straw is left open to the atmosphere. The amount of suction is determined by the depth that the long straw is immersed in the solution. One of the two short straws inserted in the remaining holes of the rubber stopper is connected by tubing to the water-seal bottle, and the other short straw is attached to a suction source. As suction is increased greater than the depth the straw is immersed, atmospheric air is drawn into the bottle, creating the vacuum. Gentle, continuous bubbling should be observed in the vacuum-control bottle. This bottle should be assessed periodically and the water replaced as necessary to keep the immersion of the long straw to the prescribed depth.

The safest way to regulate the amount of suction is through the triple-bottle setup (Fig. 5–14). The three-

bottle setup uses a drainage-collection bottle connected to a water-seal bottle that is attached to a vacuum-control bottle. As suction is added to the vacuum-control bottle and is increased greater than the depth that the straw is immersed in the solution (usually 20 cm [8 in]), atmospheric air is drawn into the bottle, creating the vacuum. The safety feature with this system is that increases in the amount of suction do not increase the amount of negative pressure in the pleural space (which would harm pulmonary tissue). Gentle, continuous bubbling should be observed in the vacuum-control bottle. (Vigorous bubbling increases the evaporation of the solution, which influences the amount of suction delivered.) This bottle should be assessed periodically and the water replaced as necessary to keep the immersion of the long straw to the prescribed depth.

A four-bottle system incorporates the features of the triple-bottle system with the addition of a bottle next to the drainage-collection bottle that serves as a vented water-seal bottle (Fig. 5–15). One of the short straws from the drainage-collection bottle is connected to the long straw (immersed 2 cm [1 in] beneath the surface of a solution of sterile water or saline) of the vented water-seal bottle. The short straw of the vented water-seal bottle is left open to air, creating the air vent. This "safety feature" bottle releases accumulated positive pressure in the event that the suction source is disconnected or obstructed.

When suction is applied to any of the bottle setups, two observations need to be made about the water-seal bottle. First, there should be no bubbling observed in the water-seal bottle (aside from a little bubbling when the suction is initially applied until air is drawn out of the system). Continuous bubbling in the water-seal bottle indicates an air leak in the system, either at the insertion site or from a loose or separated connection point in the system. Second, the solution in the water-seal bottle stays at a fixed level and does not fluctuate when suction is added. To check for fluctuations (in order to assess whether the lung has expanded), the suction source must

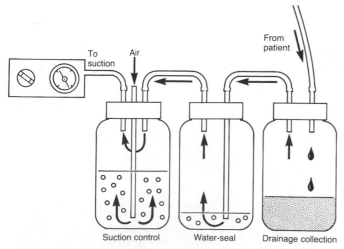

FIGURE 5–14. Triple-bottle chest drainage system. (Used with permission from J. M. Luce, M. L. Tyler, and D. J. Pierson, *Intensive Respiratory Care.* **Philadelphia: Saunders, 1984, p. 165.)**

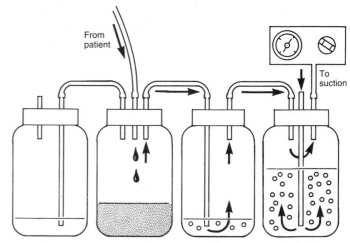

FIGURE 5–15. Four-bottle chest drainage system. (Used with permission from J. M. Luce, M. L. Tyler, and D. J. Pierson, *Intensive Respiratory Care.* **Philadelphia: Saunders, 1984, p. 166.)**

be temporarily interrupted from the drainage system so that the air vent is open (pinching off the tubing from the suction source does not open the vent to the atmosphere). Observation for fluctuations can then be made in the straw of the water-seal chamber, and subsequently, the suction source is then reconnected.

The double- and triple-bottle systems can be converted from suction to gravity drainage by disconnecting the tubing from the short straw of the water-seal bottle, creating an air-vent exit. If the suction source is disconnected for any reason (i.e., when the patient is being transported to another department), the drainage system should be converted to gravity drainage. The drainage bottles should be replaced as necessary (i.e., when they become full or in the event of breakage).

Disadvantages to the bottle systems include the risk for error during assembly due to the multiple parts and connections. Handling of the parts increases the risk for contamination. The bottles themselves are heavy and awkward, making transportation difficult and increasing the risk of breakage. The water seal can be lost if the water level is disturbed, allowing the recurrence of the pneumothorax. Likewise, if the straws are dislodged or moved, the suction or water seal can be increased or decreased. Special units are made to secure the bottles, but these take up a great deal of space at the bedside.

Disposable chest drainage units are an alternative to the traditional glass-bottle chest drainage systems (Fig. 5–16). The disposable units correlate with the triple-bottle drainage system, with collection, water-seal, and suc-

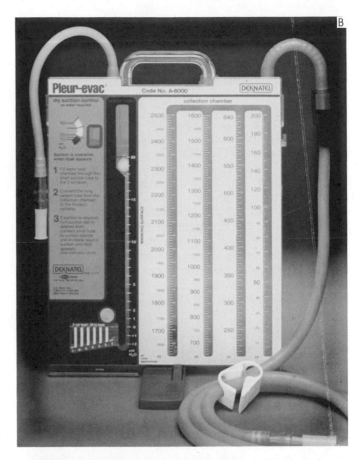

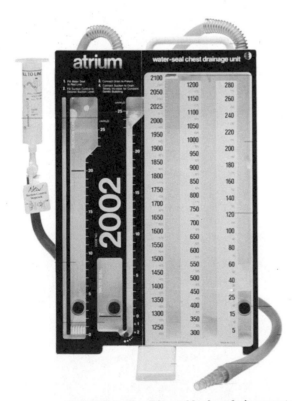

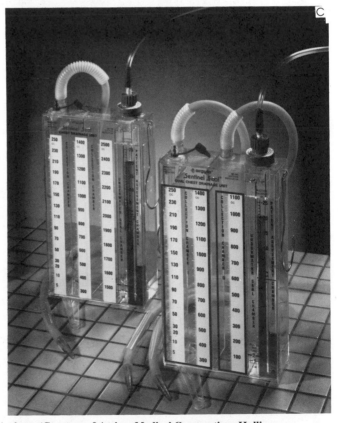

FIGURE 5–16. Disposable chest drainage systems. (*A*) Atrium. (Courtesy of Atrium Medical Corporation, Hollis, N.H.) (*B*) Pleurevac. (Courtesy of Deknatel, Inc., Fall River, Mass.) (*C*) Sentinel Seal. (Courtesy of Sherwood Medical, St. Louis, Mo.)

tion-control chambers positioned side by side in a molded plastic disposable unit (Fig. 5–17). Step-by-step instructions for setting up these units are included in the package insert and/or are printed on the unit itself. The unit hangs below the level of the chest by hanger hooks, or a floor stand can be used.

Disposable chest drainage systems have a number of safety advantages over glass-bottle systems. The chance for error in setup is decreased because multiple connections do not need to be made and straws do not need to be positioned at specific depths. Disposable systems eliminate the risk of bottle breakage, are easy to set up, and are lightweight and portable, making patient transport easier. They take up less space than bottles and can be hung out of the way at the foot of the bed. Safety valves maintain the water seal, allow venting of excess negative pressure, and prevent the accumulation of positive pressure. Fluid levels can be monitored easily using the calibrated markings on the write-on surface of the chambers. Finally, a syringe can be used to obtain specimens

from the self-sealing tubing or diaphragm at the back of the drainage-collection chamber.

Like the triple-bottle system, disposable units use gravity and/or suction to restore negative pressure and remove air, fluid, and/or blood from the pleural cavity. All connections must remain airtight in order for negative pressure to be reestablished in the pleural space. The drainage tubing from the chest tube is attached to the drainage-collection chamber. This chamber is calibrated for measurement (Fig. 5–18).

The water-seal chamber is filled to 2 cm (Fig. 5–19). As in the bottle arrangement, a short latex tube at the top of this chamber is either left open to air (by removing the connector cap) for gravity drainage or attached to a suction source. The water-seal chamber should bubble gently immediately upon insertion of the chest tube, during expiration, and with coughing. Continuous bubbling in this chamber indicates a leak in the system. Fluctuations in the water level in the water-seal chamber of 5 to 10 cm (2 to 4 in), rising (during inhalation) and falling (during expiration), should be observed with spontaneous respirations. If the patient is on mechanical ventilation, the pattern of fluctuation will be just the opposite. Additionally, if suction is being applied, this must be temporarily disconnected to correctly assess for fluctuations in the water-seal chamber. The water-seal cham-

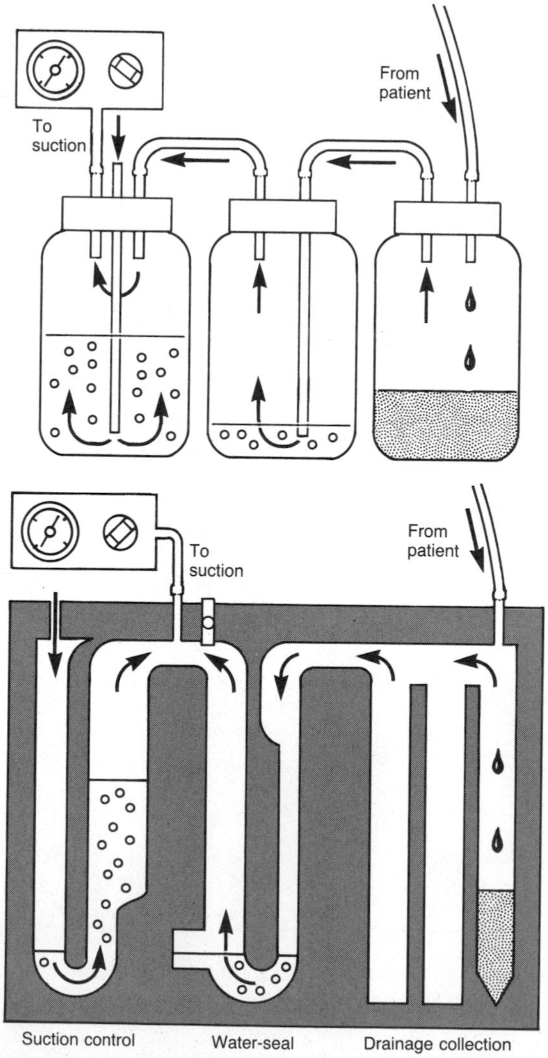

FIGURE 5–17. Disposable system correlates with triple-bottle system. (Used with permission from J. M. Luce, M. L. Tyler, and D. J. Pierson, *Intensive Respiratory Care*. Philadelphia: Saunders, 1984, p. 167.)

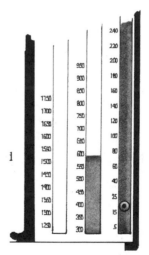

FIGURE 5–18. Calibrated drainage-collection chamber. (Courtesy of Atrium Medical Corporation, Hollis, N.H.)

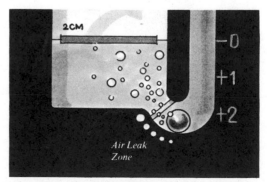

FIGURE 5–19. Water seal filled to 2 cm. (Courtesy of Atrium Medical Corporation, Hollis, N.H.)

ber may have a calibrated manometer to measure negative pressure that is referred from the pleural cavity (Fig. 5–20). As the intrapleural pressure becomes more negative, the water level in the water-seal manometer will rise.

The suction-control chamber is filled to the prescribed level, usually 20 cm (Fig. 5–21) with lower levels recommended for children or patients with fragile lung tissue (i.e., emphysema, necrotizing lung tissue). Suction is regulated by the height of the water level in this chamber. Suction should be adjusted to produce gentle, constant bubbling in this chamber. Increasing the suction level will increase the bubbling action (and evaporation of the water), but it does not increase the pressure on the pleural cavity.

Disposable systems may have some safety features such as a float valve on the water-seal chamber (Fig. 5–22) that acts to maintain the water seal in the event of high negative intrapleural pressures (i.e., milking or stripping the tubing, deep inspiration). Air-leak assessment chambers facilitate the detection of leaks in the system (Fig. 5–23). Additionally, a positive-pressure release valve opens when the pleural cavity pressure becomes positive (i.e., if the suction line becomes obstructed by kinking of the tubing or the patient lying on it). Without this feature, air could accumulate in the system, leading to a tension pneumothorax.

Some chest drainage systems are waterless (Fig. 5–24). These systems are ready to use right from the package, eliminating the need to fill any chambers. The water seal is created by a preset 1.5- to 2.0-cmH$_2$O opening of a one-way valve. This one-way valve feature allows the system to be used in the vertical or horizontal position without loss of the water seal. Thus such systems are safe even if they are accidentally tipped over. The amount of suction delivered to the suction-control chamber is regulated by an adjustable dial or knob (again eliminating the water column) that can be safely set to prevent accidental setting changes. Since the systems are waterless, they are quiet, unaffected by evaporation, and there is no danger that water can accidentally be siphoned back

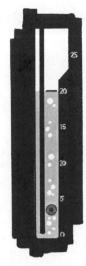

FIGURE 5–21. Vacuum-control chamber filled to 20 cm. (Courtesy of Atrium Medical Corporation, Hollis, N.H.)

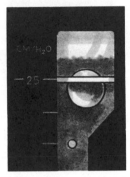

FIGURE 5–22. High-negativity release valve. (Courtesy of Atrium Medical Corporation, Hollis, N.H.)

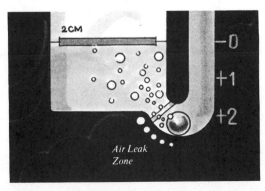

FIGURE 5–23. Air-leak assessment chamber. (Courtesy of Atrium Medical Corporation, Hollis, N.H.)

into the intrapleural space. Assessment of air leaks is accomplished by adding 15 cc of H$_2$O to the air-leak detection chamber. In the event of an air leak, bubbling will be visualized easily.

Disposable systems can be converted easily to gravity drainage by disconnecting the suction tubing and leaving the latex tubing open to air (i.e., if suction is to be discontinued during patient transport to another area or if the unit needs to be replaced).

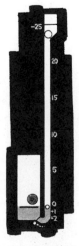

FIGURE 5–20. Water-seal chamber with calibrated manometer. (Courtesy of Atrium Medical Corporation, Hollis, N.H.)

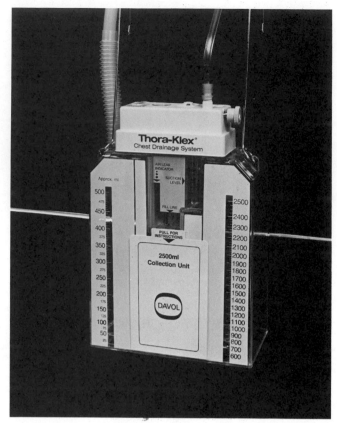

FIGURE 5–24. Thora-Klex waterless disposable chest drainage system. (Courtesy of Davol, Inc., subsidiary of C. R. Bard, Inc., Cranston, R.I.)

Milking or stripping of the drainage tubing may be required to keep the tubing patent if the drainage is thick or bloody (see Skill 5–1). Additionally, some of the disposable units may have an optional attached connector available so that blood drained from the chest can be used for autotransfusion (see Skill 27–5).

Purpose

The nurse uses closed chest drainage systems to

1. Facilitate the removal of fluid, blood, and/or air from the pleural space or the mediastinum.
2. Prevent the entrance of atmospheric air into the pleural space through the use of an underwater seal.
3. Restore negative pressure to the pleural space.
4. Promote reexpansion of a collapsed lung.
5. Relieve respiratory distress associated with a collapsed lung.
6. Improve ventilation and perfusion of the lung.
7. Assess the type and amount of drainage from the pleural space.

Prerequisite Knowledge and Skills

Prior to using a closed chest drainage system, the nurse should understand

1. Principles of aseptic technique.
2. Anatomy and physiology of the thoracic cavity and respiratory system.
3. Principles of closed chest drainage systems.

The nurse should be able to

1. Perform proper handwashing technique (see Skill 35–5).
2. Comply with universal precautions (see Skill 35–1).
3. Assess vital signs.
4. Perform respiratory/thoracic assessment.

Assessment

1. Assess for significant medical history or injury, including chronic lung disease, spontaneous pneumothorax, pulmonary disease, therapeutic procedures associated with risk of pneumothorax/hemothorax, and mechanism of injury. **Rationale:** Medical history and injury may provide the etiologic basis for the occurrence of the pneumothorax or hemothorax.
2. Assess respiratory system for tachypnea, decreased or absent breath sounds on the affected side, wheezes adjacent to the affected area, dyspnea, asymmetrical chest excursion with respirations, cyanosis, hyperresonance on the affected side (pneumothorax), subcutaneous emphysema (pneumothorax), dullness/flatness on the affected side (hemothorax, pleural effusion), sudden sharp chest pain, anxiety, restlessness, or apprehension, tachycardia, hypotension, dysrhythmias, tracheal deviation to the unaffected side (tension pneumothorax), and neck vein distension (tension pneumothorax). **Rationale:** Physical signs and symptoms that result from a pneumothorax, hemothorax, or tension pneumothorax.
3. Assess results of chest x-ray and arterial blood gases (if patient's condition does not necessitate immediate intervention). **Rationale:** Diagnostic testing confirms the presence of air and/or fluid in the pleural space, a collapsed lung, hypoxemia, and respiratory compromise.

Nursing Diagnoses

1. Impaired gas exchange related to partial or total collapse of the lung. **Rationale:** Respiratory gas exchange is decreased or absent in collapsed lung tissue.
2. Ineffective breathing pattern related to pain. **Rationale:** Pain at the site of chest tube insertion interferes with deep breathing and coughing exercises that facilitate drainage from the pleural space, promote lung reexpansion, and prevent respiratory complications.
3. Alteration in skin integrity related to insertion of a chest tube. **Rationale:** A small incision is made in the chest wall to facilitate insertion of the chest tube.
4. Potential for injury: tension pneumothorax related to unrelieved pressure within the pleural space. **Rationale:** Tension pneumothorax is a life-threatening com-

plication that can occur when air accumulates in the pleural space resulting in increased intrapleural pressure and collapse of the lung.

5. Potential for fluid volume deficit related to rapid and excessive drainage from the chest tube. **Rationale:** Rapid drainage of excessive amounts of fluid or blood may cause shock.

6. Ineffective breathing pattern related to a change in intrathoracic pressure as a result of the application of suction to the chest tube. **Rationale:** A low negative pressure within the intrathoracic cavity impedes lung expansion on inspiration, whereas a high negative pressure is traumatic to lung tissue and makes expiration difficult.

7. Potential for infection related to disruption or contamination of the system. **Rationale:** Any disruption in the airtight system due to either leaks in the connections or broken bottles disrupts the water seal, negating its effects, and allows the introduction of atmospheric air and microorganisms into the system.

Planning

Bottle Setup

1. Individualize the following goals for using a closed chest drainage with a bottle setup.
   a. Maintain effective breathing pattern. **Rationale:** Effective respirations are necessary for the exchange of oxygen and carbon dioxide.
   b. Improve gas exchange. **Rationale:** As gas exchange is improved, symptoms of respiratory distress are relieved.
   c. Promote the drainage of air, fluid, and/or blood from the intrapleural space. **Rationale:** As drainage from the intrapleural space occurs, negative intrapleural pressure will be reestablished with subsequent expansion of the lung.
   d. Absence of complications associated with disruption or contamination of the system. **Rationale:** All connections in the bottle-system setup must be airtight in order for the negative intrapleural pressure to be reestablished.
   e. For all bottle systems:
      (1) Sterile water or normal saline, 1 L.
      (2) Rack or holder for the bottles.
      (3) 1 roll of 1 in adhesive tape (used to secure all connections and/or to calibrate measurement on the bottle if bottles are not already precalibrated).
      (4) 2 rubber-tipped Kelly clamps per chest tube.
      (5) Sterile gloves.
   f. For single bottle system:
      (1) Sterile 2-L bottle.
      (2) Short straw.
      (3) Long straw.
      (4) Sterile rubber stopper with two holes.
   g. For double-bottle system:
      (1) Two sterile 2-L bottles.
      (2) Three short straws.

(3) One long straw.
(4) Two sterile rubber stoppers, one with two holes and the other with either two or three holes (depending on which type of double-bottle system is used).
(5) Sterile connecting tubing (6 ft).
(6) Suction source.

h. For triple-bottle system:
   (1) Three sterile 2-L bottles.
   (2) Five short straws.
   (3) Two long straws.
   (4) Two sterile rubber stoppers with two holes.
   (5) One sterile rubber stopper with three holes.
   (6) Sterile connecting tubing (6 ft).
   (7) Suction source.

i. For four-bottle system:
   (1) Four sterile 2-L bottles.
   (2) Seven short straws.
   (3) Three long straws.
   (4) Two sterile rubber stoppers with two holes.
   (5) Two sterile rubber stoppers with three holes.
   (6) Sterile connecting tubing (6 ft).
   (7) Suction source.

2. Prepare the patient and family.
   a. Explain how the closed chest drainage system works. **Rationale:** Explanations decrease patient and family anxiety and enhance cooperation.
   b. Administer prescribed pain medication as needed. **Rationale:** Pain medication reduces the discomfort and anxiety experienced, facilitating patient cooperation.

Disposable Setup

1. Individualize the following goals for using a disposable chest drainage system.
   a. Maintain effective breathing pattern. **Rationale:** Effective respirations are necessary for the exchange of oxygen and carbon dioxide.
   b. Improve gas exchange. **Rationale:** As gas exchange is improved, symptoms of respiratory distress are relieved.
   c. Promote the drainage of air, fluid, and/or blood from the intrapleural space. **Rationale:** As drainage from the intrapleural space occurs, negative intrapleural pressure will be reestablished with subsequent expansion of the lung.
   d. Absence of complications associated with disruption or contamination of the system. **Rationale:** All connections in the disposable chest drainage system must be airtight in order for the negative intrapleural pressure to be reestablished.

2. Prepare all necessary equipment and supplies. **Rationale:** Assembly of all the equipment and supplies facilitates quick and efficient connection of the chest drainage system to the chest tube.
   a. Disposable chest drainage system:
      (1) Disposable chest drainage unit.

(2) Suction source.

(3) Adhesive tape, 1 in, 1 roll.

(4) 1 L bottle of sterile water or normal saline for systems that use water.

(5) 50 ml irrigation syringe (for systems that use water, if not supplied with unit).

3. Prepare the patient and family.

a. Explain how the closed chest drainage system works. **Rationale:** Explanations decrease patient and family anxiety and enhance cooperation.

b. Administer prescribed pain medication as needed. **Rationale:** Pain medication reduces the discomfort and anxiety experienced, facilitating patient cooperation.

Implementation

Steps	Rationale	Special Considerations
Single-Bottle Setup (see Fig. 5–12)		
1. Wash hands.	Reduces transmission of microorganisms.	
2. Open sterile packages.	Maintain aseptic technique whenever making changes in the system.	
3. Don gloves.	Universal precautions.	
4. Fill the water-seal bottle with sterile water or saline so that the bottom of the long straw will be immersed approximately 2 cm.	Depth of solution required to establish a water seal and protect the patient from air leak or loss of water seal.	
5. Seal the bottle with the rubber stopper.	An airtight system is required to reestablish negative pressure in the intrapleural space.	
6. Insert the short straw through one of the openings in the stopper and leave open to air.	Creates the exit vent for the escape of air.	Clamping or occlusion of the exit vent may cause collapse of the lung.
7. Insert the long straw through the second opening, immersing it 2 cm (1 in) beneath the surface of the solution.	Creates the water seal and protects the patient against air leaks.	Immersing the straw deeper than 2 cm increases the work of breathing.
8. Stabilize the drainage bottle on the floor or in a special holder. The bottle must be kept below the level of the chest.	Prevents backflow of drainage into the pleural space, which interferes with lung expansion.	Disruption of the system endangers the patient by allowing the entrance of atmospheric air into the pleural space with collapse of the lung.
9. Connect the drainage tubing from the chest tube to the long straw of the water-seal bottle.	This creates the water-seal/drainage-collection bottle.	
10. Proceed with Step 25 on page 188.		
Double-Bottle Setup with a Drainage-Collection Bottle and a Water-Seal Bottle (see Fig. 5–13A)		
1. Wash hands.	Reduces transmission of microorganisms.	
2. Open sterile packages.	Maintain aseptic technique whenever making changes to the system.	
3. Don sterile gloves.	Universal precautions.	
4. Seal one bottle with a rubber stopper.	An airtight system is required to reestablish negative pressure in the intrapleural space.	
5. Insert two short straws into the rubber stopper.	Creates the drainage-collection bottle.	

Table continues on following page

Steps	Rationale	Special Considerations
6. Fill the water-seal bottle with sterile water or normal saline so that the bottom of the long straw is immersed approximately 2 cm.	Depth of solution required to establish a water seal and protect the patient from air leak or loss of water seal.	
7. Seal the bottle with a rubber stopper with two openings.	An airtight system is required to reestablish negative pressure in the intrapleural space.	
8. Insert the short straw through one of the openings in the stopper.	Creates the exit vent for the escape of air or for connection to the suction source.	
9. Insert the long straw through the second opening, immersing it 2 cm beneath the surface of the solution.	Creates the water seal and protects the patient from air leaks or loss of water seal.	Immersing the straw deeper than 2 cm increases the work of breathing.
10. Use the sterile plastic tubing to connect one of the short straws of the drainage-collection bottle to the long straw of the water-seal bottle.	Connects the drainage collection bottle to the water seal bottle.	
11. Stabilize the bottles on the floor or in a special holder. The bottles must be kept below the level of the chest.	Prevents backflow of drainage into the pleural space, which interferes with lung expansion.	Disruption of the system endangers the patient by allowing the entrance atmospheric air into the pleural space, which collapses the lung.
12. Connect the drainage tubing from the chest tube to the second short straw of the drainage-collection bottle.	Creates a drainage avenue.	
13. Leave the exit vent of the water-seal bottle open to air. *or* Connect the suction source to the exit vent and adjust to the prescribed level (usually -20 cmH$_2$O).	Increases pressure differences between the pleural space and drainage bottles which facilitate drainage from the pleural space.	Surges in suction and accidental displacement of the control knob are possible with this setup.
14. Proceed to Step 25 on page 188.		

Double-Bottle Setup with a Water-Seal/Drainage-Collection Bottle and a Vacuum-Control Bottle (see Fig. 5–13B)

1. Wash hands.	Reduces transmission of microorganisms.	
2. Open sterile packages.	Maintain aseptic technique whenever making changes to the system.	
3. Don sterile gloves.	Universal precautions.	
4. Fill the water-seal/drainage-collection bottle with sterile water or normal saline so that the bottom of the long straw is immersed approximately 2 cm.	Depth of solution required to establish a water seal and protect the patient from air leak or loss of water seal.	
5. Seal the bottle with a rubber stopper with two openings.	An airtight system is required to reestablish negative pressure in the intrapleural space.	
6. Insert the short straw through one of the openings in the stopper.	Initial step for connecting the drainage bottle to the water-seal bottle.	

Table continues on following page

Steps	Rationale	Special Considerations
7. Insert the long straw through the second opening, immersing it 2 cm beneath the surface of the solution.	Creates the water seal and protects the patient from air leaks or loss of water seal.	Immersing the straw deeper than 2 cm increases the work of breathing.
8. Add prescribed amount of sterile water or normal saline to the suction bottle (usually 20 cm).	Creates at least 20 cmH$_2$O of suction.	The amount of suction delivered to the chest tube is determined by the depth the straw is immersed in the solution.
9. Seal the suction bottle with the rubber stopper with three openings.	An airtight system is required to reestablish negative pressure in the intrapleural space.	
10. Insert the long straw through the middle opening (leaving one end immersed in the solution and the other end open to the atmosphere).	Creates an airvent.	
11. Insert the two short straws into the remaining openings of the stopper.	Creates the setup for attachment to suction and to the overflow drainage bottle.	
12. Use the sterile plastic tubing to connect the short straw from the water-seal/drainage-collection bottle to one of the short straws of the suction bottle.	Connects the water-seal bottle to the suction bottle.	
13. Attach one end of the 6-ft connecting tubing to the second short straw of the suction bottle and the other end to the suction source.	Connects the suction bottle to the suction source.	
14. Stabilize the drainage bottles on the floor or in a special holder. The bottles must be kept below the level of the chest.	Prevents backflow of drainage into the pleural space, which interferes with lung expansion.	Disruption of the system endangers the patient by allowing the entrance atmospheric air into the pleural space, which collapses the lung.
15. Connect the drainage tube from the chest tube to the long straw of the water-seal/drainage-collection bottle.	Creates the water-seal/drainage-collection bottle.	
16. Turn the suction source on to elicit gentle, constant bubbling in the suction.	Activates suction.	
17. Proceed to Step 25 on page 188.		

Triple-Bottle Setup (see Fig. 5–14)

Steps	Rationale	Special Considerations
1. Wash hands.	Reduces transmission of microorganisms.	
2. Open sterile packages.	Maintain aseptic technique whenever making changes to the system.	
3. Don gloves.	Universal precautions.	
4. Seal one of the bottles with the rubber stopper with two openings.	An airtight system is required to reestablish negative pressure in the intrapleural space.	
5. Insert two short straws into the rubber stopper.	This creates the drainage-collection bottle.	This bottle can be calibrated if it is not already by placing a piece of tape on the side so that drainage can be measured and recorded.

Table continues on following page

Steps	Rationale	Special Considerations
6. Fill the water-seal bottle with sterile water or normal saline so that the bottom of the long straw will be immersed approximately 2 cm.	Depth of solution required to establish a water seal and protect the patient from air leak or loss of water seal.	
7. Seal the bottle with a rubber stopper with two openings.	An airtight system is required to reestablish negative pressure in the intrapleural space.	
8. Insert the short straw through one of the openings in the stopper.	Creates the exit vent for the escape of air or for connection to the suction source.	
9. Insert the long straw through the second opening, immersing it 2 cm beneath the surface of the solution.	Creates the water seal and protects the patient from air leaks and loss of water seal.	Immersing the straw deeper than 2 cm increases the work of breathing.
10. Add prescribed amount of sterile water or normal saline to the suction bottle (usually 20 cm).	Creates a water seal.	The amount of suction delivered to the chest tube is determined by the depth the straw is immersed in the solution.
11. Seal the suction bottle with the rubber stopper with three openings.	An airtight system is needed to reestablish negative pressure in the intrapleural space.	
12. Insert the long straw through the middle opening (leaving one end immersed in the solution and the other end open to the atmosphere).	Creates the suction bottle.	
13. Insert the two short straws into the remaining openings.	Creates the setup for attachment to suction source and to the overflow drainage bottle.	
14. Use the sterile plastic tubing to connect the second straw of the drainage collection bottle to the long straw of the water-seal bottle.	Provides for communication between the drainage collection bottle and the water-seal bottle.	
15. Use the sterile plastic tubing to connect the short straw from the water-seal bottle to one of the short straws of the suction bottle.	Connects the water-seal bottle to the suction bottle.	
16. Attach one end of the 6-ft connecting tubing to the second short straw of the suction bottle and the other end to the suction source.	Connects the suction bottle to the suction source.	
17. Stabilize the drainage bottles on the floor or in a special holder. The bottles must be kept below the level of the chest.	Prevents backflow of drainage into the pleural space, which interferes with lung expansion.	Disruption of the system endangers the patient by allowing the entrance of atmospheric air into the pleural space, which collapses the lung.
18. Connect the drainage tube from the chest tube to the short straw of the drainage-collection bottle.	Provides a route for drainage to flow from the patient to the collection bottle.	
19. Turn the suction source on to elicit gentle, constant bubbling in the suction bottle.	Activate suction.	
20. Proceed with Step 25 on page 188.		

Implementation

Steps	Rationale	Special Considerations
Disposable Chest Drainage System (See Fig. 5–16)		
1. Wash hands.	Reduces transmission of microorganisms.	
2. Open sterile packages.	Maintain aseptic technique whenever making changes to the system.	
3. Remove the connector cap from the short tube of the water-seal chamber and use the funnel provided or a 50-cc syringe to add sterile water or normal saline to the 2-cm level (see Fig. 5–19).	Depth of solution needed to establish the water seal.	Water-seal levels more than 2 cm increase the work of breathing. Some systems color the solution for easy visibility of air-leak detection. Refill with water as necessary to the 2-cm level to replace solution lost through evaporation.
4. For gravity drainage, leave the short tube of the water-seal chamber uncapped.	Creates the exit vent for the escape of air.	Clamping or occlusion of the exit vent may cause collapse of the lung.
5. For suction drainage, remove the cap from the suction chamber, fill to the prescribed level (usually −20 cm) (see Fig. 5–21), and replace the cap.	Suction is regulated by the height of the solution level in this chamber. Decreases the noise from the bubbling when suction is applied.	Refill the solution level as necessary to the prescribed amount to replace solution lost through evaporation.
6. Hang drainage unit from bed frame or set it on a floor stand. Drainage unit must be kept below the level of the chest.	Prevents backflow of drainage into the pleural space, which interferes with lung expansion.	
7. Connect the long tube from the drainage-collection chamber to the chest tube.	Creates the drainage-collection system.	Avoid dependent or fluid-filled loops.
8. For suction drainage, connect the short tube from the water-seal bottle to the suction source.	Connects the water-seal bottle to the suction source.	
9. Turn on the suction source to elicit gentle, constant bubbling.	Activates suction.	
10. Proceed to Step 25 on page 188.		
Four-Bottle Setup (Triple-Bottle Setup with Vented Water-Seal Bottle) (see Fig. 5–15)		
1. Wash hands.	Reduces the transmission of microorganisms.	
2. Open sterile packages.	Maintain aseptic technique whenever making changes to the system.	
3. Don sterile gloves.	Universal precautions.	
4. Fill the vented water-seal bottle with sterile water or normal saline so that the bottom of the long straw will be immersed approximately 2 cm.	Depth of solution required to establish a water seal and protect the patient from air leak or loss of water seal.	
5. Seal the bottle with a rubber stopper with two openings.	An airtight system is required to reestablish negative pressure in the intrapleural space.	
6. Insert the long straw through one of the openings, immersing it 2 cm beneath the surface of the solution.	Creates the water seal and protects the patient from air leak or loss of water seal.	Immersing the straw deeper than 2 cm increases the work of respiration.

Table continues on following page

Steps	Rationale	Special Considerations
7. Insert a short straw through the second opening in the stopper and leave open to air.	Creates the vented water seal that acts as a safety feature to allow the escape of positive pressure in the event of problems with the suction source.	
8. Seal the drainage-collection bottle with a rubber stopper with three openings.	An airtight system is required to reestablish negative pressure in the intrapleural space.	
9. Insert three short straws into the rubber stopper.	This creates the drainage-collection bottle.	This bottle can be calibrated if it is not already by placing a piece of tape up the side so that drainage can be measured.
10. Fill the water-seal bottle with sterile water or normal saline so that the bottom of the long straw will be immersed approximately 2 cm.	Depth of solution required to establish a water seal and protect the patient from air leak or loss of water seal.	
11. Seal the bottle with a rubber stopper with two openings.	An airtight system is required to reestablish negative pressure in the intrapleural space.	
12. Insert the short straw through one of the openings in the stopper.	Creates the exit vent for the escape of air or for connection to the suction source.	
13. Insert the long straw through the second opening, immersing it 2 cm beneath the surface of the solution.	Creates the water seal and protects the patient from air leak and loss of water seal.	Immersing the straw deeper than 2 cm increases the work of breathing.
14. Add prescribed amount of sterile water or normal saline to the suction bottle (usually 20 cm).	Creates a water seal.	The amount of suction delivered to the chest tube is determined by the depth the straw is immersed in the solution.
15. Seal the suction bottle with the rubber stopper with three openings.	An airtight system is needed to reestablish negative pressure in the intrapleural space.	
16. Insert the long straw through the middle opening (leaving one end immersed in the solution and the other end open to the atmosphere).	Creates the manometer tube, air vent.	
17. Insert the two short straws into the remaining openings.	Creates the setup for attachment to the suction source and to the overflow drainage bottle.	
18. Use the sterile plastic tubing to connect the long straw of the vented water-seal bottle to one of the short straws of the drainage-collection bottle.	Provides for communication between the drainage system bottle and the vented water-seal bottle.	
19. Use the sterile plastic tubing to connect the second straw of the drainage-collection bottle to the long straw of the water-seal bottle.	Connects the drainage collection bottle to the water-seal bottle.	
20. Use the sterile plastic tubing to connect the short straw from the water-seal bottle to one of the short straws of the suction-control bottle.	Connects the water-seal bottle to the suction bottle.	

Table continues on following page

Steps	Rationale	Special Considerations
21. Attach one end of the 6-ft connecting tubing to the second short straw of the suction-control bottle and the other end to the suction source.	Connects the suction bottle to the suction source.	
22. Stabilize the drainage bottles on the floor or in a special holder. The bottles must be kept below the level of the chest.	Prevents backflow of drainage into the pleural space, which inteferes with lung expansion.	Disruption of the system endangers the patient by allowing the entrance of atmospheric air into the pleural space, which collapses the lung.
23. Connect the drainage tubing from the chest tube to the middle short straw of the the drainage-collection bottle.	Provides route for drainage to flow from the patient to the collection bottle.	
24. Turn the suction source on to elicit gentle, constant bubbling in the suction bottle.	Activates suction.	
25. Assess for air leaks in the system, as indicated by constant bubbling in the water-seal bottle. (Some disposable chest drainage systems have an air leak assessment chamber.)	An airtight system is required to reestablish negative pressure in the intrapleural space.	Occasional bubbling on expiration or coughing is normal and indicates that air is escaping from the pleural space. (Bubbling will occur temporarily when the suction is turned on until air in system is evacuated.)
26. Assess for fluctuations in fluid level in the long straw of the water-seal bottle or the water-seal chamber with respirations.	Indicates effective communication between the pleural space and drainage system and provides an indication of lung reexpansion.	Fluctuations will stop when the lung is reexpanded or when the tubing is obstructed by a kink, a fluid-filled loop, the patient lying on it, or a clot or tissue at the distal end. (If a suction source has been added, it must be temporarily disconnected to accurately assess for fluctuations.)
27. Tape all connection points in the chest drainage system (see Fig. 5–8A).	Maintains connections and prevents air leaks into the pleural space.	Parham bands may be used to secure connections instead of tape (see Fig. 5–8B).
a. One-inch tape is placed horizontally extending over the connections (a portion of the connector may be left unobstructed by the tape).	This technique secures the connections but allows visualization of drainage in the connector.	
b. Reinforce the horizontal tape with tape placed vertically so it encircles both ends of the connector.	Secures chest tube.	
28. In disposable chest drainage systems: Use a syringe with an 18# or 20# gauge needle to withdraw the specimen from the self-sealing latex tubing or the diaphragm on the back of the unit.	Obtains a specimen for analysis.	
29. Mark the original drainage level on the outside of the drainage-collection bottle.	Provides reference point for future measurements.	The amount of drainage should be marked in hourly/daily increments and recorded.
30. Dispose of equipment in appropriate receptacle.	Universal precautions.	
31. Wash hands.	Reduces transmission of microorganisms.	

Evaluation

1.   Compare patient's vital signs and respiratory assessment after connecting the chest tube to a closed drainage system with the baseline assessments done prior to the procedure. **Rationale:** Identifies the effects of chest tube insertion and closed chest drainage and the occurrence of developing complications.

2.   Evaluate the insertion site for the presence of subcutaneous emphysema. **Rationale:** Subcutaneous emphysema may have been present prior to insertion of the chest tube, and this should be monitored and reported to the physician if there is an increase. Subcutaneous emphysema present after the chest tube has been inserted needs to be reported immediately as it may indicate an air leak.

3.   Evaluate the chest drainage system for the type and amount of drainage. **Rationale:** Immediately after the chest tube is inserted, the sound of air escaping should be heard. Depending on the reason the chest tube was inserted, drainage may be air, fluid, blood, or a combination of these. Rapid drainage of excessive amounts of fluid or blood may result in shock, which should be reported to the physician immediately.

4.   Evaluate the chest drainage system for bubbling and fluctuations in the water-seal chamber. **Rationale:** The water level in the water-seal chamber should rise and fall with the patient's respirations until the lung is fully expanded. The absence of fluctuations immediately after the insertion of the chest tube needs to be identified and corrected. A chest x-ray will determine whether incorrect tube placement or dislodgment of the tube is the source of this problem. The chest drainage system should be checked for possible malfunction as a result of incorrect setup and/or obstruction in the tubing. Connection points should be checked and secured to ensure an airtight system.

Expected Outcomes

1.   Removal of air, fluid, or blood from pleural space. **Rationale:** Reduces the space-occupying accumulations that interfere with full lung expansion.

2.   Fluctuations noted in the water-seal chamber. **Rationale:** The water level in the water-seal chamber should rise and fall with the patient's respirations until the lung is fully expanded.

3.   Relief of respiratory distress. **Rationale:** As the lung reexpands, pulmonary exchange of gases occurs, hypoxia is relieved, and arterial blood gas results indicate improvement.

4.   Reexpansion of the collapsed lung validated by chest x-ray. **Rationale:** As negative pressure is restored to the intrapleural space, the lung reexpands and bilateral audible breath sounds are heard in all long fields.

Unexpected Outcomes

1.   Increasing respiratory distress, dysrhythmias, tachycardia, hypotension, and tracheal deviation. **Rationale:** The patient has developed a tension pneumothorax.

2.   Hypotension, tachycardia, diaphoresis, and cool skin. **Rationale:** The patient is in shock, possibly from excessive chest tube drainage.

3.   Absence of drainage and fluctuations and/or continuous bubbling in the water-seal chamber with continued respiratory distress; lung does not show evidence of reexpansion. **Rationale:** Possible equipment malfunction, incorrect tube placement, dislodgment of tube, or air leak.

4.   Fever, purulent drainage and redness around the insertion site, or purulent drainage in the chest tube. **Rationale:** Evidence of infectious process.

Documentation

Documentation in the patient record should include respiratory/thoracic and vital signs assessments before and after the procedure; date and time of connection to specific type of bottle drainage system, amount of suction, fluctuations, and the type and amount of drainage; patient's tolerance of the procedure; and completion and results of the postinsertion chest x-ray and any other diagnostic tests ordered. **Rationale:** Documents interventions, nursing care, and expected and unexpected outcomes and serves as a medical-legal record of the events.

Patient/Family Education

1.   Assess the patient and family as to their understanding of the patient's condition and the rationale for chest tube insertion and how the closed chest drainage system works. **Rationale:** Identifies patient and family knowledge deficits concerning the patient's condition, the procedure, expected benefits, and potential risks and allows time for questions to clarify information.

2.   Instruct the patient to sit in a semi-fowler's position (unless contraindicated). **Rationale:** Facilitates drainage from the lung by allowing air to rise and fluid to settle in order to be removed via the chest tube. This position also makes breathing easier.

3.   Instruct the patient to turn and position every 2 hours. **Rationale:** Turning and repositioning prevent complications related to immobility and retained secretions.

4.   Instruct the patient to cough and deep breathe, splinting the affected side. **Rationale:** Coughing and deep breathing raise intrapleural pressure, thus facilitating drainage, promoting lung reexpansion, and preventing respiratory complications associated with retained secretions. The application of firm pressure over the chest tube insertion site (i.e., splinting) decreases pain and discomfort.

5.   Instruct the patient not to lie on the tubing and to keep it free from kinks. **Rationale:** To maintain patency of tube, to facilitate drainage, and to prevent the accumulation of pressure within the intrapleural space, which interferes with lung reexpansion.

6.   Encourage active or passive range-of-motion exercises of the arm on the affected side. **Rationale:** The patient may splint the arm on the affected side to decrease discomfort at the insertion site.

7.   Instruct the patient and family about activity as prescribed while maintaining the drainage system below

the level of the chest. **Rationale:** To facilitate gravity drainage and to prevent backflow into the pleural space.

8. Instruct the patient about the availability of pre-scribed analgesic medication. **Rationale:** Alleviates pain and facilitates coughing, deep breathing, positioning, and range-of-motion exercises.

Performance Checklist
Skill 5–2: Closed Chest Drainage System (Bottle and Disposable Units)

Critical Behaviors	Complies yes	no
1. Wash hands.		
2. Use aseptic technique to open sterile packages.		
3. Don sterile gloves.		
4. Prepare single-, double-, triple-, or four-bottle setup correctly:		
a. Fill water-seal bottle to prescribed level (usually 2 cm).		
b. Fill suction-control bottle to prescribed level (usually 20 cm) for double-bottle (second type), triple-, and four-bottle setups.		
c. Ensure airtight connections of rubber stoppers.		
d. Insert straws to the correct depth.		
e. Connect the bottles together (double-, triple-, four-bottle setups), taping connections.		
f. Stabilize the drainage bottles on the floor or in a special holder.		
5. Connect the drainage tubing from the chest tube to the appropriate bottle/straw:		
a. Water-seal/drainage-collection bottle (single-, and double-bottle, second type, setups).		
b. Drainage-collection bottle (double-bottle, first type, triple- and four-bottle setups).		
c. Leave the exit vent open for gravity drainage as prescribed, *or* for suction drainage, connect to a suction source to elicit gentle bubbling.		
d. Secure connections between chest tube and chest drainage system with tape or Parham bands.		
6. Set up disposable chest drainage unit correctly:		
a. Fill water-seal chamber to prescribed level (usually 2 cm).		
b. Fill vacuum-control chamber to prescribed level (usually 20 cm) if suction is ordered.		
c. Hang drainage unit from bed frame or set it on a floor stand.		
d. Connect chest tube with drainage tubing to the drainage collection chamber:		
1. Leave the exit vent open for gravity drainage as prescribed, or for suction drainage, connect to a suction source to elicit gentle bubbling.		
2. Secure connections between chest tube and chest drainage system with tape or Parham bands.		
3. Tape all connection points securely.		
7. Assess the system for		
a. Air leaks/continuous bubbling in water-seal bottle or chamber.		
b. Fluctuations in fluid level.		
c. Drainage (amount and type).		
d. Obtain a specimen as ordered from drainage collection chamber of disposable unit.		
8. Mark original drainage level on outside of collection bottle.		
9. Dispose of equipment.		

Table continues on following page

Critical Behaviors	Complies	
	yes	no
10. Wash hands.		
11. Document procedure in patient record.		

SKILL 5–3

Chest Tube Removal

Removal of a chest tube is usually performed within 24 hours of the following indicators:

1. The drainage has decreased to 50 to 100 cc per 24 hours.

2. The patient's respiratory status has improved (i.e., nonlabored respirations, absence of shortness of breath [dyspnea] and decreased use of accessory muscles, symmetrical respiratory excursion, respiratory rate less than 24 breaths per minute, and breath sounds are audible bilaterally).

3. No fluctuations are observed in the water-seal chamber and the level of solution rises in the chamber.

4. The cessation of any air leaks that were present (assessed by the air-leak chamber or the absence of continuous bubbling in the water-seal chamber).

5. The chest x-ray indicates that the lung has reexpanded.

Placement of a chest tube for more than 7 days increases the risk for infection along the chest tube tract. Chest x-rays are done periodically to determine whether the lung has reexpanded. This and assessments that indicate improvement in the patient's respiratory status are the basis for making the decision to remove the chest tube.

Purpose

The nurse removes or assists with removal of a chest tube to

1. Facilitate its removal without the introduction of air into the pleural space.

2. Facilitate its removal without contamination and development of infection.

3. Discontinue an invasive intervention that is no longer necessary.

Prerequisite Knowledge and Skills

Prior to removing a chest tube, the nurse should understand

1. Principles of aseptic technique.

2. Anatomy and physiology of the thoracic cavity and respiratory system.

The nurse should be able to

1. Perform proper handwashing technique (see Skill 35–5).

2. Comply with universal precautions (see Skill 35–1).

3. Assess vital signs.

4. Perform respiratory/thoracic assessment.

5. Recognize indications that the lung has reexpanded.

6. Apply sterile occlusive dressing over the insertion site.

Assessment

Assess the patient for a decrease in (50 to 100 cc per 24 hours) or absence of drainage; nonlabored respirations, absence of shortness of breath (dyspnea), and decreased use of accessory muscles; symmetrical respiratory excursion, respiratory rate less than 24 breaths per minute; audible breath sounds bilaterally; absence of fluctuations in the water-seal chamber and the level of the solution rises in the chamber (problems with the drainage system have been ruled out); the cessation of any air leaks that were present (assessed by the air-leak chamber or the absence of continuous bubbling in the water-seal chamber); chest x-ray results indicate that the lung has reexpanded; stable vital signs; and improved arterial blood gases. **Rationale:** Indicates reexpansion of the lung and an improvement in the patient's respiratory status as a result of insertion of the chest tube.

Nursing Diagnoses

1. Potential for injury: respiratory distress related to recurrent pneumothorax. **Rationale:** The patient may develop a recurrent pneumothorax if the chest tube is removed before all the air, fluid, or blood in the pleural space has been drained, or pneumothorax may recur following removal of the chest tube if air is accidentally introduced into the opening in the chest wall created by removal of the chest tube.

2. Potential for infection related to contamination. **Rationale:** Prolonged insertion of a chest tube increases the risk that the tract created by the chest tube may become infected, or infection may occur following removal of the chest tube if the opening created by the removal becomes contaminated.

3. Alteration in skin integrity related to insertion and removal of a chest tube. **Rationale:** A small incision is made in the chest wall to facilitate insertion of a chest tube. Upon its removal, a suture is placed to approximate the wound edges.

Planning

1. Check institutional policy to assess the nurse's scope of practice for chest tube removal. **Rationale:** Institutional policies vary with regard to procedures that nurses are permitted to do independently and those which must be performed by the physician.
2. Individualize the following goals for removal of a chest tube.
   a. Maintain effective breathing pattern after chest tube removal. **Rationale:** Effective ventilation is necessary for the exchange of oxygen and carbon dioxide.
   b. Absence of complications associated with recurrent pneumothorax and/or infection. **Rationale:** Recurrent pneumothorax and infection complicate the patient's recovery.
3. Prepare all necessary equipment and supplies. **Rationale:** Assembly of all the equipment and supplies facilitates quick and efficient removal of the chest tube, minimizing the risk for complications.
   a. Suture removal set.
   b. Sterile gloves.
   c. Petrolatum gauze.
   d. 4 × 4 gauze pads (2 to 4).
   e. Wide tape (2 in adhesive).
   f. Bed protector (protects bed from possible drainage).
   g. Specimen collection container (if culture and sensitivity are necessary).
4. Prepare the patient and family.
   a. Explain the procedure to the patient. **Rationale:** Explanations decrease anxiety and enhance cooperation.
   b. Discuss expectations regarding the patient's participation. **Rationale:** When instructed to do so, the patient should take a deep breath and hold it as the chest tube is removed and prior to application of the occlusive dressing to prevent air from entering the chest tube tract (and consequently the pleural space).
   c. Position the patient in a semi-Fowler's position or on the unaffected side with the bed protector underneath. **Rationale:** To enhance accessibility to the insertion site of the chest tube and to protect the bed from drainage upon removal of the chest tube.
   d. Administer prescribed pain medication as needed. **Rationale:** Pain medication reduces the discomfort and anxiety experienced, facilitating patient cooperation.

Implementation

Steps	Rationale	Special Considerations
1. Wash hands.	Reduces transmission of microorganisms.	
2. Open the sterile suture removal set.	Aseptic technique is maintained to prevent contamination of the wound.	
3. Prepare a petrolatum gauze dressing and two to four 4 × 4s.	Removal of the chest tube must be accomplished rapidly with the simultaneous application of an occlusive dressing to prevent air from entering the pleural space.	
4. Assist in or perform chest tube removal.		
a. If two chest tubes are connected with a Y connector, clamp the remaining chest tube, placing Kelly clamps in opposite directions (see Fig. 5–11), while the first tube is being removed.	Prevents the introduction of air into the pleural space.	
b. Loosen the dressing over the insertion site.	Allows access to the chest tube at the skin level.	
c. Cut the sutures that secure the chest tube in place, unless the suture is a purse-string type that will be pulled to close the insertion site once the chest tube is removed.	Allows chest tube to be removed without resistance.	
d. Instruct the patient to take a deep breath and hold it.	Increases the intrathoracic pressure to prevent air from entering the pleural space.	

Table continues on following page

Steps	Rationale	Special Considerations
e. Remove the chest tube rapidly, and pull the previously tied purse-string suture closed or seal the wound with the petrolatum gauze.	Prevents the accidental entrance of air into the pleural space.	
5. Cover the entire dressing with 2 to 4 (4 × 4s gauze) and secure with occlusive tape.	Creates an airtight dressing and absorbs any drainage that may seep from the insertion site.	
6. Order a stat portable chest x-ray after chest tube removal per physician instructions or protocol.	Assesses that the lung has remained expanded.	
7. Dispose of equipment in appropriate receptacle.	Universal precautions.	
8. Wash hands.	Decreases transmission of microorganisms.	

Evaluation

Compare patient's vital signs and respiratory assessments after removal of the chest tube with those before removal of the chest tube. **Rationale:** Identifies the development of complications following chest tube removal.

Expected Outcome

Lung remains expanded following chest tube removal. **Rationale:** Upon removal of the chest tube, if air or contaminants are introduced into the pleural space, the patient may develop a recurrent pneumothorax or infection.

Unexpected Outcomes

1. Recurrent pneumothorax. **Rationale:** During removal of the chest tube, air may have inadvertently entered the pleural space.
2. Infection. **Rationale:** During removal of the chest tube, there may have been contamination of the insertion site and tract left by removal of the chest tube.

Documentation

Documentation in the patient record should include respiratory/thoracic and vital signs assessments before and after the procedure; date and time and by whom the procedure was performed; amount, color, and consistency of any drainage; application of a sterile, occlusive dressing; patient's tolerance of the procedure; completion and results of chest x-ray after chest tube removal.

Rationale: Documents interventions, nursing care, and expected and unexpected outcomes and serves as a medical-legal record of the events.

Patient/Family Education

1. Assess the patient and family as to their understanding that the lung has reexpanded and that the chest tube can be removed. **Rationale:** Identifies patient and family knowledge deficits concerning the patient's condition, the procedure, expected benefits, and potential risks and allows time for questions to clarify information.
2. Instruct the patient to turn and reposition every 2 hours after the chest tube has been removed. **Rationale:** Turning and repositioning prevent complications related to immobility and retained secretions.
3. Instruct the patient to cough and deep breathe after the chest tube has been removed, splinting the affected side. **Rationale:** Coughing and deep breathing prevent respiratory complications associated with retained secretions. The application of firm pressure over the insertion site (i.e., splinting) decreases pain and discomfort.
4. Instruct the patient as to the availability of prescribed analgesic medication. **Rationale:** Alleviates pain and facilitates coughing, deep breathing, and repositioning.
5. Instruct the patient and family to report signs and symptoms of respiratory distress or infection immediately. **Rationale:** Facilitates prompt intervention to relieve a recurrent pneumothorax or to treat an infection.

Performance Checklist
Skill 5–3: Chest Tube Removal

Critical Behaviors	Complies	
	yes	no
1. Wash hands.		

Table continues on following page

Critical Behaviors	Complies	
	yes	no
2. Open sterile suture removal set.		
3. Prepare a petroleum gauze dressing and 4 × 4s.		
4. Assist in or perform chest tube removal.		
a. Clamp one of two chest tubes if joined by a Y connector (if applicable).		
b. Loosen dressing over insertion site.		
c. Cut sutures securing chest tube unless it is a purse-string suture.		
d. Instruct patient to inhale and hold breath.		
e. Remove the chest tube rapidly, and pull purse-string suture closed *and/or* rapidly seal the wound with petrolatum gauze.		
5. Cover dressing with occlusive tape.		
6. Order stat chest x-ray per physician order or protocol.		
7. Dispose of equipment.		
8. Wash hands.		
9. Document procedure in patient record.		

SKILL 5—4

Assisting with Open Chest Thoracotomy

Blunt or penetrating chest trauma may result in a variety of injuries that necessitate the performance of an *open chest thoracotomy*, an incision into the chest wall. A hemothorax (the accumulation of blood in the pleural space) may occur as a result of a laceration to the great vessels (i.e., the aorta, inferior or superior vena cava, pulmonary or intercostal vessels) or to the mediastinal structures (i.e., the heart or lungs). The accumulation of blood and fluid in the pleural space and the loss of negative intrapleural pressure result in collapse of the lung on the affected side, decreased ventilation, hypoxia, and respiratory distress. Signs and symptoms of hypovolemic shock occur as mediastinal shifting impairs venous return and the loss of circulating blood volume results in decreased cardiac output. Ultimately, cardiac arrest occurs if the condition is not corrected.

In most cases, intrathoracic bleeding can be managed with the administration of fluids and blood via large-bore intravenous catheters along with the evacuation of blood from the pleural space via the insertion of a large-bore (i.e., 32- to 36-gauge) chest tube connected to a closed chest drainage system (see Skills 5–1, 5–2). When the chest tube is inserted, blood may drain at an extremely rapid rate. If the patient's condition improves as the blood is removed, drainage of the thoracic cavity is continued and the patient is closely monitored.

Bleeding within the thoracic cavity will slow when the pressure within the pleural cavity is equal to or greater than the pressure within the damaged vessel. Occasionally, insertion of a chest tube to treat a massive hemothorax will eliminate this tamponade effect and the patient will exsanguinate via the chest tube if this condition goes unrecognized and untreated. Further bleeding is prevented by clamping the chest tube, and an open chest thoracotomy is performed to locate and control the source of bleeding. Whenever possible, the patient is transferred to the operating room for this procedure.

Other conditions following blunt or penetrating trauma that may indicate the need for a thoracotomy include cardiac tamponade, cardiac arrest, uncontrolled air leak, esophageal injury, ruptured diaphragm, sucking chest wound, and transbronchial aspiration of blood with progressive hypoxia.

Patients with intrathoracic bleeding who require a thoracotomy are often excellent candidates for autotransfusion because there is usually no contamination of the blood in the chest cavity by intestinal fluid. The use of autotransfusion will reduce the need for banked blood to replace lost blood volume and reduce the risks to the patient (see Skill 27–5).

Purpose

The nurse assists with an open chest thoracotomy to

1. To locate the source of an intrathoracic bleed or injury.
2. To control the source of an intrathoracic bleed.
3. To repair damaged vessels or organs.

Prerequisite Knowledge and Skills

Prior to assisting with an open chest thoracotomy, the nurse should understand

1. Principles of aseptic technique.
2. Anatomy and physiology of the thoracic cavity.
3. Principles of closed chest drainage/autotransfusion systems.

The nurse should be able to

1. Perform proper handwashing technique (see Skill 35–5).
2. Comply with universal precautions (see Skill 35–1).
3. Assess vital signs.
4. Perform thoracic assessment.
5. Set up the chest drainage/autotransfusion system (see Skill 27–5).
6. Administer intravenous fluids and blood (see Skills 27–1, 33–2, 33–5).

Assessment

1. Assess for history of significant blunt, crushing, or penetrating chest trauma that results in mediastinal shifting, sucking chest wound, respiratory distress, decreased breath sounds, dullness to percussion, subcutaneous emphysema, signs and symptoms of cardiac tamponade (i.e., neck vein distension, narrowed pulse pressure, muffled heart sounds), esophageal tear, diaphragmatic rupture, cardiac arrest, or ecchymotic mask. **Rationale:** Blunt, crushing, or penetrating chest trauma may result in an intrathoracic bleed that necessitates an open chest thoracotomy.

2. Assess for signs and symptoms of hypovolemic shock: tachycardia, hypotension, tachypnea, delayed capillary refill, pallor, cool, moist skin, altered level of consciousness, decreased urinary output, delayed capillary refill, and excessive blood loss (i.e., unstable vital signs, initial chest tube drainage exceeding 1500 cc, chest tube drainage exceeding 200 cc/h for 2 or more hours, and rapid deterioration of the patient's condition after the infusion of 2 to 3 L of fluid). **Rationale:** Physical signs and symptoms of hypovolemic shock.

3. Assess for significant medical history or injury that may be a contraindication to autotransfusion, such as contaminated thoracic hemorrhage, coagulation problems, malignant neoplasms, or respiratory infection. **Rationale:** While these are not absolute contraindications to autotransfusion in cases where the need exceeds the risks, they may predispose the patient to develop complications.

4. Assessment of the results of diagnostic tests may be precluded by the nature of the emergency, but diagnostic workup may be performed as a baseline for measuring patient response and outcomes, including chest x-ray, arterial blood gases, CBC, clotting profile, blood cultures, and type and crossmatch. **Rationale:** The results of diagnostic tests confirm the need for an open chest thoracotomy and the presence of hypovolemic shock.

Nursing Diagnoses

1. Fluid volume deficit related to blood loss. **Rationale:** Excessive loss of blood from a thoracic injury results in a decreased intravascular volume.
2. Impaired tissue perfusion related to blood loss. **Rationale:** The underlying problem in hypovolemic shock is inadequate supply of oxygen and nutrients to tissues.
3. Decreased cardiac output related to blood loss and/or mediastinal shifting. **Rationale:** Mediastinal shifting and a decrease in circulating blood volume result in a decreased venous return to the heart and subsequently decreased cardiac output.
4. Impaired gas exchange related to collapse of the lung. **Rationale:** The accumulation of blood and fluid in the pleural cavity occupies the space the lungs need to expand, compressing lung tissue and causing it to collapse.
5. Alteration in skin integrity related to a wound (i.e., penetrating or surgical) or the insertion site for the chest tube. **Rationale:** A chest tube inserted before or after open chest thoracotomy, the thoracotomy incision, and the presence of a penetrating thoracic wound disrupt skin integrity.
6. Potential for injury: complications related to thoracic trauma and open chest thoracotomy. **Rationale:** Patients sustaining blunt or penetrating trauma, particularly if there is a laceration of a major blood vessel, heart, or lungs, frequently arrive in cardiac arrest and cannot be successfully resuscitated even with the performance of a thoracotomy. Complications associated with thoracotomy include empyema, bleeding, fistulas, suture-line disruption, pneumonia, and infection.

Planning

1. Individualize the following goals for assisting with an open chest thoracotomy.
   a. Restore circulating blood volume. **Rationale:** As bleeding is controlled and intravascular blood volume is restored via transfusions or autotransfusion, tissue perfusion, cardiac output, and gas exchange improve.
   b. Locate the source of an intrathoracic bleed or injury. **Rationale:** The source of the bleeding must be located in order for it to be controlled and repaired.
   c. Promote the drainage of air and/or fluid from the pleural space via chest tube and closed chest drainage system. **Rationale:** As drainage from the pleural space occurs, compression on the lungs is relieved, mediastinal shifting is corrected, and negative intrapleural pressure is reestablished with subsequent expansion of the lung.
   d. Regain skin integrity. **Rationale:** Interventions must be implemented to treat the thoracic wound and the thoracotomy incision in order to prevent contamination and promote wound healing.

e. Absence of complications associated with a thoracotomy. **Rationale:** Empyema, bleeding, fistula, suture-line disruption, pneumonia, and infection complicate the patient's recovery.

2. Prepare all necessary equipment and supplies. **Rationale:** Assembly of all the equipment and supplies facilitates performance of the thoracotomy.
   a. Thoracotomy tray.
   b. Sternal saw (if available).
   c. Sterile drapes and attire (gown, cap, mask, and gloves).
   d. Antiseptic solution (usually povidone iodine/betadine).
   e. Suture material.
   f. Suction source.
   g. Suction canister.
   h. Chest tube.
   i. Chest drainage system with autotransfusion.
   j. Sterile dressing supplies.

3. Prepare the patient and family. (Open chest thoracotomy is usually an extreme emergency, so preparation depends on the patient's condition.)
   a. Explain the procedure to the patient and family. **Rationale:** Explanations decrease patient and family anxiety and enhance cooperation.
   b. Follow hospital policy to obtain the informed consent. **Rationale:** Invasive procedures, unless performed under implied consent in a life-threatening situation, require the written consent of the patient or significant other.
   c. Establish intravenous access with large-bore catheter. **Rationale:** Large-bore IV access is required for fluid and blood or autologous infusions.
   d. Administer prescribed pain medication as needed. **Rationale:** Pain medication reduces the discomfort and anxiety experienced, facilitating patient cooperation.

Implementation

Steps	Rationale	Special Considerations
1. Wash hands.	Reduces transmission of microorganisms.	
2. Place the thoracotomy tray on the bed table.	Becomes a mobile surface for preparing the necessary equipment.	
3. Open the thoracotomy tray using sterile technique.	Maintains asepsis.	
4. Prepare the insertion site.		
a. Using aseptic technique, cleanse the insertion site with 4 × 4s soaked with providone iodine.	Inhibits the growth of bacteria at the insertion site.	Time permitting, determine that the patient has no allergies to the antiseptic.
5. Assist the physician during the thoracotomy.	Team effort assists in performing the skill in a timely fashion.	
a. Use sterile technique to pass instruments to the physician.	Reduces transmission of microorganisms.	
b. Administer IV fluids, blood, or autologous transfusions.	Restores circulating blood volume.	See Skill 27–5.
6. Assist with insertion of a chest tube and connection to a closed chest drainage system.	Drains intrathoracic blood, fluid, and air to restore negative intrapleural pressure and reexpand the lung.	See Skills 5–1 and 5–2.
7. Apply sterile dressing over the insertion site.	Reduces transmission of microorganisms.	
8. Dispose of equipment in appropriate receptacle.	Removes a potential source of injury and microorganism transmission.	
9. Wash hands.	Reduces transmission of microorganisms.	

Evaluation

1. Evaluate patient response to open chest thoracotomy, including vital signs, capillary refill, skin color, skin temperature/moisture, level of consciousness (as anesthesia wears off), urinary output, improved breath sounds, correction of mediastinal shifting, subcutaneous emphysema, neck vein distension, and heart sounds. **Rationale:** As the source of bleeding is located, corrected, and blood is evacuated from the thoracic cavity, signs

and symptoms of hemothorax should be relieved. The concomitant replacement of blood volume via intravenous infusions of blood and fluids should improve cardiac output and tissue perfusion.

2. Compare the results of baseline diagnostic tests with those done after thoracotomy, including chest x-ray, arterial blood gases, CBC (complete blood count), clotting profile, and blood cultures. **Rationale:** Diagnostic laboratory work monitors patient response and the development of complications after thoracotomy.

Expected Outcomes

1. Intrathoracic bleeding is located and controlled. **Rationale:** As bleeding is controlled and intravascular blood volume is restored via transfusions or autotransfusion, tissue perfusion, cardiac output, and gas exchange improve.

2. Fluid and blood are drained from the thoracic cavity. **Rationale:** As fluid and blood drain from the pleural space, compression of the lungs is relieved, mediastinal shifting is corrected, and negative intrapleural pressure is reestablished with subsequent expansion of the lung.

3. Improved skin integrity. **Rationale:** Interventions must be implemented to treat the thoracic wound and the thoracotomy incision to prevent contamination and promote wound healing.

4. Absence of complications associated with thoracotomy. **Rationale:** Empyema, bleeding, fistulas, suture-line disruption, pneumonia, and infection complicate the patient's recovery.

Unexpected Outcomes

1. Fever, positive blood cultures, tachycardia, and signs and symptoms of infection. **Rationale:** The patient may have developed an infection, empyema, or pneumonia.

2. Hypotension, tachycardia, diaphoresis, and cool skin. **Rationale:** The patient continues to bleed or suffer from hypovolemic shock.

3. Incisional edges separate. **Rationale:** The thoracotomy suture line is disrupted.

4. Cardiac arrest. **Rationale:** Cardiac arrest may occur if hypovolemia and the resulting alterations in tissue perfusion and cardiac output are extreme, prolonged, and cannot be corrected despite the emergency open chest thoracotomy.

Documentation

Documentation in the patient record should include thoracic and vital signs assessments before and after the procedure; date, time, and by whom the procedure was completed; insertion of the chest tube/autotransfusion/closed chest drainage system if applicable (see Skills 5–1 and 5–2, 27–5); the administration of medications and/or anesthesia; patient's tolerance of the procedure; and diagnostic workup performed before and after the procedure. **Rationale:** Documents interventions, nursing care, and expected and unexpected outcomes and serves as a medical-legal record of the events.

Patient/Family Education

Assess the patient and family as to their understanding of the patient's condition and the rationale for the open chest thoracotomy. **Rationale:** Identifies patient and family knowledge deficits concerning the patient's condition, the procedure, expected benefits, and potential risks and allows time for questions to clarify information.

Performance Checklist
Skill 5–4: Assisting with Open Chest Thoracotomy

Critical Behaviors	Complies	
	yes	no
1. Wash hands.		
2. Place thoracotomy tray on bed table.		
3. Open thoracotomy tray using aseptic technique.		
4. Prepare or assist with preparation of the operative site.		
5. Assist physician during the procedure:		
a. Use sterile technique to handle instruments.		
b. Administer intravenous fluids, blood, or autologous transfusions.		
6. Assist with insertion of a chest tube and connection to a closed chest drainage system (see Skills 5–1 and 5–2).		
7. Apply sterile dressing over incision site.		
8. Dispose of equipment.		

Table continues on following page

Critical Behaviors	Complies	
	yes	no
9. Wash hands.		
10. Document procedure in patient record.		

REFERENCES

Duncan, C., and Erickson, R. (1982). Pressures associated with chest tube stripping. *Heart and Lung* 11(2):166–171.

BIBLIOGRAPHY

Alspach, J. G. (Ed.) (1991). *AACN Core Curriculum for Critical Care Nurses*, 4th Ed. Philadelphia: Saunders.

Cardona, V. D., Hurn, P. D., Mason, P. J. B., et al. (Eds.) (1991). *Trauma Nursing from Resuscitation Through Rehabilitation*. Philadelphia: Saunders.

Erickson, R. S. (1989). Mastering the ins and outs of chest drainage, Part I. *Nursing 89* 19(5): 36–44.

Erickson, R. S. (1989). Mastering the ins and outs of chest drainage, Part II. *Nursing 89* 19(6): 46–50.

Kinney, M. R., Packa, D. R., and Dunbar, S. B. (Eds.) (1988). *AACN Clinical Reference for Critical Care Nursing*. New York: McGraw-Hill.

SPECIAL PULMONARY PROCEDURES

BEHAVIORAL OBJECTIVES

After completing this chapter, the nurse will be able to

- Define the key terms.
- Discuss the general indications for pulse oximetry and capnography.
- Outline the basic principles of pulse oximeter and capnograph operation.
- Demonstrate proper sensor site selection and sensor application for pulse oximetry.
- Demonstrate proper gas-sampling technique for capnography.
- Troubleshoot common problems associated with pulse oximetry and capnography.
- Identify indications for bronchoscopy.
- Discuss the nurse's role in the setup and performance of bronchoscopy.
- Describe various types of bronchoscopy.
- Describe methods of hyperbaric oxygen delivery.
- Identify indications for hyperbaric oxygen therapy.
- Discuss physiologic mechanism of hyperbaric oxygenation.
- Discuss safety precautions taken in patient preparation for hyperbaric oxygen treatment.

Maintenance of oxygenation, a patent airway, and the support of breathing are the primary concerns of every nurse caring for critically ill patients. Historically, nurses have relied on subjective symptomatology, clinical assessments, and intermittent arterial blood gas determinations (ABGs) to evaluate the adequacy of oxygenation and ventilation. While these are and will continue to be vital sources of information, they do not provide continuous, real-time monitoring of pulmonary gas exchange. Three devices that continuously provide these data are the pulse oximeter, the capnograph, and the continuous monitoring of mixed venous saturation.

A bronchoscopy is the passage of a rigid or flexible fiberoptic bronchoscope to gain access to the segmental bronchi for direct viewing. The bronchoscope is inserted either transnasally or through an endotracheal or tracheostomy tube. The diagnostic indications for bronchoscopy are to ascertain the cause of a cough, hemoptysis, a localized wheeze, bronchial obstruction, atelectasis, tumor, foreign body, inflammatory process, lung abscess, carcinoma, tuberculosis, bronchiectasis, diaphragmatic paralysis, or suspicious cells in the sputum. Therapeutically, bronchoscopy is used to remove foreign bodies, aspirate secretions, or arrest hemorrhage.

Another mechanism that is used to assist in tissue oxygenation is the hyperbaric chamber. Hyperbaric oxygen (HBO) is an adjunctive therapy whereby 100% oxygen is delivered to the patient in an environment of increased atmospheric pressure. This manner of oxygen delivery facilitates the treatment of selected conditions by (1) supporting angiogenesis, fibroblast formation, and the ul-

timate granulation of new tissue; (2) enhancing the bacterocidal abilities of white blood cells; (3) assisting in the rapid elimination of certain toxins, such as carbon monoxide; and (4) reducing or minimizing the effects of bubbles or emboli introduced iatrogenically or from dive-related insults.

KEY TERMS

$a\text{-}ADCO_2$	*LEDs*
airbreaks	*monoplace chamber*
alveolar plateau	*multiplace chamber*
atmospheres absolute	*optical shunt*
barotrauma	*oxygen toxicity*
bronchial brushing	*oxyhemoglobin*
bronchoalveolar lavage	$PACO_2$
CaO_2	$PaCO_2$
capnography	$PetCo_2$
CO_2 *sensor/optical bench*	*photodetector*
compression	*pulse oximeter*
decompression	SaO_2
deoxyhemoglobin	*shunt*
dysfunctional hemoglobin	SO_2
fiberoptic bronchoscopy	SpO_2
functional hemoglobin	*transtracheal biopsy*
hyperbaric oxygen therapy	$\dot{V}/\dot{Q}$ *relationship*

SKILLS

GUIDELINES

The following assessment guidelines assist the nurse in formulating a nursing diagnosis and an individualized plan of care to monitor the patient's oxygenation and ventilatory status:

1. Perform the patient's baseline respiratory assessment.

2. Obtain the patient's baseline arterial blood gases and vital signs.

3. Review the patient's current medical treatments and ventilator settings (if appropriate).

4. Obtain the patient's medical history.

5. Perform systematic respiratory assessments and equipment checks in a timely manner.

6. Master the setup, use, and troubleshooting of the equipment used for pulse oximetry, capnography, and mixed venous oxygen saturation.

7. Develop critical thinking skills for interpreting pulse oximetry measurements and for determining appropriate interventions based on findings.

8. Develop critical thinking skills for interpreting end-tidal CO_2 ($PetCO_2$) values and a-ADCO$_2$* gradients, as well as CO_2 waveforms (capnograms) and for determining appropriate interventions based on findings.

9. Know the accepted indications for bronchoscopy.

10. Know the accepted indications for hyperbaric oxygen therapy.

11. Understand the physical gas laws and their application to patients in the hyperbaric environment.

SKILL 6–1

Oxygen Saturation Monitoring by Pulse Oximetry

Pulse oximetry is a noninvasive monitoring technique used to measure arterial oxygen saturation of functional hemoglobin. A sensor that contains two light sources (red and infrared) and a photodetector is placed across a pulsating arteriolar bed such as the finger, toe, nose, or earlobe. Selected wavelengths of light are absorbed by hemoglobin and are transmitted through tissue to the photodetector. Arteriolar (pulsating) blood is registered as a fluctuating light signal by the photodetector, and the signal is transformed into a digital display of percent saturation of hemoglobin—SpO$_2$—and pulse rate. Since the venous blood, bone, tissue, and pigments are normally unchanging, they will absorb a constant amount of light and will not interfere with the measurement of SpO$_2$ (Fig. 6–1).

*Note that CO_2 diffusion occurs from blood to alveolus, creating an a-A gradient, as compared to O_2 diffusion, which occurs from alveolus to blood, creating an A–a gradient.

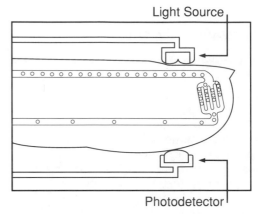

FIGURE 6–1. A sensor device that contains a light source and a photodetector is placed around a pulsating arteriolar bed, such as the finger, great toe, nose, or earlobe. Red and infrared wavelengths of light are used to determine arterial oxygen saturation. (Reprinted with permission from *Principles of Pulse Oximetry*, Hayward, CA: Nellcor, Inc., 1988.)

Patients requiring intermittent or continuous oxygen saturation monitoring by pulse oximetry should have a baseline arterial blood gas determination to check ventilation (PCO_2) and a recent hemoglobin measurement. Since pulse oximetry measures the saturation of the functional hemoglobin in the peripheral vascular bed, it is important to assess for correct sensing of the arteriolar pulse without interference from external sources or measurement of venous pulsatile blood. For this reason, pulse oximetry sensors require certain environmental conditions for optimal performance: (1) proper sensor selection and application, (2) shielding from large amounts of ambient light, (3) elimination of electrical interference, (4) reduction of motion artifacts, and (5) unimpaired venous outflow from the sensor site.

For these reasons, it is important to practice principles that ensure effectiveness of the pulse oximeter as a noninvasive monitor. Pulse oximetry principles include proper sensor site selection and application and a favorable sensor environment. When properly instituted, pulse oximetry is an effective monitor of functional hemoglobin saturation and may decrease the incidence of adverse outcomes related to occurrences of hypoxemia (Rubsamen, 1988).

Normal SpO$_2$ values (SO$_2$ as measured by pulse oximetry) are 97 to 99 percent. However, an SpO$_2$ value of 95 percent or greater generally is acceptable clinically. The oxyhemoglobin dissociation curve (Fig. 6–2) plots the relationship between SO$_2$ and PO$_2$. The term P_{50} is used to designate the PO$_2$ value that effects an SO$_2$ of 50 percent. The sigmoid shape of the oxyhemoglobin dissociation curve is physiologically advantageous to oxygen delivery. The upper portion of the curve is relatively flat, indicating that SO$_2$ is protected over a rather wide range of PO$_2$ values. In contrast, at the steep portion of the curve, a small reduction in PO$_2$ frees large amounts of previously bound oxygen to diffuse into tissues, leaving a relatively low SO$_2$ value (~75 percent) in venous blood.

Since physiologic variables other than PO$_2$ affect SO$_2$, the relationship is not fixed; that is, a PO$_2$ of 27 mmHg does not equal an SO_2 of 50 percent. Alterations in pH, PCO_2, temperature, and the 2,3-DPG level (2,3-diphosphoglycerate, a by-product of glucose metabolism that is highly efficient in the regulation of oxygen–hemoglobin binding) change the PO_2/SO_2 relationship, or "position of the curve" (Table 6–1; see Fig. 6–2). Conditions that shift the curve to the right (increased P_{50}) include decreased pH, increased temperature, increased PCO_2, and increased 2,3-DPG level. Under these conditions, oxygen–hemoglobin binding in the pulmonary circulation is impaired to some degree; however, O_2 release at the tissues is facilitated because of the reduced affinity of hemoglobin for oxygen. Conditions that shift the curve to the left (decreased P_{50}), namely, increased pH, decreased temperature, decreased PCO_2, and decreased 2,3-DPG levels, facilitate oxygen–hemoglobin binding in the pulmonary circulation yet may impair O_2 delivery to the tissues because of the increased affinity of hemoglobin for oxygen.

To quantify the content of O_2 available for transport to the tissues (CaO_2), the nurse must apply the oxygen-content equation. Neither normal PaO_2 nor normal SaO_2 values ensure a normal CaO_2; however, changes in PaO_2 and/or SaO_2 reflect changes in CaO_2. Since CaO_2 is dependent on the quantity of hemoglobin available to transport O_2, dysfunctional hemoglobins and anemia have a deleterious effect on CaO_2. Furthermore, tissue oxygen delivery is dependent on cardiac output as well as cellular ability to extract and utilize O_2. Complete assessment of oxygenation includes the evaluation of PaO_2, SpO_2, hemoglobin, and, when available, cardiac output and $S\bar{v}O_2$ (Gilboy and McGaffigan, 1989).

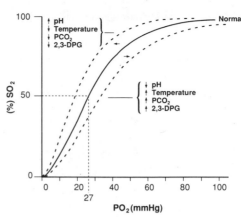

FIGURE 6–2. Oxyhemoglobin dissociation curve. (Adapted with permission from *Principles of Pulse Oximetry*. Hayward, Calif.: Nellcor, Inc., 1988.)

Purpose

The nurse implements continuous oxygen saturation monitoring by pulse oximetry to

1.   Measure the baseline SpO_2 as part of a comprehensive oxygenation assessment.
2.   Provide a mechanism for early detection of changes in SpO_2 that may progress to a critical event.
3.   Evaluate the patient's response to activities that may positively or negatively affect oxygenation (i.e., suctioning, repositioning, changes in FiO_2, changes in PEEP, etc.).

TABLE 6–1   EFFECTS OF BODY TEMPERATURE, pH, AND 2,3-DPG CHANGES ON OXYGEN–HEMOGLOBIN CONCENTRATION

Normal 2,3-DPG Levels		
Calculated SaO_2 = 85 percent (PaO_2 = 50 mmHg) Actual SaO_2:		

Body Temp.	**pH = 7.2**	**pH = 7.4**	**pH = 7.6**
30°C	90	95	97
37°C	74	85	92
40°C	65	77	89

Low 2,3-DPG Levels		
Calculated SaO_2 = 97 percent (PaO_2 = 100 mmHg) Actual SaO_2:		

Body Temp.	**pH = 7.2**	**pH = 7.4**	**pH = 7.6**
30°C	99	99	99
37°C	98	90	99
40°C	97	98	99

Potential errors in estimating oxygen saturation of hemoglobin from measurements of the partial pressure of oxygen. *Pulse Oximetry Reference Note No. 3.* Hayward, CA: Nellcor Inc., 1987.

Prerequisite Knowledge and Skills

Prior to instituting continuous oxygen saturation monitoring, the nurse should understand

1. Principles of oxygenation.
2. Anatomy and physiology of the peripheral vascular system.
3. Principles of pulse oximetry.
4. Principles of oxyhemoglobin dissociation curve.

The nurse should be able to perform

1. Proper handwashing technique (see Skill 35–5).
2. Assessment of capillary refill.
3. Palpation of peripheral pulses.
4. Cardiopulmonary assessment.
5. Simple mathematical calculations.
6. Universal precautions (see Skill 35–1).

Assessment

1. Assess the patient for indications that pulse oximetry monitoring should be instituted, i.e., borderline oxygenation (especially an FIO_2 of greater than 0.50 or PEEP greater than 10 cmH_2O), unstable or uncertain pulmonary status, diseases commonly associated with hypoxemia (including sleep disorders), and rehabilitation with increasing activity levels following respiratory failure. **Rationale:** Ensures that patients at risk for tissue hypoxia secondary to life-threatening desaturation will receive continuous monitoring and, in turn, appropriate interventions.

2. Assess the impact of the following interventions on oxygenation: changes in ventilator (or mask) FIO_2 or PEEP, suctioning, dialysis, and position changes (including chest physiotherapy and postural drainage). **Rationale:** Stated actions and therapies predispose patients to risks for increased hypoxia.

3. Assess therapeutic effects of drug on oxygenation–ventilation, including titration of inotropic agents, vasopressors, and vasodilators; muscle relaxants or neuromuscular blockades; and CNS depressants. **Rationale:** Medications affect oxygen delivery and consumption.

4. Assess the patient for frequent arterial blood gas sampling, including severe coagulopathies, extensive deep burns, arterial catheter-site infections, arterial compromise or trauma, extremely compromised immune defenses, and anatomic or physical conditions making arterial puncture very difficult. **Rationale:** Patients with unstable conditions require increased sampling of ABGs.

5. Assess for proper functioning of the pulse oximeter monitor and patient sensor, prevention of optical shunt and ambient light interference, and proper sensor

selection and application. **Rationale:** Promotes reliability of SpO_2 values and aids in effective troubleshooting.

Nursing Diagnoses

1. Potential for injury related to undetected oxygen desaturation. **Rationale:** Use of pulse oximetry allows the nurse to detect clinical events associated with abnormalities in oxygen saturation. Early detection of these events facilitates interventions to prevent hypoxemic injury to patients.

2. Potential for injury related to incorrect operational procedures (Harbage Schroeder, 1988). **Rationale:** Proper equipment use ensures accurate collection of data used for clinical decision-making. Also, correct use of the oximeter and sensors prevents injury to monitored sites, i.e., pressure ulcers, abrasions, etc.

Planning

1. Individualize the following goals for pulse oximetry:
   a. Detect oxygen desaturation. **Rationale:** Alerts the nurse to deterioration of cardiopulmonary status and elicit interventions aimed at averting a life-threatening event.
   b. Decrease the frequency of arterial blood gas sampling. **Rationale:** Frequent sampling can cause pain, anxiety, impairment to skin integrity, and reduced arterial oxygen content (CaO_2) of the blood. Pulse oximetry allows for continuous rather than intermittent monitoring.

2. Obtain a physician order for pulse oximetry *or* chart nursing rationale for initiating pulse oximetry. (Check individual institutional policy for initiating pulse oximetry.) **Rationale:** The order should include frequency of measurement, acceptable parameters for results, appropriate intervention for abnormal results, and duration of monitoring.

3. Prepare all necessary equipment and supplies. **Rationale:** Preparation of equipment and supplies contributes to the efficient initiation of pulse oximetry.
   a. Pulse oximeter with instrument cable.
   b. Pulse oximetry sensor.

5. Prepare the patient.
   a. Explain the procedure to the patient. **Rationale:** Informs the patient of the purpose of monitoring, facilitating informed consent, improving cooperation with nursing interventions, and reducing anxiety.
   b. Explain equipment to patient. **Rationale:** Facilitates patient cooperation in maintaining sensor placement.

Implementation

Steps	Rationale	Special Considerations
1. Wash hands.	Reduces transmission of microorganisms.	

Table continues on following page

Steps	Rationale	Special Considerations
2. Select appropriate pulse oximeter sensor.	Optimizes signal capture and minimizes artifact-related difficulties.	Sensors may be reusable or disposable. Sterile disposable sensors may be beneficial in reducing nosocomial infections (Szaflarski and Cohen, 1989).
3. Select sensor site by assessing digits for warmth and capillary refill. Confirm presence of arterial pulse.	SpO_2 measurements are reliant on adequate arteriolar pulse strength.	Avoid sites distal to indwelling arterial catheters, blood pressure cuffs, and MAST device or conditions predisposing to venous engorgement (i.e., A-V fistulas, blood transfusions).
4. Plug oximeter into grounded wall outlet, and plug patient cable into monitor (see Skill 36–1).	Decreases occurrence of electrical interference.	Check oximeter's battery capacity and charging time if applicable.
5. Apply sensor such that		
a. The light-emitting diodes (LEDs) oppose the photodetector (PD).	LEDs/PD send and receive optical signals; opposing positions facilitate sensing of signal.	
b. The sensor is shielded from excessive ambient light.	Optical interference occurs when light reaches the PD from an external source.	If the oximeter sensor fails to detect a pulse when perfusion seems adequate, excessive ambient light (phototherapy lights, infrared warmers, etc.) may be "blinding" the PD. Troubleshoot by shielding the sensor.
c. All sensor-emitted light comes in contact with perfused tissue beds.	Optical shunting may result in either falsely low or falsely high SpO_2 values.	Displaced sensors contribute to optical shunting (Kelleher and Ruff, 1989). Shielding the sensor will not eliminate the optical shunt.
d. The sensor does not cause restriction to arterial flow or venous return.	Pulse oximetry assumes that all pulsating blood is arteriolar in origin.	Securing sensor with extra tape may contribute to venous pulsation (VP). Physiologic sources of VP include tricuspid valve regurgitation and severe right-sided heart failure. Elevate site above heart level to eliminate physiologic VP.
6. Plug sensor into the oximeter cable.	Connects the system.	
7. Turn the instrument on, and set pulse rate and saturation alarms.	Alerts the nurse to potentially life-threatening desaturations or changes in pulse detection.	Pulse rate alarms should match the set ECG alarms. Low saturation alarms should be set within 5 percent of acceptable baseline SpO_2 or physician parameters.
8. Wash hands.	Reduces transmission of microorganisms.	

Evaluation

1. Evaluate physical assessment and laboratory results and oxygen delivery system. **Rationale:** SpO_2 results should be integrated with other assessment data to determine overall clinical picture and appropriate interventions. Shifts of the oxyhemoglobin dissociation curve affect saturation; certain conditions increasing the amount of dysfunctional hemoglobin require more in-depth assessment and oxygenation measurement.

2. Evaluate skin of sensor site every 8 hours if "wrap" style sensor is used, every 4 hours if "clip" style sensor is used (Fig. 6–3). **Rationale:** Assists in prevention of tissue damage and facilitates good hygiene. Site rotation reduces incidence of venous pulsation.

3. Warm the monitoring site if poor peripheral perfusion adversely affects ability to monitor. **Rationale:** Improves local perfusion and pulse strength. Methods include application of a warm towel or hypothermic warming system (Paulus and Monroe, 1989).

4. Eradicate the effects of motion artifact by
   a. Moving sensor to less active site using lightest-weight sensor available. **Rationale:** Lightweight sensors move with the patient and more effectively preserve signal quality. Motion artifact contributes to misidentification of phys-

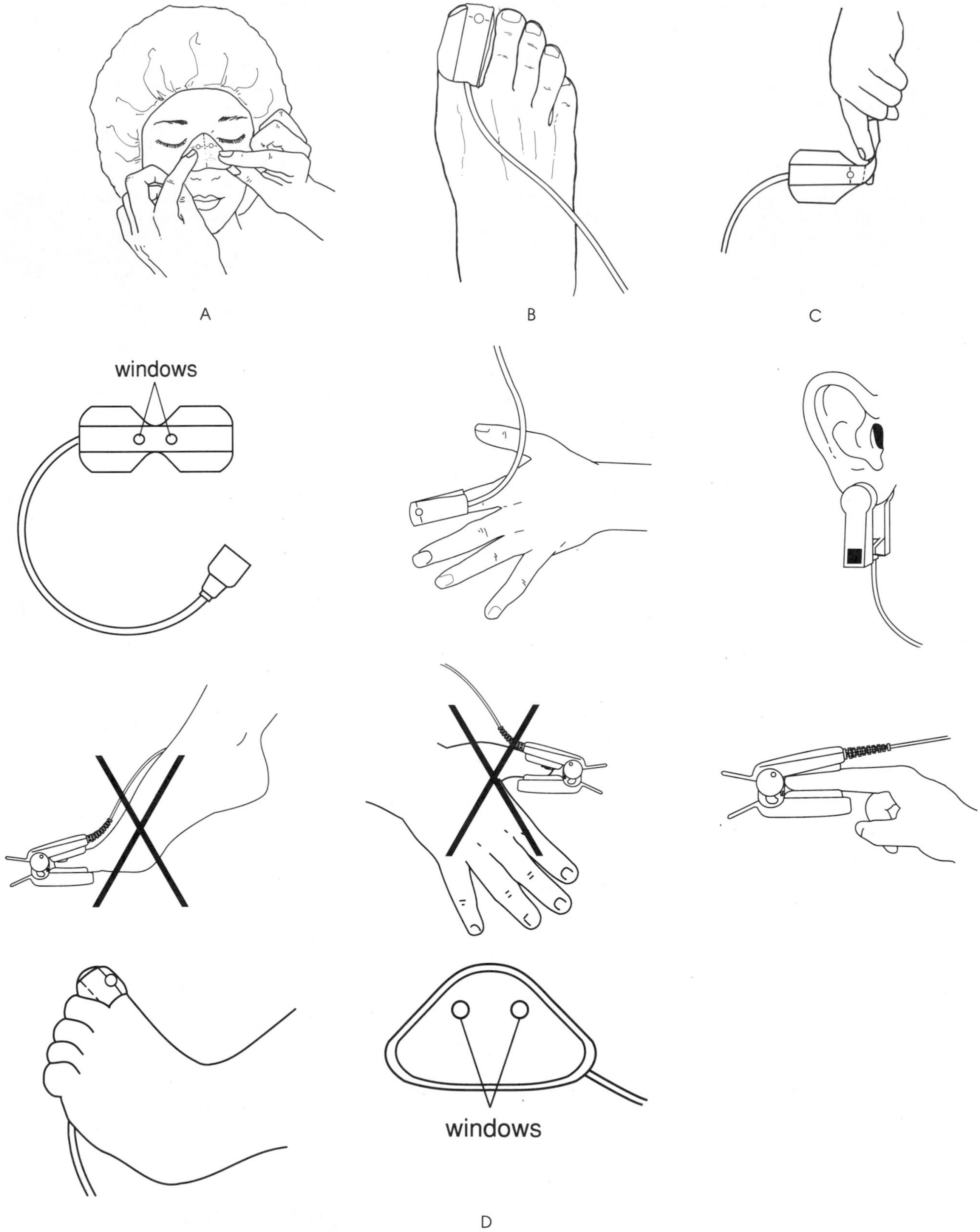

A

B

C

windows

D

FIGURE 6–3. Sensor types and sensor sites for pulse oximetry monitoring. Use "wrap" style sensors on the fingers (including thumb), great toe, and nose. The windows for the light source and the photodetector must be placed directly opposite each other on each side of the arteriolar bed to ensure accuracy of SpO_2 measurements. Choosing the correct size of sensor will help decrease the incidence of excess ambient light interferences and optical shunting. "Clip" style sensors are appropriate for fingers (except the thumb) and the earlobe. Ensuring that the arteriolar bed is well within the clip with the windows directly opposite each other will decrease the possibility of excess ambient light interference and optical shunting. (Reprinted by permission of Nellcor, Inc., Hayward, Calif., 1991.)

iologic pulses and compromises SpO_2 accuracy.
   b. Initiating ECG synchronization feature (if available). **Rationale:** ECG synchronization is a recent advance which eliminates the effects of motion artifact on SpO_2 (Barrington et al., 1988). ECG synchronization is only available on certain models of pulse oximeters.
5. Report to next caregiver those events which precipitate acute desaturations, e.g., ambulation, chest physiotherapy, etc. **Rationale:** Alerts caregiver to potentially harmful events and allows preventive interventions such as O_2 administration during activities.

Expected Outcomes

1. All desaturation events are detected. **Rationale:** Allows the nurse to respond with appropriate interventions before detrimental physiologic consequences ensue.
2. The number of adverse outcomes of oxygen desaturation are reduced. **Rationale:** Pulse oximetry allows for detection of desaturation, indicating failure of treatment modalities, changes in patient status, and need for precautionary measures or changes in therapy.
3. The need for invasive techniques for monitoring oxygenation is reduced. **Rationale:** Pulse oximetry can reduce the need for frequent invasive measurements of arterial blood gases.
4. False-positive pulse oximeter alarms are eliminated. **Rationale:** By attending to the operational procedures, false-positive alarms will be minimized, providing the nurse with continuous and reliable SpO_2 monitoring.

Unexpected Outcomes

1. Accurate pulse oximetry is not obtainable because of movement artifact. **Rationale:** Frequent movement or displacement of the sensor will result in display of inconsistent or inaccurate oximeter readings.
2. Low perfusion states or excessive edema prevents pulse oximetry measurement. **Rationale:** Low perfusion state or excessive edema may interfere with sensor signal capture.
3. In vivo SaO_2 and oximeter SpO_2 disagreement. **Rationale:** Pulse oximetry reports percent saturation of hemoglobin types that are *available to transport oxygen.*

Pulse oximeters are unable to detect the presence of dysfunctional hemoglobins. When a significant portion of the circulating hemoglobin is rendered dysfunctional, additional laboratory evaluation of blood oxygenation by CO-oximetry is indicated.

Calculated saturations, typically those reported on ABG results, may differ from pulse oximeter–measured saturations because of shifts in the oxyhemoglobin dissociation curve that were insufficiently corrected in the calculation. The accuracy of a calculated saturation is reduced, for example, when the patient's body temperature is not considered or in instances where nutritional deficiencies are associated with insufficient substrate for the manufacture of 2,3-DPG.

Documentation

Documentation in the patient record should include indications for use of pulse oximetry; patient's pulse with SpO_2 measurement; FiO_2 delivered; simultaneous ABGs, if available; recent hemoglobin measurement, if available; skin assessment at sensor site; oximeter alarm settings; events precipitating acute desaturations; and any interventions related to the patient's respiratory status. **Rationale:** Documentation should reflect proper monitoring techniques. Activities or interventions affecting SpO_2 also should be documented, including outcomes in SpO_2 values.

Patient/Family Education

1. Discuss the rationale for implementing pulse oximetry with both patient and family. **Rationale:** Facilitates informed consent and reduces patient and family anxieties associated with an additional monitor and related activities.
2. Demonstrate the equipment to the patient and family, explaining the importance of proper sensor placement. **Rationale:** Encourages patient cooperation in keeping proper and consistent placement of sensors and may assist in decreasing movement artifact.

Performance Checklist
Skill 6–1: Oxygen Saturation Monitoring by Pulse Oximetry

	Complies	
Critical Behaviors	**yes**	**no**
1. Wash hands.		
2. Select appropriate sensor.		
3. Select appropriate sensor site.		
4. Plug oximeter into grounded wall outlet and patient cable into monitor.		
5. Apply sensor appropriately.		
6. Plug sensor into oximeter cable.		
7. Set alarms appropriately and ensure proper functioning.		

Table continues on following page

	Complies	
Critical Behaviors	**yes**	**no**
8. Wash hands.		
9. Document procedure in the patient record.		

SKILL 6–2

Continuous End-Tidal Carbon Dioxide Monitoring

The *capnograph* monitors a patient's ventilatory status with displays of both waveforms and numeric measurements of inhaled and exhaled CO_2. Capnographs are often called *end-tidal CO_2 monitors* because they measure the end-tidal partial pressure of CO_2 ($PetCO_2$). An infrared capnograph passes light through an expiratory gas sample and, using a photodetector, measures absorption of that light by the gas. Then the capnograph determines the amount of CO_2 in the gas sample based on the absorption properties of CO_2. The capnograph also visually graphs the pattern in which CO_2 is exhaled and provides a display called a *capnogram* or *$PetCO_2$ waveform* (Petterson, 1990).

The capnograph samples exhaled CO_2 by one of two methods: aspiration (sidestream) or nonaspiration (mainstream) sampling (Fig. 6–4). In sidestream systems, small amounts of the expired gas are transported from the airway to the CO_2 sensor, also referred to as the *optical bench*, which may be housed either in the display unit or in a separate housing proximal to the patient. Mainstream systems mount the CO_2 sensor on the patient's airway; CO_2 is measured as the gas moves through the airway, and the data are transmitted to the display unit (Stock, 1988).

To ensure proper functioning of the capnograph, it is essential that all parts of the system be carefully assembled and checked. Problems in obtaining accurate $PetCO_2$ values and waveforms may be the result of gas leaks (poor connections or partial disconnections), airway obstructions in tubing (problems in obtaining sampling volume or in sample flow), and incorrect assembly

of the circuit. Continuous monitoring of $PetCO_2$ should include a baseline arterial blood gas determination to check oxygenation and to quantify the a-ADCO$_2$ gradient and a check of the ventilator to assess mechanical support (Carlon et al., 1988).

To use capnography effectively, the nurse must understand the components of a normal CO_2 waveform, the normal relationship between $PaCO_2$ and $PetCO_2$ values, and the physiologic basis for disruptions of this relationship. The latter is crucial when applying capnography to patients with ventilation–perfusion abnormalities within the lungs.

The normal capnographic waveform has the following characteristics (Fig. 6–5):

1. A zero baseline, which represents the beginning of exhalation of CO_2 free gas from anatomic dead space. This gas comes from the large airways, oropharynx, and nasopharynx (*A–B*).

2. A rapid, sharp upstroke as the gas from the intermediate airways, containing a mixture of fresh gas and CO_2, begins to be exhaled from the lungs (*B–C*).

3. A nearly flat alveolar plateau that occurs as exhaled flow velocity slows and mixed gas is displaced by alveolar gas (*C–D*).

4. A distinct end-tidal point that most closely reflects the concentration of CO_2 found in the alveoli (*D*).

5. A rapid downstroke as the patient inspires fresh gas that is essentially devoid of CO_2 (*D–E*).

Note that the positively deflected limbs occur with *exhalation*, whereas the negatively deflected limb occurs with inhalation. This is opposite from other respiratory waveforms, including the resprigram, spirograms, and the flow/volume loop. The capnogram will deviate from normal whenever there is a physiologic or mechanical disruption of the breath.

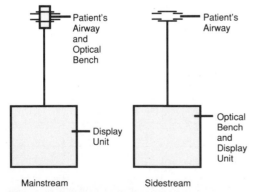

FIGURE 6–4. Mainstream and sidestream instruments differ in the position of the optical bench in relation to the display unit. (Reprinted with permission from Capnography Reference Note, No. 3. Hayward, Calif.: Nellcor, Inc., 1989.)

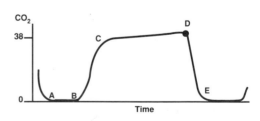

- Zero baseline (A-B)   • End-tidal value (D)
- Rapid, sharp rise (B-C) • Rapid, sharp
- Alveolar plateau (C-D)   downstroke (D-E)

FIGURE 6–5. Essentials of the normal capnographic waveform. (Reprinted with permission from W. W. Feaster, et al., *Capnography: A Quick Reference*. Hayward, Calif.: Nellcor, Inc., 1988.)

When cardiopulmonary functioning is normal and proper measurement techniques are employed,

$$PaCO_2 \approx PACO_2 \approx PetCO_2.$$

Thus $PetCO_2$ can be used as an estimate of $PaCO_2$, with $PetCO_2$ generally 2 to 5 mmHg lower than $PaCO_2$ (Skoog, 1989). Two commonly occurring physiologic conditions that result in $PetCO_2$ values greater than 5 mmHg lower than $PaCO_2$ are incomplete alveolar emptying and increased alveolar dead space. Figure 6–6 illustrates how incomplete alveolar emptying results in an abnormal waveform and a peak exhaled CO_2 level that is significantly lower than true alveolar concentrations.

Discussion of increased alveolar dead space warrants a brief review of the ventilation–perfusion relationship within the lung (Fig. 6–7). Although alveolar/capillary units differ regionally in their ventilation–perfusion ($\dot{V}/\dot{Q}$) ratios, the ideal gas exchanging unit has a $\dot{V}/\dot{Q}$ ratio of 1.0. Practically speaking, $\dot{V}/\dot{Q}$ ratio in the normal human lung is something other than 1.0 because areas of high $\dot{V}/\dot{Q}$ and low $\dot{V}/\dot{Q}$ exist within the normal physiologic realm (Lane and Walker, 1987; McCarthy, 1987; Shapiro et al., 1982).

Under normal $\dot{V}/\dot{Q}$ conditions (Fig. 6–8), $PACO_2$ and $PaCO_2$ values will be equal or nearly equal (a-ADCO$_2$ < 5 mmHg) (Skoog, 1989). Given proper sampling technique and unrestricted alveolar emptying, as determined by the shape of the capnogram, $PetCO_2$ should closely correspond to $PaCO_2$ (see Fig. 6–8).

In conditions where abnormally large numbers of alveolar/capillary units are underperfused in relation to their ventilation (high $\dot{V}/\dot{Q}$ units) or where lung units are ventilated but totally nonperfused (dead space units), transfer of CO_2 gas from blood to lung is impaired. When employing $PetCO_2$ monitoring, the nurse will observe a lower exhaled CO_2 concentration than that measured in arterial blood (widened a-ADCO$_2$). This occurs because the CO_2-free gas exhaled from nonperfused units mixes with CO_2-rich gas from perfused units, thereby diluting the overall concentration of CO_2 exhaled (Stock, 1988; Szaflarski, 1991) (Fig. 6–9).

At the opposite end of the $\dot{V}/\dot{Q}$ spectrum are the low $\dot{V}/\dot{Q}$ units and shunt units. Here perfusion exceeds ventilation. While low $\dot{V}/\dot{Q}$ and shunt units are known contributors to the development of hypoxemia (Reischman, 1988), they do not result in abnormal widening of the a-ADCO$_2$ (Swedlow, 1986) (Fig. 6–10).

The capnogram is especially useful as a visual trending tool at the bedside to monitor the following pathophysiologic changes or problems with medical management and support equipment:

1. Gradually increasing $PetCO_2$—reflective of increased metabolism, hyperthermia, sepsis, hypoventilation, neuromuscular blockade recovery, and decreases in effective alveolar ventilation (Fig. 6–11).

2. Elevated $PetCO_2$—reflective of respiratory depressant drugs, metabolic alkalosis (i.e., the body retaining CO_2 to buffer metabolic alkalosis), and inadequate minute ventilation (Fig. 6–12).

3. Transient rise in $PetCO_2$—suggestive of release of tourniquet and bicarbonate infusion (Fig. 6–13).

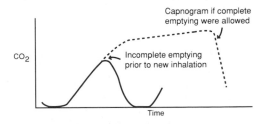

• COPD   • Upper airway obstruction
• Asthma • Partial endotracheal tube obstruction

FIGURE 6–6. Incomplete alveolar emptying. (Reprinted with permission from W. W. Feaster, et al., *Capnography: A Quick Reference.* Hayward, Calif.: Nellcor, Inc., 1988.)

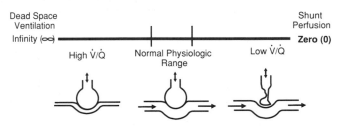

FIGURE 6–7. Ventilation-perfusion spectrum. (Reprinted with permission from W. W. Feaster, et al., *Capnography: A Quick Reference.* Hayward, Calif.: Nellcor, Inc., 1988.)

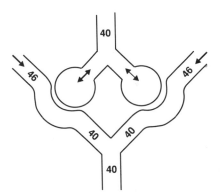

FIGURE 6–8. Lung units with matched $\dot{V}/\dot{Q}$ (a-ADCO$_2$ = 0). (Reprinted with permission from Nellcor, Inc., Hayward, Calif., 1991.)

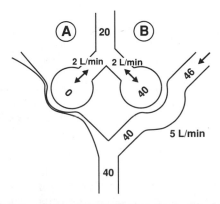

FIGURE 6–9. Dead space ventilation. Lung unit *A* is ventilated but not perfused, whereas lung unit *B* is normal. Values are for PCO$_2$ in mmHg (a-ADCO$_2$ = 20 mmHg). (Reprinted with permission from W. W. Feaster, et al., *Capnography: A Quick Reference.* Hayward, Calif.: Nellcor, Inc., 1988.)

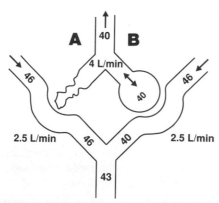

FIGURE 6–10. Shunt perfusion. Lung unit *A* is perfused but not ventilated, whereas lung unit *B* is normal. Values are for PCO_2 in mmHg (a-$ADCO_2$ = 3). (Reprinted with permission from W. W. Feaster, et al., *Capnography: A Quick Reference.* Hayward, Calif.: Nellcor, Inc., 1988.)

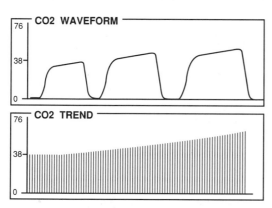

FIGURE 6–11. Gradually increasing $PetCO_2$. (Reprinted with permission from W. W. Feaster, et al., *Capnography: A Quick Reference.* Hayward, Calif.: Nellcor, Inc., 1988.)

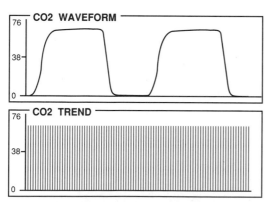

FIGURE 6–12. Elevated $PetCO_2$. (Reprinted with permission from W. W. Feaster, et al., *Capnography: A Quick Reference.* Hayward, Calif.: Nellcor, Inc., 1988.)

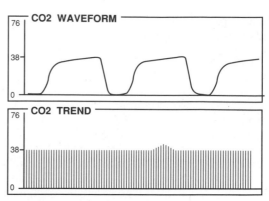

FIGURE 6–13. Transient rise in $PetCO_2$. (Reprinted with permission from W. W. Feaster, et al., *Capnography: A Quick Reference.* Hayward, Calif.: Nellcor, Inc., 1988.)

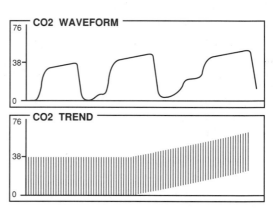

FIGURE 6–14. Gradual increase in baseline and $PetCO_2$ value. (Reprinted with permission from W. W. Feaster, et al., *Capnography: A Quick Reference.* Hayward, Calif.: Nellcor, Inc., 1988.)

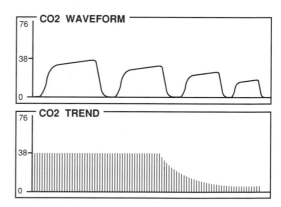

FIGURE 6–15. Exponential fall in $PetCO_2$. (Reprinted with permission from W. W. Feaster, et al., *Capnography: A Quick Reference.* Hayward, Calif.: Nellcor, Inc., 1988.)

4. Gradual increase in both baseline and $PetCO_2$ value—reflective of rebreathing of previously exhaled gas, defective exhalation valve on mechanical ventilator, and excessive mechanical dead space in the ventilator circuit (Fig. 6–14).

5. Exponential fall in $PetCO_2$—reflective of cardiopulmonary bypass, cardiopulmonary arrest, major pulmonary embolism, and severe pulmonary hypoperfusion (Fig. 6–15).

6. Decreased $PetCO_2$ (with normal waveform—reflective of high minute volume, hypothermia, and metabolic acidosis (i.e., exhaling CO_2 to buffer metabolic acidosis) (Fig. 6–16).

7. Sudden decrease in $PetCO_2$ to low values—reflective of leak in airway system, endotracheal tube in hypopharynx, partial airway obstruction, mechanical

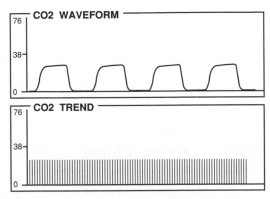

FIGURE 6–16. Decreased PetCO₂. (Reprinted with permission from W. W. Feaster, et al., *Capnography: A Quick Reference.* Hayward, Calif.: Nellcor, Inc., 1988.)

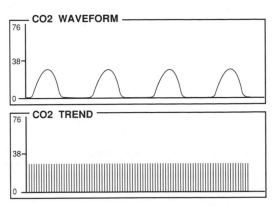

FIGURE 6–19. Low PetCO₂ without alveolar plateau. (Reprinted with permission from W. W. Feaster, et al., *Capnography: A Quick Reference.* Hayward, Calif.: Nellcor, Inc., 1988.)

ventilator malfunction, and partial disconnection of ventilator circuit (Scott, 1989) (Fig. 6–17).

8. Sudden decrease in PetCO₂ to near zero—dislodged endotracheal tube, complete airway obstruction, mechanical ventilator malfunction, airway disconnection, and esophageal intubation (Fig. 6–18).

9. Sustained low PetCO₂ without alveolar plateau—reflective of incomplete alveolar emptying, partially kinked endotracheal tube, bronchospasm, mucous plugging, improper exhaled gas sampling, and insufficient expiratory time on the ventilator (Fig. 6–19).

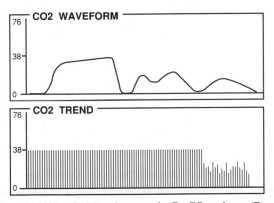

FIGURE 6–17. Sudden decrease in PetCO₂ values. (Reprinted with permission from W. W. Feaster, et al., *Capnography: A Quick Reference.* Hayward, Calif.: Nellcor, Inc., 1988.)

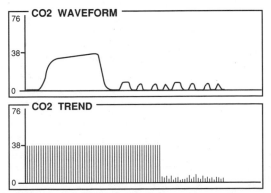

FIGURE 6–18. Sudden decrease in PetCO₂ to near zero. (Reprinted with permission from W. W. Feaster, et al., *Capnography: A Quick Reference.* Hayward, Calif.: Nellcor, Inc., 1988.)

Purpose

The nurse implements continuous end-tidal CO₂ monitoring by capnography to

1. Determine a baseline CO₂ waveform pattern and PetCO₂ value.
2. Continuously monitor the patency of the airways and presence of breathing.
3. Provide a mechanism for early detection of changes in waveform pattern and/or PetCO₂ value that may accompany a sudden or gradual change in CO₂ production or elimination.
4. Evaluate the patient's response to activities that may positively or negatively affect ventilation (i.e., suctioning, repositioning, changes in mechanical support, nutritional supplementation, etc.).

Prerequisite Knowledge and Skills

Prior to monitoring end-tidal CO₂ by capnography, the nurse should understand

1. Principles of ventilation.
2. Principles of end-tidal CO₂ monitoring.
3. Relationship between PaCO₂ and PetCO₂ and the physiologic basis of abnormalities detected.
4. Arterial blood gas determinations.
5. Anatomy and physiology of the respiratory system.

The nurse should be able to perform

1. Universal precautions (see Skill 35–1).
2. Assessment of respiratory status.

Assessment

1. Assess the patient for indications that end-tidal CO₂ (PetCO₂) monitoring should be instituted. General guidelines for capnograph use are as follows:
   a. Patients with or at risk for acute airway obstruction or apnea, including patients who are not intubated but may require monitoring via a CO₂ sampling nasal cannula (Fig. 6–20).

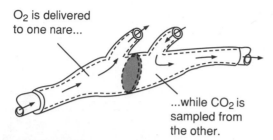

O₂ is delivered
to one nare...

...while CO₂ is
sampled from
the other.

FIGURE 6–20. Nasal cannula for sampling CO—divided style. (Reprinted with permission from Capnography Reference Note, No. 3. Hayward, Calif.: Nellcor, Inc., 1989.)

b. Patients with or at risk for dead space ventilation. Pulmonary hypoperfusion, air embolism, pulmonary thromboembolism, cardiac arrest, and PEEP may require monitoring via a divided-style sampling nasal cannula, since PEEP may result in high transalveolar pressure and decreased cardiac output.

c. Patients with or at risk for incomplete alveolar emptying, i.e., airway obstruction, COPD, asthma, and partial endotracheal tube obstructions.

Rationale: Assessment for initiation of continuous end-tidal CO_2 monitoring ensures that patients at risk for inadequate ventilation, and therefore inadequate gas exchange, will receive monitoring for such occurrences and subsequently receive appropriate interventions.

2. Assess for proper functioning of capnograph, including airway adapter, sensor, and display monitor, checking electrical grounding, accurate setup, and secure connections. **Rationale:** Ensures reliability of $PetCO_2$ values and waveforms obtained.

Nursing Diagnoses

1. Potential for injury related to undetected incidence of impaired CO_2 elimination. **Rationale:** Use of capnography may allow the nurse to detect clinical events or changes that reflect abnormalities in airways and cardiopulmonary status. Prompt detection of such conditions may prevent catastrophic injury to patients.

2. Knowledge deficit of patient and family related to implementation of $PetCO_2$ measurement by capnography. **Rationale:** Patient and family teaching promotes understanding and cooperation in use of equipment and related technical procedures.

3. Impaired gas exchange related to impaired transfer of CO_2 gas from the blood to the lung. **Rationale:** Alveolar–capillary units are underperfused in relation to their ventilation, or lungs are ventilated but nonperfused.

4. Impaired gas exchange related to $\dot{V}/\dot{Q}$ mismatch. **Rationale:** Low $\dot{V}/\dot{Q}$ shunt units cause hypoxemia.

Planning

1. Individualize the following goals for performing capnography:
   a. Early detection of impending catastrophic events. **Rationale:** Continuous $PetCO_2$ monitoring provides a mechanism for early detection of apnea, loss of airway, or changes in CO_2 elimination often before any clinical signs or symptoms are detected (Sharer and Sladen, 1988).
   b. Maintenance of normal PCO_2 and pH. **Rationale:** PCO_2 and pH values depend on the effectiveness of the lungs in eliminating CO_2 through the process of breathing; capnography monitors CO_2 elimination breath by breath; therapeutic interventions aimed at improving alveolar ventilation or CO_2 elimination can be monitored noninvasively for their effects.
   c. Reduce the frequency of arterial blood sampling. **Rationale:** Frequent blood gas sampling can cause pain, anxiety, impairment to skin integrity, reduced oxygen-carrying capacity of the blood, and decreased tissue perfusion if the artery is injured. $PaCO_2$ values provide a static view of a dynamic process. Comparisons of $PaCO_2$ and $PetCO_2$ values are useful in estimating the dead space–to–tidal volume (Vd/Vt) ratio (Yamanaka and Sue, 1987).

2. Obtain physician order for continuous $PetCO_2$ monitoring by capnography. **Rationale:** The order should provide guidelines for duration of monitoring, acceptable parameters for results, and appropriate interventions for abnormal results.

3. Prepare all necessary equipment and supplies. **Rationale:** Preparation of equipment and supplies contributes to the efficient initiation of $PetCO_2$ measurement by capnography.
   a. Capnograph.
   b. Airway adapter.

4. Explain the procedure to the patient. **Rationale:** Informs the patient of the purpose of monitoring, improves cooperation with nursing interventions, and reduces anxiety.

Implementation

Steps	Rationale	Special Considerations
1. Wash hands.	Reduces transmission of microorganisms.	
2. Plug capnograph into grounded wall outlet (see Skill 36–1), and	Decreases incidence of electrical interference.	Check capnograph's battery capacity and charging time if applicable.

Table continues on following page

Steps	Rationale	Special Considerations
plug appropriate patient cable into display monitor. Turn instrument on.		
3. Perform calibration routine if required (see operator's manual.)	Accurate measurement is dependent on proper calibration.	
4. Assemble airway adapter, sensor, and display monitor, and connect to patient circuit properly and securely (see operator's manual for details).	Decreases incidence of improper gas sampling.	Sampling errors and gas leaks in system are major causes of inaccurate readings.
5. Make sure that the sampling port is placed at a right angle to the endotracheal tube or ventilator circuit (applicable in sidestream sampling).	Decreases secretion accumulation on CO_2 port where gas is drawn for sampling.	
6. Set appropriate alarms, according to instructions in operator's manual. ($PetCO_2$ is set 5 percent below acceptable parameter or per institutional policy.)	Alerts the nurse to potentially life-threatening problems.	If monitor is interfaced with other equipment (i.e., ECG monitor, mechanical ventilator, pulse oximeter), make sure alarms are set consistently between all monitors.
7. Wash hands.	Reduces transmission of microorganisms.	

Evaluation

1. Evaluate physical assessment, check laboratory results, and check mechanical ventilator. **Rationale:** $PetCO_2$ values and waveforms should be integrated with other assessment information to evaluate overall clinical picture to determine appropriate interventions. Recall mechanical problems and pathophysiologic changes that can alter $PetCO_2$ values and waveforms, such as poor sampling technique, ventilation–perfusion mismatch (dead space ventilation, shunt perfusion), and incomplete alveolar emptying (Skoog, 1989; Szaflarski, 1991).

2. Monitor equipment setup every 8 hours: monitor sensor, airway, adapter, and ventilator. **Rationale:** Ensures accuracy of data.

Expected Outcomes

1. Significant changes in ventilatory status are detected. **Rationale:** Detection of deterioration in ventilatory status allows the nurse to respond with appropriate interventions before detrimental physiologic consequences occur.

2. Alterations in the a-$ADCO_2$ gradient are identified. **Rationale:** A normal a-$ADCO_2$ gradient indicates that an adequate ventilation–perfusion ratio exists. If a-$ADCO_2$ is large, measures can be undertaken to improve the $\dot{V}/\dot{Q}$ relationship and reduce the a-$ADCO_2$ subsequently.

Unexpected Outcomes

1. Inaccurate measurements of $PetCO_2$ are displayed. **Rationale:** Poor sampling techniques can cause inaccuracy in $PetCO_2$ measurements.

2. Inaccurate measurements resulting from calibration drift and/or contamination of optics with moisture or secretions. **Rationale:** If substances other than the respiratory gases absorb light at the sensor, CO_2 measurements may be in error.

3. Equipment malfunction. **Rationale:** Failure of the instrument to sense CO_2 when CO_2 is in fact present may be due to an occluded or fractured sample line when using an aspiration-style capnograph.

Documentation

Documentation in the patient record should include respiratory rate and $PetCO_2$ value, capnogram, mechanical ventilator settings, any ABGs, respiratory therapies, related medication doses (neuromuscular blockers, sedation, bronchodilators, etc.), respiratory assessment, and other pertinent assessments (temperature, etc.). **Rationale:** Documentation should reflect proper monitoring utilization and techniques, interventions affecting $PetCO_2$ measurement, with resulting outcomes in $PetCO_2$ measurement, and changes in patient status related to nursing interventions.

Patient/Family Education

Discuss the rationale for implementing capnography. **Rationale:** Reduces patient and family anxieties associated with an additional monitor, related interventions, or an unfamiliar procedure.

Performance Checklist
Skill 6–2: Continuous End-Tidal Carbon Dioxide Monitoring

Critical Behaviors	Complies yes	no
1. Wash hands.		
2. Plug capnograph into grounded wall outlet, plug patient cable into display monitor, and turn instrument on.		
3. Perform calibration, if required.		
4. Assemble capnography circuit correctly (airway adapter, CO_2 sensor, monitor) and correctly connect to patient.		
5. Ensure that circuit is functioning properly and accurate display is obtained on monitor.		
6. Set alarms and ensure proper functioning.		
7. Wash hands.		
8. Document procedure in the patient record.		

SKILL 6–3

Continuous Mixed Venous Oxygen Saturation Monitoring

Mixed venous oxygen saturation ($S\bar{v}O_2$) measures the oxygen saturation of the venous blood in the pulmonary artery. This parameter reflects changes in the status among global oxygen delivery, cardiac output, hemoglobin, arterial oxygen saturation, and oxygen consumption.

Whenever there is a threat to this balance, the primary compensatory mechanism is to increase delivery by increasing cardiac output. However, in the critically ill, the cardiac output may already be at the peak of potential performance. In order to meet the tissues' demand for oxygen, increased extraction occurs. This second compensatory mechanism results in a lower oxygen saturation returning to the venous side and therefore a lower $S\bar{v}O_2$.

Nursing practice is aimed at enhancing the balance between oxygen delivery and oxygen consumption. Until recently, the patient's response to nursing interventions has been assessed by changes in vital signs and other parameters. Continuous $S\bar{v}O_2$ monitoring can now provide the nurse with an on-line evaluation tool to assess the response to nursing interventions. Normal procedures such as turning, suctioning, and bathing can increase the amount of oxygen required by the tissues. If

oxygen delivery does not increase, the patient's balance may be threatened. $S\bar{v}O_2$ monitoring can assist the nurse in deciding if the compensatory reserve is sufficient to meet the increase in demand. (See Table 6–2 for factors altering oxygen consumption.) Research in the area of continuous $S\bar{v}O_2$ monitoring and standard nursing interventions is changing practice from a ritualistic program of interventions to one that is guided by the patient's response.

$S\bar{v}O_2$ does not correlate directly with any of the determinants of oxygen delivery or oxygen consumption. It only closely correlates with cardiac output if the SaO_2, hemoglobin, and oxygen consumption are constant. The critically ill patient, however, is in a dynamic state with rapidly changing oxygen demand and consumption. Therefore, $S\bar{v}O_2$ must be viewed in the light of these changing determinants and considered a global indicator of oxygen balance rather than a specific evaluation tool.

With the use of a pulmonary artery catheter, intermittent $S\bar{v}O_2$ samples from the distal port have been available to the nurse. Current technology provides the means to monitor the $S\bar{v}O_2$ value on a continuous basis at the bedside.

Continuous $S\bar{v}O_2$ monitoring is performed with a three-component system.

1. A specialized pulmonary artery catheter. The

TABLE 6–2 ALTERATIONS IN OXYGEN CONSUMPTION

Factors	Percent Change over Baseline
Temperature, 1°C	
Increase	+10–13
Decrease	−7–8
Anesthesia	−25–50
Shivering	+50–100
Endotracheal suctioning	+7–70
Position change	+31
Bath	+23
Bed-scale weighing	+36

catheter contains two fiberoptic filaments that exit at the distal port. One filament serves as a sending fiber for emission of light; the other is a receiving fiber for the light that is reflected back from the pulmonary artery.

2. The optic module. This component houses the light-emitting diodes (LEDs) that transmit various wavelengths of light and a photodetector that receives light back. Patient identification information may be stored in this component as well as previous $S\overline{v}O_2$ values.

3. A microprocessor computer. The computer converts the light information into an electrical display that is updated every few seconds for continuous monitoring.

The technology employed for $S\overline{v}O_2$ assessment is based on spectrophotometry. Transmission spectrophotometry is used in the laboratory for saturation determinations by a CO-oximeter. Various wavelengths of lights are shone through a blood sample. Desaturated, saturated (oxyhemoglobin), and dyshemoglobins (carboxyhemoglobin, methemoglobin) have different light-absorption characteristics. The ratio of hemoglobin to oxyhemoglobin is then determined and reported as a percentage value (Fig. 6–21).

Bedside $S\overline{v}O_2$ assessment employs reflection spectrophotometry. Light wavelengths transmitted through the fiberoptic filaments from the LEDs are reflected back from the pulmonary artery to the photodetector. Hemoglobin and oxyhemoglobin absorb light differently, and this reflected light is analyzed by the microprocessor to display the percentage of saturated hemoglobin, i.e., the $S\overline{v}O_2$, on a digital display and on a time/trend display screen (Fig. 6–22).

A hard-copy printer may be available, and this is used to document the $S\overline{v}O_2$ trends. Time marks can be noted on the hard copy for identifying patient events and evaluating interventions. The paper printout may be used as documentation in the patient record if desired. Institutional policies may differ with regard to the incorporation of such documentation (Fig. 6–23).

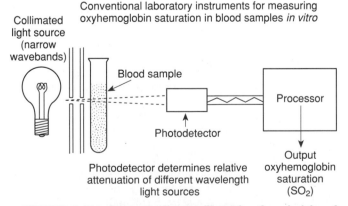

Collimated light source (narrow wavebands)

Conventional laboratory instruments for measuring oxyhemoglobin saturation in blood samples *in vitro*

Blood sample

Photodetector

Processor

Photodetector determines relative attenuation of different wavelength light sources

Output oxyhemoglobin saturation (SO_2)

FIGURE 6–21. Schematic diagram illustrating the principles of transmission spectrophotometry. (Reprinted with permission from J. F. Schweiss, *Continuous Measurement of Blood Oxygen Saturation in the High-Risk Patient*, Vol. 1. San Diego: Beach International, Inc., 1983.)

Purpose

The nurse monitors and interprets the $S\overline{v}O_2$ value to

1. Continuously assess the oxygenation balance of the patient.

2. Trend changes as they relate to the variables that affect $S\overline{v}O_2$, such as SaO_2, CO, hemoglobin, and VO_2.

3. Evaluate the effects of nursing or medical interventions on oxygen consumption.

Prerequisite Knowledge and Skills

Prior to monitoring $S\overline{v}O_2$, the nurse should understand

1. Anatomy and physiology of the cardiopulmonary system.

2. Physiologic principles related to invasive hemodynamic monitoring.

3. Technical aspects of pulmonary artery pressure monitoring.

4. Physiologic concepts of oxygen delivery and oxygen demand and consumption.

5. Basic microprocessor functions and menu activation.

The nurse should be able to perform

1. Pulmonary artery pressure monitoring (see Skills 10–5 and 10–6).

2. Mixed venous oxygen saturation blood sampling from a pulmonary artery catheter (see Skill 10–7).

3. Technically related functions of proper computer setup and maintenance.

Assessment

Institution of $S\overline{v}O_2$ monitoring is a collaborative practice. The physician determines the need for monitoring, and the nurse assists with insertion of the catheter and implements the bedside monitoring and evaluation of the data.

1. Assess patient's hemodynamic and oxygenation status. **Rationale:** Conditions that threaten the balance between oxygen delivery and demand may necessitate hemodynamic and $S\overline{v}O_2$ monitoring. Conditions that decrease delivery, such as hypoxia, anemia, hemorrhage, and decreased cardiac output, and conditions that increase demand, such as fever, shivering, seizures, and disease processes, are considered such indications.

2. Assess and monitor pulmonary artery waveforms. **Rationale:** Migration of the catheter tip may reflect postcapillary arterialized blood, which will cause an elevation in the $S\overline{v}O_2$ value. Uncorrected catheter migration also may put the patient at risk for a pulmonary infarction.

3. Assess and monitor $S\overline{v}O_2$ value and trends. **Rationale:** Normal $S\overline{v}O_2$ values range from 60 to 80 percent. Values outside this range may indicate an imbalance between oxygen delivery and consumption, as can a trending change of 5 to 10 percent over a 3- to 5-minute period of time. If, however, the patient's clinical presentation

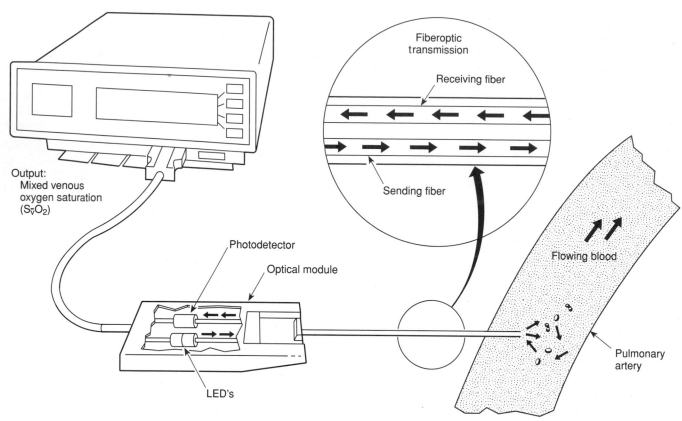

FIGURE 6–22. Example of a mixed venous oxygen saturation system using reflection spectrophotometry. (From American Edwards Laboratories, *Understanding Continuous Mixed Venous Oxygen Saturation ($S\bar{v}O_2$) Monitoring with the Swan-Ganz Oximetry TD System.* Irvine, Calif.: American Edwards Laboratories, Baxter Healthcare Corporation, 1987.)

differs from the observed $S\bar{v}O_2$ value or trends, recheck the accuracy of the monitoring system.

Nursing Diagnoses

1. Alterations in tissue perfusion: decreased related to decreased cardiac output, decreased SaO_2, and decreased hemoglobin. **Rationale:** Actions or conditions that decrease any of the delivery components may elicit a compensatory mechanism of increased tissue oxygen extraction. The result is a lower oxygen saturation level returning to the venous system and therefore a decreased $S\bar{v}O_2$.

2. Alterations in tissue perfusion: increased related to increased cardiac output, increased SaO_2, and increased hemoglobin. **Rationale:** Increasing the delivery

components to supply more oxygen than the tissues require results in a higher amount of saturated blood returning and $S\bar{v}O_2$ increases.

Planning

1. Individualize the following goals for patients requiring continuous $S\bar{v}O_2$ monitoring:
   a. Optimize oxygen delivery. **Rationale:** Provides tissues with necessary life-sustaining oxygen and decreases work of heart.
   b. Decrease oxygen demand. **Rationale:** Reduces the incidence of oxygen extraction from tissues.

2. Assemble all necessary equipment and supplies for insertion and continuous monitoring. **Rationale:** Ensures that appropriate equipment is available for assisting with catheter insertion and continuous monitoring.
   a. Continuous $S\bar{v}O_2$ computer and appropriate connecting cables.
   b. Fiberoptic $S\bar{v}O_2$ catheter (7.5 or 8.0 French).
   c. Optics module and cable.
   d. Equipment and supplies necessary for a standard pulmonary artery catheter insertion and monitoring (see Skills 10–5 through 10–8).

3. Prepare the patient. **Rationale:** Explanation of procedure to patient helps to alleviate fears and concerns and encourages cooperation.

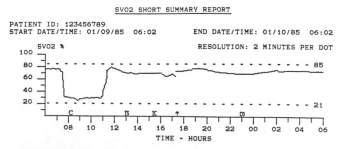

FIGURE 6–23. Example of computer hard-copy printout of $S\bar{v}O_2$ time graph.

a. Explain the procedure to the patient. **Rationale:** Reduces anxiety and encourages cooperation.

b. Explain alarms and purpose of monitoring to the patient and family.

4. Assemble all necessary equipment for mixed venous blood saturation sampling. **Rationale:** Assembly of appropriate equipment ensures efficient mixed venous blood sampling to perform in vivo calibration.

a. Heparinized blood gas syringe.
b. Syringe cap or sterile plug.
c. 5- or 10-cc syringe for drawing waste sample.
d. Basin or cup of ice.
e. Examination gloves.

Implementation

Steps	Rationale	Special Considerations
Continuous SvO₂ Monitoring		
1. Wash hands.	Reduces transmission of microorganisms.	
2. Connect computer to ac power source and turn unit on.	Allows electronics to warm up.	Manufacturers have different lengths of warm-up time required.
3. Observe the system check on the computer screen.	Confirms component function.	
4. Remove outer wrap of catheter package.	Provides access to inner package.	
5. Aseptically peel back inner wrap that covers the optic connector of the catheter.	Isolates connector from catheter tip to maintain sterility during in vitro calibration.	
6. Firmly connect the optic connector to the optic module.	Ensures that connections are tight and of proper alignment for light transmission.	
7. Perform in vitro calibration/ standardization.	Standardizes or calibrates the light source to the catheter.	Catheter lumens must be dry. *Do not flush catheter prior to performing this step or in vitro calibration will be invalid.*
8. Pull back remaining wrap covering catheter package using aseptic technique.	Prepares catheter for insertion and maintains sterility.	
9. Carefully remove catheter from tray using sterile technique.	Maintains aseptic technique.	Fiberoptics in catheter and balloon are fragile and may be damaged if not handled properly.
10. Attach pressure monitoring lines, and prime with flush solution.	Enables monitoring of chamber pressures during insertion. Maintains patency of lumens.	The use of heparin assists in decreasing fibrin deposits. Refer to hospital policy for use of heparinized solution. Some catheters are coated with heparin during the manufacturing process. At this time, the manufacturers recommend the use of heparin.
11. Assist physician with catheter insertion (see Skill 10–5 to 10–7).	Team effort assists in performing the skill in a timely fashion.	
12. Observe configuration of waveforms during insertion.	Central pulmonary artery catheter tip placement is necessary for optimal reflection of the light.	A "light intensity" or "signal" indicator verifies adequate reflection of light signals.
13. Note balloon inflation volume for optimal wedge tracing.	A 1.5-cc inflation volume is recommended for proper catheter tip placement.	Less than optimal inflation volume to obtain a wedge tracing may indicate catheter migration. The "intensity" or "signal" indicator may be activated.

Table continues on following page

Steps	Rationale	Special Considerations
		Arterialized blood may be reflected, producing an elevated $S\bar{v}O_2$ value. A rise in the $S\bar{v}O_2$ value during wedging of the catheter has been used in conjunction with balloon inflation volume and waveform evaluation to identify optimal catheter placement and accurate wedge readings.
14. Set high and low alarm limits, and activate alarms.	Individualizes alarm settings according to patient baseline. Audible alarms notify the nurse of significant changes in the $S\bar{v}O_2$ value and trends.	
15. Input patient data.	Allows for calculation of derived parameters. Provides a means for patient identification on the printed out paper strip.	
16. Apply a sterile dressing to insertion site.	Reduces transmission of microorganisms.	
17. Ensure that there are no kinks or bends in the catheter.	Fiberoptics are fragile and can break if not handled carefully. Overtightening of a Tuoghy Bourst introducer connector can cause crimping of the fiberoptics.	Subclavian approach for insertion may cause kinking in the vessel if the anatomy is tortuous. Sending/receiving light wavelengths may not be optimal, and the computer may show either a change in the light signal or values that do not reflect the patient's status.
18. Firmly secure the optic module near the patient.	Excessive tension on catheter or optic module may produce breakage of optic fibers.	
19. Continuously monitor pulmonary artery pressure tracings and $S\bar{v}O_2$ values.	Provides continuous "real time" data on patient's venous oxygen saturation. Spontaneous catheter migration may occur after insertion. As a result of reflecting postcapillary arterialized blood, the $S\bar{v}O_2$ value may rise.	
20. Perform a verification/in vivo calibration according to hospital or manufacturer's recommendations.	In vivo calibration verifies the accuracy of the $S\bar{v}O_2$ value being displayed on the computer. Typically, this should be done every 24 hours or whenever the displayed value is in question.	In vivo calibration requires a mixed venous blood sample to be drawn from the distal port of the fiberoptic catheter.
21. Wash hands.	Reduces transmission of microorganisms.	

Mixed Venous Blood Sampling and in Vivo Calibration of $S\bar{v}O_2$

Note: This step may be required to verify the accuracy of the computer and value displayed after insertion of the fiberoptic catheter. Follow specific recommendations from the manufacturer as to the frequency of calibration and specific steps to implement the process. Common to any monitoring system, the patient's hemodynamic and oxygenation status should be stable for optimal calibration. In hypothermic patients with blood samples analyzed at 37°C, a small percentage error may be introduced. It is recommended to recalibrate once the patient becomes normothermic.

1. Wash hands.	Reduces transmission of microorganisms.	
2. Don exam gloves.	Universal precautions.	
3. Aseptically attach a 5- or 10-cc syringe to the sampling stopcock on the distal port of the catheter.	Contamination of stopcock may introduce microorganisms into the system.	

Table continues on following page

Steps	Rationale	Special Considerations
4. Turn the stopcock off to the flush solution.	Stops forward flow of flush solution.	
5. Slowly (over 5 seconds) aspirate 2 to 3 cc of blood as a waste sample and discard.	Typical dead space within the lumen is approximately 1 cc. Two to three times the dead space is usually sufficient to clear the lumen of flush solution.	Dispose of blood products as biohazardous waste according to hospital policy.
6. Turn the stopcock halfway off.	Eliminates backflow of blood and forward flow of flush solution.	
7. Attach the heparinized blood gas syringe to the sample stopcock, and open stopcock to patient.	Sodium heparin is recommended as the anticoagulation medium for blood gas measurements. Provides a setup for blood withdrawal.	Typical strength of heparin: 0.1 ml of 1000 units/ml to anticoagulate 2-ml sample. Preheparinized syringes are available.
8. Aspirate slowly (over 5 seconds) 1 to 3 cc of blood.	Rapid withdrawal will cause aspiration of arterialized blood, which will produce an elevated value.	
9. Close stopcock, remove syringe, and recover the stopcock port with a sterile nonvented cap.	Maintains closed, aseptic monitoring system.	
10. Expel any excess air in syringe, and cap the syringe.	Excess air may elevate the value. Capping prevents room air contamination.	
11. Roll syringe gently between palms.	Allows for mixing of blood and heparin.	
12. Label blood sample appropriately.	Ensures proper identification of sample.	
13. Submerge blood sample in ice if it is not sent immediately to the laboratory.	Cellular metabolism alters the blood gas values if the sample is not iced. Typical time in which the blood should be analyzed without being iced is 10 minutes.	A CO-oximeter that measures saturation, rather than calculating the value, must be used for accurate verification.
14. Flush distal port until traces of blood are removed.	Clears the line of residual blood and ensures more accurate pressure waveform monitoring.	
15. Observe bedside oscilloscope for pulmonary artery tracing.	Reconfirms catheter tip placement in the pulmonary artery.	
16. Resume $S\bar{v}O_2$ monitoring after following manufacturer's procedure for laboratory $S\bar{v}O_2$ verification of accuracy.	Provides continuous "real time" monitoring.	
17. Wash hands.	Reduces transmission of microorganisms.	

Evaluation

Evaluate patient response to nursing care and therapies by monitoring $S\bar{v}O_2$ values and trends. **Rationale:** Provides data concerning oxygen delivery and oxygen consumption.

Expected Outcomes

1. $S\bar{v}O_2$ value reflects optimal oxygen delivery to meet tissue demand. **Rationale:** Cardiac output and arterial oxygenation are sufficient to meet tissue demands without eliciting the compensatory mechanism to increase extraction.

2. $S\bar{v}O_2$ trends are within 5 to 10 percent of baseline value. **Rationale:** Activities and interventions are not increasing tissue oxygen demand so as to require reliance on compensatory mechanisms to meet the increase in demand.

3. Optimal hemodynamic and oxygenation parameters. **Rationale:** $S\bar{v}O_2$ reflects the determinants of oxygen

delivery and consumption. When delivery and demand are in balance, the components should be within the normal ranges for the patient.

Unexpected Outcomes

1. $S\bar{v}O_2$ values less than 60 percent, greater than 80 percent, or continued trend change of 5 to 10 percent above or below baseline. **Rationale:** Values outside the normal range or trends within the normal range can signify that the balance between oxygen supply and demand is threatened. Alterations in the parameter alert the nurse to evaluate further the determinants of $S\bar{v}O_2$.

2. Infection from presence of an indwelling pulmonary artery catheter. **Rationale:** Invasive monitoring places the patient at risk for infection.

3. Pulmonary artery infarct or rupture. **Rationale:** Overwedging the balloon or uncorrected catheter migration may result in pulmonary artery infarct or rupture.

Documentation

Documentation in the patient record should include the $S\bar{v}O_2$ value whenever the hemodynamic profile is recorded; specific events such as suctioning, turning the patient, or titration of a vasoactive drug, especially if the events produce a marked change in the $S\bar{v}O_2$ value; and the hard-copy printout, if it is available. **Rationale:** Documenting the $S\bar{v}O_2$ response to events assists the nurse in evaluating the efficacy of the interventions. It also aids the nurse in assessing the effects of various nursing activities on oxygen supply and demand.

Patient/Family Education

Patient and family education consists of pertinent aspects of hemodynamic monitoring as well as the rationale for the additional $S\bar{v}O_2$ monitor. Special attention should be paid to the continuous on-line nature of this monitoring system as well as the significance of the alarms. **Rationale:** Additional monitors may produce increased anxiety in the patient and family.

Performance Checklist
Skill 6–3: Continuous Mixed Venous Oxygen Saturation Monitoring

Critical Behaviors	Complies	
	yes	no
CONTINUOUS $S\bar{v}O_2$ MONITORING		
1. Wash hands.		
2. Connect computer to ac power source.		
3. Confirm that $S\bar{v}O_2$ computer is functioning properly.		
4. Remove outer wrap of catheter package.		
5. Peel back inner wrap that covers optic connector.		
6. Connect optic module to catheter connector.		
7. Prior to catheter insertion, perform an in vitro calibration.		
8. Pull back remaining wrap covering catheter package.		
9. Remove catheter from tray.		
10. Attach pressure monitor lines, and prime with flush solution.		
11. Assist physician with catheter insertion.		
12. Observe configuration of waveforms during insertion.		
13. Note balloon inflation volume required for proper wedging.		
14. Set appropriate high and low alarms.		
15. Input patient data, or connect computer to hard-copy printer (if applicable).		
16. Apply sterile dressing to insertion site.		
17. Ensure that dressing does not cause kinks in the catheter.		
18. Firmly secure the optic module near patient.		
19. Continuously monitor PA pressure tracings and $S\bar{v}O_2$ values.		
20. Perform a verification in vivo calibration.		

Table continues on following page

Critical Behaviors	Complies	
	yes	no
21. Wash hands		
MIXED VENOUS BLOOD SAMPLING AND IN VIVO CALIBRATION OF $\overline{S}vO_2$ 1. Wash hands.		
2. Don exam gloves.		
3. Attach 5 or 10 cc syringe to distal port of catheter.		
4. Turn stopcock off to the flush solution.		
5. Slowly aspirate 2 to 3 cc of blood and discard.		
6. Turn stopcock halfway.		
7. Attach heparinized blood gas syringe to sample stopcock and open stopcock to patient.		
8. Slowly aspirate 1 to 3 cc of blood over 5 seconds.		
9. Close stopcock, remove syringe, and cover stopcock port with sterile nonvented cap.		
10. Expel excess air in syringe and cap syringe.		
11. Roll syringe gently between palms.		
12. Label blood sample.		
13. Submerge in ice or send immediately to lab.		
14. Flush distal port until all traces of blood are removed.		
15. Observe PA tracing.		
16. Resume $\overline{S}vO_2$ monitoring.		
17. Wash hands.		
18. Document procedure in patient record.		

SKILL 6–4

Assisting with Bronchoscopy

Therapeutic bronchoscopy involves the use of either the fiberoptic or rigid bronchoscope and has become the tool of choice in the diagnosis and management of tracheobronchial disorders. Since the rigid bronchoscope offers less flexibility than the fiberoptic bronchoscope and frequently necessitates intubation with general anesthesia, its popularity has greatly diminished. Nevertheless, because the rigid bronchoscope offers a much larger channel, it remains the preferred instrument for the removal of foreign bodies and the control of bleeding in the presence of massive hemoptysis. Other advantages of the rigid bronchoscope include more effective control of the airway and the ability to ventilate patients through the large scope.

The flexible fiberoptic bronchoscope contains high-precision lenses in both the proximal and distal ends that are aligned to provide magnification of the endobronchial tree. In addition, the polyurethane fiberoptic bronchoscope is covered with a thin rubber sheath on the distal end to provide maximum flexibility. The flexible fiberoptic bronchoscope enables exploration of segmental and subsegmental bronchi, including the upper lobes. As a result, the flexible fiberoptic bronchoscope is associated with a relative ease of insertion and better patient tolerance. Consequently, with the aforementioned exceptions, fiberoptic bronchoscopy (FOB) is considered the procedure of choice when therapeutic bronchoscopy is indicated.

The major indication for FOB is a suspected diagnosis of lung cancer. Clinical findings associated with a high index of suspicion for such a diagnosis include persistent and unexplained cough in high-risk patients, persistent hemoptysis, suspicious chest x-ray, unresolved pneumonia, abnormal sputum cytology, localized wheeze, and recurrent laryngeal nerve paralysis. Bronchial washings, brushings, and transbronchial biopsies should be taken from all suspicious areas to maximize diagnostic results when carcinoma is suspected.

The presence of a lung abscess is generally not considered an indication for FOB. When an abscess is unresponsive to conventional therapy, however, FOB may be undertaken to rule out disorders possibly potentiating the abscess, such as obstruction by neoplasms or foreign bodies. In addition to this role in ruling out hidden causes of the abscess, FOB often facilitates intrabronchial drainage of the abscess.

Hemoptysis is also a frequent indication for therapeutic bronchoscopy. In the presence of this clinical finding, FOB has both diagnostic and therapeutic benefits. As a diagnostic tool, FOB can identify the source of the bleeding, which is frequently a neoplasm. Once the source is identified, techniques to control bleeding, such as instillation of epinephrine 1:20,000 dilution at the site or tamponade using a balloon-tipped catheter placed through the suction channel of the fiberscope, can be initiated. If massive active hemoptysis occurs, obscuring the visual field, rigid bronchoscopy may be required.

As in the case of lung abscess, atelectasis and mucous plugging are not routine indications for FOB. However, when acute lobar or whole-lung atelectasis persists despite mechanical ventilation through a properly positioned endotracheal tube and initiation of conventional respiratory therapy or is associated with suspected underlying pathology or a desire for prompt improvement in oxygenation and ventilation, FOB may be instituted. Likewise, FOB may be instituted for removal of secretions or mucous plugs in cases of severe asthma or cystic fibrosis that have not responded to conventional therapy. When instituted for removal of secretions, 0.9% sodium chloride is instilled to help liquefy the secretions. Once the sodium chloride lavage is completed, Mucomyst may be instilled. The use of FOB for this particular purpose may induce or worsen existing bronchospasm, especially when Mucomyst is used in an asthmatic. In these situations, therefore, FOB should be performed under controlled conditions in the intensive care unit.

Since the incidence of acquired immunodeficiency syndrome (AIDS) and the prevalence of immunosuppressive therapy have increased, the presence of pulmonary infiltrates in immunocompromised patients has become another indication for FOB. Through FOB with bronchoalveolar lavage alone or in conjunction with transbronchial biopsy, many life-threatening opportunistic and bacterial infections can be detected and distinguished from other conditions. FOB has proved especially useful in the diagnosis of *Pneumocystis carinii*, pneumonia in patients with AIDS.

In the presence of upper airway obstruction and suspected foreign-body aspiration, the rigid bronchoscope remains the instrument of choice. However, FOB may be instituted initially for diagnostic purposes. The advent of larger forceps for the flexible fiberoptic bronchoscope makes it possible to retrieve smaller objects.

There are several indications for FOB specific to the intubated and mechanically ventilated patient. FOB may be used for emergency intubations in situations involving facial or cervical trauma, assessment of endotracheal or tracheostomy tube placement, assessment of tracheal damage following prolonged intubation, placement of double-lumen endotracheal tubes, and diagnosis of nosocomial pneumonias. When FOB is performed on an intubated patient, a special adapter called a *tracheostomy* or *T-piece* must be utilized. The purpose of this adapter is to minimize air leaks as the FOB is inserted. This is possible because of the presence of a rubber diaphragm on the open end of the T-piece that forms a seal around the FOB as it is inserted, thus allowing mechanical ventilation to continue. Since the seal formed by the dia-

phragm is so tight, lubrication of the FOB is necessary to allow free movement through the system.

An endotracheal tube with an 8.5-mm internal diameter is considered the ideal size for the standard 5- to 7-mm FOB, but 8.0-mm endotracheal tubes may be used. FOB is not generally recommended through endotracheal tubes of less than 8.0 mm diameter because it will likely result in a significant increase in peak inspiratory pressure.

Regardless of the endotracheal tube diameter, FOB during mechanical ventilation is associated with a decrease in tidal volume and PaO_2, as well as an increase in $PaCO_2$. When positive end-expiratory pressure (PEEP) is utilized, the risk of barotrauma rises, because the presence of the FOB creates additional PEEP itself. The reductions in tidal volume, functional residual capacity, and PaO_2 are further aggravated with repeated and prolonged use of suction. Consequently, if FOB is to be instituted with mechanical ventilation, the delivery of 100% oxygen and discontinuation of PEEP are recommended throughout the procedure, and suctioning is limited to short intermittent periods only.

The three most common techniques employed through the fiberoptic bronchoscope are bronchoalveolar lavage, transbronchial biopsy, and bronchial brushing. *Bronchoalveolar lavage* enables a relatively noninvasive sampling of cellular components of the lower respiratory tract for diagnostic purposes. It also enables mobilization and removal of secretions from peripheral airways for therapeutic purposes. Bronchoalveolar lavage involves the instillation of 0.9% sodium chloride in 25- to 50-cc increments through the channel of the FOB once the suspicious tissue or segment has been visualized. The solution along with cellular components is then aspirated into a sterile specimen container. This is repeated until 100 cc has been retrieved for a specimen or until a total of 400 cc of fluid has been instilled.

A *transbronchial biopsy* involves passing a flexible needle or forceps through the channel of the bronchoscope. Once visualized, suspicious areas of the trachea and bronchi can be penetrated with the needle or forceps and a specimen collected for examination. Transbronchial biopsy is contraindicated if mechanical ventilation is used because the two in combination significantly increase the risk of pneumothorax. *Bronchial brushing* involves the advancement of a catheter brush through the channel of the bronchoscope. The catheter brush is protected by a double sheath, thus allowing samples to be taken from the lower respiratory tract without contamination.

Although FOB is associated with a low incidence of major complications (less than 1 percent), some degree of risk is always present. Complications of FOB can be grouped into three major categories. The first involves complications considered secondary to premedication. These include such side effects as respiratory depression, syncope, and transient hypotension.

The second category involves complications associated with the local anesthetic agent used. Lidocaine jelly and a 4% lidocaine solution are used on the upper airway as a topical anesthetic prior to the procedure. These agents have been associated with such side effects as seizures, dysrhythmias, and laryngospasm.

The third category involves complications secondary to the procedure itself. The major complications in this category include bronchospasm, hemorrhage, and pneumothorax. Bronchospasm is most frequently associated with bronchoalveolar lavage. Hemorrhage and pneumothorax, on the other hand, are more commonly associated with transbronchial biopsy. Laryngospasm and vasovagal reactions are most likely to occur during manipulation of the bronchoscope at the level of the larynx. Hypoxemia, both during and up to 2 hours after the procedure, is a frequent finding, with the PaO_2 falling as much as 26 percent in patients receiving mechanical ventilation. Patients with severe underlying pulmonary dysfunction are especially at risk and warrant careful monitoring.

Dysrhythmias also have been reported as a complication of FOB and are most frequently associated with the period of major oxygen desaturation. Manipulation of the bronchoscope at the laryngeal level also has been associated with dysrhythmias. Fever and pulmonary infiltrates have been associated with instillation of fluid during bronchoalveolar lavage. The febrile response is generally delayed, representing a transient pyrogen effect, and is not indicative of pulmonary infection. This pyrogen effect is more likely to occur when large volumes of fluid are used or when multiple lobes are lavaged. The radiographic finding of new or increased infiltrates is also transient and is generally not associated with clinical complications. The infiltrates reflect the fluid instilled during lavage and are reabsorbed within 24 hours.

Purpose

The nurse assists with bronchoscopy for visualization of the bronchi to the segmental and subsegmental level to

1. Obtain a tissue biopsy or sputum or cytology specimens for the differential diagnosis of tracheobronchial disorders.
2. Remove secretions from the tracheobronchial tree.
3. Assess for tracheal damage resulting from prolonged intubation with mechanical ventilation.
4. Locate the source of hemoptysis.
5. Control hemoptysis.
6. Remove foreign bodies.
7. Facilitate difficult endotracheal intubations.
8. Place a double-lumen endotracheal tube.

Prerequisite Knowledge and Skills

Prior to assisting with bronchoscopy, the nurse should understand

1. Principles of aseptic technique.
2. Anatomy and physiology of the tracheobronchial tree.

3. Procedure for intubation (see Skill 1–5).
4. Procedure for endotracheal suctioning (see Skill 1–6).

The nurse should be able to perform

1. Proper handwashing technique (see Skill 35–5).
2. Universal precautions (see Skill 35–1).
3. Vital signs assessment.
4. Pulmonary assessment.
5. Assessment and management of the patient–ventilator system (see Skill 4–1).

Assessment

1. Assess for significant medical history, including foreign-body aspiration, airway obstruction, hemoptysis, immunocompromise with pulmonary infiltrates, lung abscess, lung mass, whole-lung atelectasis, retained secretions, prolonged intubation with mechanical ventilation, persistent pneumonia, and chronic unexplained cough. **Rationale:** Significant medical history indicates the need for bronchoscopy.
2. Assess for factors influencing tolerance of the procedure, including acute bronchospasm, size of endotracheal tube, peak inspiratory pressures, hypoxemia refractory to high FIO_2, use of PEEP, thrombocytopenia, coagulopathy, hemodynamic instability, and fighting the ventilator. **Rationale:** Listed conditions and disease states predispose patients to increased risk for procedural complications and discomfort.

Nursing Diagnoses

1. Ineffective breathing pattern related to airway obstruction. **Rationale:** Respiratory distress occurs as a result of increased airway resistance secondary to a decrease in the cross-sectional diameter of the airway. The obstruction may be in the form of a foreign body, retained secretions, bronchospasm, tumor, tracheal stenosis, or the bronchoscope itself.
2. Impaired gas exchange related to alveolar hypoxia. **Rationale:** Respiratory gas exchange requires adequate PAO_2 levels, which are decreased in the presence of atelectasis, retained secretions, and suctioning.
3. Potential for injury related to disruption of bronchial wall integrity. **Rationale:** Hemoptysis and pneumothorax can occur when a transbronchial biopsy is performed resulting in accumulation of air in the pleural space or blood loss.
4. Fear related to unknown outcome of procedure. **Rationale:** Lack of familiarity with the procedure or anticipation of an undesired diagnosis may result in fear.
5. Alteration in comfort related to manipulation of bronchoscope. **Rationale:** Manipulation of the bronchoscope may stimulate cough, gag, and/or irritant receptors. In addition, if mechanical ventilation is used, the peak inspiratory pressures may increase, which may be uncomfortable. Application of suction also can result in discomfort because it causes a sensation of suffocation.

Planning

1. Individualize the following goals for smooth and complication-free FOB:
   a. Optimize breathing pattern. **Rationale:** Enhances gas exchange and decreases fear and anxiety.
   b. Optimize gas exchange. **Rationale:** Enhances tissue oxygenation and relieve respiratory distress.
   c. Decrease the incidence of complications. **Rationale:** Pneumothorax and hemoptysis and bronchospasm can complicate the patient's recovery.
2. Prepare all necessary equipment for monitoring the patient during the procedure. **Rationale:** Facilitates early recognition of potential complications during an invasive procedure.
   a. Cardiac monitor (see Skill 7–1).
   b. Ventilator (see Skill 4–1).
   c. Blood pressure cuff or arterial pressure monitoring (see Skill 10–2).
   d. Pulse oximeter (see Skill 6–1).
3. Prepare all necessary equipment and supplies for the procedure. **Rationale:** Assembly of all the equipment and supplies facilitates efficient bronchoscopy.
   a. Fiberoptic or rigid bronchoscope (check with physician).
   b. Light source.
   c. Transbronchial aspiration needle.
   d. Cytology brush.
   e. Topical anesthetics.
   f. Water-soluble lubricant.
   g. Bite block.
   h. Suction apparatus.
   i. Tonsillar-type suction-tip catheter.
   j. T-piece adapter.
   k. Protective goggles.
   l. Surgical mask.
   m. Oxygen source.
   n. Gowns.
   o. Cleaning and disinfecting solutions.
   p. Specimen containers.
   q. Laboratory requisition slips.
   r. Sterile gloves for personnel performing and assisting.
4. Prepare the necessary emergency equipment. **Rationale:** Assembly of emergency equipment facilitates prompt and efficient treatment of complications.
   a. Patent IV.
   b. Bag valve mask device capable of delivery 100% oxygen and large inflation volumes.
   c. Flowmeter.
   d. Intubation equipment.
5. Prepare the patient for the procedure.
   a. Ensure that an informed consent has been obtained. **Rationale:** FOB is an invasive procedure that requires the written consent of the patient (if able) or significant other.
   b. Explain the procedure to the patient. **Rationale:** Decreases fear and anxiety as well as enhances cooperation.
   c. Position patient according to physician preference or in the supine position with the head of the bed elevated 30 degrees. **Rationale:** Provides easy access and facilitates visualization.
   d. Determine patient allergies, and then administer prescribed premedication. **Rationale:** Atropine 0.5 to 1.0 mg is given to dry secretions to promote better visualization. Use with caution in patients with heart disease because the resulting tachycardia may cause angina. Promotes better visualization of the airway.
   e. Administer sedation if prescribed. **Rationale:** Sedation, usually in the form of meperidine, midazolam, or hydroxyzine, reduces anxiety and discomfort and enhances patient cooperation. Occasionally, paralytic agents are given to patients receiving mechanical ventilation to promote patient–ventilator synchronization.
6. Collect appropriate specimens. **Rationale:** Appropriate collection of specimens enhances the diagnostic yield of this procedure.

Implementation

Steps	Rationale	Special Considerations
1. Wash hands.	Reduces transmission of microorganisms.	
2. Don protective goggles, surgical mask, protective gown, and sterile gloves.	Universal precautions.	
3. Assist physician with intubation, if necessary (see Skill 1–5).	Provides secure airway if procedure expected to be long or patient is in high-risk category.	
4. Adjust supplemental oxygen and/or ventilator settings as prescribed by physician.	Optimizes ventilation and gas exchange.	

Table continues on following page

Steps	Rationale	Special Considerations
5. Assist physician with application of topical anesthetic to upper airways (nose, pharynx).	Promotes patient comfort and tolerance as bronchoscope passes gag, irritant, and cough receptors.	If patient is intubated, viscous lidocaine may be instilled into endotracheal tube.
6. Assist physician with placement of T-piece adapter if the patient is intubated.	Provides airtight seal around bronchoscope to minimize air leak and facilitate continued mechanical ventilation.	
7. Assist physician with lubrication of the tip of the scope with a water-soluble lubricant.	Facilitates free movement and flexibility of the bronchoscope in the system.	Petrolatum-based lubricants may cause premature deterioration of the rubber sheath of the bronchoscope.
8. Assist physician with insertion of the bronchoscope. If endotracheal tube is in place, the nurse may be asked to hold tube for better stabilization.	Prevents migration of tube.	If patient is not intubated, lidocaine may be instilled through the channel of the bronchoscope at the level of the larynx. Lidocaine may be instilled at the carina on both intubated and nonintubated patients.
9. Assist physician during procedure as requested.	Team effort assists in performing the skill in a timely fashion.	
10. Assist physician with removal of the T-piece adapter and bronchoscope.	Adapter is no longer necessary once the bronchoscope is withdrawn.	
11. Obtain a stat portable chest x-ray per physician request.	Evaluates effectiveness of procedure and rules out pneumothorax as a complication.	
12. Return ventilator settings to preprocedure levels per physician instruction when appropriate.	Returns ventilator settings to original levels, especially FIO_2, tidal volume, and PEEP settings.	
13. Label specimens and send to laboratory for evaluation.	Provides identification and instruction.	
14. Dispose of equipment in appropriate receptacle.	Universal precautions.	
15. Wash hands.	Reduces transmission of microorganisms.	

Evaluation

1. Compare the patient's vital signs, respiratory assessment, and laboratory values after the FOB with the baseline assessments. **Rationale:** Identifies the effects of the FOB and the occurrence of complications.

2. Evaluate the patient's sputum after the FOB for the presence of hemoptysis. **Rationale:** A small amount of hemoptysis may result from the trauma of the procedure itself, especially if a biopsy was performed. An increase in the amount should be reported to the physician.

3. Confirm with the physician the results of the chest x-ray. **Rationale:** Identifies the effects of the FOB and the occurrence of complications.

Expected Outcomes

1. Visualization of trachea and segmental and subsegmental bronchi. **Rationale:** Identifies suspicious tissue.

2. Collection of appropriate specimens. **Rationale:** Facilitates diagnosis of tracheobronchial disorders.

3. Relief of respiratory distress. **Rationale:** Removal of tenacious secretions from the lower respiratory tree facilitates ventilation and gas exchange, which results in improved arterial blood gases and breath sounds.

4. Chest x-ray indicates resolution of consolidation. **Rationale:** Removal of secretions allows reexpansion of consolidated areas.

Unexpected Outcomes

1. Increased respiratory distress and tachycardia. **Rationale:** The patient has developed pneumothorax.

2. Hypotension and lethargy. **Rationale:** The patient has been oversedated.

3. Persistent hemoptysis. **Rationale:** The patient has experienced trauma from the bronchoscope.

4. Fever. **Rationale:** The patient has bacteremia from the bronchoscope.

5. Bradycardia. **Rationale:** The patient has experienced a vagal response.

Documentation

Documentation in the patient record should include the patient's vital signs, breath sounds, ABGs, ventilator settings, and character of sputum before and after the procedure; administration of premedication, including time, route, dosage, and response; date and time procedure was performed; name of physician performing procedure; additional procedures performed (i.e., biopsy, brushing, or lavage); patient tolerance to procedure; dispensation of specimens; and completion of postprocedure chest x-ray. **Rationale:** Records nursing care provided as well as expected and unexpected outcomes.

Patient/Family Education

1. Assess the level of understanding of the patient and family regarding the patient's condition and rationale for FOB. **Rationale:** Identifies patient and family knowledge deficits regarding the patient's condition, the procedure, and predicted outcomes and potential risks and allows for clarification of misconceptions.

2. Instruct the patient and family that drowsiness is common after the procedure and, thus, that bed rest is required. **Rationale:** Enhances patient cooperation and prevents falls.

3. Instruct patient that a sore throat, irritating cough, and small amount of hemoptysis are to be expected following the procedure. **Rationale:** The bronchoscope causes trauma to the mucosa during the procedure.

4. Instruct patient to wear supplemental oxygen as prescribed by the physician following the procedure. **Rationale:** Hypoxemia may persist for up to 2 hours after the procedure.

5. Instruct patient to cough following the procedure. **Rationale:** Coughing will facilitate removal of secretions that may be retained following lavage.

Performance Checklist
Skill 6–4:   Assisting with Bronchoscopy

Critical Behaviors	Complies yes	no
1. Wash hands.		
2. Don goggles, mask, gown, and gloves.		
3. Assist physician with intubation, if necessary.		
4. Adjust ventilator settings.		
5. Assist physician with application of topical anesthetic.		
6. Assist physician with placement of T-piece adapter.		
7. Assist physician with lubrication of scope.		
8. Assist physician with insertion of bronchoscope.		
9. Assist physician with procedure.		
10. Assist physician with removal of T-piece adapter.		
11. Order stat portable chest x-ray per physician instructions.		
12. Return ventilator settings to preprocedure level.		
13. Label and dispense specimens appropriately.		
14. Discard equipment in appropriate manner.		
15. Wash hands.		
16. Document procedure in the patient record.		

SKILL 6–5

Preparation for Hyperbaric Oxygen Therapy

Hyperbaric oxygen is administered using either a multiplace or a monoplace chamber (Figs. 6–24 and 6–25). Both chambers deliver oxygen to patients in an environment of increased atmospheric pressure.

Pressure is increased within the chamber by adding compressed gas (air in the multiplace chamber, usually oxygen in the monoplace chamber). The addition of the compressed gas is called the *compression phase* of treatment. It usually lasts 3 to 5 minutes in a multiplace chamber or as long as 30 minutes in a monoplace chamber. During compression, patients may notice a temporary rise in ambient temperature secondary to molecular fric-

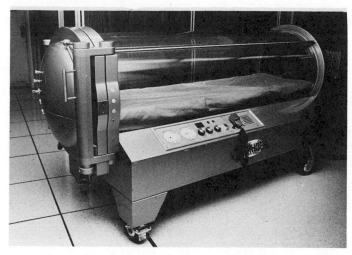

FIGURE 6–24. A monoplace chamber, in which the entire sealed chamber is usually filled with compressed 100% oxygen. The patient breathes the oxygen freely while inside the chamber, and the nurse cares for the patient's various needs from outside the chamber.

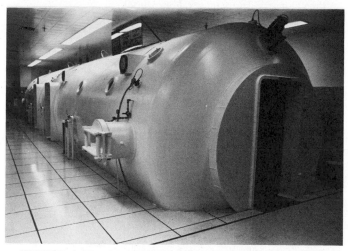

FIGURE 6–25. A multiplace chamber is larger in size, with an entire sealed chamber section filled with compressed air (approximately 21% oxygen and 79% nitrogen). The patient then receives 100% oxygen via a mask, head tent, or tracheal or endotracheal delivery system. The multiplace chamber has several compartments, each of which can be pressurized separately, allowing the transport of goods (such as blood and medications) and/or people (patients and personnel) in and out of the chamber as needed. The nurse is inside the chamber with the patient to provide uninterrupted nursing care.

tion. Barotrauma may occur if unvented gas volumes expand or contract with the accompanying changes in pressure. Potential sites for barotrauma include the middle ear space, congested sinuses, improperly sealed dental fillings, any "blockages" within the pulmonary system, or an untreated pneumothorax. Once the prescribed pressure level is achieved, hyperbaric oxygen delivery can be initiated.

Oxygen is normally transported to cells via the pulmonary system, where it is loaded onto hemoglobin for delivery through the circulatory system to tissues. The mechanism underlying hyperbaric oxygen therapy is the ability of oxygen to dissolve into solution when pressurized. By dissolving oxygen into plasma as a result of increasing atmospheric pressure around the body, a much larger "dose" of oxygen can be attained. These intermittent high doses of oxygen stimulate healing (Table 6–3).

During hyperbaric oxygen treatment, patients are encouraged to relax. Nursing care (i.e., vital signs measurements, medication, fluid and blood administration, and most interventions) proceeds as scheduled, as though the patient were still in the critical care unit.

A rare side effect of hyperbaric oxygen delivery is oxygen toxicity. Oxygen toxicity can manifest itself in the pulmonary system as pulmonary edema or neurologically as seizures. Fortunately, these complications cease with the withdrawal of hyperbaric oxygen. These side effects also can be managed by the addition of "air breaks" (scheduled interruptions of hyperbaric oxygen with air, usually 5 minutes in duration) to the hyperbaric oxygen schedule for high-risk patients.

Decompression of the chamber begins once the prescribed duration of hyperbaric oxygen is reached. The time frames are similar to those identified during compression for the respective chamber types. Chamber occupants will notice a drop in ambient temperature. Additionally, unless vented, enclosed gas spaces will expand dramatically during decompression. This phenomenon can potentially impede ventilation or cause barotrauma unless appropriate nursing interventions are employed. Patients are encouraged to breathe normally; mechanically ventilated patients are monitored to ensure lung relaxation between breaths.

Barometric pressure can be expressed in millimeters of mercury (mmHg), pounds per square inch (lb/in^2), feet of seawater (fsw), or atmospheres absolute (ATA). Sea level is the standard plane for measurement of surface barometric pressure, i.e., 760 mmHg, 14.7 lb/in^2, 0 fsw, or 1 ATA. By increasing the barometric pressure to 2 ATA or 33 fsw on an FIO_2 of 1.0, the oxygen dissolved in plasma can be increased to 4.4 vol%. The gas law governing this action is Henry's law, which states that the degree to which a gas enters into physical solution in body fluids is directly proportional to the partial pressure of the gas to which the fluid is exposed. One can see that as the partial pressure of a given gas, in this case oxygen, is increased, more oxygen is dissolved in plasma. In fact, enough oxygen can be dissolved in plasma at the pressure of 3 ATA (6.4 vol%) to sustain life in the absence of hemoglobin.

Another gas law that governs the behavior of gases under pressure is Boyle's law, which states that if the temperature remains constant, the volume of gas is inversely proportional to its pressure (i.e., the size of an intravascular air bubble will decrease in volume as barometric pressure is increased, as in a hyperbaric chamber). The gas laws involved are summarized in Table 6–4.

Purpose

The nurse prepares the patient for hyperbaric oxygen therapy to

1. Minimize patient anxiety.
2. Promote a safe patient experience.

TABLE 6–3 ACCEPTED INDICATIONS FOR HYPERBARIC OXYGEN

1. Air or gas embolism
2. Carbon monoxide poisoning and smoke inhalation, carbon monoxide complicated by cyanide poisoning
3. Clostridial myonecrosis (gas gangrene)
4. Crush injury, compartment syndrome, and other acute traumatic ischemias
5. Decompression sickness
6. Enhancement of healing in selected problem wounds
7. Exceptional blood loss (anemia)
8. Necrotizing soft-tissue infections (subcutaneous tissue, muscle, fascia)
9. Osteomyelitis (refractory)
10. Radiation tissue damage (osteoradionecrosis)
11. Skin grafts and flaps (compromised)
12. Thermal burns
13. Selected spinal cord injuries

TABLE 6–4 GAS LAWS/BASIC PHYSICS OF DIVING

Boyle's Law: In a closed system under constant temperature, as pressure increases, the volume of gas decreases, and as pressure decreases, the volume of gas increases. For example, trapped air will expand during decompression.

Charles' Law: In a closed system, the temperature of a gas is directly proportional to the pressure of the gas. For example, the patient may complain of feeling warm during compression (the first few moments of treatment) and may complain of feeling cool on decompression (the final few moments of treatment).

Henry's Law: As the partial pressure of a gas increases, more of it will be dissolved in liquid. For example, on room air (21% oxygen) at surface pressure, oxygen comprises 0.3 vol% of plasma versus oxygen levels of 6.4 to 6.9 vol% of plasma at 66 ft of sea water (fsw) on 100% oxygen.

Dalton's Law: The combined partial pressure of two or more gases equals the sum of the partial pressures of each individual gas. For example, patients receiving hyperbaric oxygen are breathing 100% oxygen only, causing a rise in oxygen concentration only. The nurse or tender in the chamber (multiplace) breathing room air will have an increase in both oxygen and nitrogen concentrations.

Prerequisite Knowledge and Skills

Prior to preparing a patient for hyperbaric oxygen therapy, the nurse should understand

1. Accepted indications for hyperbaric oxygen therapy.
2. Mechanisms of action involved in hyperbaric oxygen therapy.
3. Subjective patient responses to the treatment.
4. Special safety considerations for the hyperbaric oxygen environment.
5. Principles of pressurized gases.
6. Signs and symptoms of oxygen toxicity.

The nurse should be able to perform

1. Assessment of wound or presenting indication.
2. Assessment of the tympanic membrane mobility via the patient autoinflation technique.
3. Respiratory system assessment.
4. Assessment of additional parameters, such as basal temperature, triglyceride level, CBC, chest x-ray, and glucose level.
5. Proper handwashing technique (see Skill 35–5).
6. Universal precautions (see Skill 35–1).

Assessment

1. Assess status of wound (size, color, drainage, odor) or other presenting indication (i.e., neurologic assessment for decompression sickness or air embolism). **Rationale:** Provides baseline data to which future assessments can be compared and measures progress and efficacy of treatment.
2. Assess the mobility of the tympanic membrane in nonintubated patients. **Rationale:** Movement of the tympanic membrane allows movement of air ("venting") from the eustachian tube. By ensuring that the patient can mobilize the tympanic membrane by autoinflation

(i.e., swallowing, yawning, Valsalva maneuver, etc.), the likelihood of barotrauma within the middle ear is minimized. Patients unable to mobilize the tympanic membrane (i.e., intubated patients) will usually require myringotomies and the placement of polyethylene pressure-equalizing tubes if the patient is to have serial treatments.

3. Identify potential risk factors for pulmonary barotrauma and report them to the hyperbaric staff. Such risk factors include abnormal chest x-ray (any condition that might impede air movement), untreated pneumothorax, history of restrictive or obstructive pulmonary disease, and central venous line insertions (or attempted insertions since last treatment or within past 24 hours). **Rationale:** Awareness of risk factors facilitates necessary precautions that minimize the likelihood of pulmonary barotrauma.

4. Identify potential risk factors for oxygen toxicity and report them to the hyperbaric staff. For central nervous system oxygen toxicity, these include elevated body temperature, hyperlipidemia, history of epilepsy or seizures (i.e., after head trauma), and extreme patient agitation. For pulmonary oxygen toxicity, these include use of high FiO_2 delivery (greater than 0.5) or FiO_2 by endotracheal tube or tracheal tube in excess of 3 days. **Rationale:** Ensures that interventions to minimize the likelihood of oxygen toxicity are instituted. For example, these patients might be given additional "air breaks" during the hyperbaric treatment.

5. Trend hemoglobin and hematocrit levels. **Rationale:** During hyperbaric oxygen therapy, red blood cells are *not* actually needed, since the O_2 is being dissolved into the plasma and carried to distal tissues. However; maintenance of hemoglobin and hematocrit within the normal range promotes adequate oxygenation of healing wound tissues between hyperbaric oxygen treatments.

6. Assess respiratory system for any potential source of obstruction. **Rationale:** Minimizes the likelihood of pulmonary barotrauma.

7. Ensure that all equipment to be utilized (i.e., IV pumps) has been tested, adapted as necessary, and approved for hyperbaric use. **Rationale:** Ensures patient safety.

Nursing Diagnoses

1. Impaired tissue integrity related to altered tissue perfusion. **Rationale:** Wound healing is compromised secondary to edema, multiple trauma, negative nitrogen balance, diabetes, peripheral vascular disease, radiation therapy, invasion of the body by toxins, or sepsis.

2. Impaired gas exchange related to gas embolism. **Rationale:** Gas embolism blocks air passages mechanically; air entering the circulatory system impedes tissue perfusion.

3. Impaired gas exchange related to carbon monoxide, cyanide, or smoke exposure. **Rationale:** Carbon monoxide and cyanide have higher affinities for hemoglobin than oxygen, displacing oxygen from hemoglobin. Smoke inhalation usually results in tracheal, laryngeal, or bronchial edema, mechanically impeding air exchange. Furthermore, it can be assumed that the presence of smoke also signals concurrent exposure to carbon monoxide.

4. Sensory (visual) alterations related to subtle accommodations made by the lens in response to long-term hyperbaric oxygen exposure. **Rationale:** Long-term hyperbaric oxygen therapy causes temporary changes in visual acuity (varying in nature and in severity from patient to patient) that resolve without intervention with cessation of therapy.

5. Anxiety related to confinement, claustrophobia, and the presence of unfamiliar equipment. **Rationale:** Hyperbaric oxygen delivery requires an unusual environment and a myriad of equipment, all of which can be frightening.

Planning

1. Individualize the following goals for hyperbaric oxygen therapy:
   a. Promote wound healing. **Rationale:** Intermittent high doses of oxygen stimulate healing.
   b. Promote rapid elimination of certain toxins, such as carbon monoxide and cyanide. **Rationale:** Restoration of normal gas exchange is crucial to life. Developing a means to measure response to treatment (i.e., administration of standard neuropsychometric test battery) will help determine efficacy.
   c. Minimize effects of air or gas emboli. **Rationale:** Restoration of unimpaired tissue perfusion is crucial to life and optimal functioning.

2. Anticipate patient needs and requirements while in the hyperbaric chamber, including scheduled medications (i.e., antibiotics), pain medication, charting materials, sedation, insulin and/or patient snacks for diabetics, etc. Also provide items as necessary for comfort (pillows, blankets), and offer items such as books or puzzles. **Rationale:** Allows for care aspects and planned activities to continue.

3. Prepare the patient.
   a. Explain the procedure to the patient. **Rationale:** Minimizes risks and reduces anxiety.
   b. Explain patient's expected degree of participation and importance of swallowing, yawning, and performing the Valsalva maneuver when requested. **Rationale:** Reduces likelihood of barotrauma.
   c. Instruct patient to report feelings of claustrophobia or confinement anxiety. Provide prescribed sedation if appropriate. **Rationale:** Patient comfort promotes success of procedure.

Implementation

Steps	Rationale	Special Considerations
1. Wash hands.	Reduces transmission of microorganisms.	
2. Take necessary precautions to safeguard patient from complications related to changing atmospheric pressures:	Appropriate interventions preclude complications.	
a. If patient has endotracheal or tracheal tube, replace air in cuff with sterile water.	Volumes of gas will change as pressure changes. If inflated with air, the cuff will collapse on compression.	Maintain same cuff pressure (replace air with H_2O and follow standard procedure for ascertaining proper amount via auscultation) (see Skill 1–6).
b. Remove intravenous glass bottles (replace with plastic bags) if possible. If not possible, alert hyperbaric staff to their presence.	During pressure change, air can easily become trapped and expand into the circulatory system. Shattering of glass is also a possibility.	
c. Remove "hard" contact lenses from patient.	Corneal injury may result if the potential air space behind the contact lens contracts with compression.	
d. Determine presence of any prosthetic implants patient may have that utilize air. Deflate before treatment if possible; warn patient that the device may be damaged during treatment.	Volume of air will change as chamber pressure changes.	
e. Remove all air bubbles from IV tubings.	Small bubbles may expand on decompression to a larger, more threatening size.	
f. Avoid "clamping" of any tubes, drains, etc. Leave tubes connected to a straight drainage system (as opposed to clamping) if possible.	Increases the possibility of injury related to changing air volumes in enclosed spaces (i.e., expanding air in oral-gastric tubes resulting in vomiting and possible aspiration).	
g. Provide a mechanism for attaching chest tubes to suction or a one-way (Heimlich type) valve.	Prevents additional air from entering into pleural space with volume changes that accompany changes in pressure.	
3. Take necessary precautions to safeguard patient from injury related to use of oxygen under pressure.	Use of oxygen under pressure increases the likelihood of fire and combustion.	
a. Remove petrolatum-based products (i.e., bacitracin ointment, hairspray, petrolatum, etc.), from head and neck area for multiplace chamber use and from any body area for monoplace chamber use.	Promotes combustion under pressure.	
b. Remove cigarettes, matches, lighters, and mechanical "gadgets" (i.e., mechanical toys, personal radios, etc.) prior to the initiation of hyperbaric oxygen therapy.	Potential sources of combustion.	

Table continues on following page

Steps	Rationale	Special Considerations
c. Avoid use of hydraulic-type (using fluorocarbon as lubricant) pedal-operated stretchers.	Fluorocarbons support combustion.	Fluorocarbon lubricant can be replaced with halocarbon lubricant in order to safely adapt stretcher for chamber use (this is generally an issue relevant to multiplace chambers, since monoplace chambers utilize their own "stretchers" anyway).
4. Wash hands.	Reduces transmission of microorganisms.	

Evaluation

1. Evaluate wound healing: size, color, drainage, and odor. **Rationale:** Measures efficacy of treatment.
2. Evaluate carboxyhemoglobin and cyanide blood levels. **Rationale:** Objectively determines the presence of carbon monoxide and cyanide.
3. Evaluate neurologic status, i.e., patient's subjective complaints of fatigue, headache, lightheadedness, and other somatic complaints. **Rationale:** Improvement of somatic complaints may indicate increased oxygen levels in the plasma. Neuropsychometric tests are often performed before and after hyperbaric oxygen therapy.

Expected Outcomes

1. Wound healing: decrease in size, amount of drainage, and odor. Expect pink, healthy granulation tissue. **Rationale:** Hyperbaric oxygen promotes wound healing.
2. Normal oxygen blood levels after hyperbaric treatment for carbon monoxide, cyanide, and smoke exposure. Specifically expect improvement in ABGs, patient performance on standardized neuropsychometric tests, and patient somatic description (i.e., cessation of headache or fatigue). **Rationale:** Hyperbaric oxygen therapy restores adequate oxygen level in the tissue.
3. Elimination of air embolism. **Rationale:** Hyperbaric oxygen mechanically decreases bubble size and aids in the reabsorption of gas. It also aids in the recovery of ischemic tissues.

Unexpected Outcomes

1. Barotrauma (ears, lungs, teeth, sinus, gas-filled implant devices, etc.). **Rationale:** Volume changes of gas that accompany changes in pressure can result in adverse reactions unless appropriate precautions are taken and enforced consistently.
2. Oxygen toxicity. **Rationale:** Oxygen delivered at pressures greater than 1 ATA can have toxic effects.
3. Fire. **Rationale:** Oxygen under pressure increases the incidence for combustion.

Documentation

Documentation in the patient record should include date, time, and duration of hyperbaric oxygen therapy; assessment of wound; mobility of tympanic membrane; identified risk factors for pulmonary barotrauma and/or oxygen toxicity; assessment findings of respiratory system; safety precautions taken to reduce complications related to changing atmospheric pressures and/or injuries related to use of oxygen under pressure; elimination of toxins and/or the effects of air or gas emboli consistent with indication for use of therapy; and any unexpected outcomes and specific interventions taken. **Rationale:** Documents nursing interventions, efficacy of treatment, and expected/unexpected outcomes.

Patient/Family Education

1. Have the patient and family state their indications for hyperbaric oxygen and how hyperbaric oxygen is expected to affect the condition. **Rationale:** A realistic understanding of the treatment's effects will reduce anxiety and encourage compliance with expected participation.
2. Have the patient and family state the side effects and complications of treatment. **Rationale:** Stated side effects and complications reflect informed decision.
3. Teach patient how to clear ears (prevents tympanic membrane barotrauma), maintain normal breathing during decompression (prevents pulmonary barotrauma or air embolism), and notify the nurse of unusual sensations, "auras," or twitches (early signs of neurologic oxygen toxicity). **Rationale:** Informed patients can hopefully identify signs of early complications.
4. Determine if additional hyperbaric oxygen therapy should be continued. **Rationale:** Again, timely scheduling of activities and care will ensure delivery of services without interruption. Also, hyperbaric oxygen will have optimal effect when combined with other appropriate treatment modalities. Hyperbaric oxygen therapy may be a one-time treatment.

Performance Checklist
Skill 6–5:   Preparation for Hyperbaric Oxygen Therapy

Critical Behaviors	Complies yes	no
1. Wash hands.		
2. Take necessary precautions to protect patient from complications of changing atmospheric pressures:		
a. Replace air in endotracheal or tracheal tube cuff with sterile water.		
b. Replace glass bottles when possible; alert HBO team to their presence when unavoidable.		
c. Remove "hard" contact lenses.		
d. Remove/deflate (if possible) prosthetic implants using air.		
e. Remove air from all IV tubing.		
f. Connect tubes, drains, etc. to straight drainage system.		
3. Take necessary precautions to protect patient from injury related to use of oxygen under pressure:		
a. Remove petrolatum-based products (from head/neck for multiplace; from anywhere on body for monoplace).		
b. Remove cigarettes, lighters, matches, "gadgets" (mechanical, electrical, battery-operated).		
c. Send patients on appropriate stretcher (avoiding ones with fluorocarbon lubricant).		
4. Wash hands.		
5. Document procedure in the patient record.		

REFERENCES

American Edwards Laboratories (1987). *Understanding Continuous Mixed Venous Oxygen Saturation (S$\bar{v}$O$_2$) Monitoring with the Swan-Ganz Oximetry TD System.* Irvine, Calif.: American Edwards Laboratories, Baxter Healthcare Corporation.

Barrington, K. J., Finer, N. N., and Ryan, C. A. (1988). Evaluation of pulse oximetry as a continuous monitoring technique in the neonatal intensive care unit. *Crit. Care Med.* 16(11): 1147–1153.

Carlon, G. C., Ray, C., Jr., and Miodownik, S. (1988). Capnography in mechanically ventilated patients. *Crit. Care Med.* 16(5): 550–556.

Gilboy, N. S., and McGaffigan, P. A. (1989). Noninvasive monitoring of oxygenation with pulse oximetry. *J. Emerg. Nurs.* 15(1): 26–31.

Harbage Schroeder, C. (1988). Pulse oximetry: A nursing care plan. *Crit. Care Nurs.* 8(8): 1–12.

Kelleher, J. F., and Ruff, R. H. (1989). The penumbra effect: Vasomotion-dependent pulse oximeter artifact due to probe malposition. *Anesthesiology* 71(5): 787–791.

Lane, E. E., and Walker, J. F. (1987). *Clinical Arterial Blood Gas Analysis.* St. Louis: Mosby.

McCarthy, E. J. (1987). Ventilation–perfusion relationships. *J. Am. Assoc. Nurse Anesth.* 55(5): 437–440.

Paulus, D. A., and Monroe, M. C. (1989). Cool fingers and pulse oximetry (Letter). *Anesthesiology* 71(1): 168–169.

Petterson, M. T. (1990). Questions and answers on capnography. *Crit. Care Choices 90* 1: 12–17.

Reischman, R. R. (1988). Impaired gas exchange related to intrapulmonary shunting. *Crit. Care Nurs.* 8(8): 35–49.

Rubsamen, D. S. (1988). Hypoxic crises outside of the operating room. *Semin. Anesth.* 7(4): 307–314.

Schweiss, J. F. (1983). Introduction and Historical Perspective. In J. F. Schweiss (Ed.), *Continuous Measurement of Blood Oxygen Saturation in the High-Risk Patient,* Vol. 1 (pp. 1–12). San Diego: Beach International, Inc.

Scott, F. (1989). Nightmares can come true when circuits disconnect. *Adv. Respir. Ther.* 2(45): 1–2.

Shapiro, B. A., et al. (1982). *Clinical Application of Blood Gases,* 3d Ed. Chicago: Year Book.

Sharer, K., and Sladen, M. B. (1988). Ventilator Management by Pulse Oximetry and Capnometry after Cardiac Surgery. Paper presented at the 10th Annual Meeting of the Society of Cardiovascular Anesthesiologists, New Orleans.

Skoog, R. E. (1989). Capnography in the postanesthesia care unit. *J. Postanesth. Nurs.* 4(3): 147–155.

Stock, M. C. (1988). Noninvasive carbon dioxide monitoring. *Crit. Care Clin.* 4(3): 511–526.

Swedlow, D. B. (1986). Capnometry and capnography: The anesthesia disaster early warning system. *Semin. Anesth.* 3: 194–205.

Szaflarski, N. L., and Cohen, N. H. (1991). Use of capnography in critically ill adults. *Heart Lung* 20: 363–374.

Szaflarski, N. L., and Cohen, N. H. (1989). Use of pulse oximetry in critically ill adults. *Heart Lung* 18(5): 444–453.

Yamanaka, M. K., and Sue, D. Y. (1987). Comparison of arterial end-tidal PCO$_2$ difference and dead space/tidal volume ratio in respiratory failure. *Chest* 92(5): 832–835.

BIBLIOGRAPHY

Briones, T. L. (1988). S$\bar{v}$O$_2$ monitoring: I. Clinical case application. *Dimens. Crit. Care Nurs.* 7(2): 71–78.

Clark, A. P., et al. (1990). Effects of endotracheal suctioning on mixed venous oxygen saturation and heart rate. *Heart Lung* 19(2): 552–557.

Curley, M. D., et al. (1988). Neuropsychologic assessment of cerebral decompression sickness and gas embolism. *Undersea Biomed. Res.* 15: 223–236.

Daily, E. D. (1991). Hemodynamic Monitoring. In J. T. Dolan (Ed.), *Critical Care Nursing: Clinical Management Through the Nursing Process* (pp. 828–854). Philadelphia: F. A. Davis.

Davidson, L. J., and Brown, S. (1986). Continuous S$\bar{v}$O$_2$ monitoring:

A tool for analyzing hemodynamic status. *Heart Lung* 15(3): 287–291.

Davis, J. C., et al. (1988). Hyperbaric Medicine: Patient Selection, Treatment Procedures, and Side Effects. In J. C. Davis, T. K. Hunt (Eds.), *Problem Wounds: The Role of Oxygen* (pp. 225–235). New York: Elsevier.

Edell, E., and Cortese, D. (1989). Bronchoscope localization and treatment of occult lung cancer. *Chest* 96(4): 919–921.

Feaster, W. W., Jost, K. A., and Swedlow, D. B. (1988). *Capnography: A Quick Reference.* Hayward, Calif.: Nellcor, Inc.

Gardner, P. E., and Laurent-Bopp, D. (1987). Continuous $S\bar{v}O_2$ monitoring: Clinical application in critical care nursing. *Prog. Cardiovasc. Nurs.* 2: 9–18.

Gawlinski, A., and Henneman, E. A. (1990). Evaluating oxygen delivery and oxygen utilization with mixed venous oxygen saturation monitoring: A case study approach. *Heart Lung* 19(2): 566–570.

Gibson, A., and Davis, F. M. (1986). Hyperbaric oxygen therapy in the management of *Clostridium perfringens* infections. *N.Z. Med. J.* 99: 617–620.

Hadjimiltiades, S., et al. (1989). Coronary air embolism during coronary angioplasty. *Cathet. Cardiovasc. Diag.* 16: 164–167.

Hardy, G. R. (1988). $S\bar{v}O_2$ continuous monitoring techniques. *Dimens. Crit. Care Nurs.* 7(1): 8–17.

Hart, G. B., et al. (1987). Hyperbaric oxygen in exceptional acute blood-loss anemia. *J. Hyperbar. Med.* 2: 205–210.

Helmers, R., and Hunninghake, G. (1989). Bronchoalveolar lavage in the nonimmunocompromised patient. *Chest* 96(5): 1184–1189.

Jenkinson, S. G. (1988). Oxygen toxicity. *J. Intens. Care Med.* 3: 137–152.

Kacmarek, R., and Stoller, J. (Eds.) (1989). *Current Respiratory Care.* Philadelphia: B. C. Decker.

Mader, J. T., et al. (1987). Infectious diseases: Pathophysiology and mechanisms of hyperbaric oxygen. *J. Hyperbar. Med.* 2: 133–140.

Marx, R. E., and Johnson, R. P. (1988). Problem Wounds in Oral and Maxillofacial Surgery: The Role of Hyperbaric Oxygen. In J. C. Davis, and T. K. Hunt (Eds.), *Problem Wounds: The Role of Oxygen* (pp. 65–123). New York: Elsevier.

Mathieu, D., et al. (1985). Acute carbon monoxide poisoning: Risk of late sequelae and treatment by hyperbaric oxygen. *Clin. Toxicol.* 23: 315–324.

Measurement of Functional and Fractional Oxygen Saturation. (1987). Hayward, Calif.: Nellcor, Inc.

Mehta, A., Curtio, P., Scabzitti, A., and Meeker, D. (1990). The high price of bronchoscopy. *Chest* 98(2): 448–454.

Nelson, L. D. (1987). Mixed Venous Oximetry. In F. V. Snyder and M. R. Pinsky (Eds.), *Oxygen Transport in the Critically Ill* (pp. 235–247). Chicago: Year Book.

Pulse Oximetry Reference Note No. 3. (1987). *Potential errors in estimating oxygen saturation of hemaglobin from measurements of the partial pressure of oxygen.* Hayward, Calif.: Nellcor, Inc.

Simmons, D. (Ed.) (1990). *Current Pulmonology*, Vol. 11. Chicago: Year Book.

Stewart, F. M. (1988). $S\bar{v}O_2$ monitoring: II. Nursing research applications. *Dimens. Crit. Care Nurs.* 7(2): 79–82.

Trorrillet, J., Guiguet, M., Gibert, C., et al. (1990). Fiberoptic bronchoscopy in ventilated patients. *Chest* 97(4): 927–933.

Tyler, D. O., et al. (1990). Effects of a 1-minute back rub on mixed venous oxygen saturation and heart rate in critically ill patients. *Heart Lung* 19(2): 562–565.

White, K. (1987). Continuous Mixed Venous Oxygen Saturation. In G. O. Darovic (Ed.), *Hemodynamic Monitoring: Invasive and Noninvasive Clinical Application* (pp. 201–212). Philadelphia: Saunders.

White, K. M., et al. (1990). The physiologic basis for continuous mixed venous oxygen saturation monitoring. *Heart Lung* 19(2): 548–551.

Winslow, E. H., et al. (1990). Effects of a lateral turn on mixed venous oxygen saturation and heart rate in critically ill adults. *Heart Lung* 19(2): 557–561.

Wright, G., Matthay, M., and Matthay, R. (Eds.) (1990). *Chest Medicine: Essentials of Pulmonary and Critical Care Medicine*, 2d Ed. Baltimore: Williams and Wilkins.

UNIT II

THE CARDIOVASCULAR SYSTEM

7

ELECTRO-CARDIOGRAPHIC MONITORING

BEHAVIORAL OBJECTIVES

After completing this chapter, the nurse will be able to

- Define the key terms.
- Describe the proper lead placement for patient ECG monitoring.
- Identify the essential steps for placing a patient on a bedside ECG monitor.
- Demonstrate the procedure for obtaining a 12-lead ECG.
- Describe the setup for placing a patient on a telemetry ECG system.

Electrocardiography (commonly called *ECG*) is a display of the electric currents that are generated by the heart and are spread through the surrounding tissue to the surface of the body. Electrical impulses are picked up by the surface electrodes and are transported to and then recorded in the ECG. It is the shifting of electric charges that produces the changes in electrical voltage that can be measured and recorded at the body surface. The shifting of charges occurs with depolarization and repolarization, which is the electrical activation of the atria and ventricles. These are the major electrical events in the cardiac cycle. Thus, as an impulse travels down the specialized conduction pathway, various wave patterns or deflections are evidenced on a monitoring or recording device. These deflections have been labeled P, Q, R, S, and T waves. Electrocardiography can aid in the detection of myocardial ischemia, infarction, chamber enlargement, valve function, dysrhythmias, and conduction problems, as well as in the evaluation of the effects of electrolytes and drugs on the heart.

Continuous ECG monitoring systems include a bedside monitor (Fig. 7–1), patient cables (Fig. 7–2), lead wires (Fig. 7–3), and electrodes (Fig. 7–4). Continuous monitoring systems also include a central station (Fig. 7–5) that contains a computerized data bank. Continuous systems can be either hardwire or telemetry systems. Hardwire monitoring requires direct cable attachment from the bedside to the central station. Telemetry systems (Fig. 7–6) use radio signals to transmit information from the patient to the central station.

Diagnostic ECG monitoring equipment is comprised of the ECG recorder or monitor, cables, lead wires, and electrodes (Figs. 7–1 through 7–7). In order to obtain different views of the heart, 3 to 10 leads can be used. This equipment may be single- or multiple-channel. The single-channel monitor (Fig. 7–8) provides a recording of one lead or channel, whereas the multiple-channel monitor (Fig. 7–9) simultaneously records several leads or channels. Diagnostic electrocardiography includes the 12-lead ECG, the ambulatory ECG (or Holter monitor-

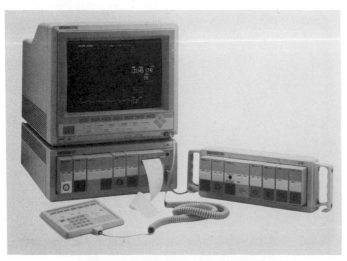

FIGURE 7–1. A bedside monitor. (Courtesy of Hewlett-Packard Company.)

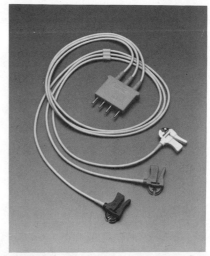

A

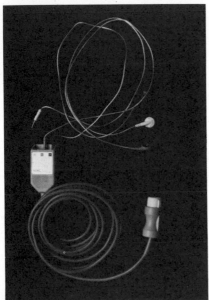

A

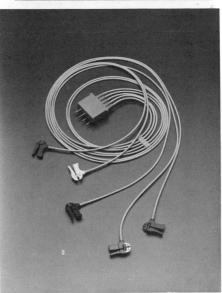

B

FIGURE 7–3. Types of lead wires: (*A*) three lead, (*B*) five lead. (Courtesy of Hewlett-Packard Company.)

ing), and exercise testing. In *echocardiography* ultrasound is added to single-lead ECG monitoring to examine cardiac structure.

Electrocardiography has provided the single most effective way to assess a patient's cardiac status. Monitoring requires interpretation and validation by nurses who are educated in dysrhythmia review. This chapter will focus on procedures used in ECG monitoring.

KEY TERMS

baseline	*lead placement*
bedside monitor	*lead selector*
central station	*lead wires*
depolarization	*midclavicular line*
electrode	*multichannel*
electrode gel	*patient cable*
frontal plane leads	*polarity*
hardwire	*recorder*
horizontal plane leads	*repolarization*
intercostal space	*single channel*
isoelectric line	*telemetry*

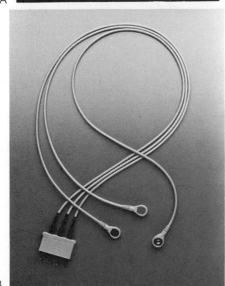

B

FIGURE 7–2. Types of patient cables: (*A*) with removable lead wires, (*B*) with permanent lead wires attached. (Courtesy of Hewlett-Packard Company.)

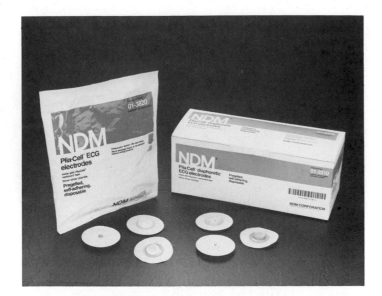

FIGURE 7–4. Electrodes used for bedside monitoring. (Courtesy of NDM Corporation.)

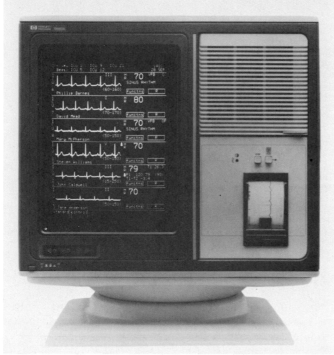

FIGURE 7–5. A central monitor. (Courtesy of Hewlett-Packard Company.)

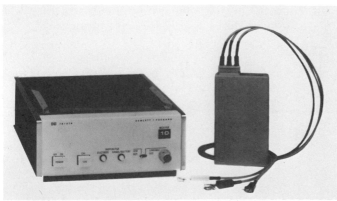

FIGURE 7–6. A telemetry system. (Courtesy of Hewlett-Packard Company.)

SKILLS

GUIDELINES

The following assessment guidelines will assist the nurse in identifying a plan of care for the patient requiring noninvasive cardiac monitoring:

1. Know the patient's pertinent medical and social history.

2. Know the patient's baseline cardiovascular assessment and follow up.

3. Determine appropriate intervention(s) for the assessed finding.

4. Become skillful using noninvasive cardiac monitoring equipment.

SKILL 7–1

Electrophysiologic Monitoring: Hardwire and Telemetry

In placing a patient on a bedside monitor, there are several lead systems that a nurse may use. It is essential for the nurse to understand the basics of lead placement in order to obtain the most accurate and appropriate information from the monitoring system. No matter which lead system is selected, electrodes should always be positioned so that they will not interfere with the care of the patient in an emergency situation.

Continuous hardwire monitoring systems use a single-channel lead to record electrical activity of the heart. The electrical activity is recorded by means of electrodes placed on specific areas of the chest that are attached to lead wires. The electrodes and lead wires transmit the electrical energy from the patient to the monitor. The two major factors that determine the contour of the ECG

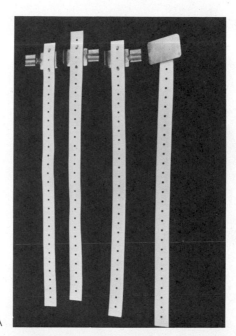

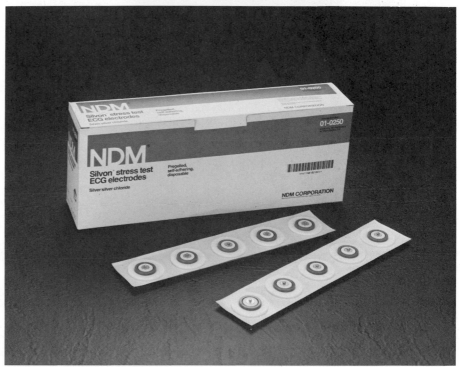

FIGURE 7–7. Electrodes used for 12-lead ECG: (*A*) plate electrodes, (*B*) disposable electrodes. (Courtesy of NDM Corporation.)

deflection on the monitor are the location of the electrodes on the body and the direction of the cardiac impulse in relation to the position of the electrode.

Lead placement in the three-lead, single-channel monitoring system requires that one of the leads is positive, one is negative, and the third is a ground. In the multiple channel systems, a five-lead placement setup is used. These wires and connections are generally coded in some way, such as by letters (RA, LL, or LA), symbols (+ or −), or colors (Fig. 7–10), so that the nurse can quickly tell the polarity of the wires.

Electrical energy flowing toward the positive electrode will be reflected on the ECG recording by a positive deflection from the isoelectric line (above the line). Energy that is directed away from the positive electrode will be seen as a negative deflection from the isoelectric line (below the line). Since placement of the leads will alter the ECG picture, the nurse must be aware of what lead is displayed in order to make appropriate judgments of cardiac rhythm.

The conventional monitoring leads that can be used are lead II and lead III. Modified chest leads MCL[1] and MCL[6] also may be selected to provide more specific information regarding dysrhythmias, bundle-branch blocks, ventricular aberration, and premature ventricular beats. These leads are modifications of leads V_1 and V_6, re-

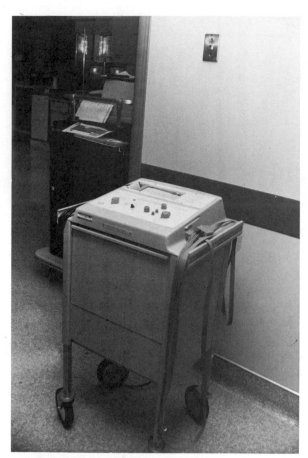

FIGURE 7–8.   A single-channel ECG machine.

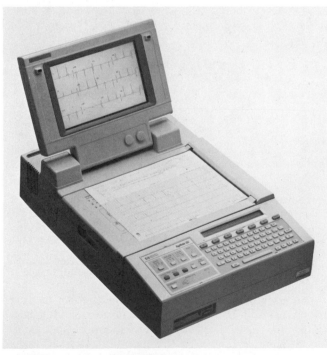

FIGURE 7–9.   A multiple-channel ECG recorder. (Courtesy of Hewlett-Packard Company.)

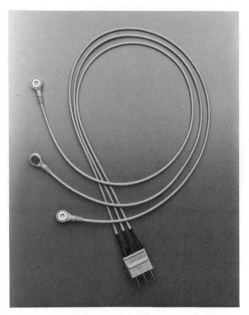

FIGURE 7–10.   Lead wires with coding (LA = −, LL = Ref, and RA = +). (Courtesy of Hewlett-Packard Company.)

spectively. A Lewis lead may be used if there is particular concern for visualization of the P waves. The lead that provides the most information regarding patient status is the best lead to monitor.

Many monitoring systems currently on the market use a lead-selector switch. This switch allows for selection of an alternate lead by simply turning a switch. This affords the nurse a quick and simple way of visualizing multiple leads without moving the leads on the chest. Some monitoring systems provide a mode for extended and diagnostic monitoring. When using such a system, three to five leads may be required. The five-lead system provides the availability of switching to multiple leads and giving a clearer and more definitive picture of the patient with regard to diagnosing specific disorders and problems of conduction.

Telemetry monitoring allows for the continuous monitoring of an ambulatory patient. It is done with a lead-to-transmitter system rather than a hardwire attachment. One advantage of this system is that the patient is not restricted by wires. Another advantage is that it will provide monitoring of the patient's tolerance to activity. As progressive ambulation is initiated, the telemetry monitor can be used to evaluate the cardiac rhythm and any dysrhythmias precipitated by activity or exercise. The equipment needed for telemetry includes electrodes (from two to five lead wires) connected to a small battery-operated radio transmitter. This transmitter relays the electrical heart pattern via radio waves to a receiver, which then forwards the information to the central station.

The disadvantage of telemetry systems is that the quality of the ECG is generally not as good as with hardwire monitoring. Distortion occurs from electrical equipment or physical structures within the hospital. There may be limitations on the distance that a patient can go and still give a good signal in the central station. Acceptable distances will vary with the manufacturer and limitations of the equipment. Most telemetry systems allow for the monitoring of only one lead. This can be a disadvantage as more views of the heart's electrical activity provide more diagnostic information. Despite these disadvantages, telemetry is a useful tool in evaluating patient status.

Purpose

The nurse places a patient on an electrocardiographic monitor to

1. Provide a continuous picture of the patient's cardiac electrical activity.
2. Record cardiac electrical activity for diagnostic or documentation purposes.
3. Anticipate and treat various dysrhythmias.

Prerequisite Knowledge and Skills

Prior to placing a patient on an ECG monitor, the nurse should understand

1. Principles of electrophysiology and dysrhythmia interpretation.
2. Anatomy of the thorax and cardiac system.
3. Principles of transthoracic resistance.
4. Principles of electrical safety (see Skill 36–1).

The nurse should be able to perform

1. Proper handwashing technique (see Skill 35–5).
2. Cardiovascular physical assessment.
3. Interpretation of dysrhythmias.
4. Basic Cardiac Life Support (BCLS).

Assessment

1. Assess for the signs and symptoms of alterations in cardiac status, including peripheral pulses, vital signs, heart sounds, level of consciousness, breath sounds, neck vein distension, complaint of chest pain or palpitations, and peripheral circulatory disorders (i.e., clubbing, cyanosis, and dependent edema). **Rationale:** Physical signs and symptoms will result from alterations in the performance of the cardiovascular system.
2. Interpret the monitor recording for rhythm, rate, presence and configuration of P waves, length of PR interval, length of QRS complex, presence and configuration of T waves, length of QT interval, presence of extra waves (such as U waves), and presence of dysrhythmias. **Rationale:** Reviews the normal conduction sequence and identifies abnormalities that may require further evaluation or treatment.

Nursing Diagnoses

1. Alteration in cardiac tissue perfusion related to reduction in blood supply to the coronary arteries secondary to spasm or occlusion of the coronary arteries. **Rationale:** Any reduction in blood supply to the myocardium will result in a decreased myocardial tissue perfusion.
2. Decreased cardiac output related to poor mechanical function of the myocardium. **Rationale:** Poor mechanical function results in decreased cardiac output and peripheral perfusion.

Planning

1. Individualize the following goals for a patient undergoing ECG monitoring.
   a. Maintain an ECG recording with a clear QRS complex, a crisp P wave, and a stable, clear baseline without artifact or distortion. **Rationale:** A clear tracing without distortion is necessary so that judgments can be made using reliable information.
   b. Record serial changes in cardiac activity. **Rationale:** Promptly treats serious dysrhythmias.
2. Prepare all necessary equipment and supplies. **Rationale:** Place the patient quickly and efficiently on the monitor so that immediate changes in the patient's cardiac rhythm can be seen immediately.
   a. ECG monitor (central and bedside monitor).
   b. Electrodes, pregelled, disposable.
   c. Gauze pads or terry cloth washcloth.
   d. Alcohol pads.
   e. Lead wires (no longer than 18 in in length).
   f. Patient cable (should adapt to monitor and lead wires).
   g. Tincture of benzoin or similar preparation, if needed.
   h. Basin and soap with shaver, if needed.
   i. Pouch or pocket gown to hold telemetry unit (for telemetry monitoring only).
3. Prepare the patient for placement on the monitor.
   a. Explain the procedure, including use of bedside and central monitoring systems. **Rationale:** Aids in reducing anxiety and ensures the patient's cooperation. This procedure is commonly done, but it may be new to the patient. Patients need to understand that there is constant viewing of the ECG picture and that any problems will be immediately acted on. Information will help allay some patients' fears.
   b. Explain actions that can make the system inoperative or set off the alarms: wire disconnect, lead displacement, excessive patient movement, and faulty connections. **Rationale:** Helps to allay fears related to use of the equipment.
   c. Emphasize that the patient should feel free to move about in bed. **Rationale:** This will encourage movement on the part of the patient and allay fears concerning disruption of the monitoring system.
   d. Explain the importance of reporting any chest discomfort or pain. **Rationale:** Ensures appropriate and timely interventions.

Implementation

Steps	Rationale	Special Considerations
1. Wash hands.	Reduces transmission of microorganisms.	
2. Turn on computerized central monitoring system.	Once activated, system will alarm to notify nurse of problems with the ECG for interpretation and attention.	Nurse must verify patterns, evaluate computer interpretations, and assess the patient to confirm findings.
3. For telemetry monitoring, insert battery into telemetry unit, matching polarity markings on transmitter.	Batteries can fail if left sitting on the shelf or in the unit. Polarity must match for proper functioning of the unit.	Manufacturers will provide recommendations on battery storage and replacement.
4. Plug monitor into grounded ac wall outlet (see Skill 36–1).	Maintains electrical safety.	
5. Turn bedside monitor on.	Equipment generally requires warmup time.	Follow manufacturer's recommendation.
6. Check cable and lead wires for fraying, broken wires, or discoloration.	Detects conditions that will give inaccurate ECG trace.	Safety must be maintained. If equipment is damaged, obtain alternative equipment and notify biomedical engineer for repair (see Skill 36–1).
7. Plug patient cable into monitor.	Hardwire systems require direct connections.	
8. Plug lead wires into patient cable, and check for secure fit. Negative wire into opening marked N, −, or RA; positive wire into opening marked P, +, LL, or LA; and ground lead into opening marked G, Neutral, or RL.	Reduces chance of disconnection, distortion, or outside interference with ECG tracing.	Manufacturers will code the lead connections so that correct attachment can be made. Often these are color coded, but they may be letter or symbol coded (see Fig. 7–10).
9. Connect electrodes to lead wires.	Placing electrodes on the chest and then attaching the lead wires can be uncomfortable for the patient and can allow air bubbles into gel, which can decrease conduction.	
10. Choose lead site.	Choice is based on constraints on chest-wall space and type of information required.	
11. Identify the sternal notch or Angle of Louis.	Palpate the upper sternum to identify where the clavicles join the sternum (suprasternal notch), then slide fingers down the center of the sternum to the obvious bony prominence. This is the sternal notch, which identifies the second rib and provides the landmark for noting the fourth ICS.	The sternal notch identifies the second rib and thereby assists in locating fourth ICS.
12. Lead sites for hardwire system: MCL[1] (Fig. 7–11).	Apply negative electrode to left midclavicular line, below clavicle. Apply positive electrode at fourth ICS, right border. Apply ground electrode inferior to right clavicle, midclavicular line.	Excellent lead for identifying bundle-branch blocks and ectopy vs. aberrancy. It produces variable P-wave polarity and a negative QRS complex. The ground lead can be placed anywhere on the chest. The location demonstrated in Fig. 7–11 is a frequent one.

Table continues on following page

Steps	Rationale	Special Considerations
MCL[6] (Fig. 7–12).	Apply negative electrode inferior to the left clavicle, midclavicular line. Apply positive electrode at fifth ICS, left midaxillary line. Apply ground electrode inferior to right clavicle, midclavicular line.	Used in telemetry and median sternotomies. It produces a tall QRS complex, so that a left ventricular ectopy and right bundle-branch block can be identified.
Lead II (Fig. 7–13).	Apply negative electrode right shoulder, close to the junction of the right arm with torso. Positive electrode should be placed well below the heart in the left abdominal region at approximately the level of the umbilicus. Apply ground electrode to the left shoulder close to the junction of the left arm with the torso.	Complexes in this lead are upright, and the P wave is positive. Can be used to see QRS changes in left anterior hemiblock. The electrodes should be placed close to the limb-torso junction to achieve as close as possible the 12-lead electrode placement. This also gets electrodes out of the way for defibrillation auscultation, CPR, etc.
Lead III (Fig. 7–14).	Apply negative electrode inferior to the left clavicle midclavicular line. Apply positive electrode below the heart on the left abdomen at approximately the level of the umbilicus. Apply ground electrode inferior to right clavicle, midclavicular line.	Provides another lead in which the complexes are positive.
Lewis lead (Fig. 7–15).	Apply negative electrode at first ICS right sternal border. Apply positive electrode to fourth ICS, right sternal border. Apply ground electrode to fourth ICS, left sternal border.	This lead system offers the best visualization of P waves.
Five-lead system (Fig. 7–16).	Apply RA electrode to the right shoulder close to the junction of the right arm and torso. Apply LA electrode to left shoulder close to the junction of the left arm and torso.	This lead system offers the rapid ECG monitoring from selected sites and can give a clearer recording. It does not replace a 12-lead ECG.

Table continues on following page

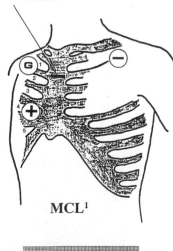

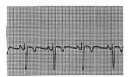

FIGURE 7–11. MCL[1] lead placement and sample strip.

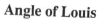

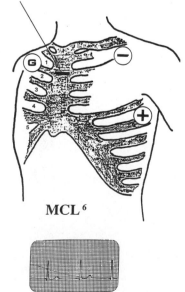

FIGURE 7–12. MCL[6] lead placement and sample strip.

Angle of Louis

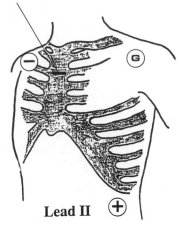

Lead II

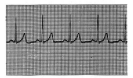

FIGURE 7–13.   Lead II lead placement and sample strip.

Angle of Louis

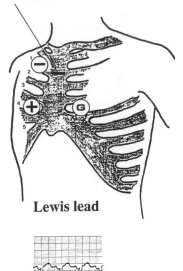

Lewis lead

FIGURE 7–15.   Lewis lead placement and sample strip.

Angle of Louis

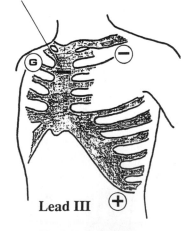

Lead III

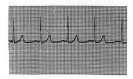

FIGURE 7–14.   Lead III lead placement and sample strip.

Angle of Louis

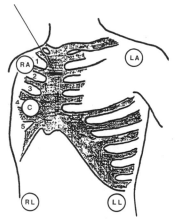

A   Five lead system

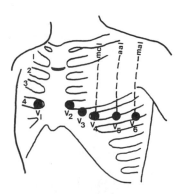

B   Precordial lead placement

FIGURE 7–16.   (A) Five-lead system lead placement. (B) Precordial lead placement.

Steps	Rationale	Special Considerations
	Apply RL electrode well below the heart in the right abdominal region approximately on the level of the umbilicus. Apply LL electrode well below the heart in the left abdominal region approximately on the level of the umbilicus. Apply the chest lead electrode on the selected site: V_1, V_2, V_3, V_4, V_5, or V_6. Set lead selector switch to appropriate lead.	Only one precordial lead can be displayed—placement of the electrode identifies the lead used.
For telemetry monitoring, two-lead system, lead II (Fig. 7–17).	Apply negative electrode to first ICS, right sternal border. Apply positive electrode to fourth ICS, left midclavicular line.	Manufacturer will recommend use of two leads.
Two-lead sites system: MCL^1 (Fig. 7–18).	Apply negative electrode left midclavicular line below clavicle. Apply positive electrode to fourth ICS, right sternal border.	
13. Prepare the skin by cleaning the area for application of leads. This can be done with soap and water, but it may require alcohol pads.	Provides for adequate transmission of electrical impulses.	Alcohol may be needed to remove oils, which can interfere with the transmission of impulses.
14. Thoroughly dry the skin.	Moist skin will not allow a surface conducive to electrode adherence.	Diaphorectic patients may require use of skin preparation solution such as tincture of benzoin.
15. Abrade skin using a washcloth, scratch pad on electrode pack, or gauze pad.	Removes dead skin cells which interfere with transmission.	
16. Shave area if needed.	Hair can interfere with conduction and is uncomfortable.	4×4 area for each electrode.
17. Remove backing from the pregelled electrode and test the center of the pad for moistness.	Gel can dry out in storage.	Gel must be moist to allow for good conduction. If not moist add gel or replace electrode.
18. Apply electrode to site assuring a seal.	Electrode must be placed tightly to prevent external influences from affecting the ECG.	

Table continues on following page

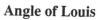
Angle of Louis

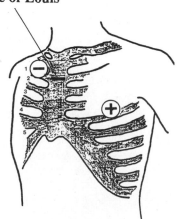

FIGURE 7–17. Lead II lead placement in two-lead system.

Angle of Louis

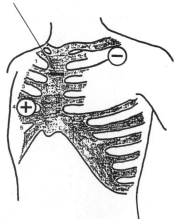

FIGURE 7–18. MCL^1 lead placement in two-lead system.

Steps	Rationale	Special Considerations
19. For hardwire monitoring, fasten lead-wire receptacle in patient cable to patient's gown.	Decreases tension on lead wires to alleviate undue stress, causing interference or faulty recordings. Minimizes pulling on electrodes, which can be uncomfortable for the patient.	
20. For telemetry monitoring, secure the transmitter in pouch or pocket in patient's gown.	Decreases tension on lead wires to alleviate undue stress, causing interference or faulty recordings. Minimizes pulling on electrodes, which can be uncomfortable for the patient. Transmitter must be secure so that it will not be dropped or damaged.	
21. Examine the ECG tracing on the monitor for size of R wave.	The R wave should be approximately twice the height of the other components of the ECG to ensure proper triggering of the machine.	Manufacturers provide for calibration of the ECG to 1 mV, and monitors have a gain control that can be used to adjust the size of the ECG.
22. Set alarms. Upper and lower alarm limits are set within 20% of patient's heart rate.	Activates the bedside or telemetry monitor system.	Monitoring systems allow for setting alarms at bedside or central console. Types of alarms may include rate (high or low), abnormal rhythms or complexes, pacer recognition, and others depending on the manufacturer. *Caution:* Turning off bedside alarms is not recommended.
23. Wash hands.	Reduces transmission of microorganisms.	

Evaluation

1. Evaluate the monitor pattern for the presence of P waves, QRS complex, a clear baseline, and an absence of artifact or distortion. **Rationale:** A clear pattern is required to make accurate judgments about the patient's status and treatment.

2. Evaluate the ECG pattern continually for dysrhythmias, assess patient tolerance of the problem, and provide prompt nursing intervention. **Rationale:** Changes in the ECG pattern can indicate significant problems for the patient and may require prompt intervention.

3. Evaluate skin integrity on a daily basis, and change electrodes as directed by the manufacturer. Rotate sites when changing electrodes. Monitor skin for any allergic reactions to the adhesive or the gel. **Rationale:** Skin integrity must be maintained in order to have a clear picture of the patient's ECG.

4. Monitor the patient for microshock (see Skill 36–1), particularly in patients having invasive lines. **Rationale:** Causes discomfort and interferes with monitoring.

Expected Outcomes

1. A clear monitor tracing is displayed (Fig. 7–19). **Rationale:** A pattern free of distortion provides a reliable picture for clinical decision-making.

2. Prompt identification and treatment of dysrhythmias. **Rationale:** Allows a constant evaluation of the patient's ECG for rapid treatment as needed.

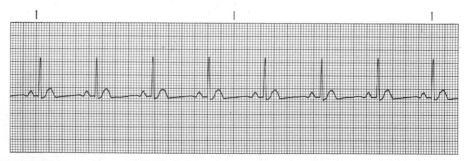

FIGURE 7–19. Clear monitor strip—lead II.

Unexpected Outcomes

1. Altered skin integrity. **Rationale:** Adhesives and electrode gels can irritate the skin.

2. Alternating-current (ac) interference, also called 60-cycle interference (Fig. 7–20). **Rationale:** Frayed wires, bad connections, improper grounding, loose electrodes, or stress on the patient cable may be the cause.

3. Wandering baseline (Fig. 7–21). **Rationale:** Due to patient movement, improper placement of electrodes, or respiratory efforts if cyclical in nature.

4. False alarms. **Rationale:** Improper gain control when the monitor detects the waves as too tall or too small, improper lead placement, and loose leads.

5. Artifact or waveform interference (Fig. 7–22). **Rationale:** Patient movement is the primary cause and may be related to problems requiring treatment, such as chills or seizures. Leads may not be attached properly or gel may not be providing effective conductivity.

6. Microshock. **Rationale:** Improperly grounded system increases patients' risk for uncomfortable sensations and potential dysrhythmia development.

Documentation

Documentation in the patient record should include an initial or baseline strip, noting the lead, interpretation, any dysrhythmias and treatments; routine strips according to the hospital's protocol, which may be every 2, 4, or 8 hours; and a monitor strip whenever there is a change in the patient's rhythm, vital signs, or mental status; the patient experiences chest pain; there is a change in lead placement; and/or when evaluating the effect of anti-dysrhythmic agents. **Rationale:** A baseline strip provides reference for future evaluations. Routine assessment of the cardiac rhythm. Monitoring when there are changes or problems may aid in the diagnosis of problems, assist in identifying the appropriate treatments, and evaluate the effects of such treatments.

Patient/Family Education

1. Assess the readiness of the patient and family to learn. **Rationale:** Anxiety and concerns the patient and family may have inhibit their ability to learn.

2. Provide explanations of the equipment and alarms to both patient and family. **Rationale:** Assists in making them feel more comfortable with monitoring and reduces anxiety.

3. Reassure the patient and family that the monitor is constantly being reviewed and that any alterations or problems will be quickly treated. **Rationale:** Reassures patient that immediate care is available.

4. Evaluate the patient's need for follow-up of any cardiac problems that are identified. **Rationale:** Provides the nurse with anticipatory planning to facilitate the patient's discharge from the hospital.

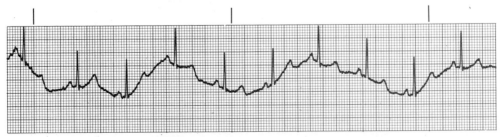

FIGURE 7–20. 60-cycle interference—lead II.

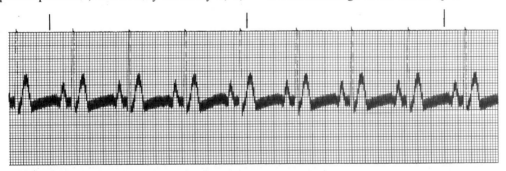

FIGURE 7–21. Wandering baseline—lead II.

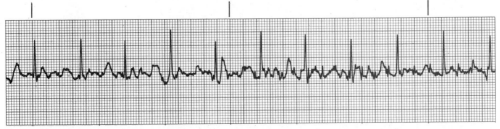

FIGURE 7–22. Artifact—lead II.

Performance Checklist
Skill 7–1:   Electrophysiologic Monitoring: Hardwire and Telemetry

Critical Behaviors	Complies	
	yes	no
1. Wash hands.		
2. Turn on computerized central monitoring system.		
3. For telemetry, insert battery into unit with proper polarity.		
4. Plug in monitor.		
5. Turn bedside monitor on.		
6. Check cables and lead wires for problems.		
7. For hardwire system, plug in patient cable.		
8. Attach lead wires to correct connections.		
9. Attach electrodes to lead wires.		
10. Choose appropriate lead site, identifying sternal notch or Angle of Louis and lead placement according to system chosen.		
11. Prepare skin using appropriate technique.		
12. Dry skin thoroughly.		
13. Abrade skin.		
14. Shave skin, if needed.		
15. Test electrode for moist gel.		
16. Apply electrodes to chest wall.		
17. Secure wires (when using hardwire unit) or secure unit in pouch pocket (when using telemetry) to reduce tension and pull.		
18. Ensure clear tracing.		
19. Set alarm.		
20. Wash hands.		
21. Document procedure in patient record.		

SKILL 7–2

Twelve-Lead Electrocardiogram

The most frequently used procedure for evaluating cardiac status is the 12-lead electrocardiogram (ECG). This tool is used primarily for identifying the presence and location of a myocardial infarction, information about the function of the conduction system, the size of the cardiac chambers, dysrhythmias, and effects of electrolytes and drugs on the heart.

The 12-lead ECG is most helpful because it gives 12 different views of the heart's electrical activity. The leads are the standard limb leads (I, II, III), the augmented limb leads (aV_R, aV_L, aV_F), and the six chest leads (V_1 to V_6). The standard and augmented leads view the heart from the vertical or frontal plane (Fig. 7–23), and the chest leads view it from the horizontal plane (Fig. 7–24).

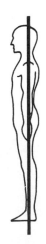

FIGURE 7–23.   Frontal plane leads—I, II, III, aV_R, aV_L, aV_F.

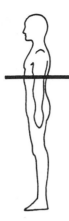

FIGURE 7–24. Horizontal plane leads—V₁ to V₆.

The machine measures the electrical potential between the leads and then amplifies and transmits it in a graphic display form to a strip-chart recorder. The graphic display consists of the P, Q, R, S, and T waves, which represent the electrical activity within the heart.

Purpose

The nurse performs a 12-lead ECG to

1. Provide information about the electrical system of the heart from 12 different views.
2. Record cardiac electrical activity for diagnostic or documentary reasons.
3. Diagnose a myocardial infarction.
4. Differentiate and identify dysrhythmias.
5. Determine effects of drugs and/or electrolytes on the heart's electrical system.

Prerequisite Knowledge and Skills

Prior to performing a 12-lead ECG, the nurse should understand

1. Principles of electrophysiology and dysrhythmia interpretation.
2. Anatomy of the thorax and cardiac system.
3. Principles of transthoracic resistance.
4. Principles of electrical safety (see Skill 36–1).

The nurse should be able to perform

1. Proper handwashing technique (see Skill 35–5).
2. Cardiovascular physical assessment.
3. Interpretation of dysrhythmias.
4. Basic Cardiac Life Support (BCLS).

Assessment

1. Assess for the signs and symptoms of an alteration in cardiac status, including peripheral pulses, vital signs, heart sounds, level of consciousness, breath sounds, neck vein distension, complaint of chest pain or palpitations, and peripheral circulatory disorders (i.e., clubbing, cy-

anosis, and dependent edema). **Rationale:** Physical signs and symptoms will result from alterations in performance of the cardiovascular system.

2. Interpret the recording for rhythm, rate, presence and configuration of P waves, length of PR interval, length of QRS complex, presence and configuration of T waves, length of QT interval, presence of extra waves (such as U waves), and identification of dysrhythmias. **Rationale:** Reviews the normal conduction sequence and identifies abnormalities that may require further evaluation or treatment.

3. Evaluate ECG for any signs of ischemia, injury, infarct, bundle-branch block, axis deviation, or hypertrophy. **Rationale:** Identifies pathophysiologic processes that may require further evaluation or treatment.

Nursing Diagnoses

1. Alteration in cardiac tissue perfusion related to reduction in blood supply to the coronary arteries secondary to spasm or occlusion of the coronary arteries. **Rationale:** Any reduction in blood supply to the myocardium from spasm or occlusion of the coronary artery will result in a decreased tissue perfusion to the myocardial tissue and cause dysrhythmias.

2. Decreased cardiac output related to poor mechanical function of the myocardium. **Rationale:** Poor mechanical function will result in decreased cardiac output and peripheral perfusion that can cause alterations in cellular function and produce dysrhythmias.

Planning

Individualize the following goal for a patient undergoing a 12-lead ECG:

1. Obtain a 12-lead ECG recording with clear waveforms, a stable baseline, and without artifact or distortion. **Rationale:** The pattern must be clear and without distortion so that judgments can be made using reliable information.
2. Prepare all necessary equipment and supplies. **Rationale:** Place the patient quickly and efficiently on the 12-lead ECG machine so that a comprehensive evaluation of the cardiac rhythm can be completed.
   a. 12-lead ECG recorder.
   b. Electrodes, pregelled, disposable, or electrode plates with straps.
   c. Gauze pads or terry cloth washcloth.
   d. Alcohol pads.
   e. Patient cable (should have from 5 to 10 lead wires).
   f. Skin prep, tincture of benzoin or similar preparation, if needed.
   g. Basin and soap with shaver, if needed.

3. Prepare the patient for the 12-lead ECG.
   a. Explain the procedure to the patient. **Rationale:** Aids in the reduction of anxiety and ensures cooperation from the patient.

b. Describe the procedure to the patient and explain actions that make the ECG difficult to read, such as wire disconnect, displacement of leads, and patient movement. **Rationale:** Identify that there are leads placed on the arms, legs and chest wall. Assure patient that there is no discomfort in the procedure and that the leads will be removed as soon as possible.

c. Emphasize that the patient should not talk, should relax, lie still, and breathe normally. **Rationale:** Sound and chest movement can distort the ECG picture. Allaying fears speeds up the procedure and ensures cooperation.

Implementation

Steps	Rationale	Special Considerations
1. Wash hands.	Reduces transmission of microorganisms.	
2. Plug ECG machine into grounded ac wall outlet (see Skill 36–1).	Maintains electrical safety.	
3. Turn recorder on.	Equipment generally requires warmup time.	Follow manufacturer's recommendation.
4. Set the lead selector to standby.	Standby mode allows warmup without running out paper or strips.	
5. Check cable and lead wires for fraying, broken wires, or discoloration.	Standby mode allows warmup without running out paper or strips. Detects conditions that will give an inaccurate ECG trace.	Safety must be maintained. If equipment is damaged, obtain alternative equipment and notify biomedical engineer for repair (see Skill 36–1).
6. Check coding on lead wires.	Lead wires must be correctly placed for accurate trace.	Manufacturers use color or symbol coding for placement of leads (i.e., RA = right arm, LL = left leg, etc.) (see Fig. 7–10).
7. Position the patient in supine position, not touching the bedrails or foot board.	Provides adequate support for limbs so that muscle activity will be minimal. Touching the bedrails or foot board may increase the chance of distortion of the trace.	Supine position is best, but Fowler's or others may be used for comfort.
8. Expose only the necessary parts of the patient's legs, arms, and chest.	Provides warmth, which reduces shivering.	Shivering may interfere with the recording.
9. Identify lead sites: Limb leads (Fig. 7–25).	Promotes correct positioning of limb leads. Ensures an accurate tracing of the heart from a view in the vertical and frontal plane.	Limb leads should be placed in "fleshy" areas and avoid bony prominences. The limb leads need to be placed equidistant from the heart and should be positioned in approximately the same place on each limb.

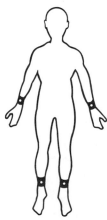

FIGURE 7–25. Limb lead placement in 12-lead ECG.

Table continues on following page

Steps	Rationale	Special Considerations
Chest leads (see Fig. 7–16B). Chest leads are placed using anatomical landmarks. Identify the Angle of Louis or sternal notch (review Skill 7–1).	Angle of Louis or sternal notch will assist with identifying the second rib for correct placement of precordial leads in appropriate ICS.	
V_1: fourth intercostal space right sternal border. V_2: fourth intercostal space left sternal border. V_3: equidistant between V_2 and V_4. V_4: fifth intercostal space at the midclavicular line. V_5: horizontal level to V_4 at the anterior axillary line. V_6: horizontal level to V_4 at the midaxillary line.	Ensures an accurate electrical tracing of the heart from a view in the horizontal plane.	
10. Cleanse the sites for electrode placement.	Adequate preparation assures a good tracing. Use soap and water to clean the skin, but alcohol pads may be needed.	Alcohol may remove oils and fat on the skin that can cause a poor trace.
11. Abrade skin using a washcloth, or gauze pad.	Removes dead skin cells which interfere with conduction and improves tracing.	
12. Shave area if needed.	Hair can interfere with conduction.	2×2 area for each electrode.
13. For pregelled-type electrodes, remove backing and test for moistness. For adhesive-type electrodes, remove backing and check the sticky, adhesive pad—it should not be moist; or prepare strap leads and chest sites by applying a small amount electrode gel or gel pads.	Allows for appropriate conduction of impulses.	Gel must be moist. If pregelled electrodes are not moist, add gel or replace electrode.
14. Apply limb electrodes securely.	Electrode must be secure and tight to prevent external influences from affecting the ECG.	Care must be taken not to overtighten straps to prevent circulatory impairment and onset of muscle spasms, which will affect tracing.
15. Fasten lead wires to limb electrodes, avoiding bending or strain on wires, and use correct lead-to-electrode connection.	Provides for correct identification of leads for accurate interpretation.	
16. Identify single- or multiple-channel machine (see Figs. 7–8 and 7–9, respectively).	Single-channel machines run one lead at a time. Multiple-channel machines will run three or more leads simultaneously.	
17. Check the settings on the ECG machine: paper speed, 25 mm/s; sensitivity, 1 or 10 mm/s; baseline at center.	Ensures an accurate trace within standard limits for proper interpretation.	Manufacturers have provided a calibration check in the machine to identify the sensitivity setting. Some machines have automatic settings that do this. If automatic calibration is not done, the nurse must calibrate the ECG at the beginning of each lead.
18. Turn the switch that begins moving the paper. Record each limb lead for 3 to 6 seconds.	ECG must be accurately marked, have a clear baseline, and absence of artifact for correct interpretation. Three to 6 seconds is all that is needed for permanent record; more may be obtained on a rhythm strip. A rhythm strip is a long lead II.	Modern systems automatically mark on the tracing strip the proper dot and dash code.

Table continues on following page

Steps	Rationale	Special Considerations
19. Record the chest leads as above. *Note:* A multiple-channel machine may run the limb and chest leads simultaneously.	The chest leads may require movement of the lead across the chest or may be set up and done with an automatic machine.	Respiratory artifact can be common in doing the chest leads and may require position changes in the stylus to ensure a good baseline. If sequential ECGs are to be obtained, chest lead sites should be marked to ensure the same lead sites will be used in the following ECG.
20. Assess the quality of the tracing.	While the patient is still hooked up to the machine, the nurse should examine the ECG to see if any leads need to be repeated.	
21. Disconnect the equipment, and clean the gel off the patient and prepare the equipment for future use.	Increases patient comfort.	
22. Wash hands.	Reduces transmission of microorganisms.	

Evaluation

Evaluate the ECG for accuracy of lead placement and any changes from previous ECGs, such as dysrhythmias, signs of ischemia, injury, or infarct, etc. **Rationale:** If the position of the limb leads is reversed, the complexes in Lead I will primarily demonstrate a negative deflection on the tracing instead of upright deflection (Fig. 7–26 A and B). If chest leads are placed below the fifth intercostal space, the horizontal plane lead may be transposed into a frontal plane lead. Changes in the ECG pattern can indicate significant problems for the patient and may require prompt intervention.

Expected Outcomes

1. A clear 12-lead recording will be obtained (Fig. 7–27). **Rationale:** A pattern free from distortion will provide a reliable picture for clinical decision-making.

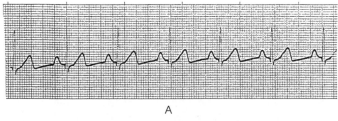

A

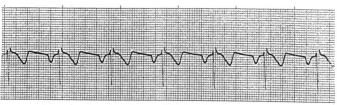

B

FIGURE 7–26. **Limb lead reversal on 12-lead ECG in lead I:** (*A*) **with correct placement,** (*B*) **with incorrect placement.**

2. Prompt identification and treatment of dysrhythmias and myocardial ischemia and infarction. **Rationale:** Provides a comprehensive picture of the electrical activity of the heart thus ensuring accurate diagnosis and rapid treatment.

Unexpected Outcomes

1. Altered skin integrity. **Rationale:** Adhesives and electrode gels can be irritating to the skin.
2. Alternating-current (ac) interference, also called 60-cycle interference (see Fig. 7–20). **Rationale:** Frayed wires, bad connections, improper grounding, loose electrodes, or stress on the patient cable may be the cause.
3. Wandering baseline (see Fig. 7–21). **Rationale:** Patient movement, improper placement of electrodes, or respiratory efforts if it is cyclical in nature may be the cause of this problem.
4. Artifact or waveform interference. **Rationale:** Patient movement is the primary cause and may be related to problems requiring treatment, such as chills or seizures. Leads may not be attached properly or gel may not be providing effective conductivity.

Documentation

Documentation in the patient record should include the fact that a 12-lead ECG was obtained; the reason for the test; any symptoms that the patient experienced, such as chest pain or palpitations; any follow up to the ECG, if indicated; and any 12-lead ECG recordings obtained in a routine or set schedule (every morning, every 6 hours, every hour for 3 hours following treatment, etc.). **Rationale:** Documents completion of the procedure, and if symptoms have occurred, provides accurate data for interpretation of the recording.

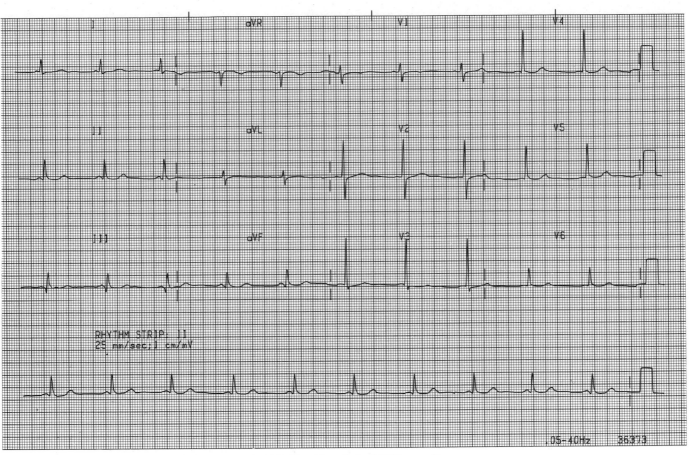

FIGURE 7–27. Clear 12-lead ECG recording.

Patient/Family Education

1. Assess the readiness of the patient to learn. **Rationale:** Anxiety and concerns of the patient and family may inhibit their ability to learn.

2. Provide explanations of the equipment and the procedure to both patient and family. **Rationale:** Information may decrease anxiety.

3. Reassure the patient and family that the 12-lead ECG will be reviewed and that any alterations or problems will be quickly treated. **Rationale:** Patients and families need to be reassured that immediate care is available if it is needed.

Performance Checklist
Skill 7–2: Twelve-Lead Electrocardiogram

Critical Behaviors	Complies	
	yes	no
1. Wash hands.		
2. Plug ECG machine in.		
3. Turn recorder on.		
4. Set lead selector to standby.		
5. Check wires for problems.		
6. Check coding on lead wires.		
7. Position the patient.		
8. Expose patient's legs, arms, and chest while covering patient as much as possible.		
9. Identify lead placement sites.		

Table continues on following page

Critical Behaviors	Complies	
	yes	no
10. Cleanse electrode placement sites.		
11. Abrade skin.		
12. Shave the skin, if necessary.		
13. Test electrodes for moistness, if gel type or stickiness, if adhesive type.		
14. Apply electrodes to sites correctly.		
15. Secure lead wires to electrodes, avoiding tension and pull.		
16. Identify single- or multiple-channel machine.		
17. Check settings on ECG machine.		
18. Run the limb leads.		
19. Run the chest leads.		
20. Assess quality of tracing.		
21. Disconnect equipment, and clean gel off patient and equipment.		
22. Wash hands.		
23. Document procedure in patient record.		

REFERENCES

Drew, B., Ide, B., and Sparacino, P. (1991). Accuracy of bedside ECG Monitoring: A Report on Current Practices of Critical Care Nurses. *Heart and Lung*, 20(6):597–609.

BIBLIOGRAPHY

Alspach, J. (1991). *Core Curriculum for Critical Care Nursing.* Philadelphia: Saunders.
Clochesy, J., et al. (1991). Electrode site preparation: A follow-up. *Heart Lung* 20(1):27–30.
Decker, S. (1987). Continuous EKG monitoring systems. *Nurs. Clin. North Am.* 22(1).

8

PRECORDIAL SHOCK

BEHAVIORAL OBJECTIVES

After completing this chapter, the nurse will be able to

- Define the key terms
- Identify indications for precordial shock therapy.
- Describe the rationale behind precordial shock.
- Describe the electrical physiology involved in precordial shock.
- Demonstrate the skills necessary to perform precordial shock.
- Describe posttreatment patient management.

Early identification and termination of potentially life-threatening dysrhythmias are essential to improve the survival of the patient at risk. When patients present with dysrhythmias, effective treatment is dependent on early identification and immediate intervention. This chapter addresses those procedures necessary in both chronic and emergent electrical management of the patient presenting with tachydysrhythmias and ventricular tachycardia.

Precordial shock is performed by passing an electric current across the chest wall and through the heart muscle, resulting in depolarization of the myocardial muscle fibers. This action causes a disruption of the chaotic electric impulses and allows for repolarization of the individual muscle fibers. The electric current delivered has the potential to restore the coordinated impulse conduction of the heart's electrical system. A single source of impulse generation can then be reestablished as the pacemaker.

Defibrillation is the most effective therapy for termination of ventricular fibrillation and ventricular tachydysrhythmias. *Defibrillation* consists of passing an electric current through a critical mass of the heart, resulting in simultaneous depolarization of the myocardial muscle fibers and the establishment of a single source of impulse generation.

In ventricular fibrillation, multiple areas of the ventricles repolarize and depolarize independent of each other. The independent initiation of impulses causes the myocardial muscle fibers to contract in a chaotic rhythm, resulting in loss of synchronization and cardiac output. During ventricular fibrillation, the heart is unable to pump blood through the cardiovascular system. The ventricles then become dilated as a result of stagnant blood flow, further compromising the situation. Organs and tissues become deprived of oxygen as hypoxemia and acidosis develop. The longer the duration of ventricular fibrillation, the greater is the damage to the myocardial muscle and the less likely is the possibility of successful conversion. Death is imminent if ventricullar fibrillation is not immediately terminated.

Sustained, recurrent ventricular dysrhythmias may represent a chronic condition for some patients despite conventional drug therapy. In this patient population, the surgical placement of an automatic implantable cardioverter–defibrillator (AICD) may be indicated.

The AICD is indicated for the patient who has survived at least one episode of cardiac arrest caused by hemodynamically unstable tachydysrhythmias unrelated to myocardial infarction. The AICD is also indicated in patients presenting with recurrent, sustained hypotensive ventricular tachycardia, ventricular fibrillation, or both in the face of current drug therapy.

Optimally, patients who are selected for AICD placement should have at least a 6-month life expectancy, have dysrhythmias with rates that exceed 155 beats per minute, demonstrate emotional security, and be able and willing to cooperate in follow-up testing and care.

KEY TERMS

action potential	*joule (J)*
arcing	*repolarization*
cardiac cycle	*synchronized cardioversion*
defibrillator (automatic	*tachydysrhythmias*
implantable device)	*ventricular fibrillation*
defibrillation (external)	*vulnerable period*
defibrillation (internal)	*watts per second (w/s)*
depolarization	

SKILLS

8–1   Cardioversion
8–2   Defibrillation (External)
8–3   Defibrillation (Internal)

GUIDELINES

The following assessment guidelines assist the nurse in identification and management of the patient presenting with potential and/or life-threatening dysrhythmias.

1. Know the patient's level of consciousness.
2. Know the patient's baseline cardiac status.

3. Know the patient's past medical history.
4. Know the patient's current laboratory data.
5. Know the patient's current medical management.

SKILL 8–1

Cardioversion

Cardioversion is the therapy of choice for termination of hemodynamically unstable tachydysrhythmias. Synchronized cardioversion is recommended for termination of unstable paroxysmal atrial tachycardia, atrial tachycardia, atrial fibrillation, atrial flutter, and unstable ventricular tachycardia with a pulse. Since ventricular tachycardia is often a precursor to ventricular fibrillation, cardioversion has the potential to prevent this life-threatening dysrhythmia.

The electric current delivered with cardioversion depolarizes the myocardium and restores the heart's coordinated impulse conduction as a single source of impulse generation is established. A countershock synchronized to the QRS complex allows for the electric current to be delivered outside the heart's vulnerable period. This synchronization occurs after the R wave but prior to the vulnerable period associated with the T wave.

Cardioversion may be implemented in the patient with either a chronic or emergent condition. Chronic dysrhythmias such as atrial fibrillation and atrial flutter are converted by elective synchronized cardioversion when the patient develops symptomology from the rapid ventricular response. In elective cardioversion, the patient is sedated to minimize discomfort.

When properly implemented, cardioversion can terminate tachydysrhythmias that compromise the patient's hemodynamic status and lead to life-threatening dysrhythmias.

Purpose

The nurse performs cardioversion to

1. Convert tachydysrhythmias that endanger the hemodynamic status.
2. Prevent the development of ventricular fibrillation in the presence of unstable ventricular tachycardia with a pulse.

Prerequisite Knowledge and Skills

Prior to performing cardioversion, the nurse should understand

1. Anatomy and physiology of the cardiovascular system.
2. Basic introductory ECG interpretation.
3. Principles of Advanced Cardiac Life Support (ACLS).
4. Principles of emergency pharmacologic agents and their dosage calculations.
5. Principles of electrical safety (Skill 36–1).

The nurse should be able to perform

1. Assessment of the cardiovascular system.
2. Basic Cardiac Life Support (BCLS).
3. Interpretation of ECG dysrhythmias.
4. Oxygen administration via bag-valve mask device (see Skill 4–2).
5. Dosage calculations for emergency pharmacologic agents.
6. Safe handling of defibrillator when testing energy levels.

Assessment

1. Assess ECG for tachydysrhythmias, including paroxysmal tachycardia, atrial fibrillation, atrial flutter, atrial tachycardia, and ventricular tachycardia, which could require synchronized cardioversion. **Rationale:** Tachydysrhythmias often precede ventricular fibrillation and precipitate deterioration of hemodynamic stability.
2. Assess patient's vital signs with each significant change in ECG rate and rhythm. **Rationale:** Deterioration of vital signs indicates hemodynamic compromise that could become life-threatening.
3. Assess serum potassium, magnesium, and digitalis levels. **Rationale:** Hypokalemia and hypomagnesemia significantly contribute to electrical instability and may potentiate postconversion dysrhythmias. Digitalis toxicity predisposes the patient to the development of life-threatening dysrhythmias after cardioversion.

Nursing Diagnoses

1. Decreased output related to supraventricular dysrhythmias. **Rationale:** Loss of the atrial kick can decrease cardiac output by 20 percent.
2. Altered cardiopulmonary tissue perfusion related to ventricular fibrillation. **Rationale:** Ventricular fibrillation is a lethal dysrhythmia that progresses to cardiopulmonary arrest and death.
3. Altered cerebral tissue perfusion related to postcardioversion therapy. **Rationale:** Cerebral emboli are a potential procedural complication of cardioversion.
4. Potential for injury related to electric current. **Rationale:** Cardioversion delivers a prescribed range of energy (from 50 to 360 joules [J]) directly to the patient's myocardium, which can cause surface burns of the chest wall.

Planning

1. Individualize the following goals for performing cardioversion:
   a. Maintain patent airway. **Rationale:** Inadequate oxygenation increases the workload of the myocardium and leads to cerebral tissue hypoxia.
   b. Maintain hemodynamic stability. **Rationale:** Deterioration of vital signs and electrical conduc-

tion of the heart can potentiate cardiopulmonary arrest.

  c.   Maintain patency of large bore venous access. **Rationale:** Emergency drugs may be administered in response to procedural complications.

  d.   Maintain skin integrity. **Rationale:** Use of appropriate conductive medium during cardioversion enhances proper conduction and reduces the potential for electrical burns.

2.   Validate that an informed consent has been obtained as per institutional policy. **Rationale:** Informed consent is advised prior to performing cardioversion unless the patient presents in a life-threatening state.

3.   Prepare all necessary equipment and supplies. **Rationale:** Proper equipment at the bedside will ensure rapid intervention for procedural complications.

  a.   Defibrillator with cardioversion mode and cable and ECG oscilloscope.

  b.   Conductive gel or saline pads.

  c.   Dry 4 × 4 gauze pads.

  d.   Administer intravenous sedative or hypnotic pharmacologic agents as prescribed. **Rationale:** Medication administered prior to the procedure helps to minimize the patient's discomfort or anxiety. An anesthesiologist CRNA (certified registered nurse anesthetist) in attendance is recommended, since short-acting anesthetics are often administered and may necessitate airway maintenance and respiratory monitoring.

  e.   Emergency pharmacologic agents:

  (1)   Lidocaine, 20 mg/cc

  (2)   Lidocaine, 2 g in 500 cc D_5W

  (3)   Bretyllium, 500 mg/10 cc

  (4)   Bretyllium, 2 g in 500 cc D_5W

  (5)   Procainamide, 20 mg/min up to 1 g total

  (6)   Procainamide, 2 g in 500 cc D_5W

  (7)   Sodium bicarbonate, 1 mEq/cc.

  f.   Flowmeter for oxygen administration.

  g.   Bag-valve mask device capable of delivering 100% oxygen and large inflation volumes. **Rationale:** Ineffective breathing patterns may develop as a result of cardioversion and subsequent cardiopulmonary complications.

4.   Prepare the patient.

  a.   Explain procedure to the patient. **Rationale:** Minimizes anxiety and promotes patient cooperation.

  b.   Establish patent intravenous access. **Rationale:** Medication administration may be required.

  c.   Position the patient. **Rationale:** Supine positioning provides the best access for procedure initiation, intervention, and management of ad-

verse effects. High Fowler's position with alternative paddle placement may be requested by the physician.

  d.   Remove all metallic objects from the patient. **Rationale:** Metallic objects are excellent conductors of electric current and could result in burns.

  e.   Connect patient's ECG hardwire to defibrillator/ECG monitor. **Rationale:** R wave must be sensed by the defibrillator to achieve synchronization for cardioversion.

  f.   Make patient NPO. **Rationale:** Decreases the risk of aspiration.

  g.   Remove loose-fitting dentures, partial plates, or other mouth prostheses. **Rationale:** Decreases the risk of airway obstruction during the procedure. Evaluate individual situation; e.g., dentures may facilitate a tighter seal for airway management.

  h.   Preoxygenate the patient as appropriate to the condition. **Rationale:** Adequate oxygenation of cardiac tissue diminishes the risk of cerebral and cardiac complications.

5.   Plug the cord from the defibrillator into the grounded wall outlet and deliver prescribed current into tester. **Rationale:** Ascertains that equipment is functioning properly. Test load ranges based on manufacturer's recommendations. Amount of energy stored in capacitator and energy indicated on meter do not always match energy delivered; therefore, routine maintenance and testing by biomedical engineering personnel are recommended (see Skill 36–1). Consult individual hospital policy for specific testing guidelines.

6.   Select monitor lead displaying an R wave of sufficient amplitude to activate the synchronization mode of the defibrillator. In most models, synchronization is achieved when the monitoring lead produces a *tall* positive R wave. **Rationale:** Synchronized cardioversion must sense the R wave so as to deliver the current outside the heart's vulnerable period. If a combination defibrillator/monitor is not being used, a convertor cable must connect the monitor to the defibrillator to achieve synchronization.

7.   Place defibrillator in synchronization mode. Ensure that the patient's QRS complex appears with a lighted blip to signify correct synchronization of the defibrillator with the patient's ECG rhythm. To confirm that synchronization has been achieved, observe for visual flashing on the screen and/or auditory beeps. **Rationale:** Synchronization prevents the random delivery of an electrical charge, which may potentiate ventricular fibrillation.

Implementation

Steps	Rationale	Special Considerations
1. Wash hands.	Reduces transmission of microorganisms.	

Table continues on following page

Steps	Rationale	Special Considerations
2. Prepare the patient and/or paddles with proper conductive agent. Conductive gel should be evenly dispersed on the defibrillator paddles and adequately cover the surface, but is not excessive so as to cause slippage or arcing of the current. *Do not* use Doppler gel. Excessive perspiration also can affect conduction, causing arcing of current.	Enhances electrical conduction through subcutaneous tissue and minimizes burns from the electric current.	Pregelled conductive pads and saline-soaked pads are available for placement in area of paddle. Never use alcohol-soaked pads because they are combustible when in contact with electric current.
3. Turn on ECG recorder for continuous printout.	Establishes a visual recording of the patient's current ECG status and response to intervention and provides a permanent record of the patient's response to intervention.	
4. Place one paddle at the heart's apex just to the left of the nipple in the midaxillary line. Place the other paddle just below the right clavicle to the right of the sternum (Fig. 8–1).	Cardioversion is achieved by passing an electric current through the cardiac muscle mass to restore a single source of impulse generation.	Alternate paddle placement in the individual with a permanent pacemaker; paddle placement is opposite site of insertion just below the clavicle and to the lateral aspect of the sternum and at least 5 in (13 cm) from the pulse generator (Fig. 8–2). Alternate paddle placement in the individual with a temporary pacemaker; disconnect the pacer wires from the pulse generator, insulate with a rubber glove prior to cardioversion, and use standard paddle placement (see Fig. 8–1). Alternate paddle placement in the individual requiring anteroposterior cardioversion (indicated when Fowler's position must be maintained or physician preference); posterior paddle is placed in the left infrascapular area behind the heart, and anterior paddle is placed in the anterior precordial area. Paddle placement in the individual with an automatic implantable defibrillator is the same as standard paddle placement for external defibrillation (see Fig. 8–1).
5. Charge defibrillator paddles as prescribed or in accordance with the recommendations of the American Heart Association.	Defibrillator is charged with the lowest energy level required to convert the tachydysrhythmia (Table 8–1).	*Pediatric recommendations:* Cardiovert with 2 J/kg of body weight with increments of 2 J/kg in subsequent attempts up to 4 J/kg.
6. Disconnect oxygen source during actual cardioversion.	Decreases the risk of combustion in the presence of electrical current.	Arcing of electric current in the presence of oxygen could precipitate an explosion and subsequent fire hazard.
7. Apply 25 lb/in² pressure to each paddle against the chest wall.	Decreased transthoracic resistance improves the flow of current across the axis of the heart.	
8. State "All clear," and visually verify that everyone is clear of contact with patient, bed, and equipment.	Maintains safety to caregivers, since electric current can be conducted from the patient to another individual if contact occurs.	

Table continues on following page

Steps	Rationale	Special Considerations
9. Depress both buttons on the paddles simultaneously, and hold until defibrillator fires. In the synchronized mode, there will be a delay before the charge is released.	Depolarizes the cardiac muscle.	Charge may also be delivered by depressing the discharge button on the defibrillator.
10. Assess for presence of a pulse, and observe monitor for conversion of the tachydysrhythmia.	Simultaneous depolarization of the myocardial muscle cells should reestablish a single source of impulse generation.	If unsuccessful in converting rhythm, proceed with repeated energy recommendations (see Table 8–1). Ventricular fibrillation may develop after cardioversion. If so, deactivate synchronizer and follow the procedure for defibrillation (see Skill 8–2).
11. Clean defibrillator, and remove any gel from paddles with dry 4 × 4 gauze pads.	Conductive gel accumulated on the defibrillator paddles impedes surface contact and increases transthoracic resistance.	
12. Discard supplies in appropriate receptacle.	Universal precautions.	
13. Wash hands.	Reduces transmission of microorganisms.	

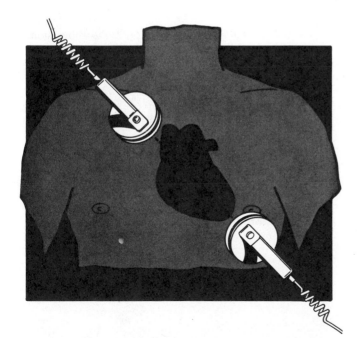

FIGURE 8–1. Standard paddle placement for synchronized cardioversion and defibrillation. (Reproduced with permission from L. Meltzer, R. Pinneo, and R. Kitchell, *Intensive Coronary Care: A Manual for Nurses*, **4th Ed. Bowie, MD: Robert J. Brady, 1983.)**

Evaluation

1. Evaluate neurologic status. Reorient patient to person, place, and time. **Rationale:** Temporary altered level of consciousness may occur following synchronized cardioversion. Cerebral emobili may develop as a post-procedure complication.

2. Evaluate respiratory status. **Rationale:** Respiratory centers of the brain may be depressed as a result of hypoxia or hypnotic or analgesic agents.

3. Evaluate cardiovascular status (blood pressure, pulse, and respiration). Continue to monitor ECG after procedure. **Rationale:** Dysrhythmias may develop cardioversion.

4. Prepare for possible IV antidysrhythmic infusion. **Rationale:** Dysrhythmias may develop after conversion.

5. Evaluate for burns. **Rationale:** Electric current in contact with subcutaneous tissue can cause loss of skin integrity.

Expected Outcomes

1. Reestablishment of a single source of impulse generation for the cardiac muscle. **Rationale:** Impulse conduction is synchronized and enables the heart to pump more effectively, maintaining hemodynamic stability.

2. Hemodynamic stabilization. **Rationale:** Synchronization of impulse conduction provides coordination of the myofibrils, resulting in improved cardiac output.

Unexpected Outcomes

1. Continued tachydysrhythmias. **Rationale:** Atrial and ventricular dysrhythmias may persist even with cardioversion.

2. Ventricular fibrillation progressing to cardiopulmonary arrest. **Rationale:** Ventricular fibrillation is a potential side effect with depolarization of the myocardial cells.

3. Pulmonary and cerebral emboli. **Rationale:** Atrial

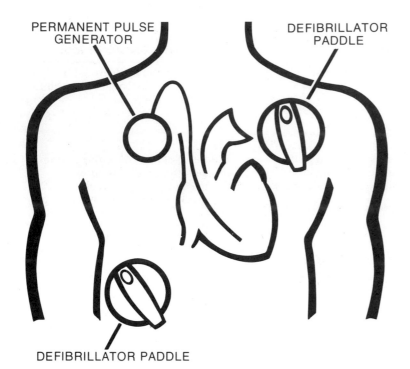

PERMANENT PULSE GENERATOR

DEFIBRILLATOR PADDLE

DEFIBRILLATOR PADDLE

FIGURE 8–2. Alternate paddle placement for synchronized cardioversion and defibrillation in the patient with a permanent pulse generator.

tachydysrhythmias predispose the patient to the development of microemboli that may be released during cardioversion.

4. Respiratory complications and hypotension. **Rationale:** Short-acting anesthetic agents administered during cardioversion as well as the intervention itself may produce respiratory depression and hypotension in the immediate postconversion period.

5. Paddle burns. **Rationale:** Cardioversion delivers electrical energy, which has the potential to disrupt skin integrity.

Documentation

Documentation in the patient record should include neurologic, respiratory, and cardiovascular assessments before and after cardioversion, nursing measures implemented to prepare the patient for cardioversion, i.e., the joules used and the number of attempts made, and patient response to cardioversion including a printout ECG tracing depicting the cardiac response. **Rationale:** Documentation provides a record of preprocedure patient status, nursing interventions, postprocedure patient sta-

TABLE 8–1. AMERICAN HEART ASSOCIATION ENERGY LEVEL RECOMMENDATIONS FOR TREATING TACHYDYSRHYTHMIAS

Ventricular tachycardia with pulse	*Ventricular tachycardia without pulse (energy recommendations are the same as for ventricular fibrillation)*	*Paroxysmal supraventricular tachycardia*
First attempt: Cardiovert with 50 J.	*First attempt:* Defibrillate with 200 J.	*First attempt:* Cardiovert with initial energy of 75 to 100 J. Subsequent attempts prescribed by physician.
Second attempt: Cardiovert with 100 J. *Third attempt:* Cardiovert with 200 J. *Subsequent attempts:* Cardiovert with up to 360 J.	*Second attempt:* Defibrillate with 200 to 300 J. *Subsequent attempts:* Defibrillate with 360 J.	

Atrial fibrillation	*Atrial flutter*
First attempt: Cardiovert with 100 J.	*First attempt:* Cardiovert with initial energy of 25 J. Subsequent attempts prescribed by physician.
Subsequent attempts: Cardiovert with 200 J, then 360 J.	

tus, and both expected and unexpected patient outcomes. Serves as a medicolegal record of the events.

Patient/Family Education

1. Assess patient and family understanding of underlying disease pathology. **Rationale:** Prepares the patient and family for both expected and unexpected outcomes.

2. Explain procedure to patient and family. **Rationale:** Decreases anxiety and promotes patient compliance.

3. Explain the signs and symptoms of hemodynamic compromise associated with preexisting cardiac dysrhythmias to both patient and family. **Rationale:** Enables the patient and family to recognize when the patient needs to contact the physician.

4. Evaluate and discuss with the patient the need for long-term pharmacologic support. **Rationale:** Allows the nurse to anticipate educational needs of the patient and family regarding specific discharge medications.

5. Assess and discuss with the patient the need for lifestyle changes. **Rationale:** Underlying pathophysiology may necessitate alterations in patient's current lifestyle and require a plan for behavioral changes.

Performance Checklist
Skill 8–1   Cardioversion

Critical Behaviors	Complies yes	no
1. Wash hands.		
2. Prepare patient and/or defibrillator paddles with proper conductive medium.		
3. Turn on ECG recorder for continuous printout.		
4. Assure defibrillator is in synchronization mode.		
5. Properly place paddles on the patient's chest wall.		
6. Charge defibrillator paddles with proper energy requirements.		
7. Apply 25 lb/in² pressure to paddles.		
8. State "All clear," and visually verify that all personnel are clear of contact with patient and equipment.		
9. Depress both buttons on paddles simultaneously until defibrillator fires.		
10. Assess for pulse.		
11. Observe monitor for conversion of tachydysrhythmia and ECG rhythm.		
12. Clean defibrillator.		
13. Discard supplies.		
14. Wash hands.		
15. Document procedure in patient record.		

SKILL 8–2

Defibrillation (External)

External defibrillation is achieved by delivering a strong electric current through electrodes placed on the surface of the patient's chest wall. Proper electrode placement ensures that the axis of the heart is directly situated between the sources of current (defibrillator paddles). Since dysrhythmias are chaotic with no coordinated ventricular response, the electric current is delivered randomly. It is through implementation of emergent defibrillation that ventricular fibrillation can be terminated and cardiac output restored.

Purpose

The nurse performs defibrillation to

1. Eradicate life-threatening ventricular fibrillation.
2. Restore cardiac output lost with ventricular fibrillation and reestablish tissue perfusion and oxygenation.

Prerequisite Knowledge and Skills

Prior to performing defibrillation, the nurse should understand

1. Anatomy and physiology as related to the cardiovascular system.
2. Basic introductory ECG interpretation.
3. Principles of Advanced Cardiac Life Support (ACLS).
4. Principles of emergency pharmacologic agents and their dosage calculations.
5. Principles of electrical safety (Skill 36–1).

The nurse should be able to perform

1. Complete cardiovascular system assessment.
2. Basic Cardiac Life Support (BCLS).
3. Interpretation of ECG dysrhythmias.
4. Oxygen administration via bag-valve mask device (see Skill 4–2).
5. Dosage calculations for emergency pharmacologic agents.
6. Safe handling of defibrillator when testing energy levels.

Assessment

1. Assess ECG for tachydysrhythmias, including paroxysmal tachycardia, atrial fibrillation, atrial flutter, atrial tachycardia, and ventricular tachycardia. **Rationale:** Tachydysrhythmias often precede ventricular fibrillation, can be life-threatening, and can precipitate deterioration of hemodynamic stability.
2. Assess ECG for ventricular fibrillation. **Rationale:** The development of ventricular fibrillation is life-threatening, and if it is not terminated immediately, death will ensue.
3. Assess vital signs with each significant change in ECG rate and rhythm. **Rationale:** Blood pressure and pulse are absent in the presence of ventricular fibrillation because of the loss of cardiac output.

Nursing Diagnoses

1. Decreased cardiac output related to ventricular fibrillation. **Rationale:** Independent contraction of myocardial muscle fibers results in a loss of synchronous pumping action of the heart.
2. Altered cardiopulmonary tissue perfusion related to ventricular fibrillation. **Rationale:** Ventricular fibrillation is a lethal dysrhythmia that progresses to complete cardiopulmonary arrest.
3. Altered cerebral tissue perfusion related to post-defibrillation therapy. **Rationale:** Cerebral emboli are a potential postprocedure complication of defibrillation.
4. Potential for injury related to live electric current. **Rationale:** Defibrillation delivers selected electrical energy directly to the patient, ranging from 200 to 360 J, which can cause surface burns of the chest wall.
5. Potential for impaired skin integrity related to live electrical current. **Rationale:** Defibrillation delivers electrical energy that has the potential to disrupt skin integrity. Improper paddle placement and/or improper use of conductive gel may precipitate electrical burns from defibrillation.

6. Potential for ineffective breathing patterns related to decreased/absent cardiac output. **Rationale:** Ventricular fibrillation alters cerebral perfusion and oxygenation, which can depress the respiratory centers in the brain.

Planning

1. Individualize the following goals for performing defibrillation:
   a. Maintain patent airway. **Rationale:** Inadequate oxygenation increases the workload of the myocardium and leads to cerebral tissue hypoxia.
   b. Restore hemodynamic stability. **Rationale:** Deterioration of vital signs and electrical conduction of the heart can potentiate cardiopulmonary arrest.
   c. Restore cardiopulmonary circulation. **Rationale:** CPR must be initiated because the heart is unable to pump while in the state of ventricular fibrillation.
   d. Maintain patency of venous access. **Rationale:** Emergency drugs may be administered in response to ventricular fibrillation.
   e. Maintain skin integrity. **Rationale:** Use of appropriate conductive medium during defibrillation enhances proper conduction and reduces the potential of electrical burns.
2. Prepare all necessary equipment and supplies. **Rationale:** Proper equipment at the bedside will ensure rapid intervention for procedural complications.
   a. Defibrillator with ECG oscilloscope.
   b. Defibrillator paddles of appropriate diameter (Table 8–2).
   c. Saline soaked 4 × 4 gauze pads or gel pads.
   d. Emergency pharmacologic agents
      (1) Lidocaine, 20 mg/cc
      (2) Lidocaine, 2 g in 500 cc D_5W
      (3) Bretyllium, 500 mg/10 cc
      (4) Bretyllium, 2 g in 500 cc D_5W
      (5) Procainamide, 20 mg/min up to 1 g total
      (6) Procainamide 2 g in 500 cc D_5W
      (7) Sodium bicarbonate, 1 mEq/cc.
   e. Flowmeter for oxygen administration.
   f. Bag-valve mask device capable of delivering 100% oxygen and large inflation volumes.
   g. Cardiac board.
   h. Insert defibrillator's electrical cord into grounded wall outlet, charge defibrillator paddles, and deliver appropriate current into tester. Test load ranges are based upon manufacturer's

TABLE 8–2. AMERICAN HEART ASSOCIATION RECOMMENDATIONS FOR EXTERNAL PADDLE/ELECTRODE DIAMETER

Infant	4 to 5 cms
Children	8 cms
Adults (optimal size unknown)	13 cms

recommendations. Amount of energy stored in capacitor and energy indicated on meter do not always match energy delivered; therefore, routine maintenance and testing by engineering personnel are recommended. Consult individual hospital policy for specific guidelines.

3. Prepare the patient.
   a. Place patient on cardiac board in supine position. **Rationale:** Supine positioning provides the best access during procedure and during intervention for and management of adverse effects. Cardiac board provides a hard surface for cardiopulmonary resuscitation.
   b. Remove all metallic objects from the patient. **Rationale:** Metallic objects are excellent conductors of electric current and may result in burns.

c. Remove loose fitting dentures, partial plates, or other prostheses. Evaluate individual situation; dentures may facilitate a tighter seal for airway management. **Rationale:** Decreases risk of airway obstruction during procedure.

4. Initiate BCLS until ready to defibrillate. **Rationale:** Cardiac output must be maintained to prevent irreversible organ and tissue damage.
5. Oxygenate the patient with bag-valve mask and 100 percent oxygen. **Rationale:** Adequate oxygenation of cardiac tissue diminishes the risk of cerebral and cardiac complications.
6. Place defibrillator in the defibrillation mode. **Rationale:** Defibrillation mode must be set in order to randomly disperse the electrical charge because the synchronization mode will not fire in the absence of a QRS complex.

Implementation

Steps	Rationale	Special Considerations
1. Wash hands.	Reduces transmission of microorganisms.	
2. Prepare the patient and/or paddles with proper conductive agent. Conductive gel is evenly dispersed on the defibrillator paddles and adequately covers surface but is not excessive so as to cause slippage or arcing of the current. Excessive perspiration also can affect conduction, causing arcing of current.	Conductive medium enhances electrical conduction through subcutaneous tissue and assists in minimizing burns from the electric current.	Pregelled conductive pads and saline-soaked pads are available for placement in area of paddle. Never use alcohol-soaked pads because they are combustible when in contact with electric current. Disposable defibrillator electrodes (DDE) are an alternative method of defibrillation. Although early in the development stage, preliminary findings with DDE suggest (1) a time reduction in actual defibrillation delivery, (2) reduced variability in defibrillation technique, (3) improved conversion rate, and (4) a reduction in loose lead artifacts.
3. Ensure that defibrillator cables are positioned to allow for adequate access to the patient.	Allows defibrillation to occur without excessive tension on cables.	
4. Turn on ECG recorder for continuous printout.	Establishes a visual recording of the patient's current ECG status and response to intervention and provides a permanent record of the patient's response to intervention.	
5. Place one paddle at the heart's apex just to the left of the nipple in the midaxillary line. Place the other paddle just below the right clavicle to the right of the sternum (see Fig. 8–1).	Defibrillation is achieved by passing an electric current through the cardiac muscle mass to restore a single source of impulse generation.	Alternate paddle placement in the individual with a permanent pacemaker: Paddle placement is opposite site of insertion, just below the clavicle, to the lateral aspect of the sternum, and at least 5 in (13 cm) from the pulse generator (see Fig. 8–2). Alternate paddle placement in the individual with a temporary pacemaker: Disconnect the pacer wires from the generator prior to defibrillation, insulate with a rubber glove, and use standard paddle placement (see Fig. 8–1). Alternate

Table continues on following page

Steps	Rationale	Special Considerations
		paddle placement in the individual requiring anteroposterior defibrillation (indicated when a high Fowler's position must be maintained or physician preference); posterior paddle is placed in the left infrascapular area behind the heart, and anterior paddle is placed in the anterior precordial area. Paddle placement in the individual with an automatic implantable defibrillator is the same as standard placement for external defibrillation (see Fig. 8–1).
6. Charge defibrillator paddles as prescribed or in accordance with recommendations of the American Heart Association.	Defibrillator is charged with the lowest energy level required to convert ventricular fibrillation.	Energy recommendations by the American Heart Association: *Ventricular fibrillation: First attempt*: defibrillate with 200 J. *Second attempt*: defibrillate with 200 to 300 J. *Subsequent attempts*: defibrillate with 360 J. *Pediatric recommendations*: Defibrillate with 2 J/kg of body weight, with increments of 2 J/kg in subsequent attempts up to 4 J/kg maximum.
7. Apply 25 lb/in^2 pressure to each paddle against the chest wall.	Decreases transthoracic resistance and improves the flow of current across the axis of the heart.	
8. State "All clear," and visually verify that all personnel are clear of contact with patient bed and equipment.	Maintains safety to caregivers, since electric current can be conducted from the patient to another individual if contact occurs.	
9. Depress both buttons on the paddles simultaneously and hold until defibrillator fires. In the defibrillation mode, there will be an immediate release of the electric charge.	Depolarizes the cardiac muscle.	Charge may be delivered by depressing the discharge button on the defibrillator.
10. Assess for the presence of a pulse, and observe for conversion of the dysrhythmia.	Simultaneous depolarization of the myocardial muscle cells reestablishes a single source of impulse generation.	
11. If unsuccessful, immediately charge paddles to 200 to 300 J and repeat Steps 5 to 10.	Immediate action increases the chance for successful depolarization of cardiac muscle.	Transthoracic resistance decreases by approximately 8 percent with the second shock.
12. If second attempt is unsuccessful, immediately charge paddles to 360 J and repeat Steps 11 to 16.	Immediate action increases the chance for successful depolarization of cardiac muscle.	BCLS must be continued between defibrillation attempts.
13. If third attempt is unsuccessful, initiate ACLS.	Actions necessary to maintain the delivery of oxygenated blood to vital organs.	
14. Clean defibrillator, and remove any gel from paddles with 4 × 4 gauze pads.	Conductive gel accumulated on the defibrillator paddles impedes surface contact and increases transthoracic resistance.	
15. Discard supplies in appropriate receptacle.	Universal precautions.	
16. Wash hands.	Reduces transmission of microorganisms.	

Evaluation

1. Evaluate neurologic status. Reorient patient to person, place, and time. **Rationale:** Temporary altered level of consciousness occurs following defibrillation. (Cerebral emboli may develop as a postprocedure complication.

2. Evaluate respiratory status. **Rationale:** Respiratory centers of the brain may be depressed as a result of hypoxia.

3. Evaluate cardiovascular status (blood pressure, pulse, and respiration). Continue to monitor the ECG after the procedure. **Rationale:** Dysrhythmias may develop after defibrillation.

4. Initiate intravenous antidysrhythmic pharmacologic therapy. **Rationale:** Ventricular fibrillation is indicative of the myocardium's state of irritability, and if antidysrhythmic therapy is not administered, recurrence of ventricular fibrillation is probable.

5. Monitor for burns. **Rationale:** Electric current in contact with subcutaneous tissue can cause loss of skin integrity.

Expected Outcomes

1. Reestablishment of a single source of impulse generation for the cardiac muscle. **Rationale:** Impulse conduction is synchronized and enables the heart to pump more effectively, maintaining hemodynamic stability.

2. Hemodynamic stabilization. **Rationale:** Coordination of impulse conduction provides synchronization of the myofibrils, resulting in restoration of cardiac output.

Unexpected Outcomes

1. Cardiopulmonary arrest and/or death. **Rationale:** Unresolved fibrillation of the cardiac muscle prevents effective pumping action of the heart and eliminates the cardiac output.

2. Cerebral anoxia and brain death. **Rationale:** Loss of cardiac output and adequate oxygenation results in death of vital body tissues and organs.

3. Respiratory complications. **Rationale:** Ventricular fibrillation alters cerebral perfusion and oxygenation, which can depress the respiratory centers in the brain.

4. Paddle burns. **Rationale:** Defibrillation delivers electrical energy, which has the potential to disrupt skin integrity. Improper paddle placement and/or improper use of conductive gel may precipitate electrical burns from defibrillation.

Documentation

Documentation in the patient record should include neurologic, respiratory, and cardiovascular assessments before and after defibrillation, nursing measures implemented to prepare the patient for defibrillation, i.e., the joules used and the number of attempts made, patient response to defibrillation, and any unexpected outcomes and the interventions taken, including a printout ECG tracing depicting the cardiac events. **Rationale:** Provides a record of preprocedure patient status, nursing interventions, postprocedure patient status, and both expected and unexpected patient outcomes. Serves as a legal medical record of the events.

Patient/Family Education

1. Assess patient and family understanding of the underlying disease pathology. **Rationale:** Prepares the patient and family for both expected and unexpected outcomes.

2. Explain the procedure to both patient and family. **Rationale:** Promotes understanding and encourages questions.

3. Explain to both patient and family the signs and symptoms of hemodynamic compromise associated with preexisting cardiac dysrhythmias. **Rationale:** Enables the patient and family to recognize when the patient needs to contact the physician.

4. Evaluate the patient's need for long-term pharmacologic support. **Rationale:** Allows the nurse to anticipate educational needs of the patient and family regarding specific discharge medications.

5. Assess and discuss with the patient the need for lifestyle changes. **Rationale:** Underlying pathophysiology may necessitate alterations in patient's current lifestyle and require a plan for behavioral changes.

6. Assess and discuss with the patient the need for an automatic implantable cardiovertor–defibrillator. **Rationale:** Life-threatening ventricular dysrhythmias may persist after initial defibrillation and pharmacologic interventions. Recurrent ventricular dysrhythmias may represent a chronic condition for the patient.

7. Assess and discuss with the patient the need for an emergency communication system. **Rationale:** Individuals with recurrent life-threatening ventricular dysrhythmias are at risk for cardiac arrest.

Performance Checklist
Skill 8–2: Defibrillation (External)

Critical Behaviors	Complies	
	yes	**no**
1. Wash hands.		
2. Prepare patient and/or defibrillator paddles with proper conductive medium.		
3. Turn on ECG recorder for continuous printout.		
4. Properly place paddles on the patient's chest wall.		

Table continues on following page

Critical Behaviors	Complies	
	yes	no
5. Charge defibrillator paddles with proper energy requirements.		
6. Apply 25 lb/in^2 pressure to paddles.		
7. State "All clear," and visually verify that all personnel are clear of contact with bed, patient, and equipment.		
8. Depress both buttons on paddles simultaneously until defibrillator fires.		
9. Assess for pulse, and identify cardiac rhythm, observing for conversion of ventricular fibrillation.		
10. If first defibrillation attempt is unsuccessful, repeat steps 5 to 10 at 200 to 300 J.		
11. If second defibrillation attempt is unsuccessful, repeat steps 5 to 6 at 360 J.		
12. If third defibrillation attempt is unsuccessful, continue BCLS and initiate ACLS.		
13. Clean defibrillator.		
14. Discard supplies.		
15. Wash hands.		
16. Document procedure in patient record.		

SKILL 8–3

Defibrillation (Internal)

Internal defibrillation is achieved by delivering an electric current directly to the myocardium's surface via an open thoracotomy approach or open sternotomy, as in the postoperative cardiovascular surgery patient. Internal defibrillation is used intraoperatively and in emergency thoracotomies. Direct internal defibrillation eliminates transthoracic resistance, so the recommended energy requirements are much lower than with external defibrillation. Energy requirements for internal defibrillation range from 5 J to as high as 60 J. Ideal energy requirements that cause minimal damage to the myocardium and are effective for defibrillation have not been established.

In a study done by Geddes et al. (1974), it was found that an energy level of 5 J was sufficient in 50 percent of the human hearts internally defibrillated. Further conclusions of the study noted that energy levels between 10 to 20 J were successful in terminating the dysrhythmias without the development of myocardial necrosis in 90 percent of the patients studied.

Internal paddle placement ensures that the axis of the heart is situated between the sources of current. Since dysrhythmias are chaotic with no coordinated ventricular response, the electric current is randomly delivered. Ventricular fibrillation can be terminated and cardiac output restored with internal defibrillation.

Purpose

The nurse assists the physician in performing internal defibrillation to

1. Convert life-threatening ventricular fibrillation.

2. Restore cardiac output lost with ventricular fibrillation and reestablish tissue perfusion and oxygenation.

Prerequisite Knowledge and Skills

Prior to defibrillating the patient internally, the nurse should understand

1. Anatomy and physiology of the cardiovascular system.
2. Principles of sterile technique.
3. Principles of universal precautions.
4. Basic introductory ECG interpretation.
5. Principles of Advanced Cardiac Life Support (ACLS).

The nurse should be able to perform

1. Proper handwashing techniques (see Skill 35–5).
2. Universal precautions (see Skill 35–1).
3. Aseptic technique.
4. Complete cardiovascular system assessment.
5. Basic Cardiac Life Support (BCLS).
6. Interpretation of ECG dysrhythmias.
7. Oxygen administration via bag-valve mask devise (see Skill 4–2).
8. Dosage calculations for emergency pharmacologic agents.
9. Safe handling of defibrillator when testing energy levels.
10. Sterile technique.

Assessment

1. Assess for ECG tachydysrhythmias, including par-

oxysmal tachycardia, atrial fibrillation, atrial flutter, atrial tachycardia, and ventricular tachycardia. **Rationale:** Ventricular dysrhythmias often precede ventricular fibrillation and precipitate deterioration of hemodynamic stability.

2. Assess ECG for ventricular fibrillation. **Rationale:** The development of ventricular fibrillation is life-threatening, and if it is not terminated immediately, death will ensue.

3. Assess vital signs with each significant change in ECG rate and rhythm. **Rationale:** Blood pressure and pulse are absent in the presence of ventricular fibrillation as a result of the loss of cardiac output.

Nursing Diagnoses

1. Decreased cardiac output related to ventricular fibrillation. **Rationale:** Independent contraction of myocardial muscle fibers results in a loss of synchronicity and pumping action of the heart.

2. Altered cardiopulmonary tissue perfusion related to ventricular fibrillation. **Rationale:** Ventricular fibrillation is a lethal dysrhythmia that progresses to complete cardiopulmonary arrest.

3. Altered cerebral tissue perfusion related to defibrillation therapy. **Rationale:** Cerebral emboli are a potential postprocedure complication of defibrillation.

4. Potential for injury related to internal defibrillation. **Rationale:** Internal defibrillation delivers selected energy levels ranging from 5 to 60 J directly to the myocardium, which can cause an electrical injury to cardiac tissue.

5. Potential for infection related to open thoracotomy or sternotomy under emergency conditions. **Rationale:** Disruption of skin integrity and/or introduction of a foreign-body allows microorganisms to enter the thoracic cavity.

Planning

1. Individualize the following goals for performing internal defibrillation:
   a. Maintain patent airway. **Rationale:** Inadequate oxygenation increases the workload of the heart and leads to cerebral tissue hypoxia.
   b. Restore hemodynamic stability. **Rationale:** Deterioration of vital signs and electrical conduction of the heart can potentiate cardiopulmonary arrest.
   c. Restore cardiopulmonary circulation. **Rationale:** CPR must be initiated because the heart is unable to pump while in a state of ventricular fibrillation.
   d. Maintain patency of venous access. **Rationale:** Emergency drugs may be administered in response to ventricular fibrillation.

2. Prepare all necessary equipment and supplies. **Rationale:** Proper equipment at the bedside will ensure rapid intervention for procedural complications.
   a. Sterile gloves, goggles, and mask.
   b. Defibrillator with ECG oscilloscope.
   c. Internal defibrillator pads (Table 8–3).
   d. Saline soaked 4 × 4s.
   e. Emergency pharmacologic agents.
      (1) Lidocaine, 20 mg/cc.
      (2) Lidocaine, 2 g in 500 cc D_5W.
      (3) Bretyllium, 500 mg/10 cc.
      (4) Bretyllium, 2 g in 500 cc D_5W.
      (5) Procainamide, 20 mg/min up to 1 g total.
      (6) Procainamide, 2 g in 500 cc D_5W.
      (7) Sodium bicarbonate, 1 mEq/cc.
   f. Flowmeter for oxygen administration.
   g. Bag-valve mask device capable of delivering 100% oxygen and large inflation volumes.

3. Prepare the patient.
   a. Place patient in supine position. **Rationale:** Supine positioning provides the best access during procedure and during intervention for and management of adverse effects.
   b. Remove all metallic objects from the patient. **Rationale:** Metallic objects are conductors of electric current and can cause burns.
   c. Prep and drape the patient. **Rationale:** Decreases the potential for nosocomial infection.
   d. Remove loose fitting dentures, partial plates, or other mouth prostheses. Evaluate individual situation; dentures may facilitate a tighter seal for airway management. **Rationale:** Decreases the risk of airway obstruction during the procedure.

4. Initiate Basic Cardiac Life Support (BCLS). **Rationale:** Decreases the risk of airway obstruction during the procedure.

5. Insert defibrillator's cord into grounded electrical wall outlet and charge. **Rationale:** Assesses electrical current. Amount of energy stored in capacitator and energy indicated on meter do not always match energy delivered; therefore, routine maintenance and testing by biomedical engineering personnel are recommended.

6. Place defibrillator in the fibrillation mode. **Rationale:** Defibrillation mode must be set in order to randomly disperse the electrical charge since the synchronization mode will not fire in the absence of a QRS complex.

7. Connect internal defibrillator paddles to the defibrillator. Maintain sterility of the internal paddles. **Rationale:** Internal paddles must be used for direct myocardial defibrillation. Paddles must be sterile prior to use.

8. Turn on ECG recorder for continuous printout. **Rationale:** Establishes a visual recording of the patient's current ECG status and provides a permanent record of the patient's response to intervention.

TABLE 8–3. RECOMMENDED INTERNAL PADDLE/ ELECTRODE DIAMETER

Infant	2.8 cms
Children	4.5 cms
Adults	6.0 or 7.5 cms

Implementation

Steps	Rationale	Special Considerations
1. Wash hands.	Reduces transmission of microorganisms.	
2. Don sterile gloves, mask, and goggles.	Maintains sterility. Provides universal precautions.	
3. Place sterile saline-soaked gauze 4 × 4 sponges between the myocardium and the defibrillator paddles.	Enhances electrical conduction and assists in minimizing burns from the electrical current.	One paddle is placed over the right atrium or right ventricle, the other paddle is placed over the apex (Fig. 8–3).
4. Charge defibrillator paddles as prescribed.	Defibrillator is charged with the lowest energy level required to convert ventricular fibrillation.	10 to 20 J is sufficient to convert ventricular fibrillation (Moore, 1986). Equipment manufacturer's operation guide provides specific recommendations.
5. State "All clear" and visually verify that all personnel are clear of contact with patient bed and equipment.	Electric current can be conducted from the patient to another individual if contact occurs.	Make sure floor area is dry.
6. Depress both buttons on the paddles simultaneously, and hold until the defibrillator fires. In the defibrillation mode, there will be an immediate release of the electric charge.	Depolarizes cardiac muscle.	Charge may also be delivered by depressing the discharge button on the defibrillator.
7. Assess for the presence of a pulse, and observe for conversion of the dysrhythmia.	Simultaneous depolarization of the myocardial muscle cells reestablishes a single source of impulse generation.	
8. If first attempt is unsuccessful, immediately charge paddles and repeat Steps 4 to 7.	Immediate action increases the chance for successful depolarization of cardiac muscle.	
9. If second attempt is unsuccessful, immediately charge paddles and repeat Steps 4 to 7.	Immediate action increases the chance for successful depolarization of cardiac muscle.	Open-chest compression of the heart must be continued between defibrillation attempts.
10. If third attempt is unsuccessful, initiate ACLS.	Actions necessary to maintain the delivery of oxygenated blood to vital organs.	
11. If successful, prepare patient for transport to the operating room.	Surgical intervention is necessary when open-chest technique is used.	Recurrent ventricular fibrillation may necessitate surgical placement of an automatic implantable defibrillator.
12. Clean defibrillator, and remove blood or body fluids. Send used paddles for resterilization with sterile paddles.	Accumulated material impedes thorough sterilization and good surface contact.	
13. Discard supplies.	Universal precautions.	
14. Wash hands.	Reduces transmission of microorganisms.	

Evaluation

1. Evaluate neurologic status. Reorient patient to person, place, and time. **Rationale:** Temporary altered level of consciousness occurs following defibrillation. (Cerebral emboli may develop as a postprocedure complication.)

2. Evaluate respiratory status. **Rationale:** Respiratory centers of the brain may be depressed as a result of hypoxia.

3. Evaluate cardiovascular status (blood pressure, pulse, and respiration). Continue to monitor ECG after procedure. **Rationale:** Dysrhythmias may develop after defibrillation.

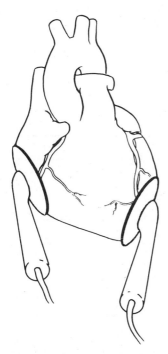

FIGURE 8–3. Paddle placement for internal defibrillation. (Reproduced with permission from S. Kinkade and J.-E. Lohrman, *Critical Care Nursing Procedures: A Team Approach*. Philadelphia: B.C. Decker, 1990.)

4. Initiate intravenous antidysrhythmia pharmacologic therapy. **Rationale:** Ventricular fibrillation is indicative of the myocardium's state of irritability, and if antidysrhythmia therapy is not administered, recurrence of ventricular fibrillation is probable.

Expected Outcomes

1. Reestablishment of a single source of impulse generation for the cardiac muscle. **Rationale:** Impulse conduction is synchronized and enables the heart to pump more effectively, maintaining hemodynamic stability.
2. Hemodynamic stabilization. **Rationale:** Coordination of impulse conduction provides synchronization of the myofibrils, resulting in restoration of cardiac output.

Unexpected Outcomes

1. Cardiopulmonary arrest and/or death. **Rationale:** Unresolved fibrillation of the cardiac muscle prevents effective pumping action of the heart and eliminates the cardiac output.
2. Cerebral anoxia and brain death. **Rationale:** Loss of cardiac output and adequate oxygenation result in death of vital body tissues and organs.
3. Respiratory complications. **Rationale:** Ventricular fibrillation alters cerebral perfusion and oxygenation, which can depress the respiratory centers in the brain.

4. Paddle burns. **Rationale:** Defibrillation delivers electrical energy, which has the potential to disrupt tissue integrity. Improper paddle placement and/or improper use of saline pads may precipitate electrical burns.
5. Infection. **Rationale:** Disruption of skin integrity and the introduction of foreign materials into the thoracic cavity predispose the patient to the risk of infection.

Documentation

Documentation in the patient record should include neurologic, respiratory, and cardiovascular assessments before and after defibrillation, nursing measures implemented to prepare the patient for internal defibrillation, i.e., joules used and number of attempts made, and patient response to defibrillation, and any unexpected outcomes and the interventions taken, including a printout ECG tracing depicting the cardiac events, and time patient sent to the operating room. **Rationale:** Documents preprocedure patient status, nursing interventions, postprocedure patient status, and both expected and unexpected patient outcomes. Serves as a legal medical record of the events.

Patient/Family Education

1. Assess patient and family understanding of the underlying disease pathology. **Rationale:** Prepares the patient and family for both expected and unexpected outcomes.
2. Explain to patient and family the signs and symptoms of hemodynamic compromise associated with preexisting cardiac dysrhythmias. **Rationale:** Enables the patient and family to recognize when the patient needs to contact the physician.
3. Evaluate the patient's need for long-term antiarrhythmic support. **Rationale:** Allows the nurse to anticipate educational needs of the patient and family regarding specific discharge medications.
4. Assess and discuss with the patient the need for lifestyle changes. **Rationale:** Underlying pathophysiology may necessitate alterations in patient's current lifestyle and require a plan for behavioral changes.
5. Assess and discuss with the patient the need for an automatic implantable defibrillator. **Rationale:** Life-threatening ventricular dysrhythmias may persist after initial defibrillation and pharmacologic interventions. Recurrent ventricular dysrhythmias may represent a chronic condition for the patient.
6. Assess and discuss with the patient the need for emergency communication system. **Rationale:** Individuals with recurrent life-threatening ventricular dysrhythmias are at risk for cardiac arrest.

Performance Checklist
Skill 8–3: Defibrillation (Internal)

Critical Behaviors	Complies yes	no
1. Wash hands.		
2. Don sterile gloves, mask, and goggles.		
3. Prepare and test defibrillator.		
4. Connect internal paddles to defibrillator.		
5. Turn on ECG recorder for continuous printout.		
6. Charge defibrillator paddles with proper energy requirements.		
7. Properly place paddles on the patient's myocardial muscle mass, or assist the physician with paddle placement.		
8. State "All clear," and visually verify that all personnel are clear of contact with patient and equipment.		
9. Depress both buttons on paddles simultaneously or discharge button on defibrillator until charge is delivered.		
10. Assess for pulse and observe monitor for conversion of ventricular fibrillation.		
11. If first attempt is unsuccessful, repeat Steps 6 to 10.		
12. If second attempt is unsuccessful, repeat Steps 6 to 10.		
13. If third attempt is unsuccessful, initiate ACLS.		
14. If successful, prepare patient for transport to operating room.		
15. Clean defibrillator.		
16. Discard supplies.		
17. Wash hands.		
18. Document procedure in patient record.		

REFERENCES

American Heart Association (1987). Electrical Therapy in the Malignant Arrhythmias. In *Textbook of Advanced Life Support*, 2d Ed. (pp. 89–95). Dallas: American Heart Association.

American Heart Association (1988). Cardiac Rhythm Disturbances. In *Textbook of Pediatric Advanced Life Support* (pp. 66–67). Dallas: American Heart Association.

Geddes, L. A., Tacker, W. A. Rosborough, J., et al. (1974). The electrical dose for ventricular defibrillation with electrodes applied directly to the heart. *J. Thorac. Cardiovasc. Surg.* 68:593–602.

Kincade, S. and Lohrman, J. E. (1990). *Critical Care Nursing Procedures: A Team Approach*. Philadelphia, B. C. Decker.

Metzer, L., Pinneo, R., and Kitchell, R. (1983). *Intensive Coronary Care: A Manual for Nurses*, 4th Ed. Bowie, MD: Robert J. Brady.

Moore, S. (1986). Jump-starting the heart: A current review of defibrillation techniques and equipment. *J.A.M.A.* 12(4):213–217.

Persons, C. B. (1987). Cardioversion. In C. B. Persons (Ed.), *Critical Care Procedures and Protocols: A Nursing Approach*. Philadelphia: Lippincott.

Spence, M. I. (1985). Defibrillation. In S. Millar (Ed.), *AACN Procedure Manual for Critical Care* (pp. 36–40). Philadelphia: Saunders.

Stults, K. R., Brown, D. D., Cooley, F., and Kerber, R. E. (1987). Self-adhesive monitor/defibrillation pads improve prehospital defibrillation success. *Ann. Emerg. Med.* 16(8):872–877.

BIBLIOGRAPHY

Kerber, R. E., Carter, J., Sanford, K., Grayzel, J., and Kennedy, J. (1980). Open chest defibrillation during cardiac surgery: Energy and current requirements. *Am. J. Cardiol.* 46:393–396.

INVASIVE VASCULAR TECHNIQUES

BEHAVIORAL OBJECTIVES

After completing this chapter, the nurse will be able to

- Define the key terms.
- Describe methods of establishing venous access.
- Discuss the indications for peripheral line placement.
- Demonstrate the skills employed in invasive vascular techniques.
- Describe potential complications of these skills and assessment findings related to each.

Many invasive vascular techniques are not unique to the critical-care setting. However, in the critical-care environment, high patient acuity, the frequency with which these procedures are performed, and the potentially life-threatening nature of side effects demand that the nurse develop proficiency in these techniques. Since critically ill patients are, by nature of their illness, at high risk for dysrhythmias or other medical emergencies, establishing and maintaining venous access are a high priority. An arterial puncture is performed selectively to obtain an arterial blood sample for immediate blood gas analysis for suspected altered respiratory function, monitoring oxygen therapy, or cardiopulmonary arrest.

The key to successfully performing invasive vascular techniques is knowing normal anatomy and physiology and selecting appropriate sites. The choice of venous access depends on the hemodynamic status of the patient, the expertise of the nurse and physician, the availability of supplies and equipment, the general condition of the vasculature, and the nature of the fluid being infused.

KEY TERMS

Allen's test
bevel
gauge
hematoma
lumen
modified Allen's test
phlebitis
stopcock
thrombosis
tourniquet
vasospasm

SKILLS

9–1 Venipuncture
9–2 Arterial Puncture

GUIDELINES

The following assessment guidelines assist the nurse in formulating a nursing diagnosis and an individualized plan of care when performing invasive vascular techniques:

1. Know the patient's baseline cardiovascular and pulmonary assessments.
2. Know the patient's baseline fluid balance status.
3. Know the patient's medical history.
4. Know the patient's current medical treatment.
5. Perform systemic cardiovascular and pulmonary assessments in a timely fashion.
6. Determine appropriate interventions for assessed findings.
7. Become adept with equipment used when performing invasive vascular procedures.

SKILL 9–1

Venipuncture

Venipuncture is performed by cannulating a superficial vein with a sterile needle/catheter and directly connecting a primed IV administration set. Direct access to the venous circulation of critically ill patients is of high priority because of the need to intervene rapidly with medications and/or fluids if life-threatening conditions (e.g., dysrhythmias or hypotension) occur. Disposable catheter needles of various lengths and lumen sizes are available. Small-gauge catheters (20 to 22 gauge) may be sufficient for IV rates less than 75 cc/h and for patients who have tortuous or fragile veins. Larger-gauge catheters (14 to 18 gauge) are necessary for patients requiring large volumes of IV fluid or blood products. Short (1 in or less) catheters may be necessary if placed over a joint or in a tortuous vein.

Purpose

The nurse performs venipuncture to

1. Obtain specimens of venous blood for laboratory determinations.
2. Maintain a patent venous route for use during emergency situations.
3. Provide a route for administration of IV fluids, medications, and blood products.
4. Provide nutritional supplements and hydration for patients unable to obtain them by other means.

Prerequisite Knowledge and Skills

Prior to performing venipuncture, the nurse should understand

1. Principles of aseptic technique.
2. Principles of universal precautions.
3. Anatomy of the vascular system.
4. General principles of IV therapy.
5. Factors affecting fluid and electrolyte balance.

The nurse should be able to perform

1. Proper handwashing techniques (see Skill 35–5).
2. Universal precautions (see Skill 35–1).
3. Cardiovascular and fluid and electrolyte assessments.
4. Administration of intravenous therapy.
5. Proper recording of intake and output.

Assessment

1. Identify patients at risk for fluid and electrolyte imbalance, such as those with cardiovascular disease, malnutrition, trauma, gastroenteritis, cancer, endocrine disorders, nasogastric suctioning, and fistulas and postoperative patients, postpartum patients, premature infants, and organ-donor patients. **Rationale:** Identify potential and actual problems that place a patient at risk for fluid and electrolyte imbalances.

2. Observe for signs and symptoms of fluid and electrolyte imbalance, including skin turgor, volume of neck veins, daily weights, intake and output totals, and mucous membranes. **Rationale:** A systematic assessment is necessary to identify fluid and electrolyte imbalances.

3. Assess patient's age, general size, skin condition, anatomy of venous system (Fig. 9–1), peripheral grafts, or shunts. **Rationale:** Assists in selection of appropriate site and catheter.

4. Obtain history of allergies, peripheral vascular disease, cellulitis, thrombosis, and vascular surgery. **Rationale:** Assists in appropriate site selection and prevents allergic reaction to prep solutions.

5. Assess the electrolyte profile and complete blood count. **Rationale:** Assists in monitoring the success or need for change in therapy.

6. Assess dietary intake. **Rationale:** Identifies alterations in nutritional and fluid requirements.

Nursing Diagnoses

1. Potential for infection related to puncture of skin. **Rationale:** Skin is the first and best line of defense against infection.

2. Anxiety related to anticipation of pain of needle stick or underlying diagnosis. **Rationale:** Excessive anxiety may decrease patient cooperation during procedure.

3. Fluid volume deficit or excess related to underlying disease process. **Rationale:** Fluid imbalance is the primary reason for IV fluid or medication administration.

4. Altered nutrition: Less than body requirements related to underlying disease process. **Rationale:** IV therapy provides an administration route for peripheral nutrition and fluid replacement when patients are unable to eat.

Planning

1. Individualize the following goals for performing venipuncture:
   a. Establish a patent venous access. **Rationale:** A patent access allows for administration of intravenous therapy, medications, and peripheral parenteral nutrition.
   b. Optimize fluid balance. **Rationale:** Venipuncture allows administration of fluids, nutrients, and medications when patients are unable to utilize an oral route.

2. Prepare all necessary equipment and supplies. **Rationale:** Assembly of all the necessary equipment at the bedside ensures that the venipuncture will be completed quickly and efficiently.
   a. Catheter of appropriate size and length.
   b. IV fluid as prescribed.
   c. IV administration set.
   d. Tourniquet.
   e. Povidone-iodine prep pads or alcohol prep pad if iodine allergy noted.
   f. Tape (1 roll of 1 in).
   g. Povidone-iodine ointment.
   h. Sterile gauze or transparent polyurethane dressing (small).
   i. Exam gloves.
   j. 3 to 5 cc normal saline flush.

3. Prepare the patient.
   a. Explain the procedure to patient. **Rationale:** Reduces anxiety.
   b. Describe patient's participation and importance of holding still during procedure. **Rationale:** Encourages cooperation and facilitates the venipuncture.
   c. Assist in positioning the patient in a comfortable position that allows easy access to the desired site. **Rationale:** Promotes comfort and reduces strain.
   d. Identify accessible veins (see Fig. 9–1). **Rationale:** Appropriate vein selection promotes success of catheter placement.

Implementation

Steps	Rationale	Special Considerations
1. Prepare IV infusion, and prime tubing.	Allows procedure to be completed expediently and maintains patency of the IV line.	

Table continues on following page

Steps	Rationale	Special Considerations
2. Wash hands.	Reduces transmission of microorganisms.	
3. Don gloves.	Universal precautions.	
4. Apply tourniquet proximal to proposed puncture site.	Increases venous pressure and allows better visualization of accessible vessels.	
5. Select appropriate venipuncture site.	Multiple factors determine the success of securing and maintaining a patent venous route.	Vein size, elasticity, and distance below skin; use most distal branch of vein selected. May need to use smaller or shorter catheters in elderly or very young patients because of the fragile nature of their veins. It may be difficult to find and access superficial veins in obese patients. Venipuncture is contraindicated in sites that show signs and symptoms of infection.
6. Release tourniquet.	Prolonged vein distension causes undue patient discomfort and impairs circulation to the extremity.	In some cases (e.g., tortuous, sclerosed veins), a tourniquet may increase venous pressure to the extent that vein may rupture when punctured.
7. Cleanse area with povidone-iodine prep pad and allow solution to dry.	Decreases number of skin microorganisms.	Note allergies and skin sensitivities. (If allergic to surface iodine, use alcohol wipes.)
8. Reapply tourniquet.	Distends venous circulation for easier puncture.	
9. Puncture skin with needle at a 45-degree angle, bevel up, parallel to the vein (Fig. 9–2A).	Causes least amount of discomfort.	
10. Reduce angle of needle, insert ⅛ to ¼ in into vein, and observe for retrograde blood flow in catheter hub.	Prevents the needle from puncturing the posterior wall of the vein.	
11. Release tourniquet.	Discourages rupture of veins as catheter is advanced.	
12. Advance catheter following appropriate procedure for needle type.		
a. Catheter over needle (Fig. 9–3):		
(1) Holding stylet in place, slowly advance catheter over the stylet to the desired position (see Fig. 9–2).	Stabilization of stylet reduces the chance of puncturing posterior aspect of vein.	
(2) Remove stylet while holding catheter hub.	Prevents dislodging catheter.	*Do not* reinsert needle into catheter if unsuccessful, since it may shear catheter.
(3) Connect primed IV administration set to catheter hub.	Provides direct entrance for IV fluids to flow through catheter.	
(4) Initiate flow of IV fluid, and assess for signs of infiltration.	If stylet has punctured back wall of vein, fluid will infuse into surrounding tissue, as evidenced by local edema and/or hematoma formation.	

Table continues on following page

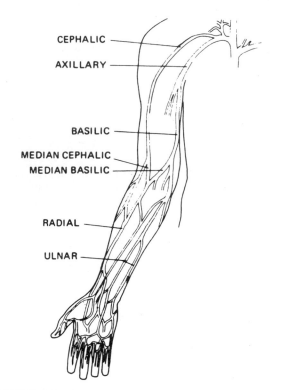

FIGURE 9–1. Anatomy of veins of the upper extremity. (Reproduced with permission from J. Donegan (Ed.), *Textbook of Advanced Cardiac Life Support*. Dallas: American Heart Association, 1987, p. 143.)

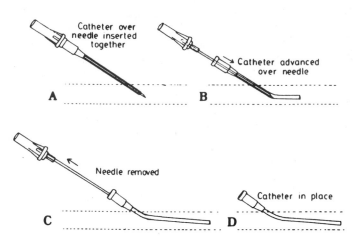

FIGURE 9–2. Insertion of catheter over the needle. (Reproduced with permission from J. Donegan (Ed.), *Textbook of Advanced Cardiac Life Support*. Dallas: American Heart Association, 1987, p. 141.)

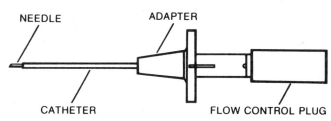

FIGURE 9–3. Components of the catheter-over-the-needle type of insertion set.

Steps	Rationale	Special Considerations
(5) Secure catheter with tape.	Prevents catheter movement, which could irritate intima of vein and lead to phlebitis.	
b. Catheter through needle (Fig. 9–4):		
(1) Stabilize stylet by holding hub, and advance catheter by applying pressure at base of catheter in plastic sleeve (Fig. 9–5).	Reduces risk of puncturing posterior aspect of vein.	If insertion of catheter through needle is unsuccessful, remove catheter and needle simultaneously.
(2) Engage needle hub into catheter hub. If catheter is inserted at least 4 in but less than its full length, it is necessary to pull needle back until it engages the catheter hub.	Connects needle to catheter.	
(3) Apply slight pressure above puncture site with nondominant hand, and use dominant hand to withdraw stylet from vein, exposing 1½ in of catheter.	Eliminates excessive bleeding or trauma.	
(4) Remove catheter guard sleeve, holding catheter hub securely.	Prevents its accidental removal.	
(5) Remove flow-control plug and stylet.	Promotes solution flow.	

Table continues on following page

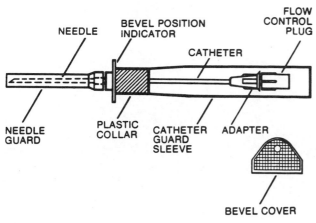

FIGURE 9–4. Components of the catheter-through-the-needle type of insertion set.

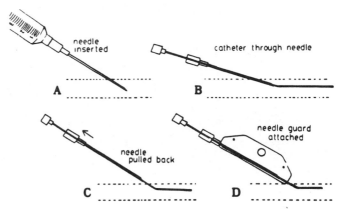

FIGURE 9–5. Insertion of catheter through the needle. (Reproduced with permission from J. Donegan (Ed.), *Textbook of Advanced Cardiac Life Support*. Dallas: American Heart Association, 1987, p. 142.)

Steps	Rationale	Special Considerations
(6) Connect primed IV fluid administration set to catheter hub.	Allows flow of solution from bag to patient.	
(7) Initiate flow of IV fluid.	Activates solution flow from bag to patient.	
(8) Apply needle guard securely over tip of needle.	The guard protects the catheter from being pierced by the needle inadvertently. Needle and catheter should be firmly in the groove of the needle guard before it is closed. If the catheter is not in the groove, infusion will cease when the guard is closed.	
(9) Secure with tape.	Prevents accidental dislodgment.	
c. Multiple-lumen peripheral catheter (Fig. 9–6):	Need for simultaneous but separate venous access sites.	If central venous access is contraindicated or unavailable.
(1) Flush the proximal port through the infusion cap with 3 to 5 cc of normal saline while holding the catheter in an upright position (Fig. 9–7).	Activates the catheter's hydrophilic coating, thereby decreasing resistance during insertion.	*Do not* allow the flush solution to go beyond the tip of the catheter because it might occlude the introducer needle and interfere with flashback.
(2) After entering the vein, advance the catheter and needle as a unit approximately ¼ to ½ in (Fig. 9–8).	Ensures that vessel dilation is complete.	
(3) Hold stylet hub in place while slowly advancing catheter over the stylet to the desired position (Fig. 9–9).	Prevents dislodging of catheter.	
(4) Remove needle while holding catheter hub.	Prevents dislodging of catheter.	
(5) Connect primed IV administration set to distal port.	Maintains patency of catheter and prevents air emboli.	*Do not* begin infusion until proximal lumen placement is verified.

Table continues on following page

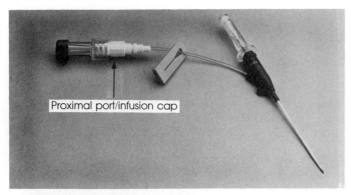

FIGURE 9–6. Multilumen peripheral catheter. (Courtesy of Arrow International, Inc.)

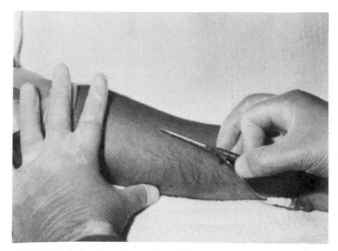

FIGURE 9–8. Insertion of multilumen peripheral catheter and needle into vein. (Courtesy of Arrow International, Inc.)

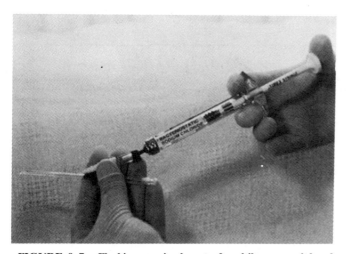

FIGURE 9–7. Flushing proximal port of multilumen peripheral catheter. (Courtesy of Arrow International, Inc.)

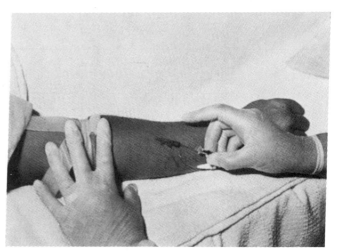

FIGURE 9–9. Advancing multilumen peripheral catheter into vein. (Courtesy of Arrow International, Inc.)

Steps	Rationale	Special Considerations
(6) Check the proximal lumen placement by aspirating blood from the proximal port through the extension line, and then attach the primed IV administration set (Fig. 9–10).	Verifies placement within the vessel lumen.	If desired, the proximal port may be heparin-locked. A slide clamp is provided to occlude flow through the proximal lumen during cap or line changes.
(7) Secure the catheter with tape.	Prevents dislodgment of catheter.	
13. Apply povidone-iodine ointment at catheter insertion site, and cover with gauze or transparent dressing and tape.	Prevents early access of microorganisms to bloodstream and irritation of intimal lining of the vessel.	
14. Regulate IV infusion as prescribed.	Provides fluid delivery as prescribed.	Types of dressings may vary according to institutional policy. Transparent dressings may be preferred when extremely close site observation is needed.

Table continues on following page

Steps	Rationale	Special Considerations
15. Label dressing with date, time, catheter gauge and length, and initials.	Alerts staff to need for routine dressing (q48h and prn) and catheter changes (q72h and prn).	
16. Discard supplies in appropriate container.	Maintains universal precautions.	
17. Remove and discard gloves.	Universal precautions.	
18. Wash hands.	Reduces the transmission of microorganisms.	

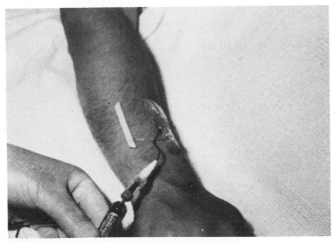

FIGURE 9–10. Checking proximal lumen placement of multilumen peripheral catheter. (Courtesy of Arrow International, Inc.)

Evaluation

1. Evaluate site for inflammation, delayed local edema, hematoma, and fluid leak. **Rationale:** May indicate infiltration or early signs of infection.
2. Evaluate extremity for impaired range of motion or circulatory compromise. **Rationale:** May indicate need to change catheter location or institute immobilization or compresses.

Expected Outcomes

1. Patent venous access. **Rationale:** Patency of the catheter is essential for rapid and efficient intervention when necessary.
2. No signs or symptoms of local or systemic inflammation or infection. **Rationale:** Local or systemic infection may predispose the patient to bacteremia/septicemia.

Unexpected Outcomes

1. Infiltration. **Rationale:** Prescribed fluid is infusing into interstitium.
2. Hematoma. **Rationale:** Indicates undue trauma to

vessel wall and/or extravasation of blood into the extravascular space.
3. Thrombosis. **Rationale:** Indicates loss of vessel patency and precludes the vessel for IV access.
4. Phlebitis. **Rationale:** Indicates inflammation of the vein from catheter trauma or early signs of infection.
5. Bacteremia. **Rationale:** Indicates presence of bacteria in the blood and possible contamination of the IV system; may progress to septicemia.
6. Septicemia. **Rationale:** Indicates systemic infection related to presence of bacteria in the blood.
7. Nerve damage. **Rationale:** Indicates trauma to adjacent or distal structures during insertion or infiltration.

Documentation

Documentation in the patient record should include date and time of insertion, insertion site, type of catheter, gauge and length of catheter, and any difficulty in performing venipuncture. **Rationale:** Provides a record of expected and unexpected outcomes and may give direction to appropriate site and catheter selection in future therapy.

Patient/Family Education

1. Discuss purpose of venipuncture, including patient in selection of site (if possible). Explain anticipated discomfort during venipuncture. **Rationale:** Encourages cooperation and understanding during procedure.
2. Answer patient and family concerns and questions regarding IV therapy. **Rationale:** Simple explanations decrease patient and family anxiety and may increase compliance with therapy.
3. Explain the signs and symptoms indicating the need for catheter site change (discomfort, burning, numbness, tingling, swelling) to both patient and family. **Rationale:** Enables the patient/family to recognize when IV is not functioning properly, and when to notify the nurse.
4. Evaluate the patient's need for long-term IV therapy. **Rationale:** Allows the nurse to anticipate the patient's needs for discharge to the floor or home.

Performance Checklist
Skill 9–1: Venipuncture

Critical Behaviors	Complies	
	yes	no
1. Prepare IV infusion, and prime tubing.		
2. Wash hands.		
3. Don gloves.		
4. Apply tourniquet proximal to proposed puncture site.		
5. Select site.		
6. Release tourniquet.		
7. Cleanse area with appropriate antiseptic solution.		
8. Reapply tourniquet.		
9. Puncture skin with needle at 45-degree angle, bevel up.		
10. Reduce angle, slowly advance needle, and observe for blood return.		
11. Release tourniquet.		
12. Insert catheter following appropriate procedure for needle type, connect primed IV administration set, and initiate flow, assessing for signs of infiltration.		
13. Secure catheter with tape.		
14. Apply povidone-iodine ointment at catheter insertion site, and secure catheter with gauze or transparent dressing and tape.		
15. Regulate infusion as prescribed.		
16. Label dressing with date, time, type of needle (gauge and length), and initials.		
17. Discard contaminated supplies.		
18. Remove and discard gloves, and wash hands.		
19. Document procedure in patient record.		

SKILL 9–2

Arterial Puncture

Arterial puncture is the percutaneous needle puncture of a peripheral artery to aspirate arterial blood for analysis. The sites most often used for arterial punctures include the radial, brachial, and femoral arteries. Arterial blood gas analysis provides a direct mechanism to assess a patient's oxygenation, acid–base balance, and to some extent, ventilation.

Disposable arterial puncture kits are available from many different manufacturers with various needle and syringe sizes. Because of the potential for patient discomfort, vasospasm, hematoma formation, or neurovascular compromise, arterial cannulation should be performed if frequent blood samples or continuous hemodynamic monitoring are needed (see Skills 10–5 and 10–7).

Purpose

The nurse performs arterial puncture to

1. Analyze arterial blood pH, oxygen tension (PaO_2), carbon dioxide tension ($PaCO_2$), arterial oxygen saturation (SaO_2), and acid–base balance.
2. Evaluate the management of altered acid–base states, metabolic acidosis and alkalosis, respiratory acidosis and alkalosis, and mixed acid–base disturbances.
3. Evaluate the management of hypoxic states.
4. Evaluate a patient's response to continuous ventilatory assistance and oxygen therapy.

Prerequisite Knowledge and Skills

Prior to performing an arterial puncture, the nurse should understand

1. Patient history of circulatory impairment of the extremities, allergies, and current medication profile.
2. Principles of aseptic technique.
3. Universal precautions.
4. Anatomy of arteries (radial, brachial, femoral) (Figs. 9–11 through 9–13).
5. Principles of arterial blood gas analysis.

The nurse should be able to perform:

1. Proper handwashing technique (see Skill 35–5).
2. Universal precautions.

3. Assessment of the respiratory system.
4. The Allen's test to select the radial artery with the best collateral circulation.

Assessment

1. Assess factors that influence ABG measurements, including anxiety, suctioning, patient positioning, body

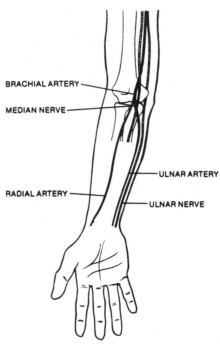

FIGURE 9–12. Anatomic landmarks for radial and brachial artery punctures.

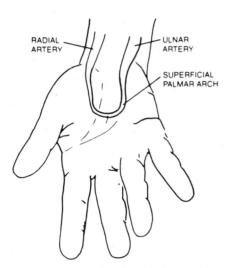

FIGURE 9–11. Anatomy of radial and ulnar arteries at wrist and superficial palmar arch. (Reproduced with permission from J. Donegan (Ed.), *Textbook of Advanced Cardiac Life Support*. Dallas: American Heart Association, 1987, p. 163.)

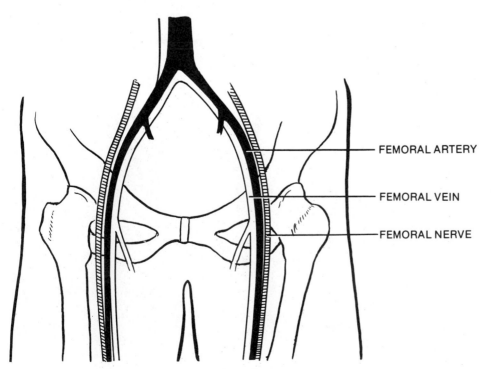

FIGURE 9–13. Anatomic landmarks for femoral artery puncture.

temperature, O_2 therapy, and metabolic rate. **Rationale:** Stated conditions or therapies can alter blood gas results.

2. Identify the need for ABG analysis. **Rationale:** Precludes unnecessary arterial puncture and allows early and appropriate intervention.

3. Evaluate history for allergies to various prep solutions, anesthetic agents, or drugs. **Rationale:** Prevents hypersensitivity reactions.

4. Obtain history of any recent surgeries. **Rationale:** Puncture of vessels or grafts may cause hematoma formation and impaired circulation.

5. Consider arterial catheter placement to facilitate obtaining serial arterial blood gas samples. **Rationale:** Repeated arterial punctures increase patient discomfort and risk of infection, hematoma, and vasospasm.

Nursing Diagnoses

1. Impaired gas exchange related to underlying disease process. **Rationale:** Arterial puncture is the most efficient method of quantifying arterial blood gas abnormalities and acid–base balance.

2. Impaired breathing patterns related to underlying disorder. **Rationale:** Understanding the presence and impact of underlying diseases may help in interpretation of ABGs.

3. Anxiety related to fear of the unknown and discomfort. **Rationale:** Anxiety may cause hyperventilation, resulting in arterial blood gas alterations.

4. Pain related to arterial puncture or potential arterial spasm. **Rationale:** Puncture of arterial wall may potentiate spasm of tunica media and alter blood flow.

5. Altered tissue perfusion related to hematoma formation or vasospasm. **Rationale:** Postprocedure hematoma and vasospasm may impair blood flow and lead to ischemia.

6. Potential for infection related to altered skin integrity. **Rationale:** Breaks in skin integrity increase the risk of nosocomial infection.

Planning

1. Individualize the following goals for performing arterial puncture:
   a. Analyze arterial blood gas status and acid–base balance. **Rationale:** Inadequate blood specimen will necessitate repeating procedure.
   b. Maintain adequate tissue perfusion. **Rationale:** Careful site selection and adequate hemostasis postprocedure will prevent complications.

2. Prepare all necessary equipment and supplies. **Rationale:** Assembly facilitates quick and efficient arterial puncture.
   a. Select a 20- to 25-gauge, ⅝- to 1½-in long hypodermic needle. Longer needles of at least 1 to 1½ in are required for brachial or femoral artery puncture.
   b. 1 to 5 cc glass or plastic syringe with a rubber stopper or cap. Many manufacturers distribute preheparinized syringes.

   c. One 1-ml ampule of sodium heparin, 1:1000 concentration, or manufacturer's preheparinized syringe.
   d. Providone iodine swabs, ×2.
   e. Alcohol wipes, ×2.
   f. Small pillow or rolled up towel.
   g. Ice-filled cup.
   h. Exam gloves.
   i. Lab slips.
   j. One or two 2 × 2 gauze pads.
   k. Tape, 1 roll of 1 in.

3. Prepare patient for puncture. **Rationale:** Decreases anxiety.

4. Select site.
   a. Use radial artery as first choice. **Rationale:** The radial artery is small and easily stabilized as it passes over a bony groove located at the wrist (Fig. 9–14).
   b. Perform Allen's test or modified Allen's test prior to radial artery cannulation. **Rationale:** Assesses collateral circulation (Fig. 9–15).
      (1) Instruct patient to form a tight fist or raise arm above heart level for several seconds to force blood from hand.
      (2) Apply direct pressure on radial and ulnar arteries to obstruct arterial blood flow to hand while patient opens and closes fist rapidly several times.
      (3) Instruct patient to open hand or keep arm above heart level with radial artery compressed.
      (4) Examine palmar surface for an erythematous blush or pallor within 6 seconds. An erythematous blush indicates ulnar artery patency and is interpreted as a *positive* Allen's test. Pallor indicates occlusion of the ulnar artery and is interpreted as a *negative* Allen's test. With a negative Allen's test, radial arterial puncture should not be done (see Fig. 9–15).
   c. Use brachial artery as second choice, except in

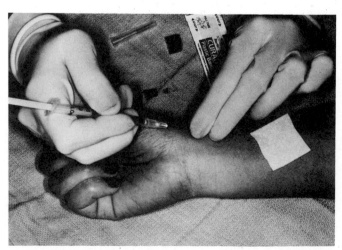

FIGURE 9–14. Radial artery puncture. (Courtesy of authors.)

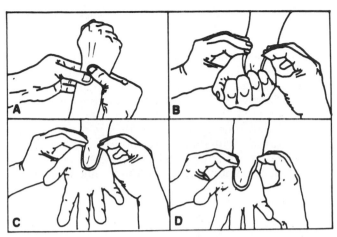

FIGURE 9–15. Modified Allen's test. (*A*) While patient's hand is held overhead with fist clenched to exsanguinate it, both radial and ulnar arteries are compressed. The hand is lowered (*B*) and opened (*C*). (*D*) Pressure is then released over the ulnar artery. (Reproduced with permission from J. Donegan (Ed.), *Textbook of Advanced Cardiac Life Support*. Dallas: American Heart Association, 1987, p. 164.)

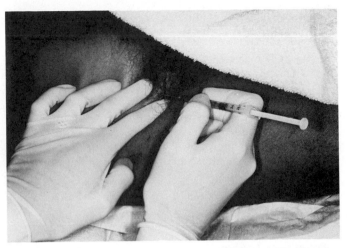

FIGURE 9–17. Femoral artery puncture. (Courtesy of authors.)

the case of poor pulsation due to shock, obesity, or sclerotic vessel (Fig. 9–16). **Rationale:** The brachial artery is larger than the radial artery. Pressure control after percutaneous puncture is enhanced by its proximity to bone if the entry point is approximately 1½ in above the antecubital fossa.

d. Use the femoral artery in the case of cardiopulmonary arrest or altered perfusion to the upper extremity arteries (Fig. 9–17). **Rationale:** The femoral artery is a large superficial artery located in the groin. It is easily palpated and punctured. Complications surrounding femoral artery puncture include hemorrhage and hematomas as bleeding is difficult to control, venous blood contamination as the femoral artery and vein lie in close proximity, infection as aseptic technique in the groin and pubic area is more difficult to maintain, and limb ischemia if the

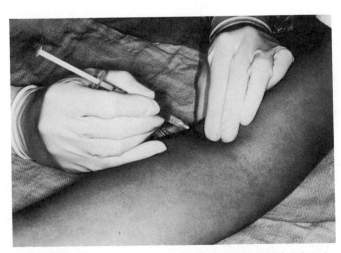

FIGURE 9–16. Brachial artery puncture. (Courtesy of authors.)

femoral artery is damaged. Femoral punctures may be utilized by physicians only. Check institutional policy for nursing utilization.

5. Position patient. **Rationale:** Enhances accessibility to the site and promotes patient comfort.
   a. Radial arterial puncture.
      (1) Semirecumbent position. **Rationale:** Position of comfort decreases anxiety.
      (2) Providing support with a small pillow, elevate and dorsiflex the wrist. **Rationale:** Moves artery closer to the skin surface making the artery easier to palpate.
      (3) Rotate hand until pulse is palpable. **Rationale:** Identification and localization of a pulse increase the chance for a successful radial artery puncture.
   b. Brachial arterial puncture.
      (1) Semirecumbent position. **Rationale:** Position of comfort decreases anxiety.
      (2) Elevate and hyperextend the arm. Support with a pillow. **Rationale:** Increases accessibility for puncture.
      (3) Rotate patient's arm until the pulse is palpable. **Rationale:** Assists with identification and localization of a pulse and increases the chance for a successful brachial artery puncture.
   c. Femoral arterial puncture. Use a supine straight leg position. **Rationale:** Provides the best position for locating the femoral pulse.

6. Heparinize syringe and needle.
   a. Assemble 22-gauge short-bevel needle on syringe. **Rationale:** Decreases the risk of overshooting the artery during entry.
   b. Prime syringe and needle with heparin, leaving only enough heparin to fill the needle and hub. **Rationale:** Prevents specimen coagulation. Excess heparin lowers pH and $PaCO_2$.
   c. Eject all air bubbles from syringe. **Rationale:** Maintains accuracy of blood gas values.

7. Wash hands and don gloves. **Rationale:** Universal precautions.
8. Prepare site.
   a. Cleanse selected site in circular motion outward with povidone-iodine or prep swabs; allow to dry. **Rationale:** Decreases risk of local infection or systemic sepsis.
   b. Cleanse site with alcohol swab; allow to dry. **Rationale:** Removes iodine coloring from skin, thereby increasing vessel visibility. Puncturing through a moist alcohol-prepared site increases pain.
9. Locally anesthetize site (optional). **Rationale:** Minimizes discomfort.
   a. Use a 1-ml syringe with 25-gauge needle and lidocaine (Xylocaine 1%) without epinephrine. **Rationale:** Increases patient comfort, decreases vessel trauma, and epinephrine decreases the incidence of peripheral vasoconstriction.
   b. Aspirate prior to injecting local anesthetic. **Rationale:** Ascertains the blood vessel has not been entered.
   c. Inject intradermally and then with full infiltration around artery. Use approximately 0.2 to 0.3 ml for an adult. **Rationale:** Decreases the incidence of localized discomfort while injecting all skin layers.

Implementation

Steps	Rationale	Special Considerations
1. Perform percutaneous puncture of selected artery.		
a. Locate pulsating artery.	Increases likelihood of correct location in artery.	
b. Stabilize artery by pulling skin taut and bracketing the area of maximum pulsation with fingertips of free hand.	Decreases chance of vessel rolling, and increases accuracy of puncture.	
c. Puncture skin slowly, holding syringe like a pencil; advance needle slowly with bevel upward at approximately 45- to 60-degree angle to the radial or brachial artery. For femoral arterial puncture, a 90-degree angle is used.	A slow, gradual thrust will promote arterial entry without passing directly through posterior wall.	Enter at an angle comfortable for stabilizing your hand. Certainty of position is more important than entry angle.
d. Observe syringe for flashback of arterial blood.	Pulsation of blood into the syringe verifies that the artery has been punctured.	Flashback occurs easily with a glass syringe. Gentle aspiration may be needed with a plastic syringe.
e. If puncture is unsuccessful, withdraw needle to skin level, angle slightly toward artery, and readvance. Do not completely withdraw needle.	Prevents necessity of another puncture and changes angle to better locate vessel.	
2. Obtain 1- to 5-cc of blood. Accurate test can be done with as little as 1 cc of blood.	This amount allows for rechecking and additional studies if necessary.	Sample volumes will vary with technology used.
3. Withdraw needle while stabilizing barrel of syringe.	Prevents inadvertant aspiration of air during withdrawal.	Especially important when using a glass syringe.
4. Apply firm continuous pressure to arterial puncture site for 5 minutes or until bleeding stops. If bleeding persists, place ice pack over site and continue firm pressure. Once bleeding stops, apply 2 × 2 gauze dressing over puncture site and secure in place with 1 in tape.	Hematomas and hemorrhage can occur if pressure is not applied correctly.	Hematoma can cause circulatory impedance and discomfort and can predispose to infection. Apply firm pressure for 10 minutes if patient has a history of increased coagulation time.
5. Protect blood sample.		
a. Hold syringe upright; express any air bubbles rapidly.	Air bubbles may alter results.	

Table continues on following page

Steps	Rationale	Special Considerations
b. Seal needle or tip of syringe immediately using rubber stopper or cap.	Keep airtight to prevent alterations in results.	
c. Roll the syringe gently.	Mixes blood and heparin. Prevents clot formation.	
d. Immerse blood sample in enough ice for transport to laboratory.	Ice decreases temperature of sample to 4°C and slows oxygen metabolism. Delays of longer than 2 minutes may alter values.	A delay longer than 2 minutes without ice will alter values.
6. Label specimen, and complete appropriate laboratory requisition. Note the percent of O_2 therapy, respiratory rate, and ventilator settings, if applicable, the temperature, and the time the specimen was drawn.	Enhances accurate analysis of results.	
7. Expedite immediate laboratory services.	No test results for any specimen, even if chilled, can be accepted as reliable if sample is tested more than 15 to 30 minutes after arterial puncture.	
8. Dispose of gloves and supplies in appropriate receptacle.	Appropriate body substance isolation measures. Reduces transmission of microorganisms.	
9. Wash hands.	Reduces transmission of microorganisms.	

Evaluation

1. Evaluate neurovascular status of extremity. Check site for delayed hematoma formation and circulation to extremity. **Rationale:** Circulatory impairment can occur for various reasons, including arteriosclerosis (increased risk of thrombosis, especially in femoral artery), large or small arterial occlusions (causes cold extremities, absent pulses, petechiae), local edema (internal hemorrhage), and neurovascular changes (tingling, pain).

2. Evaluate ABG results. **Rationale:** Provides data for evaluating oxygenation and ventilation and acid–base balance.

Expected Outcomes

1. Normal ABGs: pH = 7.35 to 7.45; $PaCO_2$ = 35 to 45 mmHg; PaO_2 = 80 to 100 mmHg; SaO_2 = 94 to 98 percent; Base excess (BE) = +2 to −2; and HCO_3 = 22 to 26 mEq/l. **Rationale:** Understanding of normal values is essential for accurate interpretation of ABG results. Normal values for COPD patients will vary.

2. ABG sample collected correctly. **Rationale:** Accuracy is directly related to the timeliness of obtaining and interpreting results.

3. Imbalances are identified and treated accordingly. **Rationale:** Early intervention is of utmost importance in medical management.

Unexpected Outcomes

1. Change in color, temperature, or pulse of extremity used for arterial puncture. **Rationale:** Signs and symptoms may indicate alteration in or impairment of circulation.

2. Hematoma or hemorrhage at the site of arterial puncture. **Rationale:** Any bleeding or hematoma formation is indicative of perforation of the vessel or bleeding dyscrasia.

3. Abnormal ABG results. **Rationale:** Patient unable to oxygenate effectively, inadequate FIO_2 delivery, or inability to excrete hydrogen ions effectively.

4. Allergy reaction to prep solution or drugs used. **Rationale:** Document allergies to prevent future administration. Administer local agents to decrease inflammatory process.

5. Sample collected incorrectly. **Rationale:** Recollection of sample leads to increased patient discomfort and a second invasive procedure.

Documentation

Documentation in the patient record should include site used, results of Allen's test, local anesthetic used (if applicable), how patient tolerated procedure, postpuncture site care, any untoward results or patient complaints, patient's temperature and O_2 therapy, disposition of sample, and results of ABG tests. **Rationale:** Provides a record of normal and abnormal results, appropriate interventions, and patient response. Serves as a legal medical record of the events.

Patient/Family Education

1. Explain the procedure and confirm patient and family understanding. **Rationale:** Understanding may improve cooperation during procedure. Need for repeated puncture may indicate need for indwelling arterial catheter.

2. Instruct patient and family to report signs and symptoms of neurovascular compromise, inflammation, or hematoma immediately. **Rationale:** Allows for early nursing and medical interventions.

Performance Checklist
Skill 9–2: Arterial Puncture

Critical Behaviors	Complies	
	yes	no
1. Select site.		
2. Position patient.		
3. Heparinize syringe and needle.		
4. Wash hands and don gloves.		
5. Prepare site.		
6. Locally anesthetize site (optional).		
7. Perform puncture.		
8. Obtain specimen.		
9. Withdraw needle while stabilizing barrel of syringe.		
10. Apply pressure to puncture site for at least 5 minutes.		
11. Expel air bubbles from syringe.		
12. Cap and roll syringe, ice sample.		
13. Label sample, and send to laboratory.		
14. Dispose of used supplies.		
15. Remove and discard gloves.		
16. Wash hands.		
17. Document procedure in patient record.		

REFERENCES

Craven, D. E., Lichtenberg, D. A., Kunches, L. M., et al. (1985). A randomized study comparing a transparent polyurethane dressing to a dry gauze dressing for peripheral intravenous catheter sites. *Infect. Control* 6(9):361–366.

Hecker, J. (1988). Improved technique in IV therapy. *Nurs. Times* 84(34):28–33.

Hoffman, K. K., Western, S. A., Kaiser, D. L., et al. (1988). Bacterial colonization and phlebitis-associated risk with transparent polyurethane film for peripheral intravenous site dressings. *Am. J. Infect. Control* 16(3):101–106.

Millam, D. A. (1988). Mastering arterial punctures. *Am. J. Nurs.* 99:1213–1224.

Miller, K. M. (1985). Arterial Puncture. In S. Millar, L. K. Sampson, and M. Soukup (Eds.), *AACN's Procedure Manual for Critical Care*, 2d Ed. (pp. 54–61). Philadelphia: Saunders.

Miller, K. M. (1985). Venipuncture. In S. Millar, L. K. Sampson, and M. Soukup (Eds.), *AACN's Procedure Manual for Critical Care*, 2d Ed. (pp. 41–46). Philadelphia: Saunders.

Potter, P. A., and Perry, A. G. (1989). Fluid, Electrolyte and Acid–Base Balances. In *Fundamentals of Nursing*, 2d Ed. (pp. 1022–1073). St. Louis: Mosby.

Thee, K. G., and Bednarczyk, L. (1988). Two-lumen peripheral IV catheter evaluation and overall clinical acceptance. *Journal of Intravenous Nursing*, 11(6):368–371.

BEHAVIORAL OBJECTIVES

After completing this chapter, the nurse will be able to

- Define the key terms.
- Discuss the equipment required for setup of a single or multiple pressure transducer system.
- Discuss care of the pulmonary artery catheter, arterial catheter, left atrial catheter, and central venous catheter.
- Identify normal and abnormal waveforms for hemodynamic pressures measured.
- Describe the nurse's role in removal of hemodynamic lines.
- Demonstrate the skills involved in hemodynamic monitoring.
- Develop a teaching plan for the patient who is being monitored hemodynamically.

HEMODYNAMIC MONITORING

Invasive hemodynamic monitoring is an essential technique for assessing the critically ill patient. When used properly, hemodynamic monitoring aids in the early identification of life-threatening conditions, in the evaluation of a patient's immediate response to therapy, and in medical diagnosis determination. The nurse prepares and cares for the hemodynamic monitoring equipment, evaluates the waveforms, interprets the data, and makes clinical decisions regarding changes in therapy. Invasive monitoring is not without risks to the patient; therefore, the nurse also must know how to detect and prevent complications of this clinical tool.

This chapter focuses on procedures for the various types of hemodynamic monitoring. Techniques discussed include setup and care of the pressure monitoring system, how to monitor central venous, right atrial, pulmonary artery, pulmonary wedge, left atrial, and arterial pressures, cardiac output techniques, and hemodynamic waveform analysis.

KEY TERMS

calibration
cardiac output
central venous pressure
left atrial pressure
leveling
pulmonary artery pressure

pulmonary artery wedge pressure
right atrial pressure
right ventricular pressure
transducer
zeroing

SKILLS

GUIDELINES

The following assessment guidelines assist the nurse in formulating a nursing diagnosis and an individualized plan of care to perform hemodynamic monitoring:

1. Know the patient's baseline and current cardiovascular assessment.
2. Know the patient's baseline and current vital signs, laboratory results, and fluid balance.
3. Know the patient's medical history.
4. Know the patient's current medical therapy and rationale for hemodynamic monitoring.
5. Know when hemodynamic monitoring catheters were placed.
6. Assess the location and patency of hemodynamic lines.
7. Assess all hemodynamic waveforms.
8. Continuously monitor ECG and hemodynamic pulse pressure waveforms.
9. Assess the patient's mental status and ability to comprehend verbal/written instructions.
10. Determine appropriate nursing diagnoses and interventions based on preceding assessments.

SKILL 10–1

Single and Multiple Pressure Transducer Systems (Reusable and Disposable)

A pressure transducer, when connected to a monitoring system, allows the nurse to continuously view intravascular and intracardiac pressures. The transducer detects dynamic signals from the intravascular pressure changes and transmits these signals to the bedside monitor. Reusable transducers are now in limited use because of the advantages of disposable transducers. In addition, it is difficult to measure more than one pressure from a reusable transducer without the use of a manifold. This skill will discuss the assembly of single and multiple, reusable and disposable pressure transducer systems (Figs. 10–1 to 10–3), and the procedures for leveling, zeroing, and calibration.

A multiple pressure transducer system is used when a patient requires monitoring of more than one or two pressures. A single pressure transducer system can be used to monitor one or two pressures. Arterial pressure monitoring requires a single pressure transducer, but when a PA catheter is added, a multiple transducer system is necessary.

Examples of the combinations of lines that may be monitored with a multiple pressure transducer system include:

- Arterial, pulmonary artery pressure (PAP), pulmonary artery wedge pressure (PAWP), and right atrial pressures (RAP).
- Arterial, left atrial (LAP), RA pressures (direct catheter into RA).
- Arterial, PAP (directly into PA), and RA pressures (directly into RA).

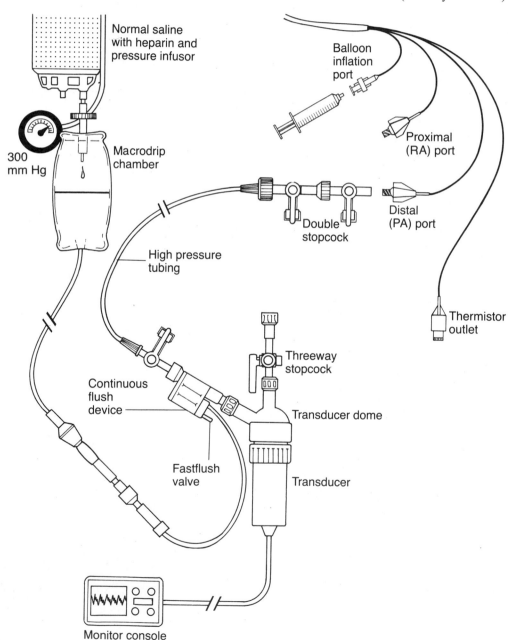

FIGURE 10–1. Single reusable pressure transducer system. (From G. O. Darovic, *Hemodynamic Monitoring*: Invasive and Noninvasive Clinical Application. Philadelphia: Saunders, 1987, p. 142, with permission.)

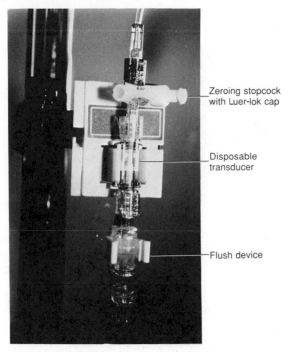

FIGURE 10–2. **Single disposable pressure transducer. (A). Schematic, (B). Actual setup. (Courtesy of Baxter Corporation, Edwards Division.)**

- Arterial, PA/PAW, RA, and left ventricular pressures (LVP, direct catheterization).
- Intraaortic balloon (IAB) catheter, arterial, radial arterial, PA/PAW, and RA pressures.

The combination of lines is determined by the patient's diagnosis and the rationale for monitoring. Pediatric and adult patients who undergo surgery for heart disease will often have anatomy that does not allow passage of a PA catheter. In these instances, the surgeon places an LA line, an RA line or both during surgery and brings these out through the abdomen wall via a subxiphoid incision. When patients undergoing cardiac transplantation have higher than normal PA pressures postoperatively, a direct catheter into the PA may be inserted. Patients on certain types of heart-assist devices require continuous direct monitoring of LV pressure. The IAB has a pressure lumen that opens in the arch of the aorta. This provides information on central arterial pressure, while the radial artery catheter provides information on peripheral perfusion pressures.

To ensure accuracy of the hemodynamic values obtained from any transducer system, four procedures are performed prior to monitoring: leveling, zeroing, instrument calibration, and transducer calibration. *Leveling* is performed to eliminate the effects of hydrostatic pressure on the transducer. It should be done before and after connecting the pressure system to the patient, with every change in bed height or changes in elevation of the head of the bed, with any significant change in the patient's hemodynamic variables, and prior to zeroing and calibration.

Zeroing is performed to eliminate the effects of atmospheric pressure on the transducer. Zeroing should be performed before and after connecting the pressure system to the patient, with any leveling change, and whenever there is significant change in the hemodynamic variables.

Instrument calibration is the third step in preparing a pressure transducer system. Calibration of the internal electronics of the monitor ensures that the pressure readings are accurate. Calibration is usually performed at the time of equipment setup, after the patient has been connected to the system, and at least once every 12 hours. Since newer monitoring systems are more accurate, the reader is referred to individual manufacturers' recommendations for whether or not calibration is necessary and how often to calibrate.

Transducer calibration is the final step in preparing a pressure transducer system. Transducer calibration is performed at the initiation of hemodynamic monitoring and whenever there is suspected damage to the transducer.

Purpose

The nurse assembles the equipment and maintains a pressure transducer system to

1. Ensure accurate measurement of intravascular pressures.
2. Prevent complications of pressure monitoring systems.

Prerequisite Knowledge and Skills

Prior to working with a single pressure transducer system, the nurse should understand

1. Purpose of a pressure bag.
2. Principles of aseptic technique.
3. Principles of signal transmission within a fluid coupling system.
4. Effects of patient position on pressure measurement.
5. Principles and rationale for a continuous flush device.

The nurse should be able to perform

1. Stopcock manipulation.
2. Zeroing, leveling, and calibration of the monitor and pressure transducer system.
3. Proper handwashing technique (see Skill 35–5).
4. Universal precautions (see Skill 35–1).

Assessment

1. Observe patient for signs and symptoms of critical illness that warrant use of a single pressure transducer system, including gradual or acute hypotension, dysrhythmias, circulatory collapse, cardiac arrest, hemorrhage, hypertension, hypoxemia, metabolic acidosis/alkalosis, respiratory acidosis/alkalosis, positive fluid

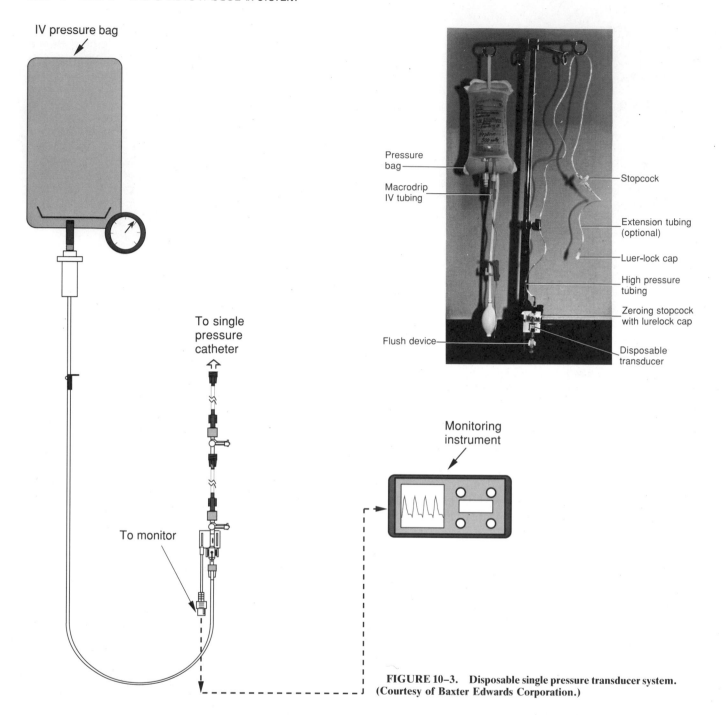

FIGURE 10–3.   Disposable single pressure transducer system. (Courtesy of Baxter Edwards Corporation.)

balance, oliguria, anuria, diminished mental alertness, and laboratory abnormalities (leukocytosis, hyperbilirubinemia, hyper- or hypoglycemia, liver function abnormalities, etc.). **Rationale:** The earlier signs and symptoms of critical illness are identified, the sooner an appropriate catheter can be placed for pressure measurement. Prompt treatment of critical illness is associated with improved chances for survival.

2.   Assess patient for history of catheter placement. Has the patient ever had an intravascular catheter? Did he or she experience any complications with the insertion or during the catheter's existence? Was the catheter placement recent (i.e., within the same hospitalization)? **Rationale:** A patient who had a difficult insertion in the

past will likely experience difficulty again. If a patient had an arterial line placed previously, within the same hospitalization, insertion into the same site should be avoided. Knowing that a patient experienced vascular complications from a previous catheter insertion would alert the nurse to be especially observant for circulatory problems again.

Nursing Diagnosis

Potential for infection related to disruption of the skin and access to the vascular system. **Rationale:** Pressure monitoring devices have been associated with the development of bacteremia (Tafuro and Ristuccia, 1984).

Planning

1. Individualize the following goals for assembling a single pressure transducer system:
   a. Maintain hemodynamic pressure(s) within prescribed parameters. **Rationale:** A single pressure transducer system is most commonly inserted for an acute physiologic crisis. The nurse should be prepared to assemble this system rapidly.
   b. Maintain a closed, aseptic monitoring system. **Rationale:** Bacteremia can result from contamination of the system, either during assembly or while in operation.
2. Prepare all necessary equipment and supplies and bring to bedside. **Rationale:** Assembly of all equipment facilitates the efficient monitoring of the hemodynamic profile.
   a. 500 ml of normal saline with or without heparin, as prescribed by physician.*
   b. Pressure bag for each intravenous flush bag.
   c. IV pole or other hook at the bedside.

   *The question of whether or not heparin is to be used in the flush solution is under investigation by AACN's "Thunder Project."

   d. IV tubing with macro drip chamber for each hemodynamic line.
   e. Pressure transducer for each hemodynamic line (or two lines can be monitored off one transducer).
   f. Transducer dome for reusable transducer only.
   g. Several three-way stopcocks. +
   h. Continuous flush device, one for each hemodynamic line. +
   i. Pressure tubing, one for each hemodynamic line. +
   j. Extension pressure tubing with stopcock, if desired.
   k. Bedside monitor.
   l. Transducer holder for IV pole or strap for securing transducer to arm or body.
   m. Syringe-type pump or microinfusion pump for pediatric patients *only*.
   n. Carpenter's level.

   +It is common now for these items to be assembled by the company who makes the tubing into a kit that is prepackaged, sterile, and ready to go. Kits such as these can be custom ordered to meet individual unit needs.

Implementation

Steps	Rationale	Special Considerations
Transducer Setup		
1. Wash hands.	Reduces transmission of microorganisms.	
2. Turn on bedside monitor 5 to 15 minutes prior to use.	Allows time to warm up.	
3. Plug transducer cable into monitor.	For signal transmission to oscilloscope.	
4. Turn on monitor screen that corresponds to the hook-in location of the transducer cables.	For waveform display.	Usually the monitor screen display has been programmed to show the waveforms in an order that corresponds to a particular jack for the cable; i.e., the top cable position corresponds to the first waveform position on the screen, etc.
5. Set or program the appropriate scale for the pressure being measured.	Necessary for visualization of the complete waveform and to obtain accurate readings.	PAP usually is measured on a 60-mmHg scale, RAP on a 30-mmHg scale, and arterial pressure on a 300-mmHg scale.
6. Flush solution: Draw up prescribed amount of heparin, and inject into a collapsible IV bag via the medication port. Prepare all bags in this manner.	Collapsible bag allows IV fluid to be pressurized. Heparin is thought to prevent the development of clots in the catheter, although further research is necessary to substantiate this practice.	The AACN Thunder Project is currently studying the issue of heparinization of arterial lines.
7. Label IV bags indicating dose of heparin, the date and time of addition, and your initials.	Documents when the IV solution was prepared and validates proper dilution.	

Table continues on following page

Steps	Rationale	Special Considerations
8. Label IV bags with IV tapes and mark the date and time each solution is hung.	Provides a method to account for the amount of flush solution delivered each shift.	One study (Von Rueden, 1984) found that the volume of flush solution delivered to cardiac surgery patients increased the 24-hour intake by 16 percent.
9. Remove all air from each bag using a 22-gauge needle inserted in the medication port, with bag in an inverted position (Fig. 10–4).	Prevents entry of air into the pressure transducer system.	
10. Spike outlet port of each flush solution with macrodrip IV tubing.	Accesses IV flush solution.	
11. Open the IV roller clamps, squeeze the drip chambers, and fill with IV solution to about one third.	Primes drip chamber.	It is important not to overfill this chamber. When the pressure is applied, it will fill more. Also, the nurse will want to be able to see that solution is flowing when performing a manual flushing of the invasive catheter.
12. Close the roller clamps and insert the IV bags into the pressure bags on IV pole. Flush the line under gravity and close the roller clamps.	Primes IV tubing.	By not pumping the bag up, there is less likelihood of turbulence from the high pressure and less chance of micro air bubble formation with flushing system. Air should never be allowed to develop in a hemodynamic system. Micro or macro air emboli can migrate to major organs and present a life-threatening blockage. This is especially important when catheters are in the heart or pulmonary artery. An undetected atrial septal defect or other congenital heart defect can allow passage of air emboli from the right side of the heart to the left side and then to the brain.

Table continues on following page

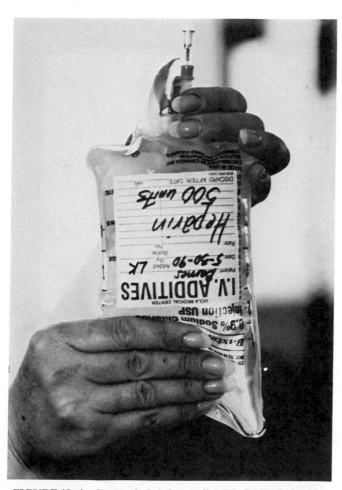

FIGURE 10–4. Removal of air from collapsible flush solution bag.

Steps	Rationale	Special Considerations
13. Following manufacturer's directions, attach transducers to holder/manifold and place on an IV pole.	Secures transducer.	It is not accurate or safe to leave a transducer lying on the bed.
For Single Reusable Transducer		
14. Remove protective cover from transducer. Draw up 1 ml of sterile water and drip onto transducer diaphragm. Do *not* overfill (Fig. 10–5).	Establishes an interface between the dome membrane and the diaphragm surface.	Saline may damage the delicate diaphragm. Maintain sterility of internal dome and diaphragm.
15. Screw sterile transducer dome onto diaphragm. Assemble the hemodynamic transducer, pressure tubing, and stopcock as shown in Fig. 10–1.	Pressure tubing conducts dynamic signals from patient's vessels to transducer. The dome is an essential part of the system.	The upper dome chamber (if present) will be flushed with the flush solution.
For Single Disposable Transducer:		
16. Open prepackaged single pressure transducer kit on clean surface, and check all connections to be sure that they are secure. *Or* assemble the hemodynamic transducer, pressure tubing, and stopcocks.	Prepackaged systems often have loose connections for sterilization purposes. Loose connections provide an entry point for bacteria and air.	If monitoring two pressures from one transducer, two stopcocks will be needed here, one for opening the transducer to air and one to connect to the second pressure tube (Fig. 10–6).
For Multiple Pressure Transducer System		
16. Assemble the hemodynamic transducer pressure tubing, stopcock, flush device, and transducer dome for each line as illustrated in Fig. 10–7.	Entire system should be assembled prior to flushing.	

Table continues on following page

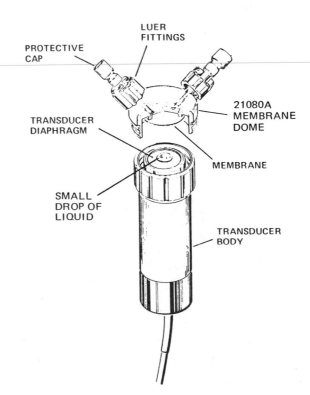

FIGURE 10–5. The components of the reusable pressure transducer. A drop of sterile water is placed on the diaphragm to establish a fluid interface between the dome chamber and the transducer diaphragm. (From Hewlett-Packard Operating Guide, *Physiological Pressure Transducer Series 1280, 1286*. Monterey Park, California, 1976, with permission.)

Steps	Rationale	Special Considerations
17. Flush entire system, including transducer, all stopcocks, and pressure tubing. Replace any vented caps with Luer-lok or "deadend" caps, and tighten securely.	Eliminates air from the system.	Many disposable pressure monitoring kits come with vented caps to allow for thorough sterilization. However, these vented caps will allow bacteria and air into the system.
18. Pump up pressure bag to 300 mmHg.	Pressure is required for most flush devices.	At 300 mmHg pressure, most flush devices deliver 3 cc/h.
19. Wash hands.	Reduces transmission of microorganisms.	

Leveling of Transducer

1. Wash hands.	Reduces transmission of microorganisms.	

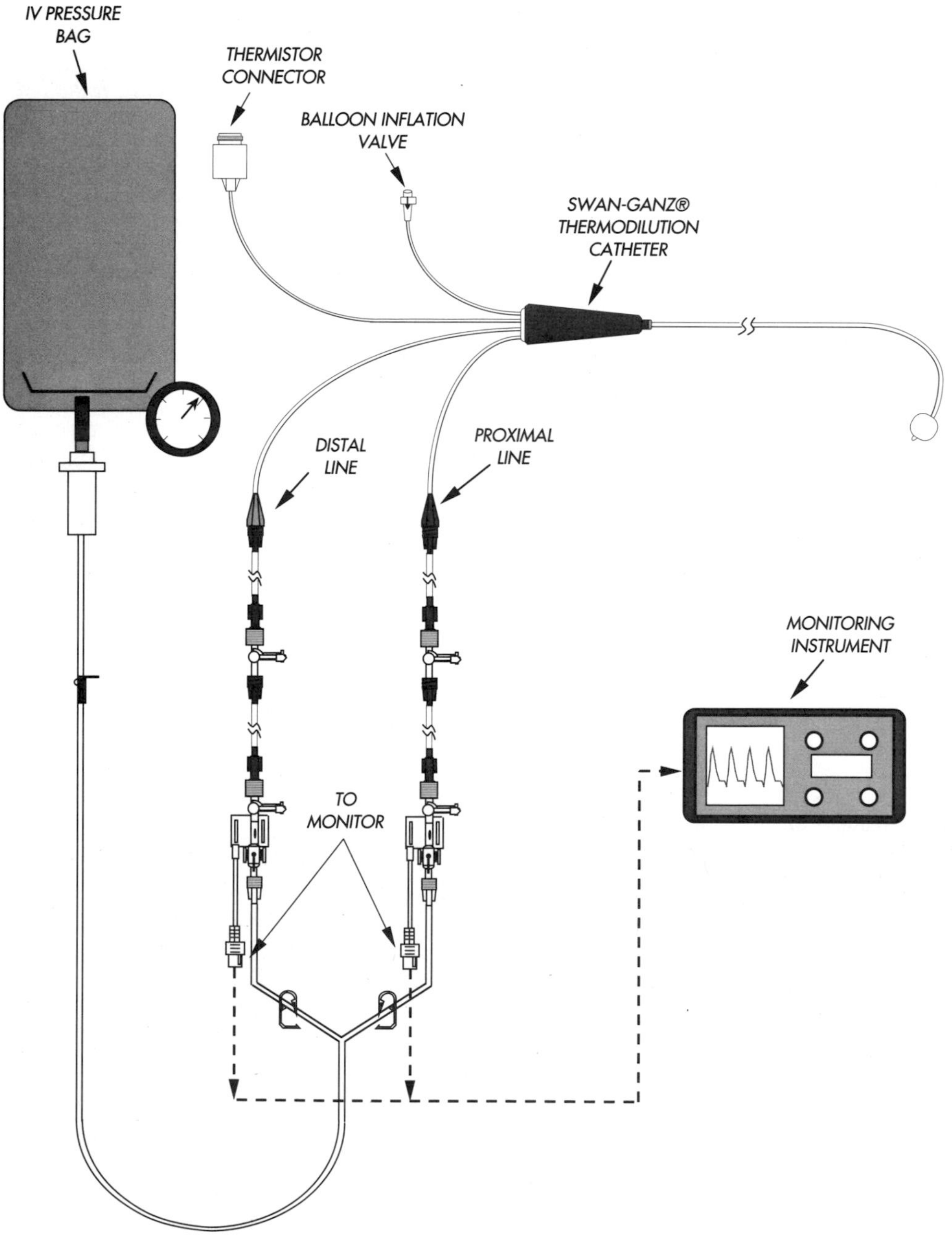

FIGURE 10–6. Monitoring two pressures from two transducers with a multiple pressure transducer system. (Courtesy of Baxter Edwards Corporation.)

Figure continues on following page

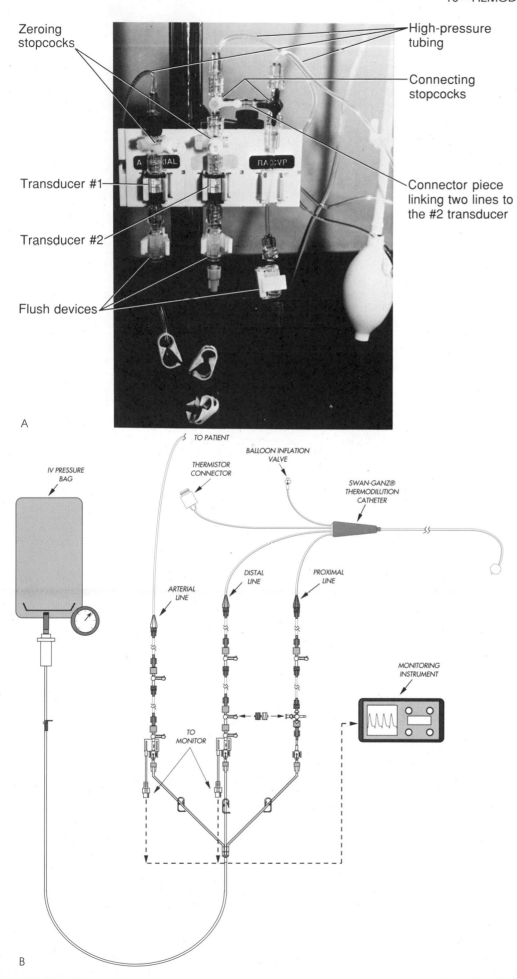

Zeroing stopcocks

High-pressure tubing

Connecting stopcocks

Transducer #1

Connector piece linking two lines to the #2 transducer

Transducer #2

Flush devices

A

TO PATIENT

IV PRESSURE BAG

THERMISTOR CONNECTOR

BALLOON INFLATION VALVE

SWAN-GANZ® THERMODILUTION CATHETER

ARTERIAL LINE

DISTAL LINE

PROXIMAL LINE

MONITORING INSTRUMENT

TO MONITOR

B

FIGURE 10–7A and B. Monitoring three pressures from two transducers with a multiple pressure transducer system. (Courtesy of Baxter Edwards Corporation.)

Steps	Rationale	Special Considerations
2. Position the bed so that the patient is in a 0 to 45 degrees, supine position.	Ensures accuracy of readings.	A number of research studies have supported the taking of PAP in a supine position with the head of the bed (HOB) elevated. (Ahlberg et al., 1989; Chulay and Miller, 1984; Laulive, 1982; Woods et al., 1982). The taking of readings with the HOB greater than 45 degrees has been studied, but further research is needed. Research on lateral positioning for PAP and PCW pressure readings remains controversial (Groom et al., 1990; Keating et al., 1986; Kennedy et al., 1984; Osika, 1989; Wild, 1984).
3. Locate the phlebostatic axis (Fig. 10–8): a. Locate the fourth intercostal space (ICS) on the edge of the sternum. b. Draw an imaginary line along the fourth ICS laterally, along the chest wall. c. Draw a second line from the axilla downward, midway between the anterior and posterior chest wall.	Serves as the reference point for the level of the transducer, which ensures accuracy in heart pressures (at the level of right atrium) by eliminating the effect of hydrostatic forces on the transducer. For example, if the transducer were located at a level above the right atrium, the hydrostatic forces would be moving away from the transducer and result in a falsely low reading. Ensures consistency of hemodynamic readings. The difference in measured values is approximately 2 mmHg per inch.	When the patient is in a lateral position, the exact location of the phlebostatic axis can be unclear. Some have advocated that the midsternum is the correct location, while others maintain that it is unchanged from the standard midaxillary location (Groom et al., 1990). Further research is needed to guide the nurse on how and when to take measures in a lateral position.

Table continues on following page

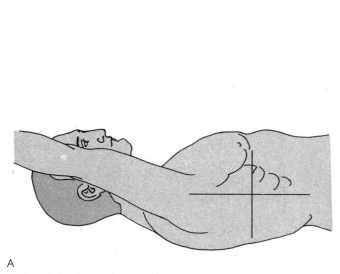

A

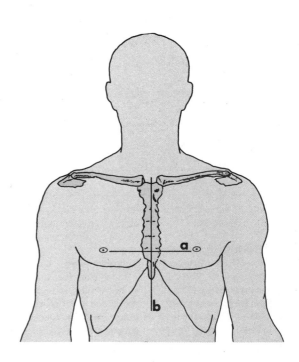

B

FIGURE 10–8. Transducer leveling from different positions. (*A*) Phlebostatic axis in the supine patient. (*B*) Transducer leveling position in the anterior lateral position.

Figure continues on following page

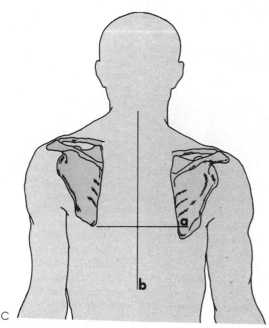

C

FIGURE 10–8. Cont'd. (*C*) **Transducer leveling position in the posterior lateral position.** (From T. Taylor, Monitoring left atrial pressures in the open-heart surgical patient. *Crit. Care Nurs.* 6(2):64–65, 1985, with permission.)

Steps	Rationale	Special Considerations
d. Where these two lines cross is the level of the right atrium (phlebostatic axis).		
e. Mark and maintain this line with skin marker.		
4. Place the carpenter's level between the phlebostatic axis and the air–fluid interface of the transducer. Move the transducer up or down the IV pole until the bubble is centered (Fig. 10–9).	Ensures that the transducer is level with the phlebostatic axis or the tip of the catheter.	Some have advocated the "eyeball" method of leveling the transducer, i.e., the performance of the leveling without the carpenter's level (Kolodychuk et al., 1989). Further research is needed to substantiate this method. In addition, there are new devices that utilize a light beam attached to the transducer to level to the phlebostatic axis. This device would replace the carpenter's level.

Zeroing the Transducer

Steps	Rationale	Special Considerations
1. Wash hands.	Prevents bacterial contamination.	
2. Open the stopcock located on the transducer to air.	So monitor can use atmospheric pressure as a reference for zero.	
3. Push and release the zeroing button on the bedside monitor. Observe the digital reading to fall to a "zero" value display. If the value is greater than 2, the transducer may be defective.	So monitor can automatically adjust itself to zero. Zeroing negates the effects of atmospheric pressure so that the only pressure values that are measured are the ones within the blood vessel or within the heart.	On older models, the zero button may need to be turned and adjusted manually.
4. Turn stopcock back to open position and resume pressure monitoring.	Pressure monitoring cannot occur if stopcock is not in open position.	

Table continues on following page

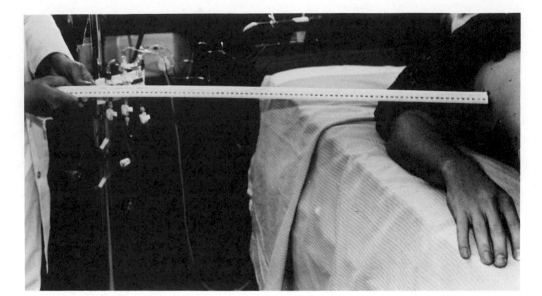

FIGURE 10–9. Leveling transducer to phlebostatic axis.

Steps	Rationale	Special Considerations
Calibration of Monitor		
1. Wash hands.	Reduces transmission of microorganisms.	
2. Open stopcock next to the transducer to air. Observe the digital display on the bedside monitor to ensure that it reads zero.	Transducer should be zeroed prior to calibration.	
3. Depress the "cal" button on the bedside monitor.	Activates the calibration procedure, which is a totally internal process.	Always consult the manufacturer's guidelines for how to perform calibration. Newer equipment does not require manual calibration.
4. After the number stabilizes, adjust the control knob until the appropriate calibration factor is reached (refer to manufacturer's guidelines for the calibration factor).	Minor adjustments in calibration may need to be performed manually.	
5. Release the control knob, and observe that the digital display returns to zero. If it does not, notify biomedical engineer.	The digital display should return to zero.	
Calibration of Reusable Transducer		
1. Wash hands.	Reduces transmission of microorganisms.	
2. Attach a mercury manometer to one of the Luer-lok fittings of the transducer dome (Fig. 10–10).	The mercury manometer serves as the calibration reference.	
3. Attach a hand bulb to the other Luer-lok.	The bulb is used to apply pressure to the transducer.	
4. Turn off hand-bulb control knob (as in manual blood pressure procedure).	Allows air to move into system under pressure.	

Table continues on following page

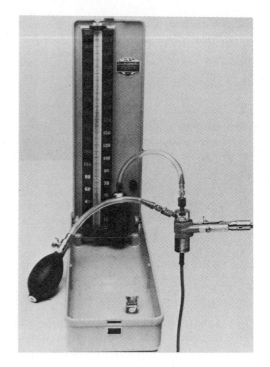

FIGURE 10–10. Calibration of reusable transducer. (From E. K. Daily and J. S. Schroeder, *Techniques in Bedside Hemodynamic Monitoring*, 4th Ed. St. Louis: Mosby, 1989, p. 43, with permission.)

Steps	Rationale	Special Considerations
5. Pump bulb until the mercury column in the manometer reads 200 mmHg.	200 mmHg is used as calibration factor, but any number could be used.	
6. Simultaneously observe the bedside monitor, which also should read 200 ± 2 mmHg.	If the digital readout corresponds with the mercury manometer, then the transducer is functioning properly and can be used.	
7. Release the hand-bulb control knob, and observe for return of digital readout to zero.	Ensures that transducer is sensitive in reading lower values.	
8. Prior to patient monitoring, remove dome used for calibration and replace with a new sterile dome.	Maintains sterility of system.	

Calibration of Paper Printout

Steps	Rationale	Special Considerations
1. During the zeroing procedure of the monitor as stated above, turn paper printer on a slow speed and adjust stylus to the bottom line on the paper grid.	Since it is rare that a pressure will be less than zero, it is appropriate for the first line on the grid to be zero. It is important that a consistent zero point on the paper be used; making the bottom line zero is easy for all medical personnel to remember.	On newer monitoring equipment, the bottom line is preset as zero, and the pressure scale is preset. (Refer to manufacturer's directions for how to adjust this.)
2. Press the calibration button and simultaneously adjust the stylus to the line where you want the calibration factor value to be measured.	An accurate adjustment of the scale is necessary to obtain an accurate documentation of pressure readings.	Again, this may be automatically preset on newer monitoring equipment.
3. Release calibration button, and the paper will now be ready for printing hemodynamic waveforms.	The stylus returns to zero, and you now have a scale for reading pressures from the paper printout.	

Evaluation

Evaluate for hemodynamic stability before and after instituting hemodynamic monitoring. **Rationale:** Hemodynamic monitoring provides data concerning the patient's physiologic functioning on which clinical decisions are based.

Expected Outcomes

1. Proper performance of the pressure transducer system: clearly visible waveform on the oscilloscope without dampening; a clear and accurate waveform on paper printout from which pressure measurements can be made. **Rationale:** If the transducer and monitor are properly connected, zeroed, leveled, and calibrated and the system is without air, the waveforms should be clear and accurate and should print out on the bedside monitor. Contact biomedical engineering to evaluate waveforms that are of poor quality and which you cannot troubleshoot.

2. Patient will not exhibit any symptoms or signs of infections, i.e., fever, chills, increased white blood cell count (WBC), or redness at catheter site. **Rationale:** Aseptic technique used in the setup and handling of the system decreases the risk of infection.

Unexpected Outcomes

1. Loss of or dampened waveform or the scale on the paper printout is incorrect, resulting in incorrect values and improper treatment of the problem. **Rationale:**

Loss of or dampened waveforms occur when air is in the system, a stopcock has been left closed, connections are loose, or the system is not properly zeroed, leveled, and calibrated.

2. Patient develops a catheter-related sepsis, with fever, chills, increased systemic vascular resistance, decreased cardiac output (CO), positive blood cultures, and increased WBC. **Rationale:** There are multiple entry sites for bacteria in pressure transducer systems.

Documentation

Documentation in the patient record should include the date and time of setup, the time the system is zeroed, leveled, and calibrated, the type of flush solution used, the amount of heparin used, and the amount of flush solution infused. **Rationale:** Documents nursing care given.

Patient/Family Education

Instruct the patient and family about the purpose of pressure transducer system. Show them the bedside waveform, and explain how it assists the nurse in making decisions about the patient's care. **Rationale:** Reduces patient and family anxiety about the multiple pieces of equipment at the bedside.

Performance Checklist
Skill 10–1: Single and Multiple Pressure Transducer Systems (Reusable and Disposable)

Critical Behaviors	Complies	
	yes	no
1. Wash hands.		
2. Turn on bedside monitor.		
3. Plug transducer cable into monitor.		
4. Turn on appropriate monitor oscilloscope.		
5. Set oscilloscope scale for pressure being measured.		
6. Inject prescribed amount of heparin into collapsible IV bag.		
7. Label IV bag with heparin dose, date, and time.		
8. Label IV bag with IV tape and mark date and time hung, and initial.		
9. Remove all air from IV bag.		
10. Spike outlet port of flush bag with IV tubing.		
11. Fill drip chamber one third full with flush solution.		
12. Insert flush solution into high-pressure bag, and flush IV tubing.		
13. Attach transducer holder/manifold to IV pole, and attach transducer to holder.		
FOR REUSABLE TRANSDUCER 1. Draw up sterile water and apply to transducer diaphragm.		
2. Attach sterile transducer dome.		

Table continues on following page

Critical Behaviors	Complies	
	yes	no
3. Assemble pressure transducer system (or open kit), and tighten all connections.		
4. Document in patient record.		
FOR MULTIPLE TRANSDUCER 1. Assemble hemodynamic system.		
2. Flush entire system and replace vented caps with deadend caps.		
3. Pump pressure bag to 300 mmHg.		
4. Wash hands.		
5. Document in patient record.		
LEVELING OF TRANSDUCER 1. Position patient with HOB 0 to 45 degrees, supine.		
2. Locate phlebostatic axis.		
3. Use carpenter's level to level air–fluid interface of transducer with phlebostatic axis.		
4. Document in patient record.		
ZEROING THE TRANSDUCER 1. Wash hands.		
2. Open stopcock nearest to transducer to air.		
3. Push and release zeroing button, observing bedside monitor to see that zero has been reached.		
4. Turn stopcock back to open position.		
5. Document in patient record.		
CALIBRATION OF MONITOR 1. Wash hands.		
2. Open transducer stopcock to air to be sure it is zeroed.		
3. Depress ''cal'' button on bedside monitor.		
4. Adjust calibration according to monitor manufacturer's recommendations.		
5. Release ''cal'' button and observe to be sure digital display returns to zero.		
6. Document in patient record.		
CALIBRATION OF REUSABLE TRANSDUCER 1. Wash hands.		
2. Attach mercury manometer to one of the Luer-lok fittings of transducer dome.		
3. Attach hand bulb to other Luer-lok.		
4. Tighten hand-bulb control knob.		
5. Pump bulb up until mercury manometer reads 200 mmHg.		
6. Observe bedside monitor to see that it reads 200 mmHg.		
7. Release hand-bulb control knob, and observe for return of digital readout to zero.		
8. Remove dome and replace with new sterile dome prior to initiating patient monitoring.		
9. Document in patient record.		
CALIBRATION OF PAPER PRINTOUT 1. During zeroing, adjust paper printer stylus to read zero on the bottom line of grid.		
2. Press calibration button, and adjust paper printer stylus.		

Table continues on following page

Critical Behaviors	Complies	
	yes	no
3. Release calibration button.		
4. Document in patient record.		

SKILL 10-2

Insertion and Care of Arterial Pressure Line

Arterial pressure represents the forcible ejection of blood into the aorta. Because of the intermittent pumping action of the heart, the arterial pressure is generated in a pulsatile manner (Fig. 10–11). The ascending limb of the aortic pressure wave represents left ventricular (LV) ejection, and the peak of this ejection is the *peak systolic pressure*, which is normally 100 to 140 mmHg in adults. After reaching this peak, the ventricular pressure declines to a level below aortic pressure, and the aortic valve closes with a small rebound wave that makes a notch, the *dicrotic notch*, marking the end of ventricular systole. *Diastole* occupies the rest of the descending limb of the curve and is characterized by a long, declining pressure wave, during which the aortic wall recoils and propels blood into the arterial network. The diastolic pressure is measured as the lowest point of the descending limb of the curve and is normally 60 to 80 mmHg. The difference between the systolic and diastolic pressures is termed the *pulse pressure*, with a normal value of 40 mmHg. Pulse-pressure changes represent changes in stroke volume or arterial compliance.

The average arterial pressure during a cardiac cycle is termed the *mean arterial pressure*. It is not the average of the systolic plus diastolic pressures because during the cardiac cycle, the pressure remains closer to diastole for a longer period of time than to systole (at normal heart rates). Therefore, the true mean is calculated by determining the area under the pulse-pressure curve. This is done automatically by most patient monitoring systems. The mean arterial pressure also can be roughly calculated by using the following formula:

$$MAP = \frac{1(\text{systolic pressure}) + 2(\text{diastolic pressure})}{3}$$

Mean arterial pressure is important because it is the pressure that represents the driving force (perfusion pressure) for blood flow through the cardiovascular system. Mean arterial pressure is at its highest point in the aorta. As blood travels through the circulatory system, systolic pressure increases and diastolic pressure decreases, with an overall decline in the mean pressure (Fig. 10–12).

Arterial pressure is determined by the relationship between cardiac output (flow) and resistance to ejection. The arterial pressure is therefore affected by any factors

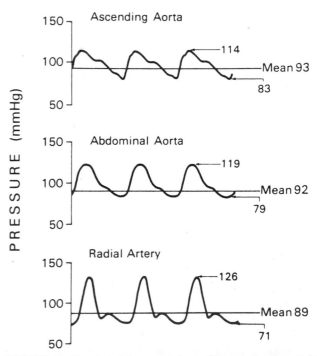

FIGURE 10–12. Arterial pressure from different sites in arterial tree. The arterial pressure waveform will vary in configuration depending on the location of the catheter. With transmission of the pressure wave into the distal aorta and large arteries, the systolic pressure increases and the diastolic pressure decreases, with a resulting heightening of the pulse pressure. However, the mean arterial pressure declines steadily. (From J. J. Smith and J. P. Kampine, *Circulatory Physiology: The Essentials.* Baltimore: Williams and Wilkins, 1980, p. 57, with permission.)

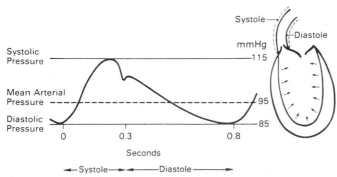

FIGURE 10–11. The generation of a pulsatile waveform. This is an aortic pressure curve. During systole, the ejected volume distends the aorta and aortic pressure rises. The peak pressure is known as the *aortic systolic pressure.* After the peak ejection, the ventricular pressure falls, and when it drops below the aortic pressure, the aortic valve closes, which is marked by the dicrotic notch, the end of systole. During diastole, the pressure continues to decline and the aortic wall recoils, pushing the blood toward the periphery. The trough of the pressure wave is the *diastolic pressure.* The difference between systolic and diastolic pressure is the *pulse pressure.* (From J. J. Smith and J. P. Kampine, *Circulatory Physiology: The Essentials.* Baltimore: Williams & Wilkins, 1980, p. 55, with permission.)

that change either resistance offered by the arterial network or changes in cardiac output. In children, arterial pressure is a particularly sensitive indicator of changes in cardiac output and blood volume.

When a patient requires continuous monitoring of arterial pressure, or when arterial pressure is unobtainable by other methods (cuff, Doppler), a rigid plastic catheter will be inserted by the physician into an artery to provide for direct pressure readings. The pressure waveform is transmitted via a fluid-filled high-pressure tube to a transducer that converts the pressure signal into an electrical signal seen on an oscilloscope as the pulse waveform (see Skill 10–1). Once inserted, the arterial catheter causes little or no discomfort to the patient and allows continuous blood pressure assessment without disturbing the patient. Blood samples also can be withdrawn from this catheter in a painless manner.

The location of the arterial catheter depends on the patient's age, the condition of the arterial vessels, and the presence of other catheters (i.e., the presence of a dialysis shunt is a contraindication for placing an arterial catheter in the same extremity). In adults, arterial catheters may be placed in the radial, brachial, femoral, or dorsalis pedis arteries. In pediatric patients, arterial catheters are placed in the radial, dorsalis pedis, posterior tibial, femoral, and umbilical (in neonates) arteries. When an intraaortic balloon (see Skill 12–1) is in place, arterial pressure may be monitored from the tip of the balloon in the aortic arch.

Arterial pressure monitoring carries certain risks. Infection at the insertion site can develop and spread to the bloodstream. Clots can form in the catheter and be carried into the circulation. The catheter can perforate the vessel wall and cause extravasation of flush solution into the tissues. Circulation to the extremity distal to the catheter can be impaired. The nurse therefore plays a major role not only in monitoring the information obtained from the arterial catheter, but also in preventing catheter complications.

Purpose

The nurse assembles the equipment, monitors, and maintains the arterial pressure system to

1. Identify changes in arterial pressure.
2. Evaluate medical therapy (i.e., titration of vasoactive drugs, fluid administration).
3. Obtain blood samples for laboratory analysis.

Prerequisite Knowledge and Skills

Prior to working with an arterial pressure system, the nurse should understand

1. Anatomy and physiology of the cardiovascular system.
2. Principles of leveling, zeroing, and calibrating a monitoring system. (see Skill 10–1)
3. Physiology of arterial pressure.

4. Aseptic technique.
5. Universal precautions.
6. Principles of hemodynamic monitoring.

The nurse should be able to perform

1. Proper handwashing technique (see Skill 35–5).
2. Stopcock manipulation and management techniques for catheter patency.
3. Recording of pressures from a bedside or central station monitor (see Skill 10–5).
4. Sterile technique.
5. Universal precautions (see Skill 35–1).
6. Peripheral vascular assessment.
7. Assessment of fluid balance.

Assessment

1. Observe for signs and symptoms that warrant use of arterial pressure monitoring: gradual or acute hypotension (etiology known or unknown), circulatory collapse, cardiac arrest, hemorrhage, hypertensive crisis, shock (due to any etiology), neurologic injury, postoperative complications, multiple trauma, respiratory failure, sepsis, and obstetrical emergencies or complications. **Rationale:** Arterial pressure monitoring provides continuous readouts, which facilitates immediate intervention or titration of existing therapy.
2. Assess peripheral circulation (i.e., color and warmth of extremities, presence and fullness of pulses, capillary refill, and motor function). An Allen's test is performed prior to insertion of a radial catheter (see Skill 9–2). Assess cuff or Doppler pressure in both arms. Assess heart sounds and ECG pattern. Assess mental status. Assess medical history for diabetes, hypertension, and peripheral vascular disease. **Rationale:** Identifies any circulatory impairment in the extremity where the arterial line is to be placed.

Nursing Diagnoses

1. Decreased cardiac output related to a decreased preload, an increased afterload, a change in heart rate, or the effects of cardiovascular pharmacology. **Rationale:** Any factors that alter cardiac output will result in a change in arterial pressure.
2. Potential for altered tissue perfusion related to catheter insertion in the arterial vasculature. **Rationale:** One of the most common complications of arterial catheters particularly in children is impaired circulation to the extremity distal to the insertion site.
3. Hemorrhage related to blood loss with line disconnect. **Rationale:** In restless patients or when the arterial catheter has not been sutured in place, there is a danger of the line disconnecting with rapid blood loss.
4. Potential for infection related to presence of an invasive catheter. **Rationale:** Any invasive catheter is a potential source of infection, particularly catheters that are entered repeatedly for blood sampling. Any infection that begins at this catheter could enter the bloodstream and result in a life-threatening bacteremia.

5. Potential for fluid volume overload related to excessive volume delivery with catheter flushing. **Rationale:** In pediatric and geriatric patients, and in patients with labile congestive heart disease, fluid volume overload can occur.

Planning

1. Individualize the following goals for performing invasive arterial pressure monitoring:
    a. Provide accurate, continuous readings of arterial pressure. **Rationale:** Arterial pressure monitoring allows for the early identification of complications of critical illness and continuous evaluation of the patient's response to medical and nursing therapy.
    b. Provide a method of atraumatic blood withdrawal. **Rationale:** In the patient with problems of gas exchange and/or acid–base imbalance, the arterial catheter allows for frequent nontraumatic blood withdrawal.
2. Prepare all necessary equipment and supplies for insertion of arterial catheter. **Rationale:** Equipment and supplies need to be readily available and functional to initiate and care for arterial pressure lines.
    a. Povidone-iodine solution.
    b. 1% Xylocaine solution.
    c. 10 ml syringe.
    d. 1- to 2-in (2.5 to 5 cm) over-the-needle catheter

(14 to 18 gauge for adults, 22 gauge for children, and 24 gauge for newborns).
    e. Antibacterial ointment.
    f. Transparent dressing.
    g. Arm board.
    h. 4 × 4 gauze.
    i. Pads.
    j. Soft restraints.
    k. Assembled pressure transducer system (see Skill 10–1).
    l. Two pairs of exam gloves.
3. Level, zero, and calibrate the equipment (see Skill 10–1). **Rationale:** Evaluates waveform and arterial pressure.
4. Prepare the patient.
    a. Explain rationale and procedure for arterial catheter placement. **Rationale:** Reduces patient anxiety and obtains cooperation during insertion.
    b. Explain that once the catheter is inserted, there will be minimal discomfort from the catheter, but that the insertion site will need to be immobilized. **Rationale:** Reduces anxiety and prevents dislodgment of catheter.
    c. Position patient comfortably, with adequate exposure and lighting of insertion site. **Rationale:** Facilitates accurate insertion.
    d. Immobilize as needed the extremity to be cannulized on an arm board. **Rationale:** Insures accuracy of hemodynamic measures.

Implementation

Steps	Rationale	Special Considerations
Assisting with Insertion		
1. Wash hands.	Reduces transmission of microorganisms.	
2. Don exam gloves.	Universal precautions.	
3. Immobilize site during catheter insertion.	Prevents needle from lacerating vessel wall during insertion.	
4. Assist with catheter insertion as directed.	Allows for smooth cooperative effort.	
5. Once catheter is positioned, connect high pressure tubing with Luer-lok adapter to arterial catheter.	Allows signal to be transmitted to monitor. Physician will hold catheter in place while nurse makes connection. Catheter is at risk of coming dislodged until it has been secured.	
6. If dampened (Fig. 10–13), attempt to withdraw blood, and then flush. Try repositioning arm board. Catheter position may need to be adjusted if these procedures are unsuccessful.	Ensures accuracy of pressure waveform.	
7. Once catheter is secured in place by physician, apply antimicrobial ointment and transparent dressing.	Prevents bacterial growth. A clear dressing enables the nurse to view insertion site for bleeding, drainage, or erythema.	

Table continues on following page

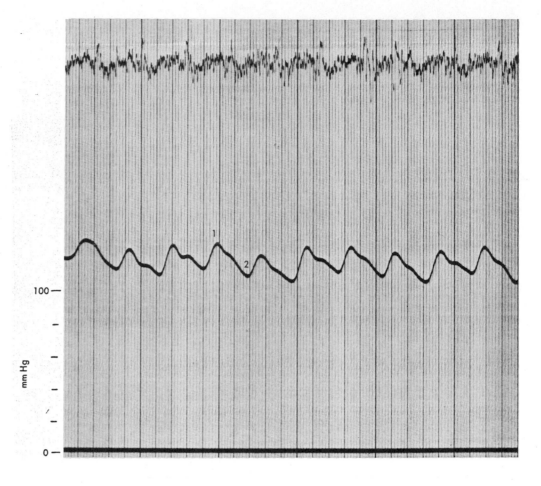

FIGURE 10–13. Dampened arterial waveform (*1* = systole; *2* = diastole). (From E. K. Daily and J. S. Schroeder, *Hemodynamic Waveforms: Exercises in Identification and Analysis*. St. Louis: Mosby, 1990, p. 101, with permission.)

Steps	Rationale	Special Considerations
8. Remove and discard gloves in appropriate receptacle.	Universal precautions.	
9. Wash hands.	Reduces transmission of microorganisms.	

Catheter Care/Troubleshooting

Steps	Rationale	Special Considerations
1. Check arterial line flush system q12h:	Ensures accuracy of pressure waveform and functioning of system.	
a. Ensure that pressure bag is inflated to 300 mmHg.	Necessary for proper function of flush device and to prevent blood backflow.	
b. Ensure that fluid is present in flush bag.	Catheter will clot off if fluid is not continuously infusing.	
c. Ensure that flush system is delivering 1 to 3 ml/h.	Maintains catheter patency and prevents fluid overload.	
2. Continuously observe arterial waveform quality. If waveform becomes dampened, the nurse should	Dampening should be troubleshooted immediately to prevent clotting of catheter.	
a. Check the patient.	A sudden hypotensive episode can look like a dampened waveform (Fig. 10–14).	
b. Check the arterial line insertion site for catheter positioning.	In radial site, wrist movement, and in the femoral site, leg flexion can cause catheter kinking or dislodgment and result in dampened waveform.	

Table continues on following page

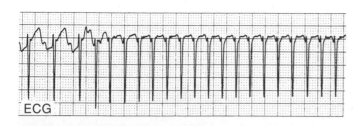

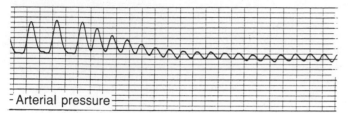

FIGURE 10–14. Arterial pressure tracing in a 9-month-old child after Senning procedure. Patient developed a supraventricular tachycardia (SVT) with a fall in arterial pressure. Note how the arterial line appears dampened but is in fact reflecting a severe hypotensive episode associated with the tachycardia.

Steps	Rationale	Special Considerations
c. Attempt to aspirate and flush catheter as follows:	Assists with the withdrawal of any clots that may be at catheter's tip. A catheter with a dampened tip should *always* be aspirated prior to flushing.	
(1) Attach a 10-cc syringe to stopcock closest to patient.	10-cc syringe generates less pressure.	
(2) Turn stopcock off to flush bag.	Opens the system from the patient to the syringe.	
(3) Gently attempt to aspirate; if resistance is felt, stop and notify physician.	Allows check on catheter patency. Normally blood should be aspirated into the syringe.	
(4) If blood is withdrawn, remove 3 cc of blood, turn stopcock off to syringe, and discard the 3-cc sample.	Removes any clot material within catheter.	All blood wastes should be disposed of according to institutional policies/ procedures.
(5) Return syringe to stopcock, and turn stopcock off to patient.	Prepares for hand irrigation with syringe.	
(6) Squeeze fast-flush device, and fill syringe with 2 ml solution.	This solution will be used to irrigate catheter.	
(7) Turn stopcock off to pressure tubing system, and open to syringe and patient.	Opens syringe to patient in preparation for flushing.	
(8) Keep hand on syringe barrel at all times, and *gently* inject solution into arterial line with syringe.	Controls backpressure from artery, which could force barrel out of syringe.	
d. Turn stopcock off to patient, flush clear, and then turn stopcock off to opening (where syringe was) and replace with deadend cap.	Removes blood residue from stopcock, where it would be a reservoir for bacterial growth.	
e. Record amount of flush solution used.	Measures intake for fluid balance status.	

Table continues on following page

Steps	Rationale	Special Considerations
3. Change arterial line dressing; frequency is determined by type of dressing material used and unit policy; generally q24h:	Prevents infection of insertion site.	Clear dressings do not need to be changed as often as a gauze dressing and may be more cost-effective.
a. Wash hands.	Reduces transmission of microorganisms.	
b. Don exam gloves.	Universal precautions.	
c. Gently remove old dressings, being careful not to place tension on arterial catheter.	Prevents inadvertent dislodgment of catheter.	If excessive tape is used, a second nurse may be needed to assist with dressing removal, one nurse to secure catheter while the second nurse removes the tape. Accidental dislodgment or removal of arterial catheter can occur.
d. Observe site for signs of infection. Infected catheters are removed and cultured.	Prevents bacteremia.	
e. Cleanse insertion site with povidone-iodine solution.	Prevents growth of bacteria at insertion site.	
f. Allow to dry, and apply povidone-iodine ointment.	Iodine solutions need to air dry for maximum effectiveness.	
g. Replace dressing using aseptic technique.	Decreases risk of infection.	
h. Remove and discard gloves in appropriate receptacle.	Universal precautions.	
i. Wash hands.	Reduces transmission of microorganisms.	

Evaluation

1. Evaluate arterial waveform on oscilloscope following insertion. Document a recorded strip every 12 hours or according to unit policy. **Rationale:** Ensures that catheter is in position, without excessive movement in the vessel (fling); that it is not easily dampened by the patient's position; and that the catheter has not become disconnected.

2. Evaluate arterial line site daily for signs of infection (i.e., redness, localized edema, drainage, and heat). **Rationale:** Early identification of infection decreases the risk of bacteremia and sepsis.

3. Monitor extremity distal to insertion site every 2 hours for color, warmth, capillary refill, presence and fullness of pulses, and presence or absence of pain. **Rationale:** A complication of arterial catheters is clot formation and embolization to the extremity where the catheter is located. A clot to the extremity could result in impaired circulation.

4. Evaluate configuration of arterial waveform continuously. **Rationale:** Identifies early dampening or changes that indicate catheter misplacement within the vessel; ensures accuracy of the pressure waveforms. Any changes in the waveform should be evaluated promptly to be sure that dampening is not due to a change in the patient's condition.

5. Monitor fluid intake from the flush solution every shift. **Rationale:** Ensures that the patient is not receiving too much solution with the fast flushes being performed.

6. Record arterial, systolic, diastolic, and mean pressures as indicated for the patient's condition or according to unit protocol. The arterial waveform for a child is identical to that of an adult, with the only difference being that the child's pressure is lower than an adult's (Table 10–1). The blood pressure in an elderly individual (over 65 years) will normally be higher than that in a younger adult. **Rationale:** Documents line patency and identifies complications or abnormal waveforms early.

Expected Outcomes

1. Minimal discomfort from arterial catheter. **Rationale:** If catheter is within the vessel, and if it is stabilized by an arm board or other device, there should be no irritation.

2. Patient will remain infection-free. **Rationale:** If the site is cared for with antibacterial ointment, the dressing changed regularly (according to type of dressing material used), and the health care personnel use sterile technique during insertion, the catheter should remain infection-free.

3. Patient will have a normal hemoglobin and hematocrit and will not suffer injury as a result of blood loss from the arterial catheter. **Rationale:** If catheter has

TABLE 10–1 NORMAL BLOOD PRESSURE RANGES FOR CHILDREN

Age	Systolic Pressure	Diastolic Pressure
Neonate (1 month)	85–100	51–65
Infant (6 months)	87–105	53–66
Toddler (2 years)	95–105	53–66
School age (7 years)	97–112	57–71
Adolescent (15 years)	112–128	66–80

Source: Blood pressure tables taken from the 50th to 90th percentile ranges extrapolated from graphs published by M. J. Horan, Chairman, Task Force on Blood Pressure Control in Children, Report of the second task force on blood pressure in children, Pediatrics 79:1, 1987. These blood pressure ranges were derived by the task force from a sampling of more than 70,000 children.

been secured in place and the nurse continuously observes the arterial catheter and waveform, then excessive blood loss from a disconnect should not occur.

4. Adequate circulation to extremity distal to catheter insertion site. **Rationale:** Signs of impaired circulation should be reported to the physician in a timely manner to prevent irreversible changes in tissue perfusion.

5. Euvolemic. **Rationale:** The nurse monitors the intake from the flush solution to prevent fluid volume overload.

Unexpected Outcomes

1. Pain and/or discomfort from arterial catheter insertion site. **Rationale:** Catheter is against vessel wall or has punctured vessel wall with infiltration of fluid into tissues or catheter has become infected.

2. Redness at the insertion site, pain, edema, drainage from site, elevated temperature, or elevated WBC. **Rationale:** Catheter site has become infected.

3. Impaired peripheral tissue perfusion (i.e., edema of fingers, color changes of fingers, painful fingers, coolness of extremity, pale color of extremity, and slow capillary refill). **Rationale:** Catheter is occluding circulation to extremity. A clot has formed and traveled distal to catheter. Local edema at insertion site has reduced circulation to extremity.

4. Catheter disconnect and loss of a significant amount of blood. **Rationale:** Catheter has remained hidden from the nurse's view and has become disconnected; catheter was not secured to skin; a Luer-lok or other tight connection was not used between the catheter and high-pressure tubing; the patient is very restless and has caused catheter to disconnect.

5. Fluid volume overload. **Rationale:** The catheter has been used for excessive blood draws, and the patient has received an excessive amount of flush solution.

Documentation

Documentation in the patient record should include recorded waveform labeled with date, time, and systolic and diastolic pressures; peripheral vascular assessment; insertion-site condition; date and time of insertion; patient response to insertion procedure; and amount of flush solution infused. **Rationale:** Provides a record of nursing care given and expected and unexpected outcomes.

Patient/Family Education

1. Instruct patient and family on rationale for arterial pressure system and how the arterial pressure is monitored on bedside scope. Explain that patient movement may affect digital numbers displayed. **Rationale:** Alleviates patient and family anxiety.

2. If use of restraints or sedation of patient is required, explain to patient and family the danger in an arterial line becoming inoperable or dislodged. **Rationale:** Seeing a loved one restrained or sedated can be frightening for families. Elderly patients will often react to use of physical restraints, so it is always important to explain repeatedly why they are necessary.

Performance Checklist
Skill 10–2: Insertion and Care of Arterial Pressure Line

Critical Behaviors	Complies yes	no
ASSISTING WITH INSERTION 1. Wash hands.		
2. Don exam gloves.		
3. Immobilize insertion site.		
4. Connect high-pressure tubing, with Luer-lok adapter, to arterial catheter.		
5. Assess quality of arterial waveform, if dampened troubleshoot.		

Table continues on following page

Critical Behaviors	Complies	
	yes	**no**
6. Apply antibacterial ointment and transparent dressing to arterial catheter insertion site.		
7. Remove and discard gloves.		
8. Wash hands.		
9. Document in patient record.		
CATHETER CARE/TROUBLESHOOTING 1. Observe arterial line flush system q12h:		
a. Ensure that pressure bag is inflated to 300 mmHg.		
b. Ensure that fluid is present in flush bag.		
c. Ensure that flush system is delivering 1 to 3 ml/h.		
2. Continuously observe quality of arterial waveform, taking appropriate steps to troubleshoot dampened arterial waveform:		
a. Check the patient.		
b. Check insertion site for catheter position.		
c. Flush catheter gently using a syringe and flush solution.		
d. After flushing, close system properly.		
e. Record amount of flush solution in patient record.		
3. Change arterial line dressing q24h or according to unit policy.		
a. Wash hands.		
b. Don nonsterile gloves.		
c. Use care in removing old dressing.		
d. Observe for signs of infection at insertion site.		
e. Cleanse insertion site.		
f. Apply antibacterial ointment to insertion site.		
g. Replace dressing using aseptic technique.		
h. Remove and discard gloves.		
i. Wash hands.		
4. Document in patient record.		

SKILL 10–3

Central Venous Pressure/Right Atrial Pressure

The central venous pressure (CVP) is the pressure measured at the tip of a catheter placed within the right atrium (RA). There are three methods for measuring pressure in the right atrium: (1) use of a water manometer attached to a central venous catheter, (2) use of the proximal lumen of a PA catheter (see Skill 10–7), and (3) use of a line placed directly into the right atrium and attached to a transducer system. Measurement of the CVP provides information about the body's volume status and right ventricular (RV) function. For the purpose of this skill, CVP and RAP will be used interchangeably, and the water manometer and mercury transducer methods of reading will be described.

CVP influences and is influenced by venous return and cardiac function. Physiologically, right atrial pressure (or CVP) represents right-side heart preload, or the volume of blood found in the right ventricle at the end of diastole. Although CVP is used as a measure of changes in RV volume, the relationship is not linear. Because of the ventricle's ability to expand and alter its compliance, changes in volume can occur with little change in pressure. Consequently, a decreased CVP does not rule out the possibility of depressed cardiac function. Additionally, a single measurement of CVP cannot accurately predict end-diastolic volume, and therefore, monitoring trends in CVP is more meaningful.

The CVP waveform normally has three components: *a* wave, *c* wave, and *v* wave (Fig. 10–15). The *a* wave represents the atrial pressure during atrial contraction. The *c* wave is associated with the transient pressure rise during tricuspid valve closure, and the *v* wave represents the filling of the atria that occurs during ventricular systole. The *a* wave is followed by a fall in pressure called the *x* descent, and the *v* wave followed by the *y* descent. Changes in the height of the waves or the slope of the *x* or *y* descent signal the presence of cardiac disease. When monitoring CVP/RAP from a catheter attached to a transducer system, the nurse is responsible for monitoring the mean pressure, which normally is 0 to 7 mmHg.

When measured by a water manometer, CVP is reported in centimeters of water (cmH_2O) pressure as opposed to millimeters of mercury (1 mmHg = 1.36 cmH_2O pressure). The advantage of the water manometer method is its simplicity, so that this technique remains useful in the critical-care setting. The significance of an increase or decrease in CVP can be seen in Table 10–2.

Purpose

The nurse performs CVP monitoring to

1. Evaluate right-side heart hemodynamics.
2. Evaluate patient response to therapy.

Prerequisite Knowledge and Skills

Prior to performing CVP measures, the nurse should understand

1. Cardiac anatomy and physiology.
2. Physiology of fluid balance.
3. Pathophysiology of renal failure and heart failure.
4. Pathophysiology of the diseases for which CVP measurements are indicated.
5. Aseptic technique.
6. Universal precautions.
7. Principals of hemodynamic monitoring.

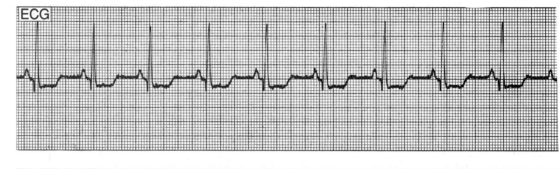
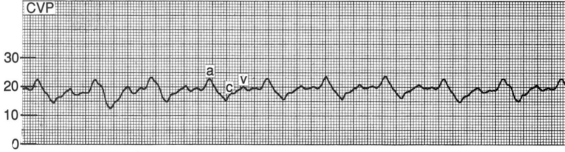

FIGURE 10–15. CVP waveform with *a*, *c*, and *v* waves present. The *a* wave is usually seen just after the P wave of the ECG. The *c* wave appears at the time of the RST junction on the ECG. The *v* wave is seen in the TP interval.

TABLE 10–2 CENTRAL VENOUS PRESSURE

Conditions Causing Increased CVP
    Elevated vascular volume
    Increased cardiac output (hyperdynamic cardiac function)
    Depressed cardiac function (RV infarct, RV failure)
    Cardiac tamponade
    Constrictive pericarditis
    Pulmonary hypertension
    Chronic left ventricular failure
Conditions Causing Decreased CVP
    Reduced vascular volume*
    Decreased mean systemic pressures (e.g., as in late shock states)
    Venodilation (drug induced)

*Be aware that while the measured CVP is low, cardiac function may be depressed, normal, or hyperdynamic when there is reduced vascular volume.

The nurse should be able to perform

1. Proper handwashing techniques (see Skill 35–5).
2. Sterile technique.
3. Universal precautions (see Skill 35–1).
4. Stopcock manipulation.
5. Single pressure transducer setup (see Skill 10–1).
6. Cardiovascular system assessment.
7. Assessment of fluid balance.

Assessment

1. Assess for signs and symptoms of fluid volume deficit, including weakness, thirst, decreased urine output, increased urine specific gravity, output greater than intake, sudden weight loss or gain, decreased PWP, hemoconcentration, hypernatremia, postural hypotension, tachycardia, decreased skin turgor, dry mucous membranes, decreased pulse pressure, weak and thready pulse, depressed fontanelle (infant), and altered mental status (AACN, 1990). **Rationale:** The patient's clinical picture should be correlated with CVP value. Fluid volume deficit will most usually result in a decreased CVP.

2. Assess for signs and symptoms of fluid volume excess, including dyspnea, orthopnea, anxiety, sudden weight gain, intake greater than output, pulmonary congestion, abnormal breath sounds (e.g., rales, crackles), S3 heart sound, dependent edema, pleural effusion, anasarca, tachypnea, dilutional decrease in hemoglobin and hematocrit, tachycardia, dysrhythmias, blood pressure changes, increased PAP or PWP, JVD, oliguria, urine specific gravity changes, altered electrolytes, and altered mental status (AACN, 1990). **Rationale:** The patient's clinical picture should be correlated with CVP value. Fluid volume overload will most usually result in an elevated CVP.

3. Assess for signs and symptoms of air embolus, including sucking sound on inspiration, dyspnea, tachypnea, hypoxia, hypercapnia, wheezing, bell-shaped air bubble in pulmonary outflow track per chest x-ray film, increased pulmonary artery pressure, tachycardia, cyanosis, JVD, hypotension, increased SVR, substernal chest pain, ST-segment depression on ECG, cor pulmonale, cardiac arrest, lightheadedness, confusion, anxiety, fear of dying, aphasia, localized neurologic deficits, hemiplegia, unresponsiveness, and seizures. **Rationale:** Air embolus is a rare but fatal (40 to 50 percent mortality) complication of CVP catheterization (Thielen, 1990). This may develop during insertion, with an accidental disconnect of catheter, and during removal. With this complication, CVP will be elevated.

4. Assess for history of heart failure, renal disease, or liver disease. **Rationale:** These diseases are frequently accompanied by fluid imbalances that will cause an increase or decrease in CVP.

Nursing Diagnoses

1. Fluid volume overload related to excess fluid ingestion or infusion, nonadherence to a fluid intake limit, increased sodium intake, drug therapy, and hypoproteinemia. **Rationale:** Fluid volume overload will result in an elevated CVP.

2. Fluid volume deficit related to abnormal fluid loss (vomiting, drains, diarrhea, wound drainage, extreme diaphoresis), hemorrhage, burns, fever, increased metabolic rate, imposed fluid restriction, decreased motivation to drink liquids, difficulty or inability in swallowing or in feeding self, excessive use of diuretics or laxatives, and hypoproteinemia. **Rationale:** Fluid volume deficit will result in a decreased CVP.

3. Potential for injury: cardiac air embolus due to improper catheter handling during insertion, maintenance, and removal. **Rationale:** Air embolus is a rare but fatal complication of CVP catheterization.

4. Potential for decreased cardiac output related to decreased myocardial contractility. **Rationale:** RV infarct will result in decreased contractility of RV, decreased stroke volume, increased preload, and increased CVP.

5. Potential for infection related to improper catheter care or contamination during insertion, maintenance, and removal. **Rationale:** Infection is a complication of any invasive line. If bacteria enter the bloodstream from an infected catheter, the mortality is very high.

Planning

1. Individualize the following goals for performing CVP measures:
   a. Maintain intact, aseptic CVP monitoring system. **Rationale:** Proper care and use of equipment should make complications preventable.
   b. Maintain CVP within an acceptable range (to be determined jointly with the physician for the individual patient). **Rationale:** If appropriate therapy is administered in a timely manner, the patient should maintain a CVP appropriate for his/her clinical picture.

2. Prepare all necessary equipment and supplies. **Rationale:** Assembly of all the necessary equipment at the bedside ensures that CVP measures can be completed quickly and efficiently.
   a. Pressure transducer setup (flushed and ready to connect), or
   b. IV solution, IV tubing, a water manometer, and extension tubing assembled, flushed, and ready to connect (Fig. 10–16).
   c. Carpenter's level.

3. Prepare the patient.
   a. Explain procedure. **Rationale:** Reduces anxiety.
   b. Place the patient flat. **Rationale:** Eliminates the effects of increased or decreased venous return from the head or lower extremities.

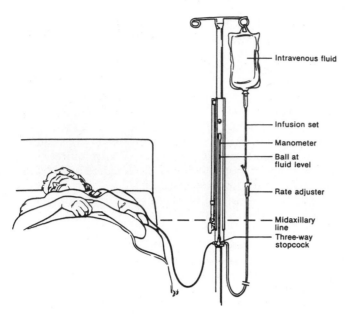

- Intravenous fluid
- Infusion set
- Manometer
- Ball at fluid level
- Rate adjuster
- Midaxillary line
- Three-way stopcock

FIGURE 10–16. CVP water manometer flush system. This manometer is attached to the IV pole, and the height is adjusted to the phlebostatic axis using a carpenter's level. (From C. Hudak, *Critical Care Nursing: A Holistic Approach*. Philadelphia: Lippincott, 1989, p. 123, with permission.)

Implementation

Steps	Rationale	Special Considerations
CVP Measurement Using Water Manometer Method		
1. Wash hands.	Reduces transmission of microorganisms.	
2. Locate the phlebostatic axis (see Skill 10–1).	All CVP measures are to be taken as close to the right atrial pressure as possible. The phlebostatic axis is approximately at the level of the right atrium.	
3. Place the zero level of the water manometer at the level of the phlebostatic axis (Fig. 10–17).	This is the level from which all CVP readings will be taken.	The nurse may want to tape the manometer to an IV pole to use with each measure. In this instance, the nurse will need to use a carpenter's level to ensure that the zero level of the manometer is level with the phlebostatic axis (see Fig. 10–16).
4. Turn water manometer stopcock open to the flush bag (Fig. 10–18, System A).	To be sure that manometer is not open to patient, which would allow blood backup into the tubing.	
5. Open IV tubing roller clamp so that fluid flows from the flush bag into the water manometer, fill the manometer two-thirds full or above the level of the expected CVP, and close off roller clamp.	If fluid is allowed to overflow the top of the manometer, contamination will result. Underfilling will result in an inaccurate reading.	
6. Turn water manometer stopcock open to the patient and closed to the flush solution (Fig. 10–18, System B).	Allows fluid to flow into the patient until the fluid column equalizes with the pressure in the RA.	

Table continues on following page

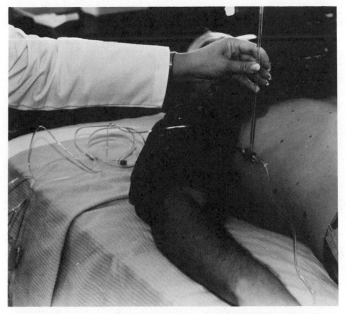

FIGURE 10–17. Water manometer placed at phlebostatic axis on patient.

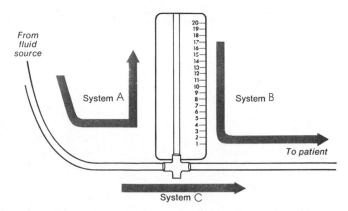

FIGURE 10–18. Central venous pressure measurement. (*A*) Stopcock closed to patient for filling of manometer. (*B*) Stopcock closed to fluid source and open to patient. (*C*) Stopcock closed to manometer and fluid system opened to patient. (Adapted from C. Hudak, *Critical Care Nursing: A Holistic Approach.* Philadelphia: Lippincott, 1989, p. 122, with permission.)

Steps	Rationale	Special Considerations
7. Watch the fluid column closely, since it will often fall rapidly, and do not allow all the fluid to flow out.	If the manometer is allowed to empty, air may enter the patient.	
8. The fluid column should fall quickly and then fluctuate at the point where the fluid column equalizes with the RA pressure. This is the CVP (Fig. 10–18, System C).	The pressure within the manometer equalizes with the pressure in the RA. The height of the fluid column reflects the RA pressure.	
9. Turn the water manometer stopcock open to the flush solution and the patient, and regulate the roller clamp for the prescribed drip rate.	Prevents clotting of catheter and reestablishes IV flow.	
10. Wash hands.	Reduces transmission of microorganisms.	
11. Record the CVP reading in centimeters of water pressure on the appropriate part of the patient record.	Ensures consistency in readings and interpretation.	

Calibrated Transducer Method of Reading RAP

1. Wash hands.	Reduces transmission of microorganisms.	
2. Validate waveform as RAP on bedside monitor.	Ensures that catheter is still in proper location.	
3. Fast flush catheter for 2 seconds.	Ensures patency of catheter.	
4. Level transducer to the phlebostatic axis (see Skill 10–1). Patient should be in a supine position, with the head of the bed no higher than 45 degrees.	Eliminates effects of hydrostatic pressure artifact from a transducer that is higher or lower than the level of the RA.	

Table continues on following page

Steps	Rationale	Special Considerations
5. Print out RAP on bedside or central station recorder that has been zeroed and calibrated (see Skill 10–1).	A printed pressure tracing is the most accurate method of reading hemodynamic pressures. Also, current risk-management guidelines for many hospitals require at least one hardcopy of waveforms every shift. (Check individual institutional policies as shifts may vary from 8 to 10 to 12 hours.)	More recent models of hemodynamic monitoring equipment may not require paper printout for readings. It is recommended that a trial of paper printout readings versus digital display readings be conducted and results documented by biomedical department prior to relying on digital display numbers.
6. Allow printer to record three respiratory cycles of RA.	Allows the nurse to identify the end-expiratory phase, which is when pressure values should be read.	
7. Identify the end-expiration phase for each respiratory cycle, and find two cycles where this point is the same. This is where the RAP is to be read (Fig. 10–19).	Two out of three cycle agreements ensure greater accuracy in reading values.	
8. Record the location where the reading was taken on the printout, the patient's body position, the pressure value (in mmHg), the patient's name, the date and time of the strip, and place in patient record.	Ensures that others will interpret the RAP value using the same technique. Careful labeling allows for the review of the waveform for comparison to subsequent readings.	

Evaluation

Compare assessments before and after reading of CVP. **Rationale:** Identifies any complications related to the procedure.

Expected Outcomes

1. Absence of air embolus or catheter contamination. **Rationale:** Proper technique should prevent these complications of CVP reading.

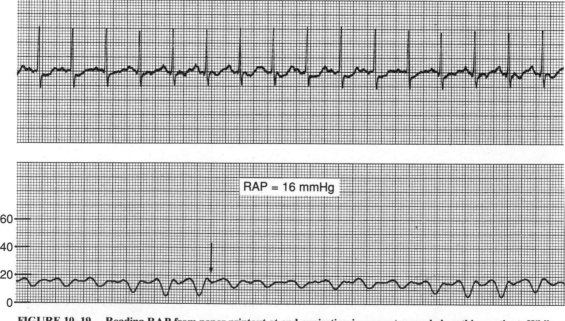

FIGURE 10–19. Reading RAP from paper printout at end-expiration in a spontaneously breathing patient. While observing the patient, identify inspiration. The point just prior to inspiration is end-expiration. Arrow indicates points of end-expiration. Reading is taken as a mean value. The RAP value for this patient is 16 mmHg.

2. Absence of infection at insertion site. **Rationale:** Aseptic technique used in daily dressing changes should prevent bacterial contamination.

3. CVP readings correlate with physical findings. **Rationale:** Proper technique in taking readings and maintaining hemodynamic system should provide accurate readings.

Unexpected Outcomes

1. Air embolus. **Rationale:** Air embolism may occur when taking readings, when flushing or setting up hemodynamic system, or during insertion or removal of CVP catheter. It is important to note that air comes out of solution with time much the same as bubbles form in a glass of water left sitting on a table. When the patient's body temperature is elevated, the air comes out of solution at a rate greater than normal. This can also occur when the room temperature is elevated. Therefore, lines should be observed for air bubble formation and air flushed out through a stopcock.

2. Patient develops redness, drainage, edema at insertion site, pain, fever, or elevated WBC. **Rationale:** Catheter insertion site has become infected.

Documentation

Documentation in the patient record should include cardiopulmonary assessment, labeled CVP waveform (see above), assessment of catheter insertion site, the date and time monitoring lines are changed, dressing change dates and times, the amount of flush solution intake and the assessment of fluid balance. **Rationale:** Documents nursing care given, patient's cardiopulmonary status, and expected and unexpected outcomes.

Patient/Family Education

1. Discuss rationale for CVP catheter with both patient and family. **Rationale:** Reduces anxiety.

2. Discuss rationale for CVP monitoring with patient and family. **Rationale:** Reduces anxiety.

3. If patient is to be discharged home soon after removal of CVP catheter, the patient and family should be instructed to observe catheter insertion site for 2 days following removal for signs of new drainage, edema, or redness, at which time their physician should be notified immediately. **Rationale:** Late infection of catheter insertion site is a rare but possible complication following removal.

Performance Checklist
Skill 10–3:   Central Venous Pressure/Right Atrial Pressure

Critical Behaviors	Complies yes	no
WATER MANOMETER METHOD 1. Wash hands.		
2. Place patient flat.		
3. Locate phlebostatic axis.		
4. Place the zero level of water manometer at level of phlebostatic axis.		
5. Open manometer to flush bag.		
6. Fill manometer two-thirds full.		
7. Open manometer to patient.		
8. Observe fall in fluid column until fluid level fluctuates.		
9. Turn stopcock off to manometer, and resume IV fluid infusion to patient.		
10. Wash hands.		
11. Document in patient record.		
CALIBRATED TRANSDUCER METHOD 1. Wash hands.		
2. Observe RAP waveform.		
3. Fast flush catheter.		
4. Level transducer to phlebostatic axis.		
5. Print out three respiratory cycles of RAP.		
6. Identify end-expiratory period for each cycle.		

Table continues on following page

Critical Behaviors	Complies	
	yes	no
7. Find two cycles with same end-expiration period and record location of reading on strip.		
8. Document in patient record.		

SKILL 10-4

Left Atrial Pressure

Left atrial pressure (LAP) is measured with a polyvinyl catheter placed in the left atrium during open heart surgery. There are two methods of insertion: needle puncture of the right superior pulmonary vein with subsequent threading into the LA or direct cannulation of the LA through a needle puncture at the intraatrial groove (Recker, 1985). The catheter is then brought through the chest wall or through the inferior end of the sternal incision where it is connected to a pressure transducer system (Skill 10–1) for continuous bedside monitoring (Taylor et al., 1990).

Left atrial pressure provides the same information as the PAWP, and the waveforms have a very similar configuration (Fig. 10–20). The normal LAP is 4 to 12 mmHg. Some reasons why an LA line is inserted include the following: it is easy to obtain continuous readings from the LA line; it can be used in patients with prosthetic tricuspid or pulmonic valves where a PA catheter is contraindicated; it can be used in patients with abnormal heart anatomy (i.e., single ventricle, tricuspid atresia); it can be used in patients with high PAPs, which interfere with the accuracy of the PAWP; it is an accurate indicator of LV pressures; and it provides accurate information when vasoconstricting medications are infused in conjunction with pulmonary vasodilator medications (Bojar, 1989).

One danger with the use of this catheter is the potential for air or blood clot emboli to enter the left atrium and be carried to the brain or other body organs. Close attention to line maintenance and monitoring of the waveform is imperative.

Purpose

The nurse performs LAP monitoring to

1. Assess for complications following open heart surgery.
2. Evaluate response to treatment.
3. Evaluate progression of postoperative recovery.

Prerequisite Knowledge and Skills

Prior to performing LAP monitoring, the nurse should understand

1. Cardiovascular anatomy and physiology.
2. Pathophysiology of the diseases for which LAP monitoring is indicated.

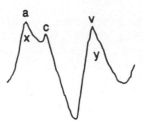

FIGURE 10–20. LAP waveform and its components—a wave—the presystolic wave resulting from atrial contraction; x descent—the down slope of the a wave caused by atrial relaxation; c wave—a sharp inflection caused by mitral valve closure; v wave—an atrial pressure wave rising to a peak during late ventricular systole caused by filling of the atrium while the mitral valve is closed; y descent—the down slope of the v wave caused by early diastolic runoff through the mitral valve. Changes in the waveform configuration may indicate valve or myocardial disease. For example, an elevated a wave is seen in mitral stenosis and an elevated v wave in mitral insufficiency. Both the a and v waves are elevated in cardiac tamponade.

3. Signs and symptoms of cardiac tamponade.
4. Physiology of fluid balance.
5. Aseptic technique.
6. Universal precautions.
7. Principles of hemodynamic monitoring.

The nurse should be able to perform

1. Proper handwashing technique (see Skill 35–5).
2. Sterile technique.
3. Universal precautions (see Skill 35–1).
4. Pressure transducer system setup (see Skill 10–1).
5. Zeroing, leveling, and calibrating of hemodynamic monitoring system (see Skill 10–1).
6. Stopcock manipulation.
7. Cardiovascular system assessment.
8. Assessment of fluid balance.

Assessment

1. Assess LAP waveform continuously. **Rationale:** Ensures that it is in proper position and has not migrated into LV (Fig. 10–21) or come out of LA (i.e., slipped into pericardial space). Dampened waveform would indicate air or clot in system and should not be used for readings until corrected.
2. Assess patient's vital signs, cardiac output (CO) (if available), RAP, PAP (if available), fluid balance, heart sounds, breath sounds, pulse fullness, skin temperature and color, fontanels (infant), and skin turgor in relation to LAP. **Rationale:** Physical findings should correlate with LAP value.

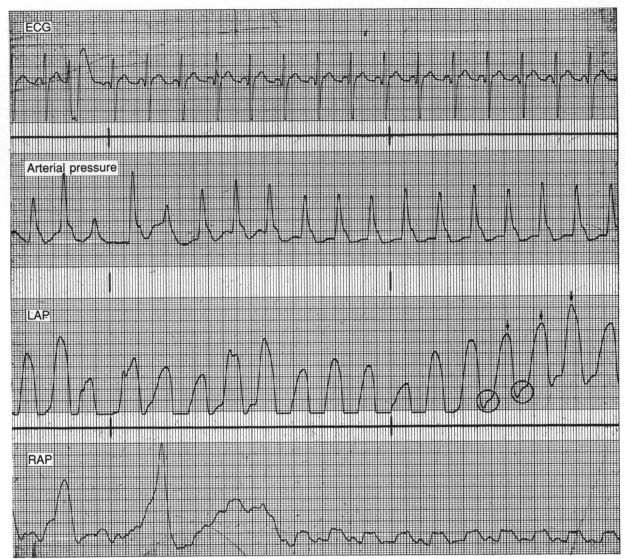

FIGURE 10–21. LAP catheter that has slipped into LV. Note anacrotic notch on upstroke of LV waveform (*circled*). Note also that paper was not calibrated in this example.

Nursing Diagnoses

1. Decreased cardiac output related to altered preload, afterload, or contractility. **Rationale:** The LAP is used to evaluate changes in cardiovascular hemodynamics that affect cardiac output. Changes in LAP and potential etiologies for these are listed in Table 10–3.

TABLE 10–3 ETIOLOGIES FOR CHANGES IN LAP

Decreased LAP
  Fluid volume deficit
Increased LAP
  Fluid volume overload
  Decreased myocardial contractility
  Increased cardiac afterload
  Dysrhythmias
  Cardiac tamponade

2. Potential for decreased cardiac output related to cardiac tamponade following LA line removal. **Rationale:** When the catheter is removed, a small hole is present in the LA tissue that must clot and self-seal. If this does not occur, the patient will bleed into the pericardial space and develop cardiac tamponade (Table 10–4).

3. Potential for altered cerebral, myocardial, or peripheral arterial tissue perfusion related to clot or air emboli from LA line. **Rationale:** Blood clots can form on the tip of the LA line if it is not properly flushed. Air bubbles that enter the pressure transducer system can travel through the left side of the heart and to other body organs.

Planning

1. Individualize the following goals for performing LAP measures:

TABLE 10-4 SIGNS AND SYMPTOMS OF CARDIAC TAMPONADE

Early Signs
  CVP/RAP elevation
  Neck vein distension
  Pressure plateau
  Sinus tachycardia
Late Signs
  Pulsus paradoxus
  Widened mediastinum on radiograph
  Decreased cardiac output
  Hypotension
  Signs of circulatory collapse
  Electromechanical dissociation (EMD)

a. Maintain cardiac output within individual patient's normal limits. **Rationale:** If the LAP is used appropriately to determine treatment, the CO should return to normal prior to removal. If there is no bleeding following removal, the patient maintains his/her CO.

b. Maintain normal cerebral, myocardial, and peripheral arterial tissue perfusion. **Rationale:** With proper catheter care and observations for air bubbles, the patient will not develop bleeding or air emboli.

2. Prepare all necessary equipment and supplies. **Rationale:** Ensures that LAP will be monitored quickly and efficiently.
    a. Carpenter's level.
    b. Single pressure transducer assembled and setup.

3. Prepare the patient.
    a. Explain the procedure to the patient. **Rationale:** Reduces anxiety.
    b. Sedate the patient as prescribed. **Rationale:** The restless patient could accidentally pull the LA line out. It is best during this time of intensive monitoring to keep the patient comfortable and quiet.
    c. Explain to the patient the importance of not putting tension on this line. This is especially important in the pediatric patient or the confused elderly patient who may want to play with or pull out this catheter. **Rationale:** Prevents accidental removal of catheter.

Implementation

Steps	Rationale	Special Considerations
1. Wash hands.	Reduces transmission of microorganisms.	
2. Zero, level, and calibrate equipment (Skill 10–1).	Ensures accuracy of readings.	
3. Turn on bedside recorder, and record three respiratory cycles of LA waveform.	Allows the nurse to identify end-expiration, which is when pressure values should be read.	
4. Identify the end-expiratory period for each respiratory cycle, and locate two cycles where this point is similar. The mean value of the LAP is read here.	Ensures greater accuracy in reading values.	
5. Record on strip *a* and *v* waves, inspiration and expiration, location where LAP was read, the patient's name, and date and time of the recording, and place in patient record.	Provides reference for other health care practitioners. Promotes consistency of waveform interpretation.	
6. Continuously monitor waveform for any changes in configuration (i.e., dampening, LV waveform, absence of waveform), and correlate any changes with physical findings. Arterial blood gas values will confirm position of LA catheter, i.e., in LA rather than in RA.	Indicative of problems with the catheter that require troubleshooting.	Dampening means clot in catheter, air in system, or hypovolemic state. LV waveform means forward migration of catheter. Absent waveform means clotted catheter or perforation of LV. It is important in all these situations *not* to irrigate the catheter (Taylor, 1985).

Table continues on following page

Steps	Rationale	Special Considerations
7. *Do not* use LAP line for blood withdrawal, administration of medications, or IV therapy. It is present for pressure monitoring purposes only.	Each time the line is entered, there is a risk of introducing air emboli or bacteria.	Bacterial contamination of this line is of great concern, since it sits within the heart, in close proximity to suture lines.
8. Change entire LAP pressure monitoring system q48h or as per unit policy.	Decreases risk of infection.	
9. Wash hands.	Reduces transmission of microorganisms.	

Evaluation

1. Compare assessments before and after reading of LAP. **Rationale:** Identifies complications related to the procedure.

2. Prior to removal, assess prothrombin time (PT), partial thromboplastin time (PTT), and platelets. **Rationale:** It is important to be sure that the patient will not have any difficulty forming a clot at the LAP insertion site following removal. Failure to form a clot can lead to cardiac tamponade. PT and PTT must be normal prior to removal. Platelets must be at least 60,000/mm^3 prior to removal.

3. Following removal of LA line, keep patient in bed and monitor chest tube drainage, vital signs, and heart rate hourly for 2 hours. **Rationale:** Excessive chest tube drainage (>3 ml/kg/h in pediatric patients and >100 ml/h in adults) suggests that the insertion site has not clotted off and that the patient is hemorrhaging.

4. Evaluate catheter insertion site daily for signs of infection (i.e., heat, redness, drainage, or edema). **Rationale:** Prevents adverse infectious sequelae.

5. Change dressing daily using aseptic technique, and apply antibacterial ointment to insertion site. **Rationale:** Decreases risk of infection.

6. Monitor LAP pressure transducer system for the presence of air bubbles. **Rationale:** Air entering the LAP line has a direct route to the brain and could result in stroke or death. If air is observed, turn off LA line to patient and flush air from catheter.

7. Evaluate daily chest x-ray for catheter location. **Rationale:** To be sure it has not moved forward or backward, resulting in inaccurate measures.

Expected Outcomes

1. Normal cerebral, myocardial, and peripheral arterial perfusion. **Rationale:** Proper handling and technique in LAP pressure readings should prevent air embolus, cardiac tamponade, and hemorrhage.

2. LAP readings correlate with physical findings (see Table 10–3). **Rationale:** Proper technique in taking readings and maintaining hemodynamic monitoring system should result in accurate readings.

3. Absence of infection. **Rationale:** Proper infection control practices will maintain an infection-free LAP.

Unexpected Outcomes

1. Infection. **Rationale:** Patient develops redness, drainage, edema at insertion site, pain, fever, or elevated WBC.

2. Hemorrhage. **Rationale:** Clot formation at the insertion site does not occur once the catheter has been removed. Monitor for excessive chest tube drainage (>3 ml/kg/h in pediatric patients and >100 ml/h in adults).

3. Air embolus. **Rationale:** The pressure transducer system creates a direct avenue for air bubbles to travel to the left side of the heart.

4. Cardiac tamponade. **Rationale:** Failure of the LA tissue to self-seal following LA line removal followed by bleeding into the pericardial space results.

Documentation

Documentation in the patient record should include date and time the monitoring line is changed, the amount of intake of flush solutions, cardiopulmonary assessment, labeled LAP waveform, assessment of catheter insertion site, and dressing change dates and times. **Rationale:** Documents nursing care given, patient's cardiopulmonary status, and expected and unexpected outcomes.

Patient/Family Education

Discuss rationale, catheter location, and the importance of not touching this line with both patient and family. **Rationale:** Reduces patient and family anxiety, and prevents line contamination and inadvertent line removal.

Performance Checklist
Skill 10–4: Left Atrial Pressure

Critical Behaviors	Complies	
	yes	no
1. Wash hands.		

Table continues on following page

Critical Behaviors	Complies	
	yes	no
2. Zero, level, and calibrate equipment.		
3. Record three respiratory cycles of LAP waveform.		
4. Identify the end-expiratory period of each respiratory cycle, and read LAP at this point.		
5. Document on strip the *a* and *v* waves, inspiration and expiration, location where LAP was read, patient's name, date, and time of recording, and place in patient record.		
6. Monitor waveform for any changes in configuration.		
7. Change entire pressure monitoring system q48h.		
8. Record date catheter was inserted in patient record, and monitor length of time catheter is present.		
9. Prior to LAP removal, assess PT, PTT, and platelet value.		
10. Following LAP line removal, keep patient in bed and keep chest tubes present for at least 2 hours.		
11. Wash hands.		
12. Document in patient record.		

SKILL 10–5

Pulmonary Artery and Pulmonary Artery Wedge Pressures

The pulmonary artery pressure (PAP) is one of many hemodynamic measures that are used in the evaluation and treatment of critically ill patients. It is obtained with a PA catheter (Fig. 10–22), which is passed through the right side of the heart into a pulmonary artery branch vessel (Fig. 10–23). The PA pressure is monitored through the distal lumen in the pulmonary capillary bed. When the 1.5-cc balloon on the distal tip is inflated, the pulmonary artery wedge pressure (PAWP) can be obtained. Proximal to the PA lumen is an opening in the right atrium (RA) through which right atrial pressure (RAP) can be monitored (see Skill 10–3).

The PA waveform consists of two phases: systole and diastole (Fig. 10–24). Systole begins with pulmonic valve opening. Blood is rapidly ejected to a peak, and then pressure falls as volume declines. The peak of ejection is the systolic PAP. When right (RV) ventricular pressure falls below the PA pressure, the pulmonic valve closes and a dicrotic notch appears on the downslope of the waveform. The pressure continues to fall until the next RV systole. The PA end-diastolic pressure is the value just before systole (PA valve opening). The normal values for PA systolic pressure are 15 to 28 mmHg, for diastolic pressure 5 to 16 mmHg, and for mean pressure 10 to 22 mmHg. In the absence of pulmonary disease, the PAD pressure closely approximates left ventricular end-diastolic pressure. The significance of high and low PA pressures can be seen in Table 10–5.

The PAWP is obtained by inflation of the balloon located at the tip of the catheter. Balloon inflation allows the catheter to float into a wedged, or occlusive, position, where the pressure behind the balloon is obstructed and the tip of the catheter (distal to balloon) can read the antegrade pressure. The value of the PAWP is that it is an indirect measure of mean left atrial (LA) pressure, which in turn is an indirect measure of left ventricular end-diastolic pressure (LVEDP) or left ventricular preload. During diastole, when the balloon is inflated, a static fluid column created within the pulmonary circulation allows the distal balloon lumen to detect a pressure that is continuous into the left ventricle.

The PAWP waveform consists of two distinct pressure peaks and troughs. The first pressure peak, the *a* wave, represents the increase in atrial pressure during atrial contraction at the end of diastole. This deflection correlates with the PR interval on the ECG. The *a* wave is followed by a fall pressure called the *x* descent. The second peak is the *v* wave, which represents passive filling of the left atrium (LA) that occurs during ventricular systole. It corresponds with the TP interval on the ECG and is followed by the *y* descent. The LVEDP occurs at that point in time on the pulse pressure trace when the mitral valve is open and the pressures in the LA and LV are equal. This is just prior to ventricular systole, or as seen on the PAWP waveform, just prior to the *v* wave, (Fig. 10–25). The normal wedge pressure value is 6 to 15 mmHg. The significance of high and low PAWP values can be seen in Table 10–6.

The PA catheter provides information about right- and left-sided intracardiac pressures, cardiac output by thermodilution method, and mixed venous blood for gas and chemical analysis. In addition, newer models of this catheter allow for continuous measurement of venous oxygen saturation (see Skill 6–3), atrial and ventricular pacing, diagnosis of complex dysrhythmias, and right ventricular volume. It can be used in a variety of situations to evaluate the course of such critical conditions as CHF, shock, pulmonary disease, renal failure, multiple organ failure, preshock syndrome, trauma, life-threatening dysrhythmias, eclampsia, etc. While most hemo-

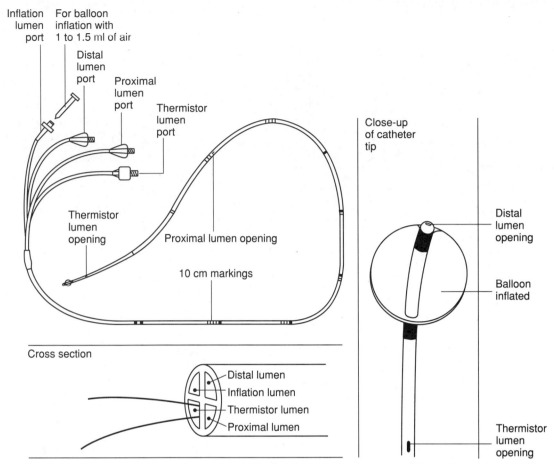

Inflation lumen port

For balloon inflation with 1 to 1.5 ml of air

Distal lumen port

Proximal lumen port

Thermistor lumen port

Thermistor lumen opening

Proximal lumen opening

10 cm markings

Close-up of catheter tip

Distal lumen opening

Balloon inflated

Thermistor lumen opening

Cross section

Distal lumen
Inflation lumen
Thermistor lumen
Proximal lumen

FIGURE 10–22. Anatomy of the PA catheter. The standard no. 7 French thermodilution PA catheter is 110 cm in length and contains four lumens. It is constructed of radiopaque polyvinyl chloride. In 10-cm increments there are black markings on the catheter beginning at the distal end. At the distal end of the catheter is a latex rubber balloon of 1.5-cc capacity, which, when inflated, extends slightly beyond the tip of the catheter without obstructing it. Balloon inflation cushions the tip of the catheter and prevents contact with the RV wall during insertion. The balloon also acts to float the catheter into position and allows measurement of the PAWP. Note black bands on catheter which indicate length of insertion. Narrow black bands represent 10 cm lengths and wide black bands indicate 50 cm lengths. (From F. Visalli and P. Evans, The Swan-Ganz catheter: A program for teaching safe, effective use. *Nursing 81* 11[1], 1981, with permission.)

FIGURE 10–23. PA catheter location within heart. Pulmonary artery wedge pressure (PAWP) is an indirect measure of left atrial and left ventricular end-diastolic pressure. (From L. D. Kersten, *Comprehensive Respiratory Nursing: A Decision-Making Approach*. Philadelphia: Saunders, 1989, p. 758, with permission.)

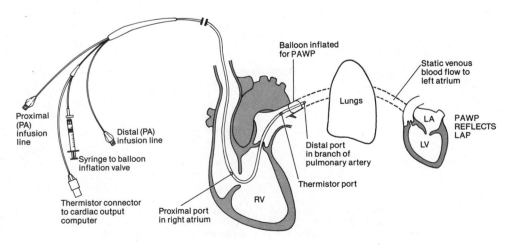

Proximal (PA) infusion line

Distal (PA) infusion line

Syringe to balloon inflation valve

Thermistor connector to cardiac output computer

Proximal port in right atrium

Balloon inflated for PAWP

Lungs

Static venous blood flow to left atrium

LA

LV

PAWP REFLECTS LAP

Distal port in branch of pulmonary artery

Thermistor port

RV

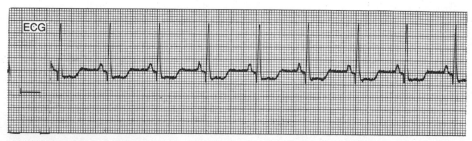
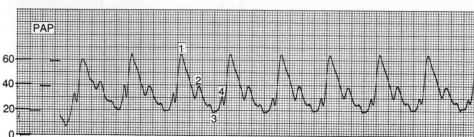

FIGURE 10–24. PA waveform and components. 1 = PA systole, 2 = dicrotic notch, 3 = PA end-diastole, 4 = anacrotic notch of PA valve opening.

TABLE 10–5 ETIOLOGIES FOR CHANGES IN PAP

Decreased PAP
 Fluid volume deficit
 Pulmonary artery vasodilation (i.e., drug induced)
Increased PAP
 Pulmonary hypertension
 Pulmonary disease
 Mitral valve disease
 Left ventricular failure
 Atrial or ventricular left-to-right shunt
 Hypoxia
 Pulmonary emboli

ECG

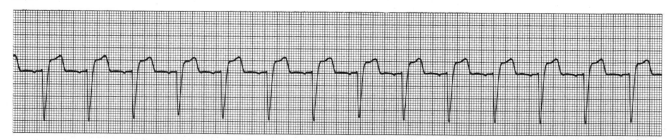
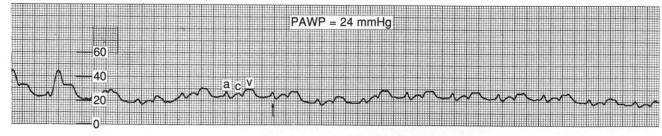

FIGURE 10–25. Normal PAWP waveform and components. Note delay in *a*, *c*, and *v* waves due to time it takes for the mechanical events to show a pressure change. This waveform is from a spontaneously breathing patient. The arrow indicates end-expiration, where the height of *a* wave pressure is measured.

TABLE 10–6 ETIOLOGIES FOR CHANGES IN PAWP

Decreased PAWP
  Fluid volume deficit
  Venodilation (i.e., due to drug therapy)
Increased PAWP
  Left ventricular failure
  Cardiac tamponade
  Mitral valve disease
  Constrictive pericarditis
  Fluid volume overload

dynamic monitoring occurs in critical care areas, recent applications in patients with chronic heart failure have included such monitoring in the cardiac stepdown area (Kern, 1990).

The PA catheter has proved to be an important guide for the management of the critically ill. However, a number of complications have been reported with its use, including PA thrombosis, jugular vein thrombosis, PA rupture, PA hemorrhage, RA thrombosis, sepsis, atrial and ventricular dysrhythmias, and endocarditis, to name a few (Hines and Barash, 1990, Masters, 1989; Robin, 1985). One study (Gore et al., 1985) of more than 3000 patients with acute myocardial infarction demonstrated prolonged hospitalizations and a higher mortality rate with use of the PA catheter.

The patient who has a PA catheter present is usually restricted to bed rest. With bed rest, the patient is prone to pulmonary, skin, cardiac, and musculoskeletal complications. Frequent position changes, pulmonary toilet, and skilled assessment help to minimize pulmonary complications associated with bed rest during monitoring (Mariani, 1989).

One nursing study by Pierson and Funk (1989) demonstrated that nurses caring for postoperative cardiac surgery patients relied on clinical assessment data for fluid management decisions despite the presence of the PA catheter. The authors rightfully question the need for this catheter in these patients and also point out that the PA catheter is often left in place for longer periods of time than necessary. The longer the catheter is in place, the greater is the risk for infection and thrombotic complications (Conners et al., 1985, Tafuro and Ristuccia, 1984).

Many complications are prevented when the catheter is appropriately used and cared for. The nurse is the primary user of the PA catheter and therefore is responsible for controlling the environmental conditions that can alter the accuracy of PA readings. Lack of regular leveling and calibration of equipment (see Skill 10–1) contributes to inaccuracies. Dampening of the waveform can occur if the catheter tip becomes clogged with fibrin clot material as a result of dysfunctional flush system. The PA catheter estimation of LA pressures can be affected when the catheter is placed in West's lung zones 1 or 2 (Fig. 10–26) and the position is not checked with a postinsertion chest x-ray. These are just a few of the environmental conditions that affect PA values.

Patient factors also can alter PAP and PAWP readings. Patients with pulmonary hypertension, a dilated pul-

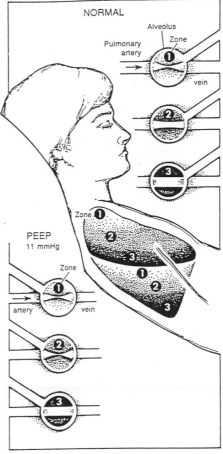

FIGURE 10–26. Lung zones. Source: Daily, E. K., in Dolan, J. T., *Critical Care Nursing: Clinical Management Through the Nursing Process*. Philadelphia: FA Davis Co., 1990, p. 840, with permission.

monary artery, or dilated cardiomyopathy frequently exhibit catheter "whip" or "fling" on the tracing. Muscular blockade with paralyzing agents can result in substantial changes in PAP and a 20 percent decrease in CO during paralysis. Patients with decreased left ventricular compliance (due to LV hypertrophy, septal displacement, acute MI, myocardial fibrosis, and amyloidosis) will exhibit higher PAWP values that overestimate left ventricular end-diastolic volume (LVEDV) (Enger, 1989). An increase in juxtacardiac pressures (as a result of ascites, MAST suit application, cardiac tamponade, pericardial disease, or increased intrathoracic pressures) also can result in an increased PAWP in the presence of a stable LVEDV. The nurse therefore assesses the patient for underlying pathology so that threats to the validity of these numbers can be anticipated.

Purpose

The nurse performs PAP and PAWP monitoring to

1. Assess the underlying disease process.
2. Evaluate response to treatment.
3. As a research tool.

Prerequisite Knowledge and Skills

Prior to performing PAP and PAWP measures, the nurse should understand

1. Cardiovascular anatomy and physiology.
2. Respiratory anatomy and physiology.
3. Pathophysiology of the disease(s) for which the PAP and PAWP measures are indicated.
4. Treatment of life-threatening dysrhythmias.
5. Physiology of fluid balance.
6. Aseptic technique.
7. Universal precautions.
8. Principles of hemodynamic monitoring.

The nurse should be able to perform

1. Proper handwashing technique (see Skill 35–5).
2. Sterile technique.
3. Universal precautions (see Skill 35–1).
4. Pressure transducer system setup (see Skill 10–1).
5. Zero, leveling, and calibrating of hemodynamic monitoring system (see Skill 10–1).
6. Stopcock manipulation.
7. Basic dysrhythmia recognition.
8. Defibrillation (see Skill 8–2).
9. PA catheter care (see Skill 10–6).

Assessment

1. Assess the patient's vital signs, blood pressure, heart and breath sounds, skin color and temperature, mentation, peripheral pulses, and laboratory data. **Rationale:** The patient's clinical picture should correlate with pulmonary artery pressure readings.

2. If the patient is being mechanically ventilated, note type of support, ventilator mode, and presence of PEEP or CPAP. Observe rate of mode being delivered and whether or not patient is contributing any spontaneous breaths. **Rationale:** The presence of mechanically ventilated breaths will alter physiology.

3. Assess recent chest x-ray results. **Rationale:** Identifies catheter position within pulmonary artery and evaluates patient's pulmonary status and cardiac disease.

Nursing Diagnoses

1. Decreased cardiac output related to altered pre-load, altered afterload, or altered contractility. **Rationale:** The pulmonary artery and wedge pressures are used to evaluate changes in cardiopulmonary function that affect cardiac output. An adequate cardiac output is needed to provide blood flow to body tissues to meet metabolic demands. Decreased cardiac output related to decreased preload is evidenced by a decreased PAP and PAWP (decreased LV preload) or decreased RAP (decreased RV preload). Decreased cardiac output related to increased afterload would be evidenced by an increased systemic vascular resistance (SVR). Decreased cardiac output related to decreased contractility would be evidenced by a corrected PAWP (with drug therapy) and a corrected afterload (with drug therapy/mechanical support) in the presence of a continuing low cardiac output (Kern, 1990).

2. Potential for injury: PA rupture related to insertion complication or improper wedging technique. **Rationale:** Patients with advanced age (>60 years), pulmonary hypertension, anticoagulation therapy, and Coronary Artery Bypass surgery are at risk for PA rupture (Barash et al., 1981; Chun and Ellestad, 1971; Daily and Schroeder, 1989; Golden et al., 1975). PA rupture can occur with distal migration of catheter, overinflation of balloon, eccentric inflation of balloon, and manual flushing of a wedged catheter.

Planning

1. Individualize the following goals for performing PAP and PAWP measurements:
   a. Achieve a normal or improved CO. **Rationale:** PAP monitoring provides continuous data regarding the patient's physical well-being on which therapy is based.
   b. Maintain adequate pre-load, after load, and contractility. **Rationale:** If accurate, PAP, RAP, and PAWP values will provide physiological parameters on which therapy is based.

2. Prepare and check all equipment prior to PAP and PAWP measures. **Rationale:** Prevents inaccuracies in pressure measurement.
   a. Multiple pressure transducer system assembled and setup.
   b. Carpenter's level.

3. Inspect hemodynamic system to ensure that there are no air bubbles in the pressure tubing, stopcocks, or transducers. **Rationale:** Air will dampen waveform and result in false readings.

4. Zero, level, and calibrate equipment before performing pressure measurements. **Rationale:** Ensures accuracy of readings.

5. Prepare the patient by explaining the purpose for measuring PAP and PAWP values. **Rationale:** Reduces anxiety.

Implementation

Steps	Rationale	Special Considerations
Reading PAP from Paper Printout		
1. Wash hands.	Reduces transmission of microorganisms.	
2. Observe PA waveform on bedside monitor.	Ensures that catheter tip is in PA prior to recording waveform.	
3. Turn on paper printout, and record PAP for three respiratory cycles (Fig. 10–27A).	The digital readout is an unreliable method for reading PAP and PAWP because it reflects the average taken over a period of time or a number of beats. Three respiratory cycles allow the nurse to accurately identify the end-expiration waveform where readings are taken. This is particularly helpful when there is catheter fling or dysrhythmias present that make interpretation of end-expiration difficult (Cenzig et al., 1983; Enger, 1989).	Newer monitoring equipment takes readings at end-expiration for the digital display. It is recommended that these values be compared with paper printout values prior to reliance solely on digital display.
4. While recording waveform, note how patient's inspiration correlates with PA waveform fluctuation on the printed waveform; i.e., is expiration at the high point of the waveform or the low point?	Simultaneous observation of both patient's respirations and the waveforms will aid in the accurate identification of end-expiration.	The pattern of respiratory variation will be different for spontaneous breaths versus mechanically ventilated breaths versus the mode of mechanical ventilation.
5. Locate the three inspiration points on each wave (Fig. 10–27B). For spontaneous inspiration, this will usually be the lowest point, since spontaneous inspiration causes a *decrease* in intrapulmonary pressures while expiration causes an *increase*.	Location of inspiration is usually easier than expiration and will enable the nurse to identify the end-expiratory point.	
6. The waveform prior to inspiration is the *end-expiratory pressure*. This is the reference point where the PAP is measured (Fig. 10–27C).	Changes in intrathoracic pressure have the least hemodynamic effects at end-expiration (Enger, 1989). Changes in airway pressure during mechanical ventilation are at a minimum (Kersten, 1989).	
7. For PAP, the pressure is interpreted by taking the systolic pressure at end-expiration and the diastolic pressure *preceding* the measured systolic peak.	For consistency, it is best to measure the diastolic pressure preceding the systolic peak.	The diastolic pressure following end-expiration will vary because of the changing intrapulmonary pressures with inspiration.
8. The mean PAP, if required, can be calculated by the following formula: $$\frac{1(PAS) + 2(PAD)}{3}$$	Mean PAP can be a useful value to monitor in the patient with pulmonary hypertension.	
9. Wash hands.	Reduces transmission of microorganisms.	
Pulmonary Artery Wedge Pressure Procedure and Precautions		
Note: Refer to manufacturer's instructions for wedging procedure for individual PA catheters.	The guidelines here are general guidelines that should apply to most catheters.	

Table continues on following page

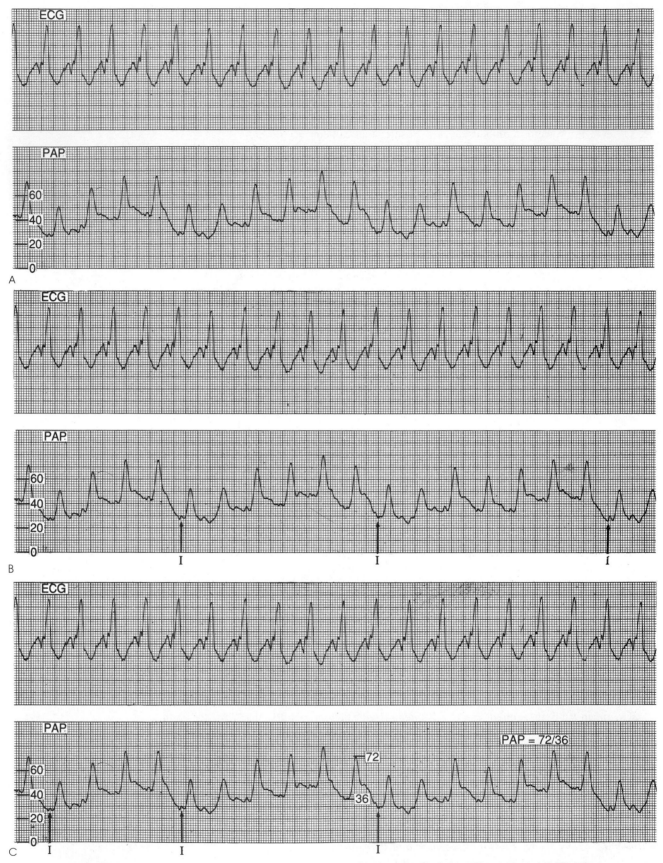

FIGURE 10–27. Respiratory fluctuations of PAP waveform in a spontaneously breathing patient. (*A*) Waveform as it is printed out. (*B*) The location of inspiration (*I*) is marked on the waveform. (*C*) The points just prior to inspiration are end-expiration, where readings will be taken.

Steps	Rationale	Special Considerations
1. Wash hands.	Reduces transmission of microorganisms.	
2. Observe PA waveform on bedside monitor.	The nurse must have a good PA waveform in order to observe wedging of the catheter.	If the PA waveform is dampened with whip or fling (Fig. 10–28), then the catheter must be repositioned prior to wedging.
3. Fill a 3-cc syringe with 1.5 cc of air or CO_2 (or maximum amount recommended by manufacturer).	It is important not to inject more air than the balloon can hold. Overfilling of balloon may result in rupture.	CO_2 may be used in patients with known congenital heart defects and right-to-left shunting of blood.
4. Attach syringe with air to the balloon lumen of the catheter.	Prepares for injection of air.	
5. Align gate-valve arrow to open position (Fig. 10–29), if this is present.	Gate valve is kept closed (arrows offset) at all times to prevent inadvertent injection of air or fluid into balloon lumen.	
6. Inflate balloon with air slowly while observing PA pressure waveform. Inflate balloon with the minimum volume needed to obtain PAWP waveform (Fig. 10–30). It should take 1.25 to 1.5 cc of air to wedge catheter. Any amount less than this indicates that catheter is too far into PA (Enger, 1990).	Avoids PA rupture.	Figure 10–31 demonstrates the possible mechanisms for PA rupture.
7. Record PAWP waveform for a minimum of two to three respiratory cycles. (Reading pressure off paper is discussed further down.)	Two to three cycles will allow enough recording to observe for respiratory variations in pressure. The PAWP is read at end-expiration.	When wedging catheter in elderly (>60 years) patient or patient with pulmonary hypertension, wedge for no longer than 10 to 15 seconds. These patients are at increased risk for PA rupture.
8. Disconnect syringe and allow balloon to deflate passively.	Withdrawal of air with syringe will weaken the balloon and result in early leaks.	
9. Close gate valve to off position (arrows offset).	Prevents accidental air injection.	
10. Keep number of PAWP readings to a minimum. If PAD and PAWP are similar values (<4 mmHg difference), then PAD can be substituted for PAWP.	Frequent balloon inflations increase wear on the balloon and increase the risk for balloon deterioration.	
11. If strong resistance is met during inflation, *do not* inflate balloon. Notify the physician.	Catheter may be knotted.	
12. If air goes in freely (without any resistance), or if blood comes back from balloon, disconnect syringe and close off lumen. Label gate valve with sign that says, "Do not inject air." Notify physician.	Balloon is very likely ruptured. Air into this lumen can enter pulmonary circulation as an embolus and is life-threatening.	
13. *Never flush catheter when in a wedged position.*	Flushing a wedged catheter has resulted in PA rupture.	

Table continues on following page

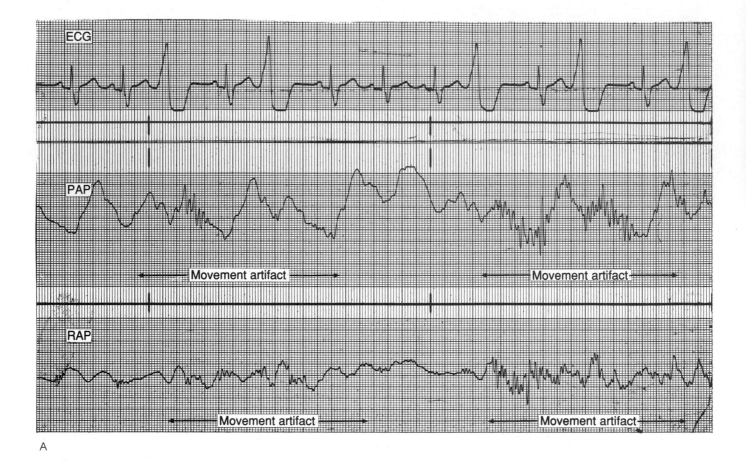

A

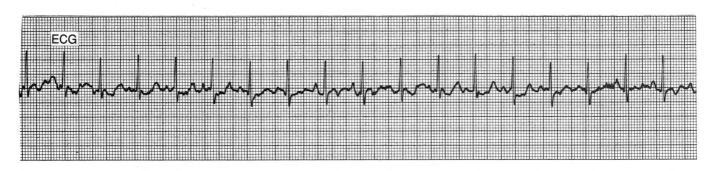

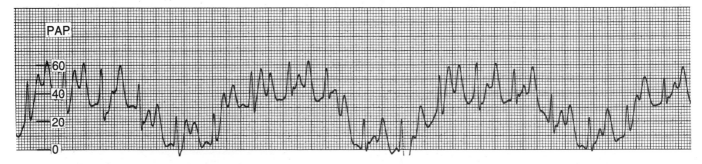

B

FIGURE 10–28. Variations in the PAP waveform. (*A*) PAP and RAP have evidence of catheter fling and patient movement artifact, making reading of the waveform impossible. (*B*) Waveform artifact and respiratory variation make this waveform difficult to interpret. The artifact was not due to the catheter position (which was checked on x-ray), but was thought to be due to a malfunction with the hemodynamic lines (compliance problem with high-pressure tubing).

Figure continues on following page

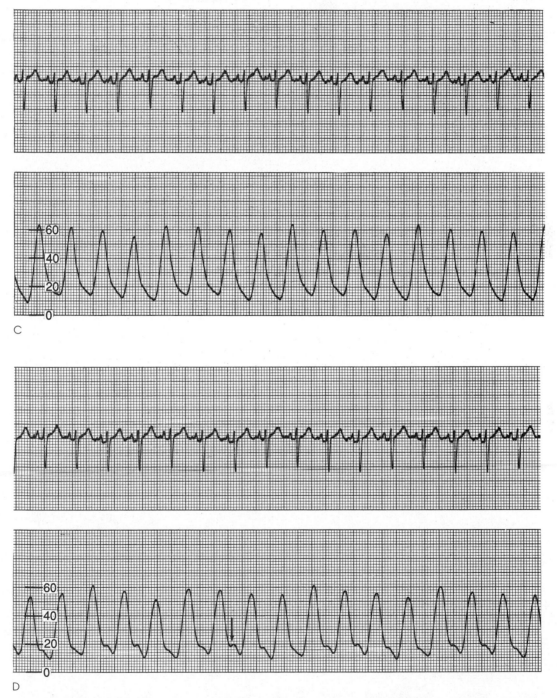

FIGURE 10–28. Cont'd. (*C*) **A dampened PAP waveform in a patient with pulmonary hypertension.** (*D*) **Cause of dampening in *C* was found to be small air bubbles in pressure system. Once removed, the dicrotic notch (*arrow*) again became apparent.**

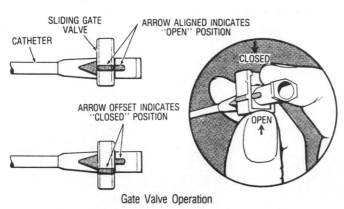

FIGURE 10-29. Gate valve in open position on PA (distal) lumen of PA catheter. (Courtesy of Baxter Edwards Corporation.)

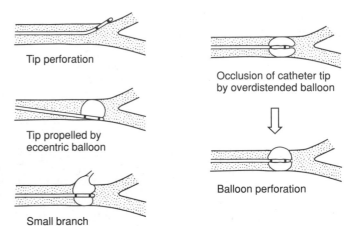

FIGURE 10-30. Mechanisms for PA perforation. (From P. G. Barash, D. Nardi, G. Hammon, et al., Catheter-induced pulmonary artery perforation: Mechanism, management, and modifications. *J. Thorac. Cardiovasc. Surg.* 82:5-12, 1981, with permission.)

Steps	Rationale	Special Considerations
14. Spontaneous catheter tip migration toward the periphery of the pulmonary bed may occur. Therefore, it is important to monitor the PAP tracing continuously. Report the appearance of a PAWP waveform to physician immediately.	Migration of catheter into a wedge position will result in pulmonary infarct. A wedged catheter must be pulled back immediately.	
15. Wash hands.	Reduces transmission of microorganisms.	

Reading PAWP from Paper Printout

1. Wash hands.	Reduces transmission of microorganisms.	

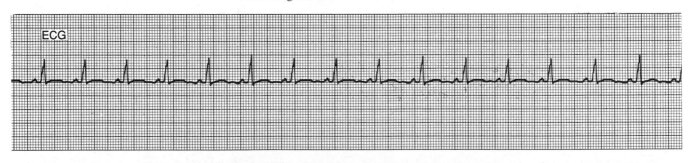

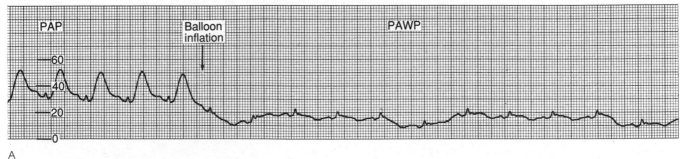

A

FIGURE 10-31. Change in PAP waveform to PAWP waveform with balloon inflation. The balloon is inflated while observing the bedside monitor for the change in waveform. (*A*) Balloon inflation (*arrow*) in patient with normal PAWP.

Figure continues on following page

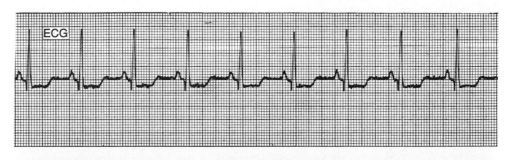

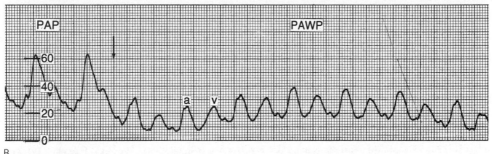

B

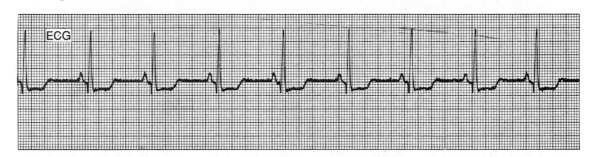

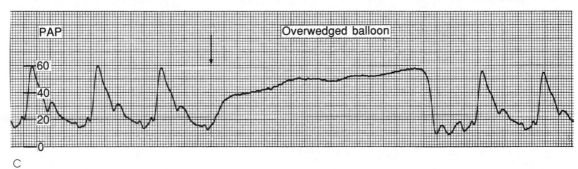

C

FIGURE 10–31 Cont'd. (*B*) Balloon inflation (*arrow*) in patient with elevated wedge pressure and predominant *a* and *v* waves. (*C*) Overwedging of balloon (balloon has been overinflated). The danger of overinflating balloon is that the PA vessel may rupture from the pressure of the balloon.

Steps	Rationale	Special Considerations
2. Record three respiratory cycles of PAWP waveform as described above.	Three respiratory cycles allow the nurse to accurately identify the end-expiration waveform, which is where readings are taken.	
3. Identify the point of inspiration for each waveform. The point just prior to inspiration is end-expiration, where readings will be taken (Fig. 10–32).	Location of inspiration is usually easier than expiration and will enable the nurse to identify the end-expiratory point.	

Table continues on following page

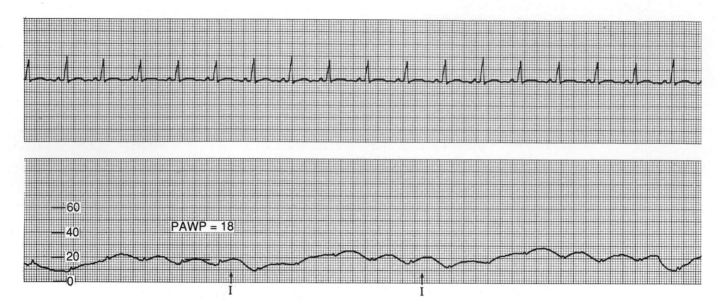

FIGURE 10–32. Respiratory variations in a PAWP waveform (*I*-inhalation). The PAWP reading is taken at end-expiration (see text for explanation).

Steps	Rationale	Special Considerations
4. Locate the *a* and *v* waves on the PAWP waveform. The PAWP mean pressure is measured by measuring the height of the *a* wave and bottom of the *a* wave and taking an average, when waveform is normal (Fig. 10-33).	Multiple research studies have supported the value of the *a* wave in estimating LVEDP. In addition, when a large *v* wave is present (as in mitral regurgitation) PAWP measures of the *a* and *v* wave components together will result in falsely elevated pressure measures.	As a general rule, the *a* wave method is most accurate. One exception is the patient with mitral stenosis, which causes increased resistance to LV filling and an elevated *a* wave. This elevated *a* wave will therefore not be an accurate indicator of LVEDP. In this instance, the *v* wave may be the most accurate reflection of LVEDP.

Table continues on following page

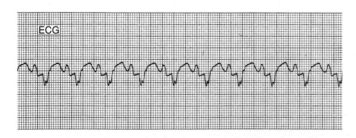

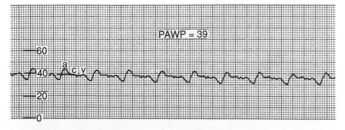

FIGURE 10–33. PAWP waveform without respiratory variation. The mean PAWP is measured by taking the top of the *a* wave (here, 44 mmHg) and the bottom of the *a* wave (here, 34 mmHg), and dividing the sum by 2. The PAWP here is 39 mmHg.

Steps	Rationale	Special Considerations
5. If the patient has an abnormal waveform (i.e., an elevated *a* wave, an elevated *v* wave, or both), then values obtained may not be an accurate reflection of LVEDP. Table 10–7 demonstrates how the PAWP waveform is to be interpreted when there are variations in the *a* or *v* wave. Figure 10–34 illustrates a patient with increased *a* and *v* waves and how this waveform is read.	Elevation of the *a* or *v* wave indicates a cardiac abnormality. Measurement of each waveform will provide information about the degree of abnormality present and is clinically useful to the nurse. For example, in mitral regurgitation (MR), an elevated *v* wave is measured and monitored. As the MR improves, the nurse will see a decrease in the height of the *v* wave.	
6. On the recorded waveform, document the following information: patient's name, date and time, waveform, body position, inspiration/expiration, and pressure values obtained, and place in patient record.	Enables others to follow trends in pressure values and waveform changes.	
7. Wash hands.	Reduces transmission of microorganisms.	

Table continues on following page

TABLE 10–7   INTERPRETATION OF PAWP WAVEFORMS

	Increased *a* Wave	Increased *v* Wave	Both Increased
PAWP	Mean *a* wave recorded as $PAWP_a$.*	Mean *v* wave recorded as $PAWP_v$	Both recorded separately as $PAWP_a$ and $PAWP_v$

*Whenever there is elevation of a wave component, the *mean* pressure of that wave component is taken and recorded with a subscript letter designating the wave.

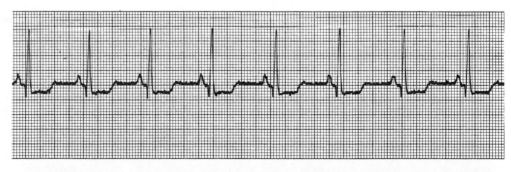
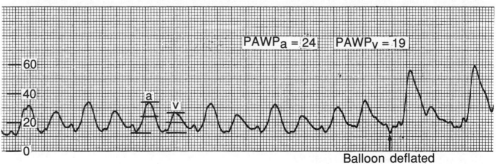

FIGURE 10–34. Elevated *a* and *v* waves on a PAWP waveform. See Table 10–7 for explanation of how to record these readings.

Steps	Rationale	Special Considerations
PAP/PAWP Measures with Control-Mode Ventilation		
1. Wash hands.	Reduces transmission of microorganisms.	
2. Record PA and PAW waveforms for three respiratory cycles.	Allows the nurse to accurately identify the end-expiration period for more than one period of time.	
3. Locate inspiration and end-expiration. The change in pressure with control-mode ventilation will be the opposite of spontaneous breathing (Fig. 10–35).	With controlled ventilation, PA/PAW pressures rise during mechanical inspiration (as the ventilator delivers a positive-pressure breath) and fall with mechanical expiration.	The positive-pressure breath given by the mechanical ventilator increases intrapulmonary pressures, while passive expiration of the ventilator breath returns intrapulmonary pressures to zero (or whatever level of PEEP has been added to the ventilator system). PA, PAW, and RA pressure waveforms therefore generally *increase* with ventilator cycling and return to a stable baseline between ventilator breaths.
4. Record end-expiratory pressure values, and place in patient record.	Documents where readings are taken so that others will be consistent in their readings.	
5. Wash hands.	Reduces transmission of microorganisms.	
SIMV Ventilation		
1. Wash hands.	Reduces transmission of microorganisms.	
2. Record PA/PAWP waveforms for three respiratory cycles.	Allows the nurse to be accurate in determining where end-expiration is located.	

Table continues on following page

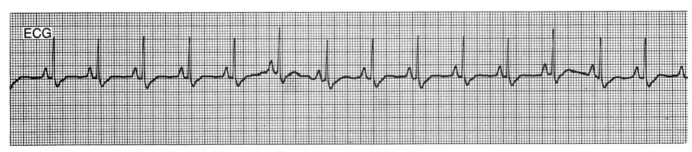

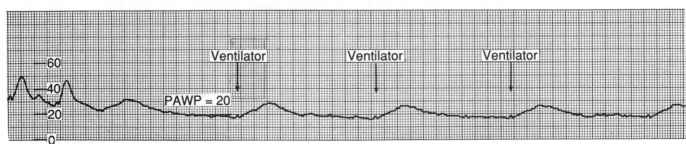

FIGURE 10–35. Mechanically ventilated patient (on pressure support-type ventilator) who had no spontaneous respirations because of neuromuscular blocking agent (vecuronium). The point of end-expiration is located just prior to the ventilator artifact.

Steps	Rationale	Special Considerations
3. Locate the points of spontaneous end-expiration. This will be just prior to a large increase in pressure that is associated with ventilator cycling.	In the SIMV mode, the patient receives a ventilator breath that is timed to occur with his or her own inspiratory efforts. The spontaneous end-expiration is the most stable time to take readings.	
4. Pressures are recorded as measured at the spontaneous end-expiration point and are placed in the patient record.	Provides reference for other health care professionals; promotes consistency in readings.	
5. Wash hands.	Reduces transmission of microorganisms.	

IMV Ventilation

1. Wash hands.	Reduces transmission of microorganisms.	
2. Record PA/PAWP waveforms for three respiratory cycles.	Allows accurate identification of spontaneous end-expiration.	
3. Locate patient's spontaneous breaths on waveform tracing (Fig. 10–36). Locate spontaneous breath end-expiration.	Pressure values will be the least affected by hemodynamic changes at the spontaneous breath end-expiration.	
4. Pressures are recorded as measured from the end-expiration of the spontaneous breath and are placed in the patient record.	Provides reference for other health-care professionals; promotes consistency in measurements.	
5. Wash hands.	Reduces transmission of microorganisms.	

PAWP Measurement in Mitral Regurgitation

1. Wash hands.	Reduces transmission of microorganisms.	
2. Record three respiratory cycles of PAWP waveform with corresponding ECG tracing.	Allows for accurate identification of the end-expiratory point.	
3. Using the ECG as a reference, locate the *a* and *v* waves of the PAWP waveform.	Accurate identification of the *a* and *v* waves is important because each wave will be read separately.	

Table continues on following page

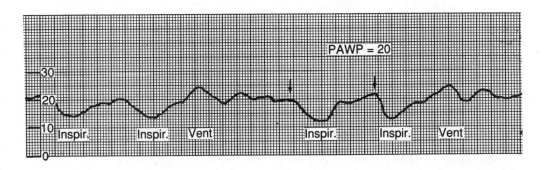

FIGURE 10–36. A mechanically ventilated patient on IMV. PAWP decreases with each spontaneous inspiration and increases with each ventilator cycle. The point of spontaneous end-expiration is located just before the pressure decrease with spontaneous inspiration. The areas in the waveform where ventilator cycling causes an increase in pressures should be avoided or erroneously high hemodynamic values will result. Arrows indicate where reading is taken (*Inspir* = inspiration by patient; *Vent* = ventilator giving a breath to patient).

Steps	Rationale	Special Considerations
4. Locate the end-expiration periods for the three respiratory cycles. Locate the *a* waves for these end-expiratory points.	The *a* wave is an accurate reflection of LVEDP. Readings are taken at end-expiration, where changes in intrathoracic pressure are minimal.	
5. Read the PAWP *a* wave at end-expiration, and record in patient record when *a* wave is elevated. (Fig. 10–37A).	Provides reference for other health-care professionals. Promotes consistency in readings.	In patients with unstable hemodynamics, it is important to know LVEDP in order to optimize cardiac output.
6. Locate *v* waves at end-expiration for each respiratory cycle. The height of the *v* wave is measured as the distance from the *a* wave to the top of the *v* wave divided in half. This gives a mean reading of the *v* wave (Fig. 10–37B). Record in patient record as PAWP*v*.	The calculation of the *v* wave into the mean PAWP is not an accurate reflection of the LVEDP; therefore, it is read separately. Since we measure the mean PAWP, a mean of the *v* wave is also taken, but this is recorded separately from the *a* wave mean value.	The *v* wave reflects LAP and PAWP, but not LVEDP, when it is elevated.
7. Wash hands.	Reduces transmission of microorganisms.	

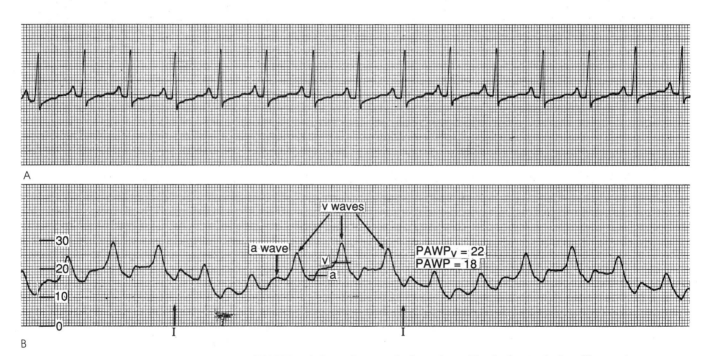

FIGURE 10–37. Measurement of PAWP and elevated *v* waves in the patient with mitral regurgitation. The mean pressure of *a* and *v* waves are measured. Both measures are taken at end-expiration in this spontaneously breathing patient. The PAWP for this patient would be recorded as follows: PAWP = 18 mmHg, PAWPv = 22 mmHg. Arrows indicate inspiration.

Evaluation

1. Compare cardiac assessments before and after PAP/PAWP measurement. **Rationale:** Identifies effects of measurement procedure.
2. Evaluate PAP waveform after measurement. **Rationale:** Ensures that the balloon is deflated and that the catheter remains in the proper location.
3. Evaluate daily chest x-ray results. **Rationale:** Monitors catheter location.

Expected Outcome

Absence of complications of PA pressure measurement (i.e., absence of hemoptysis, chest pain, tachypnea, hypotension, tachycardia, and ventricular ectopy). **Rationale:** PAP/PAWP measurement, when performed correctly, should not result in complications.

Unexpected Outcome

Catheter-related problems, e.g., continuous wedging,

looped catheter in RV position, and/or balloon rupture. **Rationale:** Patient becomes tachypneic, tachycardic, has hemoptysis, ventricular ectopy, chest pain, or hypotension during PAP or PAWP monitoring.

Documentation

Documentation in the patient record should include a copy of the PAP and PAWP waveform each shift or with every significant change that is labeled with patient name, date, time waveform inspiration/expiration phases, and pressure readings. **Rationale:** Documents where and how readings were taken, and promotes consistency in waveform interpretation.

Patient/Family Education

Explain to both patient and family the purpose of PAP and PAWP measures and how these numbers assist in the provision of care. **Rationale:** Reduces patient and family anxiety.

Performance Checklist
Skill 10–5: Pulmonary Artery and Pulmonary Artery Wedge Pressures

Critical Behaviors	Complies yes	Complies no
READING PAP FROM PAPER PRINTOUT 1. Wash hands.		
2. Observe PA waveform on bedside monitor.		
3. Record PA waveform for three respiratory cycles.		
4. Observe and correlate patient's respirations with waveform fluctuations.		
5. Identify three inspiration points on paper printout.		
6. Identify the end-expiration point for each respiratory cycle.		
7. Take PAP reading at end-expiration.		
8. Calculate mean PAP.		
9. Wash hands.		
10. Document in patient record.		
PULMONARY ARTERY WEDGE PRESSURE PROCEDURE AND PRECAUTIONS 1. Wash hands.		
2. Observe PA waveform on bedside monitor.		
3. Fill 3-cc syringe with 1.5 cc air.		
4. Attach syringe to balloon lumen of catheter.		
5. Align gate-valve arrow to open position.		
6. Slowly inflate balloon with air while watching waveform on bedside monitor, inflating balloon to minimal volume.		
7. Record PAWP waveform.		
8. Disconnect syringe and allow balloon to passively deflate.		
9. Close gate valve to off position.		
10. Keep number of PAWP readings to a minimum.		
11. If resistance is met during balloon inflation, do not continue to try to inflate, notify physician.		
12. If air goes into balloon freely or blood returns from balloon lumen, close gate valve, label valve "Do not inject air," and notify physician.		
13. Never flush catheter when it is wedged.		
14. Recognize PAWP waveform, and notify physician if catheter spontaneously wedges.		

Table continues on following page

Critical Behaviors	Complies	
	yes	no
15. Wash hands.		
16. Document in patient record.		
READING PAWP FROM PAPER PRINTOUT 1. Wash hands.		
2. Record three respiratory cycles of PAWP waveform as described in wedging procedure.		
3. Identify end-expiratory points.		
4. Locate *a* and *v* waves on PAWP waveform.		
5. Take measure of mean *a* wave for PAWP reading at end-expiration.		
6. Document appropriate information on all strips, and place in patient record.		
7. Wash hands.		
PAP/PAWP MEASURES WITH CONTROL-MODE VENTILATION 1. Wash hands.		
2. Record PA/PAWP waveforms for three respiratory cycles.		
3. Locate inspiration and end-expiration on waveforms, and note differences in cycle with control-mode ventilation.		
4. Record end-expiration values, and place in patient record.		
5. Wash hands.		
SIMV VENTILATION 1. Wash hands.		
2. Record PA/PAWP waveforms for three respiratory cycles.		
3. Locate the points of spontaneous end-expiration, just prior to ventilator cycling.		
4. Record pressures as measured at end-expiration values, and place in patient record.		
5. Wash hands.		
IMV VENTILATION 1. Wash hands.		
2. Record PAP/PAWP waveforms for three respiratory cycles.		
3. Locate patient's spontaneous breaths on waveform tracing, and locate spontaneous breath end-expiration.		
4. Record pressures as measured from the end-expiration of the spontaneous breath, and place in patient record.		
5. Wash hands.		
PAWP MEASURE IN MITRAL REGURGITATION 1. Wash hands.		
2. Record three respiratory cycles of PAWP waveform with corresponding ECG.		
3. Identify *a* and *v* waves of the PAWP waveform.		
4. Locate the end-expiratory period for each respiratory cycle.		
5. Read the PAWP *a* wave at end-expiration, and record in patient record as PAWP$_a$.		
6. Locate and measure mean *v* wave value, and record in patient record as PAWP$_v$.		
7. Wash hands.		

SKILL 10-6

Care and Troubleshooting of Pulmonary Artery Catheter

Pulmonary artery catheterization is performed in the critical-care setting to provide hemodynamic data that can be used to make a diagnosis of disease, to make decisions about therapy, to monitor a patient's progress of disease, to monitor a patient's response to therapy, and as a tool of research. The data that can be generated from this catheter include RAP, PAP, PAWP, $S\bar{v}O_2$ (in selected PA catheters), CO, and heart rate. From these direct data, derived parameters can be calculated, such as systemic vascular resistance (SVR), stroke volume (SV), stroke volume work index (SVWI), cardiac index (CI), etc.

Pulmonary artery catheterization can be performed in age groups from pediatrics through the elderly. Its primary benefit is that clinical decision making and diagnostic accuracy are greatly improved with knowledge of the data derived from this catheter. In numerous situations, a treatment regimen has been changed when the PA and PAW pressures became known. In this respect, then, the PA catheter is cost-effective. Through continuous monitoring of these pressures, the nurse and physician can detect early changes in cardiac and vascular hemodynamics and appropriately intervene.

Patients are usually uncomfortable with the presence of this catheter, particularly when it is inserted in the external jugular vein in the neck. In the past it was felt that patients must remain in bed with a PA catheter. This is no longer true. In selected situations, patients have ambulated to the bathroom and cycled at the bedside with this catheter in place.

Complications can occur during insertion and advancement of the catheter as well as during maintenance. Technical problems with the catheter can provide inaccurate information. Technical problems are common, because of the location of the catheter, the type of hemodynamic systems currently used, and the fact that the patient may move about in bed or even ambulate with the catheter present. Thus, troubleshooting becomes an important nursing responsibility. The nurse plays a vital role in identifying problems and intervening when technical and patient complications occur. When properly cared for, the PA catheter is an invaluable tool for managing the critically ill patient.

Purpose

The nurse performs PA catheter care and troubleshooting to

1. Maintain catheter patency to provide accurate data.
2. Prevent the development of catheter-related and patient-related complications (i.e., thrombosis, pulmonary infarction, PA rupture, and ventricular ectopy sepsis).
3. Maximize patient comfort with a PA catheter.

4. Ensure that displayed waveforms are clear and accurate.

Prerequisite Knowledge and Skills

Prior to performing PA catheter care and troubleshooting, the nurse should understand

1. Cardiovascular anatomy and physiology.
2. Normal values for intracardiac pressures (see Skills 10–1 to 10–5).
3. Waveform configurations for RA, RV, PA, and PAW pressures (see Skills 10–2 to 10–5).
4. Venous access routes and procedure for venous catheterization (see Skill 9–1).
5. Principles of sterile technique.
6. Universal precautions.
7. Treatment of life-threatening dysrhythmias.

The nurse should be able to perform

1. Hemodynamic waveform interpretation (see Skill 10–5).
2. Basic dysrhythmia recognition.
3. Multiple pressure transducer setup (see Skill 10–1).
4. Proper handwashing technique (see Skill 35–5).
5. Zeroing, leveling, and calibrating the hemodynamic monitoring system (Skill 10–1).
6. Stopcock manipulation.
7. Basic Cardiac Life Support/Advanced Cardiac Life Support (BCLS/ACLS).
8. Cardiopulmonary assessment.
9. Universal precautions (see Skill 35–1).

Assessment

1. Assess PA pressure waveform continuously. **Rationale:** The catheter may migrate forward into a wedged position, which could result in a pulmonary infarction. A migration foward is evidenced by a change in waveform from PAP to PAWP waveform (see Fig. 10–30A). In addition to migration foward, the catheter may loop around and fall into the right ventricle (RV) as evidenced by an RVP waveform (Fig. 10–38).

2. Perform physical assessment including heart and breath sounds, skin color and temperature, fluid balance, mentation, urinary output, jugular vein distension, peripheral pulses, and daily chest x-ray. **Rationale:** The patient's clinical picture should correlate with data derived from the catheter. When there is a discrepancy, the hemodynamic monitoring system should be assessed for mechanical problems.

3. Assess the patient daily for signs and symptoms of infection (i.e., increased WBC, fever, chills, tachycardia, decreasing SVR, increased CO, induration at catheter insertion site, assess temperature q4h during insertion). **Rationale:** Infection can develop at the catheter insertion

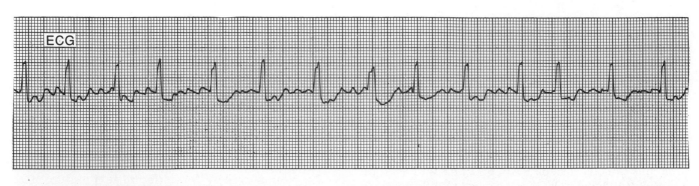

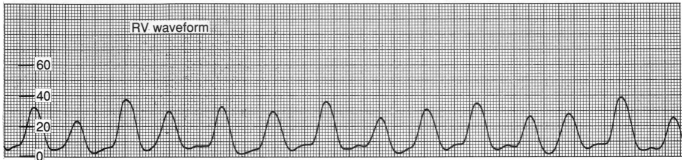

FIGURE 10–38. RVP waveform. This was seen coming from the PA (distal) lumen of a PA catheter. The catheter had become coiled in the RV.

site or with a nonsterile entry into the hemodynamic monitoring system.

4. Assess the patient's comfort at the PA catheter insertion site. **Rationale:** Patients may experience a neck ache or headache from the catheter. Anxiety and pain can contribute to sympathetic stimulation, which may aggravate a primary cardiac condition.

5. Assess the configuration of PAP, RAP, and PCWP waveforms with each measurement. **Rationale:** Thrombus formation at the catheter lumen may be evidenced by a dampened waveform (Fig. 10–39b).

6. Assess pertinent laboratory tests (i.e., venous oxygen saturation, arterial blood gases, electrolytes, BUN/creatinine, WBC, and PT and PTT). **Rationale:** Laboratory result changes will be observed with some mechanical complications of the PA catheter. For example, hypoxemia and decreased venous oxygen saturation will be observed with obstruction of pulmonary blood flow or infarction.

Nursing Diagnoses

1. Potential for impaired gas exchange: hypoxemia related to catheter-induced pulmonary infarction. **Rationale:** The PA catheter can migrate into a wedged position, can perforate the artery wall, or can develop clots at the tip that can break free into the pulmonary circulation. Inadvertent prolonged wedging of catheter can result in pulmonary infarction.

2. Potential for infection related to invasive line. **Rationale:** Infection has been associated with PA catheterization (Applefeld et al., 1978; Boyd et al., 1983; Damen, 1985; Elliott et al., 1979; Greene et al., 1975; Pinilla et al., 1983; Samsoondar et al., 1985; Singh et al., 1982).

The risk of infection increases each time the line is entered (i.e., for blood withdrawal, manual flushing) and if the catheter is in place longer than 72 hours (Applefeld et al., 1978).

3. Potential for dysrhythmias related to catheter insertion or migration of catheter into RV. **Rationale:** Right bundle-branch block, ventricular ectopy, or ventricular fibrillation may occur during PA catheter insertion (Cairns and Holder, 1975; Sprung et al., 1981, 1982; Thomson et al., 1979). If the patient has a preexisting left bundle-branch block, a complete heart block may occur. PA catheter migration into the RV can cause irritation to the endocardium, resulting in ectopy.

4. Potential for impaired tissue perfusion: cerebral related to inadvertent injection of air or clots into the circulation. **Rationale:** Improper care of the PA catheter can result in air or blood clot emboli entering the circulation. Even with the catheter positioned in the PA, it is possible for these emboli to go on to the left side of the heart or pass through an undetected atrial septal defect to the left side of the heart and on to the brain.

Planning

1. Individualize the following goals for catheter care and troubleshooting:
   a. Maintain hemodynamic monitoring system without complications. **Rationale:** PA rupture, embolism, and dysrhythmias are complications of this catheter. All are potentially fatal, and all are preventable with proper catheter use.
   b. Prevent infection. **Rationale:** All invasive catheters are a source of infection. Infection carries a high mortality rate in critically ill patients.
   c. Promote comfort while catheter is in place. **Ra-**

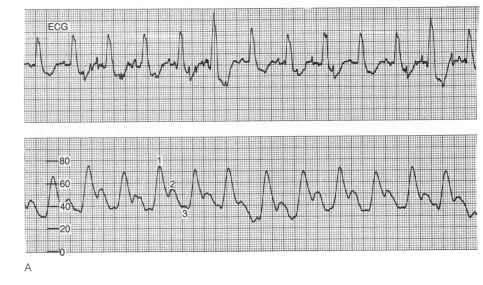

A

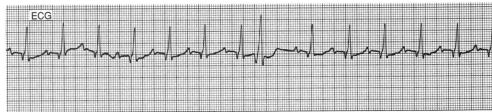

B

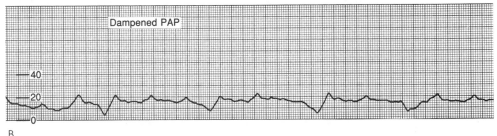

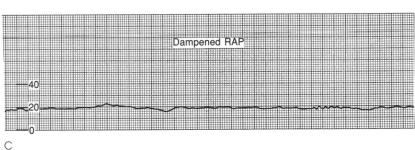

C

FIGURE 10–39. Effects of dampening on PAP and RAP waveforms. (*A*) Normal PAP waveform. (*I* = PA systole; *2* = dicrotic notch; *3* = PA diastole). (*B*) Dampened PAP waveform. (*C*) Dampening of RAP waveform. Dampening of the waveform may be due to clots at catheter tip, catheter against vessel or heart wall, air in lines, stopcock partially closed, deflated pressure bag, or actual patient hypotension.

tionale: Pain leads to increased anxiety, insomnia, and increased body stress response.

d. Maintain clear and accurate PAP and PAWP waveforms. **Rationale:** If the catheter is monitored appropriately and troubleshooting is performed in a timely manner, the patient should have clear and accurate waveforms.

e. Maintain normal heart rhythm without catheter-related dysrhythmias. **Rationale:** If catheter displacement into the RV is detected and rapidly corrected, the patient should have minimal or no dysrhythmias.

2. Prepare all necessary equipment and supplies. **Ra-**

tionale: Facilitates rapid intervention to promote catheter life.

a. 3-cc syringe.

b. Sterile 4 × 4 or 2 × 2 pads.

c. Povidone-iodine ointment.

d. IV labels.

e. Deadend caps.

f. Replacement IV flush bag, IV tubing, pressure tubing, stopcocks, and disposable transducers.

3. Prepare the patient.

a. Explain purpose and location of PA catheter. **Rationale:** Reduces anxiety.

b. Explain catheter care procedures. **Rationale:** Many patients become anxious when they know a procedure is about to be performed.

c. Explain that mechanical problems with PA catheters are common and easily corrected. **Rationale:** Reduces anxiety.

Implementation

Steps	Rationale	Special Considerations
System Care and General Precautions		
1. Wash hands.	Reduces transmission of microorganisms.	
2. Following insertion, check to see that catheter has been sutured to skin.	As the catheter warms to body temperature, it tends to migrate into PA.	
3. Obtain chest x-ray after insertion, after manipulation, and daily (or according to unit protocol).	Ensures proper position of catheter.	The tip of the catheter should not be evident beyond the silhouette of the mediastinal structures (Darovic, 1987).
4. Validate date of insertion and how far catheter was initially inserted.	Catheter should be changed every 72 hours. Detects catheter movement.	
5. Check and tighten all connections and stopcocks q4h.	Loose connections may develop with constant tension on the line. Loose connections provide for the entry of air and bacteria.	
6. Place sterile deadend caps on all stopcocks. Replace with new sterile caps whenever these are removed.	Stopcocks are a major source of contamination.	When deadend caps are removed, they are easily contaminated.
7. Continuously monitor hemodynamic lines, transducer dome, and stopcocks for air.	Air emboli are potentially fatal, particularly if a right-to-left intracardiac shunt is present.	In patients with known right-to-left shunt, CO_2 is recommended for balloon inflation. Patients may have an undetected atrial or ventricular septal defect.
8. Change IV tubing, stopcocks, and disposable transducers q48h.	Decreases risk of infection.	
9. Label tubing with date and time hung.	Identifies tubing change and indicates when the next change will occur.	
10. Maintain pressure bag at 300 mmHg.	Ensures proper functioning of flush device, which will deliver 2 to 5 cc/h. Prevents clot formation within the catheter.	
11. Do not fast flush catheter for longer than 2 seconds (Daily and Schroeder, 1989, p. 409).	Pulmonary artery rupture may occur with prolonged flushing of high-pressure fluid.	
12. Use aseptic technique when withdrawing from or flushing catheter (see Skill 10–7).	Prevents bacterial contamination of system.	
13. Remove all traces of blood from catheter, tubing, and stopcocks after blood withdrawal, and flush completely.	Blood can become a medium for bacterial growth. Clots may be flushed into line next time stopcock is entered.	
14. Maintain sterility of plastic sleeve over catheter, and avoid placing tape on sleeve.	Any tear in the sleeve will break the sterile barrier, making catheter manipulation no longer possible.	
15. Do not infuse viscous fluids (i.e., whole blood, albumin) via catheter lumens.	Flow is slow and may occlude catheter.	The largest lumen of the PA catheter is too small for blood administration and will damage RBCs and reduce the effectiveness of the transfusion.

Steps	Rationale	Special Considerations
16. Wash hands.	Reduces transmission of microorganisms.	
PA Catheter Site Care		
1. Change dressing daily using aseptic technique, and apply povidone-iodine ointment to insertion site.	Decreases risk of infection at catheter insertion site.	The frequency of dressing changes also depends on the type of dressing material used. Gauze dressings require daily changes; other materials may require less frequent changes.
2. Date, time, and initial dressing, and document in patient record.	Ensures consistency in daily change. Identifies dressing change and indicates when next change will occur.	
Troubleshooting Absent Waveform		
1. Wash hands.	Reduces transmission of microorganisms.	
2. Check all connections to be sure that they are tight. Be sure all stopcocks have deadend (not vented) caps.	Loose connections or vented caps will allow air into system, dampening waveforms or eliminating waveform from view on oscilloscope.	Prepackaged pressure monitoring kits often have vented caps to allow for sterilization.
3. Check stopcocks to be sure that they are open to transducer.	Closed stopcocks will prevent waveform transmission to oscilloscope.	
4. Check transducer to be sure it is securely plugged into monitor.	If transducer is not plugged in, there will be no waveform.	
5. Check to see that monitor is turned on.	Required for monitor functioning.	
6. Make sure that correct scale on bedside monitor has been chosen for the pressure being measured; i.e., a 40-mmHg scale is used for PAP monitoring.	A large scale will cause the waveform to be much smaller and possibly not visible on the oscilloscope in the space provided.	
7. Replace transducer and cable with new ones.	A faulty transducer or cable will result in an absent waveform.	Transducer can be checked against a known value with a mercury manometer (see Skill 10–1).
8. Aspirate through catheter to check for blood return. If unable to aspirate, do not flush. Notify the physician.	A clotted catheter will have no waveform and no blood return when aspirated.	
9. Wash hands.	Reduces transmission of microorganisms.	
Troubleshooting Dampened Waveform		
1. Wash hands.	Reduces transmission of microorganisms.	
2. Check all connections to be sure that they are tight, and check stopcocks to be sure that all vented caps have been replaced with deadend caps.	Loose connections and vented caps allow air into system, which causes dampening of waveform.	
3. Check all tubing for air bubbles, including transducer dome. If air is present, troubleshoot in the following way:		
a. Open to flush the stopcock that is closest to the air but between the air and the patient.	Allows air movement out of tubing and prevents air from going into patient.	

Table continues on following page

Steps	Rationale	Special Considerations
b. Compress the fast-flush device, and observe air movement out of tubing. If air bubbles are not moving, flick tubing with a finger and hold stopcock above levels of bubbles.	Air will rise upward when suspended in fluid. Changing the tubing position will facilitate this.	
c. If this procedure is unsuccessful, using same stopcock, attach a syringe and attempt to aspirate air bubbles while compressing flush device.	Assists in manually aspirating air from the system.	
4. Check pressure bag to be sure that it is inflated to 300 mmHg.	Low counter pressure from bag will result in dampened waveform.	
5. Check patient to be sure there has not been a change in condition resulting in a fall in PAP. Check vital signs, pulses, and patient's mentation.	Rapid onset of hypovolemia or shock could lead to a fall in PAP that mimics a dampened waveform. Administration of IV vasodilating drugs (such as sodium nitroprusside) for the first time also can result in a sudden fall in pressures.	
6. Attempt to aspirate blood from catheter; if unable to aspirate, do not flush catheter. Notify physician.	Catheter may be clotted; flushing could result in pulmonary or systemic embolus.	There has been one report of a clot from a PA catheter traveling through an unknown ventricular septal defect to the brain and causing a stroke (Devitt et al., 1982).
7. If blood is aspirated, discard a 2 cc sample, flush the stopcock until clear, then open catheter to flush, and compress fast-flush device to clear tubing.	Blood is discarded because it may contain clot material. The line must then be flushed to prevent clotting.	
8. Wash hands.	Reduces transmission of microorganisms.	

Troubleshooting Continuously Wedged Waveform

Steps	Rationale	Special Considerations
1. Wash hands.	Reduces transmission of microorganisms.	
2. Recognize that the catheter is wedged and the balloon is deflated.	Flushing of the catheter in the wedged position is associated with PA rupture and hemorrhage (Baele et al., 1982; Hardy et al., 1982).	SvO$_2$ readings, if available, will increase when catheter gets close to a spontaneously wedged position.
3. *Do not flush catheter!* Notify physician.	The catheter will need to be pulled back.	Usually a 3- to 5-cm pullback of catheter is sufficient.
4. Have patient change his or her position or cough while observing oscilloscope.	This may help catheter to float out of wedge position.	
5. Obtain order for chest x-ray to check positioning after pulling back catheter.	Confirms PA position in proper lung field and distance in PA.	
6. Wash hands.	Reduces transmission of microorganisms.	

Troubleshooting Catheter in RV

Steps	Rationale	Special Considerations
1. Wash hands.	Reduces transmission of microorganisms.	

Table continues on following page

Steps	Rationale	Special Considerations
2. Recognize catheter in RV waveform: rapid upstroke and downstroke waveform with a diastolic pressure lower than PA diastolic pressure (Fig. 10–38).	The RV has more dynamic pressure changes than PA.	Patients with enlarged hearts and decreased CO are more prone to having catheter migration into RV.
3. Inflate balloon with 1.5 ml of air.	Cushions catheter tip and prevents endocardial irritation.	
4. Observe waveform for catheter movement back into PA position. Have patient move around with balloon inflated. If catheter does not return to PA position, notify physician.	If catheter does not move back immediately into PA position, physician will need to reposition catheter manually.	
5. Obtain an order for a chest x-ray to confirm position after repositioning.	Catheter has returned to a good position in PA.	
6. Wash hands.	Reduces transmission of microorganisms.	

PAP Waveform Visible; PAWP Waveform Absent with Balloon Inflation

1. Wash hands.	Reduces transmission of microorganisms.	
2. Check to be sure balloon has been inflated with maximum amount of air, 1.5 ml.	Insufficient air can prevent wedging.	
3. Observe for resistance with balloon inflation. If no resistance is felt or if blood is aspirated from the balloon lumen, discontinue balloon inflations and notify physician. Tape off balloon so others cannot use it and label "DO NOT INJECT AIR."	If balloon is ruptured, no resistance will be felt during attempted inflation. Blood also may come back through balloon lumen.	The balloon may rupture due to overinflation, frequent inflations, or repeated aspiration of air from balloon rather than allowing it to passively deflate. Absorption of blood lipoproteins also may be a factor.
4. Compare present PA waveform with past PA waveforms. Consult with physician to reposition catheter if necessary.	Catheter tip may not be distal enough in PA to float into wedged position.	
5. Obtain chest x-ray after repositioning.	Validates that proper position has been obtained.	
6. Wash hands.	Reduces transmission of microorganisms.	

PAWP Achieved by Using a Smaller Volume to Inflate Balloon

1. To prevent problem:	Catheter may have moved from its position in main PA to a more distal position in a peripheral vessel.	
a. Inflate balloon only as necessary.	The more the balloon is inflated, the greater is the chance of migration.	
b. Observe and record amount of air being used to inflate balloon each day (should take at least 0.8 cc of air).	Monitors for catheter migration which would be evident by decreasing amounts of air required.	
c. Keep patient on bed rest for at least 1 hour following PA catheter insertion.	Allows catheter to settle into a secured position in PA.	Nursing research is needed to confirm the value of this practice.

Table continues on following page

Steps	Rationale	Special Considerations
d. Observe waveforms after patient has been out of bed.	Patient movement may contribute to catheter displacement.	Nursing research is needed to evaluate the effects of patient mobility on catheter location.
2. Record any interventions in the patient record.	Provides a record of troubleshooting interventions.	

Unexpected Changes in PAP

1. Wash hands.	Reduces transmission of microorganisms.	
2. Check to be sure transducer is level with the phlebostatic axis (see Skill 10–1).	If transducer is higher than phlebostatic axis, pressures will be falsely low. If transducer is lower, pressures will be falsely high (Woods and Mansfield, 1976).	
3. Recalibrate equipment.	Calibration may be incorrect, particularly if patient was transferred from one area to another.	
4. Check for air bubbles in pressure monitoring system.	Air will dampen waveform, resulting in lower readings (Hathaway, 1978; Woods and Mansfield, 1976).	
5. Wash hands.	Reduces transmission of microorganisms.	

Blood Backup into PA Catheter

1. Wash hands.	Reduces transmission of microorganisms.	
2. Turn stopcock off to patient.	Prevents blood from going into transducer dome.	If blood reaches transducer, the transducer diaphragm may be damaged. Replace transducer.
3. Check all connections, and make sure that all stopcocks are closed to air and have deadend caps present.	Loose connections will cause a decrease in pressure within the fluid-filled system, and blood may begin to exert a backpressure into the pressure tubing.	
4. Check pressure bag to ensure that inflation is at 300 mmHg.	Low backpressure from bag will result in blood backup.	
5. Once source of problem is located, flush entire line using fast-flush device. Flush repeatedly for 2-second intervals, rather than as one long flush.	Prevents clot formation within hemodynamic system.	
6. Wash hands.	Reduces transmission of microorganisms.	

Patient Coughs up Blood or Develops Bloody Secretions from Endotracheal Tube during PA Catheter Monitoring

1. Notify physician immediately.	PA perforation with hemorrhage is a lethal complication of PA catheter. The amount of hemorrhage can be from 5 ml of coughed up blood to massive bleeding from the lungs (Barash et al., 1981, Kelly et al., 1981, Paulson et al., 1980, Rosenbaum et al., 1981).	Perforation and hemorrhage are most commonly seen in the elderly, patients with hypothermia or pulmonary hypertension, female patients, patients with a distally placed catheter, or when flushing a wedged catheter.
2. Maintain patency of airway (see Chapter 1).	Prevents hypoxemia and respiratory arrest.	

Table continues on following page

Steps	Rationale	Special Considerations
3. Be prepared for the following possible actions:		
a. Clotting studies and chest x-ray.	Checks for coagulopathies that may be contributing to the problem; x-ray evaluates anatomical problems.	
b. Prepare for intubation and mechanical ventilation (see Skill 1–5).	Establishes an airway and provides ventilation.	If patient is being mechanically ventilated, ambulate patient and secure help. This is a medical emergency.
c. Send blood specimen for type and crossmatch for blood transfusion.	Blood loss from lungs can be significant.	
4. Stay with patient at all times and reassure him or her that bleeding will be controlled.	Reduces anxiety and fear.	

Evaluation

1. Evaluate RAP, PAP, and PAWP waveform configurations. **Rationale:** As evidence that system care measures have been successful.
2. Evaluate vital signs, physical cardiopulmonary signs and symptoms, and ECG. **Rationale:** As evidence that there have not been catheter-related complications.
3. Evaluate for catheter-related infection. **Rationale:** As evidence that catheter care has been successful.
4. Evaluate the patient's comfort with a PA catheter. **Rationale:** As evidence that pain reduction and education measures have been successful.
5. Assess hemodynamic waveforms and pressure values before and after troubleshooting. **Rationale:** Identifies that troubleshooting has been effective.

Expected Outcomes

1. Normal pulmonary tissue perfusion: *absence* of chest pain, hemoptysis, sudden increase in PAP, shortness of breath (SOB), hypotension, hypoxemia on blood gas, and decreasing oxygen saturation. **Rationale:** Pulmonary infarction and/or rupture should not occur if the catheter is not overwedged, the catheter is immediately pulled back into proper position when it migrates to a wedged position, and there is no attempt to flush a wedged catheter.
2. Absence of catheter-related dysrhythmias: ventricular ectopy. **Rationale:** Dysrhythmias should rarely be present during catheter maintenance if the catheter remains in proper position or if deviations are detected and treated immediately.
3. Absence of signs of catheter-related infection: increased WBC, fever, chills, induration at insertion site, positive culture on catheter tip upon removal, tachycardia, unexplainable decreasing SVR, and unexplainable increase in CO. **Rationale:** Daily dressing changes, infrequent entry into the PA catheter, changing of the PA pressure transducer system q48h, and use of aseptic technique when handling all components of the pressure monitoring system will aid in the prevention of infection.
4. Absence of discomfort associated with catheter. **Rationale:** Patient will have minimal discomfort if he or she has been educated about the catheter and has received appropriate pain medication.
5. Clear and accurate PAP, RAP, and PAWP waveforms. **Rationale:** Catheter is performing as expected, and troubleshooting has been successful.

Unexpected Outcomes

1. Pulmonary infarction or rupture of pulmonary artery: patient develops acute, sharp, chest pain, hemoptysis, hypotension, tachycardia, hypoxia, and a sudden increase in PAP. **Rationale:** Excessive wedging of catheter, inadvertent continuous wedging of catheter, or flushing of wedged catheter has resulted in pulmonary infarction or rupture of pulmonary capillary.
2. Ventricular tachycardia unresponsive to antidysrhythmic drugs (i.e., lidocaine, procainamide). **Rationale:** Catheter tip is in right ventricle and is irritating endocardial tissue.
3. Catheter-related infection with resultant septicemia. **Rationale:** Risk of infection increases with improper care during insertion placement for more than 72 hours.
4. Severe neck, arm, or groin discomfort at the PA catheter insertion site. **Rationale:** Catheter is irritating surrounding tissues, and patient has not obtained relief from pain medication.

Documentation

Documentation in the patient record should include date of PA catheter insertion; RAP, PAP, and PAWP waveforms, ECG, cardiopulmonary physical assessment, VS, fluid balance, patient's subjective comfort level, condition of PA catheter insertion site, daily dressing change, patient teaching, and daily chest x-ray and laboratory results. **Rationale:** Documents nursing care given, patient's cardiopulmonary status, and expected and unexpected outcomes.

Patient/Family Education

1. Assess the patient's knowledge of current condition and understanding of the PA catheter. **Rationale:** Patients requiring a PA catheter are often critically ill and anxious about their prognosis. They may be afraid to move because of the catheter's presence.

2. With use of visual aids, instruct patient and family on purpose of PA catheter, location, insertion procedure, patient responsibilities during procedure, postprocedure care, and normal sensations to be experienced from the catheter's presence (i.e., achiness at catheter insertion site). **Rationale:** Patient comfort and cooperation are enhanced with knowledge of procedures. Providing patients with sensory information reduces fear and anxiety (Johnson et al., 1978).

3. Instruct patient and family about signs and symptoms to report to nurse: chest pain, palpitations, new cough, tenderness at insertion site, and chills. **Rationale:** Patients may ignore or not recognize signs of PA complications as important.

Performance Checklist
Skill 10–6: Care and Troubleshooting of Pulmonary Artery Catheter

Critical Behaviors	Complies yes	no
SYSTEM CARE AND GENERAL PRECAUTIONS 1. Wash hands.		
2. Following insertion, observe that catheter has been sutured in place.		
3. Obtain chest x-ray after insertion, after manipulation, and daily.		
4. Document catheter insertion date and depth of insertion in patient record.		
5. Check and tighten all connections and stopcocks q4h.		
6. Place sterile deadend caps on all stopcocks. Replace with new sterile caps whenever they are removed.		
7. Continuously observe hemodynamic lines, transducer dome, and stopcocks for air.		
8. Change IV tubing, stopcocks, and disposable transducers q48h.		
9. Label tubing with date and time hung.		
10. Keeps pressure bag pumped up to 300 mmHg.		
11. Perform fast flush in less than 2 seconds.		
12. Use aseptic technique when withdrawing blood from or flushing fluid into catheter manually.		
13. Remove all traces of blood from catheter, tubing, and stopcocks after blood withdrawal, and flush system completely.		
14. Maintain sterility of plastic sleeve over catheter.		
15. Do not infuse viscous fluids via catheter lumens.		
16. Wash hands.		
PA CATHETER SITE CARE 1. Change dressing daily using aseptic technique.		
2. Date, time, and initial dressing, and document in patient record.		
TROUBLESHOOTING ABSENT WAVEFORM 1. Wash hands.		
2. Check all connections to be sure that they are tight and all stopcocks to be sure no vented caps are present.		
3. Check stopcocks to be sure that they are open to transducer.		
4. Check transducer to be sure it is plugged into monitor.		

Table continues on following page

Critical Behaviors	Complies	
	yes	no
5. Check to see that monitor is turned on.		
6. Check to be sure scale on monitor is correct.		
7. Try use of a new transducer and cable.		
8. Aspirate catheter for blood return.		
9. Wash hands.		
10. Document in patient record.		
TROUBLESHOOTING DAMPENED WAVEFORM 1. Wash hands.		
2. Check all connections to be sure that they are tight.		
3. Check all tubing for air bubbles.		
a. Flush air out of tubing through stopcock turned off to patient.		
b. Aspirate air out of tubing when it does not flush out.		
4. Check pressure bag to be sure it is inflated to 300 mmHg.		
5. Check patient to be sure that there is no change in condition.		
6. Attempt to aspirate blood from catheter, and notify physician if unable to aspirate blood.		
7. If blood is aspirated, discard specimen and flush entire pressure transducer system.		
8. Wash hands.		
9. Document in patient record.		
TROUBLESHOOTING CONTINUOUSLY WEDGED WAVEFORM 1. Wash hands.		
2. Identify wedged waveform and note that balloon is deflated.		
3. *Do not flush catheter!* Notify physician.		
4. Have patient change position or cough while observing waveform on oscilloscope.		
5. Obtain order for chest x-ray following troubleshooting.		
6. Wash hands.		
7. Document in patient record.		
TROUBLESHOOTING CATHETER IN RV 1. Wash hands.		
2. Identify catheter in RV waveform.		
3. Inflate balloon with 1.5 ml of air.		
4. Observe waveform for catheter movement back into position in PA, or notify physician if catheter does not move back into position.		
5. Obtain chest x-ray to confirm position after troubleshooting.		
6. Wash hands.		
7. Document in patient record.		
PAP WAVEFORM VISIBLE; PAWP WAVEFORM ABSENT WITH BALLOON INFLATION 1. Wash hands.		
2. Check to be sure balloon is inflated with maximum amount of air.		

Table continues on following page

Critical Behaviors	Complies	
	yes	no
3. Observe for resistance with balloon inflation. If no resistance is felt or if blood is coming from balloon lumen, notify physician.		
4. Compare present PA waveform with past PA waveforms. Consult with physician regarding catheter position.		
5. Obtain chest x-ray after repositioning.		
6. Wash hands.		
7. Document in patient record.		
PAWP Achieved by Using Smaller Volume to Inflate Balloon 1. Prevent problem by		
a. Inflating balloon only as necessary.		
b. Observing and recording the amount of air required for balloon inflation.		
c. Keeping the patient on bed rest for 1 hour after PA catheter insertion.		
d. Observing waveform after patient has been out of bed.		
2. Document any interventions in patient record.		
Unexpected Changes in PAP 1. Wash hands.		
2. Check to be sure transducer is level with phlebostatic axis.		
3. Check calibration of equipment.		
4. Check for air bubbles in pressure monitoring system.		
5. Wash hands.		
6. Document in patient record.		
Blood Backup into PA Catheter 1. Wash hands.		
2. Turn stopcock off to patient.		
3. Check all connections to be sure that they are tight and all stopcocks to be sure they are open to the patient and have deadend caps.		
4. Check pressure bag to ensure that inflation is at 300 mmHg.		
5. After problem source is located, flush entire system using several brief (<2 seconds) flushes.		
6. Wash hands.		
7. Document in patient record.		
Patient Coughs up Blood or Develops Bloody Secretions from Endotracheal Tube during PA Catheter Monitoring 1. Notify physician immediately.		
2. Maintain patency of airway.		
3. Be prepared for:		
a. Clotting studies and chest x-ray.		
b. Intubation and mechanical ventilation.		
c. Obtain blood for type and crossmatch.		
4. Document in patient record.		

SKILL 10–7

Blood Sampling from Pulmonary Artery Catheter

One of the advantages of PA catheterization is that samples of mixed venous blood can be taken for the purposes of evaluating venous blood oxygen saturation.

The technique for blood withdrawal is not without complications and therefore requires knowledge of the proper procedure. Blood withdrawal from PA catheters should be done only when the data to be obtained are essential for patient therapy rather than as a routine route of blood withdrawal. If continuous monitoring of mixed venous oxygen saturation is indicated, the adult patient should have an $S\bar{v}O_2$ catheter inserted (see Skill 6–3).

Aseptic technique and universal precautions are also important with this procedure. Stopcocks are a source of infection and should be flushed thoroughly and not allowed to gather blood residue. A number of closed system blood withdrawal units have been developed to protect health care personnel from direct contact with a patient's blood. One such unit is pictured in Figure 10–40.

Following blood removal, flushing of the catheter becomes important to prevent fibrin clot buildup within the lumen(s), which would result in dampening of waveforms or total catheter occlusion.

Purpose

The nurse performs PA catheter blood removal to

1. Determine mixed venous oxygen saturation.

2. Provide a blood sample for laboratory analysis as a route of last resort.

Prerequisite Knowledge and Skills

Prior to performing PA blood removal, the nurse should understand

1. Principles of aseptic technique.
2. Cardiac anatomy and physiology.
3. Pulmonary anatomy and physiology.
4. Principles of gas exchange.
5. Principles of acid–base balance.
6. PA catheter purpose, location, and normal waveforms (see Skill 10–7).
7. Principles of hemodynamic monitoring (see Skill 10–1).
8. The effect of heparin on various blood tests and appropriate discard volumes.
9. Universal precautions.

The nurse should be able to perform

1. Proper handwashing technique (see Skill 35–5).
2. Stopcock manipulation.
3. PA catheter troubleshooting (see Skill 10–6).
4. Proper withdrawal technique for data validity.
5. Universal precautions (see Skill 35–1).

Assessment

Perform cardiopulmonary physical assessment and evaluate patient for signs and symptoms of cardiac or pulmonary disease, including abnormal heart/breath

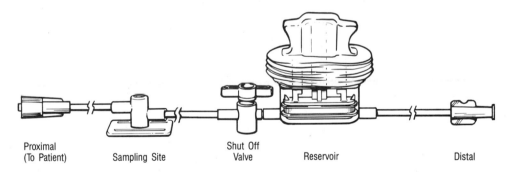

Proximal (To Patient) — Sampling Site — Shut Off Valve — Reservoir — Distal

FIGURE 10–40. VAMP system for needleless blood withdrawal from hemodynamic lines. (Courtesy of Baxter-Edwards Laboratories.)

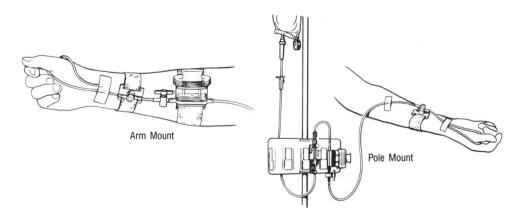

Arm Mount

Pole Mount

sounds, dysrhythmias, rales in lungs, diminished pulses, decreased mentation or agitation, skin color changes, peripheral edema, liver enlargement, jugular vein distension, clubbing of fingernails, positive or negative fluid balance, increased or decreased respirations, abnormal chest-wall excursion, rib retractions with respirations, nasal flaring, shortness of breath, dyspnea, orthopnea, paroxysmal nocturnal dyspnea, chest pain, cough, mucus production, and fever. **Rationale:** These are the signs and symptoms that would necessitate blood sampling for venous oxygenation or other laboratory tests.

Nursing Diagnosis

Decreased cardiac output related to decreased preload, increased afterload, or decreased contractility. **Rationale:** Mixed venous blood samples are used to evaluate changes in cardiopulmonary function that affect cardiac output (see Skill 6–3). A mixed venous oxygen saturation less than 75 percent *may* indicate a low cardiac output state.

Planning

1. Individualize the following goals for performing PA blood sampling:
   a. Maintain sterility of closed system. **Rationale:** Prevents infection.
   b. Maintain catheter patency. **Rationale:** With repeated blood sampling from the PA catheter, clots may form within the lumen.
2. Prepare all necessary equipment and supplies. **Rationale:** Preparation of equipment in advance reduces the risk of error and saves time.
   a. Exam gloves.
   b. 5 cc syringe.
   c. Two 10 cc syringes.
   d. 2 × 2 gauze pad.
   e. Appropriate laboratory tubes and slips.
3. Prepare the patient by explaining why blood withdrawal is being performed. Explain that it will not cause patient discomfort, that the amount of blood to be removed is minimal, and that the patient will not require a blood transfusion to replace blood taken for laboratory tests. **Rationale:** Reduces patient and family anxiety.

Implementation

Steps	Rationale	Special Considerations
1. Wash hands.	Reduces transmission of microorganisms.	
2. Don exam gloves.	Universal precautions.	
3. Attach a 5-cc syringe to top port of the stopcock closest to the catheter. Turn stopcock off to pressure tubing.	Allows access for blood sampling.	
4. Aspirate, noticing when blood enters the syringe, and withdraw about 2½ times the dead space of the catheter.	Clears the catheter lumen of heparinized solution.	
5. Turn stopcock one-quarter turn. Remove syringe and discard in appropriate receptacle.	Stops blood flow and closes all ports of stopcock. Universal precautions.	
6. Connect syringe for blood sample to top port of stopcock. Turn stopcock off to pressure tubing. Slowly aspirate the necessary amount of blood.	Opens syringe to catheter.	For $S\bar{v}O_2$ measurement, slow aspiration is important to prevent contamination of the mixed venous sample with arterial blood from PA capillary.
7. Turn stopcock one-quarter turn. Remove syringe and fill appropriate test tubes.	Turns all ports of stopcock off.	
8. Attach a 10-cc syringe to top port of stopcock. Turn stopcock off to catheter. Fill syringe with approximately 5 ml of flush solution.	Opens syringe to flush solution.	

Table continues on following page

Steps	Rationale	Special Considerations
9. Turn stopcock off to pressure tubing. Aspirate until blood enters the syringe. No clots should be visible, and plunger should be pulled back easily. Then, flush catheter with the flush solution in the syringe.	Opens syringe to catheter. Checks patency of catheter and prevents flushing of clots into patient.	If clots are aspirated, turn stopcock one-quarter turn, discard syringe, and begin again with a new syringe.
10. Turn stopcock one-quarter turn. Remove syringe and discard in appropriate receptacle.	Clears top port of stopcock of any bloody residue. Universal precautions.	
11. Turn stopcock off to catheter, flush through top port of stopcock onto a 2 × 2 gauze pad. Turn stopcock off to top port. Attach new, sterile deadend cap to top port of stopcock.	Maintains sterility of system.	
12. Remove and discard gloves in appropriate receptacle.	Universal precautions.	
13. Wash hands.	Reduces transmission of microorganisms.	

Evaluation

1. Evaluate the RA, PA, and PAW pressure waveforms. **Rationale:** Prevents catheter-related complications.
2. Correlate venous oxygen saturation results with measured thermodilution cardiac output (CO). **Rationale:** Decreased $S\bar{v}O_2$ will be seen when CO is decreased.

Expected Outcome

Patient will have an improved or normal CO and show improvement in tissue perfusion (i.e., improved mentation, increased urinary output, decrease in SVR, normal PAWP, normal acid–base balance, normal respirations, normal heart and breath sounds, normal cardiac rhythm, and improved or normal peripheral perfusion). **Rationale:** If PA blood sampling is not performed properly or in a timely manner, the patient's clinical condition will not improve. Also, if too much blood is taken from patient, the patient's clinical condition may actually deteriorate.

Unexpected Outcome

Patient does not show an improvement in CO and continues to exhibit signs of decreased tissue perfusion. **Rationale:** If blood sample from PA is taken in a timely manner and using proper technique, interventions will be appropriate and timely. Also, if too much blood is taken from patient, the patient may suffer hypovolemia and have a further decrease in cardiac output.

Documentation

Documentation in the patient record should include the date and time that the blood sample was taken and what tests were performed. **Rationale:** Documents nursing interventions performed and blood loss.

Patient/Family Education

Explain purpose of blood withdrawal, that it will not cause patient discomfort, that minimal amounts of blood will be removed, and that patient will not require a blood transfusion to replace blood. **Rationale:** Reduces anxiety and fear.

Performance Checklist
Skill 10–7: Blood Sampling from Pulmonary Artery Catheter

Critical Behaviors	Complies yes	no
1. Wash hands.		
2. Don exam gloves.		

Table continues on following page

Critical Behaviors	Complies	
	yes	no
3. Attach a 5-ml syringe to top port of stopcock closest to catheter, and turn stopcock off to pressure tubing.		
4. Aspirate and withdraw 3 ml.		
5. Turn stopcock one-quarter turn. Remove and discard syringe.		
6. Connect 10 ml blood-sampling syringe to top port of stopcock, turn stopcock off to pressure tubing, and aspirate necessary amount of blood.		
7. Turn stopcock one-quarter turn. Remove syringe and fill appropriate test tubes.		
8. Attach a 10-ml syringe to top port of stopcock, turn stopcock off to catheter, and fill syringe with 5 ml of flush solution.		
9. Turn stopcock off to pressure tubing, aspirate on syringe until blood enters the syringe, observe for clots in aspirate, and flush catheter with flush solution using gentle pressure.		
10. Turn stopcock one-quarter turn, remove and discard syringe, turn stopcock off to catheter, flush through top port of stopcock, and attach new deadend cap to top port of stopcock.		
11. Send samples to laboratory.		
12. Observe waveform on bedside oscilloscope.		
13. Remove and discard gloves, and wash hands.		
14. Document procedure in patient record.		

SKILL 10–8

Removal of Pulmonary Artery Catheter

Pulmonary artery (PA) catheterization and monitoring of intracardiac pressures are described in Skills 10–5 and 10–6. As the patient's condition improves and the PA catheter is no longer necessary, the nurse may be asked to remove this catheter according to institutional policy (Baird et al., 1990). This skill describes PA catheter removal.

Purpose

The nurse performs PA catheter removal

1. When the patient's condition is improved such that PA monitoring is no longer necessary.
2. To reduce the risk of complications from the presence of the catheter (i.e., dysrhythmias, pulmonary infarction).
3. To reduce the risk of infection, which is associated with prolonged use of intravascular lines.

Prerequisite Knowledge and Skills

Prior to performing PA catheter removal, the nurse should understand

1. Cardiovascular anatomy and physiology.
2. Normal values for intracardiac pressures.
3. Waveform configurations for RA, RV, PA, and PAW pressures.
4. Venous access routes and procedure for venous cannulation.
5. Principles of aseptic technique.
6. Treatment of life-threatening dysrhythmias.
7. Normal PT and PTT values.
8. Universal precautions.

The nurse should be able to perform

1. Hemodynamic waveform interpretation.
2. Inflation and deflation of balloon (see Skills 10–5 and 10–6).
3. Basic dysrhythmias recognition.
4. Stopcock manipulation.
5. Defibrillation (see Skill 8–2).
6. Cardiovascular assessment.
7. Universal precautions (see Skill 35–5).
8. Proper handwashing technique (see Skill 35–1).

Assessment

1. Perform cardiovascular physical assessment. **Rationale:** Complications of removal are evidenced by cardiovascular changes.
2. Observe PA waveform on bedside monitor for configuration. **Rationale:** Assesses current catheter location and patency. It is customary to observe waveform changes while catheter is being removed.
3. Assess current PT, PTT, and WBC values. **Rationale:** If patient has prolonged coagulation times, there could be difficulty in obtaining hemostasis at insertion site. An elevated WBC could indicate possible infection,

in which case the physician may want the nurse to save the catheter tip for culture and sensitivity studies.

4. Determine whether the patient is receiving anti-coagulant medications. **Rationale:** Anticoagulants increase the risk for bleeding from PA catheter insertion site.

5. Assess the patient for knowledge of PA catheter rationale and understanding of why it is no longer indicated. **Rationale:** Ensures that the patient does not become alarmed by removal and obtains patient cooperation during procedure and reduces anxiety.

Nursing Diagnoses

1. Potential for injury related to debris embolization with catheter removal. **Rationale:** Thrombus can form on catheter and be embolized with removal. This is especially true after catheter has been in place more than 36 hours (Connors et al., 1985).

2. Potential for injury related to removal of an inflated balloon or knotted catheter. **Rationale:** Removal of catheter with balloon inflated or removal of knotted catheter could result in tricuspid or pulmonic valve damage.

3. Potential for fluid volume deficit related to hemorrhage at introducer insertion site. **Rationale:** Since PA catheter is inserted into a large vein, there is always a risk of excessive bleeding once catheter is removed.

4. Potential for impaired skin integrity related to improper removal technique. **Rationale:** If sutures are not removed and the introducer is pulled on during catheter removal, there could be skin injury.

Planning

1. Individualize the following goals for PA catheter removal:

a. Prevent complications of catheter removal, including embolization, hemorrhage, skin injury, or valve injury. **Rationale:** If the nurse follows the proper technique for catheter removal, these complications should not occur.

b. Promote patient cooperation during PA catheter removal. **Rationale:** If the patient has received proper preparation, he or she should be still during the removal. If the patient is restless during the procedure, the nurse may accidentally cause injury to the valve structure or vessel lumen with catheter removal.

2. Prepare all necessary equipment and supplies:
a. Two suture removal kits.
b. Two pairs exam gloves.
c. 1.5-cc syringe.
d. Appropriate receptacle for disposal of contaminated materials.
e. Antibacterial ointment.
f. 4 × 4 gauze pads.
g. 1-in (2.5 cm) tape.
h. One barrier proof absorbent pad.

3. Prepare the patient.
a. Explain the procedure and why catheter is no longer necessary. **Rationale:** Reduces anxiety and fear.
b. Explain to patient the importance of lying still during removal. **Rationale:** Encourages patient's cooperation and prevents complications of a disruptive removal.

4. Secure written physician order for PA catheter removal. **Rationale:** PA catheter removal is a physician decision and therefore requires a written order.

Implementation

Steps	Rationale	Special Considerations
1. Wash hands.	Reduces transmission of microorganisms.	
2. Don exam gloves.	Universal precautions.	This is a clean procedure. Sterile gloves are not necessary.
3. Position patient so that PA catheter and introducer are readily visible; i.e., turn head away from insertion site if catheter is in jugular vein. If catheter is in the jugular vein, Trendelenberg position may be desirable.	Prevents accidental removal of introducer while removing PA catheter. Prevents entry of air into vein during catheter removal.	If PA catheter is in femoral vein, extend leg and be sure groin area is adequately exposed. Consider use of sedation if necessary to keep patient still.
4. Attach 1.5-cc syringe to balloon lumen, and pull back on plunger to be sure balloon is deflated.	Prevents injury to valve tissues during removal.	
5. Lock balloon lumen.	Ensures that balloon remains deflated.	

Table continues on following page

Steps	Rationale	Special Considerations
6. Place barrier-proof absorbent pad under catheter and catheter insertion site.	Contains any bloody drainage associated with removal and serves as a receptacle for the contaminated catheter.	
7. Open suture removal kit and remove scissors and forceps. Locate skin sutures that are securing the PA catheter.	Prepares for suture removal.	
8. Grasping suture with forceps with non-dominant hand, use the dominant hand to clip suture, being careful not to cut PA catheter or patient's skin.	Frees the PA catheter for removal.	
9. Pick up any loose suture material with forceps, and discard according to institutional policy. Discard scissors and forceps in appropriate receptacle.	Universal precautions.	
10. While securing introducer with non-dominant hand, gently pull on PA catheter to remove. Keep watch on the cardiac monitor for the presence of dysrhythmias. (If resistance is encountered, do not try to pull any further. Stay with patient and have another nurse call the physician for further instructions.) Continue with catheter withdrawal until it is completely out in a smooth, continuous motion.	The PA catheter should be removed as quickly as possible to prevent intraventricular irritation and ectopy. If resistance is encountered, this may be due to catheter knotting or wedging, which requires a special procedure for safe removal.	
11. Lay PA catheter on barrier proof absorbent pad until disposed. Check to be sure all of catheter has been removed.	Universal precautions.	
12. Observe for any bleeding through outlet.	Sometimes the introducer entry port (outlet) may wear and develop a leak that becomes apparent following PA catheter removal.	
13. Dispose of PA catheter, flush solution, tubing, and gloves in appropriate receptacle.	Universal precautions.	
14. Apply dressing to introducer if it is not removed at this same time.	Prevents infection of introducer insertion site.	
15. To remove introducer, turn off all IVs infusing through the side port of introducer.	These IVs will no longer be able to be infused.	It is important that the nurse not disconnect vasoactive or cardiotonic IV drugs.
16. Obtain a new suture removal kit.	Removes suture.	
17. Position patient with HOB flat and introducer visible.	Prevents air entry with removal of introducer.	
18. Put on a new pair of exam gloves.	Universal precautions.	
19. Cut away any suture material holding introducer in place. Dispose of this in an appropriate receptacle.	Universal precautions.	

Table continues on following page

Steps	Rationale	Special Considerations
20. Open sterile 4 × 4 pad, and place a small amount of antibacterial ointment on center of pad.	Makes ready for placement over introducer insertion site.	
21. With 4 × 4 pad in non-dominant hand, grasp introducer with dominant hand and gently pull to remove. (If resistance is encountered, notify physician and wait for further instructions.) As introducer is coming out, place 4 × 4 pad over insertion site and apply pressure.	4 × 4 is ready for quick placement.	
22. Continue applying pressure at insertion site with 4 × 4 until bleeding has ceased, usually 5 to 10 minutes.	Stops bleeding. Since a large vein is used for insertion, it may take up to 10 minutes for hemostasis to occur.	
23. Apply a sterile dressing to insertion site.	Decreases risk of infection at insertion site.	
24. Monitor site q15min × 4 for bleeding through dressing. After 1 hour, lift up dressing and, with gloved hand, gently palpate skin around insertion site to assess for any hematoma formation. Observe to ensure that bleeding has ceased.	Even if bleeding appears to have stopped, it may begin again and appear as a slow ooze. A hematoma can develop if the skin has closed and there is still bleeding from the vessel.	
25. Date, time, and initial dressing.	Indicates when dressing was placed.	
26. Remove and discard gloves, and wash hands.	Reduces transmission of microorganisms.	

Evaluation

Compare patient assessment before and after removal. **Rationale:** Identifies untoward effects of PA catheter and introducer removal.

Expected Outcomes

1. Removal of PA catheter without embolization. **Rationale:** If PA catheter is removed in a timely manner and is not forced when resistance is felt, the patient will have a decreased risk of developing clots/emboli in the bloodstream.

2. Removal of PA catheter without valve injury. **Rationale:** There should be no complications of removal if procedure is followed.

3. Hemostasis. **Rationale:** By not removing catheter in a patient with a coagulopathy and by closely observing the insertion site, this problem should be averted.

Unexpected Outcomes

1. Embolization of clot material to lungs: hemoptysis, chest pain, tachycardia, hypotension, and hypoxia. **Rationale:** Catheter has been in place longer than 72 hours or when removed has been pulled on despite resistance.

2. Cardiac valve injury progressing to heart failure: new murmur heard, falling blood pressure, tachycardia, diminished pulses, possible decreased mental alertness, and possible decreased urinary output. **Rationale:** Catheter has been removed with balloon inflated or with a knot.

3. Hemorrhage. **Rationale:** Significant fluid volume deficit could occur if bleeding from the insertion site is not controlled.

Documentation

Documentation in the patient record should include assessments before and after removal, patient's response to procedure, and date and time of removal. **Rationale:** Documents nursing care given, patient's cardiac status, and expected and unexpected outcomes.

Patient/Family Education

1. Instruct the patient and family about the rationale for catheter removal, the procedure for catheter removal, the importance of lying still during catheter removal, and the rationale for continued monitoring of the insertion

site. **Rationale:** Reduces fear and anxiety and secures the patient's cooperation during the procedure.

2. If the patient is being discharged within 12 hours of catheter removal, the patient and family should be instructed to observe for and report any bloody drainage on the dressing, bloody drainage around the dressing, and new pain or pressure at the insertion site and to remove the dressing the next day. **Rationale:** Bleeding may start up with excessive patient activity. If the patient has any coagulopathy, he or she may have significant bleeding requiring physician intervention. These instructions also will relieve the patient and family anxiety about what to do for the insertion site.

Performance Checklist
Skill 10–8: Removal of Pulmonary Artery Catheter

Critical Behaviors	Complies yes	no
1. Obtain physician order for catheter removal.		
2. Wash hands.		
3. Don exam gloves.		
4. Position patient properly.		
5. Deflate balloon.		
6. Lock balloon lumen.		
7. Place barrier-proof pad under PA catheter.		
8. Open suture kit, and locate sutures.		
9. Cut away suture material.		
10. Pick up and dispose of suture material in proper container.		
11. Pull PA catheter with one swift, continuous movement. Notify physician if resistance is felt and wait for instructions.		
12. Lay catheter on pad, and check that all of catheter has been removed.		
13. Observe for bleeding through outlet.		
14. Dispose of PA catheter, flush solution, and gloves in proper receptacle.		
15. Apply dressing to introducer if it is not being removed.		
16. If removing introducer, turn off all IVs or select another IV site for infusion of vasoactive drugs.		
17. Obtain a new suture removal kit.		
18. Position patient properly.		
19. Don new gloves.		
20. Remove suture material, and dispose of properly.		
21. Open and prepare sterile 4 × 4 with antibacterial ointment.		
22. Remove introducer gently. If resistance is felt, notify physician and wait for instructions.		
23. Keep pressure on insertion site until bleeding ceases.		
24. Apply a sterile dressing.		
25. Monitor site q15min × 4 for bleeding. After 1 hour, check for hematoma formation at insertion site.		
26. Date, time, and initial dressing.		
27. Remove and discard gloves, and wash hands.		
28. Document procedure in patient record.		

SKILL 10-9

Cardiac Output Measurement Techniques

Cardiac output is defined as the amount of blood pumped by the heart per minute. Each ventricle has a cardiac output of 4 to 6 L/min. Four physiologic factors directly affect cardiac output. These factors are preload, afterload, contractility, and heart rate. Contractility and heart rate are inherent to the cardiac tissues but can be influenced by neural and humoral mechanisms. *Preload*, the load or volume that stretches the LV myocardium just prior to contraction, is measured by the pulmonary wedge pressure (see Skill 10-5). *Afterload*, the load the heart muscles must move after the heart starts to contract, is a critical determinant of cardiac performance and is also influenced by cardiac and vascular conditions. Left-side heart afterload is clinically evaluated by calculating the systemic vascular resistance (SVR). The normal SVR is 900 to 1400 $dyn/s/cm^{-5}$.

Cardiac output measures are so essential to critical-care nursing that all newer hemodynamic monitoring equipment has the capability of displaying CO curves, CO trends, and data on all hemodynamic parameters, both direct and derived. The nurse measures CO according to the patient's needs. At times it will be necessary to measure CO every hour, and at other times it will be required only once or twice a day. CO measures not only confirm the physical assessment of the patient, but aid the nurse in assessing whether or not an intervention has been successful.

The technique for bedside measurement of CO, known as the *thermodilution method*, is a relatively recent development, having been based on the previously popular indicator-dilution technique. With the indicator-dilution method, a dye injected into a vein was followed along its pathway through the heart to determine the rate of blood flow. The thermodilution method requires the presence of a PA catheter (see Skill 10-6), and the indicator used to follow the blood flow is a fluid (either dextrose or saline) with a known volume and temperature. The CO solution is injected into the RA lumen of the PA catheter and exits in the RA, where it mixes with blood and travels through the heart. At the distal end of the catheter, 4 cm from the tip, sits a thermistor that detects the temperature change and sends a signal to the CO computer to which the catheter is connected. The thermistor actually measures the body temperature first, then the injectate altered blood temperature, and then back to body temperature. This change in temperature over time is plotted as a curve (Fig. 10-41). The area under the curve is then used to mathematically calculate the cardiac output, which is digitally displayed. This area is inversely proportional to the flow rate of blood. Thus a high cardiac output is associated with a small area under the curve, whereas a low cardiac output is associated with a large area under the curve (Fig. 10-42).

This procedure can be performed in pediatric patients who have a PA catheter present. The major difference being that a smaller volume of injectate must be used in pediatric patients, who cannot tolerate large-volume injections (Hazinski, 1989). Because of the smaller volume

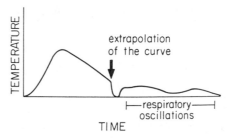

FIGURE 10-41. Cardiac output (CO) curve. The normal curve has a smooth, rapid upslope to peak temperature and a gradual downslope to the point where computer data processing ends and extrapolation of the remainder of the curve occurs. Baseline respiratory oscillations are also evident on this curve recording. (From B. J. Loveys and S. L. Woods, Current recommendations for thermodilution CO measurement. *Prog. Cardiovasc. Nurs.* 1[1]:25, 1986, with permission.)

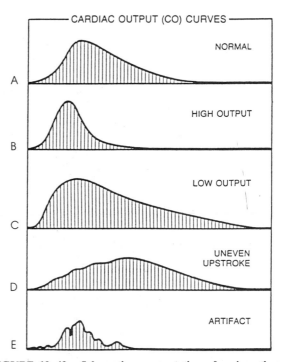

FIGURE 10-42. Schematic representation of various thermodilution CO curves. (*A*) Normal curve. (*B*) Small area beneath the curve as seen in patients with high COs. (*C*) Large area beneath the curve as seen in patients with low cardiac output. (*D*) Uneven injection indicated by uneven upstroke on curve. (*E*) Artifact in both upstroke and decline of curve resulting in erroneous cardiac output measurement. (From A. Tilkian and E. K. Daily, *Cardiovascular Procedures.* St. Louis: Mosby, 1986, p. 95, with permission.)

used, there is greater risk of error in measures, and therefore, an iced injectate is preferred. Impeccable technique is an absolute necessity in pediatric patients.

There are limitations to the use of the thermodilution method (Riedinger, 1984). It cannot, for example, be used in patients with large intracardiac shunts, in whom a PA catheter may pose a danger. It cannot be performed with a ventricular septal defect (VSD) present because of improper mixing of the thermal indicator with blood. It cannot be performed in the setting of tricuspid regurgitation because of blood regurgitation prolonging the mixing time and movement of the thermal indicator.

Because of these limitations, and because of the complications associated with PA catheterization, other noninvasive techniques for CO measurement are being developed. An example of such a method is Doppler cardiac output determination. This technique uses the Doppler principle by measuring aortic blood flow velocity through a known aortic diameter to obtain CO (Taylor et al., 1990). The Doppler transducer placed in the suprasternal notch aims the ultrasound beam toward the aortic root to measure blood velocity (Fig. 10–43). It is currently still in an evaluative phase, but if it is successful, it will greatly reduce the hazards of cardiac output determination via an invasive line.

One additional major limitation of the thermodilution technique includes a required injection of the thermal indicator that is intermittently performed, so continuous measurement of CO is not possible. This can increase the risk of infection if the nurse does not follow strict aseptic technique. In addition, there is the high possibility of errors in the CO valve if the technique is not strictly adhered to. The training of new nurses to perform this procedure properly is time-consuming. It also requires nursing time to perform each injection and wait for the result.

As a result of these shortcomings, a new type of catheter, the *heat-exchange cardiac output catheter*, is being tried. This catheter has a membrane that allows for heat exchange with blood in the vena cava. Continuous measurement of cardiac output can be performed without the need for injected fluid, as is presently required. Should this method have a high correlation with the thermodilution method of obtaining cardiac output, it could possibly replace thermodilution. This device also would eliminate the risk of fluid overload from numerous CO injections and minimize the risk of infection and air emboli.

Other techniques being tried for CO measurement include bioimpedance CO, pulsed-heat CO, and CO by arterial morphology.

The one commercially available closed system CO delivery set (CO-Set, Fig. 10–44) can be used with both iced or room-temperature (RT) injectate. The advantages of this system over the syringe method are the closed system reduces the number of times a stopcock must be entered and therefore reduces the risk of contamination; it saves staff times required to gather and prefill the syringes; it saves in patient costs, particularly if CO syringes are prepared by a pharmacist as is done in some hospitals; and it may be more accurate, since an in-line temperature probe reads the injectate temperature as it enters the patient.

Studies have been done to compare the results with prefilled syringes versus those with the CO-Set. Barcelona et al. (1985) evaluated the two methods in 21 cardiac care unit patients with congestive heart failure (CHF) or low cardiac output states. In 17 of the patients, CO measurements using 10-ml iced prefilled syringes was compared with 10 ml of RT CO-Set injectate. Regression analysis showed a moderate correlation ($r = 0.71$). In a group of 10 patients, a high correlation ($r = 0.935$) was found between CO values obtained with iced prefilled syringes and RT prefilled syringes. The investigators concluded that the closed system cardiac output technique would not give reliable results when an RT injectate was used.

Gardner et al. (1987) also evaluated the prefilled syringe technique and the CO-Set. They compared the iced prefilled syringe methods with both RT and iced CO-Set preparations. Fifty-seven critically ill patients with a wide range of CO measures were studied. Although statistically significant differences were found in the closed (iced and RT) method versus the iced prefilled syringe method, this difference was found not to be clinically significant. The investigators concluded that CO-Set technique results were reproducible and that, for most patients, this method will be accurate. The investigators also suggested that if results obtained by the CO-Set seem inaccurate, they should be checked against the prefilled syringe method. Clearly, further research is needed to evaluate the validity of closed systems.

Purpose

The nurse performs CO measurement to

1. Assess a patient's cardiovascular status.
2. Evaluate vasoactive drug therapy and other interventions that affect hemodynamic status.
3. Identify early complications of the hemodynamic derangements.

Prerequisite Knowledge and Skills

Before performing CO measurements, the nurse should understand

1. Cardiovascular anatomy and physiology.
2. Principles of hemodynamic monitoring.
3. Rationale for CO measurements.
4. Aseptic technique.

The nurse should be able to perform

1. Stopcock manipulation.
2. PAP, RAP, and PAWP waveform interpretation.

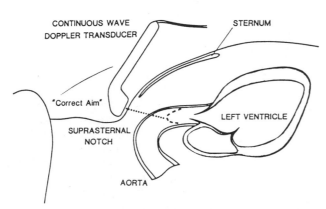

FIGURE 10–43. Doppler CO technique. (From R. W. Taylor, et al., *Techniques and Procedures in Critical Care*. Philadelphia: Lippincott, 1990, p. 80, with permission.)

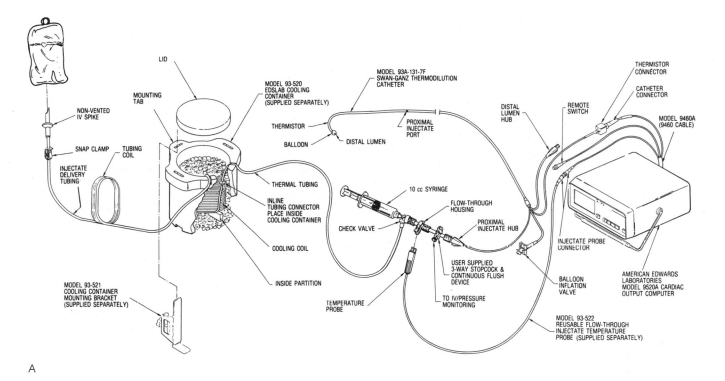

A

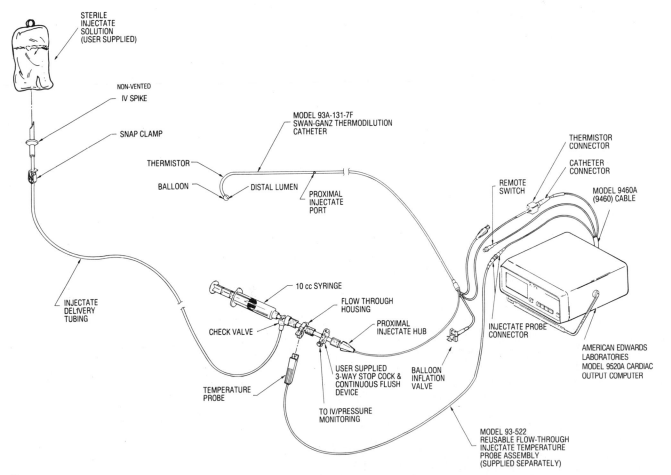

B

FIGURE 10–44. CO-Set preparations for CO measurement. (*A*) Iced injectate preparation. (*B*) Room-temperature injectate preparation. (Courtesy of Baxter Edwards Corporation.)

3. Proper handwashing technique (see Skill 35–5).
4. Universal precautions (see Skill 35–1).

Assessment

1. Assess the patient's vital signs, blood pressure, fluid balance, heart and breath sounds, skin color and temperature, mentation, peripheral pulses, and 12-lead ECG and hemodynamic variables. **Rationale:** Clinical information provides data regarding blood flow and tissue perfusion.

2. Assess medical history for (i.e., presence of coronary artery disease, presence of valvular heart disease, intracardiac pressures, ejection fraction, and overall ventricular function). **Rationale:** Provides information regarding cardiovascular status.

3. Assess pertinent laboratory results (i.e., CBC, PT and PTT, arterial blood gases, BUN, creatinine, electrolytes, and urine electrolytes). **Rationale:** Provides data regarding coagulations, blood volume, fluid status, oxygen transport. Patient laboratory findings correlate with CO values.

4. Assess PAP, RAP, and PAWP waveforms. **Rationale:** Assures PA catheter is in the proper location.

5. Assess the patient's medical history for cardiac disease, cardiac surgery, infection, neurologic disorders, renal disease, pulmonary disease, recent trauma, and hospitalizations within past year, no matter what the diagnosis. **Rationale:** Commonly associated with an alteration in CO.

6. Assess the patient's neurologic status (i.e., level of consciousness, motor ability of all extremities, and ability to follow instructions). A more indepth neurologic assessment should be performed if the patient is semiconscious or unconscious. **Rationale:** A rare but possible complication of CO measures is air embolism to the brain. This can occur particularly in the setting of congenital heart disease with intracardiac shunting of blood. Air emboli can result in stroke or other abnormalities of neurologic function.

Nursing Diagnoses

1. Decreased cardiac output related to decreased preload, increased afterload, impaired cardiac contractility, myocardial ischemia, drug effects, anatomic alterations from cardiac surgery. **Rationale:** Causes alterations in either the amount of blood entering the heart, the resistance the heart must pump against, the ability of the heart to pump adequate blood, or the cardiovascular system as a whole. They will all result in changes in CO.

2. Potential for fluid volume overload related to repeated CO measures and injection of large amounts of solution. **Rationale:** CO may be performed hourly. If 10 cc of injectate is used and the nurse performs three injections with each measure, the patient can receive over 700 cc fluid per day from CO measures. This can be problematic for the patient with heart failure who cannot tolerate excess crystalloid infusions.

3. Potential for impaired cerebral perfusion related to air embolism. **Rationale:** With the syringe bath preparation or the closed system, there is opportunity for air to accidentally be drawn into the CO flush system.

Planning

1. Individualize the following goals for performing CO measurements:
   a. Obtain CO measures. **Rationale:** Erroneous readings will result in delays or mistakes in interventions.
   b. Maintain fluid balance. **Rationale:** If CO measures are performed only when necessary and with consideration to the amount of fluid being administered, the patient should remain normovolemic.
   c. Maintain intact, closed cardiac output measurement system. **Rationale:** Proper handling of injectate syringes should prevent air embolism or infection.

2. Prepare all necessary equipment and supplies. **Rationale:** Assembly of all the necessary equipment at the bedside ensures that CO measurements will be completed quickly and efficiently.

For Syringe Bath Method:

   a. Three 10-cc syringes.
   b. Three Luer-lok caps.
   c. One polyethylene plastic bag, large enough to contain all three syringes, or ice bath preparation.
   d. Plastic beaker, 1-L size.
   e. Sterile 5% dextrose or normal saline solution.
   f. Three 1-in 20-gauge needles.
   g. Alcohol swabs.
   h. Cardiac output computer and cable.
   i. Temperature probe for ice bath.

For Closed System Technique:

   a. 500 ml of D_5W or normal saline (NS).
   b. Two stopcocks.
   c. One IV pole.
   d. One 10-ml syringe.
   e. One cooling bucket with IV pole bracket (for iced injectate).
   f. One CO-Set (iced or RT, according to unit policy).
   g. In-line temperature probe.
   h. Cardiac output computer with connecting cable.
   i. Crushed iced and water (for iced injectate).
   Note: Syringes for iced injections should be prepared at least 1 hour prior to using in order to be sure they are cooled to the proper temperature, 1 to 5°C.

3. Prepare the patient.
   a. Explain the procedure to patient. **Rationale:** Minimizes risks and reduces anxiety.

b. Explain to the patient that he or she may feel a cold sensation within the thoracic cavity if an iced injectate is used. **Rationale:** It is not unusual for the patient to feel an iced injectate. This can be frightening if the patient has not been warned ahead of time.

Implementation

Steps	Rationale	Special Considerations
Preparation of Syringes		
1. Wash hands.	Reduces transmission of microorganisms.	
2. Attach a 20-gauge needle to four 10-cc syringes.	Saves time and reduces risk of needle sticks from connect/disconnect procedure.	
3. Cleanse injection port of normal saline bag or D_5W bag with alcohol swab.	Reduces bacterial contamination.	
4. Withdraw solution into each syringe. Be sure amount withdrawn into syringe is accurate.	2.5 ml is used for pediatric patients; 5 or 10 ml can be used in adult patients. Accuracy is important because an error of 0.5 ml in a 5-ml injection will cause a 10 percent measurement error.	Repeated high correlations of 10 ml of iced versus room-temperature (RT) injectate have been found. The reliability of 5 ml has not been totally resolved, although many have recommended 5 ml for fluid-restricted patients (Gardner, 1989; Groom et al., 1990; Loveys and Woods, 1986).
5. Replace needles with sterile luer-loc caps.	Prevents bacterial contamination.	
6. Place all three syringes into a polyethylene bag and close bag by zip locking or by applying a wire closure.	Prevents syringe contamination.	Some institutions have special trays for holding prepared CO syringes or will place one beaker within another.
7. Store syringes in medication refrigerator (for later use as iced injectate) or store in patient's medication tray (for RT injectate).	Storing syringes in refrigerator allows them to cool so that less time for cooling is required at the bedside.	The research on RT versus iced injectate supports the accuracy of either temperature when a 10-ml volume is used; 5-ml volumes remain controversial (Gardner, 1989; Groom et al., 1990; Loveys and Woods, 1986).
8. When it is time to set up CO computer, place bagged syringes into a sterile beaker.	Sterile beaker serves as a storage place for syringes at bedside. Syringes should not be left lying about.	
9. For an iced injectate, fill beaker with sterile water and ice, forming a slush solution. For RT injectate, leave beaker empty.	Iced slush is used to cool syringes.	RT injectate holds several advantages over iced: Less time is required to reach equilibration; there is less chance of erroneous measures due to syringe warming; and RT injectate reduces the risk of possible dysrhythmias associated with iced injectate.
10. Open polyethylene bag, remove the plunger from one syringe, and place a temperature probe into this syringe and its contents.	Serves as the test syringe to be sure injectate is cooled to 0 to 5°C.	
11. Carefully reseal polyethylene bag around the temperature probe wire.	Prevents bacterial contamination.	

Table continues on following page

Steps	Rationale	Special Considerations
12. Place the polyethylene bag with syringes into the beaker. If using iced injectate, polyethylene bag should be in a vertical position and securely closed so that slush solution does not enter the bag.	Bacterial contamination of syringes may occur if they are not sealed tightly (Riedinger et al., 1985).	
13. Allow iced injectate to cool 30 to 45 minutes or until temperature probe reads 0 to 5°C. Syringes are now ready for use.	It is important that the temperature be within the required range to ensure accuracy of values obtained.	Store syringes in an environment where the temperature will be maintained (i.e., not in front of a sunny window).
14. Wash hands.	Reduces transmission of microorganisms.	

Syringe Measurement Technique

Steps	Rationale	Special Considerations
1. Wash hands.	Reduces transmission of microorganisms.	
2. Turn on CO computer, and connect CO cable to PA catheter thermistor.	Gives computer adequate time to warm up. Interfaces CO computer to catheter thermistor.	
3. Position patient in supine position, HOB no higher than 20 degrees.	Research has demonstrated that results may differ when the patient is in a lateral position. There is no research that has evaluated the effects of HOB elevation greater than 20 degrees (Grose et al., 1979; Kleven, 1984; Whitman et al., 1982).	If CO measures are being taken hourly, it may not be practical or safe to constantly change the patient's position for these readings. Most important, the patient should be resting and should have been in his or her current position for at least 20 minutes prior to taking CO measures.
4. Dial in the appropriate computation constant.	An accurate computation constant is essential to obtain accurate CO measures.	Catheter size and type, volume and temperature of injectate, and injectate preparation will determine which constant is used. Refer to operation manual.
5. Verify PA waveform on oscilloscope. Note patient's ECG.	Ensures PA catheter is in proper position. If patient is having frequent ectopy, CO measures may be inaccurate.	Improper catheter position will result in erroneous values (Gardner, 1989).
6. Check to be sure CO computer is ready. Have start button within easy reach.	Avoids wasting injectate or erroneous measures.	
7. Locate stopcock nearest to patient on PA catheter proximal lumen; the lumen RAP is being monitored.	This stopcock will be used for injection. It is important to be sure the proper stopcock is identified and that no IV fluids are being administered through the RA lumen.	If the patient is receiving IV fluids through the RA lumen, they should be discontinued while CO measures are being performed. It is recommended that no cardiotonic or vasoactive drugs be given through this lumen because of the risks (i.e., cardiac arrest, hypotension) of bolusing of these medications during CO measurements.
8. Observe the patient's inspiratory and expiratory chest excursion.	Prepares for injection on expiration.	Performing CO measurements during a particular time of the respiratory cycle will promote consistency in measures.
9. Open polyethylene bag, and take out one syringe, being careful not to handle barrel if using iced solution. Work quickly.	Handling of the barrel can result in warming of syringe and errors in CO values.	

Table continues on following page

Steps	Rationale	Special Considerations
10. Remove cap and connect syringe to RA lumen stopcock. Turn stopcock off to transducer.	Opens injectate syringe to patient.	
11. At end-expiration, press the start button on the computer and manually inject the syringe contents rapidly and smoothly within a 4-second period.	Each injection should be timed to occur at the same point in the respiratory cycle to ensure comparability of measurements.	End-expiration has been recommended, based on research, to be the best time for CO measures (Armengol et al., 1981; Ehlers et al., 1986; Jansen et al., 1981; Levett and Replogle, 1979; Loveys and Woods, 1986; Okamoto et al., 1986; Stevens et al., 1985; Swinney et al., 1980; Tajiri et al., 1984), particularly in mechanically ventilated patients.
12. Observe CO thermodilution curve on bedside oscilloscope (if available) or strip recorder. It should have a rapid upstroke and gradual, smooth return to baseline (see Fig. 10–40).	Observation of the curve is important in order to identify problem sources. Abnormal curves and their etiologies can be seen in Figure 10–41.	
13. Record the value displayed on the computer (if computer does not automatically store values).	This is the computed CO value.	
14. Repeat the injections two additional times.	Three CO measures are taken for averaging values.	
15. Average all three values together *if* they are within 10 to 15 percent of the medial value. If they are not close to the medial value, discard any spurious value and average the remaining two.	Errors in measurement are common and can result in erroneous numbers. At least one study has demonstrated that the first value is often the inaccurate one (Kadota, 1986), but since this is not always the case, all three values need to be observed and the spurious value discarded.	
16. Return the RA lumen stopcock to its original position and be sure it is capped with a Luer-lok cap.	Decreases the risk of infection.	
17. Verify again the PA waveform on the oscilloscope, and observe ECG waveform.	Ensures that there has been no change in waveform. Ensures no new dysrhythmias have developed.	The development of bradycardia has been observed to occur during iced injection CO measures.
18. Wash hands.	Reduces transmission of microorganisms.	

Special Considerations and Troubleshooting

1. If variations in serial readings are observed:		
a. Be sure injections are smooth, over a 4-second period.	Uneven injections may result in varying values.	
b. Limit patient movement during procedure.	Prevents varying results.	
c. Use 10 ml of iced injectate to increase signal-to-noise ratio.	In patients with labile hemodynamics or especially high or low CO values, iced injectate may give more consistent results (Gardner, 1989).	
d. Inject solution at same point in respiratory cycle, end-expiration.	Increases comparability of results, particularly in mechanically ventilated patients.	
e. Check computation constant.	Wrong constant will result in incorrect values.	

Table continues on following page

Steps	Rationale	Special Considerations
f. Observe ECG for dysrhythmias.	Frequent ectopic beats may contribute to variations in CO measures.	
g. Observe CO curve for variations indicating a problem.	CO curve is useful in determining cause of problem readings.	
2. If RA lumen becomes clotted or nonfunctional:		
a. Notify physician.	Other alternatives need to be discussed.	
b. Discuss with physician the possibility of using the venous infusion port (VIP lumen), introducer side port, or centrally placed catheter that exits into a central vein for CO measures.	Research has supported the use of these other lumens for CO injections (Gibney and Ryan, 1984; Lee and Stevens, 1985; Martin et al., 1983; Mault et al., 1983; Vicari and Ogle, 1987).	Whichever lumen is used, it must be beyond the introducer sheath to avoid retrograde flow from an IV line connected to the introducer side port (Gardner, 1989).
c. Make note in patient record and carefully label catheter as to which line is being used for CO measures.	Ensures consistency in measures.	

Closed System Technique

Steps	Rationale	Special Considerations
1. Wash hands.	Reduces transmission of microorganisms.	
2. Hang IV flush solution on IV pole, and attach ice bucket holder and bucket to pole.	Flush must be hanging to promote fluid movement to the patient.	Bucket and holder are not used for RT injectate.
3. Remove CO-Set from package.	Prepares for assembly.	RT method packaging is very different from iced method packaging.
4. Close the snap clamp.	Prevents rapid fluid flow when the bag is spiked.	
5. Remove protective cap from IV spike, and insert nonvented spike into flush solution.	Accesses flush solution.	
6. Pull apart the tubing coil (*not* the cooling coil in iced setup) to obtain desired tubing length between the IV container and ice bucket.	Tubing coil is designed to be separated for added length. Cooling coil is not.	
7. Place cooling coil in bucket (Fig. 10–45).	Injectate solution will be cooled by coils.	
8. Add ice to cover coil in bucket, add enough water to make a slush (the water should be visible above the ice level), and place the lid on the bucket.	A slush is necessary to ensure that there are no air pockets in the ice. Air pockets will result in uneven cooling.	
9. Connect the 10-ml CO syringe (in CO-Set package) to the check valve (Fig. 10–46).	Syringe will be used to clear tubing of air as well as for measures.	*Caution: Do not* connect the syringe to the catheter side of the flow-through housing. Pressurization or flushing from the wrong side of the flow-through housing may result in damage to the check valve.
10. Check to make sure all connections are tight and secure.	Loose connections will allow air into system and give inaccurate measures.	
11. Open the snap clamp and allow solution to flow from the flush bag into a discard container.	Clears tubing of air.	

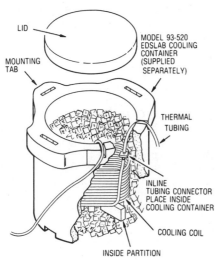

FIGURE 10-45. Tubing and cooling coil for CO-Set. (Courtesy of Baxter Edwards Corporation.)

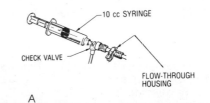

A

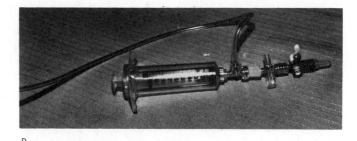

B

FIGURE 10-46. Syringe and check valve, close-up view. (A) Diagram. (B) Photograph. (Courtesy of Baxter Edwards Corporation.)

Steps	Rationale	Special Considerations
12. *Slowly* pull the syringe plunger to prime the system, and then push the plunger in. Repeat procedure five to six times until the system is free from air.	Rapid pulling may cause turbulence in the system and air bubble formation.	
13. Return the syringe plunger to the fully depressed position.	Prevents fluid from being accidentally injected into patient.	
14. Close the snap clamp.	Prevents syringe from filling with fluid.	
15. Attach two three-way stopcocks directly to the proximal lumen of the PA catheter. Pressure tubing should lead away from the stopcocks to the transducer (i.e., be distal to the stopcocks).	One will be used for CO measures; the other for blood withdrawal, clearing of lines, etc. This allows the CO-Set to remain a closed system.	
16. Attach the CO-Set flow-through housing to the three-way stopcock on the proximal lumen (Fig. 10-47).	The CO injections should be performed through the stopcock closest to the patient to reduce the resistance to injection.	
17. Insert injectate temperature probe into flow-through housing (Fig. 10-48).	This probe will measure injectate temperature as it is injected into the patient.	

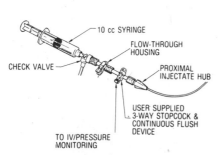

FIGURE 10-47. CO-Set attached to proximal stopcock. (Courtesy of Baxter Edwards Corporation.)

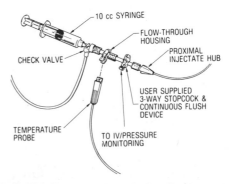

FIGURE 10-48. Temperature probe into flow-through housing of CO-Set. (Courtesy of Baxter Edwards Corporation.)

Steps	Rationale	Special Considerations
18. Connect injectate temperature probe cable to the "injectate probe" lead of computer cable.	Enables computer to read temperature and display it.	
19. Position patient in supine position, HOB no higher than 20 degrees.	Research has demonstrated that results may differ when the patient is in a lateral position. There is no research that has evaluated the effects of HOB elevation greater than 20 degrees (Grose et al., 1979; Kleven, 1984; Whitman et al., 1982).	If CO measures are being taken hourly, it may not be practical or safe to constantly change the patient's position for these readings. Most important, the patient should be resting and should have been in the same position for 20 minutes prior to taking CO measure.
20. Dial in the appropriate computation constant.	An accurate computation constant is essential to obtain accurate CO measures.	Catheter size and type, volume and temperature of injectate, and injectate preparation will determine which constant is used.
21. Verify PA waveform on oscilloscope. Note patient's ECG.	Ensures PA catheter is in proper position. If patient is having frequent ectopy, CO measures may be inaccurate.	Improper catheter position will result in erroneous values (Gardner, 1989).
22. Check to be sure CO computer is ready. Have start button within easy reach.	Avoids wasting injectate or erroneous measure.	
23. Observe the patient's inspiratory and expiratory chest excursion.	Prepares for injection on expiration.	See discussion below on why CO is performed on end-expiration.
24. Open snap clamp.	Fills syringe with injectate.	
25. Turn the stopcock at the catheter injectate hub to close the IV flush and to open the fluid path between the syringe and catheter.	Allows for measure of CO.	
26. Push the CO button on the computer, and slowly withdraw 10 ml of injectate into the 10-ml syringe.	Prepares for injection.	
27. At end-expiration, press the start button on the computer, manually inject the syringe contents rapidly and smoothly, within a 4-second period, and observe injectate temperature during injection.	Each injection should be timed to occur at the same point in the respiratory cycle to ensure comparability of measurements.	End-expiration has been recommended, based on research, to be the best time for CO measures (Armengol et al., 1981; Ehlers et al., 1986; Jansen et al., 1981; Levett and Replogle, 1979; Loveys and Woods, 1986; Okamoto et al., 1986; Stevens et al., 1985; Swinney et al., 1980; Tajiri et al., 1984), particularly in mechanically ventilated patients.
28. Observe CO thermodilution curve on bedside oscilloscope (if available) or strip recorder. It should have a rapid upstroke and gradual, smooth return to baseline.	Observation of the curve is important to identify problem sources. Abnormal curves and the underlying problem can be seen in Figure 10–47.	
29. Record the value displayed on the computer in the patient record.	This is the computed CO value.	
30. Repeat the injections two additional times.	Three CO measures are taken for the purpose of averaging values.	Space injections at least 1 minute apart to improve reproducibility.
31. Average all three values if they are within 10 to 15 percent of the medial value. If they are not close	Errors in measurement are common and can result in erroneous numbers. At least one study has demonstrated	

Table continues on following page

Steps	Rationale	Special Considerations
to the medial value, discard any spurious value and average the remaining two.	that the first value is often the inaccurate one (Kadota, 1986), but since this is not always the case, all three values need to be observed and the spurious value discarded.	
32. Return the RA lumen stopcock to its original position.	Resumes continuous monitor of RA and to open line to IV flush.	
33. Close the snap clamp.	Prevents solution flow.	
34. Verify again the PA waveform on the oscilloscope. Observe ECG waveform.	Ensures that there has been no change and to be sure that no new dysrhythmias have developed.	
35. Wash hands.	Reduces transmission of microorganisms.	

Source: Adapted from American Edwards Laboratories, *Closed Injectate Delivery System for Cold Injectate, Model 93-500* and *Closed Injectate Delivery System for Room Temperature Injectate, Model 93-510*. Irvine, CA., 1990.

Evaluation

Compare patient's cardiovascular and neurologic assessments before and after CO measurement. **Rationale:** Identifies patient responses to CO procedure and CO-based interventions.

Expected Outcomes

1. Accurate, consistent CO measurements. **Rationale:** Adherence to CO technique will support reproducibility and comparability of CO values.
2. Fluid balance maintained. **Rationale:** Patient does not develop fluid overload from excessive CO measures.
3. Patient will have the same neurologic findings before and after CO measurement. **Rationale:** Patient has not had air emboli to the brain.

Unexpected Outcomes

1. Variable of inconsistent CO measurements. **Rationale:** CO measurement technique may not be accurate. Measurements are being performed with RT injectate when ice may be preferred for this patient. The etiology for the decreased CO has not been correctly identified. The interventions for decreased CO have not been successful or are not appropriate. The patient's condition is unresponsive to medical therapy.
2. Fluid volume overload. **Rationale:** Too many CO measures may have been taken. The nurse has not used

clinical discretion in performing CO measures. Only 5 ml of injectate may be needed in light of fluid balance status, but the results should be compared with 10-ml results prior to using 5 ml of injectate.
3. Decreased mental alertness, motor weakness, communication impairment, or other signs of a neurologic event. **Rationale:** Patient has had an embolic event to the brain, possibly related to CO technique.

Documentation

Documentation in the patient record should include CO value after averaging, computed cardiac index (CI), hemodynamic values and vital signs at the time of CO measurement, patient position for CO, and any unusual responses (i.e., neurologic changes, bradycardia). **Rationale:** Documents nursing care given and patient's response to procedure.

Patient/Family Education

Discuss with patient and family the rationale for CO measures. **Rationale:** Reduces fear of unknown and anxiety about bedside procedure.

Performance Checklist
Skill 10–9:   Cardiac Output Measurement Techniques

Critical Behaviors	Complies	
	yes	no
PREPARATION OF SYRINGES 1. Wash hands.		
2. Attach 20-gauge needles to four 10-ml syringes.		

Table continues on following page

Critical Behaviors	Complies	
	yes	**no**
3. Cleanse injection port of injectate bag.		
4. Withdraw proper volume of injectate into syringes.		
5. Replace needles with Luer-lok caps.		
6. Place syringes into polyethylene bag, and securely close bag.		
7. Store syringes in refrigerator for iced injectate, medication tray for RT injectate.		
8. When ready to set up CO computer, place syringes into sterile beaker.		
9. For iced injectate, fill beaker with water and ice; for RT injectate, leave beaker empty.		
10. Place temperature probe into test syringe.		
11. Reseal polyethylene bag around temperature probe wire.		
12. Place polyethylene bag in vertical position in slush solution.		
13. Check to be sure iced syringes are cooled to 0 to 5°C.		
14. Wash hands.		
SYRINGE MEASUREMENT TECHNIQUE 1. Wash hands.		
2. Turn on CO computer and allow to warm up.		
3. Position HOB no higher than 20-degrees supine.		
4. Dial in appropriate computation constant.		
5. Verify PA waveform on oscilloscope, and note ECG.		
6. Check to be sure CO computer is ready.		
7. Locate stopcock where CO injections will be made.		
8. Observe patient's respiratory excursion.		
9. Remove syringe from iced bag without handling barrel.		
10. Quickly connect syringe to stopcock, and open stopcock to syringe.		
11. At end-expiration, push start button, and rapidly and smoothly inject CO injectate over 4 seconds.		
12. Observe CO curve.		
13. Record CO value.		
14. Repeat procedure two additional times, recording each value.		
15. Discard spurious values and average similar values.		
16. Return stopcock to original position.		
17. Verify again that there is no change in PA waveform, and observe ECG for changes.		
18. Wash hands.		
19. Document procedure and patient response in patient record.		
CLOSED SYSTEM TECHNIQUE 1. Wash hands.		
2. Hang IV flush solution on IV pole, and attach ice bucket holder and bucket to pole (for iced injectate).		
3. Remove CO-Set from package.		

Table continues on following page

Critical Behaviors	Complies	
	yes	no
4. Close snap clamp.		
5. Remove cap from IV spike, and insert into flush solution.		
6. Prepare tubing coil.		
7. Place cooling coil in bucket.		
8. Add ice and water to fill bucket, and put lid on bucket.		
9. Connect the CO syringe to the check valve.		
10. Check to make sure all connections are tight.		
11. Open snap clamp and allow solution to flow from flush bag into discard container.		
12. Slowly pull the syringe plunger to prime the system, and repeat this procedure three times.		
13. Return the syringe plunger to fully depressed position.		
14. Close snap clamp.		
15. Attach two stopcocks to proximal lumen of PA catheter.		
16. Attach the CO-Set flow-through housing to the proximal stopcock on PA lumen.		
17. Insert injectate temperature probe into flow-through housing.		
18. Connect injectate temperature probe cable to the computer cable.		
19. Position patient supine, HOB no higher than 20 degrees.		
20. Dial in correct computation constant.		
21. Verify PA waveform on oscilloscope, and note ECG.		
22. Check to be sure computer is ready.		
23. Observe patient's inspiratory and expiratory chest excursion.		
24. Open snap clamp.		
25. Open fluid path between syringe and catheter.		
26. Push CO button on the computer, and slowly withdraw 10 ml of injectate into the 10-ml syringe.		
27. At end-expiration, rapidly and smoothly inject solution, making injection in less than 4 seconds.		
28. Observe CO curve on bedside oscilloscope.		
29. Record CO value displayed on computer.		
30. Repeat injections two additional times.		
31. Average the two closest values (all three if they are within 10 to 15% of the medial value).		
32. Reopen stopcock so that PA lumen is open to transducer.		
33. Close snap clamp.		
34. Observe PA waveform again to ensure that it is unchanged, and observe ECG.		
35. Wash hands.		
36. Document procedure in patient record.		
SPECIAL CONSIDERATIONS AND TROUBLESHOOTING 1. Observe for variations in serial readings.		
2. Observe for patency of RA lumen.		

REFERENCES

AACN (1990). *Outcome Standards for Nursing Care of the Critically Ill.* Laguna Nigel, Calif.: AACN.

Ahlberg, J., Wallace, S. H., Dobbin, K., and Chulay, M. (1989). PA pressure measurement in pulmonary hypertension (Abstract). *Heart Lung* 18(3):300–301.

Applefeld, J. J., Caruthers, T. E., Reno, D. J., and Civetta, J. M. (1978). Assessment of the sterility of long-term cardiac catheterization using thermodilution Swan-Ganz catheter. *Chest* 74(4):377–380.

Armengol, J., Man, G. C. W., and Balsys, A. J. (1981). Effects of the respiratory cycle on cardiac output measurements: Reproducibility of data enhanced by timing the thermodilution injection in dogs. *Crit. Care Med.* 9(12):852–854.

Baele, P. L., McMichan, J. C., Marsh, H. M., Sill, J. C., and Southorn, P. A. (1982). Continuous monitoring of mixed venous oxygen saturation in critically ill patients. *Anesth. Analg.* 61(6):513–517.

Baird, M. S., Raud, B., and Adkinson, M. P. (1990). Nursing responsibility levels for cardiac surgical procedures. *Dimens. Crit. Care Nurs.* 9(2):98–106.

Barash, P. G., Nardi, D., Hammon, G., et al. (1981). Catheter-induced pulmonary artery perforation: Mechanisms, management, and modifications. *J. Thorac. Cardiovasc. Surg.* 82:5–12.

Barcelona, M., Patague, L., Bunoy, M., et al. (1985). Cardiac output determination by the thermodilution method: Comparison of ice-temperature injectate contained in prefilled syringes or a closed injectate delivery system. *Heart Lung* 14(3):232–235.

Bojar, R. M. (1989). *Manual of Perioperative Care in Cardiac and Thoracic Surgery* (pp. 17, 233). Boston: Blackwell Scientific Publications.

Boyd, K. D., Thomas, S. J., Gold, J., and Boyd, A. D. (1983). A prospective study of complications of pulmonary artery catheterization in 500 consecutive patients. *Chest* 84(3):245–249.

Cairns, J. A., and Holder, D. (1975). Ventricular fibrillation due to passage of a Swan-Ganz catheter (Letter). *Am. J. Cardiol.* 35:589.

Cenzig, M., Crapo, R. D., and Gardner, R. M. (1983). The effect of ventilation on the accuracy of pulmonary artery and wedge pressure measurement. *Crit. Care Med.* 11:502.

Chulay, M., and Miller, T. (1984). The effect of backrest elevation on pulmonary artery and pulmonary capillary wedge pressures in patients after cardiac surgery. *Heart Lung* 13(2):138–140.

Chun, G. M., and Ellestad, M. H. (1971). Perforation of the pulmonary artery by a Swan-Ganz catheter. *N. Engl. J. Med.* 284:1041.

Connors, A. F., Castele, R. J., Farhat, N. Z., and Tomashefski, J. F. (1985). Complications of right heart catheterization: A prospective autopsy study. *Chest* 88(4):567–572.

Daily, E. K. (1990). Hemodynamic Monitoring. In J. T. Dolan (Ed.), *Critical Care Nursing: Clinical Management Through the Nursing Process* (pp. 828–855). Philadelphia: F. A. Davis.

Daily, E. K., and Schroeder, J. S. (1989). *Techniques in Bedside Hemodynamic Monitoring,* 4th Ed. (pp. 138, 289, 306, 409). St. Louis: Mosby.

Damen, J. (1985). Ventricular arrhythmias during insertion and removal of pulmonary artery catheters. *Chest* 88(2):190–193.

Darovic, G. O. (1987). *Hemodynamic Monitoring: Invasive and Noninvasive Clinical Application.* Philadelphia: Saunders.

Devitt, J. H., Noble, W. H., and Byrick, R. J. (1982). A Swan-Ganz catheter-related complication in a patient with Eisenmenger's syndrome. *Anesthesiology* 57(4):335–337.

Ehlers, K. C., Mylrea, K. C., and Waterson, C. K. (1986). Cardiac output measurements: A review of current technique and research. *Ann. Biomed. Eng.* 14(3):219–239.

Elliott, C. G., Zimmerman, G. A., and Clemmer, T. P. (1979). Complications of pulmonary artery catheterization in the care of critically ill patients. *Chest* 76(6):647–652.

Enger, E. L. (1989). Pulmonary artery wedge pressure: When it's valid, when it's not. *Crit. Care Nurs. Clin. North Am.* 1(3):603–618.

Gardner, P. E. (1989). Cardiac output: Theory, technique, and troubleshooting. *Crit. Care Nurs. Clin. North Am.* 1(3):577–587.

Gardner, P. E., Monat, L. A., and Woods, S. L. (1987). Accuracy of the closed injectate delivery system in measuring thermodilution cardiac output. *Heart Lung* 16(5):552–561.

Gibney, R. T., and Ryan, H. (1984). Thermodilution cardiac output measurements. *Crit. Care Med.* 12(7):614–615.

Golden, M. S., Pinder, T., Anderson, W. T., and Cheitlin, M. D. (1975). Fatal pulmonary artery hemorrhage complicating use of the flow-directed balloon-tipped catheter in a patient receiving anticoagulant therapy. *Am. J. Cardiol.* 32(6):865–867.

Gore, J. M., Alpert, J. S., Benotti, J. R., et al. (1985). *Handbook of Hemodynamic Monitoring.* Boston: Little, Brown.

Greene, J. F., Jr., Fitzwater, J. E., and Clemmer, T. P. (1975). Septic endocarditis and indwelling pulmonary artery catheter. *J.A.M.A.* 233:891.

Groom, L., Elliott, M., and Frisch, S. (1990). Injectate temperature: Effects on thermodilution cardiac output measurements. *Crit. Care Nurs.* 10:112–120.

Grose, B. L., Woods, S. L., and Laurent, D. J. (1979). Effects of backrest position on thermodilution cardiac output measurements in 30 acutely ill patients. *Circulation* 60:248.

Hathaway, R. (1978). The Swan-Ganz catheter: A review. *Nurs. Clin. North Am.* 13(3):389–407.

Hardy, U., Ward, D. R., and Gilliliau, R. (1982). Fatal pulmonary hemorrhage complicating Swan-Ganz catheterization. *Surgery* 91:24.

Hazinski, M. F. (1989). Hemodynamic Monitoring in Children. In E. K. Daily and J. S. Schroeder (Eds.), *Techniques in Bedside Hemodynamic Monitoring* (p. 306). St. Louis: Mosby.

Hines, R., and Barash, P. G. (1990). Pulmonary Artery Catheterization. In C. D. Blitt (Ed.), *Monitoring in Anesthesia and Critical Care Medicine* (p. 227). New York: Churchill-Livingstone.

Hook, M. L., Reuling, J., Luettgen, M. L., et al. (1987). Comparison of the patency of arterial lines maintained with heparinized and non-heparinized infusions. *Heart Lung* 16(6):693–699.

Hudak, C. (1989). *Critical Care Nursing: A Holistic Approach.* Philadelphia: Lippincott.

Jansen, J. R. C., Schrueder, J. J., and Bogaard, J. M. (1981). Thermodilution technique for measurement of cardiac output during artificial ventilation. *J. Appl. Physiol.* 51:584–591.

Johnson, J. E., Fuller, S. S., Endress, M. P., and Rice, V. H. (1978). Altering patient's responses to surgery: An extension and replication. *Res. Nurs. Health* 1(3):111–121.

Kadota, L. T. (1986). Reproducibility of thermodilution cardiac output measurements. *Heart Lung* 15(6):618–622.

Keating, D., Bolyard, K., Eichler, J., and Reed, J. (1986). Effect of sidelying positions on pulmonary artery pressures. *Heart Lung* 15(6):605–610.

Kelly, T. F., Jr., Morris, G. C., Jr., Crawford, E. S., et al. (1981). Perforation of the pulmonary artery with Swan-Ganz catheters. *Ann. Surg.* 193(6):686–692.

Kennedy, G. T., Bryant, A., and Crawford, M. H. (1984). The effects of lateral body positioning on measurements of pulmonary artery and pulmonary artery wedge pressures. *Heart Lung* 13(2):155–158.

Kern, L. (1990). Manual for Advanced Cardiac Evaluation Unit. Unpublished manual. Los Angeles: UCLA Medical Center.

Kersten, L. D. (1989). Hemodynamic Monitoring: Respiratory Applications. In L. D. Kersten (Ed.), *Comprehensive Respiratory Nursing.* Philadelphia: Saunders.

Kleven, M. R. (1984). Effect of backrest position on thermodilution cardiac output in critically ill patients receiving mechanical ventilation with positive end-expiratory pressure. *Heart Lung* 13(3):303–304.

Kolodychuk, G. R., Joiner, G., and Barnhouse, A. H. (1989). The accuracy of leveling hemodynamic pressure monitoring transducers by the "eyeball" and "carpenter's level" methods (Abstract). *Heart Lung* 18(3):303–304.

Laulive, J. L. (1982). Pulmonary artery pressures and position changes in the critically ill adult. *Dimens. Crit. Care Nurs.* 1(1):28–34.

Lee, D. W., and Stevens, G. H. (1985). Comparison of thermodilution cardiac output measurement by injection of the proximal lumen versus side port of the Swan-Ganz catheter. *Heart Lung* 14(2):126–127.

Levett, J. M., and Replogle, R. L. (1979). Thermodilution cardiac output: A critical analysis and review of the literature. *J. Surg. Res.* 27:392–404.

Loveys, B. J., and Woods, S. L. (1986). Current recommendations for thermodilution cardiac output measurement. *Progr. Cardiovasc. Nurs.* 1(1):24–32.

Mariani, J. J. (1989). Postoperative atelectasis: Pathophysiology, clinical importance, and principles of management. *Respir. Care* 29:516–522.

Martin, C., Saux, P., Auffray, P., et al. (1983). Thermodilution cardiac output measurements by injection in pulmonary artery vs. CVP catheter. *Crit. Care Med.* 11(6):460–461.

Masters, S. (1989). Complications of pulmonary artery catheters. *Crit. Care Nurs.* 9(9):82–91.

Mault, J. R., Bartlett, R. H., Decher, R. E., and Clark, S. F. (1983). Central venous catheter versus proximal port injection site for thermodilution cardiac outputs. *Crit. Care Med.* 11(3):224.

Okamoto, K., Komatsu, T., Kumar, V., et al. (1986). Effects of intermittent positive-pressure ventilation on cardiac output measurements by thermodilution. *Crit. Care Med.* 14(11):977–980.

Osika, C. N. (1989). Measure of pulmonary artery pressures: Supine versus side-lying head elevated position (Abstract). *Heart Lung* 18(3):298–299.

Paulson, D. M., Scott, S. M., and Sethi, G. K. (1980). Pulmonary hemorrhage associated with balloon flotation catheters: A report of a case and review of the literature. *J. Thorac. Cardiovasc. Surg.* 80:453.

Pierson, M. G., and Funk, M. (1989). Technology vs. clinical evaluation of fluid management decisions in CABG patients. *Image: J. Nurs. Scholarship* 21(4):192–195.

Pinilla, J. C., Ross, D. F., Martin, T., and Crump, H. (1983). Study of the incidence of intravascular catheter infection and associated septicemia in critically ill patients. *Crit. Care Med.* 11(1):21–25.

Recker, D. H. (1985). Procedure for left atrial catheter insertion. *Crit. Care Nurs.* 5(4):36–41.

Retailliau, M. A., Leding, M., and Woods, S. L. (1985). The effect of backrest position on the measurement of left atrial pressure in patients after cardiac surgery. *Heart Lung* 14(5):477–483.

Riedinger, M. S., and Shellock, F. G. (1984). Technical aspects of the thermodilution method for measuring cardiac output. *Heart Lung* 13(3):215–222.

Riedinger, M. S., and Shellock, F. G. (1985). Sterility of prefilled thermodilution cardiac output syringes maintained at room and ice temperatures. *Heart Lung* 14(1):8–11.

Robin, E. D. (1985). The cult of the Swan-Ganz catheter: Overuse and abuse of pulmonary flow catheters. *Ann. Intern. Med.* 103(3):445–449.

Rosenbaum, L., Rosenbaum, S. H., Askanazi, J., and Hyman, A. I. (1981). Small amounts of hemoptysis as an early warning sign of pulmonary artery rupture by a pulmonary arterial catheter. *Crit. Care Med.* 9(4):319–320.

Samsoondar, W., Freeman, J. B., Coultish, I., and Oxley, C. (1985). Colonization of intravascular catheters in the intensive care unit. *Am. J. Surg.* 149(6):730–732.

Singh, S., Melson, N., Acosta, I., and Check, F. E. (1982). Catheter colonization and bacteremia with pulmonary and arterial catheters. *Crit. Care Med.* 10(11):736–739.

Sprung, C. L., Jacobs, L. J., and Caralis, P. V. (1981). Ventricular arrhythmias during Swan-Ganz catheterization of the critically ill. *Chest* 79:413.

Sprung, C. L., Pozen, R. G., Rozanski, J. J., et al. (1982). Advanced ventricular arrhythmias during bedside pulmonary artery catheterization. *Am. J. Med.* 72(2):203–208.

Stevens, J. H., Raffin, T. A., Mihm, F. G., et al. (1985). Thermodilution cardiac output measurement: Effects of the respiratory cycle on its reproducibility. *J.A.M.A.* 253(15):2240–2242.

Swinney, R. S., Davenport, M. W., Wagers, P.W., et al. (1980). Iced versus room temperature injectate for thermodilution cardiac output. *Crit. Care Med.* 8(4):265.

Tafuro, P., and Ristuccia, P. (1984). Recognition and control of outbreaks of nosocomial infections in the intensive care setting. *Heart Lung* 13(5):486–495.

Tajiri, J., Katsuya, H., and Okamoto, K. (1984). The effects of the respiratory cycle by mechanical ventilation on cardiac output measured by the thermodilution method. *Jpn. Circ. J.* 48:328–330.

Taylor, R. W., Civetta, J. M., and Kirby, R. R. (1990). *Techniques and Procedures in Critical Care* (pp. 79–81). Philadelphia: Lippincott.

Taylor, T. (1985). Monitoring left atrial pressures in the open-heart surgical patient. *Crit. Care Nurs.* 6(2):62–68.

Thielen, J. B. (1990). Air emboli: A potentially lethal complication of central venous lines. *Focus Crit. Care* 17(5):374–383.

Thomson, I. R., Dalton, B. C., Lappas, D. G., and Lowenstein, E. (1979). Right bundle-branch block and complete heart block caused by Swan-Ganz catheter. *Anesthesiology* 51(4):359–362.

Tilkian, A., Dailey, E. K. (1986). *Cardiovascular Procedures* (p. 95). St. Louis: Mosby.

Urban, N. (1986). Integrating hemodynamic parameters with clinical decision making. *Crit. Care Nurs.* 6(2):48–59.

Vicari, M., and Ogle, V. (1987). Comparison of measurements of cardiac output from the side port versus the proximal lumen of the Swan-Ganz catheter: Follow-up study. *Heart Lung* 16(4):379–380.

Von Rueden, K. (1984). The effect of flush solution on the fluid status of cardiac surgery patients (Abstract). *Heart Lung* 13(3):300–301.

Ward, C. R., Constancia, P. E., and Kern, L. (1990). Nursing interventions for families of cardiac surgery patients. *J. Cardiovasc. Nurs.* 5(1):34–42.

Whitman, G. R., Howaniak, D. L., and Verga, T. S. (1982). Comparison of pulmonary artery catheter measurements in 20° supine and 20° right and left lateral recumbent positions. *Heart Lung* 11(3):256–257.

Wild, L. (1984). Effect of lateral recumbent position on the measurement of pulmonary artery and pulmonary artery wedge pressures. *Heart Lung* 13:155.

Woods, S. L., and Mansfield, L. (1976). Effect of patient position upon the pulmonary capillary wedge pressures in nonacutely ill patients. *Heart Lung* 5(1):83–90.

Woods, S. L., Grose, L., and Laurent-Bomp, D. (1982). Effect of backrest position on pulmonary artery pressure in critically ill patients. *J. Cardiovasc. Nurs.* 18:19.

11

ARTIFICIAL CARDIAC PACEMAKERS

BEHAVIORAL OBJECTIVES

After completing this chapter, the nurse will be able to

- Define the key terms.
- Describe the indications for artificial cardiac pacing.
- Describe artificial pacemaker components.
- Explain the concepts of sensing and capture.
- Demonstrate the skills involved in cardiac pacing.

Electrical activity in the myocardium is controlled by a very specialized conduction system that initiates and conducts impulses in an orderly and synchronous fashion. Artificial cardiac pacemakers may be required when either the normal mechanism of impulse formation fails or the normal mechanism of impulse conduction fails. Normal myocardial impulse formation and conduction result in activation of the atria prior to activation of the ventricles. This provides the opportunity for the atria to contract and empty blood into the ventricles prior to ventricular contraction. This atrial contribution to the cardiac output may be as much as 25 to 30 percent. Artificial pacing may be performed in a manner maintaining A-V synchrony, as in dual-chamber A-V sequential pacing, or it may be performed in such a manner as to eliminate A-V synchrony, as single-chamber ventricular pacing.

Cardiac pacing is a therapeutic modality used in a variety of clinical situations. It is often a lifesaving intervention in situations where bradycardia or tachycardia is producing hemodynamic compromise. The use of temporary cardiac pacemakers can be therapeutic in producing an adequate heart rate in the setting of brady-dysrhythmias or in the termination of tachydysrhythmias. Pacemakers may be used prophylactically in the setting of acute myocardial infarction (MI) or other pathophysiologic states to prevent high-grade or complete A-V block and bradycardia-dependent tachydysrhythmias. Pacemakers also may be used diagnostically to evaluate cardiac electrophysiologic function, such as evaluating conduction abnormalities or abnormalities of impulse formation.

Cardiac pacing is a method of artificially stimulating the myocardium utilizing a pacing lead and a pulse generator. The characteristics of lead systems vary considerably, but in general, they consist of an insulated lead wire with electrodes located at the tip of the wire. Pulse generators provide the energy source and the control settings for cardiac pacemakers. The components of pulse generators also vary considerably, but in general, they consist of controls to establish the desired pacing rate, the level of energy to be delivered to the myocardium, and the amount of intrinsic myocardial electrical activity that will be sensed. Additional controls may determine the variety of modes of pacemaker response in varying clinical situations.

Two basic concepts inherent in the understanding of artificial cardiac pacing are the concepts of sensing and capture. *Sensing* refers to the ability of the artificial pacemaker to recognize electrical activity generated by the myocardium. While not present in all artificial pacemakers, the ability to sense intrinsic electrical activity allows for pacemaker activity to be either inhibited or stimulated depending on the clinical situation. *Capture* refers to the successful stimulation of the myocardium by the pacemaker impulse. It is evidenced on the ECG by a pacemaker artifact followed by either an atrial or ventricular complex depending on the chamber being paced.

KEY TERMS

alligator clip	*milliamperes (mA)*
antitachycardiac pacing	*mode*
A-V interval	*output or current*
A-V sequential	*overdrive suppression*
bipolar	*pacing artifact or spike*
connecting cable	*pulse generator*
demand or synchronous	*refractory period*
electrode	*(pacemaker)*
electromagnetic interference	*stimulation threshold*
(EMI)	*transcutaneous external*
epicardial pacemaker	*pacemaker*
fixed-rate	*transvenous endocardial*
intrinsic rate	*pacemaker*
intrinsic rhythm	*unipolar*
lead	*V-A interval*
microshock	

SKILLS

11–1   Emergency Application of Temporary External Chest Pacing
11–2   Initiating Temporary Pacing
11–3   Overdrive Atrial Pacing
11–4   Atrial Electrograms
11–5   Permanent Pacing: Assessing the Modes

GUIDELINES

The following assessment guidelines will assist the

nurse in formulating nursing diagnoses and planning care for patients requiring pacemaker therapy:

1. Assess laboratory data, including arterial blood gases, electrolytes, complete blood count, drug levels.

2. Assess patient's pharmacologic treatment, including, antidysrhythmics, anesthetic agents, sedatives, analgesics, antibiotics, anticoagulants.

3. Know the nursing and medical history. If permanent pacemaker has been previously implanted, obtain pertinent information regarding reason for implantation, programmed settings, last pacemaker check, last battery change, and unusual symptoms.

4. Review results of diagnostic tests, including electrophysiologic tests, exercise treadmill tests, tilt-table tests, electrocardiogram, ambulatory ECG monitoring.

5. Assess current rhythm with rhythm strip or 12-lead ECG.

SKILL 11–1

Emergency Application of Temporary External Chest Pacing

External or transcutaneous pacing is a method of stimulating myocardial contraction through the chest wall via two large pacing patches. The patches are placed on the anterior and posterior chest wall and are attached by cable to an external pulse generator that houses the pacemaker controls.

Once the external pulse generator is activated, a specific level of energy then travels from the external pulse generator through the pacing patches to the myocardium, stimulating contraction. A critical mass of myocardium must be stimulated before contraction will occur. The efficacy of external pacing is influenced by a number of variables: the position and adherence of the pacing electrode patches, the level of energy delivered to the myocardium, the presence of acidosis or electrolyte imbalances, concomitant drug therapy, and anatomic features of the patient (i.e., barrel chest). Frequently, the external pulse generator is combined with a cardiac monitor to allow detection of the patient's cardiac rhythm and evaluation of pacemaker function (Fig. 11–1).

External pacing can be used in a variety of clinical settings and is applicable to the pediatric population with the use of special pacing patches. It is indicated for both acute and chronic conditions in both the in-hospital and prehospital settings and has several advantages over placement of an endocardial transvenous pacing wire. Application of transcutaneous pacing is relatively simple, requires less skill and time to initiate, and has fewer risks and complications than transvenous pacing. Patients may experience mild to severe discomfort depending on the level of energy required to pace and the technique of the operator. Adherence to external pacing guidelines helps minimize the degree of discomfort and maximizes the potential for capture to occur.

Temporary external (transcutaneous) chest pacing is indicated for asystolic cardiac arrest, symptomatic bradycardia (including A-V block), overdrive suppression and/or termination of supraventricular and ventricular tachydysrhythmias (via underdrive pacing or burst overdrive pacing), and prophylaxis in high-risk conduction disturbances (i.e., MI, drug toxicity) in patients for whom invasive techniques are contraindicated (immunosuppression, severe vascular disease, pretransplant candidates, high bleeding risk). Discontinuation of tempo-

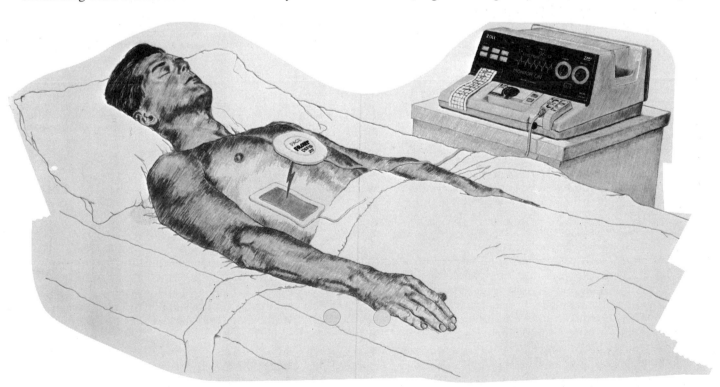

FIGURE 11–1. Temporary external pacing. (Reprinted with permission from ZOLL Medical Corporation, Woburn, Mass.)

rary external pacing is appropriate in a variety of clinical circumstances, including resolution of the bradydysrhythmia with restoration of a reliable intrinsic rhythm, upon insertion of a temporary transvenous pacing electrode, patient intolerance, and evidence of noncapture or failure to sense the patient's intrinsic rhythm.

Purpose

The nurse initiates external cardiac pacing to

1. Stimulate the myocardium to contract in the absence of an intrinsic rhythm.
2. Establish an adequate cardiac output and blood pressure to ensure tissue perfusion to vital organs.
3. Reduce the possibility of ventricular dysrhythmias in the presence of bradycardia (overdrive suppression).
4. Interrupt a tachydysrhythmia to allow the normal sinus mechanism to pace the heart.

Prerequisite Knowledge and Skills

Before initiating external pacing, the nurse should understand

1. Anatomy and physiology of the cardiovascular system.
2. Principles of cardiac pacing.
3. Principles of electrical safety.

The nurse should be able to perform

1. Basic Cardiac Life Support/Advanced Cardiac Life Support (BCLS/ACLS).
2. Basic dysrhythmia interpretation.
3. Cardiovascular physical assessment.
4. 12-lead ECG (see Skill 7–2).
5. Vital signs assessment.
6. Handwashing techniques (see Skill 35–5).
7. Universal precautions.
8. Electrical safety techniques (see Skill 36–1).

Assessment

1. Assess cardiac rhythm for the presence of bradydysrhythmias (including A-V block), bradydysrhythmias with associated premature ventricular contractions, tachydysrhythmias, or asystole. **Rationale:** May warrant the initiation of transcutaneous pacing.
2. Assess the hemodynamic response to the dysrhythmia, such as blood pressure less than 90 mmHg systolic; altered level of consciousness; complaints of dizziness, shortness of breath, nausea, and vomiting; cool, clammy skin; and the development of ischemic chest pain. **Rationale:** The decision to intervene once specific cardiac dysrhythmias are noted is dependent on the effect of the dysrhythmia on the patient's cardiac output. Assessment of clinical parameters that reflect a decreased cardiac output will allow the health care team to determine whether pacing is indicated.

Nursing Diagnoses

1. Altered tissue perfusion (cardiopulmonary and peripheral) related to decreased cardiac output. **Rationale:** Bradydysrhythmias reduce cardiac output and systemic tissue perfusion because the heart is not beating a sufficient number of times per minute to sustain an adequate blood flow. Tachydysrhythmias reduce cardiac output and systemic tissue perfusion because the heart is beating too rapidly and stroke volume is reduced secondary to decreased ventricular filling.
2. Fear of dying related to verbalization of panic or apprehension or actions such as increased questioning, crying, withdrawal, or inability to concentrate. **Rationale:** The occurrence of potentially life-threatening dysrhythmias creates a state of real threat to personal well-being.
3. Alteration in comfort related to delivery of energy through the chest wall. **Rationale:** Relatively high levels of energy must travel from the external pacing electrodes through the chest wall to stimulate cardiac tissue. Cutaneous nerve endings are also stimulated, thus eliciting a pain response.

Planning

1. Individualize the following goals for external pacing:
   a. Maintain adequate cardiac output. **Rationale:** A sustained reduction in cardiac output will result in decreased systemic tissue perfusion.
   b. Decrease fear of death. **Rationale:** Fear decreases the ability of an individual to cope with situations and activates physiologic responses that may potentiate the dysrhythmias.
   c. Promote comfort. **Rationale:** Pain activates physiologic responses that may potentiate the dysrhythmia. The level of discomfort experienced will directly influence the patient's tolerance of the procedure.
2. Prepare all necessary equipment for external pacing (Fig. 11–2). **Rationale:** Assembly of all the equipment necessary for external pacing will ensure efficient initiation.
   a. Pulse generator and monitor unit.
   b. Pacing cable.
   c. Pacemaker patches.
   d. ECG electrode patches.
   e. ECG monitor and cable.
   f. Soap and water for skin prep (optional in emergency).
3. Prepare the patient as the clinical situation permits. **Rationale:** Preparation of the patient and family will promote compliance with the procedure, reduce anxiety and misconceptions about the care being delivered, and ensure that the patient and family are informed participants.
   a. Explain the purpose of the external pacemaker.
   b. Describe the equipment used for external pacing.
   c. Describe the potential sensations the patient

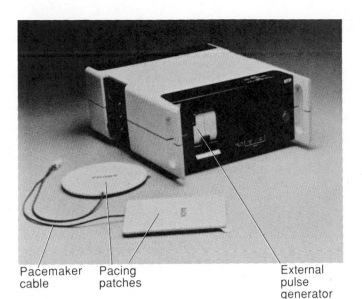

Pacemaker cable   Pacing patches   External pulse generator

FIGURE 11–2. Temporary external pacemaker. (Reprinted with permission from ZOLL Medical Corporation, Woburn, Mass.)

might experience (muscular twitching, discomfort).

d. Explain the procedure.

e. Discuss the possible interventions to alleviate the discomfort (i.e., adequate preparation of skin, proper placement of patches avoiding bony structures or open areas in skin, use of lowest level of energy to achieve consistent capture, repositioning of patches, and use of medication to sedate or diminish level of pain).

Implementation

Steps	Rationale	Special Considerations
1. Wash hands.	Reduces transmission of microorganisms.	
2. Turn on pulse generator/monitor.	Ensures that equipment is functional.	Many devices work on battery or ac (alternating current), power.
3. Apply ECG electrodes in the conventional 3-lead, single channel monitoring system or the 5-lead multichannel system (see Skill 7–1, Figs. 7–13, 7–16).	Check intrinsic rhythm and pacer function.	
4. Connect ECG cable to monitor inlet of pulse generator.	Allows pulse generator to sense the intrinsic rhythm.	
5. Adjust ECG lead and size to maximum R-wave size.	Detection of intrinsic rhythm is necessary for proper demand pacing.	Lead II usually provides most prominent R wave (unnecessary step with asystole) (see Skill 7–1).
6. Obtain prepaced rhythm strip.	Provides documentation of baseline rhythm requiring intervention.	
7. Prepare the skin for pacing electrode placement by washing with soap and water and trimming chest hair with scissors, if appropriate (see Skill 7–1).	Removal of skin oils, lotion, and moisture will improve patch adherence and maximize delivery of pacing energy through the chest wall.	Optional step in an emergency. Skin preparation is an important consideration if high levels of energy are required for capture. Avoid use of flammable liquids to prep skin (alcohol, tincture of benzoin) because of increased potential for burns. Avoid shaving chest hair, since the presence of nicks in the skin under the pacing patches greatly increases patient discomfort.
8. Apply the back (posterior, +) pacing electrode between the spine and left scapula at the level of the heart (Fig. 11–3).	Placement of pacing patches in the recommended anatomic location will enhance the potential for successful pacing.	Avoid placement over bone, because this increases the levels of energy required to pace, causing greater discomfort and the possibility of noncapture.

Table continues on following page

Steps	Rationale	Special Considerations
9. Apply the front (anterior, −) pacing electrode at the left fourth intercostal space, midclavicular line (V₃ or V₄ position depending on the manufacturer) (Fig. 11–4).	Placement of pacing patches in the recommended anatomic location will enhance the potential for successful pacing.	Adjust position of electrode below or lateral to breast tissue to ensure optimal adherence.
10. Connect pacing electrodes to external pulse generator.	Necessary for the delivery of electrical energy.	
11. Set pacemaker settings as prescribed by the physician, including rate, level of energy (output, mA), and mode, if available (demand, nondemand) (Fig. 11–5).	Each patient may require different pacemaker settings to provide safe and effective external pacing.	Nurses may initiate pacing per established protocols. Check specific state practice act and institutional policy, since policies governing this practice may vary. Attempt to use the lowest level of energy necessary to pace consistently if the patient is conscious. Use demand mode if available, nondemand only in the absence of an intrinsic rhythm.
12. Initiate pacing by slowly increasing the rate until capture occurs.	Stimulates myocardial contraction.	
13. Monitor ECG tracing pacer artifact and associated capture (Fig. 11–6).	Ensures adequate functioning of the pacer.	It is possible to see pacer artifact without cardiac stimulation. Increase level of energy (output, mA) to encourage capture. Ensure proper placement of electrodes.
14. Palpate patient's carotid or femoral pulse.	Ensures adequate blood flow with paced beats.	It is possible to have electrical activity without the associated mechanical contraction.
15. Wash hands.	Reduces transmission of microorganisms.	

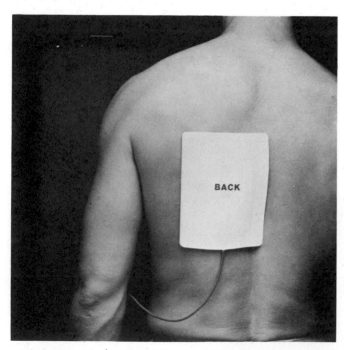

FIGURE 11–3. Location of the posterior (back) pacing electrode. (Reprinted with permission from ZOLL Medical Corporation, Woburn, Mass.)

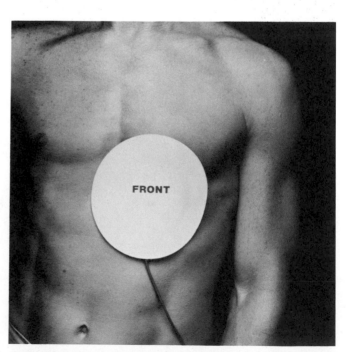

FIGURE 11–4. Location of the anterior (front) pacing electrode. (Reprinted with permission from ZOLL Medical Corporation, Woburn, Mass.)

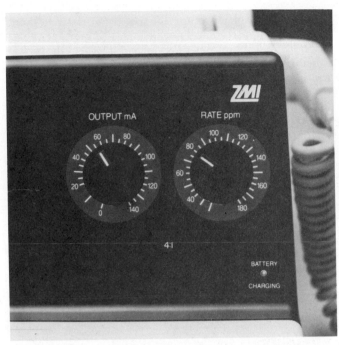

FIGURE 11–5. Pacemaker settings for external pacing. (Reprinted with permission from ZOLL Medical Corporation, Woburn, Mass.)

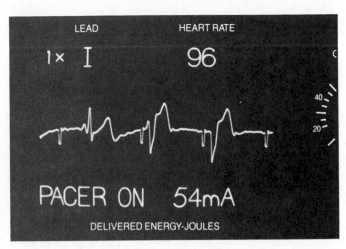

FIGURE 11–6. ECG tracing of external pacing. (Reprinted with permission from ZOLL Medical Corporation, Woburn, Mass.)

Evaluation

1. Monitor vital signs hourly. **Rationale:** Ensures adequate tissue perfusion with paced beats. Adjustments in pacing rate may need to be made based on the vital signs.
2. Evaluate level of comfort. **Rationale:** If the patient is conscious, external delivery of energy through the chest wall may cause varying degrees of discomfort.
3. Administer pain medication/sedation if adjustment in level of energy is not possible. **Rationale:** Increases patient tolerance of the procedure. Assess blood pressure and respiratory status prior to the administration of medication.
4. Obtain ECG strip to document pacing. **Rationale:** Documentation of pacemaker efficacy is necessary for the patient record.
5. Evaluate pacemaker function (capturing and sensing) with any changes in patient condition or at least every 4 hours. **Rationale:** Ensures continued functioning of pacer. Introduction of other variables such as acidosis or electrolyte imbalance may alter the level of energy required to pace effectively.
6. Monitor vital signs for resolution of the hemodynamically significant dysrhythmia that warranted treatment. For bradydysrhythmias, this may require turning the external pacemaker off if the intrinsic rate is less than the pacing rate. **Rationale:** Indicates whether external pacing has been an effective method of treatment.
7. Evaluate the hemodynamic response to pacing, and compare with baseline. **Rationale:** Evaluates the patient's physiologic response to pacing and ensures that it is consistent with the level of functioning prior to the change that warranted intervention.

Expected Outcomes

1. Adequate systemic tissue perfusion and cardiac output as evidenced by blood pressure greater than 90 mmHg systolic, alert and oriented patient, absence of dizziness, absence of shortness of breath, absence of nausea and vomiting due to hypotension, and absence of ischemic chest pain. **Rationale:** Prevents dysfunction of key organ systems within the body.
2. Stable cardiac rhythm. **Rationale:** Promotes an adequate cardiac output.

Unexpected Outcomes

1. Failure of the pacemaker to sense patient's underlying rhythm with the possibility of R-on-T phenomenon (initiation of ventricular tachydysrhythmias as a result of an improperly timed pacer spike on the T wave). **Rationale:** Inability of the pacemaker to detect the patient's underlying rhythm may cause inadvertent electrical competition and may potentiate life-threatening ventricular dysrhythmias.
2. Failure of the pacemaker to capture the myocardium. **Rationale:** Inability of the pacemaker to actually stimulate the heart to contract will prevent the pacemaker from supplementing or interrupting the dysrhythmia, allowing the clinical condition to persist.
3. Failure of the pacemaker to pace. **Rationale:** Inability of the pacemaker to deliver an electric stimulus will prevent the pacemaker from supplementing or interrupting the dysrhythmia, allowing the clinical condition to persist.
4. Discomfort, including skin irritation or burns from the delivery of high levels of energy through the chest wall. **Rationale:** If the patient is conscious, delivery of high levels of energy through the chest wall may make the procedure intolerable.

Documentation

Documentation in the patient record should include the date and time of initiation and completion of the procedure; a description of events warranting intervention; pre- and postpacing vital signs and physical assessment; a sample of prepacing and postpacing ECG strips; a description of patient tolerance of the procedure; any medications administered, rationale for administration, and response; current pacemaker settings; and patient education provided and evaluation of the patient's and family's level of understanding. **Rationale:** Documentation of the clinical events leading to initiation of pacing and a description of the procedure and the outcome serve as a legal document to identify care rendered.

Patient/Family Education

1. Assess learning needs, readiness to learn, and factors that will influence learning. **Rationale:** Individualizes teaching in a manner that will be meaningful to the patient and family.
2. Discuss basic facts about the normal conduction

system, such as structure of the conduction system, source of heart beat, normal and abnormal heart rhythms, and symptoms of abnormal heart rhythms. **Rationale:** Understanding of the normal conduction system will assist the patient and family in recognizing the seriousness of the patient's condition and the need for external pacing.

3. Discuss basic facts about the external pacemaker, such as reason for pacemaker, explanation of the equipment, what to expect during the procedure, what to expect after the procedure, and adjuncts to pacing (medications). **Rationale:** Understanding of pacemaker functioning and expectations of the procedure will assist the patient and family in developing a realistic perception of the procedure and how it will help the patient.

4. Evaluate patient's need for permanent pacing support. **Rationale:** If permanent pacing is required, the patient and family will need further instruction regarding possible lifestyle modifications, follow-up visits, and specifics about the pacemaker to be implanted.

Performance Checklist
Skill 11–1:   Emergency Application of Temporary External Chest Pacing

Critical Behaviors	Complies yes	no
1. Wash hands.		
2. Turn on external pulse generator/monitor.		
3. Apply ECG electrodes in conventional 3- or 5-lead configuration.		
4. Connect ECG cable to monitor.		
5. Adjust ECG size to maximize R wave.		
6. Obtain prepared rhythm strip.		
7. Prepare skin for pacing patch placement.		
8. Apply posterior pacing electrode.		
9. Apply anterior pacing electrode.		
10. Connect pacing electrodes to external pulse generator.		
11. Set pacemaker settings.		
12. Initiate pacing.		
13. Monitor ECG tracing for pacer functioning.		
14. Palpate patient's pulse.		
15. Wash hands.		
16. Document procedure in nurse's notes.		

SKILL 11–2

Initiating Temporary Pacing

The insertion of a temporary transvenous pacemaker is performed in both emergency and elective clinical situations. The therapeutic goal of temporary cardiac pac-

ing is to ensure an adequate heart rate. The clinical indications for insertion of a temporary transvenous pacing electrode include symptomatic bradycardia, asystole, overdrive suppression/termination of ventricular tachydysrhythmias, second- or third-degree A-V block, and prophylaxis during cardiac surgery. Temporary cardiac pacing also may play a role as a diagnostic modality in evaluating cardiac electrophysiologic function.

In temporary transvenous pacing, the pulse generator is externally attached to a pacing lead that is inserted through a vein into the right atrium or ventricle. In emergency situations requiring temporary cardiac pacing, the goal is to establish an adequate heart rate as quickly as possible. In this situation, single-chamber ventricular pacing is generally the most appropriate. Insertion of the pacing lead can be done at the patient's bedside or under fluoroscopy. The pacing lead is an insulated wire with one or two electrodes at the tip of the wire. It can be a hard-tipped or balloon-tipped pacing catheter that is placed in direct contact with the endocardium. Most temporary leads are bipolar, with the distal tip electrode separated from the proximal ring electrode by 1 to 2 cm (Figs. 11–7 and 11–8).

The lead may be inserted into the heart via an antecubital, femoral, jugular, or subclavian approach. The risks and benefits of each insertion site must be considered in the context of the clinical situation. In an emergency situation in which there is significant hemodynamic compromise, the subclavian vein may be the best insertion site because of the relative constancy of this anatomic site from person to person, the relative ease of insertion, and lead stability at this insertion site. The jugular vein is also a preferred site in an emergency for similar reasons, with a decreased risk of pneumothorax.

During insertion of a temporary transvenous pacemaker, it is essential that emergency equipment be readily available. The introduction of a pacing lead into the cardiac chambers predisposes the patient to the development of potentially lethal dysrhythmias as well as other serious complications, such as pneumothorax, myocardial perforation, or cardiac tamponade. Because of its ease and ability for quick insertion, a balloon-tipped flotation pacing lead is often used in emergencies. If longer-term pacing is anticipated, a stiffer lead may be selected because the flotation lead tends to soften when exposed to body temperature and is displaced from its

original position. The risk of complications is related to the stiffness of the lead, the skill of the physician, and the clinical circumstances under which the lead is being placed.

In temporary A-V sequential pacing, the pulse generator is attached to two electrode catheters that are positioned in the right atrium and right ventricle. The electrodes may be positioned in the endocardium, or they may be positioned on the epicardium, during cardiothoracic surgical procedures. If the electrodes are placed in the endocardium, the procedure for insertion is similar to that of temporary transvenous ventricular pacemaker insertion.

The presence of atrial and ventricular pacing electrodes allows for a variety of pacing modalities, including asynchronous atrial or ventricular pacing, demand atrial or ventricular pacing, asynchronous A-V sequential pacing, and demand A-V sequential pacing (Fig. 11–9). The A-V sequential mode of pacing paces the atria and ventricles in sequence, allowing for atrial contribution to ventricular filling. This mode of pacing generally provides a greater stroke volume and subsequent cardiac output, which allows for adequate heart rate without a compromise in hemodynamic status.

The use of a thermodilution pulmonary artery (PA) catheter for temporary atrial and/or ventricular pacing can be done with catheters specifically designed for temporary pacing. Several companies manufacture pulmonary artery catheters with ventricular pacing and A-V sequential pacing capabilities. Older products were made with the pacing electrodes as a part of the catheter itself, whereas newer models consist of a standard PA catheter with additional ports through which pacing electrodes can be inserted into the right atrium and/or the right ventricle (Figs. 11–10 and 11–11).

Indications for temporary cardiac pacing with a PA catheter include bradydysrhythmias, tachydysrhythmias, A-V blocks, and decreased cardiac output. Use of a PA catheter combines the capabilities of PA pressure monitoring, thermodilution cardiac output measurement,

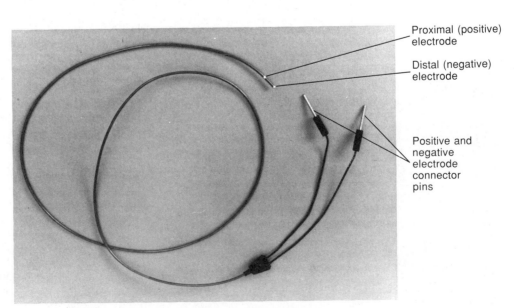

FIGURE 11–7. Bipolar lead wire.

Proximal (positive) electrode

Distal (negative) electrode

Positive and negative electrode connector pins

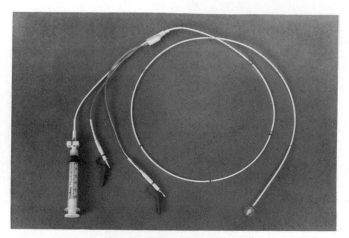

FIGURE 11–8. Balloon-tipped bipolar lead wire.

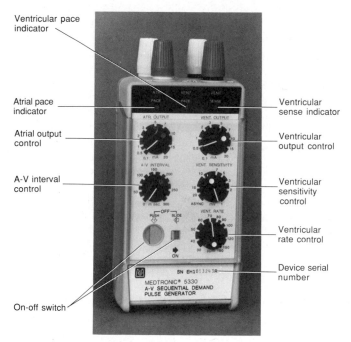

Ventricular pace indicator

Atrial pace indicator

Atrial output control

A-V interval control

On-off switch

Ventricular sense indicator

Ventricular output control

Ventricular sensitivity control

Ventricular rate control

Device serial number

MEDTRONIC® 5330
A-V SEQUENTIAL DEMAND
PULSE GENERATOR

SN EH1013243R

FIGURE 11–9. Demand A-V sequential pulse generator.

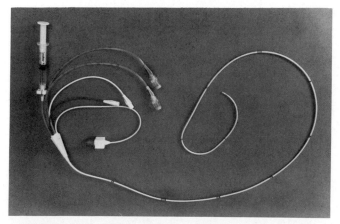

FIGURE 11–10. Pulmonary artery catheter with atrial and ventricular pacing lumens.

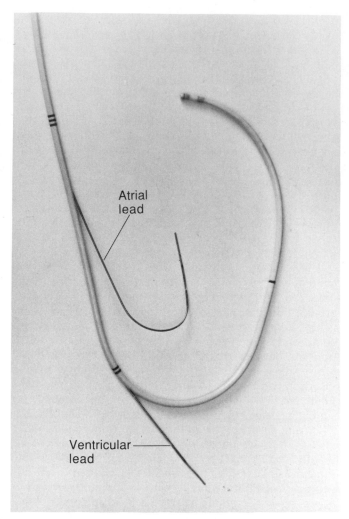

Atrial lead

Ventricular lead

FIGURE 11–11. Pulmonary artery catheter with atrial and ventricular leads in place.

fluid infusion, and mixed venous oxygen sampling. The simultaneous measurement of pulmonary artery wedge pressure (PAWP) and pacing, however, is sometimes not possible. While such catheters are designed to perform both pacing and the measurement of PAWP, in some patients, the measurement of PAWP causes pacing to become intermittent because of repositioning of the pacing electrode with catheter movement during balloon inflation.

Temporary epicardial pacing is a method of stimulating the myocardium through the use of Teflon-coated stainless steel wires that are attached to the epicardium during open heart surgery. These wires may be attached to the right atrium for atrial pacing, the right ventricle for ventricular pacing, or both for A-V sequential pacing. Once implanted on the epicardial surface, the wire is brought through the chest wall before the chest is closed. Typically, the atrial wires are located to the right of the sternum, whereas the ventricular wires exit to the left of the sternum (Figs. 11–12 and 11–13). An external temporary pulse generator is then connected to the epicardial pacing wires to provide the power source and the controls to initiate pacing.

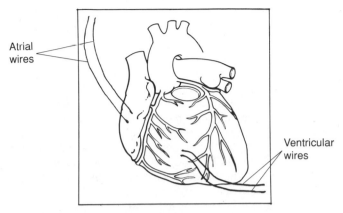

FIGURE 11–12. Location of atrial and ventricular epicardial wires. (Reprinted with permission from L. S. Baas and C. L. Schneider, Temporary epicardial electrodes. *Dimens. Crit. Care Nurs.* 5(2):81, 1986.)

Epicardial pacing wires are indicated in the postoperative cardiac surgical patient to provide supplemental bradycardia pacing, to improve hemodynamic status, and to suppress ventricular ectopy. This patient population is prone to dysrhythmias because of a variety of conditions that can occur prior to or during the operative experience, some of which are listed in Table 11–1.

Epicardial pacing most commonly occurs within the first 48 hours after surgery and can be accomplished using either a unipolar or bipolar configuration. To pace the heart, only one electrode needs to directly communicate with myocardial tissue. The other electrode can be attached to the heart or to the skin to complete the electric circuit required for current flow. The negative electrode delivers the energy to the heart, and the positive electrode returns the energy to the pulse generator.

A *unipolar* pacing system is one in which there is only one electrode (the negative electrode) in contact with the chamber being paced. The positive, or indifferent, electrode is commonly sewn to the subcutaneous tissue of the chest wall. A *bipolar* pacing system is one in which both the negative and positive electrodes directly communicate with the myocardial tissue in the chamber being paced. Bipolar pacing is the preferred method because it provides reliable delivery of energy and can be con-

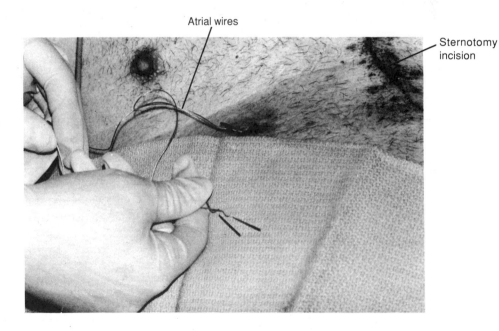

FIGURE 11–13. Atrial epicardial wires exiting the chest wall to the right of the sternotomy incision. (Reprinted with permission from L. S. Baas and C. L. Schneider, Temporary epicardial electrodes. *Dimens. Crit. Care Nurs.* 5(2):81, 1986.)

TABLE 11–1 CONDITIONS THAT PROMOTE POSTOPERATIVE DYSRHYTHMIAS

Effects of anesthetics and medications
Ischemia of myocardial tissue
Injury to myocardial tissue
Hypothermia
Electrolyte imbalances
Hypoxia
Reduced oxygen-carrying capacity
Transient myocardial depression
Preoperative myocardial dysfunction
Prior history of dysrhythmias

verted to a unipolar system should failure of one electrode occur. Therefore, it is most common for two atrial and two ventricular epicardial pacing wires to be placed during surgery to allow for bipolar pacing.

The temporary pulse generator houses the controls and energy source for epicardial pacing (Fig. 11–14). There are pulse generators that can be used for single-chamber pacing or with dual-chamber pacing. With single-chamber pacing, there is one set of terminals at the top of the pulse generator into which the pacing wires are inserted. A dual-chamber pacemaker requires two sets of terminals for the atrial and ventricular wires. Pacing rate is determined by the rate dial. For dual-chamber pacing, a singular rate dial controls both the atrial and ventricular pacing rate. The amount of time between atrial and ventricular stimulation is controlled by the A-V interval dial on a dual-chamber pulse generator. The energy delivered to the myocardium is determined by setting the output dial on the pulse generator. With dual-chamber pacing, separate selections are required for each chamber, necessitating two output dials. The ability of the pacemaker to detect the patient's intrinsic rhythm is determined by the sensitivity dial. When the dial is turned to the asynchronous setting, the pacemaker is not able to sense any of the patient's own cardiac activity and will function as a fixed-rate pacemaker. When the dial is turned to the lowest setting (fully clockwise), the pacemaker is able to sense the patient's intrinsic activity.

One limitation of the temporary pulse generator is its inability to adequately sense intrinsic atrial activity. Therefore, when the atria are being paced alone, they are paced in the asynchronous mode (Fig. 11–15). When the ventricles are paced alone, the operator has the option of pacing in the asynchronous or demand (VVI) mode. Because of the risk of R-on-T phenomenon with ventricular asynchronous pacing, this mode is not recommended if the patient has any underlying rhythm. When A-V sequential pacing occurs, the pacemaker functions in the DVI mode (dual chamber pacing, ventricular sensing, inhibition of atrial and ventricular pacing with sensed ventricular events).

As with any method of pacing, the ability of the pacemaker to stimulate the myocardium to contract is dependent on a number of variables: the position of the electrode and degree of contact with viable myocardial tissue; the level of energy delivered through the pacing wire; the presence of hypoxia, acidosis, or electrolyte imbalances; and concomitant drug therapy. An understanding of pacing principles and an awareness of the total patient condition are necessary to ensure that epicardial pacing is successful when needed.

Purpose

The nurse assists in initiating cardiac pacing to

1. Stimulate the myocardium to contract in the absence of an intrinsic rhythm.
2. Establish an adequate cardiac output and blood pressure to ensure blood flow and tissue perfusion to vital organs.
3. Reduce the possibility of ventricular dysrhythmias in the setting of bradycardia.
4. Interrupt a tachydysrhythmia to allow the normal sinus mechanism to pace the heart.

Prerequisite Knowledge and Skills

Before initiating temporary pacing, the nurse should understand

1. Anatomy and physiology of the cardiovascular system.
2. Principles of cardiac pacing.
3. Principles of hemodynamic monitoring.
4. Principles of electrical safety.
5. Principles of asepsis.
6. Principles of universal precautions.

The nurse should be able to perform

1. Basic Cardiac Life Support/Advanced Cardiac Life Support (BCLS/ACLS).

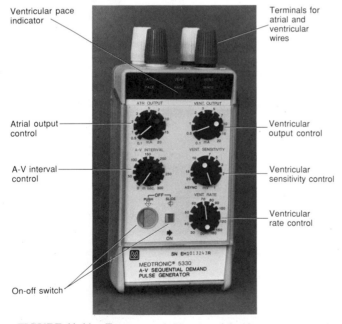

FIGURE 11–14. Temporary A-V sequential pulse generator with two sets of terminals.

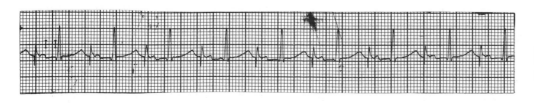

FIGURE 11–15. ECG tracing showing asynchronous atrial pacing via temporary A-V sequential pulse generator.

2. Basic dysrhythmia interpretation.
3. Cardiovascular physical assessment.
4. 12-lead ECG (see Skill 7–2).
5. Vital signs assessment.
6. Hemodynamic monitoring (see Chapter 10).
7. Sterile technique.
8. Battery insertion and check of pulse generator.
9. Universal precautions (see Skill 35–1).
10. Handwashing techniques (see Skill 35–5).
11. Electrial safety techniques (see Skill 36–1).

Assessment

1. Assess cardiac rhythm for the presence of brady-dysrhythmias, A-V block, tachydysrhythmias, or asystole. **Rationale:** Baseline assessment of cardiac rhythm is necessary to evaluate the patient's response to the temporary pacing and to identify changes in rhythm during and after the procedure.

2. Assess the hemodynamic response to the dysrhythmia. Rhythm disturbances such as bradycardia, asystole, A-V block, or tachydysrhythmias may significantly reduce the amount of blood ejected from the heart and circulated to vital organs. **Rationale:** Baseline assessment of the hemodynamic status is necessary to evaluate the patient's response to temporary pacing.

3. Assess the immediate environment for electrical safety (see Skill 36–1). **Rationale:** Because the pacing electrode is in direct contact with the heart, special care must be taken to avoid conducting stray electric current from surrounding equipment through the pacing electrode to the myocardium.

Nursing Diagnoses

1. Potential for infection related to insertion of the pacing electrode through the skin's surface. **Rationale:** Localized infection at the site of electrode insertion, systemic infection, or endocarditis may occur as a result of the invasive procedure.

2. Anxiety related to potentially life-threatening dysrhythmia, fear of death, fear of pain experienced during the procedure, or other real or potential threats to self. **Rationale:** Acute illness and potentially painful or harmful procedures may precipitate a state of anxiety.

3. Potential for injury related to microshock, as evidenced by the precipitation of a lethal dysrhythmia (see Skill 36–1). **Rationale:** The pacing electrode is in direct contact with the myocardium and may conduct stray electric current from surrounding equipment.

Planning

1. Individualize the following goals for temporary transvenous pacing:

a. Increase cardiac output. **Rationale:** To improve tissue perfusion to vital organs.
b. Prevent infection. **Rationale:** Invasive nature of temporary pacemaker disrupts the natural skin barrier and predisposes patient to infection.
c. Prevent microshock. **Rationale:** The pacing electrode will be in direct contact with the myocardium and may conduct stray electric current to the myocardium, potentially causing lethal dysrhythmias.
d. Decrease anxiety. **Rationale:** Patient may experience anxiety related to experiencing life-threatening dysrhythmia, fear of death, fear of pain, or other real or imagined threats to self.
e. Achieve A-V synchrony. **Rationale:** A primary goal of A-V sequential pacing is to stimulate the atria to contract and empty blood into the ventricle during ventricular diastolic filling. This increases stroke volume and maximizes cardiac output.

2. Prepare all necessary equipment for insertion of pacing electrode. **Rationale:** Assembly of all the equipment and supplies at the bedside ensures that the procedure will be completed quickly and efficiently.
a. Antiseptic skin preparation solution (povidone-iodine).
b. Local anesthetic.
c. Sterile drapes, towels, masks, gowns, gloves, and dressings.
d. Pacing lead.
e. Pulse generator.
f. Nine-volt battery for pulse generator.
g. Connecting cable (Fig. 11–16).
h. Percutaneous introducer or 14-gauge needle.
i. Alligator clips (Fig. 11–17).
j. Sutures (3-0 silk or surgeon's preference).
k. ECG monitor and recorder.
l. Emergency pharmacologic agents (as per current ACLS protocol).
m. Exam gloves.
n. Supplies for dressing at insertion site.

3. Prepare the patient.
a. Explain the need for temporary pacing and describe the procedure. **Rationale:** Explanations may help to alleviate anxiety.
b. Validate informed consent signed. **Rationale:** Temporary pacing is an invasive technique.
c. Administer pain medication or sedation as prescribed. **Rationale:** May be indicated depending on patient's level of anxiety and pain.
d. Explain precautions and restrictions necessary, such as limitation of mobility and electrical safety. **Rationale:** Excessive mobility may contribute to electrode dislodgment. Use of personal electrical equipment such as shavers or radios and unprotected handling of pacemaker equipment may predispose to microshock hazard.

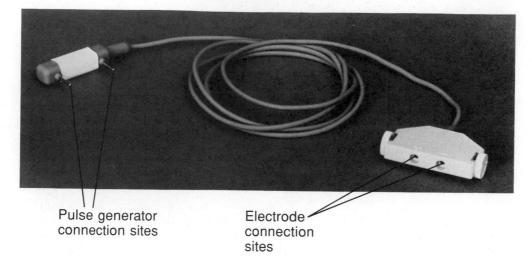

Pulse generator connection sites

Electrode connection sites

FIGURE 11–16. Connecting cable.

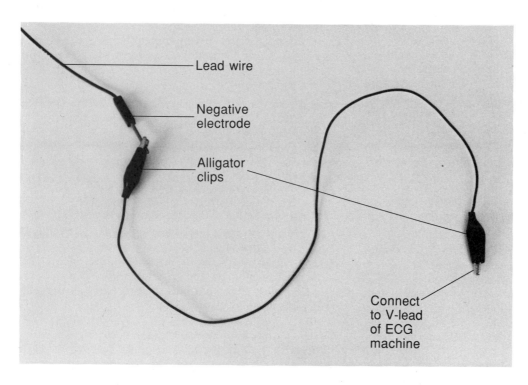

Lead wire

Negative electrode

Alligator clips

Connect to V-lead of ECG machine

FIGURE 11–17. Alligator clips.

Implementation

Steps	Rationale	Special Considerations
1. Wash hands.	Reduces transmission of microorganisms.	
2. Connect patient to ECG machine and monitor ECG continuously.	Monitor intrinsic rhythm as well as rhythm during and after the procedure to evaluate for adequate rate and pacemaker function.	

Table continues on following page

Steps	Rationale	Special Considerations
3. Test battery function in pulse generator.	Equipment should be operational because the patient's condition may deteriorate, necessitating immediate intervention. Failure of the indicators to flash indicates that battery voltage is low, and the battery should be replaced.	A new battery or one that has been checked to ensure function should be inserted in the pulse generator. The pulse generator may have a battery test button that provides for a battery voltage check. As an example, in one model with the test button depressed, both sense and pace indicators flash simultaneously to indicate that the battery voltage is sufficient for use. Failure of the indicators to flash indicates that battery voltage is low, and the battery should be replaced. The switch must be in the on position during a battery check. Check manufacturer's recommendations for specific instructions.
4. If necessary, replace battery. A 9-volt alkaline battery is commonly used. Check specific manufacturer's manual of pulse generator model (Figs. 11–18 through 11–21).	Battery life is dependent on a variety of factors, including type, pacemaker settings, and length of use.	At typical rate and output settings of 70 beats per minute and 10 mA, projected battery life is approximately 500 hours. It is recommended that the battery be replaced each time the pulse generator is used for a different patient. Except for emergency situations, changing the battery while pacing a patient is not recommended.

Table continues on following page

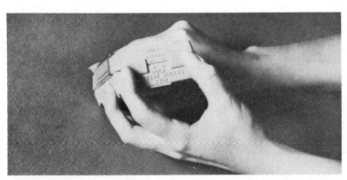

FIGURE 11–18. Battery change: Disengage battery cartridge by moving latch buttons inward as indicated. (From *Pulse Generator 5375 Technical Manual*, Minneapolis, Minn., Medronic, Inc., 1988, p. 30. Reprinted with permission.)

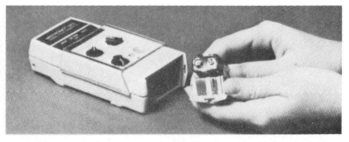

FIGURE 11–20. Battery change: Remove battery from cartridge and replace. Observe voltage polarity markings on battery and cartridge. (From *Pulse Generator 5375 Technical Manual*, Minneapolis, Minn., Medronic, Inc., 1988, p. 30. Reprinted with permission.)

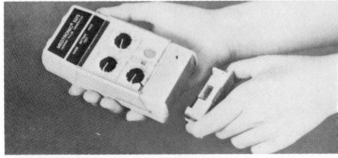

FIGURE 11–19. Battery change: Remove battery cartridge from pulse generator. (From *Pulse Generator 5375 Technical Manual*, Minneapolis, Minn., Medronic, Inc., 1988, p. 30. Reprinted with permission.)

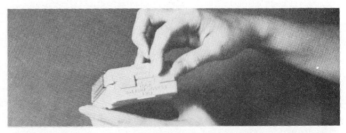

FIGURE 11–21. Reinstall battery cartridge in pulse generator. Engage cartridge by moving latch buttons outward as indicated. (From *Pulse Generator 5375 Technical Manual*, Minneapolis, Minn., Medronic, Inc., 1988, p. 30. Reprinted with permission.)

Steps	Rationale	Special Considerations
For Epicardial Pacing		
1. Don exam gloves.	Exam gloves should be worn whenever handling the epicardial wires to prevent conduction of stray electric current to the patient.	
2. Expose the epicardial pacing wires, and identify the chamber of origin (see Fig. 11–13).	It is important to determine which wires are originating from the atrium and which from the right ventricle to ensure that the appropriate chamber is paced.	
3. Identify the method of pacing desired.	A variety of pacing modes may be achieved using epicardial wires (atrial asynchronous, ventricular asynchronous, ventricular demand, A-V sequential demand). Use of unipolar configuration versus bipolar configuration needs to be established.	
4. Connect the pericardial wires to the terminals on the pulse generator.	The wires must be connected to a power source to be able to pace the heart.	The wire connected to the negative terminal determines where the energy will be delivered. The wire connected to the positive terminal determines how the energy will return to the pulse generator. With A-V sequential pacing, be sure to place both atrial wires in the terminals labeled "atrium" and both ventricular wires in the terminals labeled "ventricle." With single-chamber pacing, be sure that either the atrial wires or the ventricular wires are placed into the terminals. With bipolar pacing, either wire can be the negative electrode. With unipolar pacing, the epicardial wire must be the negative electrode and the skin wire must be the positive electrode.
5. Set the pacemaker rate, level of energy, output (mA), and sensitivity ("demand" or "asynchronous") as prescribed and initiate pacing.	Determination of pacemaker settings is based on patient response and the threshold of capture measured after the epicardial wires are connected.	Atrial pacing is always asynchronous because of the inability of the temporary pulse generator to consistently sense intrinsic atrial activity. For ventricular pacing, the demand mode is most frequently used to avoid competing with the patient's intrinsic rate and to avoid stimulating the heart during the vulnerable phase of repolarization (latter half of T wave). The output is set to ensure consistent capture of the myocardium. For A-V sequential pacing, separate output settings are necessary to ensure capture of the atrium and ventricle. There is only one sensitivity dial in the standard A-V sequential pacemaker for detection of intrinsic ventricular activity (DVI).
6. Monitor ECG tracing for signs of pacer artifact and associated capture.	Validates adequate functioning of the pacer.	It is possible to see pacer artifact without cardiac stimulation. Increase level of energy (output mA) to encourage capture. Ensure proper settings and connections with epicardial wires.

Table continues on following page

Steps	Rationale	Special Considerations
For Temporary Transvenous/A-V Sequential Pacing		
1. Prepare insertion site by clipping hair close to the skin in the area surrounding the insertion site.	Essential to prevent infection.	Shaving of hair should be avoided because nicks in the skin may predispose patient to infection.
2. Mask, gown, cap, and glove all persons performing and assisting with the procedure.	Prevents infection and maintains universal precautions.	
3. Cleanse site with antiseptic solution, such as a povidone-iodine based solution.	Prevents infection.	
4. Provide local anesthetic to anesthetize the insertion site.	A large gauge introducer is used, which may cause discomfort during the insertion procedure.	
5. Assist with the insertion procedure as requested by the physician.		
a. A percutaneous puncture through a vein is performed at the jugular, subclavian, antecubital, or femoral site.	Allows for direct placement of introducer.	Selection of an appropriate site should consider patient mobility and comfort, potential for infection, ease of insertion, risk of pneumothorax, and other risks and benefits associated with specific sites.
b. A pacing electrode is passed through the introducer.	Introducer provides an avenue for ease of insertion.	
c. The pacing electrode is positioned in the right ventricle. This is done either under fluoroscopy or with the use of an ECG machine. If a balloon-tipped pacing lead is being utilized, balloon inflation occurs when the tip of the pacing lead is in the vena cava. The air-filled balloon allows the blood flow to carry the catheter tip into the desired position in the right ventricle.	Ideally, fluoroscopy is utilized to visualize placement of the electrode to reduce manipulation of the catheter within the cardiac chambers.	If fluoroscopy is utilized, all personnel must be shielded from the radiation with lead aprons or be positioned behind lead shields. If an ECG machine is used, the patient must be connected to the limb leads. The distal electrode is then attached to the chest lead of the electrocardiograph with an alligator clip or a specially made connector that is available with some insertion kits. The ECG machine is then set to continuously record the "V" lead. The ECG is then derived directly from the pacing electrode, and the position of the catheter tip is verified by the unipolar intracavitary electrogram (Figs. 11–22 through 11–25).
6. After the pacing electrode is properly positioned in the right ventricle, attach the electrodes to the pulse generator. Connect the proximal and distal electrodes to the respective positive and negative connectors of the pulse generator (Fig. 11–26).	The electrode must be connected securely to the pacemaker to ensure appropriate sensing and capture as well as to prevent inadvertent disconnection.	Not all lead wires have "positive" and "negative" marked on them. The distal electrode is always negative and the proximal electrode is always positive. A connecting cable may be used between the electrode and the pacemaker to provide added length for increased mobility or convenience.

Table continues on page 385

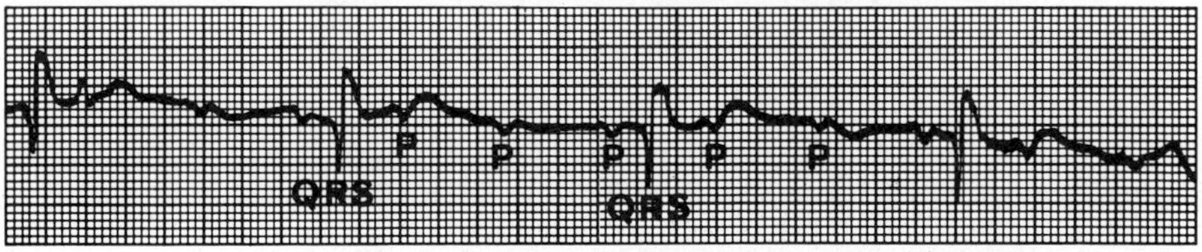

FIGURE 11–22. ECG rhythm in the vena cava: Small inverted P waves when pacing electrode is in vena cava. (Reprinted with permission from L. E. Meltzer, R. Pinneo, and J. R. Kitchell, *Intensive Coronary Care*, 4th Ed. Bowie, Md.: Robert J. Brady Co., 1983, p. 233.

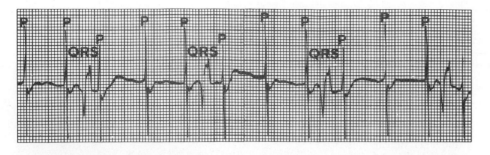

FIGURE 11-23. ECG rhythm recorded in the right atrium: Tall biphasic P waves when pacing electrode is in right atrium. (Reprinted with permission from L. E. Meltzer, R. Pinneo, and J. R. Kitchell, *Intensive Coronary Care*, 4th Ed. Bowie, Md.: Robert J. Brady Co., 1983, p. 233.

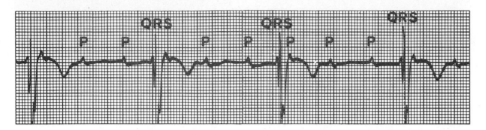

FIGURE 11-24. ECG rhythm recorded in the right ventricle: Large QRS complexes and progressively smaller P waves when pacing electrode is in right ventricle. (Reprinted with permission from L. E. Meltzer, R. Pinneo, and J. R. Kitchell, *Intensive Coronary Care*, 4th Ed. Bowie, Md.: Robert J. Brady Co., 1983, p. 233.

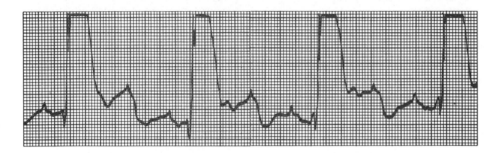

FIGURE 11-25. ECG rhythm recorded in the right ventricle: Elevated ST segments when pacing electrode is wedged against the endocardial wall of the right ventricle. (Reprinted with permission from L. E. Meltzer, R. Pinneo, and J. R. Kitchell, *Intensive Coronary Care*, 4th Ed. Bowie, Md.: Robert J. Brady Co., 1983, p. 233.

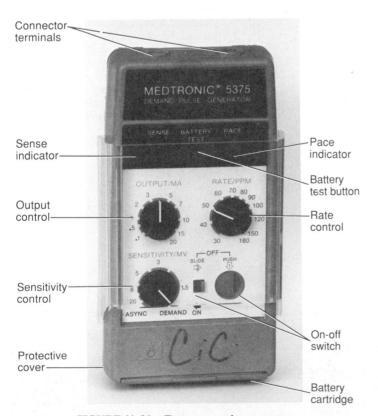

FIGURE 11-26. Temporary pulse generator.

Steps	Rationale	Special Considerations
For A-V Sequential Pacing		
1. Connect atrial electrode to atrial output terminals, connecting positive and negative electrode terminals to respective positive and negative output terminals.	Secure connections are essential for proper conduction of pacemaker energy.	
2. Connect ventricular electrode to ventricular output terminals, connecting positive and negative electrode terminals to respective positive and negative output terminals.	Secure connections are essential for proper sensing and conduction of pacemaker energy.	The method for securing connections varies with different models. Screw-type connectors and clip-type connectors are the most common.
Pacing with a Pulmonary Artery Catheter		
1. Assist physician with insertion of PA catheter, and perform hemodynamic monitoring as per Skills 10–5 and 10–6. Pacing electrodes may be inserted at the time of PA catheter insertion, or they may be inserted at a later time when temporary pacing is required because of change in rhythm status.		
2. If the pacing electrode probe is not already inserted, obtain the appropriate electrode for insertion.	Only probes specifically manufactured for use with the PA catheter should be used. Check manufacturer's recommendations. Never attempt to interchange probes from one manufacturer to the other, since all catheters differ in design and probe specifications. Continuous monitoring of the right ventricular pressure waveform via the pacing lumen is recommended prior to electrode insertion to ensure correct placement of the right ventricular port 1 to 2 cm distal to the tricuspid valve.	
3. Assist physician with insertion of the pacing probe(s).	Close monitoring of the ECG during insertion of the probes is necessary to detect lethal dysrhythmias as well as proper electrode placement.	Follow specific manufacturer's instructions regarding electrode insertion and securing electrodes in place within the catheter lumen. Catheters vary in the types of adapters, protective sterile sheaths, etc. that are used at the insertion site. Electrodes may be positioned under fluoroscopy or with the use of an ECG machine. Depending on physician preference, the electrodes may be attached to the V lead of the ECG machine for recording of an intracardiac ECG for electrode positioning, or ECG monitoring for appropriate capture to determine positioning is utilized.

Table continues on following page

Steps	Rationale	Special Considerations
4. After the electrode(s) are properly positioned in the right atrium and/or ventricle, attach the electrode(s) to the pulse generator. Connect the positive and negative electrodes to the respective positive and negative output terminals of the pulse generator.	The electrode must be securely connected to the pulse generator to ensure appropriate sensing and capture as well as to prevent inadvertent disconnection.	A connecting cable may be used between the electrode and the pacemaker to provide added length for increased mobility or convenience.
For all Methods of Temporary Pacing		
1. Determine stimulation threshold:		
a. Set pacing rate above patient's intrinsic rate.	The output dial regulates the amount of electric current (milliamperes, or mA) that is delivered to the myocardium to initiate depolarization. Ventricular pacing (stimulation threshold) should be established at less than 1 mA current output whenever possible. The maintenance threshold is set at 1.5 to 2 times above the stimulation threshold to allow for increases in the stimulation threshold without the loss of ventricular capture.	Nurses are generally permitted to test the stimulation threshold, but individual institutional policies governing this procedure may vary. Threshold may increase or decrease within hours of electrode placement as a result of fibrosis around the tip of the electrode, medication administration, underlying pathology (including electrolyte imbalance), or alteration of electrode position. There will be separate output controls for both the atrium and the ventricle when an A-V sequential pulse generator is used. The threshold for each must be determined.
b. Gradually decrease output (mA) from 20 mA until capture is lost.		
c. Gradually increase output (mA) until 1:1 capture is established. This is the stimulation threshold.		
d. Set output (mA) at least 1.5 to 2 times higher than the stimulation threshold. This output setting is sometimes referred to as the *maintenance threshold*.		
2. Determine sensitivity threshold:		
a. Set rate at least 10 beats per minute below patient's intrinsic heart rate.	*Sensitivity threshold* is the level at which intrinsic ventricular activity is recognized by the sensing electrodes. For demand pacing, the sensitivity must be measured and set.	Some physicians prefer to set sensitivity settings all the way to the demand mode or all the way to the asynchronous mode regardless of the sensitivity threshold. The demand mode is most frequently used to avoid competing with the patient's intrinsic rate and to avoid stimulating the heart during the repolarization phase (the vulnerable phase or the ST segment on the ECG). The initial rate is set above the patient's intrinsic rate to determine threshold measurements and to ensure proper pacemaker function. The rate may then be set below the patient's intrinsic rate if the patient's own rate is adequate. Nurses are generally allowed to test the sensitivity threshold. Institutional policies governing this procedure may vary. When determining the sensitivity threshold, there is the possibility of the pacemaker stimulus occurring during the T wave (R-on-T phenomenon). The output may be turned down during this procedure, to avoid inducing potentially lethal dysrhythmias.
b. Set sensitivity control to most sensitive setting (fully demand or lowest numerical setting). Sense indicator light should flash with each intrinsic R wave.		

Table continues on following page

Steps	Rationale	Special Considerations
3. Set the pacemaker rate, output (mA), and sensitivity (demand or asynchronous), as prescribed or as determined by threshold testing.	Determination of pacemaker settings is based on the patient's response and the threshold of capture and sensitivity measured after electrode insertion. A-V interval (similar to an intrinsic PR interval) should be set for optimal ventricular filling, usually between 150 to 250 ms.	
4. Assess rhythm for appropriate pacemaker function: a. Capture: Is there a QRS complex for every ventricular pacing artifact? b. Rate: Is the rate at or above the pacemaker rate if in the demand mode? c. Sensing: Does the sensitivity light indicate that every QRS complex is sensed?	ECG tracing should reflect appropriate response to pacemaker settings if pacemaker is functioning properly.	
5. After settings are adjusted for optimal patient response, place protective plastic cover over pacemaker controls.	Pacemaker settings may be inadvertently altered by patient movement or handling if controls are not covered.	If a plastic cover is missing, tape may be used to cover controls. Although not ideal, this method may serve to avoid inadvertent alteration of control settings.
6. Check institutional policy or obtain specific physician orders regarding the purposeful wedging of the PA catheter to obtain pulmonary artery wedge pressure (PAWP) readings during pacing.	When pacing with a PA catheter, many physicians prefer not to wedge the catheter to obtain pulmonary capillary wedge pressure measurements. Intermittent capture has been noted during the wedging procedure as a result of movement of the electrode with catheter migration into the PAWP position.	
7. Assess patient response to pacing including blood pressure, level of consciousness, heart rhythm, and other hemodynamic parameters, if available.	Pacemaker settings are determined by patient response.	When ventricular pacing is used, a higher rate may be necessary to compensate for the loss of atrial contribution to cardiac output.
8. After the pacing lead is sutured into place, apply an occlusive sterile dressing over the insertion site.	Prevents infection.	Epicardial electrodes placed during cardiothoracic surgical procedures may not require occlusive dressings. Because of the smaller size of the electrodes, the insertion sites may remain open to air and require only cleansing with an iodine-based antiseptic.
9. Throughout the procedure, assess the patient's need for sedative or analgesic medication, and administer as necessary.	The procedure may be anxiety producing as well as uncomfortable for the patient.	Close monitoring of hemodynamic status, such as blood pressure, heart rate, respiratory rate, and level of consciousness, should be performed with the administration of medication.
10. Secure necessary equipment, such as hanging pulse generator on attached IV pole, strapping pulse generator to patient's torso, or hanging pulse generator around patient's neck (if ambulatory), whichever is more appropriate to the clinical situation.	The pulse generator should be protected from falling or becoming inadvertently detached by patient movement. Disconnection or tension on the pacing electrode may lead to pacemaker malfunction.	

Table continues on following page

Steps	Rationale	Special Considerations
11. Wash hands.	Reduces transmission of microorganisms.	
12. Obtain a chest x-ray as prescribed.	In the absence of fluoroscopy, an x-ray is essential to detect potential complications associated with insertion as well as to visualize lead position.	

13. Selectively restrict patient mobility depending on the insertion site.
 	
  a. Antecubital approach: An armboard should be used to immobilize the arm. The pulse generator may be secured to the patient's arm with gauze or a commercial immobilizer. Abduction of the arm should be avoided by instructing the patient or securing the arm to the torso.
 	
  b. Femoral approach: The pulse generator may be fastened to the thigh or waist or suspended from an IV pole in a secure bag. The leg may be moved, but frequent abduction of the hip should be avoided.
 	
  c. Jugular or subclavian approach: The pulse generator is attached to the patient's waist or suspended from an IV pole. Mobility of both arms is permissible. If the patient is ambulatory, the pulse generator may be hung around the patient's neck.
	Prevents electrode dislodgment.	Some institutions will not allow ambulation with a temporary transvenous pacemaker. Check institutional policy. An extension cable adds additional length, allowing for greater versatility in pulse generator location. The use of an extension cable increases the number of connection sites. Check connection sites frequently for loosening, and secure or tighten as needed.

Evaluation

1. Evaluate ECG for presence of paced rhythm or resolution of initiating dysrhythmia. **Rationale:** Proper pacemaker functioning is assessed by observing the ECG for pacemaker activity consistent with the parameters set on the pacemaker.

2. Evaluate patient's hemodynamic response to paced rhythm. **Rationale:** Purpose of cardiac pacing is to improve cardiac output by increasing heart rate or overriding other life-threatening dysrhythmias.

3. Evaluate pacemaker function and surrounding equipment for any evidence of electrical hazards. **Rationale:** Stray electric current may be conducted through the pacemaker electrode causing lethal dysrhythmias (see Skill 36–1).

4. When pacing with a PA catheter, if PAWP measurements are to be taken per physician order, observe the ECG for pacemaker function during the wedge procedure. **Rationale:** Intermittent pacing (loss of capture) may occur during the wedge procedure as a result of movement of the pacing electrode during catheter wedging.

Expected Outcomes

1. ECG will show paced rhythm consistent with parameters set on pacemaker, as evidenced by appropriate heart rate, proper sensing, and proper capture. Capture is indicated by a ventricular response after each pacemaker impulse. Sensing is indicated by the sensing indicator lighting with each intrinsic ventricular beat. **Rationale:** Proper pacemaker functioning is evaluated by analyzing the ECG tracing.

2. Patient will show hemodynamic stability, as evidenced by having a systolic blood pressure greater than 90 mmHg, a mean arterial blood pressure greater than 60 mm Hg, being alert and oriented, and not being dizzy. **Rationale:** Adequate cardiac output and systemic tissue perfusion will be attained with an adequate blood pressure.

3. Pacemaker electrode will be isolated from other electric equipment by maintaining secure connections into pulse generator. If disconnected from pulse generator, the electrode should be covered by a rubber glove or finger cot. **Rationale:** Stray electric current may be conducted to the heart via the pacemaker electrode, potentially causing lethal dysrhythmias.

4. When pacing with a PA catheter, proper pacemaker function will be maintained during hemodynamic monitoring procedures. **Rationale:** Pulmonary artery catheters made with additional lumens for the introduction of pacing electrodes should function as both pressure monitoring catheters and temporary pacemakers under optimal conditions.

Unexpected Outcomes

1. Failure of the pacemaker to sense and/or capture. **Rationale:** This may be due to improper positioning of the electrode or the underlying pathologic condition, loose connections, lead fracture, or battery failure.

2. Pacemaker oversensing. **Rationale:** The oversensing of unwanted signals will cause the pacing rate to slow or cease firing completely as a result of inhibition of the pulse generator output. Unwanted signals may be generated by T waves, P waves, the environment, movement of the extension cable, or wire fractures.

3. Stimulation of diaphragm of chest wall causing hiccups. **Rationale:** Lead wire position, perforation, or normal lead wire position with the output (mA) being set too high may contribute to this condition.

4. Development of phlebitis, thrombosis, embolism, and bacteremia. **Rationale:** Invasive nature of temporary pacemaker placement in the venous system predisposes patient to these potential complications. The incidence of complications increases with the length of time the catheter is left in place.

5. Ventricular dysrhythmias. **Rationale:** Ventricular irritability may result from manipulation of the electrode within the cardiac chamber.

6. Pneumothorax or hemothorax. **Rationale:** During the insertion procedure, the pleura or major vessels may be punctured. A chest x-ray obtained after electrode insertion may assist in diagnosing.

7. Myocardial perforation and cardiac tamponade. **Rationale:** The myocardium may be perforated during insertion of particularly stiff temporary electrodes. The incidence of myocardial perforation ranges from 2 to 30 percent, with the incidence of cardiac tamponade much lower.

8. Air embolism. **Rationale:** May occur during insertion of the venous dilator and introducer sheath. Use of the Trendelenburg position, catheter introduction during the expiratory phase of respiration, and ensuring that the introducer sheath is not left open to air help to prevent air from entering the central circulation.

9. Lead dislodgment. **Rationale:** Patient movement may contribute to lead dislodgment, or the lead may spontaneously dislodge. This is the most common complication of temporary transvenous cardiac pacing, occurring in up to 27 percent of patients.

10. Failure to sense in the demand mode. **Rationale:** May be related to electrode position, sensitivity setting too high (unable to sense intrinsic beat), fibrosis around tip of lead wire, or other reasons. The lower the millivolt setting on the sensitivity dial, the more sensitive the pacemaker is to the patient's intrinsic heart rhythm. The higher the millivolt setting, the less sensitive the pacemaker is to intrinsic electrical activity.

11. Pacemaker syndrome. **Rationale:** In single-chamber ventricular pacing, there is loss of atrioventricular (A-V) synchrony. This may result in a decrease in cardiac output as a result of nonsynchronized atrial activity occurring during ventricular pacing.

12. Pacing with a PA catheter: Intermittent pacing during wedging procedure. **Rationale:** The pacing electrodes may move during the wedging procedure because of catheter migration.

Documentation

Documentation in the patient record should include the date and time the procedure was initiated; a description of events warranting temporary pacemaker insertion; hemodynamic parameters before, during, and after the procedure; ECG monitor rhythm strip before and after pacemaker insertion; a description of the patient's response to the procedure; medications administered and patient response to medication; pacemaker settings, including rate, output, sensitivity, threshold measurements, and whether turned on or off; patient and family education and response to education; and the date and time that pacing was discontinued.

Patient/Family Education

1. Provide a basic description of cardiac dysrhythmias and the need for temporary pacemaker. **Rationale:** Patient and family should understand why the procedure is necessary and what potential risks and benefits will be derived from undergoing this invasive procedure.

2. Provide a basic description of the temporary pacemaker insertion procedure. **Rationale:** Patient and family should be informed of the invasive nature of the procedure and any risks associated with the procedure. An understanding of the procedure may reduce anxiety associated with the procedure.

3. Provide a basic description of temporary pacemaker function. **Rationale:** Patient and family should understand how the pacemaker is expected to work and the temporary nature of the pacemaker.

4. Describe the precautions and restrictions required while the temporary pacemaker is in place, such as limitation of movement, avoiding handling the pacemaker or touching exposed portion of electrode, and the inability to use electrical equipment such as a shaver. **Rationale:** Understanding potential limitations may improve patient compliance with restrictions and precautions.

5. Anticipate the patient's need for a permanent pacemaker. **Rationale:** The need for a permanent pacemaker will be dependent on whether the condition necessitating temporary pacing is transient or can be corrected by other treatment modalities, such as medications or correcting underlying abnormalities.

Performance Checklist
Skill 11–2: Initiating Temporary Pacing

Critical Behaviors	Complies	
	yes	no
1. Wash hands.		
2. Connect patient to ECG machine, maintain continuous monitoring.		
3. Test battery function in pulse generator.		
4. If needed, replace battery.		
FOR EPICARDIAL PACING 1. Don exam gloves.		
2. Expose pacing wires and identify chamber of origin.		
3. Identify desired pacing method.		
4. Connect pericardial wires to the pulse generator.		
5. Set pacer parameters as prescribed and initiate pacing.		
6. Monitor ECG tracing.		
FOR TEMPORARY TRANSVENOUS/A-V SEQUENTIAL PACING 1. Prepare insertion site.		
2. Mask, gown, cap, and glove all persons performing and assisting with procedure.		
3. Cleanse site with antiseptic solution.		
4. Provide local anesthetic for insertion site.		
5. Assist physician with insertion.		
6. Once electrodes are positioned attach electrodes to pulse generator.		
FOR A-V SEQUENTIAL PACING 1. Connect atrial electrode to atrial output terminal.		
2. Connect ventricular electrode to ventricular output terminal.		
PACING WITH A PULMONARY ARTERY CATHETER 1. Assist physician with insertion of PA catheter and initiate hemodynamic monitoring (see Skills 10–5 and 10–6).		
2. Secure appropriate pacing electrode for insertion.		
3. Assist physician with insertion of pacing probe(s).		
4. Once positioned, attach electrode(s) to pulse generator.		
FOR ALL METHODS OF TEMPORARY PACING 1. Determine stimulation threshold.		
2. Determine sensitivity threshold.		
3. Set pacemaker rate, output, and sensitivity as prescribed.		
4. Assess ECG rhythm for pacemaker function.		
5. Apply protective plastic cover over pacemaker controls.		
6. Obtain physician's orders regarding wedging of a PA catheter during pacing.		
7. Assess patient response to pacing.		
8. Apply occlusive sterile dressing over insertion site.		
9. Throughout procedure, assess patient's need for sedation/analgesic.		
10. Secure protective equipment for pulse generator.		

Table continues on following page

Critical Behaviors	Complies	
	yes	no
11. Wash hands.		
12. Obtain prescribed chest x-ray.		
13. Restrict patient mobility according to insertion site.		
14. Document procedure in nurses notes.		

SKILL 11–3

Overdrive Atrial Pacing

Overdrive atrial pacing is a method of terminating supraventricular tachydysrhythmias that most commonly uses temporary epicardial pacing wires placed during open heart surgery. Overdrive atrial pacing also can be accomplished using a transvenous wire located in the atrium. The atrium is paced at rates exceeding the tachycardia's atrial rate for brief periods of time in an attempt to interrupt the tachycardia circuit and restore normal sinus rhythm.

This technique is effective for a variety of supraventricular tachydysrhythmias, including atrial flutter type I (atrial rate less than 340 beats per minute, with uniform flutter waves), paroxysmal atrial tachycardia, and dysrhythmias associated with Wolff-Parkinson-White (WPW) syndrome. Overdrive atrial pacing (or rapid atrial pacing) is not effective with atrial fibrillation, atrial flutter type II (flutter rate greater than 340 beats per minute), sinus tachycardia, or ventricular dysrhythmias.

This technique offers several advantages over cardioversion of the supraventricular dysrhythmia. It can be initiated immediately after the dysrhythmia has been noted, with little patient discomfort. It avoids the use of sedatives and anesthetics, commonly used during cardioversion. If the patient has received digoxin, it avoids the potential ventricular dysrhythmias that often arise with cardioversion. It is less traumatic for the patient and eliminates the potential for skin burns on the chest.

The disadvantages of overdrive atrial pacing include the inability of the pacemaker to capture the atrium and successfully interrupt the tachydysrhythmia, the potential dislodgment of the epicardial wire, its specificity for select tachydysrhythmias, and the potential for acceleration of the atrial rate. An alternate end point to treatment with overdrive atrial pacing is the conversion to atrial fibrillation, which can then have the ventricular rate controlled or be converted to normal sinus rhythm.

The technique of overdrive atrial pacing is similar to the use of epicardial pacing wires for temporary bradycardia support (see Skill 11–2) in the sense that atrial epicardial wires are connected to a temporary pulse generator, which provides the energy and controls to manipulate pacing. The pulse generator for overdrive atrial pacing is unique in that the rate dial has a maximum capacity of 800 pulses per minute. The output dial is capable of delivering a maximum of 20 mA to the atrial myocardium (Fig. 11–27). The pacemaker will pace the atrium asynchronously.

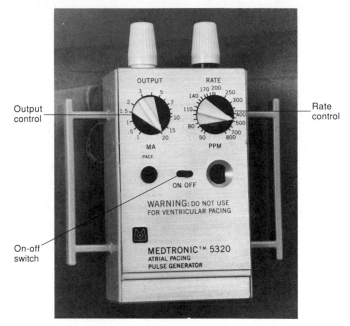

FIGURE 11–27. High-rate temporary atrial pulse generator for overdrive atrial pacing.

Because of the ability to pace the atrium at extraordinarily high rates, it is essential that the pulse generator be used for atrial pacing only. Inadvertent pacing of the ventricles at these rapid rates will cause ventricular tachycardia or fibrillation. It is possible for the atrial pacing impulses to conduct to the ventricles, creating ventricular dysrhythmias. Therefore, this technique is typically initiated by a physician with assistance from the nurse.

Purpose

The nurse assists in the initiation of overdrive atrial pacing to

1. Terminate supraventricular tachydysrhythmias.
2. Allow for restoration of normal sinus rhythm.
3. Allow for conversion to atrial fibrillation with a controlled ventricular response.

Prerequisite Knowledge and Skills

Before assisting with the initiation of overdrive atrial pacing, the nurse should understand

1. Anatomy and physiology of the cardiovascular system.
2. Principles of cardiac pacing.
3. Principles of electrical safety (see Skill 36–1).

The nurse should be able to perform

1. Physical assessment.
2. 12-lead ECG (see Skill 7–2).
3. Vital signs assessment.
4. Basic Cardiac Life Support/Advanced Cardiac Life Support.
5. Basic dysrhythmia interpretation.
6. Universal precautions (see Skill 35–1).
7. Handwashing techniques (see Skill 35–5).
8. Defibrillation (see Skill 8–1).

Assessment

1. Assess the cardiac rhythm for the presence of supraventricular tachydysrhythmias. **Rationale:** May warrant overdrive atrial pacing.
2. Identify a compromised hemodynamic response to the tachydysrhythmia, such as blood pressure less than 90 mmHg systolic, mean arterial blood pressure less than 60 mmHg, altered level of consciousness, complaints of dizziness, shortness of breath, nausea and vomiting, cool or clammy skin, or development of ischemic chest pain. **Rationale:** The decision to intervene once specific cardiac dysrhythmias are noted is dependent on the effect of the dysrhythmias on the cardiac output. Assessment of clinical parameters that reflect a decreased cardiac output allows the nurse to anticipate whether pacing is indicated.

Nursing Diagnoses

1. Altered tissue perfusion (cardiopulmonary and peripheral) related to inadequate cardiac output. **Rationale:** Tachydysrhythmias reduce cardiac output and systemic tissue perfusion because the heart is beating too rapidly and stroke volume is reduced secondary to decreased ventricular filling.
2. Potential for infection related to the presence of an epicardial pacing wire. **Rationale:** The presence of epicardial pacemaker wires provides a pathway for microorganisms to bypass the protective skin barrier and enter the myocardium.
3. Potential for injury (microshock) related to epicardial pacemaker wires (see Skill 36–1). **Rationale:** Direct connection of the heart to the outside environment

via the epicardial pacing wire predisposes the patient to increased risk of inadvertent microshock and the development of ventricular dysrhythmias.

Planning

1. Individualize the following goals for overdrive atrial pacing:
   a. Provide a cardiac output adequate for tissue perfusion to vital organs. **Rationale:** A sustained reduction in cardiac output will cause dysfunction of key organ systems.
   b. Promote healing of incision. **Rationale:** Reduction of possible sources of infection, improvement in nutritional state, and meticulous insertion-site care will reduce the risk of infection via the pacemaker wires.
   c. Maintain an electrically-safe environment (see Skill 36–1). **Rationale:** Extreme caution when manipulating the pacemaker wires and attention to possible sources of environmental hazard will greatly reduce the risk of microshock.
2. Prepare all necessary equipment and supplies. **Rationale:** Assembly of all the equipment and supplies ensures overdrive atrial pacing will be initiated quickly and efficiently.
   a. Atrial pacing pulse generator.
   b. Battery for pulse generator.
   c. Exam gloves.
   d. Emergency drug box and equipment.
   e. ECG monitor and recorder.
   f. Materials for site care (i.e., gauze pads, povidone-iodine ointment, paper tape, finger cots, or test tubes).
3. Prepare the patient.
   a. Explain the need for overdrive atrial pacing and describe the steps in the procedure. **Rationale:** Promotes compliance with the procedure, reduces anxiety and misconceptions about the care being delivered, and ensures that the patient is an informed participant.
   b. Connect patient to ECG monitor, and monitor ECG continuously. **Rationale:** Evaluates for adequate pacemaker function and expected response to intervention. Ensures that equipment is grounded and poses no electrical hazard to the patient. It is possible for the rhythm to either accelerate or terminate in a severe bradydysrhythmia with overdrive pacing.

Implementation

Steps	Rationale	Special Considerations
1. Wash hands.	Reduces transmission of microorganisms.	
2. Don exam gloves.	Prevents microshock. Universal precautions.	

Table continues on following page

Steps	Rationale	Special Considerations
3. Expose the epicardial pacing wires, and identify the chamber of origin.	It is essential to determine which wires are originating from the atrium and which from the ventricle to ensure that the appropriate chamber is paced.	*Inadvertent high-rate pacing of the ventricle can cause lethal ventricular dysrhythmias.* Typically, the atrial wires exit the chest to the right of the sternum and the ventricular wires exit to the left of the sternum (see Fig. 11–13).
4. Assist the physician in connecting the epicardial atrial wires to terminals on the atrial pacing pulse generator.	Power source to pace the atrium.	The physician confirms that the wires are of atrial origin either by performing an electrogram (see Skill 11–4) or by pacing at a rate of 80 to 100 beats per minute and noting the ECG rhythm. The pacemaker is connected to the ventricular wires if ventricular capture occurs.
5. Assist the physician in establishing rate and output settings for overdrive atrial pacing.	Determination of pacemaker settings is based on the characteristics of the patient's tachydysrhythmia and the threshold of capture.	Pacing is initiated either by slowly increasing atrial pacing rate to approximately 125 percent of the patient's intrinsic atrial rate or by immediately initiating atrial pacing at a rate exceeding the intrinsic atrial rate (Fig. 11–28). It commonly requires greater levels of energy to capture the atrium with overdrive atrial pacing.

Table continues on following page

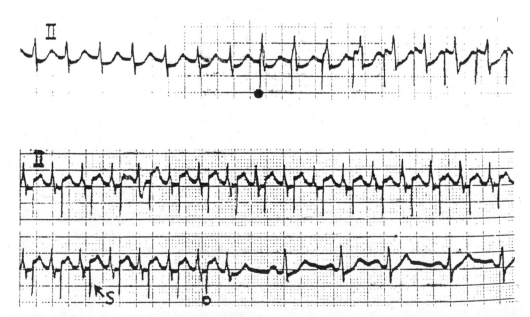

FIGURE 11–28. The top trace shows ECG lead II recorded during an episode of paroxysmal atrial tachycardia at a rate of 150 beats per minute. Beginning with the eighth beat in this trace (black dot), rapid atrial pacing at a rate of 165 beats per minute was initiated. In the middle trace, which begins 12 seconds after the top trace, atrial capture is demonstrated clearly. In the bottom trace, which is continuous with the middle trace, sinus rhythm appears when atrial pacing is terminated abruptly (open circle). S = stimulus artifact. Paper recording speed 25 mm/s. (Reprinted with permission from T. B. Cooper, W. A. H. MacLean, and A. L. Waldo, Overdrive pacing for supraventricular tachycardia: A review of theoretical implications and therapeutic techniques. *PACE* 1:200, 1978.)

Steps	Rationale	Special Considerations
6. Pace the myocardium for a brief period of time (several beats or up to 1 minute), and then abruptly terminate pacing.	The pacemaker must be able to capture the atrium and interrupt the ectopic activity to allow for restoration of sinus node activity.	It is possible for the atrial rate to accelerate or for the atrial pacing to conduct to the ventricles causing hemodynamically compromising dysrhythmias. It is also possible for the sinus node to be suppressed for a brief period after pacing is terminated, predisposing the patient to severe bradydysrhythmias (i.e., sinus bradycardia, junctional escape, ventricular escape, asystole). It may be necessary to immediately initiate either atrial or ventricular temporary epicardial pacing for bradycardia support after termination of overdrive atrial pacing.
7. Apply a dry sterile dressing to the exit sites of the epicardial wires. Protect exposed wires with finger cots or glass test tubes. Place gauze beneath the wires and cover with a dry sterile dressing. Label each dressing or test tube to identify the location of the atrial and ventricular wires.	Prevents infection and microshock. Gauze padding beneath the wires helps maintain skin integrity.	Wear exam gloves whenever handling pacemaker wires to prevent microshock. If bradycardia pacing is required following overdrive atrial pacing, follow the procedure for temporary epicardial pacing (see Skill 11–2).
8. Wash hands.	Reduces transmission of microorganisms.	

Evaluation

1. Observe the ECG for resolution of the dysrhythmia that warranted treatment and the presence of a hemodynamically stable rhythm. **Rationale:** Indicates effectiveness of overdrive atrial pacing.

2. Observe the patient's hemodynamic response to pacing and compare with baseline. **Rationale:** Allows the nurse to evaluate the patient's physiologic response and ensures that the cardiac output is improved.

3. Periodically assess the patient's rhythm and observe for the recurrence of the tachydysrhythmia (i.e., atrial flutter, paroxysmal supraventricular tachycardia. **Rationale:** Although overdrive atrial pacing is extremely effective in interrupting the tachycardia, it is not uncommon for the rhythm to recur without supplemental antidysrhythmic therapy.

Expected Outcomes

1. Hemodynamically stable rhythm. **Rationale:** Return of rhythm stability promotes an adequate cardiac output.

2. Adequate systemic tissue perfusion and cardiac output as evidenced by having a blood pressure greater than 90 mmHg systolic, being alert and oriented, without complaints of dizziness, shortness of breath, nausea and vomiting due to hypotension, or ischemic chest pain. **Rationale:** Prevents dysfunction of vital organ systems.

Unexpected Outcomes

1. Failure to capture. **Rationale:** Inability of the pacemaker to actually stimulate the heart to contract will prevent the pacemaker from interrupting the dysrhythmia, allowing for the offending condition to persist.

2. Conversion to severe bradydysrhythmia or asystole. **Rationale:** Abrupt termination of rapid atrial pacing may cause suppression of sinus node activity, predisposing the patient to bradydysrhythmias.

3. Conversion to atrial fibrillation. **Rationale:** Overdrive atrial pacing may accelerate the atrial rate, causing conversion to atrial fibrillation. It is hoped that the ventricular response rate is controlled should this occur. Administration of antidysrhythmics and/or cardioversion may be warranted.

4. Microshock, resulting in ventricular dysrhythmias. **Rationale:** The potential for stray current to communicate with the myocardium via epicardial wires always exists.

Documentation

Documentation in the patient record should include a description of events warranting overdrive atrial pacing; prepacing and postpacing vital signs and physical assessments; a sample of the prepacing and postpacing ECG strips; a description of the patient's response to the procedure; medications administered, rationale for administration, and patient response; pacemaker settings required for interruption of the tachydysrhythmia and number of attempts required for successful conversion; and patient education provided and an evaluation of patient and family understanding. **Rationale:** Provides a record of the clinical events leading to initiation of pacing and a description of the procedure and the outcome and serves as a legal record of the events.

Patient/Family Education

1. Assess learning needs, readiness to learn, and factors that influence learning. **Rationale:** Allows the nurse to individualize teaching in a manner that will be meaningful to the patient and family.
2. Provide basic information about the normal conduction system, such as structure of the electrical system, source of the heart beat, normal and abnormal heart rhythms, and symptoms of abnormal heart rhythms. **Rationale:** Assists the patient and family in recognizing the seriousness of the patient's condition and the need for overdrive atrial pacing.
3. Provide basic information about overdrive atrial pacing, such as reason for pacing, explanation of the equipment, and what to expect during overdrive atrial pacing. **Rationale:** Assists the patient and family in developing a realistic perception of the procedure and its benefits.
4. Anticipate the patient's need for permanent antitachycardiac pacing support or antidysrhythmic therapy. **Rationale:** If permanent pacing or drug therapy is required, the patient and family will need further instructions regarding possible lifestyle modifications, medications, follow-up visits, and specifics about the pacemaker to be implanted.

Performance Checklist
Skill 11–3:   Overdrive Atrial Pacing

Critical Behaviors	Complies	
	yes	no
1. Wash hands.		
2. Don exam gloves.		
3. Expose epicardial wires and identify the chamber of origin for each.		
4. Assist with the connection of epicardial wires to pulse generator.		
5. Assist with the establishment of the rate and output settings.		
6. Monitor patient during pacing and abrupt cessation.		
7. Apply dressing to epicardial wire exit sites.		
8. Wash hands.		
9. Document procedure in the nurses notes.		

SKILL 11–4

Atrial Electrograms

An *atrial electrogram* (AEG) is a method of recording electrical activity originating from the atria by using temporary atrial epicardial pacing wires placed during open-heart surgery. Atrial electrograms are indicated in situations where atrial activity is not clearly reflected on the standard 12-lead ECG and assists in identifying the origin of the rhythm. This information is important in determining the course of treatment for the dysrhythmia. Differentiation of wide complex rhythms, such as ventricular tachycardia and a supraventricular tachycardia with aberrant ventricular conduction, is one indication for AEG. Another clinical event that commonly requires clarification in the patient following open heart surgery is the presence of a narrow complex supraventricular tachycardia that could either be sinus tachycardia, atrial tachycardia, paroxysmal supraventricular tachycardia, atrial flutter, atrial fibrillation with relatively regular R-to-R intervals, or junctional tachycardia.

The standard 12-lead ECG records electrical events from the heart using electrodes located on the surface of the patient's body, which is a considerable distance from the myocardium. One limitation of the standard 12-lead ECG is its inability to detect P waves effectively, particularly when atrial activity coincides with ventricular activity or in the presence of a tachydysrhythmia, when the various waves of the cardiac cycle tend to merge together. Atrial electrograms detect electrical events directly from or in close proximity to the atria, providing a greatly enhanced tracing of atrial activity. This allows for comparison of atrial events with ventricular events and determination of the relationship between the two.

Atrial electrograms can be performed using a standard 12-lead ECG machine or can be recorded on special multichannel ECG machines that allow for simultaneous display of the atrial electrogram along with the surface ECG

(Fig. 11–29). Two types of atrial electrograms may be obtained from the epicardial pacing wires if two wires are attached to the right atrium. A *unipolar* electrogram measures electrical activity between one atrial epicardial wire and an indifferent electrode some distance from the myocardium (i.e., surface limb electrode). A *bipolar* electrogram detects electrical activity between the two atrial epicardial wires attached to the myocardium.

Because the electrograms detect electrical activity over different areas, the tracings for unipolar and bipolar atrial electrograms reflect these differences. The unipolar AEG is able to measure electrical events originating from a much larger area, since it has a broader detection range between the two sensing electrodes. Therefore, it displays deflections representing both atrial and ventricular activity. The atrial activity is significantly enhanced as compared with a surface 12-lead ECG, and the ventricular events are still clearly discernible (Fig. 11–30). The bipolar AEG predominantly detects atrial activity, since both sensing electrodes are attached to the atrium. The bipolar tracing displays amplified atrial deflections with minimal or absent ventricular deflections (Fig. 11–31). Ideally, it is helpful to obtain either a unipolar and bipolar electrogram or a bipolar electrogram and a surface ECG for comparison to identify clearly the presence of atrial activity and its relationship with the ventricular events.

Purpose

The nurse obtains an atrial electrogram to

1. Determine the presence of atrial activity in a dysrhythmia.
2. Identify the relationship between atrial and ventricular depolarizations.

Prerequisite Knowledge and Skills

Before obtaining an atrial electrogram, the nurse should understand

1. Anatomy and physiology of the cardiovascular system.
2. Principles of cardiac conduction.

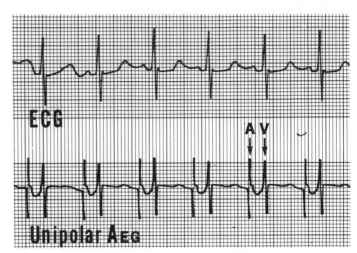

FIGURE 11–30. Monitor ECG lead recorded simultaneously with a unipolar atrial electrogram (AEG) recorded during regular sinus rhythm. Although the atrial (A) and ventricular (V) complexes in the unipolar atrial electrogram are approximately the same amplitude in this tracing, this is not a constant finding. Rather, there is considerable variation, in that the atrial complex may be larger or smaller than the ventricular complex. (Reprinted with permission from A. L. Waldo and W. A. H. MacLean, *Diagnosis and Treatment of Cardiac Arrhythmias Following Open Heart Surgery.* New York: Futura, 1980, p. 22.)

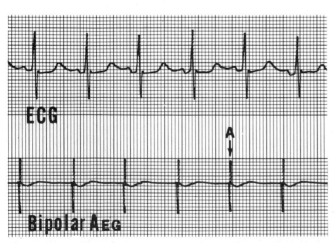

FIGURE 11–29. Monitor ECG lead recorded simultaneously with a bipolar atrial electrogram (AEG) during regular sinus rhythm in the same patient as Figure 11–32. Although the atrial complex (A) is the only discrete deflection recorded in the bipolar atrial electrogram, a small ventricular complex also may be recorded. (Reprinted with permission from A. L. Waldo and W. A. H. MacLean, *Diagnosis and Treatment of Cardiac Arrhythmias Following Open Heart Surgery.* New York: Futura, 1980, p. 83.)

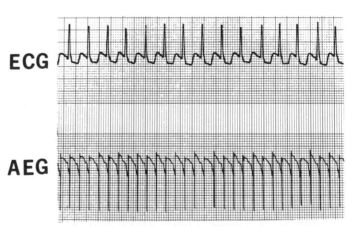

FIGURE 11–31. Monitor ECG lead recorded simultaneously with a bipolar atrial electrogram (AEG) during type II atrial flutter. Note that from the ECG alone, the nature of atrial activation and its relationship to ventricular activation cannot be discerned. In fact, the ventricular rate of 180 beats per minute in the presence of a narrow QRS complex tachycardia had suggested a diagnosis of paroxysmal atrial tachycardia. However, the bipolar atrial electrogram clearly identifies atrial activation at a rate of 360 beats per minute, thereby establishing a diagnosis of type II atrial flutter with 2:1 A-V conduction. (Reprinted with permission from A. L. Waldo and W. A. H. MacLean, *Diagnosis and Treatment of Cardiac Arrhythmias Following Open Heart Surgery.* New York: Futura, 1980, p. 23.)

3. Principles of basic dysrhythmia interpretation.
4. Principles of electrical safety.

The nurse should be able to perform

1. Handwashing technique (see Skill 35–5).
2. Vital signs assessment.
3. Physical assessment.
4. 12-lead ECG (see Skill 7–2).
5. Basic dysrhythmia interpretation.
6. Basic Cardiac Life Support/Advanced Cardiac Life Support (BCLS/ACLS).
7. Electrical safety techniques (see Skill 36–1).

Assessment

1. Assess the cardiac rhythm for the presence of dysrhythmias in which atrial activity is unclear. **Rationale:** The presence of these dysrhythmias may warrant obtaining an atrial electrogram to assess whether atrial activity is actually occurring.
2. Assess the cardiac rhythm for the presence of dysrhythmias in which the relationship between atrial and ventricular activity is unclear. **Rationale:** The presence of these dysrhythmias may warrant obtaining an atrial electrogram to assess whether the atria and ventricles are functioning in a coordinated fashion.
3. Assess the compromised hemodynamic response to the dysrhythmias, such as systolic blood pressure less than 90 mmHg, mean arterial pressure less than 60 mmHg, altered level of consciousness, complaints of dizziness, shortness of breath, or nausea and vomiting, cool or clammy skin, or development of ischemic chest pain. **Rationale:** The decision to intervene once specific cardiac dysrhythmias are noted is dependent on the effect of the dysrhythmia on the cardiac output. Clinical parameters that reflect a decreased cardiac output indicate a need for interventions.

Nursing Diagnoses

1. Altered tissue perfusion (cardiopulmonary and peripheral) related to inadequate cardiac output. **Rationale:** Tachydysrhythmias may reduce cardiac output and systemic tissue perfusion because the heart is beating too rapidly and stroke volume is reduced secondary to decreased ventricular filling.

2. Potential for injury (microshock) related to the presence of stray electric current with exposed epicardial wires. **Rationale:** Direct connection of the heart to the outside environment via the epicardial pacing wires predisposes the patient to increased risk of inadvertent microshock and the development of ventricular dysrhythmias (see Skill 36–1).

Planning

1. Individualize the following goals for performing an atrial electrogram:
   a. Maintain cardiac output adequate for tissue perfusion to vital organs. **Rationale:** A sustained reduction in cardiac output will cause dysfunction of vital organ systems.
   b. Maintain an electrically safe environment. **Rationale:** Extreme caution when manipulating the pacemaker wires and attention to possible sources of environmental hazard will greatly reduce the risk of microshock via the pacemaker wires.
2. Prepare all necessary equipment and supplies. **Rationale:** Assembly of all the equipment and supplies necessary for initiation of an atrial electrogram will ensure that the procedure is initiated efficiently.
   a. 12-lead ECG machine.
   b. Two alligator clips.
   c. ECG monitor and recorder.
   d. Materials for site care (i.e., gauze pads, povidone-iodine ointment, tape, finger cots, and glass test tubes).
   e. Emergency drugs and cart.
3. Prepare the patient.
   a. Explain the need for an atrial electrogram and describe the procedure. **Rationale:** Promotes compliance with the procedure, reduces anxiety and misconceptions about the care being delivered, and ensures that the patient is an informed participant.
   b. Connect the patient to ECG monitor, and monitor ECG continuously. **Rationale:** Monitor intrinsic rhythm during atrial electrogram recording for changes. Ensure that equipment is grounded and poses no electrical hazard.

Implementation

Steps	Rationale	Special Considerations
General AEG Setup		
1. Wash hands.	Reduces transmission of microorganisms.	
2. Don exam gloves.	Exam gloves should be worn whenever handling the epicardial wires to prevent microshock (see Skill 36–1). Universal precautions.	

Table continues on following page

Steps	Rationale	Special Considerations
3. Expose the epicardial pacing wires, and identify the chamber of origin.	It is important to determine which wires are originating from the atrium and which from the ventricle to ensure that the appropriate chamber is recorded.	Typically, the atrial wires exit the chest to the right of the sternum and the ventricular wires exit to the left of the sternum (see Fig. 11–13).
4. Connect the patient to the limb leads of the 12-lead ECG machine, and run a recording.	Obtaining a baseline ECG of the limb leads will provide the nurse with a surface tracing for comparison.	Ensure that the ECG machine has been inspected recently and sanctioned safe for use with epicardial wires.
Bipolar AEG		
5. Connect one of the atrial epicardial pacing wires to the left arm (LA) limb lead and the other to the right arm (RA) limb lead of the 12-lead ECG machine with alligator clips.	Connection to the limb leads of the ECG machine allows for the detection and recording of atrial electrical activity.	
6. Select lead I on the ECG machine lead selector, and record a tracing.	Lead I measures the electrical potential between the right and left arm limb leads, which are sensing atrial activity from both epicardial wires, providing a bipolar tracing (Fig. 11–32).	
Unipolar AEG		
7. Connect one of the atrial epicardial pacing wires to the left arm (LA) limb lead and the other to the right arm (RA) limb lead of the 12-lead ECG machine with alligator clips.	Connection to the limb leads of the ECG machine allows for the detection and recording of atrial electrical activity.	

Table continues on following page

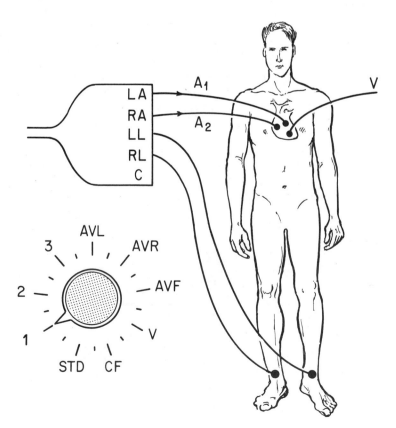

FIGURE 11–32. Connection for bipolar atrial lead. Attach two limb leads of ECG as usual. Using two alligator clip wires, attach each of the atrial pacing wires (A$_1$ and A$_2$) to the remaining limb leads. Run a rhythm strip in that limb lead position, i.e., lead I. (Adapted by permission of the American Heart Association, Inc., from K. S. Wulff, Use of temporary epicardial electrodes for atrial pacing and monitoring. *Cardiovasc. Nurs.* 18:1, 1982.)

Steps	Rationale	Special Considerations
8. Select lead II or lead III with the lead selector on the ECG machine, and run a tracing.	Lead II detects electrical activity between the right arm limb lead and the left leg. Since only one epicardial pacing wire is connected to the right arm lead, the atrial electrical activity recorded will occur from a unipolar configuration. Lead III detects electrical activity between the left arm limb lead and the left leg. Since only one epicardial pacing wire is connected to the left arm lead, the atrial electrical activity will be recorded from a unipolar configuration (Fig. 11–33).	

Alternate Method for Unipolar AEG

Steps	Rationale	Special Considerations
9. Connect one of the atrial epicardial wires to the V (precordial) lead of the 12-lead ECG machine with an alligator clip.	Connection of the epicardial wire to the ECG machine allows for the detection and recording of atrial electrical activity.	
10. Select the V lead on the lead selector of the 12-lead ECG machine, and record a tracing.	Use of the precordial lead will allow detection of the atrial electrical activity between the V lead and an indifferent limb lead in a unipolar configuration (Fig. 11–34).	

Table continues on following page

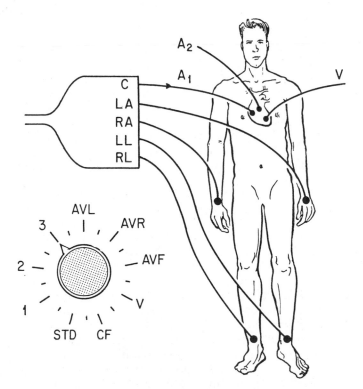

FIGURE 11–33. Connection of unipolar atrial lead. Attach four ECG limb leads. Use an alligator clip to connect the metal end of the atrial pacing wire (A₁) to the chest (C) lead cable of the ECG machine. Obtain rhythm strip with the dial in the 2- or 3-lead position. (Adapted by permission of the American Heart Association, Inc., from K. S. Wulff, Use of temporary epicardial electrodes for atrial pacing and monitoring. *Cardiovasc. Nurs.* 18:1, 1982.)

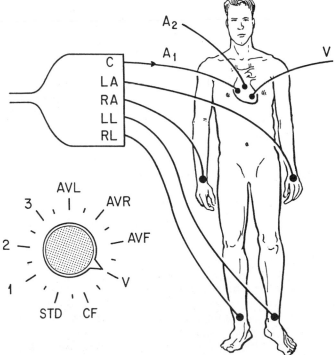

FIGURE 11–34. Connection of unipolar atrial lead. Attach four ECG limb leads. Use an alligator clip to connect the metal end of the atrial pacing wire (A₁) to the chest (C) lead cable of the ECG machine. Obtain rhythm strip with the dial in the V-lead position. (Adapted by permission of the American Heart Association, Inc., from K. S. Wulff, Use of temporary epicardial electrodes for atrial pacing and monitoring. *Cardiovasc. Nurs.* 18:1, 1982.)

Steps	Rationale	Special Considerations
General AEG Care		
11. Apply a dry sterile dressing to the exit sites of the epicardial wires, and label atrial and ventricular locations. If only one set of wires is used, protect all exposed wire ends with finger cots or other nonconductive material and place gauze beneath the wires and cover with a dry sterile dressing.	Prevents infection and microshock. Use of gauze padding beneath the wires helps maintain skin integrity.	Wear exam gloves whenever handling the pacemaker wires to prevent microshock.
12. Wash hands.	Reduces transmission of microorganisms.	

Evaluation

1. Evaluate the atrial electrogram for the presence of atrial activity and its relationship to ventricular activity. Compare with surface ECG for interpretation. **Rationale:** Atrial electrograms will enhance the atrial activity often masked on the surface ECG, allowing for clarification of the dysrhythmia's origin.

2. Monitor the ECG tracing for changes in the patient's rhythm. **Rationale:** The underlying dysrhythmia may change during the recording of the atrial electrogram.

3. Implement interventions based on the physician's interpretation of the atrial electrogram. **Rationale:** Treatment of the dysrhythmia will be based on its identified origin.

4. Evaluate the patient's response to the atrial electrogram and the interventions, including pulse, blood pressure, level of consciousness, and heart rhythm. **Rationale:** Ensures adequate tissue perfusion with the current rhythm.

5. Monitor the patient's rhythm for the development of dysrhythmias that require an atrial electrogram for clarification. **Rationale:** A dysrhythmia may recur, warranting differentiation with an AEG.

6. Evaluate the need for ongoing treatment of the dysrhythmia. **Rationale:** Prompt identification and treatment of dysrhythmias generally improve the patient's outcome.

Expected Outcomes

1. Adequate systemic tissue perfusion and cardiac output, as evidenced by having a blood pressure greater than 90 mmHg systolic, a mean arterial pressure greater than 60 mmHg, being alert and oriented, without complaints of dizziness, shortness of breath, nausea and vomiting due to hypotension, or ischemic chest pain. **Rationale:** Adequate systemic perfusion and cardiac output will prevent dysfunction of vital organ systems.

2. Absence of hemodynamically significant dysrhythmias. **Rationale:** Return of rhythm stability promotes an adequate cardiac output.

3. Absence of dysrhythmias in which atrial activity is unclear or the relationship between atrial and ventricular activity is unclear. **Rationale:** Ensures that the rhythm can be clearly interpreted by the surface ECG.

Unexpected Outcome

Microshocks, causing ventricular dysrhythmias. **Rationale:** The potential for stray current to the myocardium via epicardial wires exists.

Documentation

Documentation in the patient record should include date and time of atrial electrogram, a description of the events warranting recording of an atrial electrogram; vital signs and physical assessments prior to the atrial electrogram; rhythm strip prior to and following the AEG; a tracing from the atrial electrogram with an interpretation; any interventions that were done based on the interpretation of the atrial electrogram, rationale, and patient response; and patient education provided and an evaluation of the patient and family understanding. **Rationale:** Provides a record of the clinical events requiring an atrial electrogram, a description of the procedure, and the outcome of treatment and serves as a legal document to identify nursing care rendered.

Patient/Family Education

1. Assess learning needs, readiness to learn, and factors that influence learning. **Rationale:** Allows the nurse to individualize teaching in a manner that will be meaningful to the patient and family.

2. Provide information about the normal conduction system, such as structure of the electrical system, source of heart beat, normal and abnormal heart rhythms, and symptoms of abnormal heart rhythms. **Rationale:** Understanding of the normal conduction system assists the patient and family in recognizing the seriousness of the patient's condition and the need to perform an atrial electrogram.

3. Provide information about the atrial electrogram, such as reason for the AEG, explanation of the equipment, and what to expect during the AEG. **Rationale:** Assists the patient and family to develop a realistic perception of the procedure and how it will help the patient.

Performance Checklist
Skill 11–4: Atrial Electrograms

Critical Behaviors	Complies yes	Complies no
GENERAL AEG SETUP 1. Wash hands.		
2. Don exam gloves.		
3. Expose the epicardial pacing wires, and identify the chamber of origin.		
4. Connect the patient to the limb leads of the 12-lead ECG machine, and run a recording.		
BIPOLAR AEG 5. Connect one of the atrial epicardial wires to the left arm limb lead and the other to the right arm limb lead.		
6. Select lead I on the ECG machine, and record a tracing.		
UNIPOLAR AEG 7. Connect one of the atrial epicardial wires to the left arm limb lead and the other to the right arm limb lead.		
8. Select lead II or lead III on the ECG machine, and record a tracing of each.		
ALTERNATE METHOD FOR UNIPOLAR AEG 9. Connect one of the atrial epicardial wires to the V lead on the ECG machine.		
10. Select the V lead on the ECG machine, and record a tracing.		
GENERAL AEG CARE 11. Apply dressing, and cover exposed pacer wires.		
12. Document procedure in patient record.		
13. Wash hands.		

SKILL 11–5

Permanent Pacing: Assessing the Modes

Permanent pacing is a method of stimulating the myocardium utilizing a transvenous pacing lead and a pulse generator implanted subcutaneously within the chest. The transvenous electrode may be positioned in the right atrium, the right ventricle, or both depending on the type of pacing required. The pulse generator is typically made of stainless steel or titanium and contains the electronic components as well as the batteries necessary to sustain pacing (Fig. 11–35).

The transvenous pacing leads may be unipolar or bipolar in configuration. Unipolar leads have the negative electrode in direct contact with the myocardium and the positive electrode located on the pulse generator so that electrical activity flows to the myocardium via the pacemaker lead and returns to the pulse generator by traveling through the patient's chest. Bipolar pacing leads have both the negative and positive electrodes located

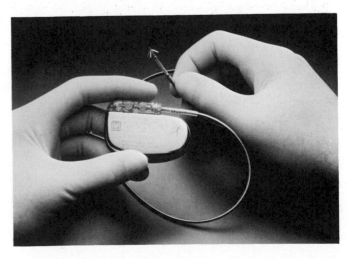

FIGURE 11–35. Permanent pacemaker pulse generator with lead wire. (Reprinted with permission from Medtronic, Inc.)

at the tip of the lead wire in contact with the myocardium so that the electric circuit remains within the heart. Bipolar leads tend to have fewer problems with inappropriate inhibition of pacing from muscular activity. Unipolar leads are thought to sense intrinsic electrical activity more accurately.

Permanent pacemakers are indicated for clinical conditions that necessitate supplemental bradycardia support, such as A-V block, sick sinus syndrome, hypersensitive carotid sinus syndrome, interventricular conduction defects, severe bradydysrhythmias, and A-V nodal disease. Permanent pacemakers also may be indicated for the treatment of tachydysrhythmias by providing either overdrive suppression or acute intervention with antitachycardic pacing when a tachydysrhythmia is detected. This method of pacing is applicable to both atrial and ventricular tachydysrhythmias and may be used in conjunction with supplemental bradycardia pacing.

Permanent pacemakers may be programmed to respond in a variety of ways to complement the intrinsic rhythm. The pacemaker can function in a single chamber, pacing either the atrium or the ventricle, or both chambers. The ability of the pacemaker to detect the underlying rhythm may be manipulated to maximize the effect on the hemodynamic state. Other features that can be programmed into the pacemaker include the pacing rate (both upper and lower rate limits), the amount of time the pacemaker waits between atrial activity and ventricular activity, the period of time during which the pacemaker is unable to detect intrinsic activity, how the pacemaker should respond if the upper rate limit is reached, and the amount of energy delivered to the myocardium with each paced event.

Because of the variety of ways a pacemaker can be programmed to respond, an international code was developed by the Intersociety Commission for Heart Disease (ICHD) to communicate this information in clinical practice. The ICHD code contains five letters that represent specific features of the pacemaker (Table 11–2).

Most recently, the North American Society of Pacing and Electrophysiology (NASPE) and the British Pacing and Electrophysiology Group (BPEG) have updated the ICHD code to accommodate the expanding functions of permanent pacemakers (NBG code) (Table 11–3). The codes are very similar, with the first three letters representing identical features, and are used solely for anti-bradydysrhythmia functions.

Because of the complexity of today's permanent pacemakers, it is essential for the nurse to be able to assess whether the device is functioning correctly. The nurse should be able to determine the programmed mode using the ICHD or NBG code and troubleshoot failure to pace, failure to sense, and failure to capture. *Failure to pace* means that the pacemaker has not discharged a pacing stimulus to the myocardium and is recognized on the ECG as absence of a pacing stimulus where expected (Fig. 11–36). *Failure to sense* means that the pacemaker has either detected signals that mimic intrinsic electrical

TABLE 11–2 ICHD PACEMAKER CODE

First letter:	Chamber paced	V = ventricle A = atrium D = double (atrium and ventricle)
Second letter:	Chamber sensed	V = ventricle A = atrium D = double (atrium and ventricle) 0 = none (no sensing)
Third letter:	Mode of response	I = inhibited T = triggered* D = double (both inhibited and triggered) 0 = none (no response)
Fourth letter:	Programmable functions	P = simple programmable M = multiprogrammable 0 = none
Fifth letter:	Tachydysrhythmic functions	B = burst N = normal rate competition S = scanning E = external 0 = none

Examples: VVI = Paces the ventricle, senses intrinsic ventricular activity, and is inhibited by the sensed beats.
DVI = Paces both the atrium and ventricles in the absence of a ventricular rhythm, senses only ventricular activity, and inhibits both atrial and ventricular pacing when ventricular beats are sensed.
DDD = Paces both the atrium and ventricle, senses both atrial and ventricular activity, pacing is inhibited by sensed atrial or ventricular beats, and sensed atrial activity will trigger a ventricular paced response.

*Triggered: A sensed event causes a paced stimulus.

TABLE 11–3 NBG CODE (NASPE/BPEG GENERIC PACEMAKER CODE)

First letter:	Chamber paced	0 = none A = atrium V = ventricle D = dual (A + V)
Second letter:	Chamber sensed	0 = none A = atrium V = ventricle D = dual (A + V)
Third letter:	Response to sensing	0 = none T = triggered I = inhibited D = dual (T + I)
Fourth letter:	Programmability rate modulation	0 = none P = simple programmable M = multiprogrammable C = communicating R = rate modulation
Fifth letter:	Antitachyarrhythmia functions	0 = none P = pacing (antitach.) S = shock D = dual (P + S)

activity (oversensing) or did not accurately identify intrinsic activity (undersensing) (Fig. 11–37). Oversensing is recognized on the ECG by pauses where paced beats were expected and prolongation of the interval between paced beats. Undersensing is recognized on the ECG by inappropriate placement of pacemaker spikes in relationship to the intrinsic waveforms (within the P wave, QRS complex, or T wave) and shortened distances between paced beats. *Failure to capture* means that the pacemaker has delivered a pacing stimulus that was unable to initiate depolarization of the myocardium and the subsequent contraction (Fig. 11–38). This problem is recognized on the ECG by pacemaker spikes that are not followed by a P wave for an atrial pacemaker or a QRS complex for a ventricular pacemaker.

Purpose

The nurse assesses permanent pacemakers to

1. Monitor the patient's response to permanent pacemaker therapy.
2. Evaluate pacemaker function.

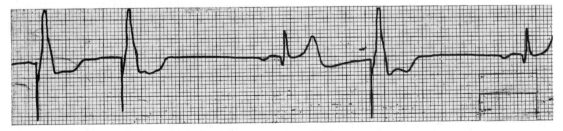

FIGURE 11–36. Example of failure to pace.

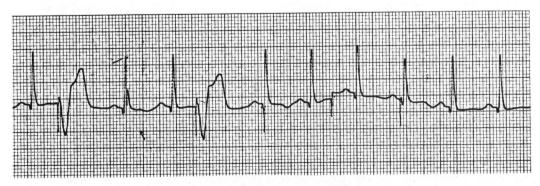

FIGURE 11–37. Example of failure to sense.

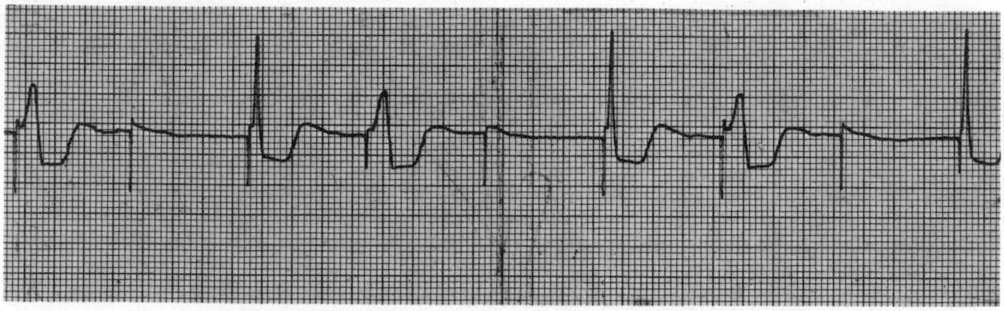

FIGURE 11–38.   Example of failure to capture.

Prerequisite Knowledge and Skills

Before assessing permanent pacemaker function, the nurse should understand

1. Anatomy and physiology of the cardiovascular system.
2. Principles of the cardiac conduction system.
3. Principles of cardiac pacing.
4. The ICHD code.
5. The NASPE/BPEG generic pacemaker code.

The nurse should be able to perform

1. Physical assessment.
2. 12-lead ECG (see Skill 7–1).
3. Vital signs assessment.
4. Basic dysrhythmia interpretation.
5. ECG interpretation of a paced rhythm.
6. Universal precautions (see Skill 35–1).

Assessment

1. Identify the programmed mode of the pacemaker. **Rationale:** Knowledge of how the pacemaker is intended to respond is necessary to detect inappropriate function.
2. Identify the reason for permanent pacemaker support. **Rationale:** Knowledge of the clinical indication will provide the nurse with baseline data when evaluating pacemaker function and patient response.
3. Determine the patient's pacemaker history (the date of insertion, the last battery change, when the pacemaker was last checked, and whether the patient has been experiencing any unusual symptoms, such as palpitations or dizziness). **Rationale:** The pacemaker history will provide clues to any potential problems that might be occurring.
4. Assess the cardiac rhythm for the presence of pacemaker activity. **Rationale:** Evidence of pacemaker activity will allow for the determination of appropriate function.

5. Assess the patient's hemodynamic response to the paced rhythm, such as systolic blood pressure greater than 90 mmHg, mean arterial blood pressure greater than 60 mmHg, level of consciousness, complaints of dizziness, shortness of breath, or nausea and vomiting; cool or clammy skin, or complaints of pain. **Rationale:** The patient's response will indicate how effective the pacemaker is in maintaining an adequate cardiac output.

Nursing Diagnoses

1. Potential alteration in tissue perfusion (cardiopulmonary and peripheral) related to inappropriate pacemaker function. **Rationale:** If the pacemaker is not functioning correctly, the patient may exhibit a variety of cardiac rhythms that may adversely affect the cardiac output.
2. Fear of death related to dependence on a mechanical device. **Rationale:** The possibility of pacemaker malfunction creates a state in which the individual experiences a real threat to personal well-being.

Planning

Individualize the following goals for assessing permanent pacing:
1. Maintain cardiac output adequate for tissue perfusion to vital organs. **Rationale:** A sustained reduction in cardiac output will cause dysfunction of key organ systems in the body.
2. Decrease fears of death. **Rationale:** Fear decreases the ability of an individual to cope with situations and activates physiologic responses that may potentiate the dysrhythmia.

Implementation

Steps	Rationale	Special Considerations
1. Assess the cardiac rhythm for the presence of pacemaker activity.	Allows for the determination of pacemaker function.	

Table continues on following page

Steps	Rationale	Special Considerations
a. Identify atrial activity. Is the pacemaker programmed to detect intrinsic atrial activity? Was the atrial activity sensed? What is the pacemaker programmed to do once atrial activity is detected? If the pacemaker is programmed to trigger ventricular pacing with sensed atrial activity, is there a ventricular paced complex at the programmed A-V interval? If not, is there an intrinsic QRS complex that occurred before the A-V interval has been completed?	Troubleshoots programming of the pacemaker as well as the electrical response of the atria and ventricules.	
b. If there is no intrinsic atrial activity present, determine whether the pacemaker is programmed to pace the atrium. If atrial pacing should be occurring, determine the lower rate limit that the pacemaker will stimulate atrial activity (a paced atrial event should occur at the end of the VA interval). Evaluate whether the pacemaker is firing at this rate. If pacemaker spike is present but evidence of atrial capture is not present, attempt to assess the presence of atrial contraction by looking at the CVP waveform (if available).	Troubleshoots programming of the pacemaker and atrial response.	
c. Look for ventricular activity. Is the pacemaker programmed to detect intrinsic activity? Is it sensed appropriately? What is the pacemaker programmed to do once ventricular activity is sensed? Does inhibition of ventricular pacing occur?	Determines the presence of ventricular activity and response to pacemaker actions.	
d. If there is no intrinsic ventricular activity, determine whether the pacemaker is programmed to pace the ventricles. If pacing should occur, identify the lower rate limit and determine whether ventricular pacing spikes are occurring at this rate. If ventricular pacing spikes are occurring at intervals that are longer than the lower rate limit, evaluate for oversensing of unwanted signals. If ventricular pacing spikes are occurring at intervals that are shorter than the lower rate limit, determine whether there is hidden atrial activity that is triggering a ventricular output (if appropriate for the	Troubleshoots the relationship between pacemaker programming and ventricular response.	

Table continues on following page

Steps	Rationale	Special Considerations
programmed mode) or suspect undersensing. Determine whether each ventricular pacing spike is followed by a QRS complex. If the pacemaker has an upper rate limit, determine whether the patient is being paced appropriately once that limit has been reached.		
e. If antitachycardic pacing is programmed, determine whether the tachycardia detection criterion has been met and if the pacemaker intervened appropriately.	Determines appropriate pacemaker function.	
2. Assess the patient's hemodynamic response.	It is possible for the patient to have electrical activity of pacing occurring without the associated mechanical activity of cardiac contraction (electromechanical dissociation).	
3. If inappropriate pacemaker function is detected, notify the physician immediately.	Inappropriate pacemaker function may compromise the cardiac output and require immediate adjustment of settings and/or replacement of malfunctioning components.	

Evaluation

1. Monitor the ECG continuously for the presence of a rhythm that is consistent with the programmed pacing parameters. **Rationale:** Indicates ongoing functioning of the permanent pacemaker.

2. Evaluate the hemodynamic response to pacing, and compare with baseline. **Rationale:** Allows the nurse to evaluate the patient's physiologic response to pacing.

Expected Outcomes

1. Adequate systemic tissue perfusion and cardiac output, as evidenced by having a blood pressure greater than 90 mmHg systolic, mean arterial blood pressure greater than 60 mmHg; being alert and oriented, without complaints of dizziness and shortness of breath, nausea and vomiting due to hypotension, or ischemic chest pain. **Rationale:** Adequate systemic perfusion and cardiac output promote function of vital organs.

2. Absence of hemodynamically significant dysrhythmias. **Rationale:** Return of rhythm stability promotes an adequate cardiac output.

3. Appropriate heart rate and proper sensing and proper capture demonstrated on ECG. **Rationale:** Ensures pacing is being delivered consistent with set parameters.

Unexpected Outcomes

1. Failure to sense with the possibility of R-on-T phenomenon (initiation of ventricular tachycardia as a result of an improperly timed pacer spike). **Rationale:** Inability of the pacemaker to detect the patient's underlying rhythm may cause inadvertent electrical competition and may potentiate life-threatening ventricular dysrhythmias.

2. Failure to capture. **Rationale:** Inability of the pacemaker to stimulate the heart to contract will prevent the pacemaker from supplementing or interrupting the dysrhythmias, allowing the clinical condition to persist.

3. Failure to pace. **Rationale:** Inability of the pacemaker to deliver an electric stimulus will prevent the pacemaker from supplementing or interrupting the dysrhythmia, allowing the clinical condition to persist.

4. Pacemaker-mediated tachycardia. **Rationale:** With pacemakers in which atrial triggering occurs, it is possible that retrograde conduction of a ventricular impulse to the atria can cause initiation of a reentrant tachycardia in which the patient is paced at the upper rate limit.

5. Pacemaker syndrome. **Rationale:** With single-chamber pacing, the patient may not be paced at a rate consistent with metabolic need. Coordination of atrial and ventricular activity is absent, creating symptoms of decreased cardiac output.

Documentation

Documentation in the patient record should include pacemaker history; programmed parameters; ECG rhythm strip; an evaluation of pacemaker function; vital signs, physical assessment parameters, and subjective comments; any interventions and the patient's response; and patient education provided and evaluation of patient and family understanding. **Rationale:** Provides a record of the clinical events associated with assessment of permanent pacing and nursing care rendered.

Patient/Family Education

1. Assess learning needs, readiness to learn, and factors that will influence learning. **Rationale:** Allows the nurse to individualize teaching in a meaningful manner.

2. Provide information about the normal conduction system, such as structure of the electrical system, source of heart beat, normal and abnormal heart rhythms, and symptoms of abnormal heart rhythms. **Rationale:** Understanding of the normal conduction system will assist the patient and family in recognizing the seriousness of the patient's condition and the need for permanent pacing.

3. Provide information about permanent pacing, such as reason for pacing, explanation of the equipment, what to expect during permanent pacing, precautions and restrictions in activities of daily living, signs and symptoms of complications and instruction when to call the physician or seek assistance, and information on patient follow-up. **Rationale:** Understanding of pacemaker functioning and expectations after discharge assists the patient and family in developing realistic perceptions of permanent pacing and in being able to manage effectively after discharge.

4. Provide information about transtelephonic monitoring. **Rationale:** Periodic pacemaker checks over the phone may be required for routine monitoring or if there is a change in the patient's condition.

Performance Checklist
Skill 11–5: Permanent Pacing: Assessing the Modes

Critical Behaviors	Complies	
	yes	no
1. Assess the rhythm for pacemaker activity.		
2. Assess the hemodynamic response to pacing.		
3. Communicate findings to physician (if inappropriate function is detected).		
4. Document findings and ECG strip in patient record.		

REFERENCES

Altamura, G., et al. (1989). Treatment of ventricular and supraventricular tachyarrhythmias by transcutaneous cardiac pacing. *PACE* 12:331–337.
Bass, L. S., and Schneider, C. L. (1986). Temporary epicardial electrodes. *Dimens. Crit. Care Nurs.* 5(2):80–92.
Medtronic, Inc. (1988). *Pulse Generator 5375 Technical Manual.* Minneapolis, Minn.: Medtronic.

BIBLIOGRAPHY

American Heart Association (1987). *Textbook of Advanced Cardiac Life Support.* Dallas: American Heart Association.
Baxter Healthcare Corporation, Edwards Critical-Care Division (1986). *Clinical Evaluation of the Swan-Ganz Thermodilution Paceport Catheter and Chandler Transluminal V-Pacing Probe: Results in 100 Patients.* Santa Ana, Calif.: Baxter.
Berstein, A. D., Camm, A. J., Fletcher, R. D., et al. (1987). The NASPE/BPEG generic code for antibradyarrhythmia and adaptive-rate pacing and antitachyarrhythmia devices. *PACE* 10:794–799.
Birdsal, C. (1987). When is A-V sequential pacing used? *Am. J. Nurs.* 87(5):598–599.
Camm, J., and Ward, D. (1983). Overdrive and Underdrive Stimulation for Tachycardia Termination. In *Pacing and Tachycardia Control* (pp. 59–84). Englewood, Colo.: Telectronics.
Carpenito, L. J. (1987). *Nursing Diagnosis: Application to Clinical Practice*, 2d Ed. Philadelphia: Lippincott.
Colardyn, F., Vandenbogaerde, J., DeNiel, C., et al. (1986). Ventricular pacing via a Swan-Ganz catheter: A new mode of pacemaker therapy. *Acta Cardiol.*, 41:23–29.
Conover, E. L. (1986). Electrical Hazards. In A. G. Tilkian and E. K. Daily (Eds.), *Cardiovascular Procedures* (pp. 466–476). St. Louis: Mosby.
Conover, M. B. (1988). Supraventricular Ectopics. In M. B. Conover

(Ed.), *Understanding Electrocardiography*, 5th Ed. (pp. 97–132). St. Louis: Mosby.
Conover, M. B. (1988). Electrograms. In M. B. Conover (Ed.), *Understanding Electrocardiography*, 5th Ed. (pp. 351–360). St. Louis: Mosby.
Conover, M. B. (1988). Pacemakers. In M. B. Conover (Ed.), *Understanding Electrocardiography*, 5th Ed. (pp. 387–414). St. Louis: Mosby.
Crockett, P., and McHugh, L. G. (1988). *Noninvasive Pacing: What You Should Know.* Redmond, Wash.: Physiocontrol Corporation.
Eitel, D. R., et al. (1987). Noninvasive transcutaneous cardiac pacing in prehospital cardiac arrest. *Ann. Emerg. Med.*, 16:531–534.
Finkelmeier, B. A., and O'Mara, S. R. (1984). Temporary pacing in the cardiac surgical patient. *Crit. Care Nurs.* 5(3):21–24, 108–114.
Finkelmeier, B. A., and Salinger, M. H. (1984). The atrial electrogram: It's diagnostic use following cardiac surgery. *Crit. Care Nurs.* 00:42–46.
Fisher, J. D., Matos, J. A. and Kim, S. G. (1984). Antitachycardia Pacing and Stimulation. In M. E. Josephson and H. J. J. Wellens (Eds.), *Tachycardias: Mechanisms, Diagnosis, Treatment* (pp. 413–425). Philadelphia: Lea and Febiger.
Haskin, J. B. (1989). Pacemakers. In S. L. Underwood, S. L. Woods, E. S. Sivarajan, Froelicher, and C. J. Halpenny (Eds.), *Cardiac Nursing*, 2d Ed. (pp. 766–812). Philadelphia: Lippincott.
Haywood, D. L. (1985). Temporary A-V sequential pacing using an epicardial lead system. *Crit. Care Nurs.* 5(3):21–24.

Waldo, A. L., and MacLean, W. H. (1983). *Diagnosis and Treatment of Cardiac Arrhythmias Following Open Heart Surgery: Emphasis on the Use of Atrial and Ventricular Epicardial Wire Electrodes.* New York: Futura.
Wulff, K. S. (1982). Use of temporary epicardial electrodes for atrial pacing and monitoring. *Cardiovasc. Nurs.* 18(1):1–5.

Heiselman, D. E., Maxwell, J. S., and Petno, V. (1986). Electrode displacement from a multipurpose Swan-Ganz catheter. *PACE* 9:134–136.

Huang, S. H., Kessler, C., McCulloch, C., and Dasher, L. A. (1989). *Coronary Care Nursing.* Philadelphia: Saunders.

Instromedix, Inc. (1990). *Lifesigns Receiving Center, Operation and Service Manual.* Hillsboro, Ore.: Instromedix.

Instromedix, Inc. (1986). *A + V Super Transmitter, Operation and Service Manual.* Hillsboro, Ore.: Instromedix.

Luck, J. C., and Davis, D. (1987). Termination of sustained tachycardia by external noninvasive pacing. *PACE* 10:1125–1129.

Macander, P. J., Kuhnlein, J. L., Buteweg, J., et al. (1986). Electrode detachment: A complication of the indwelling pacing Swan-Ganz catheter. *N. Engl. J. Med.* 314:1711.

Mickus, D., Monahan, K. J., and Brown, C. (1986). Exciting external pacemakers. *Am. J. Nurs.* 86(4):403–405.

Mills, N. L., and Oschener, J. L. (1973). Experience with atrial pacemaker wires implanted during cardiac operations. *J. Thorac. Cardiovasc. Surg.* 66(6):878–885.

Monico, L. M. (1990). Artificial Cardiac Pacing. In C. M. Hudak, B. M. Gallo, and J. J. Benz (Eds.), *Critical Care Nursing: A Holistic Approach* (pp. 144–161). Philadelphia: Lippincott.

Morelli, R. L., and Goldschlager, N. (1987). The technique of inserting a transvenous pacing catheter. *J. Crit. Illness* 2(3):63–73.

Morelli, R. L., and Goldschlager, N. (1987). Temporary transvenous pacing: Resolving postinsertion problems. *J. Crit. Illness* 2(4):73–80.

Moses, H. W., Taylor, G. J., Schneider, J. A., and Dove, J. T. (1987). *A Practical Guide to Cardiac Pacing*, 2d Ed. Boston: Little, Brown.

Pennock, R., and Snyder, S. (1984). Pacemaker Follow-Up. In A., A-HadiHakki (Ed.), *Ideal Cardiac Pacing* (pp. 182–194). Philadelphia: Saunders.

Person, C. B. (1987). Transcutaneous pacing: Meeting the challenge. *Focus Crit. Care* 14(1):13–19.

Pierce, C. D. (1989). Transcutaneous cardiac pacing: Expanding clinical applications. *Crit. Care Clin. North Am.* 1(2):423–435.

Powe, A., and Conover, M. (1988). Troubleshooting DDD Electrograms. In M. B. Conover (Ed.), *Understanding Electrocardiography*, 5th Ed. (pp. 415–427). St. Louis: Mosby.

Pride, H. B., and McKinley, D. F. (1990). Third-degree burns from the use of an external cardiac pacing device. *Crit. Care Med.* 18(5):572–573.

Purcell, J. A., and Burrows, S. G. (1985). A pacemaker primer. *Am. J. Nurs.* 85(5):553–568.

Sager, D. P. (1987). Current facts on pacemaker electromagnetic interference and their application to clinical care. *Heart Lung* 16(2):211–221.

Schultz, C. K., and Woodall, C. E. (1989). Using epicardial pacing electrodes. *J. Cardiovasc. Nurs.* 3(3):25–33.

Strickland, R. A., and Reves, J. G. (1983). Uses of temporary pacemakers in the perioperative period. *Semin. Anesth.* 2(4):276–286.

Sulzbach, L. M. (1985). The use of temporary atrial wire electrodes to record atrial electrograms in patients who had cardiac surgery. *Heart Lung* 14(6):540–548.

Thelan, L. A., Davie, J. K., and Urden, J. D. (1990). *Textbook of Critical Care Nursing: Diagnosis and Management.* St. Louis: Mosby.

Trankina, M. F., and White, R. D. (1989). Perioperative cardiac pacing using an atrioventricular pacing pulmonary artery catheter. *J. Cardiothorac. Anesth.* 3(2):154–162.

Vitello-Cicciu, J. M., et al. (1987). Profile of patients requiring the use of epicardial pacing wires after coronary artery bypass surgery. *Heart Lung* 16(3):301–305.

Waldo, A. L., MacLean, W.A.H., Cooper, T. B., et al. (1978). Use of temporarily placed epicardial atrial wire electrodes for the diagnosis and treatment of cardiac arrhythmias following open-heart surgery. *J. Thorac. Cardiovasc. Surg.* 76(4):500–505.

Waldo, A. L., Ross, S. M., and Kaiser, G. A. (1971). The epicardial electrogram in the diagnosis of cardiac arrhythmias following cardiac surgery. *Geriatrics* 00:108–112.

Wiener, I., and Conover, M. B. (1986). Pacemakers. In A. G. Tilkian and E. K. Daily (Eds.), *Cardiovascular Procedures* (pp. 290–313). St. Louis: Mosby.

Zaidan, J. R., and Freniere, S. (1983). Use of a pacing pulmonary artery catheter during cardiac surgery. *Ann. Thorac. Surg.* 35(6):633–636.

Zoll, P. (1987). Noninvasive temporary cardiac pacing. *J. Electrophysiol.* 1(2):156–161.

CIRCULATORY ASSIST DEVICES: CONTROL TECHNIQUES

BEHAVIORAL OBJECTIVES

After completing this chapter, the nurse will be able to

- Define the key terms.
- Describe the devices for circulatory assistance.
- Identify the indications and contraindications for circulatory assist devices.
- Identify troubleshooting techniques for circulatory assist devices.

Adequate circulation is essential to support the myocardium and systemic perfusion. When patients present with inadequate circulation and altered hemodynamics as a result of hypovolemia, fluid overload, myocardial ischemia, depressed myocardial activity, and mechanical defects, the key to successful management is problem identification and rapid intervention. The choice of therapy depends on the cause of the circulatory deficit and the degree of hemodynamic instability.

Improvement in cardiac output is achieved through the use of circulatory assist devices to augment venous return and venous resistance. The goal of therapy is to promote adequate myocardial and cerebral perfusion.

The left ventricular assist device (LVAD) also is being used with increased frequency in patients with severe cardiogenic shock. The LVAD is more effective than the IABP and is capable of pumping total systemic blood flow.

KEY TERMS

cardiac output
congestive heart failuure
diuretics
inatropic agents
interstitial tissue
neurovascular status
peripheral vascular
  resistance
pneumatic counterpressure
preload

pulmonary artery wedge
  pressure
pulmonary edema
pulsus alternans
right atrial pressure
sequester
tourniquet
vasodilators
venous return

SKILLS

12–1   Intraaortic Balloon Pump Management
12–2   External Counterpressure with Pneumatic Antishock Garments
12–3   Rotating Tourniquets

GUIDELINES

The following assessment guidelines assist the nurse in formulating nursing diagnoses and an individualized plan of care for the patient with a circulatory assist device:

1. Know the patient's baseline hemodynamic and respiratory status.
2. Know the patient's baseline neurovascular examination.
3. Know the patient's medical history.
4. Know the patient's medical and nursing treatment plan.
5. Know the indications and contraindications for instituting a specific circulatory assist device.
6. Perform systematic cardiovascular, respiratory, and neurovascular assessments.
7. Determine appropriate interventions based on assessment findings.
8. Know the equipment and become adept in performing the skills used for assisting circulation.

SKILL 12–1

Intraaortic Balloon Pump Management

Cardiac assistance via the intraaortic balloon pump (IABP) is performed to improve myocardial oxygen supply and reduce cardiac workload. It is an acute, short-term therapy for patients with reversible left ventricular failure or as an adjunct to other therapies for irreversible heart failure.

Initiation of IABP therapy is indicated in cardiogenic shock, mechanical defects, refractory angina, recurrent ventricular dysrhythmias due to ischemia, prophylaxis prior to cardiac surgery, failure to wean from cardiopulmonary bypass, and left ventricular failure after cardiopulmonary bypass. Contraindications to balloon pump therapy are moderate to severe aortic insufficiency and thoracic and abdominal aortic aneurysms. The relative value of IABP therapy in the presence of severe aortoiliac disease, major coagulopathies, and terminal disease should be evaluated individually.

Intraaortic balloon pumping is based on the principles of counterpulsation (Fig. 12–1). The events of the cardiac cycle provide the stimulus for balloon function, and the movement of helium or CO_2 gas between the balloon and the control console gas source produces inflation and deflation of the balloon. Recognition of the R wave or QRS complex on the ECG is the most commonly used trigger for balloon deflation. Deflation should occur just prior to ventricular systole or ejection. This decreases

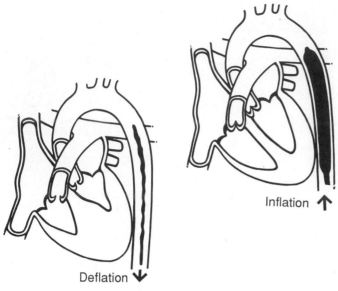

FIGURE 12–1. Counterpulsation. (Reprinted with permission from Datascope Corp., Montvale, New Jersey.)

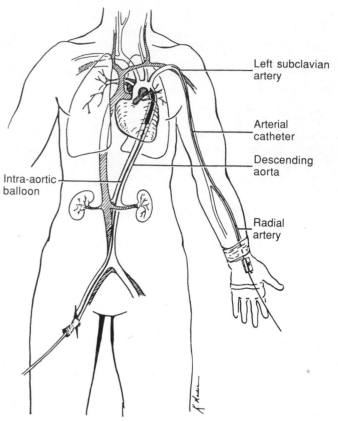

FIGURE 12–2. Correct intraaortic balloon catheter placement. (Reprinted with permission from S. J. Quaal, *Comprehensive Intraaortic Balloon Pumping*. St. Louis: Mosby, 1984.)

the pressure within the aortic root, reducing afterload and cardiac workload. Inflation occurs during ventricular diastole, causing an increase in aortic pressure. This increased pressure displaces blood proximally to the coronary arteries and distally to the rest of the body. The result is an increase in myocardial oxygen supply and subsequent improvement in cardiac output.

The IAB catheter can be placed in the femoral artery via percutaneous puncture or arteriotomy. Surgical placement via the transthoracic approach also may be used. Fluoroscopy may be used to aid in proper IAB catheter positioning, especially with a tortuous aorta. Correct catheter position must be verified via radiography if fluoroscopy is not used during catheter insertion. The IAB catheter should lie inferior to the subclavian artery and superior to the renal arteries (Fig. 12–2). This position allows for maximum balloon effect without occlusion of other arterial supply.

Single- or double-lumen catheters may be used. The majority of IAB catheters are wrapped by the manufacturer for ease of insertion. The central lumen of many IAB catheters provides a means for monitoring aortic pressure. The mechanics of the control console vary from manufacturer to manufacturer. Specific information concerning controls, alarms, troubleshooting, and safety features is available from each manufacturer and should be read thoroughly by the nurse prior to use of the equipment.

Purpose

The nurse maintains intraaortic balloon pump therapy to

1. Increase coronary artery perfusion.
2. Increase systemic perfusion.
3. Decrease myocardial workload.
4. Decrease afterload.

Prerequisite Knowledge and Skills

Prior to caring for a patient undergoing IABP therapy, the nurse should understand

1. Principles of aseptic technique.
2. Anatomy and physiology of the cardiovascular and peripheral vascular systems.
3. Principles of hemodynamic monitoring.
4. Principles of coagulation.
5. Principles of counterpulsation.

The nurse should be able to perform

1. Proper handwashing technique (see Skill 35–5).
2. Vital signs assessment.
3. Cardiovascular and peripheral vascular assessment.
4. Hemodynamic assessment.
5. Blood sampling for hematologic and coagulation profiles.
6. Pain assessment.
7. Cardiac output and cardiac index determinations (see Skill 10–9).
8. Titration of vasoactive agents.
9. Universal precautions (see Skill 35–1).

Assessment

1. Assess for signs and symptoms of cardiac failure requiring IABP therapy, including systolic blood pres-

sure less than 90 mmHg, cardiac index less than 2.5, pulmonary artery wedge pressure greater than 18 mmHg, MAP less than 70 mmHg with vasopressor support, inadequate peripheral perfusion, urine output less than 0.5 cc/kg per minute, altered mental status, heart rate greater than 110 beats per minute, dysrhythmias, decreased mixed venous oxygen saturation, and unstable angina. **Rationale:** Physical signs and symptoms result from the heart's inability to adequately contract and/or inadequate coronary artery perfusion.

2. Assess extremity for quality and strength of femoral popliteal, dorsalis pedal, and posterior tibial pulses. **Rationale:** The IAB catheter will be inserted into the vasculature of the extremity exhibiting the best perfusion.

Nursing Diagnoses

1. Altered cardiac output (decreased) related to left ventricular failure, increased afterload, and/or myocardial ischemia. **Rationale:** A decrease in myocardial contractility, an increased resistance to ejection, and a decreased myocardial oxygen supply will diminish the heart's ability to meet the tissue's oxygen demands adequately.

2. Alteration in comfort related to angina, incisional pain, catheter insertion, and/or immobility. **Rationale:** Angina will result if the myocardial oxygen requirements are greater than the oxygen supply. Patients who have the IAB catheter inserted before or after cardiac surgery will additionally experience postoperative incisional discomfort. Pain may be experienced at the insertion site, especially initially after insertion. Bed rest and relative immobility of the extremity with the IAB catheter may create generalized discomfort.

3. Alteration in mobility related to required bed rest and immobilized extremity with the balloon in place. **Rationale:** Bed rest and immobilization of the affected extremity are important so that the IAB catheter is not kinked, disconnected, or dislodged.

4. Potential alteration in tissue perfusion (cerebral, renal, mesenteric, or extremity) related to thrombus formation and/or particle emboli or migration of the IAB catheter. **Rationale:** If the IAB catheter is advanced too far, circulation to the left arm can be altered if the left subclavian artery is occluded. If the IAB catheter is too low, it may occlude the mesenteric or renal arteries. Air emboli from a ruptured balloon or dislodged thrombi from the insertion site or IAB catheter may cause altered perfusion to the cerebral, renal, mesenteric, or peripheral circulation.

5. Potential fluid volume deficit, hemorrhage related to mechanical trauma of IABP therapy, and blood loss. **Rationale:** Platelet integrity may be disrupted because of mechanical trauma from the balloon inflating and deflating. Anticoagulation also may contribute to blood loss.

6. Potential for infection related to invasive IAB catheter. **Rationale:** Because of the location of the insertion site (femoral artery), the urgent manner in which the IAB catheter is usually inserted, and the patient's debilitated condition, the patient is at increased risk for infection.

7. Knowledge deficit related to the purpose and need for IABP therapy. **Rationale:** Often IABP therapy is initiated emergently. Both the patient and family will need information regarding the reasons for insertion and how the therapy supports the myocardium.

8. Potential ineffective patient and family coping related to IABP therapy. **Rationale:** The patient and family may be disappointed by the patient's need for IABP therapy. The critical nature of the illness may be difficult for the patient and family to cope with.

Planning

1. Individualize the following goals for IABP management:
   a. Identify patient need for IABP therapy and perform a baseline physical assessment. **Rationale:** Early initiation of IABP therapy is essential to prevent cardiac decompensation and death. Baseline assessment is necessary in order to identify further physiologic changes.
   b. Effective IABP therapy that will increase oxygen supply to the myocardium, decrease myocardial workload, and increase cardiac output. **Rationale:** During diastole, the balloon inflates, which increases intraaortic pressure and blood flow to the coronary arteries and to the periphery. Deflation of the balloon occurs just prior to systole, resulting in a reduction of afterload or resistance to left ventricular ejection.
   c. Maintain accurate IABP timing. **Rationale:** If timing is not accurate, cardiac output may be decreased rather than increased.
   d. Identify parameters that will demonstrate clinical readiness to wean from IABP therapy. **Rationale:** Close observation of the patient's tolerance to weaning procedures is necessary to ensure that the body's oxygen demands can be met.

2. Prepare all necessary equipment and supplies. **Rationale:** Assembly of all the necessary equipment at the bedside ensures that IABP therapy will be initiated quickly and efficiently.
   a. IAB catheter, size range is 8.5 to 12 French for adults. Prepare console and check gas supply and console.
   b. Povidone-iodine solution.
   c. IAB catheter insertion kit.
   d. ECG and arterial pressure monitoring supplies (see Skills 7–1 and 10–2).
   e. Caps, masks, sterile gowns, gloves, and drapes.
   f. Sterile dressing supplies.
   g. O-silk suture on a cutting needle, used to suture catheter to skin.
   h. No. 11 scalpel, used for skin entry.
   i. 1% lidocaine without epinephrine, one 30-cc vial.
   j. Emergency drugs and resuscitation equipment.

k. Stopcocks, one 2-way and one 3-way.
l. Specimen syringe.
m. Vasopressors as prescribed.
n. Prescribed IV solutions.
o. 500 cc normal saline with 1000 U heparin or flush solution recommended in your institution.
p. Hemodynamic monitoring tubing with transducer (see Skill 10–5).
q. Analgesics/sedatives as prescribed.
r. Heparin infusion or dextran if prescribed.
s. Antibiotics if prescribed.
t. Lead apron.
u. 1 Luer-lok plug.

3. Prepare the patient.
   a. Explain the procedure. **Rationale:** Teaching provides information and may decrease anxiety and fear.
   b. Explain the patient's expected participation during the procedure. **Rationale:** Encourages patient compliance.
   c. Explain the importance of keeping the affected extremity immobile. **Rationale:** Encourages patient compliance.

d. Validate patency of central and peripheral venous line. **Rationale:** Central access is needed for vasopressor administration; peripheral access is needed for fluid administration.
e. Obtain current lab profile including CBC, platelet count prothrombin time (PT), partial thromboplastin time (PTT), and bleeding time. **Rationale:** Baseline coagulation studies are helpful in determining an increased risk for bleeding. Platelet function may be affected by the mechanical trauma from balloon inflation and deflation.
f. Place patient in a supine position and shave and prep both groins with povidone iodine solution. **Rationale:** Provides for site access and patient comfort.
g. Drape the patient with sterile sheets from neck to feet. **Rationale:** Prepares the sterile field.
h. Assist with 1% lidocaine administration. **Rationale:** Anesthetizes the surrounding skin and subcutaneous tissue.

Implementation

Steps	Rationale	Special Considerations
1. Wash hands.	Reduces transmission of microorganisms.	
2. Provide and don caps, masks, sterile gowns, and gloves for the physician, all assistants, and patient.	Universal precautions.	
3. Turn on gas supply of either helium or carbon dioxide.	Activates the gas driving balloon pump.	Check manufacturer's recommendations.
4. Sedate the patient as needed; the affected extremity may need to be restrained.	Movement of the lower extremity may inhibit insertion of the catheter.	
5. Establish ECG input to IABP console and obtain ECG configuration with optimal R wave amplitude and absence of artifact. Indirect ECG input can be obtained via "slave" of bedside ECG to IABP console.	The R wave, QRS complex, or arterial pressure waveform may be the trigger for balloon inflation and deflation. Patient cable from console establishes ECG.	A secondary ECG source is desirable in the event of lead disconnection or loss of trigger. Review manufacturer's instructions for selecting the appropriate trigger control. If the patient has a pacemaker, the trigger should be set to reject the pacemaker artifact.
6. Assist physician with placement of hemodynamic lines if not already present (see Skill 10–2).	Hemodynamic monitoring is necessary for assessment and management of a patient requiring IABP therapy.	Radial arterial line if the central lumen arterial pressure will not be used. The arterial tracing is used to optimize timing and also may be used as a trigger source.
7. Complete IABP console preparation. Refer to instruction manual.	Ensures adequate functioning of the IABP device.	Models of the pump console vary. Review of manufacturer's instructions is recommended.

Table continues on following page

Steps	Rationale	Special Considerations
8. Remove from sterile packing and place on the sterile field the balloon catheter and insertion tray.	Makes available supplies while maintaining sterility.	
9. Administer heparin bolus prior to arterial puncture, if prescribed.	Anticoagulation may decrease the incidence of thromboemboli related to the indwelling IAB catheter.	Systemic anticoagulation may not be used in all patients.
10. Attach a stopcock and 50 cc syringe to the Luer tip of the distal end of the balloon lumen.	Creates a device for air removal from the balloon device.	Maintains wrap of balloon for insertion.
11. Open the stopcock system from the balloon to the syringe.	Allows for air aspiration from the balloon.	
12. Pull back slowly on the syringe until all air is aspired.	Creates a vacuum and removes air from the balloon.	
13. Turn the stopcock off to the balloon and disconnect syringe.	Prevents air entry back into balloon.	
14. Lubricate the catheter with sterile saline.	Decrease "drag" on the catheter during insertion.	
15. The central lumen of the IAB catheter may be flushed with heparinized saline prior to insertion.	Removes air from the central lumen.	If the catheter is not flushed prior to insertion, allow backflow of arterial blood before connection to the flush system.
16. Assist the physician with introducer sheath/dilator assembly and insertion.	Prepares for balloon catheter entry.	
17. Assist the physician with balloon catheter insertion through the introducer sheath.	Catheter placement is necessary part of IAB setup.	
18. Assist the physician with stopcock removal and balloon unwrapping according to the manufacturer's recommendations.	Releases the vacuum and readies the balloon for counterpulsation.	
19. If the central lumen of a double-lumen catheter is used to monitor arterial pressure, attach a three-way stopcock with continuous heparinized flush and transducer to the monitor. Set the alarms.	Monitors arterial pressure.	The central lumen, if used, must be attached to an alarm because undetected disconnection could cause life-threatening bleeding.
20. Avoid fast flush and blood sampling from the central aortic lumen.	Some manufacturers and institutions recommend hourly manual flush of central lumen lines. However, the risk of air embolus entry or dislodging a thrombus at the lumen tip is a major concern. Refer to your institution's policy in regard to fast flush or manual flushing of central lumen catheters.	Some institutions do not recommend the use of the central lumen for blood sampling because of the risk of air entry or potential dislodgment of emboli or formation of thrombus. Refer to your institution's policy.
21. If the central aortic lumen is not used to monitor arterial pressure, aspirate 3 to 5 cc of blood from the lumen and cap with a Luer-lok plug.	Allows clotting of the central lumen and prevents air or thrombus entry into the aorta.	
22. Attach the balloon-lumen tubing to the pump console.	Attachment is necessary as the console programs and operates balloon counterpulsation.	

Table continues on following page

Steps	Rationale	Special Considerations
23. Follow steps for timing, standard care, and troubleshooting (pp. 414–419).	Provides for appropriate operation of counterpulsation.	
24. Zero and calibrate pressure transducers.	Ensures accurate timing, maintenance, and functioning of the IABP.	
25. Order a portable chest x-ray as soon as possible.	Correct IAB catheter position must be confirmed to prevent complications associated with interference with arterial blood supply.	If fluoroscopy is used for insertion of the catheter, x-ray immediately after placement will not be necessary.
26. Apply dressing to catheter insertion site.	Allows for aseptic management.	
27. Remove and discard gloves, mask, gown, etc., and wash hands.	Reduces transmission of microorganisms.	
Timing of IABP		
1. Select an ECG lead that optimizes the R wave and decreases other artifacts.	The R wave triggers the balloon to deflate.	An alternate trigger also can be used if necessary.
2. Time the IABP using the arterial waveform.	The arterial waveform assists in identifying accurate IAB inflation and deflation.	
3. Set the IABP frequency to the every other beat setting (1:2) (Fig. 12–3).	Comparison can be made between the assisted and unassisted arterial waveforms.	IABP manufacturers may recommend another timing method (i.e., Kontron: initiating with 1:1 pumping using a feature that compares the patient's unassisted arterial waveform to the assisted arterial waveform).
4. Inflation:		
a. Identify the dicrotic notch of the assisted systolic waveform (Fig. 12–4).	The dicrotic notch represents closure of the aortic valve.	
b. Adjust inflation later to expose the dicrotic notch of the unassisted systolic waveform.	Ensures accurate inflation.	
c. Slowly adjust inflation earlier until the dicrotic notch disappears and a sharp V wave forms (see Fig. 12–3).	Balloon augmentation should occur after the aortic valve closes.	

Table continues on following page

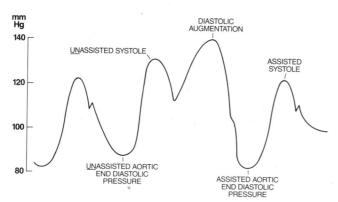

FIGURE 12–3. 1:2 intraaortic balloon pump frequency. (Reprinted with permission from Datascope Corp., Montvale, New Jersey.)

Timing Errors
Late Inflation

Inflation of the IAB markedly after closure of the aortic valve

Waveform Characteristics:
- Inflation of the IAB after the dicrotic notch.
- Absence of sharp V
- Sub-optimal diastolic augmentation

Physiologic Effects:
- Sub-optimal coronary artery perfusion

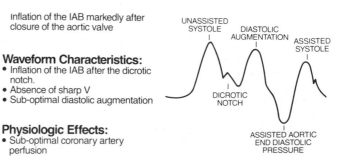

FIGURE 12–4. Late inflation. (Reprinted with permission from Datascope Corp., Montvale, New Jersey.)

Steps	Rationale	Special Considerations
d. Compare the diastolic augmentation to the unassisted systole.	Balloon augmentation should be equal to or greater than the patient's unassisted systolic blood pressure.	If the balloon augmentation is less than the patient's systolic pressure, consider that balloon is positioned too low, there is hypovolemia or tachycardia, or the balloon volume is set too low.
e. Adjust inflation if needed.	Necessary to achieve optimal diastolic augmentation.	Timing of inflation will vary slightly depending on the location of the arterial line. Aortic root: Inflate after exposing the dicrotic notch. Radial: Inflate 40 to 50 ms prior to the dicrotic notch. Femoral: Inflate 120 ms prior to the dicrotic notch (Fig. 12–5). Because of the distance of the radial and femoral arteries from the actual closure of the aortic valve, the arterial pressures are delayed.

Table continues on following page

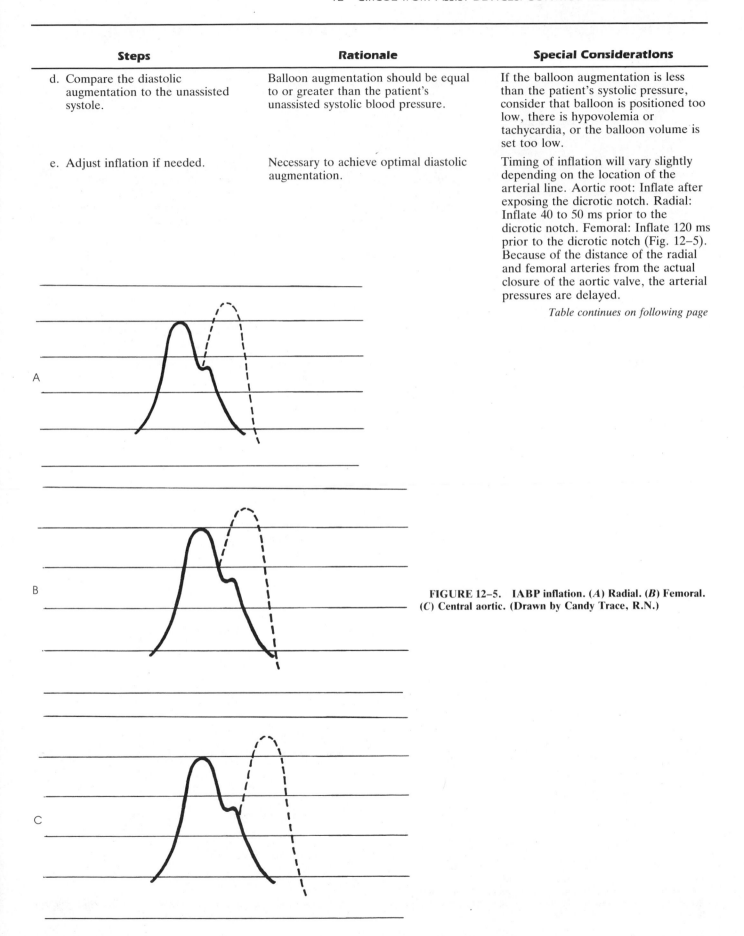

FIGURE 12–5.   IABP inflation. (*A*) Radial. (*B*) Femoral. (*C*) Central aortic. (Drawn by Candy Trace, R.N.)

Steps	Rationale	Special Considerations
5. Deflation:		
a. Identify the assisted and unassisted aortic end-diastolic pressures and the assisted and unassisted systolic pressures. Ratio is usually 1:1 or 1:2.	These landmarks are important in determining accurate IAB deflation.	
b. Set the balloon to deflate so that the balloon-assisted aortic end-diastolic pressure is as low as possible while still maintaining optimal diastolic augmentation and not impeding on the next systole.	The assisted systolic pressure will be less than the unassisted systolic pressure due to a decrease in afterload, thus reducing the myocardial workload.	Reduction of afterload will decrease the energy required by the heart during systole. It is important to achieve afterload reduction without diminishing diastolic augmentation.
6. Set the IABP frequency to 1:1 (Fig. 12–6).	Ensures that each heart beat is assisted.	
7. Assess timing every 1 hour and whenever heart rate increases or decreases by more than 10 beats per minute or rhythm changes.	Inappropriate timing prevents effective IABP therapy.	The computerized IABPs vary in the degree of adjustment to changes in heart rate and rhythm. Refer to specific manufacturer's guidelines for automatic timing adjustment.
8. Assess and intervene to correct inappropriate timing:	Ensures accurate timing and optimal functioning of the IABP.	
a. Early inflation (Fig. 12–7). Move inflation later.	Inflation occurs prior to closure of the aortic valve, leading to premature aortic valve closure, increased left ventricular volume, and decreased stroke volume.	
b. Late inflation (see Fig. 12–4). Move inflation earlier.	A delay in inflation leads to a decrease in coronary artery perfusion.	
c. Early deflation (Fig. 12–8). Move deflation later.	Deflation occurs prior to the aortic valve opening, leading to low balloon augmentation and less or no afterload reduction; coronary artery perfusion is also decreased.	Note the sharp diastolic wave after augmentation and the increase in the assisted systolic pressure.

Table continues on following page

1:1 IABP Frequency

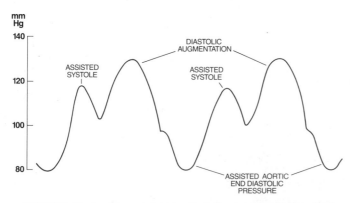

FIGURE 12–6. Correct intraaortic balloon pump timing (1:1). (Reprinted with permission from Datascope Corp., Montvale, New Jersey.)

Timing Errors
Early Inflation

Inflation of the IAB prior to aortic valve closure

Waveform Characteristics:
- Inflation of IAB prior to dicrotic notch.
- Diastolic augmentation encroaches onto systole (may be unable to distinguish)

Physiologic Effects:
- Potential premature closure of aortic valve
- Potential increased in LVEDV and LVEDP or PCWP
- Increased left ventricular wall stress or afterload
- Aortic Regurgitation
- Increased MVO_2 demand

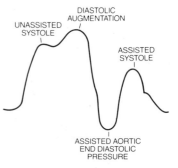

FIGURE 12–7. Early inflation. (Reprinted with permission from Datascope Corp., Montvale, New Jersey.)

Timing Errors
Early Deflation

Premature deflation of the IAB during the diastolic phase

Waveform Characteristics:
- Deflation of IAB is seen as a sharp drop following diastolic augmentation
- Suboptimal diastolic augmentation
- Assisted aortic end diastolic pressure may be equal to or less than the unassisted aortic end diastolic pressure
- Assisted systolic pressure may rise

Physiologic Effects:
- Sub-optimal coronary perfusion
- Potential for retrograde coronary and carotid blood flow
- Angina may occur as a result of retrograde coronary blood flow
- Sub-optimal afterload reduction
- Increased MVO_2 demand

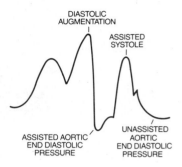

FIGURE 12–8. Early deflation. (Reprinted with permission from Datascope Corp., Montvale, New Jersey.)

Timing Errors
Late Deflation

Deflation of the IAB late in diastolic phase as aortic valve is beginning to open

Waveform Characteristics:
- Assisted aortic end-diastolic pressure may be equal to or greater than the unassisted aortic end diastolic pressure
- Rate of rise of assisted systole is prolonged
- Diastolic augmentation may appear widened

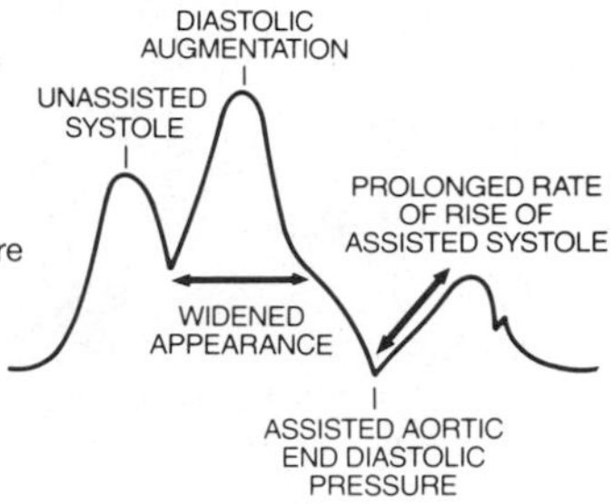

Physiologic Effects:
- Afterload reduction is essentially absent
- Increased MVO_2 consumption due to the left ventricle ejecting against a greater resistance and a prolonged isovolumetric contraction phase
- IAB may impede left ventricular ejection and increase the afterload

FIGURE 12–9. Late deflation. (Reprinted with permission from Datascope Corp., Montvale, New Jersey.)

Steps	Rationale	Special Considerations
d. Late deflation (Fig. 12–9). Move deflation earlier.	Deflation occurs after the aortic valve has opened, leading to an increase in the aortic end-diastolic pressure and an increase in afterload.	Note the delayed diastolic wave after augmentation and the diminished assisted systole.
9. Wash hands.	Reduces transmission of microorganisms.	
Standard Care		
1. Wash hands.	Reduces transmission of microorganisms.	
2. Perform a systematic cardiovascular, peripheral vascular, and hemodynamic assessment.		
a. Level of consciousness (LOC), assess every 15 to 60 minutes.	Assesses adequate cerebral perfusion; thrombi may develop and dislodge during IABP therapy.	
b. Vital signs and pulmonary artery pressures, assess every 15 to 60 minutes.	Demonstrates effectiveness of IABP therapy.	
c. Cardiac output and cardiac index determinations, assess every 15 to 60 minutes during unstable periods.	Demonstrates effectiveness of IABP therapy.	
d. Circulation to the extremities, assess every 15 to 60 minutes.	Validates adequate peripheral perfusion.	
e. Urine output, assess every 15 to 60 minutes.	Validates adequate perfusion of kidneys.	
f. Assess heart and lung sounds every 4 hours and as needed.	Abnormal heart and lung sounds may indicate the need for additional treatment.	When patient's condition permits, place IABP on standby to accurately assess heart and lung sounds.

Table continues on following page

Steps	Rationale	Special Considerations
3. Maintain head of bed at less than 45 degrees.	Prevents kinking of the IAB catheter and migration of catheter.	
4. Logroll patient every 2 hours. Prop pillows to support patient and to maintain alignment.	Promotes comfort and skin integrity and prevents kinking of the IAB catheter.	
5. Immobilize the cannulated extremity with a draw sheet tucked under the mattress or a soft ankle restraint or other leg immobilizer.	Prevents migration of the IAB catheter.	Assess skin integrity and perfusion distal to the restraint every 2 hours.
6. Institute passive and active range-of-motion exercises every 2 hours to extremities that can be mobilized.	Prevents venous stasis and muscle atrophy.	
7. Assess the area around the IAB catheter insertion site every 2 hours and as needed for evidence of hematoma bleeding, or infection.	IAB catheter inflation and deflation traumatizes RBCs. Anticoagulation therapy may alter hemoglobin and hematocrit and coagulation values.	
8. Change the dressing every 24 to 48 hours.	Decreases the incidence of infection and provides an opportunity for site assessment.	Sterile dressing change may include the following: Cleanse site with alcohol, then cleanse site with povidone iodine solution for 1 minute; place povidone ointment on insertion site and cover site with a dry, sterile, occlusive dressing; label with the date, time, and initials.
9. Maintain anticoagulation as prescribed.	The IAB catheter is antithrombogenic, yet prophylactic anticoagulation may be used to prevent thrombi and emboli development.	
Troubleshooting		
1. Atrial fibrillation: Set the IABP to inflate and deflate the majority of the patient's beats.	IABP therapy will not be 100 percent effective during atrial fibrillation (AF) due to the irregular rhythm.	The underlying cause of the AF should be treated. IABPs will automatically deflate the balloon on the R wave. Use the atrial fibrillation trigger mode if available.
2. Tachycardia:		
a. Use helium instead of CO_2.	Helium shuttles faster than CO_2.	
b. Change IABP frequency to 1:2.	Since diastole is shortened during tachycardia, the balloon augmentation time is shortened. Pumping every other beat may improve mean arterial pressure.	
c. Decrease balloon volume and maintain 1:1 frequency.	Decreasing balloon volume will decrease gas shuttle time.	
d. Use delay out if needed and available on the IABP console.	Removes the preset inflation delay.	
3. Asystole:		
a. Switch the trigger to arterial pressure.	This trigger can be used if there is at least a 15 mmHg rise in arterial pressure.	This feature may be available on specific consoles. Refer to the operator's manual for this information.
b. Set inflation to provide diastolic augmentation and deflation to occur prior to upstroke of the next systole.	Programs the machine for appropriate preset timing.	

Table continues on following page

Steps	Rationale	Special Considerations
c. If chest compressions do not provide an adequate trigger:		
(1) Turn to internal trigger.	Internal trigger will keep the catheter fluttering so clot formation is prevented.	
(2) Set the rate at 60 to 80 beats per minute.	Maintains rapid movement of IAB catheter.	
(3) Set the IABP frequency to 1:2.	1:2 frequency is adequate to prevent thrombus formation on the IAB catheter.	
(4) Turn the balloon augmentation down enough to see slight movement of gas in and out of the safety chamber.	Slight inflation and deflation of the IAB catheter will prevent clot formation.	
4. Ventricular tachycardia and ventricular fibrillation:		
a. Ensure that personnel are cleared from the patient and equipment prior to cardioverting or defibrillating (see Skill 8–1, 8–3).	Prevents spread of energy to health care personnel. Maintains electrical safety (See Skill 36–1).	
b. Cardiovert or defibrillate as necessary.	Converts rhythm.	The IABP console is electrically isolated.
5. Loss of vacuum:		
a. Check connections on pneumatic tubing.	A loose connection may have contributed to loss of vacuum.	
b. Check the compressor power source.	Ensures that power is available to drive helium.	
c. Use backup CO_2 or helium tank if available.	Ensures that gas is available to fill the IAB catheter.	Some IABP manufacturers use helium tanks only.
d. Hand inflate and deflate the balloon every 5 minutes with half of the total amount the balloon holds if necessary.	Prevents clot formation along the dormant balloon.	
6. Suspected balloon rupture:		
a. Observe for loss of augmentation.	Gas may be gradually leaking from the balloon catheter.	Always set the alarms so the alarm will sound if there is a 10-mmHg drop in diastolic augmentation.
b. Observe safety chamber for wrinkled appearance.	If gas is lost, the chamber will not be full.	
c. Check for blood in the catheter tubing.	Blood in the tubing indicates the balloon has ruptured and arterial blood is present.	
7. Balloon rupture:		
a. Place the IABP on standby.	Prevents further IAB pumping and continued gas exchange.	Some IABP consoles will automatically shut off if a leak is detected. The balloon should be removed within 15 to 30 minutes.
b. Clamp the IAB catheter.	Prevents arterial blood backup.	
c. Notify the physician.	The IAB catheter will need to be removed or replaced immediately.	
d. Prepare for IAB catheter removal.	The IAB catheter should not lie dormant longer than 30 minutes.	
e. Discontinue anticoagulation therapy.	Clotting will occur more readily if anticoagulation is stopped.	

Table continues on following page

Steps	Rationale	Special Considerations
Weaning and IAB Catheter Removal		
1. Assess clinical readiness for weaning:	Optimal clinical and hemodynamic parameters validate readiness for weaning.	
a. Heart rate less than 110 beats per minute.		
b. Absence of lethal or unstable dysrhythmias.	Patient hemodynamic status should be optimal prior to weaning of IABP therapy.	
c. Mean arterial pressure greater than 70 mmHg with little or no vasopressor support.		
d. Pulmonary artery wedge pressure less than 18 mmHg.		
e. Cardiac index greater than 2.5.		
f. Capillary refill less than 3 seconds.		
g. Urine output greater than 0.5 cc/kg per minute.		
h. Mixed venous oxygen saturation between 70% and 80%.		
2. Change assist ratio to 1:2, and monitor patient response for 1 to 6 hours or as noted per protocol.	Length of time required to wean from IABP therapy depends on hemodynamic response of patient and length of time patient has been on IABP therapy.	
3. If hemodynamic parameters remain satisfactory, further change ratio from 1:3 to 1:8 depending on patient and balloon console assist frequencies or as prescribed per protocol.	IABP consoles vary in assist ratios.	When using weaning ratios of 1:3 through 1:8, some manufacturers recommend returning the IABP to 1:1 for 5 minutes every hour to decrease the possibility of clot formation on the balloon. Refer to your institution's policy on weaning procedures.
4. Turn the IABP to standby or off.	Ensures deflation of IAB catheter.	
5. Discontinue heparin or dextran 4 to 6 hours prior to IAB catheter removal or reverse heparin with protamine just prior to catheter removal as prescribed.	This will decrease the likelihood of bleeding after balloon removal.	
6. Assist the physician with removal of percutaneous balloon.	Facilitates removal.	
7. Ensure that hemostasis is obtained after pressure is held on the insertion site for 30 to 45 minutes after the IAB catheter is withdrawn.	Decreases incidence of bleeding and hematoma formation.	
8. Monitor vital signs and hemodynamic parameters every 15 minutes × 4, every 30 minutes × 2, then every 1 hour as the patient's condition warrants.	Validates patient stability or identifies hemodynamic compromise.	

Table continues on following page

Steps	Rationale	Special Considerations
9. Assess the quality of perfusion to the decannulated extremity immediately after removal and every 1 hour × 2, then every 2 hours.	Removal of the IAB catheter may dislodge thrombi on the catheter and lead to arterial occlusion.	
10. Assess insertion site for signs of bleeding or hematoma formation prior to application of a sterile pressure dressing.	Assists in the detection of bleeding.	
11. Apply pressure dressing to the insertion site for 2 to 4 hours. A 5- to 10-lb sand bag also may be applied to the site for 2 to 4 hours.	Decreases bleeding from insertion site.	
12. Maintain immobility of decannulated extremity and bed rest with the head of the bed no greater than 45 degrees for 24 hours.	Promotes healing and decreases stress at the insertion site.	

Evaluation

1. Monitor for signs and symptoms of impaired perfusion to the extremity with the IAB catheter in place, including capillary refill greater than 2 seconds, diminished or absent pulses (popliteal, tibial, pedal), color pale, mottled, or cyanotic, cool or cold to touch, diminished or absent sensation, diminished or absent movement, and calf tenderness. **Rationale:** Signs and symptoms indicative of catheter obstruction of blood flow, thromboembolus, or anterior compartment syndrome, which impair circulation to the extremity.

2. Monitor for signs and symptoms of balloon rupture, including obvious blood or brown flecks in the tubing, loss of IABP augmentation, and control console alarm activation (e.g., gas loss). **Rationale:** If the balloon ruptures, helium or CO_2 will continue to be released into the patient's thoracic aorta, potentially causing an embolic event.

3. Monitor for signs and symptoms of IABP misplacement, including decreased perfusion to the left arm (i.e., capillary refill greater than 2 seconds, diminished or absent pulses, e.g., antecubital and radial, color pale, mottled, or cyanotic, diminished or absent sensation, diminished or absent movement, dampened or flat radial artery tracing, or IAB waveform changes specific to IABP manufacturer), and decreased perfusion to the mesentery and renal arteries (i.e., diminished or absent bowel sounds, increased abdominal girth, abdomen firm to touch, tympany, abdominal pain, decreased urine output, less than 5 cc/kg per minute, increased osmolality of urine, increased BUN/creatinine, or in some cases, reduced IABP augmentation). **Rationale:** The IAB catheter may be positioned too high or too low, thus occluding the left subclavian artery, or the celiac artery, the inferior or superior mesenteric artery, and/or the renal arteries.

4. Monitor for signs and symptoms of pain, including increased heart rate, increased or decreased blood pressure, increased respirations, verbalization of pain, nonverbal responses (restlessness, grimacing, clenching of teeth), and ECG changes. **Rationale:** The patient may experience pain due to angina, IAB catheter placement, or limited mobility.

5. Monitor for signs and symptoms of bleeding and coagulation disorders, including bleeding at the balloon insertion site, incisions, and mucous membranes, petechiae and ecchymoses, positive guiac of nasogastric aspirate or stool specimens, hematuria, decreased hemoglobin and hematocrit, decreased filling pressures, increased heart rate, and retroperitoneal hematoma. **Rationale:** Hematologic and coagulation profiles may be altered as a result of blood loss during balloon insertion, anticoagulation, and platelet dysfunction due to mechanical trauma by balloon inflation and/or deflation.

6. Monitor for signs and symptoms of aortic dissection, including acute back, flank, testicular, and/or chest pain, decreased pulses, variation in blood pressure between left and right arms, decreased cardiac output, increased heart rate, decreased hemoglobin and hematocrit, and decreased filling pressures. **Rationale:** Repeated mechanical inflation and deflation of the IAB catheter may traumatize the aorta.

Expected Outcomes

1. Decreased myocardial oxygen demands. **Rationale:** Afterload is reduced.

2. Increased myocardial oxygen supply. **Rationale:** The coronary arteries receive augmented perfusion during diastole, thus decreasing or preventing chest pain.

3. Increased cardiac output. **Rationale:** Afterload reduction decreases the pressure in the aorta against which the left ventricle contracts.

4. Increased tissue perfusion, including cerebral,

renal, and peripheral circulation. **Rationale:** Increase in cardiac output will improve oxygen supply to all tissues.

Unexpected Outcomes

1.   Labile hemodynamics continue. **Rationale:** Severe left ventricular or biventricular failure may be unresponsive to counterpulsation.

2.   Balloon rupture or gas leak. **Rationale:** Possible damage to the balloon catheter during insertion or pumping against atherosclerotic plaque can cause balloon rupture and possible gas leak.

3.   Ischemia to the affected limb. **Rationale:** Placement of the IAB catheter in a femoral artery may decrease or occlude circulation distal to the insertion site.

4.   Emboli. **Rationale:** Thrombus formation on the balloon catheter can occur despite the antithrombogenic property of the catheter and/or the use of systemic anticoagulation.

5.   Infection. **Rationale:** Patients requiring IABP therapy are already debilitated and can be further compromised by the invasive procedure.

Documentation

Documentation in the patient record should include vital signs every hour or as condition dictates, IABP assist ratio with corresponding blood pressures and IABP pressure and other hemodynamic parameters, vasoactive drug titration, quality of peripheral pulses, tolerance to insertion/removal procedure as appropriate, complaints of pain and measures to relieve pain and patient response, assessment of timing cycle and afterload reduction, response to vasoactive agents and changes in assist ratio, perfusion to the affected extremity, appearance of insertion site with the every 24-hours and any event that affected IABP function, such as a change in rhythm or heart rate. **Rationale:** Provides a record of nursing interventions and patient responses and serves as a legal document of the events.

Patient/Family Education

1.   Assess patient and family understanding of physician explanation of IABP therapy and reason for its use. **Rationale:** Clarification or reinforcement of information is an expressed family need during times of stress and anxiety.

2.   Explain standard care to the patient and family, including explanations of alarms, dressings, need for immobility of affected extremity, expected length of therapy, and parameters for discontinuation of therapy. **Rationale:** Encourages patient and family to ask questions and voice specific concerns about the procedures.

3.   After catheter removal, instruct patient to report any warm or wet feeling on leg and any dizziness or lightheadedness. **Rationale:** Indicative of bleeding at insertion site.

Performance Checklist
Skill 12–1:   Intraaortic Balloon Pump Management

Critical Behaviors	Complies	
	yes	no
INITIATION OF **IABP** THERAPY		
1. Wash hands, don mask, cap, gowns and gloves.		
2. Maintain aseptic environment, and turn on gas supply.		
3. Consider patient sedation and restraint.		
4. Establish ECG tracing to IABP console.		
5. Prepare hemodynamic monitoring equipment.		
6. Complete IABP console preparation:		
a. Establish a power source.		
b. Check gas supply.		
7. Open sterile packing and place catheter and insertion tray on a sterile field.		
8. Administer heparin bolus, if prescribed.		
9. Attach a one-way valve to the balloon, and withdraw all the air.		
10. Lubricate the catheter with sterile saline.		
11. Flush central lumen of catheter with heparinized saline, if necessary.		
12. Purge the system of air.		
13. Initiate IABP timing.		

Table continues on following page

Critical Behaviors	Complies	
	yes	**no**
14. Zero and calibrate pressure transducers.		
15. Obtain chest x-ray.		
16. Attach three-way stopcock to catheter tube if it is to be used for arterial pressure monitoring, flush with heparinized saline, and attach to transducer and monitor.		
17. Avoid fast flush and blood sampling from central lumen.		
18. If not used for arterial pressure monitoring, aspirate 3 to 5 cc of blood and cap line.		
19. Remove and discard gloves, mask, gown, etc., and wash hands.		
20. Document in patient record.		
TIMING OF IABP		
1. Select an ECG lead that optimizes the R wave.		
2. Time the IABP using the arterial waveform.		
3. Set the IABP frequency to 1:2 or as recommended by the IABP manufacturer.		
4. Set inflation to occur at the dicrotic notch, and adjust inflation to achieve optimal diastolic augmentation.		
5. Set deflation to occur so that the balloon-assisted aortic end-diastolic pressure is as low as possible while still maintaining optimal diastolic augmentation and not impeding on the next systole, and adjust deflation to optimal reduction of afterload.		
6. Set IABP frequency to 1:1.		
7. Reverify timing hourly.		
8. Assess and intervene to correct		
a. Early inflation.		
b. Late inflation.		
c. Early deflation.		
d. Late deflation.		
9. Document in patient record.		
STANDARD CARE		
1. Wash hands.		
2. Perform cardiovascular, peripheral vascular, and hemodynamic assessments every 15 to 60 minutes.		
3. Maintain HOB elevated less than 45 degrees.		
4. Turn patient every 2 hours, and maintain alignment.		
5. Logroll extremity with the IAB catheter.		
6. Perform active or passive range-of-motion exercises every 2 hours.		
7. Assess IAB catheter insertion site every 2 hours for evidence of hematoma or bleeding.		
8. Change the dressing every 24 hours.		
9. Maintain two means of obtaining ECG tracings.		
10. If central aortic lumen is patent, maintain heparin flush, maintain monitor alarms on, and flush and withdraw blood according to hospital policy.		
11. Obtain coagulation blood samples every 8 to 12 hours.		
12. Maintain anticoagulation as prescribed.		

Table continues on following page

Critical Behaviors	Complies	
	yes	no
13. Maintain and titrate vasoactive agents as prescribed.		
14. Wash hands.		
15. Document in patient record.		
TROUBLESHOOTING 1. Be able to identify and perform interventions to correct IABP timing for patient's developing		
a. Atrial fibrillation.		
b. Tachycardia.		
c. Asystole.		
d. Ventricular tachycardia and ventricular fibrillation.		
e. Loss of vacuum.		
f. Suspected balloon rupture.		
g. Balloon rupture.		
2. Document in patient record.		
WEANING AND IAB CATHETER REMOVAL 1. Assess for readiness to wean.		
2. Decrease IABP assist ratio and assess response.		
3. If patient is stable, further decrease assist ratio as per protocol.		
4. Assist physician with removal of balloon.		
5. Turn IABP to standby or off.		
6. Discontinue heparin 4 to 6 hours before removal.		
7. Maintain aseptic technique during removal.		
8. Ensure hemostasis of insertion site.		
9. Monitor vital signs and hemodynamic parameters.		
10. Assess perfusion of affected extremity.		
11. Assess insertion site for bleeding or hematoma.		
12. Apply a pressure dressing to insertion site.		
13. Maintain leg immobility and bed rest.		
14. Continue physical assessments.		
15. Instruct patient about symptoms of deterioration in cardiac function.		
16. Document in patient record.		

SKILL 12–2

External Counterpressure with Pneumatic Antishock Garments

External counterpressure is a noninvasive form of circulatory assistance. These devices are referred to as antishock garments, military antishock trousers (MASTs), or pneumatic antishock garments (PASGs). For the purpose of this skill, they will be referred to as PASGs.

PASGs are indicated in the resuscitative phase in acute trauma patients for early management of hemorrhagic shock and for splinting of pelvic and lower extremity fractures.

The mechanism of action of the PASG is the application of pneumatic counterpressure to the abdomen and legs, which is transferred to the capillaries, veins, and arteries. This causes an increase in peripheral vascular resistance and prevents further expansion of capacitance vessels. This reduction in intravascular capacity improves cardiac, pulmonary, and cerebral blood flow as well as blood pressure while reducing blood flow to the abdomen and lower extremities. Original theories stated that approximately 750 to 1000 cc of autologous blood is redistributed, creating an autotransfusion effect, but this remains controversial. The clinical results should be control of hemorrhage, improvement in blood pressure, and increased cerebral and cardiac perfusion.

PASGs have three independently controlled compartments, each with its own high-pressure tubing and pressure-control valve. The garment is made of heavy-duty nylon or polyvinyl fabric that encases the abdomen and both legs. Velcro fasteners are used to secure the trousers around the patient. The abdominal compartment extends from the costal margin to the pubis, and each leg compartment extends from the groin crease to the ankle. PASGs are manufactured in sizes appropriate for adults and for children over 6 years of age. The incorrect size for a pediatric trauma patient can cause respiratory compromise as a result of excessive pressure on the chest cavity.

Each compartment is connected to a separate tubing for air flow and pressurization; each individual compartment tubing is interconnected to a single connection that is attached to a foot pump. Each tube contains two valves: (1) an on/off flow valve, which allows independent pressurization of the compartment, and (2) a pressure-relief or pop-off valve, which is a safety device to prevent inflation pressure from exceeding 104 mmHg (Fig. 12–10).

The PASG is a short-term intervention for support of hemorrhage until definitive care can be initiated. Fluid support and control of bleeding are necessary for resuscitation. The PASG *cannot* and *should not* be used as a long-term support device because of such potential complications as impaired peripheral tissue perfusion, compartment syndrome, skin breakdown, respiratory impairment, bleeding, exacerbation of pulmonary edema, and congestive heart failure.

Purpose

The nurse utilizes a PASG to

1. Stabilize arterial blood pressure.
2. Redistribute blood flow from compressed areas to the vital organs.
3. Tamponade bleeding site.
4. Splint fractures of the pelvis and lower extremities (especially femoral fractures).
5. Provide short-term therapy until definitive treatment is initiated.

Prerequisite Knowledge and Skills

Prior to applying a PASG, the nurse should understand

1. Physiology of hemodynamics (blood pressure, preload, afterload).
2. Effects of external thoracic pressure on the cardiorespiratory system.
3. Physiology of tissue perfusion.
4. Pathophysiology of hemorrhagic shock.
5. Complications associated with application of PASGs.

The nurse should be able to perform

1. Assessment of cardiac and respiratory status.
2. Neurovascular examination.
3. Measurement of hemodynamic parameters.
4. Assessment of skin integrity (see Skill 29–1).
5. Venipuncture (see Skill 9–1).
6. Rapid fluid administration.
7. Proper handwashing technique (see Skill 35–5).

Assessment

1. Assess for signs and symptoms of hemorrhagic shock, including tachycardia, hypotension, decreased urine output, cool and clammy skin, decreased cardiac

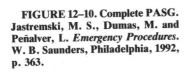

FIGURE 12–10. Complete PASG. Jastremski, M. S., Dumas, M. and Peñalver, L. *Emergency Procedures.* W. B. Saunders, Philadelphia, 1992, p. 363.

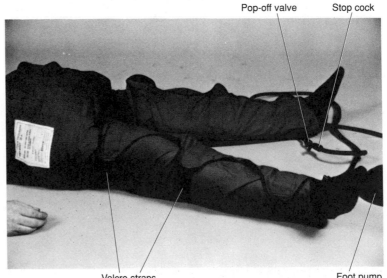

filling pressures, decreased hematocrit, and altered level of consciousness. **Rationale:** Physical signs and symptoms result from major blood volume loss.

2. Assess for signs and symptoms of compartment syndrome (see Skill 26–1), including pain, pallor, swelling, tenderness, decreased capillary refill, decreased sensation, decreased movement, and loss of peripheral pulse (late sign). **Rationale:** Physical signs and symptoms are indicative of increased external pressure secondary to the PASG and decreased tissue perfusion.

3. Assess for signs and symptoms of respiratory compromise, including tachypnea, cough, rales, distended neck veins, and hypoxia. **Rationale:** Physical signs and symptoms are indicative of increased intrathoracic pressure and increased workload to the heart.

4. Monitor arterial blood gas and lactate values. **Rationale:** Metabolic acidosis can develop as a result of muscle necrosis and tissue ischemia.

Nursing Diagnoses

1. Fluid volume deficit related to major hemorrhage. **Rationale:** Blood loss from major abdominal injury or pelvic and lower extremity fractures decreases intravascular volume.

2. Altered peripheral tissue perfusion related to increased extracompartmental pressure. **Rationale:** Increased pressure around the compartment caused by the PASG results in occlusion of microcirculation, with muscle ischemia and necrosis.

3. Impaired skin integrity related to irritation over pressure areas. **Rationale:** Increased pressure over bony areas results in skin irritation, increasing the potential for breakdown.

4. Ineffective breathing pattern related to increased intrathoracic pressure. **Rationale:** Inflation of the abdominal section increases intrathoracic pressure, resulting in respiratory compromise.

Planning

1. Individualize the following goals for PASG therapy:
   a. Control intravascular volume loss into the abdomen, pelvis, and lower extremities. **Rationale:** Maintenance of intravascular volume is necessary for vital organ perfusion.
   b. Maintain adequate tissue perfusion. **Rationale:** PASG decreases peripheral perfusion and may cause muscle ischemia and necrosis.

2. Assemble and prepare all necessary equipment and supplies. **Rationale:** Access to necessary equipment and supplies ensures that PASG therapy will be completed quickly and efficiently.
   a. PASG with foot pump.
   b. PASG tubing with stopcocks.
   c. Blood pressure monitoring equipment.
   d. PASG pressure gauge (present with some devices).
   e. Venipuncture equipment.

3. Prepare the patient.
   a. Explain the procedure. **Rationale:** Decreases anxiety and promotes cooperation.
   b. Ensure patient has a decompressed bladder and stomach and patent airway. **Rationale:** Increased abdominal and intrathoracic pressure can result in compromised airway, aspiration, and bladder rupture.

Implementation

Steps	Rationale	Special Considerations
1. Wash hands.	Reduces transmission of microorganisms.	
2. Apply blood pressure cuff, and obtain baseline measurement.	Provides baseline data for measuring effectiveness of device.	
3. Confirm that the patient meets the blood pressure criterion for PASG application.	Supports appropriate usage.	Definite indication: systolic blood pressure (SBP) $\leq$ 90 mmHg. Possible indication: SBP 80 to 100 mmHg and signs of shock (see Assessment).
4. Remove all clothing.	Prevents tissue damage from pressure on clothing.	Thorough assessment and documentation of skin integrity are essential prior to PASG application.
5. Completely unfold the PASG, and lay it flat (it should be smoothed of wrinkles).	Prepares the device for immediate use.	
6. Position the patient on the trousers by log rolling or lifting.	Maintenance of C-spine immobilization is essential in the trauma patient.	If there is suspected spinal cord injury, log roll patient onto trousers.

Table continues on following page

Steps	Rationale	Special Considerations
7. Position the PASG so that the abdominal section ends just below the costal margin and the leg sections end at the ankle.	Supradiaphragmatic compression interferes with thoracic movement.	
8. Check for a dorsalis pedis/ posterior tibial pulse, wrap trousers around left leg, and secure with Velcro fasteners. Repeat with right leg and then the abdomen.	Proper placement of trousers prevents respiratory compromise.	
9. Attach foot pump and air tubes to the PASG. Be sure all stopcocks are open.	Allows for trouser compartment inflation.	
10. Inflation: a. Open the valve(s) of the compartment(s) to be inflated and close the valve(s) of the compartment(s) that are not to be inflated. b. Inflate the leg segment(s). c. After both leg segments have been inflated, inflate the abdominal segment. d. Closely monitor blood pressure for desired response throughout inflation.	Allows for proper inflation of device. Inflation should mobilize blood from lower extremities to the abdomen first and then from the abdomen to heart, brain, and pulmonary circulation. Positions valves for inflation of compartments. Assesses effectiveness of therapy and monitors hemodynamic stability.	Leg inflation is contraindicated if there is an impaled object in leg. Both extremity compartments must be inflated before inflation of abdominal section. Abdominal inflation is contraindicated in pregnant patients and patients with an impaled object in abdomen, evisceration, tension pneumothorax, penetrating chest trauma, or diaphragmatic rupture.
11. Insert an IV, and infuse fluid volume as prescribed to maintain pressure.	The PASG is not a substitute for fluid volume replacement.	
12. Continue inflation until a. Desired blood pressure is achieved. b. Maximal suit pressure is reached and pop-off valve is activated.	Minimal pressure at which arterial pressure is stabilized should be used to prevent complications.	a. Inflation occurs until SBP is 90 to 100 mmHg. b. Pop-off pressure is 104 mmHg. Continue to inflate until Velcro fasteners begin to crackle or pressure-relief valves begin to vent.
13. When optimal blood pressure is obtained, close all valves.	Prevents air leakage from valves.	
14. Assess and document pedal pulses, color, temperature, and sensory and motor function of lower extremities.	Detects early signs of compartment syndrome.	PASG should not be used longer than 24 hours. Definitive treatment should be instituted immediately after resuscitation.
15. Closely monitor vital signs, observe patient for evidence of respiratory impairment, and auscultate breath sound for rales, rhonchi, or wheezing.	Respiratory impairment can occur as a result of increased intrathoracic pressure from abdominal inflation.	Auscultate breath sounds; if decreased or rales are present, notify physician. Pulmonary edema is an absolute contraindication.

Table continues on following page

Steps	Rationale	Special Considerations
16. Monitor the patient for indications of discontinuation of PASG, including blood pressure and pulse within normal limits, urine output 0.5 cc/kg per hour, adequate tissue perfusion, and normal cardiac filling pressures.	Required for deflation. Sudden deflation without adequate volume replacement may cause blood pressure to fall precipitously. Sequential release of compartments, starting with the abdomen, prevents hemodynamic instability. This allows for a gradual return of blood flow from the central circulation back into the extremities.	Stop deflation if systolic blood pressure falls 5 mmHg. Administer volume and inflate trousers as ordered.
17. Deflation: a. Obtain a written physician's order prior to deflating the trousers that includes increments of deflation and parameters for fluid resuscitation. b. Deflate the PASG slowly while monitoring blood pressure at time of deflation and every 5 to 10 minutes thereafter. (1) Deflate the abdominal section first by opening the valve. (2) After hemodynamic stabilization, deflate the extremity compartments, one leg at a time, by opening the valve.	Validates hemodynamic stability.	Leave PASG under patient until patient is hemodynamically stable. Should the patient experience a fall in blood pressure, reinflate the device until fluid resuscitation can be instituted and/or surgical intervention.
18. After deflation, continue monitoring vital signs every 15 minutes for 1 hour and then every hour for 24 hours.	Inflation of trousers may cause altered peripheral perfusion and skin breakdown.	
19. Monitor neurovascular status and skin integrity.	In case of hemodynamic instability in transport, the trousers can be reinflated.	
20. Leave suit on (deflated) until definitive treatment is instituted.	Maintains suit in readiness.	

Evaluation

Compare the patient's hemodynamic status before and after application of PASG.

Expected Outcomes

1. Stop or control bleeding. **Rationale:** Counterpressure tamponades bleeding and stabilizes long bone and pelvic fractures.
2. Correct placement of PASG. **Rationale:** Correct placement is necessary to ensure that adequate pressure is maintained and complications are prevented.
3. Stable hemodynamic status. **Rationale:** Increased peripheral resistance and possible redistribution of blood to vital organs; increasing cerebral and cardiac perfusion.

Unexpected Outcomes

1. Acute hypotension. **Rationale:** Rapid deflation of PASG may cause altered hemodynamic status.

2. Compartment syndrome. **Rationale:** Compartment syndrome may occur as a consequence of prolonged use. Inflation of PASG increases pressure external to the extremity collapse of the microcirculation, decreased perfusion, and muscle ischemia, leading to necrosis.
3. Respiratory compromise. **Rationale:** Increased respiratory rate, decreased breath sounds, and rales may occur if abdominal compartment of trousers is inflated.
4. Impaired skin integrity. **Rationale:** Pressure on bony prominence from PASG may result in skin breakdown.
5. Metabolic acidosis. **Rationale:** Impaired tissue perfusion may cause buildup of metabolic waste (acid) that may reenter circulation after deflation.

Documentation

Documentation in the patient record should include

rationale for institution of device, blood pressure, pulse, assessment of respiratory status, neurovascular assessment (i.e., pulses, skin, color, sensation, movement, temperature), assessment of skin integrity, PASG compartments that are inflated, time of inflation, time of deflation, and intake and output. **Rationale:** Provides a record of patient status before procedure, nursing and medical interventions, postprocedure patient status, and expected and unexpected patient outcomes and serves as a legal record of the events.

Patient/Family Education

Explain the indications and the procedure for institution of PASG to both patient and family. **Rationale:** Encourages patient cooperation and understanding of procedure.

Performance Checklist
Skill 12-2: External Counterpressure with Pneumatic Antishock Garments

Critical Behaviors	Complies yes	Complies no
1. Wash hands.		
2. Confirm that patient meets blood pressure criterion for application of PASG.		
3. Apply blood pressure cuff, and obtain baseline values.		
4. Remove all clothing from patient.		
5. Unfold PASG and lay flat.		
6. Carefully slide PASG under the patient, maintaining C-spine immobilization.		
7. Position PASG properly.		
8. Check pedal pulses, and fold the PASG about the left leg and fasten, right leg and fasten, abdomen and fasten.		
9. Attach air tubes to the compartments and foot pump.		
10. Inflate PASG properly, and document time, date, and patient response.		
11. Insert an IV and infuse fluid as prescribed.		
12. Check vital signs and observe for respiratory compromise.		
13. Deflate PASG properly:		
a. Review physician order for deflation.		
b. Deflate slowly, in increments.		
14. Monitor vital signs every 15 minutes for 1 hour and then every hour for 24 hours.		
15. Closely monitor neurovascular status and skin integrity.		
16. Document procedure in patient record.		
17. Leave PASG on patient until patient is hemodynamically stable.		

SKILL 12-3 _____

Rotating Tourniquets

Rotating tourniquets are a temporary intervention utilized to reduce venous return to the heart in the event of life-threatening congestive heart failure with pulmonary edema. This method of preload reduction is generally used in conjunction with pharmacotherapeutic therapies such as diuretics, vasodilators, antihypertensives, morphine sulfate, and inotropic agents. Other electromechanical therapies that may be used are the intraaortic balloon pump and slow continuous ultrafil-tration (SCUF). Supportive care includes oxygen therapy, bed rest with the head of the bed elevated to 45 degrees, and restriction of sodium and fluids.

Rotating tourniquets are a technique whereby pressure cuffs on the extremities are sequentially inflated and deflated to sequester blood in the limbs. The pressure cuffs are inflated sufficiently to isolate venous blood in the limbs, thereby reducing preload. Inflation of the pressure cuffs should never impede arterial blood supply to the extremities; therefore, the maximum inflation pressure should be kept at the diastolic blood pressure so that distal pulses are always palpable.

While the necessary equipment used for this procedure is relatively inexpensive, the nursing time required and patient discomfort may be considerable.

Purpose

The nurse uses rotating tourniquets to temporarily reduce venous return to the heart in patients with pulmonary edema and severe congestive heart failure.

Prerequisite Knowledge and Skills

Prior to utilizing rotating tourniquets, the nurse should understand

1. Anatomy and physiology of the circulatory system.
2. Pathophysiology of congestive heart failure and pulmonary edema.
3. Principles of preload reduction.
4. Principles of arterial and venous blood flow.

The nurse should be able to perform

1. Cardiovascular and vital signs assessment.
2. Peripheral vascular assessment.
3. Proper handwashing techniques (see Skill 35–5).

Assessment

1. Assess for signs and symptoms of congestive heart failure and acute pulmonary edema necessitating rotating tourniquets: (1) *neurologic*, including decreased level of consciousness, dizziness, syncope, insomnia, and/or fatigue (moderate to severe); (2) *respiratory*, including dyspnea, orthopnea, diffuse rhonchi, moist rales, crackles, wheezing, and cough with frothy or blood tinged sputum; (3) *cardiac*, including tachycardia, weak thready pulse, hypertension, narrowed pulse pressure, S3 and S4 gallop, systolic murmur, pulsus alternans, pallor, cool skin, diaphoresis, peripheral edema (pitting), hepatomegaly, ascites, splenomegaly, and dilation of peripheral veins (particularly jugular); (4) *renal*, including decreased urine output. **Rationale:** Physical signs and symptoms indicative of decreased myocardial contractility and subsequent fluid retention.
2. Evaluate serial diagnostic studies, including chest x-ray (i.e., increased pulmonary congestion, interstitial edema, and pleural effusion), electrocardiogram (i.e., tachycardia, dysrhythmias, left and right ventricular hypertrophy, and atrial hypertrophy), and hemodynamic monitoring (i.e., decreased cardiac output, elevated pulmonary artery pressure, left ventricular end-diastolic pressure, pulmonary capillary wedge pressure, and right atrial pressure). **Rationale:** Cardiac and respiratory failure will be reflected in objective parameters.

Nursing Diagnoses

1. Fluid volume excess related to pulmonary and peripheral interstitial edema. **Rationale:** Decreased cardiac output results in interstitial fluid retention.
2. Impaired gas exchange related to pulmonary interstitial and alveolar edema. **Rationale:** Interstitial and alveolar edema decreases the diffusion of oxygen and carbon dioxide across alveolar membranes.
3. Potential for impaired skin integrity of extremities related to pressure cuff inflation. **Rationale:** Pressure cuff inflation decreases peripheral capillary blood flow, preventing oxygen delivery to tissue.
4. Anxiety related to dyspnea and exhaustion. **Rationale:** Respiratory distress and physical exhaustion may lead to patient's feeling of impending doom.
5. Potential for extremity pain related to pressure cuff inflation. **Rationale:** The pressure from rotating tourniquet cuffs may compress nerve fibers and/or vessels supplying blood to nerve fibers, thereby creating a painful sensation.

Planning

1. Individualize the following goal for utilizing rotating tourniquets to reduce venous return to the heart. **Rationale:** Decreased preload will enhance cardiac performance and decrease pulmonary congestion.
2. Gather all necessary equipment and supplies. **Rationale:** Assembly of essential supplies ensures rapid and efficient initiation of the rotating tourniquets.
   a. Four blood pressure cuffs or automatic rotating tourniquet device.
   b. Four small towels.
   c. Clock to time sequential rotation of manual cuffs.
   d. Marking pen (water soluble).
3. Prepare the patient. **Rationale:** Reduces anxiety.
   a. Explain procedure and rationale for treatment to the patient and family.
   b. Explain patient's participation and the importance of limiting physical activity. **Rationale:** Promotes cooperation.

Implementation

Steps	Rationale	Special Considerations
1. Position patient with head of bed elevated to 45 degrees.	Enhances respiratory effort and reduces circulating volume.	

Table continues on following page

Steps	Rationale	Special Considerations
2. Wash hands.	Reduces transmission of microorganisms.	
3. Apply pressure cuffs 4 inches (10 cm) below groin and axillas over small towel (Fig. 12–11). Cuff should be snug but able to accommodate two fingerbreadths.	Cuff application should be comfortable and should not impede arterial circulation.	Do not apply pressure cuffs to extremities with IVs or signs of ischemia or infection.
4. Assess and mark peripheral pulses with water-soluble pen.	Facilitates arterial pulse monitoring.	

Manual Rotating Tourniquets

Steps	Rationale	Special Considerations
5. Inflate three pressure cuffs to patient's diastolic blood pressure level.	Prevents tissue damage to extremities while reducing preload.	*Do not* inflate pressure cuffs enough to impede arterial blood flow (distal pulses must be palpable).
6. Sequentially inflate/deflate pressure cuffs in clockwise fashion every 5 to 15 minutes (Fig. 12–12).	Venous outflow should not be restricted more than 45 minutes in each extremity.	Rotation schedule may vary according to physician order.

Table continues on following page

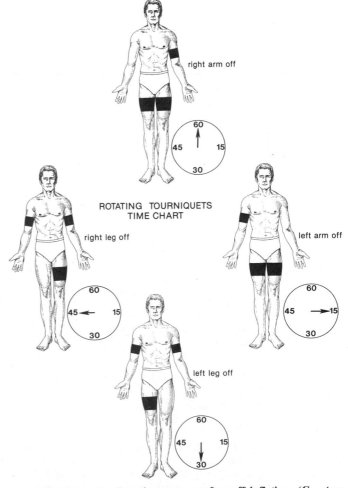

FIGURE 12–12. Rotation sequence for cuff inflation. (Courtesy of the author.)

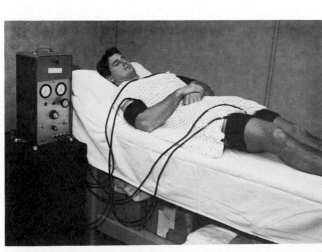

FIGURE 12–11. Correct placement of rotating tourniquet cuffs. (Courtesy of the author.)

Steps	Rationale	Special Considerations
Automatic Rotating Tourniquets		
5. Secure cuffs to proper hoses on automatic machine, and clamp off any unused cuffs.	For correct operation of device, and ensures correct sequencing.	Be prepared to use manual cuffs in the event of machine failure.
6. Turn on machine, set maximum inflation pressure at patient's diastolic blood pressure level, and set rotation timing sequence for 5- to 15-minute intervals.	Prevents tissue damage to extremities while reducing preload. Venous outflow should not be restricted more than 45 minutes in each extremity.	Do not set inflation pressure high enough to impede arterial blood flow (distal pulses must be palpable). Rotation schedule may vary according to physician order.
7. Monitor and record blood pressure every 15 minutes in unused extremity.	Rotating tourniquets may cause hypotension in some patients.	
8. Assess neurovascular status of extremities every 15 minutes.	Maintain flow sheet for accurate record of nursing actions and patient response.	
9. When no longer needed, remove one pressure cuff at a time during deflation cycle.	Prevents sudden increase in circulating blood volume.	
10. Assess extremities for warmth, palpable pulses, skin integrity, and peripheral ischemia.	Enables identification of any complications.	
11. Wash hands.	Reduces transmission of microorganisms.	

Evaluation

Compare the patient's signs, symptoms, physical findings, and diagnostic tests before and after therapy. **Rationale:** Treatment effectiveness will be demonstrated by trends documented in patient record and by serial physical examinations.

Expected Outcomes

1. Improved gas exchange demonstrated by clear breath sounds, reduced orthopnea and dyspnea, absence of cough or frothy sputum production, and absent hypoxemia and hypercarbia. **Rationale:** Pulmonary congestion is effectively reduced or eliminated when cardiac performance is improved.

2. Reduction of preload and improved ventricular function, demonstrated by increased cardiac output, decreased pulmonary capillary wedge pressure, increased urine output, decreased heart rate and dysrhythmias. **Rationale:** The effectiveness of cardiac pump action is increased by improved myocardial contractility.

3. Decreased anxiety demonstrated by the patient's ability to rest and verbalize concerns. **Rationale:** Resolution of dyspnea and orthopnea.

Unexpected Outcomes

1. Hypotension. **Rationale:** The use of rotating tourniquets results in decreased circulating volume.

2. Arterial emboli. **Rationale:** Resulting from prolonged arterial pressure and clot formation in extremities.

3. Circulatory overload at end of procedure. **Rationale:** Due to rapid return of sequestered volume to systemic circulation.

4. Peripheral ischemia. **Rationale:** Pressure cuffs may impede capillary blood flow.

5. Impaired skin integrity. **Rationale:** Results from mechanical trauma related to cuff application, inflation, deflation, and removal.

Documentation

Documentation in the patient record should include patient assessment prior to implementation; date, time, and length of procedure; rotation schedule; quality of pulses in all extremities before, during, and after procedure; and patient's response to procedure (i.e., respiratory rate and effort, presence of productive cough, anxiety level). **Rationale:** Documents nursing assessment, care given, and expected and unexpected outcomes.

Patient/Family Education

1. Assess understanding of congestive heart failure and pulmonary edema. Describe disease process, causes, and various therapeutic modalities. **Rationale:** Provides a basis for discussion of procedure.

2. Explain to patient and family the procedure, the rationale for use, and the goal of therapy with regard to

rotating tourniquets. **Rationale:** Encourages understanding and cooperation and reduces anxiety.

3. Keep patient and family informed of progress. **Rationale:** Decreases anxiety and promotes trust.

4. When appropriate, provide patient and family with information concerning limited physical activity, sodium restriction, daily weights to evaluate fluid accumulation, and name, dose, and potential side effects of prescribed medications. **Rationale:** Education is directed toward understanding and compliance with short- and long-term therapeutic goals.

Performance Checklist
Skill 12–3:   Rotating Tourniquets

Critical Behaviors	Complies	
	yes	no
1. Place patient in high Fowler's position.		
2. Wash hands.		
3. Apply pressure cuffs 4 inches (10 cm) below groin and axilla.		
4. Assess and mark peripheral pulses.		
MANUAL ROTATING TOURNIQUETS		
5. Inflate all but one cuff to patient's diastolic blood pressure.		
6. Sequentially inflate/deflate cuff pressure every 5 to 15 minutes		
AUTOMATIC ROTATING TOURNIQUETS		
5. Secure cuffs to proper hoses, and clamp unused cuffs.		
6. Set rotation sequence time and inflation pressure, activate device, and monitor accuracy.		
7. Monitor and document patient's vital signs every 15 minutes.		
8. Assess extremities every 15 minutes.		
9. Remove pressure cuffs one at a time during deflation cycle.		
10. Assess extremities for warmth, palpable pulses, skin integrity, and peripheral ischemia.		
11. Wash hands.		
12. Document in patient record.		

REFERENCES

Datascope Corp (1989). *Mechanics of Intraaortic Balloon Counterpulsation.* Montvale, New Jersey.

Jacobs, L. and Bennett, B. (1983). *Emergency Patient Care: Prehospital, Ground, and Air Procedures.* New York: Macmillan, page 165.

Quaal, S. J. (1984). *Comprehensive Intraaortic Balloon Pumping.* St. Louis: Mosby.

BIBLIOGRAPHY

Cardona, V. D., Editor, *Trauma reference manual.* Bowie, Brady Communications Company, Inc. 1985.

Daily, E. K. and Tilkian, A. G. (1986). Intraaortic Balloon Pumping. In E. K. Daily and A. G. Tilkian (Eds.), *Cardiovascular Procedures.* St. Louis: Mosby.

Fenton, M. (1985). Intraaortic balloon pump therapy. *Crit. Care Nurs.* 15:54–60.

Funk, M., Gleason, J., and Foell, D. (1989). Lower limb ischemia related to the use of the intraaortic balloon pump. *Heart & Lung* 18:542–552.

Goran, S. (1989). Vascular complications of the patient undergoing intraaortic balloon pumping. *Crit. Care Nurs. Clin. North Am.* 1(3):459–467.

Hudak, C. M., Gallo, B. M., and Benz, J. J. (1990). *Critical Care Nursing,* 5th Ed. Philadelphia: Lippincott.

Joseph, D. L. and Bates, S. (1990). Intraaortic balloon pumping: how to stay on course. *Am. J. Nurs.,* 90(9):42–47.

Mattox, K. L., Bickell, W., Pepe, P., Burch, J., Feliciano, D. (1989). Prospective MAST study in 911 patients. *Trauma* 29(8): 1104–1112.

Millar, S., Sampson, L. K., and Soukup, M. (1985). *AACN Procedure Manual for Critical Care.* Philadelphia: Saunders.

Patacky, M. G., Garvin, B. J., and Schwirin, P. M. (1985). Intraaortic balloon pumping and stress in the coronary care unit. *Heart & Lung* 14:142–148.

Soukup, M. (1988). Plan of care for the patient requiring intraaortic balloon pump therapy in the nursing diagnosis framework. *Cardiac Assists* 4:1–6.

Webster, H. and Veasy, L. G. (1985). Intraaortic balloon pumping in children. *Heart & Lung* 14:548–555.

Whitman, G. (1978). Intraaortic balloon pumping and cardiac mechanics: A programmed lesson. *Heart & Lung* 7:1034–1050.

Vitello-Cicciu, J., Stewart, S. L., and Griffin, E. L. (1988). Coronary Artery Disease. In M. R. Kinney, D. R. Packa, and S. B. Dunbar (Eds.), *AACN's Clinical Reference for Critical Care Nursing,* 2 Ed. New York: McGraw-Hill Book Company.

13

LIFESAVING TECHNIQUES

BEHAVIORAL OBJECTIVES

After completing this chapter, the nurse will be able to

- Define the key terms.
- Assist with pericardiocentesis.
- Identify clinical indicators suggesting cardiac tamponade.
- Monitor the patient's hemodynamic status throughout the procedure.

The pericardium is the sac that encloses the heart and portions of the great vessels. This sac consists of an outer fibrous layer and an inner serous layer. The space between these two layers is the pericardial cavity. This cavity normally contains 10 to 30 ml of clear fluid that facilitates the movement of the two layers (Randall, 1989). The abnormal accumulation of more than 50 ml of fluid in the pericardial sac is a pericardial effusion. A pericardial effusion can be noncompressive or compressive. The heart usually functions normally with a noncompressive pericardial effusion. As the effusion becomes compressive, there is increased pressure within the pericardial sac, which results in cardiac tamponade and resistance to cardiac filling. Symptoms of cardiac tamponade are not specific, and patients may exhibit signs and symptoms of an associated disease. As a result of a decrease in cardiac output, the patient often develops tachypnea, tachycardia, pallor, cyanosis, impaired cerebral and renal function, and sweating. Most patients are hypotensive and demonstrate neck vein distension and pulsus paradoxus (Spodick, 1989). Three important factors contributing to the development of cardiac tamponade are

1. The rapidity with which the fluid collects in the pericardial space.
2. The total amount of fluid within the space.
3. The physical makeup of the pericardium itself (Muirhead, 1989).

The presence and amount of fluid in the pericardium are evaluated through chest roentgenogram, two-dimensional echocardiogram, and clinical findings. Once tamponade is verified, a pericardiocentesis is performed to remove fluid from the pericardial sac.

KEY TERMS

cardiac output   pericardiocentesis
cardiac tamponade   pulse pressure
pericardial effusion   pulsus paradoxus
pericardial sac

SKILL

13–1   Assisting with Pericardiocentesis

GUIDELINES

The following assessment guidelines assist the nurse in formulating a nursing diagnosis and an individualized plan of care to assist with a pericardiocentesis:

1. Know the baseline cardiovascular status.
2. Know the baseline 12-lead ECG.
3. Know the medical history, pharmacologic profile, and current treatment plan.

SKILL 13–1

Assisting with Pericardiocentesis

Pericardiocentesis is performed in order to remove excess fluid from the pericardial sac. Some institutions have found two-dimensional echocardiography–guided pericardiocentesis to be effective, but Pandian and colleagues have found this technique to be underused (Pandian et al., 1988). Usually, the pericardiocentesis is performed by the physician with the nurse's assistance. The chest is prepped and draped using sterile technique with 1% lidocaine (without epinephrine) used as the local anesthesia. A three-way stopcock connects the pericardial aspiration needle to a 50-cc syringe. Using an alligator clip, the V lead (precordial lead) of the ECG is attached to the needle. The physician then slowly inserts a needle until fluid is obtained (Fig. 13–1). By using the 12-lead ECG, injury to the heart may potentially be avoided. If the needle contacts the ventricle, ST depression should be seen. With atrial contraction, PR-segment elevation will occur. When ECG changes are seen, the physician will need to reposition the needle (Yeston and Niehoff, 1988).

The nurse plays an important and active role in this procedure by acting as an assistant in the actual withdrawal of fluids and by monitoring the patient throughout the procedure.

Purpose

Pericardiocentesis is performed to

1. Remove fluid from the pericardial sac.
2. Provide a specimen for the differential diagnosis of pericardial effusion.

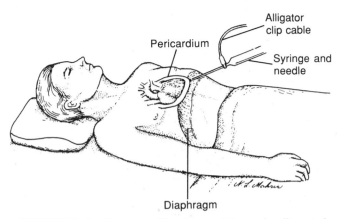

FIGURE 13–1. Proper needle placement for pericardiocentesis. Reprinted with permission from Yeston, N. and Niehoff, J. *Critical Care.* Philadelphia, Lippincott, 1988, p. 267.

3. Improve cardiac output.
4. Prevent or treat cardiac tamponade.

Prerequisite Knowledge and Skills

Before assisting with pericardiocentesis, the nurse should understand

1. Anatomy and physiology of the cardiovascular system.
2. Principles of aseptic technique.
3. Principles of ECG monitoring.
4. Principles of hemodynamic monitoring.
5. Universal precautions.

The nurse should be able to perform

1. Aseptic technique.
2. Universal precautions (see Skill 35–1).
3. Assessment of cardiovascular system.
4. Interpretation of dysrhythmias.
5. Basic Cardiac Life Support/Advanced Cardiac Life Support
6. Hemodynamic monitoring (see Chapter 10).
7. Monitor and interpret an ECG tracing (see Skill 7–2).

Assessment

Assess baseline heart rate, cardiac rhythm, heart sounds (S_1, S_2, rubs), blood pressure, pulse pressure, venous pressure, and respiratory status. **Rationale:** Establishes baseline parameters to assess changes during or after procedure.

Nursing Diagnoses

1. Decreased cardiac output related to increased fluid in pericardial sac. **Rationale:** Accumulation of fluid within the pericardial sac restricts ventricular diastolic filling, which, in turn, reduces cardiac output, stroke volume, and arterial blood pressure.

2. Anxiety related to uncertainty of the cause of illness and prognosis, unfamiliarity of the environment, and possible fear of death. **Rationale:** Critical illness and the unknown associated with illness and hospital procedures result in a state of helplessness, which then causes anxiety.

Planning

1. Individualize the following goals for the patient undergoing pericardiocentesis.
   a. Improve cardiac output. **Rationale:** Prevents or eliminates cardiac tamponade.
   b. Promote patient comfort. **Rationale:** Improves cardiac output and alleviates signs and symptoms of cardiac tamponade.

2. Obtain all necessary supplies, medications, and equipment. **Rationale:** Facilitates the smooth and orderly progression of the procedure.
   a. Pericardiocentesis tray (or thoracentesis tray).
   b. 2- and 3-in tape.
   c. 16- or 18-gauge cardiac needle or catheter over the needle, 3 in in length.
   d. J-Guidewire, 35 mm diameter, vessel dilator, no. 7 French, pigtail catheter, no. 7 French, tubing and drainage bag (for continuous drainage setup).
   e. 30 cc Povidone iodine.
   f. Two packs of 4 × 4 gauze pads.
   g. Sterile 10-cc, 5-cc, and 3-cc syringes (2 each).
   h. Gowns, gloves, mask, and surgical cap for all personnel.
   i. Alligator clip cable.
   j. Two three-way stopcocks.
   k. 1% lidocaine (topical).
   l. Emergency drug box.
   m. Emergency cart and equipment.
   n. 12-lead ECG machine.

3. Prepare the patient.
   a. Provide step-by-step description of the procedure. **Rationale:** Decreases anxiety and encourages questions.
   b. Validate that the informed consent form has been signed. **Rationale:** Protects rights of patient and makes competent decision possible for patient; however, under emergency circumstances, time may not allow form to be signed.
   c. Position patient comfortably in supine position with head of bed elevated 30 degrees. **Rationale:** Facilitates aspiration of fluids and breathing.
   d. Medicate patient as prescribed. **Rationale:** Reduces anxiety, promotes comfort, and decreases myocardial workload.

4. Apply limb leads of 12-lead ECG. **Rationale:** ECG changes may indicate injury to heart.

Implementation

Steps	Rationale	Special Considerations
1. Wash hands.	Reduces transmission of microorganisms.	
2. Open pericardiocentesis tray and appropriate supplies using aseptic technique (other supplies are opened as needed).	Minimizes potential for infection.	
3. Don gown and mask.	Maintains aseptic technique.	
4. Prep skin by scrubbing with antibacterial solution.	Minimizes potential for infection.	Shaving the area may be necessary prior to scrubbing.
5. Assist personnel with donning mask, gown, and gloves.	Maintains aseptic technique.	
6. Help physician connect one end of alligator clip to the needle and the other end to the lead of the ECG. Turn machine on (Fig. 13–1).	Provides the mechanism to identify myocardial injury. Maintains aseptic technique.	
7. Continuously monitor ECG, vital signs, and venous pressures during needle insertion, fluid withdrawal, and withdrawing of needle.	Detects myocardial injury.	
8. Once the needle has been withdrawn, cleanse antiseptic solution from skin, and apply sterile dressing.	Minimizes skin breakdown and minimizes infection.	
9. Send specimens to laboratory for evaluation.	Provides diagnoses of organism involved in the pericardial effusion.	Usual tests include body fluid cytology, cell count, and electrolytes.
10. Wash hands.	Reduces transmission of microorganisms.	

Evaluation

1. Continuously monitor ECG, vital signs, venous pressure, and heart sounds after procedure. **Rationale:** Changes may indicate injury to heart or cardiac tamponade. Be prepared for chest exploration.
2. Observe for bloody fluid with presence of indwelling drainage tube. **Rationale:** Continuous bleeding may indicate injury to heart.
3. Monitor dressing for excess bleeding; change as condition indicates. **Rationale:** Excess bleeding may indicate injury to heart.
4. Treat dysrhythmias as prescribed. **Rationale:** Dysrhythmias may lead to cardiac decompensation and/or arrest.
5. Notify physician of deterioration in patient's condition. **Rationale:** Deterioration may indicate cardiac tamponade as quantified by decreased blood pressure, dysrhythmias, increased venous pressure, change in mental and respiratory status, sweating, and distant heart sounds. Be prepared for chest exploration.

Expected Outcomes

1. Fluid is removed from pericardial sac. **Rationale:** Reduces pericardial effusion.
2. Improved cardiac output. **Rationale:** Pressure within pericardial sac has been reduced.
3. Blood pressure, venous pressure, heart sounds, pulse pressure, and cardiac rhythm are within normal limits. **Rationale:** Cardiac tamponade has been averted.

Unexpected Outcomes

1. Drop in blood pressure, rise in venous pressure, cardiac rhythm changes, ST depression, PR-segment elevation, or excessive bleeding. **Rationale:** Indicate myocardial injury in the presence of cardiac tamponade.
2. Dysrhythmias. **Rationale:** Insertion of foreign object and removal of fluid may cause cardiac irritation.
3. Shortness of breath with increasing apprehensiveness. **Rationale:** Pneumothorax or hemothorax has occurred.
4. Recurring cardiac tamponade. **Rationale:** Fluid may reaccumulate.

Documentation

Documentation in the patient record should include preprocedure instruction and patient's response; pre- and postprocedure blood pressure, venous pressure, heart sounds, level of consciousness, respiratory status, and cardiac rhythm; medications administered, amount and consistency of pericardial drainage; and site of pericardiocentesis. **Rationale:** Documents nursing care given, expected and unexpected outcomes, and interventions taken.

Patient/Family Education

1. Assess the ability of the patient and family to comprehend the necessity for performing the procedure. **Rationale:** Different social, economic, education, and stress levels of families affect their ability to process information.

2. Reinforce the reason pericardiocentesis is needed, give a description of the procedure, and explain expected outcomes and possible complications. **Rationale:** The unknown increases anxiety and apprehension for the patient and family.

3. Instruct patient and family on potential signs and symptoms of recurrent pericardial effusion (i.e., dyspnea, dull ache or pressure within the chest, dysphagia, cough, tachypnea, hoarseness, hiccups, or nausea) (Muirhead, 1989). **Rationale:** Early detection of pericardial effusion may prevent complications from heart compression.

4. Instruct patient and family as to patient's risk for recurrent pericardial effusion. **Rationale:** Predicting pericardial effusion may help with early detection of life-threatening problem.

Performance Checklist
Skill 13–1: Assisting with Pericardiocentesis

Critical Behaviors	Complies yes	no
1. Wash hands.		
2. Open pericardiocentesis tray and appropriate supplies onto sterile field.		
3. Don gown and mask.		
4. Shave chest as needed and scrub with antibacterial solution.		
5. Assist personnel with donning of mask, gown, and gloves.		
6. Assist with the connection of one end of alligator clip to the needle and other end to the V-lead.		
7. Assist physician with procedure.		
8. Monitor patient's ECG, vital signs, and venous pressure continuously during procedure.		
9. Cleanse antiseptic solution from skin, and apply sterile dressing.		
10. Send specimens to laboratory.		
11. Wash hands.		
12. Document procedure in patient record.		

REFERENCES

Muirhead, J. (1989). Pericardial Disease. In S. L. Underhill, S. L. Woods, E. S. Savarajan Froelicher, and C. J. Halpenney (Eds.), *Cardiac Nursing*, 2d Ed. (pp. 916–917). Philadelphia: Lippincott.

Pandian, N., Brockway, B., Simonetti, J., et al. (1988). Pericardiocentesis under two-dimensional echocardiographic guidance in loculated pericardial effusion. *Ann. Thorac. Surg.* 45:99–100.

Randall, E. M. (1989). Recognizing cardiac tamponade. *J. Cardiovasc. Nurs.* 3:42–48.

Spodick, D. (1989). Pericarditis, pericardial effusion, cardiac tamponade, and constriction. *Crit. Care Clin.* 5:455–476.

Yeston, N., and Niehoff, J. (1988). Pericardiocentesis. In J. M. Civetta, J. W. Taylor, and R. R. Kirby (Eds.), *Critical Care* (pp. 266–268). Philadelphia: Lippincott.

UNIT III

THE NEUROLOGIC SYSTEM

14

TEMPERATURE REGULATING DEVICES

BEHAVIORAL OBJECTIVES

After completing this chapter, the nurse will be able to

- Define the key terms.
- Describe methods for attaining a normothermic state.
- Discuss indications for use of temperature regulating devices.
- Demonstrate the skills involved in regulating a patient's temperature.

Thermoregulatory balance, balance of the body's temperature, is controlled by the hypothalamus. A variety of factors including hypothermia and hyperthermia affect multisystem morbidity and mortality (Fig. 14–1). Hypothermia occurs when the body's temperature is less than 95°F (35°C). Hyperthermia occurs when the body's temperature is above 106°F (38.3°C). A state of fever exists when the body's temperature rises above the normal temperature (96.6 to 99.6°F or 35.9 to 37.5°C), which varies with each individual.

Causes of hypothermia are categorized into three areas: metabolic, pharmacologic, and mechanical (Table 14–1).

Hypothermia can lead to profound physiologic consequences (Fig. 14–2). Shivering, the body's attempt to warm itself through the contractions of skeletal muscle, can double oxygen consumption and increase cardiac output three to four times. An increase such as this may weaken the myocardium. Thus the elderly individual whose heart may already be compromised is at particular risk for cardiovascular problems associated with hypothermia.

During hyperthermia, body metabolism generates heat, and retains more than it expels. At temperatures greater than 106°F (41°C), cellular metabolism is so high

that the body is unable to provide enough oxygen and nutrients to the cells. Thus cells, and eventually the body as a whole, may die.

This chapter centers on the techniques needed to assist the critically ill patient in attaining and maintaining a normothermic state.

KEY TERMS

bradycardia	hypovolemia
cardiac dysrhythmias	intracranial pressure
Celsius	morbidity
cellular metabolism	mortality
cerebral edema	myocardium
core temperature	normothermia
crystalloid fluid	pathophysiologic
electrolyte	phlebitis
enzyme	shivering
Fahrenheit	thermal burn
fever	thermoregulatory balance
gastric motility	thyrotoxicosis
hypothyroidism	vasodilator
hyperthermia	ventricular fibrillation
hypothermia	

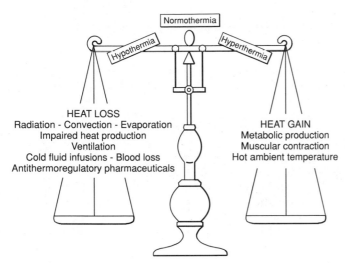

FIGURE 14–1. Factors responsible for thermoregulatory balance. Reproduced with permission from *Geriatric Nursing*. Biddle, C. J., and Biddle, W. L. A Plastic Head Cover to Reduce Surgical Heat Loss. *Geriatric Nursing*, 6(1):39–41, 1985, p. 41.

TABLE 14–1. CAUSES OF HYPOTHERMIA

Metabolic Causes
Burns
Trauma
Malnutrition
Hypoglycemia
Central nervous system disease
Neuromuscular disease
Hypothyroidism
Hypoadrenalism
Diabetic ketoacidosis
Anorexia nervosa

Mechanical Causes
Cold fluid infusion
Wet dressings/linen/clothing
Open body cavities/wounds
Cool environmental temperature
Inspiration of cool gases
Cold irrigating solutions
Air draft exposures
Active perspiration
Extremes in age
Tachypnea

Pharmacologic Causes
Morphine
Diazepam
Barbiturates
General anesthetics
Ethanol
Phenothiazines
Vasodilators—nitroprusside, nitroglycerin
Reserpine

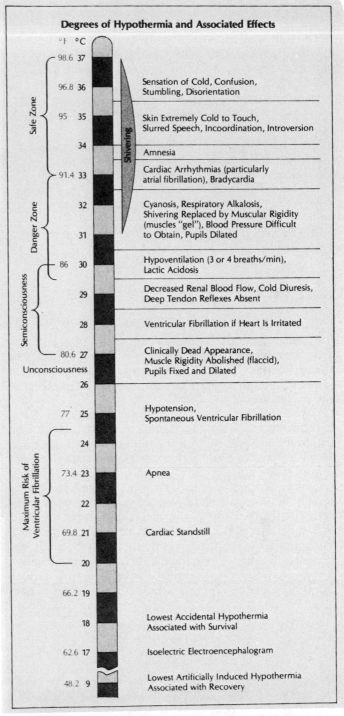

FIGURE 14–2. Degrees of hypothermia and associated effects. Reproduced with permission from Matz, R., Hypothermia: Mechanisms and Countermeasures, *Hospital Practice*, Jan. 30, 1986, pg. 47.

SKILLS

14–1 Use of Hypothermia/Hyperthermia Blanket
14–2 Fluid Warming Devices
14–3 Microwaved Solutions

GUIDELINES

The following assessment guidelines assist the nurse in identifying nursing diagnoses and a plan of care for the patient experiencing thermoregulatory imbalance:

1. Know the patient's baseline temperature.
2. Know the patient's baseline vital signs, including heart rate and rhythm, blood pressure, and respiratory rate.
3. Know the patient's baseline level of consciousness.
4. Know the patient's past medical history.
5. Know the patient's current medical regimen.
6. Know methods for accurate temperature taking.
7. Determine appropriate intervention for assessed finding.
8. Become skillful in the use of temperature regulating devices.

SKILL 14–1

Use of Hypothermia/Hyperthermia Blanket

At times, external measures to maintain a patient's body temperature within a desired range are indicated. Use of a hypothermia/hyperthermia blanket promotes generalized body cooling or heating in an efficient, non-invasive manner.

Cooling of the body to a normothermic state is useful in reducing the body's metabolic demands and oxygen requirements. Hypothermia blanket therapy is preferred over ice packs or tepid water and alcohol baths for temperatures over 102°F (38°C) because the body is cooled in a more steady and efficient manner. Generalized body heating via hyperthermia blanket therapy is used to elevate the temperature to a normal level, but not to induce a state of fever. Hyperthermia blanket therapy provides more rapid and efficient body heating than can be achieved by simply applying blankets or warming lights.

Hypothermia/hyperthermia blanket therapy utilizes the principle of *conduction*, which is the transfer of heat or cold through contact with another surface. The blanket is constructed of coils covered with plastic or synthetic fibers that are easy to handle, clean, and apply to the body. The thermal blanket or pad is either disposable or reusable. The blanket itself is attached to tubing that connects to the main unit. Each unit contains a pump that circulates a water and/or alcohol solution from a reservoir through the thermal blanket or pad, which is in turn warmed or cooled. A control panel contains the indicator lights, control knobs, and thermometers (Figs. 14–3, 14–4).

Many units have both automatic and manual modes. The automatic control unit monitors the patient's temperature via a rectal or skin probe and sends this information to the control system, which, in turn, regulates

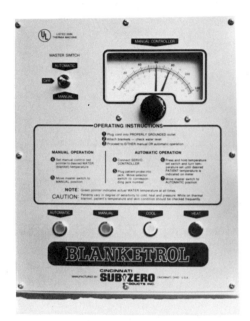

FIGURE 14–3. Control panel with needle temperature indicator. (Courtesy of Cincinnati Sub-zero Products, Inc.)

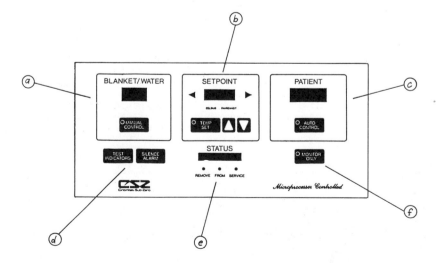

BLANKETROL II CONTROL PANEL

FIGURE 14–4. Control panel with digital temperature indicators: a = actual temperature of circulating water; b = desired temperature of water or patient; c = actual temperature of patient; d = test indicators/silence alarm; e = reports status of unit; f = monitors patient temperature only. (Courtesy of Cincinnati Sub-zero Products, Inc.)

heating or cooling within preset limits. The manual mode does not utilize this feedback system. The same unit can be used for both hypothermia and hyperthermia therapy.

Purpose

The nurse applies a hypothermia blanket to

1. Decrease body temperature.
2. Decrease cellular metabolism.

The nurse applies a hyperthermia blanket to

1. Rewarm the body.
2. Achieve a normothermic state to assess brain wave activity (evaluation for brain death).

Prerequisite Knowledge and Skills

Prior to using a hypothermia/hyperthermia blanket, the nurse should understand

1. Principles of temperature taking.
2. Effects of hypothermia and hyperthermia on body systems.
3. Adverse effects of cooling or warming the patient's body too rapidly.
4. Principles of conduction.

The nurse should be able to perform

1. Proper temperature taking.
2. Vital signs assessment.
3. Level of consciousness assessment.
4. Skin assessment (see Skill 29–1).
5. Cardiac monitoring.
6. Cardiopulmonary assessment.

Assessment

1. Assess temperature, heart rate and rhythm, blood pressure, respiratory rate, and level of consciousness. **Rationale:** Baseline data necessary to identify the changes effected by therapy. Level of consciousness is the best indicator of neurologic status.
2. Assess skin integrity for areas of redness, breakdown, and decubiti, especially over areas of bony prominences. **Rationale:** Externally applied thermic devices can cause skin damage.
3. Assess the type and length of temperature exposure. **Rationale:** Assists in anticipating specific patient problems. Determines the type and course of treatment.
4. Assess prothrombin time, partial prothromboplastin time, platelet count, and cultures of bodily fluids. **Rationale:** Hypothermia can disrupt the clotting cascade. Microbacterial cultures may determine the etiology of fever.

Nursing Diagnoses

1. Hypothermia related to environmental exposure

to cold. **Rationale:** Trauma and surgery may induce hypothermia.
2. Hyperthermia related to neurohumoral changes, hypothalmic disturbances, pharmacologic interventions, and/or an infectious process. **Rationale:** These conditions affect the body's ability to maintain thermoregulation.
3. Potential impaired skin integrity related to use of a hypothermia/hyperthermia blanket. **Rationale:** Prolonged or improper use may lead to ischemia and/or burns.

Planning

1. Develop individualized goals for the use of a hypothermia/hyperthermia blanket: Patient will attain and maintain a state of normothermia. **Rationale:** Hypothermia/hyperthermic states affect body systems and metabolic demands (see Fig. 14–2).
2. Prepare all necessary equipment and supplies. **Rationale:** Assembly of necessary equipment enhances efficient institution of thermoregulatory therapy.
   a. Hypothermia/hyperthermia unit and detachable blanket or pad.
   b. Two sheets or bath blankets.
   c. One rectal thermometer or skin probe if rectal probe is contraindicated.
   d. One bottle of lubricating fluid (mineral oil or lanolin).
3. Prepare the patient.
   a. explain the rationale for instituting use of hypothermia/hyperthermia blanket therapy. **Rationale:** Minimizes anxiety and provides education regarding therapy.
   b. Discuss the procedure and possible discomfort that may be experienced. **Rationale:** Minimizes anxiety and facilitates having the patient alert the nurse when a side effect is experienced.
4. Review individual manufacturer's instructions to become adept with using your particular hypothermia/hyperthermia unit. **Rationale:** Each manufacturer's unit functions differently.
5. Inspect the hypothermia/hyperthermia unit:
   a. Be sure that the reservoir in the machine is filled with the appropriate fluid to the level recommended by the manufacturer. **Rationale:** The reservoir must be filled to the proper level for the machine to perform properly.
   b. Ensure that the unit has been inspected and approved for use by biomedical engineering or the appropriate hospital personnel. **Rationale:** Electrical safety precaution.
   c. Attach hoses from the thermal pad to the device. Make sure that the hoses are not kinked. **Rationale:** Allows flow of warmed/cooled fluid to the pad.
   d. Plug the device into a grounded outlet. **Rationale:** A grounded outlet is necessary for electrical safety.
   e. Check for leaks, and ensure that all connections are secure. **Rationale:** Allows for smooth equip-

ment operation and promotes a safe environment.

6. Verify physician's order for hypothermia/hyperthermia therapy. Physician's order should include: the desired temperature range and length of time patient is to be on/off therapy. **Rationale:** Prevents error in augmenting thermoregulatory mechanisms.

Implementation

Steps	Rationale	Special Considerations
1. Wash hands.	Reduces transmission of microorganisms.	
2. Place one sheet or bath blanket between patient and thermal pad. If additional thermal pad is placed over patient, place a sheet between patient and pad.	Protects the skin by decreasing the possibility to exposure to ice on the pad, which may form with condensation.	Avoid use of additional lifter sheets, since more efficient heating or cooling occurs with maximal contact between the thermal pad and skin.
3. Activate the hyperthermia/hypothermia unit.	To warm or cool patient.	
Manual Control		
a. Push the start and manual control switches.	Initiates therapy.	
b. Set the temperature dial to the desired thermal pad/fluid temperature.	To achieve/maintain normothermic state.	Desired thermal pad temperature refers to the temperature in the reservoir and thermal pad.
To Warm Patient		
(1) Set temperature dial to 100°F for approximately 5 minutes.	Allows device time to warm up.	Control panels on individual devices vary. *Temperature dial* thus refers to needle display or digital display of temperature.
(2) Then reset temperature dial to setting between 80 to 108°F.	Warms patient.	Body should be warmed no faster than 1°F per hour.
(3) Turn off machine when patient's temperature is 1 to 2°F below the desired patient temperature.	Patient's actual temperature tends to drift 1 to 2°F above the desired patient temperature.	
To Cool Patient		
(1) Set temperature dial to 40°F for approximately 5 minutes.	Allows device time to cool down.	Freeze burns and ischemia to pressure areas of skin may occur with prolonged periods of cooling at 40°F.
(2) Then reset temperature dial to setting between 40 to 60°F.	Cools patient.	Avoid drops of more than 1°F every 15 minutes. If continued cooling is desired, set the temperature dial to 20 to 25°F below the desired patient temperature.
(3) Turn off machine when patient's temperature is 1 to 2°F above the desired patient temperature.	The patient's actual temperature tends to drift 1 to 2°F below the desired patient temperature.	
Automatic Control		
a. Push start and manual control switch.	Initiates therapy.	Device needs to be warmed up or cooled down by manual mode before automatic temperature control can be initiated.

Table continues on following page

Steps	Rationale	Special Considerations
b. Set the temperature dial to the desired thermal pad/fluid temperature.	To achieve/maintain normothermia.	
To Warm Patient		
(1) Set temperature dial to 100°F for approximately 5 minutes.	Allows device time to warm up.	
To Cool Patient		
(1) Set temperature dial to 40°F for approximately 5 minutes.	Allows device time to cool down.	
c. Activate the automatic control switch.	Initiates autoregulating function within the device.	
d. Then set the temperature dial to the desired patient temperature.	To achieve/maintain normothermia.	Most automatic devices can regulate patient's temperature ±1°F of desired temperature.
4. Insert the lubricated temperature probe 3 to 4 in into the patient's rectum and tape securely into place.	Decreases incidence of injury to the rectal mucosa.	Use a water-based lubricant instead of a petroleum-based lubricant because it dissolves more readily in the rectum. An axillary skin probe may be substituted if a rectal probe is contraindicated.
5. Attach the other end of the probe into the probe adapter on the device.	For temperature monitoring.	Fluid circulating through the thermal pad will be heated or cooled in response to the patient's temperature. Lights on control panel will indicate whether device is heating or cooling fluid at one particular time.
6. Obtain patient's temperature from device readout.	Indicates patient's actual body temperature.	
7. Take patient's rectal temperature manually and compare with device readout.	Validates the temperature from the device.	
8. If both manual thermometer and device readout correlate, proceed with automatic temperature control.	Accuracy of temperature readout from device is essential for safe use of automatic temperature control.	
9. Wash hands.	Reduces transmission of microorganisms.	

Evaluation

1. Evaluate patient's temperature using consistent route every 15 to 30 minutes. Avoid temperature decreases exceeding 1°F every 15 minutes. **Rationale:** Use of consistent route is essential in trending temperature changes. Overly rapid cooling can induce shivering and cardiac insufficiency.

2. With manual mode, shut device off once actual body temperature reaches 1°F above (when cooling) or below (when heating) desired temperature. **Rationale:** Provides for expected "drift" in temperature; usually takes 3 to 4 hours to bring patient's temperature to desired range using one thermal pad. Also provides for a break in blanket use.

3. Evaluate heart rate and rhythm, blood pressure, capillary refill, lip color, and respiratory rate every 15 to 30 minutes. **Rationale:** Cardiac irregularities ranging from bradycardia to ventricular fibrillation can occur with rapid rewarming; hypotension may occur with rapid warming; rapid cooling may induce shivering, thus increasing metabolic needs and cardiac demand.

4. Evaluate patient's level of consciousness every 15 to 30 minutes. **Rationale:** Neurologic function can be affected by temperature extremes. Level of consciousness is the best indicator of neurologic function.

5. Measure urine output hourly. **Rationale:** During hypothermia, metabolism decreases, thus kidney function is diminished.

6. Inspect skin every 30 to 60 minutes for changes; reapply lubrication, massage pressure areas, and reposition patient. **Rationale:** Hypothermia/hyperthermia blanket therapy can predispose exposed areas of skin to thermal burns or frostbite. Areas of bony prominences such as the sacrum and scapulae are more prone to injury.

7. Assess for shivering on an ongoing basis; notify physician and adjust the temperature of blanket accordingly or discontinue use. **Rationale:** Shivering may indicate that the body is being cooled too rapidly. It markedly elevates the body's temperature and metabolic rate.

8. Assist the awake patient in coughing and deep breathing exercises at least every 2 hours. Suction the intubated patient whenever necessary. **Rationale:** Cold, immobilized patients tend to retain respiratory secretions; measures to prevent hypostatic pneumonia.

9. Perform range-of-motion exercises for unconscious patients or instruct the alert patient to perform them twice daily unless contraindicated. **Rationale:** Prevents circulatory stasis.

10. Avoid use of pins or needles near the thermal pad. **Rationale:** Pins and needles may puncture the pad and cause leakage of fluid.

Expected Outcome

Normothermia is achieved. **Rationale:** The process of conduction has assisted in effecting a temperature change.

Unexpected Outcomes

1. With a hypothermia blanket, frostbite, shivering, cardiac dysrhythmias. **Rationale:** Frostbite occurs as constricted peripheral blood vessels cause decreased blood flow to the skin. Shivering occurs with rapid body cooling as an attempt to increase the body's temperature. Cardiac dysrhythmias may result from this sudden increase in metabolic rate.

2. With hyperthermia blanket, burns, cumulative effect of drugs, cardiac insufficiency. **Rationale:** Cool, poorly perfused skin is at an increased risk for thermal burns. In hypothermia, the metabolism of drugs is decreased owing to inefficient liver and kidney function. As the body warms up, effects of the drugs may increase. With warming, peripheral blood vessels dilate, causing cold blood to shift to the heart. This may irritate the myocardium, causing ventricular fibrillation. As the periphery dilates with warming, blood is shunted away from the heart, reducing cardiac output. Hypotension may be a response to vasodilation with warming.

Documentation

Documentation in the patient record should include date and length of therapy; mode used (hypothermia vs. hyperthermia); assessment data before, during, and following therapy, including body temperature and route, heart rate and rhythm, blood pressure, respiratory rate, skin condition, level of consciousness, urine output, laboratory values (especially platelet count, prothrombin time, partial thromboplastin time, and cultures results); and any unexpected outcomes and the interventions taken. **Rationale:** Documents nursing care given and expected and unexpected outcomes.

Patient/Family Education

Explain to both patient and family the necessity to promptly report possible side effects, including pain, especially to areas exposed to thermal pad, lethargy or confusion, shivering, changes in skin condition, and bleeding. **Rationale:** Encourages patient and family participation in care; potentially prevents serious sequelae from side effects.

Performance Checklist
Skill 14–1: Use of Hypothermia/Hyperthermia Blanket

Critical Behaviors	Complies	
	yes	no
1. Wash hands.		
2. Appropriately place one sheet or bath blanket.		
3. Activate unit.		
MANUAL MODE a. Push start switch and manual control switch.		
b. Cool down or warm up device by setting dial to 40°F or 100°F.		
AUTOMATIC MODE a. Activate the manual control switch.		
b. Cool down or warm up device by setting dial to 40°F or 100°F.		
c. Activate the automatic control switch.		
d. Set temperature dial to desired patient temperature.		

Table continues on following page

Critical Behaviors	Complies	
	yes	no
4. Insert the rectal temperature probe.		
5. Attach rectal probe to probe adapter on device.		
6. Obtain temperature readout on device.		
7. Take patient's temperature manually.		
8. Compare temperature readout on device with manual reading.		
9. Wash hands.		
10. Document procedure in patient record.		

SKILL 14-2

Fluid Warming Devices

Intravenous (IV) infusion of cold banked blood or cold fluids can induce hypothermia and cardiac dysrhythmias, particularly in small children and elderly adults. The average temperature of banked blood products is 39.2°F (4°C) when dispatched from the blood bank. Fluid warming devices heat blood products and intravenous fluids to over 86°F (30°C), which can assist in preventing inadvertent hypothermia and dysrhythmias. Most fluid warming devices require a specific type of infusion tubing, which increases the cost of fluid delivery. Fluid warming devices that utilize a standard size IV tubing and smaller-gauge venous catheters are helpful in treating the hypothermic patient who does not require massive fluid volume replacement. When large volume replacement is required a fluid warmer utilizing larger-diameter tubing and venous catheters may be preferred.

Two types of fluid warming devices are discussed here, both of which utilize standard size IV tubing and can be attached to any size intravenous catheter. The first device (Fig. 14-5) contains an in-line system with an electronically powered warmer that holds and warms a disposable plastic bag between two warming plates. During infusion, the fluid flows through a series of channels within the bag (Fig. 14-6), descending into a bubble trap/drip chamber and through tubing into the patient. The second type of device contains an electrically powered aluminum cylindrical heating unit (Fig. 14-7). A fluid cuff is applied around this cylinder that contains the intravenous solution or blood product to be administered. Fluid is then purged into a bubble trap/drip chamber through the IV tubing and into the patient (Fig. 14-8). Most manufacturers provide a one-piece fluid bag or cuff administration set, to which standard IV or blood administration tubing can be attached. All units contain safety systems that ensure that the fluid temperature will not exceed 104°F (40°C), preventing thermal burns to the patient.

Purpose

The nurse uses a fluid warming device to

1. Provide warmed IV solutions or blood products.

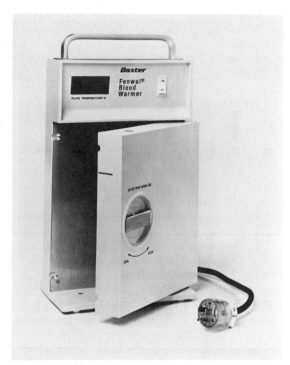

FIGURE 14-5. In-line, dry-heat fluid warming device. (Courtesy of Travenol Laboratories.)

2. Restore normothermia and fluid balance.
3. Prevent and/or treat physiologic malfunctions precipitated by a hypothermic state.

Prerequisite Knowledge and Skills

Prior to using a fluid warming device, the nurse should understand

1. Principles of temperature taking.
2. Principles of intravenous therapy.
3. Principles of fluid balance.
4. Principles of aseptic technique.
5. Pathophysiologic alterations associated with hypothermia and fluid imbalance.

The nurse should be able to perform

1. Proper handwashing technique (see Skill 35-5).

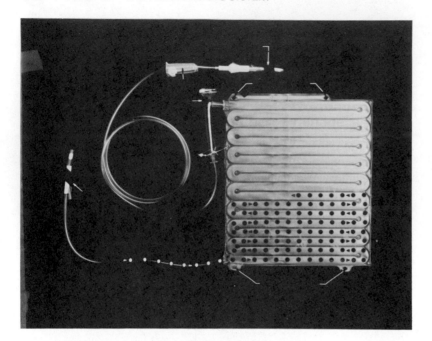

FIGURE 14–6. The blood warmer is used only with a FENWAL® blood warming bag to form a dry heat warming system. During use, blood enters the blood warmer through the disposable blood warming bag, which is positioned within the blood warmer unit. Operation of the combined units keeps the retained blood volume to a minimum within the bag and maintains a precise temperature range while the blood passes through the system at flow rates up to 150 ml/minute. (Courtesy of Travenol Laboratories.)

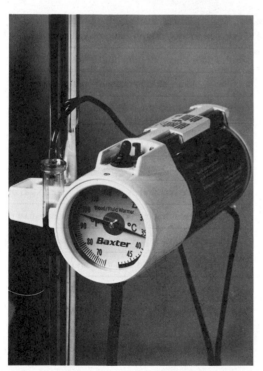

FIGURE 14–7. Aluminum cylindrical fluid warming device. (Courtesy of Baxter Healthcare Corporation.)

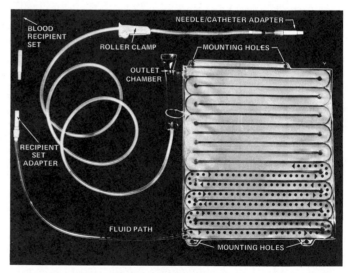

FIGURE 14–8. Blood warming bag with adapters and fluid path indicated. During operation, blood passes through a recipient set that has been connected to the warming bag positioned within the blood warmer. Blood enters the bag through a lower side inlet port, where it is channeled upward through the fluid path of the bag. A warming plate on each side of the bag transfers heat to maintain a blood temperature range of 30 to 37°C. Warmed blood exits the system through an outlet chamber on the upper side of the bag. (Courtesy of Travenol Laboratories.)

2. Administration of IV therapy and blood products.
3. Temperature taking.
4. Vital signs assessment.
5. Respiratory system assessment.
6. Cardiovascular system assessment.
7. Assessment of fluid balance status.

Assessment

1. Assess the patient's body temperature for hypothermia (less than 95°F or 35°C) and vital signs, including heart rate and rhythm, blood pressure, and respiratory rate. **Rationale:** Data necessary to identify the changes effected by therapy.

2. Assess for signs and symptoms of hypothermia (see Fig. 14–2), including cardiac dysrhythmias ranging from bradycardia to ventricular fibrillation, decreased urine output less than 0.5 cc/h per kilogram of body weight, and decreased level of consciousness. **Rationale:** Necessary to identify the changes effected by therapy.

3. Assess fluid balance status, including central venous pressure (normal range 2 to 14 mmHg), pulmonary artery capillary wedge pressure (normal range 4 to 12 mmHg), urine output, breath sounds (crackles may indicate fluid overload), skin and mucous membranes (dry, cracked skin and mucous membranes may indicate hypovolemia), and heart rate and blood pressure (tachycardia and hypotension may indicate hypovolemia). **Rationale:** Reliable indicators of fluid balance.

4. Assess venous catheter insertion site for patency and signs of infiltration or phlebitis. *Infiltration:* edema, pain, leakage of fluid at site. *Phlebitis:* local redness, edema, pain, warmth, red streak over distribution of vein. **Rationale:** Intravenous therapy should be instituted only when the insertion site is patent and free from signs of infiltration or phlebitis.

5. Obtain the patient's medical history, especially the type and length of cold exposure or surgery. **Rationale:** Assists in anticipating specific patient problems and provides direction for treatment selection.

Nursing Diagnoses

1. Hypothermia related to metabolic states, mechanical causes, and pharmacologic interventions (Table 14–1). **Rationale:** Causes of hypothermia can be classified into three major categories.

2. Potential for injury related to rapid infusion of cold IV solutions or blood products. **Rationale:** Rapid infusion of cold fluids can predispose the patient to hypothermia and cardiac dysrhythmias.

3. Potential for fluid volume excess related to aggressive intravenous fluid or blood administration. **Rationale:** Patient is at risk for fluid overload with aggressive fluid resuscitation.

Planning

1. Develop individualized goals for administering IV fluids or blood products through a warming device to attain or maintain normothermia and/or normovolemia. **Rationale:** Hypothermia can lead to multisystems pathophysiologic malfunctioning.

2. Prepare all necessary supplies and equipment. **Rationale:** Assembly of necessary equipment ensures that fluid warming device will be set up quickly and efficiently.
   a. Fluid warming device.
   b. Prescribed IV fluid or blood product.
   c. One device-specific administration set.
   d. One standard intravenous or blood tubing.
   e. One 19-gauge or larger needle.
   f. One roll 1-in tape.

3. Review manufacturer's instructions for specific device to be used. **Rationale:** To prevent errors in administration and damage to equipment.

4. Ensure that the device has been inspected and approved for use by the appropriate hospital personnel (see Skill 36–1). **Rationale:** For the safety of the nurse and patient.

5. Prepare the patient by explaining the rationale for use of a fluid warming device. **Rationale:** Reduces anxiety.

Implementation

Steps	Rationale	Special Considerations
1. Wash hands.	Reduces transmission of microorganisms.	
2. Verify physician order for administration of warmed blood products or fluid.	Prevents errors in blood product or IV fluid administration.	Physician's order should include type of blood product or IV solution, rate of infusion, and actual patient temperature at which time warm fluid therapy should be discontinued.
3. Plug device into outlet, and turn it on.	Activates device.	
4. Perform all function and alarm checks as per manufacturer's instructions.	Safety precautions. Validates proper equipment function.	
5. Wait for temperature readout to reach operating temperature.	Prevents administration of cold fluids.	Operating range is usually 30 to 37°C (66 to 98.6°F).
6. Open the door(s) of the device.	To access warming mechanism.	

Table continues on following page

Steps	Rationale	Special Considerations
In-Line, Dry-Heat Device		
7. Mount the fluid bag into the device as per manufacturer's instructions.	Required for fluid warming.	
8. Close the door.	Device will not operate with open door.	
9. Spike standard blood or IV tubing into the prescribed blood product or IV solution.	Allows priming of the fluid warming device to occur.	
10. Attach the male Luer-lok of the standard blood product or IV tubing to the female Luer-lok of the fluid bag.	Continues assembly.	
11. Attach needle onto patient end of tubing.	To initiate IV fluid therapy.	Red blood cells should be infused via a 19-gauge or larger needle and intravenous catheter in order to prevent cell breakage.
12. Open the roller clamps on both the standard blood or IV tubing and the tubing that extends from the fluid bag, and purge the entire system of air.	Primes the system and reduces the incidence of air embolus.	Each drip chamber/bubble trap should be approximately halfway full.
Aluminum Cylindrical Device		
7. Wrap fluid cuff around the aluminum cylinder.	Allows heat conduction to fluid bag.	
8. Close the doors.	Device will not operate with open doors.	
9. Spike the standard blood or IV tubing into the prescribed blood product or IV fluid.	Allows priming of the fluid warming device to occur.	
10. Attach the male Luer-Lok of the standard blood or IV tubing to the female Luer-Lok of the fluid bag.	Continues assembly.	
11. Attach needle to patient end of tubing.	Initiates IV fluid therapy.	
12. Open the roller clamps on both the standard blood or IV tubing and the tubing that extends from the fluid bag, and purge the entire system of air.	Primes the system and reduces the incidence of air embolism.	Some manufacturers require that drip chamber/bubble trap of the fluid cuff tubing be inverted while priming.
For Both Types of Fluid Warmer		
13. After the system has been purged of air, place the drip chamber/ bubble trap in the position or slot indicated by the manufacturer.	For proper administration of fluid.	
14. Piggyback the needle into the primary infusion line, and secure connection with tape.	Prevents accidental disconnection.	
15. Adjust the rate and temperature as prescribed.	To attain or maintain normothermia and/or fluid balance.	
16. Wash hands.	Reduces transmission of microorganisms.	

Evaluation

1. Evaluate patient's temperature using consistent route every 30 to 60 minutes. **Rationale:** Use of consistent route is essential in trending temperature changes. Monitors efficacy of therapy.

2. Evaluate heart rate and rhythm, blood pressure, capillary refill, lip color, and respiratory rate every 15 to 30 minutes. **Rationale:** Cardiac dysrhythmias ranging from bradycardia to ventricular fibrillation can occur with rapid rewarming; hypotension may occur with rapid warming; and rapid cooling may induce shivering, thus increasing metabolic needs and cardiac demand.

3. Evaluate patient's level of consciousness every 15 to 30 minutes. **Rationale:** Neurologic function can be affected by temperature extremes.

4. Measure urine output hourly. **Rationale:** During hypothermia, metabolism decreases, and kidney function is diminished.

5. Evaluate fluid status every 30 minutes using assessment measures in Step 3 (p. 447). **Rationale:** These assessment parameters, when used in combination, can be reliable indicators of fluid balance.

Expected Outcomes

1. Normothermia is achieved (temperature greater than 95°F or 35°C). **Rationale:** Infusion of warmed fluids has assisted in effecting a temperature change.

2. Fluid balance is achieved, as evidenced by the following parameters within normal limits (see Assessment Step 3, p. 447), central venous pressure, pulmonary capillary wedge pressure, urine output, blood pressure and heart rate, condition of skin and mucous membranes, and chest x-ray and breath sounds. **Rationale:** Infusion of fluids has assisted in restoring fluid balance. The state of fluid balance may vary with each individual.

Unexpected Outcomes

1. Persistent hypothermia (temperature less than 95°F or 35°C). **Rationale:** Infusion of warmed fluids alone may not be sufficient to restore normothermia.

2. Fluid overload, as evidenced by increased central venous pressure and pulmonary capillary wedge pressure, jugular vein distension, and auscultation of crackles. **Rationale:** In attempting to restore fluid balance and normothermia, patient may have received an excess of fluid.

Documentation

Documentation in the patient record should include date and time fluid warming device was initiated, heart rate and rhythm, blood pressure, respiratory rate and breath sounds, level of consciousness, urine output, central venous pressures and pulmonary capillary wedge pressures, volume and type of IV solution or blood product, temperature of infusion, and any unexpected outcomes and the interventions taken. **Rationale:** Documents nursing care given, expected and unexpected outcomes.

Patient/Family Education

Reinforce to the patient and family the rationale for warming blood products and IV fluids. **Rationale:** Decreases patient and family anxiety.

Performance Checklist
Skill 14–2: Fluid Warming Devices

Critical Behaviors	Complies	
	yes	no
1. Wash hands.		
2. Verify physician's order.		
3. Plug device into outlet, and turn device on.		
4. Perform all function and alarm checks.		
5. Wait for temperature to reach operating range.		
6. Open device door(s).		
In-Line, Dry-Heat Device 7. Mount the fluid bag into device.		
8. Close door.		
9. Spike standard IV or blood tubing into bag of prescribed IV solution or blood product.		
10. Attach male Luer-lok of standard IV tubing to female Luer-lok of fluid bag.		
11. Attach needle to patient end of fluid bag or tubing.		
12. Open roller clamps to purge entire system of air.		

Table continues on following page

	Complies	
Critical Behaviors	**yes**	**no**
13. Place drip chamber/bubble trap in recommended position or slot.		
14. Attach needle into well-established venous catheter, and secure with tape.		
15. Begin infusion, and adjust rate and temperature.		
16. Wash hands.		
17. Document procedure in patient record.		
ALUMINUM CYLINDRICAL DEVICE 7. Wrap fluid cuff around aluminum cylinder.		
8. Close doors.		
9. Spike standard IV or blood tubing into bag of prescribed IV solution or blood product.		
10. Attach male Luer-lok of standard IV tubing to female Luer-lok of fluid bag.		
11. Attach needle to patient end of fluid bag or tubing.		
12. Open roller clamps to purge entire system of air.		
13. For both types of fluid warmers, place bubble trap/drip chamber in proper position.		
14. Attach needle into well-established venous catheter, and secure with tape.		
15. Begin infusion, and adjust rate and temperature.		
16. Wash hands.		
17. Document procedure in patient record.		

SKILL 14–3

Microwaved Solutions

Microwaving intravenous solutions is a practical and efficient method for core rewarming of the hypothermic and volume-depleted patient. It is performed by warming crystalloid fluids in a maximum output of 600- to 650-W, 2450-mHz microwave oven. Blood should not be warmed by the microwave because the uneven heating and poor mixing that occurs can lead to breakage of red blood cells and other cell changes. Precise duration of heating and accurate monitoring of solution temperature are imperative to ensure safe and adequate rewarming. The microwave oven must operate at an exact power level.

Purpose

Solutions are microwaved to

1. Warm solutions rapidly and efficiently.
2. Restore normothermia.
3. Prevent and/or treat physiologic conditions related to a hypothermia.

Prerequisite Knowledge and Skills

Prior to microwaving solutions, the nurse should understand

1. Principles of temperature taking.
2. Principles of intravenous therapy.
3. Principles of fluid balance.
4. Principles of aseptic technique.
5. Pathophysiologic complications associated with hypothermia and fluid imbalance.
6. Danger of thermal burns related to overheated solutions.

The nurse should be able to perform

1. Proper handwashing technique (see Skill 35–5).
2. Administration of IV therapy.
3. Temperature taking of the patient and of IV fluids.
4. Vital signs assessment.
5. Respiratory system assessment.
6. Cardiovascular system assessment.
7. Assessment of fluid balance status.
8. Identification of appropriate microwave oven for use.
9. Operation of available microwave oven.

Assessment

1. Assess body temperature for hypothermia (less than 95°F or 35°C) and vital signs, including heart rate and rhythm, blood pressure, and respiratory rate. **Rationale:** Data are necessary to identify changes effected by therapy.
2. Assess for signs and symptoms of hypothermia

(see Fig. 14–2). **Rationale:** Necessary to identify the changes effected by therapy.

3. Assess fluid balance status, including central venous pressure (normal range 2 to 14 mmHg), pulmonary artery capillary wedge pressure (normal range 4 to 12 mmHg), urine output, breath sounds (crackles may indicate fluid overload), skin and mucous membranes (dry, cracked skin and mucous membranes may indicate hypovolemia), and heart rate and blood pressure (tachycardia and hypotension may indicate hypovolemia). **Rationale:** Reliable indicators of fluid balance.

4. Obtain the patient's medical history, especially the type and length of cold exposure or surgery. **Rationale:** Assists in anticipating specific patient problems.

Nursing Diagnoses

1. Hypothermia related to metabolic states, mechanical causes, and pharmacologic interventions (Table 14–1). **Rationale:** Causes of hypothermia can be classified into three major categories.

2. Potential for injury related to infusion or application of solutions greater than 101°F (38.1°C). **Rationale:** Improper monitoring of solution's temperature may predispose the patient to thermal burns. Red blood cell hemolysis can occur with infusion of overly warmed solutions.

Planning

1. Develop individualized goals for microwaving solution to attain or maintain normothermia. **Rationale:** Hypothermia affects thermoregulation and metabolic demands.

2. Prepare all necessary supplies and equipment. **Rationale:** Ensures efficient heating of solution.
   a. Microwave oven (600 to 650 W, 2450 mHz).
   b. Digital display thermometer.
   c. Prescribed nondextrose solution contained in a plastic polyvinyl chloride container (glass bottle or container with metal parts is contraindicated).
   d. One intravenous administration set.
   e. One 18- to 22-gauge needle.
   f. One roll 1-in tape.

3. Ensure that microwave oven has been inspected and approved for safe use by the appropriate hospital personnel (see Skill 36–1). **Rationale:** For safety of nurse and patient.

Implementation

Steps	Rationale	Special Considerations
1. Wash hands.	Reduces transmission of microorganisms.	
2. Verify physician's order for microwaving solution(s).	Prevent errors in solution(s) preparation.	Physician's order should include type of solution, rate of infusion, and actual patient temperature at which time warm fluid therapy should be discontinued.
3. Obtain 1-L bag of prescribed nondextrose solution.	Dextrose caramelizes at high temperatures.	Polyvinyl chloride plastic containers are safe for use in microwave ovens.
4. Establish baseline temperature of solution by using closed-bag technique: fold plastic bag over thermometer.	Closed-bag technique ensures sterility of solution. Knowledge of baseline solution temperature is essential in predicting fluid temperature after microwaving.	Average temperature of solutions at room temperature is 70°F.
5. Place solution in center of microwave oven 1 L at a time.	In this position, heating is most efficient. Adequate heating is not ensured when more than 1 L is heated at one time.	
6. Heat bag for 60 seconds on high power.	Provides mechanism for initial heating of solution.	
7. Shake bag and turn over.	Ensures mixing of unevenly heated solution.	
8. Heat bag for an additional 60 seconds.	Clinical trials demonstrate that fluid temperatures increase 31°F after 120 seconds of heating.	
9. Shake bag vigorously at end of heating for approximately 5 seconds.	Ensures mixing of unevenly heated solution.	

Table continues on following page

Steps	Rationale	Special Considerations
10. Measure temperature of bag immediately prior to administration of fluid using closed-bag technique.	Fluid may rapidly lose heat in transport to patient's bedside.	Do not administer fluids with temperature greater than 101°F. High fluid temperature may cause burns to patient or may hemolyze red blood cells.
11. Spike IV administration set or tubing into prescribed solution.	Prepares setup for priming.	
12. Attach needle onto patient end of tubing, and prime line.	Continues assembly and prevents air embolism.	
13. Piggyback into primary infusion, and tape connection.	Prevents accidental disconnection.	
14. Adjust rate as prescribed.	To attain or maintain normothermia and/or fluid balance.	
15. Wash hands.	Reduces transmission of microorganisms.	

Evaluation

1. Evaluate patient's temperature using consistent route every 30 to 60 minutes. **Rationale:** Use of consistent route is essential in trending temperature changes. Monitors efficacy of therapy.

2. Evaluate heart rate and rhythm, blood pressure, capillary refill, lip color, and respiratory rate every 15 to 30 minutes. **Rationale:** Cardiac dysrhythmias ranging from bradycardia to ventricular fibrillation can occur with rapid rewarming; hypotension may occur with rapid warming.

3. Evaluate patient's level of consciousness every 15 to 30 minutes. **Rationale:** Neurologic function can be affected by temperature extremes.

4. Measure urine output hourly. **Rationale:** During hypothermia, metabolism decreases and kidney function is diminished.

5. Evaluate fluid status every 30 minutes using assessment measures mentioned earlier (see Steps 2 and 3, p. 450–451). **Rationale:** These assessment parameters, when used in combination, are reliable indicators of fluid balance.

Expected Outcomes

1. Normothermia is achieved (temperature greater than 95°F or 35°C) and maintained. **Rationale:** Administration or application of warmed fluids affects core body temperature.

2. Fluid balance is achieved, as evidenced by the following parameters within normal limits: central venous pressure, pulmonary capillary wedge pressure, urine output, blood pressure and heart rate, condition of skin and mucous membranes, and chest x-ray and breath sounds. **Rationale:** Infusion of fluids has assisted in restoring fluid balance. The state of fluid balance may vary with each individual.

Unexpected Outcomes

1. Persistent hypothermia (temperature less than 95°F or 35°C). **Rationale:** Warmed fluids alone may not be sufficient to restore normothermia.

2. Fluid overload, as evidenced by increased central venous pressure and pulmonary capillary wedge pressure, jugular vein distension, and auscultation of crackles. **Rationale:** Patient may have received an excess of fluid.

3. Thermal burn or hemolysis. **Rationale:** Overheated solutions may cause tissue damage on lysis of red blood cells.

Documentation

Documentation in the patient record should include date and time warmed fluid via microwave was administered or applied, heart rate and rhythm, blood pressure, respiratory rate and breath sounds, level of consciousness, urine output, central venous pressures and pulmonary capillary wedge pressures, volume and type of IV solutions, temperature of infusion, and any unexpected outcomes and the interventions taken. **Rationale:** Documents nursing care given and expected and unexpected outcomes.

Patient/Family Education

Explain to patient and family the need to promptly report possible side effects, such as pain, redness, or swelling at IV insertion site. **Rationale:** Encourages participation in care and facilitates prompt intervention.

Performance Checklist
Skill 14–3: Microwaved Solutions

Critical Behaviors	Complies yes	no
1. Wash hands.		
2. Verify physician's order.		
3. Obtain prescribed IV fluid or solution.		
4. Take baseline temperature of fluid using closed-bag technique.		
5. Place solution in center of microwave oven.		
6. Heat 1 L of solution for 60 seconds on high power.		
7. Shake bag and turn it over.		
8. Heat bag for another 60 seconds on high power.		
9. Shake bag at end of heating.		
10. Measure temperature of bag immediately prior to administration of fluid.		
11. Spike IV solution with IV tubing or administration set.		
12. Attach needle onto tubing, and prime line.		
13. Piggyback fluid into patent primary infusion line, and tape connection.		
14. Adjust rate as prescribed.		
15. Wash hands.		
16. Document procedure in patient record.		

BIBLIOGRAPHY

Biddle, C. (1985). Hypothermia: Implications for the critical care nurse. *Crit. Care Nurs.* 5(2):34–38.

Biddle, C. J., and Biddle, W. L. (1985). Factors responsible for thermoregulatory balance. *Geriatric Nurs.* 6(1):41.

Cincinnati Sub-Zero Products, Inc. (1979). *The Blanketrol System for Hyper-Hypothermia* (Operation, Service, and Technical Manual). Cincinnati, Ohio.

Hospital of the University of Pennsylvania, Department of Nursing (1985). *Applications of Heat and Cold* (Nursing Policy Manual). Philadelphia, Pa.

Hospital of the University of Pennsylvania, Department of Nursing (1990). *Use of Blood/Fluid Warmers in Adult Transfusion Therapy* (Nursing Policy Manual). Philadelphia, Pa.

Kenney, C. V., Guzzetta, C. E., and Dossey, B. M. (1985). *Critical Care Nursing: Mind–Body–Spirit*, 2d Ed. Boston: Little, Brown.

Leaman, P. L., and Martyak, G. G. (1985). Microwave warming of resuscitation fluids. *Ann. Emerg. Med.* 14(9):876–879.

Matz, Robert (1986). Hypothermia: Mechanisms and countermeasures. *Hosp. Pract.* Jan. 30, p. 47.

Morgan, S. P. (1990). A comparison of three methods of managing fever in the neurologic patient. *J. Neurosci. Nurs.* 22(1):19–24.

Ricci, M. M. (1985). Hypothermia and Hyperthermia. In S. Millar, L. K. Sampson, and M. Soukup (Eds.), *AACN Procedure Manual for Critical Care*, 2d Ed. (pp. 346–351). Philadelphia: Saunders.

Rueler, J. B. (1978). Hypothermia: Pathophysiology, clinical settings, and management. *Ann. Intern. Med.* 89(4):876–879.

Seymour, G. (1986). *Medical Assessment of the Elderly Surgical Patient.* Rockville, Md.: Aspen Publications.

Travenol Laboratories, Inc. (1981). *Fenwal Blood Warmer* (Operator's Manual). Deerfield, Ill.

Werwath, D. L., Schwab, C. W., Scholten, J. R., and Robinett, W. (1986). Warming nondextrose crystalloid in a microwave oven. *Ann. Emerg. Med.* 15(2):228–230.

15

TRACTION DEVICES

BEHAVIORAL OBJECTIVES

After completing this chapter, the nurse will be able to

- Define the key terms.
- Identify populations requiring cervical traction.
- Discuss, describe, and facilitate safe application and maintenance of traction.
- Identify potential complications of cervical traction.
- Demonstrate the skills involved in the use of traction devices.

Skeletal traction is applied to the cervical spine when it has become unstable as a result of spinal injury, degenerative disease, or surgery. Cervical alignment and reduction are the goals of treatment. Immobilization reduces the risk of further injury to the vertebrae, ligaments, and underlying soft neural tissue. Reduction achieves realignment of the vertebrae, verified by serial x-rays. The definitive method used to treat cervical fractures depends on the injury classification but may be physician- or institution-specific.

This chapter focuses on the nursing skills required to care for a patient in cervical traction.

KEY TERMS

autonomic dysreflexia
autonomic nervous system
CT scan
halo: ring, struts, vest
  (Halo external fixator)
hyperextension
hyperflexion
immobilization
insensate
MRI
myelogram
neurogenic bladder
neurogenic bowel
orthosis (orthotic device)

osteomyelitis
outer table (of the skull)
overdistraction
poikilothermia
reduction
spinal injury
spinal cord injury
spine stabilization
sympathetic nervous system
tenodesis
tomogram
tongs: Gardener-Wells,
  Crutchfield, Vinke
torque

SKILLS

15–1 Assisting with Insertion of External Fixation Devices
15–2 Maintenance of Desired Traction
15–3 Tong and Pin Care
15–4 Halo Traction Care

GUIDELINES

The following assessment guidelines assist the nurse in formulating a nursing diagnosis and an individualized plan of care to maintain desired cervical traction in a safe, effective manner:

1. Know the patient's baseline motor and sensory function.
2. Identify associated injuries that may contraindicate tong application (i.e., skull fracture).
3. Know the patient's baseline vital signs.
4. Know the patient's past medical history, including specifically allergies, previous bony fractures requiring traction, and previous motor or sensory deficits.
5. Predict multisystem response to spinal cord injury.
6. Know the goals of traction.
7. Determine appropriate interventions if assessment findings indicate motor or sensory deterioration.
8. Assess for unexpected outcomes of cervical tong/pin placement.
9. Anticipate patient's tolerance of the procedure and ability to cooperate.
10. Become adept with equipment required to initiate and maintain cervical traction.
11. Anticipate potential complications related to immobility.

SKILL 15–1

Assisting with Insertion of External Fixation Devices

External fixation devices (tongs) are applied to the skull to align the cervical spine. Tongs consist of a stainless steel body with pins attached at each end or a graphite body with titanium pins (used in institutions where MRI is available) (Fig. 15–1). The pin insertion for tong placement may vary slightly, but the care is essentially the same.

The insertion of Crutchfield and Vinke tongs necessitates an incision to expose the skull. Two holes are made in the outer table of the skull with a twist drill, and the pins are inserted and tightened until there is a firm fit. Gardener-Wells tongs are inserted by placing the razor-sharp pin edges to the prepared areas of the scalp and tightening the screws until the spring-loaded mechanism indicates that the correct pressure has been

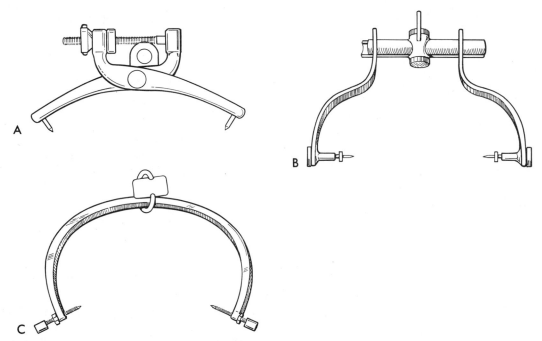

FIGURE 15–1. All three types of cervical tongs consist of a stainless steel body and a pin with a sharp tip attached to each end. (*A*) Crutchfield tongs are placed about five inches apart in line with the long axis of the cervical spine. (*B*) Vinke tongs are placed at the parietal bones, near the widest transverse diameter of the skull. (*C*) Gardener-Wells tongs are inserted slightly above the patient's ears.

achieved. All types of pins are well seated in the outer table of the skull and angle inward to decrease the possibility of tong displacement.

After the tongs are inserted, traction is applied by the serial addition of weights to a rope-and-pulley device attached to the tongs (Fig. 15–2). Serial x-rays are taken to document vertebral alignment at specific weight intervals. Serial neurologic examinations are performed with the addition or subtraction of weights to assess the effects of cervical traction on underlying neural structures. Excessive traction may cause stretching of and damage to the spinal cord. Once these tongs are in place,

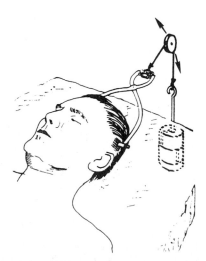

FIGURE 15–2. Continuous traction provided by weight applied to a cervical external fixation device via a rope-and-pulley system. (Reprinted with permission from R. McRae, *Practical Fracture Treatment*, 2d Ed. Edinburgh: Churchill-Livingstone, 1989, p. 184.)

the patient is maintained on bed rest with mobility restriction, which may necessitate the use of a specialty bed such as a Roto-Rest or Stryker frame.

Cervical traction also may be applied using a halo ring device. This is a stainless steel or graphite ring that is attached to the skull by four stabilizing pins (two anterior and two posterolateral) (Fig. 15–3). The pins are threaded through holes in the ring, screwed into the outer table of the skull, and locked in place. Direct traction may be applied to the ring device with rope and pulley or by attaching the ring to a body vest, which allows for increased mobility of the patient.

Purpose

The nurse assists with the application of a cervical external fixation device to

1. Assess motor or sensory function.
2. Assess vital signs.
3. Assess the integument at the insertion sites.
4. Provide comfort measures to the patient.
5. Support the physician with tong placement.

Prerequisite Knowledge and Skills

Prior to assisting the physician with tong application, the nurse should understand

1. Anatomy of the cranium and overlying soft tissue.
2. Goals and principles of traction.
3. Pathophysiology of vertebral and spinal cord injury.

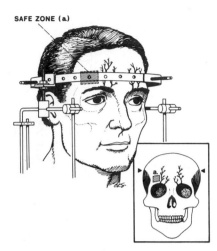

SAFE ZONE (a)

FIGURE 15–3. Diagram illustrating placement of halo pins and ring. The anterior pins are placed anterolaterally 1 cm above the orbital ridge. This "safe zone" avoids the temporalis muscle laterally and an orbital nerve plexus and frontal sinus medially. (Reprinted with permission from M. Botte, S. Garfin, T. Byrne, et al., The halo skeletal fixator: Principles of applications and maintenance. *Clin. Orthop.* 239:14, 1989.)

4. Neurologic innervation and function of specific spinal levels.

The nurse should be able to perform

1. Motor and sensory assessment.
2. Neurologic assessment.
3. Vital signs assessment.
4. Pulmonary assessment.
5. Skin assessment.
6. Pain and discomfort assessment.
7. Aseptic technique.
8. Setup and application of traction.
9. Proper handwashing technique (see Skill 35–5).
10. Log-rolling techniques.

Assessment

See Table 15–1 for assessment parameters specific to spinal cord injury.

1. Perform motor/sensory assessment. **Rationale:** Establishes baseline motor/sensory status to identify any deviations (Figs. 15–4 and 15–5 and Table 15–2). Improving motor/sensory assessment may indicate proper spinal/vertebral alignment; deteriorating examinations may indicate poor spinal/vertebral alignment, an ex-

TABLE 15–1 PHYSIOLOGIC RESPONSES TO IMMOBILITY AND SPINAL CORD INJURY

Body System	Physiologic Response to Immobility	Physiologic Response to Spinal Cord Injury	Assessment Parameters
Integumentary	Pressure → ischemia → integumentary disruption	Protective motor and sensory functions lost or impaired below the level of the lesion.	Inspect bony prominences. Identify preexisting skin disruptions. Assess specific pressure areas related to traction devices and positioning.
Pulmonary	Decreased chest expansion Secretions pool CO_2 retention → respiratory acidosis	Lost or impaired neuromuscular stimulus to diaphragm, internal and external intercostals, abdominal muscles, and accessory muscles	Thoracic inspection. Identify breathing patterns. Auscultate breath sounds. Respiratory parameters (NIF/FVC). Supplemental O_2. ABG/pulse oximetry. Identify associated pulmonary injury.
Cardiovascular	Increased cardiac workload Thrombus formation Orthostatsis	Decreased vasomotor tone Loss of sympathetic response Poor venous return Poikilothermia Spinal shock → autonomic dysreflexia	Vital signs and rhythm interpretation. Hemodynamic parameters. Body/skin temperature. Organ perfusion assessment: Level of consciousness. Urine output.
Musculoskeletal	Muscle atrophy Joint immobility → contractures	Loss/impairment of voluntary motor function Flaccid → spastic paralysis	Identify level of lesion. Serial motor/sensory examinations. Assess joint mobility (flaccidity/spasticity). Identify traction and applied weights.

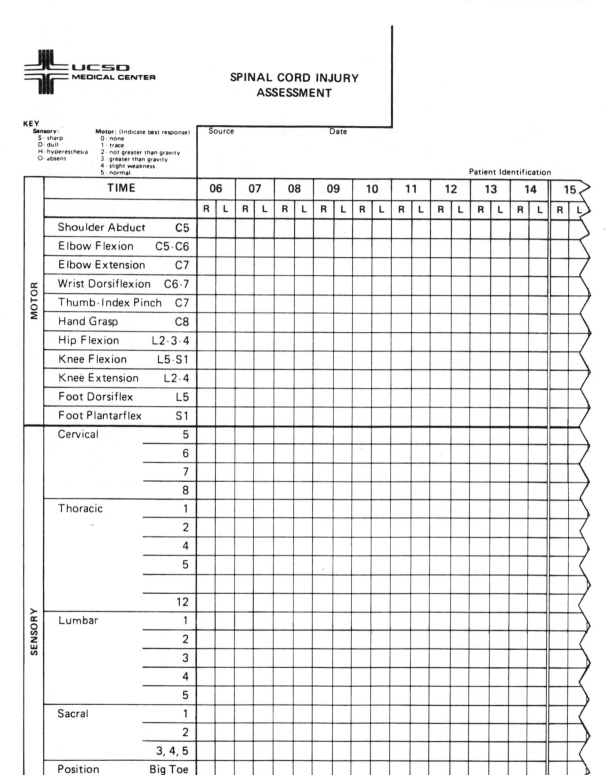

FIGURE 15–4. Sample of flowsheet documentation for motor and sensory testing. Courtesy of University of California, San Diego (UCSD) Medical Center.

panding process within the spinal cord, evolving or ascending spinal cord injury, and poor patient compliance with testing (this may be volitional or related to a de-

creasing level of consciousness or the administration of pain medications).

2. Perform neurologic assessment, including level of

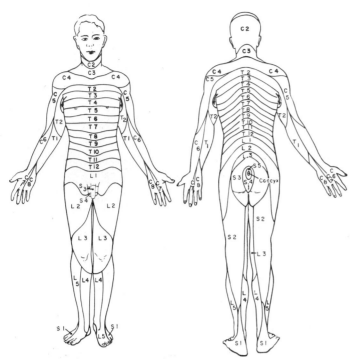

FIGURE 15–5. Sensory dermatomes; guidelines for sensory testing. (Reprinted with permission from M. L. Barr and J. A. Kiernan, *The Human Nervous System: An Anatomical Viewpoint,* 5th Ed. Philadelphia: Lippincott, 1988, p. 81.)

consciousness, mentation, and patient's ability to understand and cooperate with instructions. **Rationale:** Establishes baseline neurologic function, identifies deviations from baseline, and predicts patient's tolerance of and cooperation with tong placement.

3.　Assess vital signs. **Rationale:** Establishes baseline vital signs to identify deviations from the baseline. Patients with spinal cord lesions above the sixth thoracic level are at risk to experience spinal shock, resulting from a loss of sympathetic innervation below the level of the

TABLE 15–2　ASSESSMENT OF MUSCLE STRENGTH

Motor Score	Indicators
5	Normal muscle strength; can maintain high degree of function against maximal resistance.
4	The muscle can go through its normal range of motion, but it can be overcome by increased resistance.
3	The muscle can go through its normal range of motion against gravity only; it cannot tolerate external resistance.
2	The muscle contracts weakly; it does not have sufficient strength to overcome gravity.
1	Visible or palpable muscle contractions may be seen or felt, but there is no movement in the limb.
0	Complete paralysis; no evidence of motor function.

Source: Adapted from J. Hickey, *The Clinical Practice of Neurological and Neurosurgical Nursing,* 2d Ed. Philadelphia: Lippincott, 1986, with permission.

lesion. Spinal shock results in severe bradycardia, profound hypotension, warm dry skin, and absent reflexes below the level of the lesion. The symptoms of spinal shock should be recognized as potentially life-threatening and require immediate intervention.

4.　Assess the pulmonary status. **Rationale:** Spinal cord injury interferes with normal pulmonary function (see Table 15–1).

5.　Assess the patient's skin. **Rationale:** Establishes a baseline of any preexisting skin irritation or breakdown (Table 15–3). To identify any open areas interfering with pin placement.

6.　Assess the patient's level of pain and discomfort. **Rationale:** The patient may require sedation or pain medication in order to safely perform pin placement with the patient's full cooperation.

Nursing Diagnoses

1.　Potential for injury related to pin placement. **Rationale:** Both bitemporal and halo pins pierce the skin, underlying soft tissue, and outer table of the skull. Any structure in the pathway of the pin is at risk for disruption, including facial and skull muscles, veins, arteries, and nerves. Specific anatomic landmarks are identified to avoid venous, arterial, and nervous structures.

2.　Impairment in skin integrity related to pin or tong insertion. **Rationale:** Pin placement disrupts the integrity of the skin. Local care and assessment are integral to preventing or identifying superficial infections.

3.　Pain related to tong or pin insertion, injury, application of weights, and muscle spasm. **Rationale:** Although a local anesthetic is injected prior to pin/tong insertion, most patients describe local discomfort as the pins are secured to the outer table of the skull. The patient also may be experiencing pain related to the injury itself or as a result of cervical muscle spasm, which may be relieved by the administration of a muscle relaxant, such as diazepam.

4.　Anxiety related to anticipatory pain and pin placement. **Rationale:** Anxiety heightens the perception of pain, interferes with information processing, and disrupts cooperation during the procedure.

Planning

1.　Individualize the following goals for the patient undergoing pin insertion and application of cervical traction:
　　a.　Verbalization of comfort. **Rationale:** Administration of systemic narcotics relieves pain and promotes cooperation.
　　b.　Cervical spine immobilization. **Rationale:** Cervical immobility reduces the risk of additional injury to the bony elements, ligaments, spinal cord, and spinal nerves.

2.　Prepare all necessary equipment and supplies. **Rationale:** Facilitates efficient insertion of external fixation device.

TABLE 15–3   HIGH-RISK FOCUS-AREA SKIN ASSESSMENT GUIDE

High-Risk Skin Areas

Devices/Positions	Forehead	Occiput	Chin	Ear	Clavicle	Scapula	Shoulder	Upper Arm	Elbow	Forearm	Wrist	Thumb Webbing	Axilla	Sternum	Ribs	Iliac Crest: Ant.	Iliac Crest: Post	Sacrum	Groin	Trocanter	Thigh	Knee	Calf	Ankle	Heel	Toe	Pin Sites
Halo vest device		√		√	√	√							√	√											√		
High-top sneakers																							√	√	√		
Resting arm splints								√	√	√	√																
Resting foot splints																						√	√	√	√		
Rotating kinetic table		√		√	√	√	√				√		√		√	√		√		√				√	√		
Stryker frame: prone	√	√	√		√	√	√								√	√				√				√	√		
Stryker frame: supine		√				√											√	√							√		
Tenodesis splints									√	√	√																
Tongs:																											
Gardener-Wells		√																									√
Crutchfield		√																									√
Vinke		√																									√

a. Tongs or halo ring insertion tray, including either specific type of tongs to be utilized or halo ring with insertion pins.

b. Razor/clipper.

c. Local anesthetic: Lidocaine 1% to 2% with or without epinephrine depending on physician's preference. Lidocaine with epinephrine may be preferred for scalp injection because of the scalp's vascularity.

d. Povidone-iodine scrub or solution (100 cc).

e. 4 × 4 sponges (four packages or one tub).

f. Syringe (1 to 3 cc).

g. Needles: 18 gauge for withdrawing medication from vial; 23 gauge for subcutaneous injection.

h. Sterile gloves (two to three pairs).

i. Traction assembly.

j. Rope.

k. S or C hook (to attach to distal end of rope for weight application).

l. Sandbag weights (desired amount will vary; verify with physician).

m. Halo-ring head positioner (Hershey jig).

n. Torque wrench.

3. Set up traction on regular or specialty bed (Stryker frame or rotating kinetic table). **Rationale:** Allows for immediate application of traction once the tongs/pins are inserted.

   a. Obtain/identify pulley device. Pulley device must be applied to a regular bed or rotating kinetic table. Pulley is usually contained within the Stryker frame. **Rationale:** Functions as a fulcrum for traction forces.

   b. Thread rope through pulley device. **Rationale:** Allows for the application of (1) rope to tongs and (2) rope to weights.

   c. Knot connecting hook to distal end of rope. **Rationale:** Provides mechanism to attach weights to rope.

4. Prepare the patient.

   a. Explain tong/pin application to the patient. **Rationale:** Reinforces information given by the physician and allows the patient to ask appropriate questions.

   b. Review expectations regarding positioning and mobility with the patient. **Rationale:** It is imperative that the patient understand positioning restrictions prior to pin/tong placement.

   c. Review need for radiographs. **Rationale:** Multiple radiographs may be required to verify vertebral positioning.

   d. Maintain patient supine with head in a neutral position. **Rationale:** Facilitates tong/pin placement.

   e. Medicate the patient with pain-relieving agent as prescribed. **Rationale:** To promote comfort during procedure. Administration of analgesia and anti-anxiety agents to the spinal cord-injured population must be done prudently to avoid side effects such as respiratory depression.

   f. Clip/shave selected pin sites or assist physician with same. **Rationale:** Prepares area for pin insertion.

Implementation

Steps	Rationale	Special Considerations
1. Wash hands.	Reduces transmission of microorganisms.	
2. Cleanse selected pin sites with povidone-iodine solution.	Decreases skin surface bacteria.	Specific preparation may vary; check institutional guidelines.
3. Assist the physician with tong insertion by	Facilitates the procedure.	
a. Assisting with local anesthesia administration.	Decreases discomfort during tong/pin application.	
b. Donning sterile gloves.	Decreases bacteria in prepared areas.	
c. Stabilizing the patient's head during the procedure.	Maintains alignment of the cervical spine and provides support to the injured areas.	Cervical stability also can be maintained by the use of a hard collar, Philadelphia collar, or any device that limits head rotation and neck flexion/extension. A soft collar is *not* considered a stabilizing device. *Utmost care should be taken to prevent head rotation and neck flexion/extension.*
4. Assess the patient's tolerance to pin insertion.	Discomfort or anxiety may interfere with the patient's ability to cooperate with procedure.	The patient may require repeated explanation, reassurance, sedation, or pain medication.
5. Wash hands.	Reduces transmission of microorganisms.	

Evaluation

1. Evaluate motor/sensory function with each application or subtraction of cervical weights and routinely every 2 to 4 hours. **Rationale:** Evaluates the patient's response to and tolerance of a change in traction and identifies any untoward effects of continued traction. The patient should continue to demonstrate either baseline or improved neurologic function during the course of vertebral realignment. Occasionally, when significant reduction is required, the physician applies a large amount of weight (greater than 50 lbs). As cervical traction weight increases, the chance of overdistracting the spine and spinal cord occurs. In these cases, the patient will demonstrate deteriorating motor/sensory function. *The physician must be notified immediately if a neurologic deterioration is identified.*

2. Monitor vital signs every 1 to 2 hours. **Rationale:** To identify potential physiologic changes occurring with traction application (see Table 15–1).

3. Evaluate pin sites immediately after insertion and every 4 hours thereafter. **Rationale:** Ensures pin integrity and facilitates timely identification of complications, such as hematoma, irritation, swelling, and infection. (See Skill 15–3 for tong and pin care.)

4. Ensure that serial radiographs have been obtained after the tongs and traction are placed and with each change in traction weight. **Rationale:** Radiographs are required to demonstrate alignment of the cervical spine. The physician adds or removes the weights.

5. Evaluate tolerance to pin and weight application.

Rationale: Assists with the achievement of proper cervical reduction and alignment.

Expected Outcomes

1. Immobilization and alignment of the cervical spine. **Rationale:** Reduces further risk of injury and provides stability to the cervical spine.

2. Motor/sensory function improves or remains stable. **Rationale:** Indicates that no further injury has been incurred as a result of traction application.

3. Skin is free from irritation at pin sites. **Rationale:** Validates continuation of traction and absence of infection.

Unexpected Outcomes

1. Skin beneath the pins is "tented" or pulled as weights are applied to or maintained in the traction setup. **Rationale:** Indicates that tongs have not been set in or are out of the outer table of the cranium. If this occurs upon initial weight application, ask the physician to reassess tong placement. If this occurs during traction maintenance, the physician must be notified. (See Skill 15–2 for maintaining cervical traction.)

2. Deterioration of motor/sensory function. **Rationale:** May indicate overdistraction, cervical malalignment, or evolution of spinal cord injury. The physician must be notified immediately that the patient has declining motor/sensory capabilities. The physician should confirm the assessment findings, evaluate cervical alignment by use of a lateral radiograph, and remove weights if indicated.

3. Tong/pin sites become reddened, swollen, or have purulent discharge. **Rationale:** Indicates local infection with bacterial colonization. This may advance to osteomyelitis if not identified and treated.

4. The patient does not tolerate pin insertion or application of weights. **Rationale:** The patient may require further sedation, analgesia, or muscle relaxant. Most patient's require repeated reinforcement of the need for the procedure and continuous emotional support throughout the procedure to ensure cooperation.

Documentation

Documentation in the patient record should include date, time, and physician inserting tongs; sites of insertion; types of tongs/pins used; amount of weight applied; patient's motor/sensory examination before and after the procedure; patient's general tolerance of the procedure; vital signs; skin, respiratory, and neurologic assessments, with emphasis on changes from the baseline; completion of radiograph(s); appearance of pin sites; method of maintaining traction; specialty bed utilized; and effectiveness of methods or agents used for pain and anxiety control. **Rationale:** Provides a record of nursing interventions and expected and unexpected outcomes and serves as a legal document of the events.

Patient/Family Education

1. Review with the patient and family the pathology of the disease or injury, such as displaced vertebra, spinal instability, and effects of spinal cord injury. **Rationale:** Provides knowledge base for further education.
2. Discuss with the patient and family the immediate goals of traction, such as to provide support to the spine, to align the spine, and to ensure immobilization, and emphasize the importance of cervical immobilization. **Rationale:** Enhances understanding of treatments and mobility restrictions.
3. Describe the type of bed the patient will be on in order to maintain traction and immobility, the process of inserting tongs/pins, and the importance of cooperation with serial motor/sensory examinations.

Rationale: Decreases anxiety and ensures cooperation with serial testing.
4. Review the following restrictions:
   a. Nothing should be placed under the patient's head or shoulders *unless* it is approved by the physician. **Rationale:** Pillows and towel rolls placed under the patient's head or shoulders interfere with spinal alignment and cervical flexion/extension. *However*, in some instances, orthopedic alignment is enhanced by placement of a towel roll or other device to achieve a specific position. This must be evaluated by a radiograph, and care must be taken not to disturb devices placed to achieve improved vertebral alignment.
   b. The patient may not turn independently while affixed to cervical traction. **Rationale:** Physically repositioning the patient may be contraindicated because of spinal instability. Specialty beds, such as a rotating kinetic table, Stryker frame, or CircOlectric bed, negate the need to reposition the patient from side to side (Fig. 15–6). Nevertheless, skin and pulmonary issues are critical and must be addressed. The patient on a rotating kinetic table must undergo at least 20 hours of rotation daily to benefit from kinetic therapy. The patient in a Stryker frame or CircOlectric bed must be turned supine/prone every 2 hours. Log-rolling techniques are best utilized to ensure neutrality and provide support to the spine when manual repositioning is necessary.
   c. The patient and family must be instructed *not* to handle traction equipment. **Rationale:** Handling or manipulating the traction apparatus in any way could cause further injury to the patient. Patients who are confused or who have poor short-term memory require repeated instructions and emotional support to ensure their safety while in cervical traction. The patient and family require concrete information regarding the nature of the injury and potential implications of unauthorized traction manipulation; however, severe reprimands predicting further paralysis or worsening injury are not therapeutic and are discouraged in the care of these patients.

Performance Checklist
Skill 15–1: Assisting with Insertion of External Fixation Devices

Critical Behaviors	Complies yes	no
1. Wash hands.		
2. Perform or assist with povidone-iodine scrub to elected areas.		
3. Assist physician with tong insertion:		
a. Assist with local anesthesia or sedation administration.		
b. Don sterile gloves.		

Table continues on following page

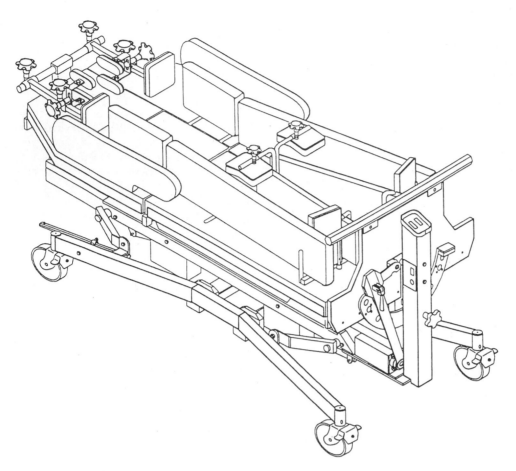

FIGURE 15–6. The Rotating Kinetic Treatment Table®. The patient is positioned and balanced on the table. The motor mechanism allows the patient to be rotated side to side, thereby displacing weight and assisting to relieve pressure areas. Cervical traction may be applied via a tension system at the head of the bed. Kinetic Therapy^SM can also facilitate pulmonary care of the patient, allowing easy access to the thoracic area for physiotherapy and coughing. (Courtesy of Kinetic Concepts Incorporated, San Antonio, Texas.)

Performance Checklist
Skill

Critical Behaviors	Complies	
	yes	no
c. Stabilize patient's head through procedure.		
d. Administer pain/anxiety medications.		
4. Assess patient's tolerance to pin insertion.		
5. Assess pin sites and motor/sensory function after pin/tong insertion.		
6. Ensure that radiograph has been completed.		
7. Wash hands.		
8. Document procedure in patient record.		

SKILL 15–2

Maintenance of Desired Traction

Once cervical tongs or a halo ring has been applied, it is the nurse's responsibility to maintain the traction. General guidelines for traction maintenance include

1. Allowing the weights to hang freely.
2. Preventing knots in the rope from getting caught in the pulley device.
3. Ensuring proper body alignment.
4. Centering rope on pulley device.

The rope-and-pulley system can be attached to a hospital bed frame, but it is more likely that the patient will be cared for in a specialty bed, such as a Stryker frame, a Rotating Kinetic Treatment Table®, or a CircOlectric frame (see Fig. 15–6). These beds provide stability to the spine yet allow for patient mobility to facilitate pulmonary, integumentary, cardiovascular, bowel, and bladder care. The CircOlectric bed may be contraindicated for use in patients with cervical trauma because of orthostatic hypotension and excessive tension on the fracture produced when the bed is manipulated to change the patient's position.

Purpose

The nurse cares for the patient in cervical traction to

1. Maintain continued reduction, alignment, and immobilization of the cervical spine.
2. Prevent/minimize complications of continued immobility (see Table 15–1).
3. Evaluate the patient's tolerance to therapy.
4. Evaluate the effect of traction on the patient's motor/sensory examination.
5. Provide comfort measures to the patient.

Prerequisite Knowledge and Skills

In order to maintain cervical traction, the nurse should understand

1. Principles of traction.
2. Anatomy and physiology of the spine and spinal cord.
3. Principles of cervical immobility.
4. Signs, symptoms, and complications of overdistraction.
5. Multisystem response to immobility and spinal cord injury (see Table 15–1).

Prior to caring for the patient in cervical traction, the nurse should be able to perform

1. Motor/sensory assessment.
2. Pulmonary assessment.
3. Vital signs assessment.
4. Cardiovascular assessment.
5. Skin assessment.
6. Musculoskeletal assessment.
7. Proper handwashing technique (see Skill 35–5).
8. Neurologic assessment.
9. Traction maintenance.
10. Pain/discomfort assessment.
11. Techniques facilitating patient positioning to maintain spinal neutrality.
12. Passive range-of-motion exercises and other interventions to minimize development of contractures.
13. Gastrointestinal assessment.
14. Genitourinary assessment.

Assessment

1. Perform motor/sensory assessment. **Rationale:** To identify deviation from the baseline assessment. Deterioration may indicate overdistraction, a stretching of the spinal cord resulting from increased weight application to the traction apparatus. Improvement may indicate improved spinal alignment and restored neurologic function postinjury (see Table 15–2 and Fig. 15–4).
2. Perform pulmonary assessment (see Table 15–1 for specific pulmonary indicators). **Rationale:** Immobility and spinal cord injury can cause serious compromise in the patient's pulmonary/ventilatory function.
3. Assess vital signs. **Rationale:** To identify the pa-

tient's continued physiologic response to immobility and spinal cord injury.
4. Perform cardiovascular assessment (see Table 15–1 for specific cardiovascular indicators). **Rationale:** Immobility and spinal cord injury can seriously compromise homeostatic cardiovascular responses, specifically sympathetic responses.
5. Assess the skin every 2 hours. **Rationale:** Impaired mobility and lack of protective sensation predispose spinal cord–injured patients to skin breakdown. Particular attention should be given to all bony prominences and the skin beneath specific equipment and devices (see Table 15–3).
6. Perform musculoskeletal assessment (see Table 15–1). **Rationale:** Immobility and spinal cord injury affect normal musculoskeletal tone and function. Efforts must be taken to identify joint immobility and contractures.
7. Assess neurologic status. **Rationale:** Continued assessment of neurologic function is necessary to predict patient's continued tolerance of and cooperation with cervical traction.
8. Assess for pain/discomfort. **Rationale:** Pain/discomfort may occur as a result of continued traction and immobility and cervical muscle spasm.
9. Assess patient's body alignment/positioning. **Rationale:** Maintain cervical spine neutrality to prevent further injury and to promote optimal joint mobility.
10. Assess urine output. **Rationale:** Immobility is associated with urinary retention; spinal cord injury may result in neurogenic bladder.
11. Assess bowel motility. **Rationale:** Immobility is associated with constipation; spinal cord injury may result in paralytic ileus and neurogenic bowel.
12. Assess mastication (with bitemporal tong placement) or eye closure (with halo ring and pin placement). **Rationale:** Bitemporal tong pins pierce the masseter muscle and may interfere with mastication (Garfin et al., 1986). Anterior halo pin placement may impair complete eye closure (Nazaroff et al., 1989).
13. Assess traction setup for kinks, knots, or malpositioning of the rope; pin placement and integrity; rope position; amount of weight; and freely hanging weights. **Rationale:** To detect problems that may impair proper traction.

Nursing Diagnoses

1. Potential for injury related to improper application and maintenance of traction. **Rationale:** Results in motor/sensory deterioration, pulmonary and cardiovascular compromise, and jeopardizes long-term rehabilitative potential.
2. Impaired physical mobility related to imposed mobility restrictions and concurrent neuromuscular dysfunction. **Rationale:** See Table 15–1 for complications of immobility. Physical immobility must be restricted to maintain proper alignment with restoration of neurologic function.
3. Self-care deficits related to enforced positioning

and neuromuscular impairment. **Rationale:** The patient is likely to be dependent for all self-care needs because of motor impairments and prescribed immobility to maintain cervical traction.

4. Potential for impaired skin integrity related to immobility and tong placement. **Rationale:** Maintaining cervical traction restricts mobility; spinal cord injury also renders the patient immobile to some degree. See Table 15–3 for high-risk skin assessment areas.

5. Potential for impaired gas exchange related to immobility. **Rationale:** The physiologic response to immobility is associated with specific pulmonary complications. Neuromuscular dysfunction also impairs normal pulmonary function (see Table 15–1).

6. Urinary retention related to immobility and spinal cord injury. **Rationale:** Both immobility and spinal cord injury can impair normal bladder-emptying mechanisms.

7. Constipation related to immobility and spinal cord injury. **Rationale:** Poor gastric motility and impairments in neuromuscular innervation to the gut (neurogenic bowel) result in ineffective bowel emptying.

8. Potential for alteration in nutrition: less than body requirements. **Rationale:** The patient may exhibit difficulty with chewing related to bitemporal pin placement. Soft foods and high-protein/calorie supplements may be offered to increase caloric intake if needed.

9. Potential for injury related to incomplete eye closure. **Rationale:** Incomplete eye closure may occur with anterior halo pin placement. Specific eye care (as prescribed) may be performed to avoid corneal injury.

Planning

1. Individualize the following goals for the patient in cervical traction:

    a. Maintain cervical traction. **Rationale:** Provides support for cervical spine alignment.
    b. The patient will be turned every 2 hours *or* the kinetic table will be rotated 20 of every 24 hours. **Rationale:** Decreases the risk of immobility-related complications and provides a means for skin assessment and care.
    c. Minimize the complications of immobility (see Table 15–1). **Rationale:** Decreases risk of additional patient morbidity.
    d. Maintain neutral spine positioning. **Rationale:** Minimizes the risk of further spinal injury.
    e. Minimize pain/discomfort. **Rationale:** Optimizes patient comfort and ensures continued cooperation with maintenance of cervical traction.

2. Gather all equipment and supplies needed to perform care while patient is in traction. **Rationale:** Facilitates efficient performance of care.
    a. Towels, washcloths, linen.
    b. Lotion, powder, soap.

3. Prepare the patient prior to any procedure or related care. **Rationale:** Promotes cooperation with maneuvers.
    a. Reinforce the need for maintaining cervical traction. **Rationale:** Emphasizes importance of cervical traction and provides an opportunity for questions.
    b. Review method of repositioning the patient. **Rationale:** This may involve either rotating, flipping, or turning the patient depending on the type of bed the patient is on. These maneuvers can be very stressful to the patient and frequently require review of what to expect during turning procedure.

Implementation

Steps	Rationale	Special Considerations
1. Wash hands.	Reduces transmission of microorganisms.	
2. Perform pin care (see Skill 15–3).	Decreases risk of local infection and identifies pin-related problems.	
3. Reposition the patient.	Prevents or minimizes the risk of immobility-related complications.	
4. Perform pulmonary toilet, including chest physiotherapy, cough/deep breathing, and quad-assist cough (when indicated).	Mobilizes secretions and maintains effective airway clearance.	It is generally *not recommended* that patients in cervical traction be placed in postural drainage positions for pulmonary toilet because of the risk of traction malfunction.
5. Perform active/passive range-of-motion exercises on all extremities.	Decreases the occurrence of joint immobility and contracture formation.	
6. Apply orthotic devices as prescribed.	Provides intermittent support to areas at risk for contracture development.	Leather high-top sneakers, resting foot splints, tenodesis splints, resting arm splints, and soft restraints may be used to prevent contractures associated with immobility and spinal cord injury.

Table continues on following page

Steps	Rationale	Special Considerations
7. Wash hands.	Reduces transmission of microorganisms.	

Evaluation

1. Evaluate motor/sensory function every 2 to 4 hours routinely. **Rationale:** To assess the effects of traction and repositioning of the patient. Motor/sensory function should be evaluated with any addition or subtraction of 1cervical weights.

2. Evaluate vital signs (i.e., heart rate, rhythm, respiratory rate, and blood pressure). **Rationale:** To determine if there is any deviation from the baseline resulting from traction manipulation or repositioning of the patient. The patient on a Stryker frame with a spinal cord injury may *not* tolerate a face-down position because of a loss of sympathetic function below the level of the lesion. These patients must be monitored closely until positioning tolerance has been achieved.

3. Auscultate breath sounds every 2 to 4 hours. **Rationale:** To determine effects of traction and repositioning on the pulmonary system.

4. Evaluate patient's perception of pain and discomfort. **Rationale:** To identify the effects of repositioning and interventions aimed at relieving pain and discomfort, such as specific positioning, medications, and relaxation techniques.

5. Evaluate the patient's body position and alignment. **Rationale:** Maintenance of cervical traction weight may cause the patient to be slowly and inadvertently pulled up in bed. Repositioning the patient also may result in a change in body alignment.

6. Evaluate effectiveness of bowel and bladder elimination. **Rationale:** Many patients require Foley catheterization for complete bladder emptying and stool softeners to ease bowel movements. Spinal cord–injured patients *must* be placed on a bowel program as soon as possible to avoid impaction and facilitate gastrointestinal function.

7. Evaluate the patient's nutritional status (see Skill 32–2). **Rationale:** Nutritional support is essential to promote healing.

Expected Outcomes

1. Cervical alignment. **Rationale:** Immobilization of the cervical spine prevents further deterioration of neurologic function until surgery is performed or a halo-vest is applied.

2. Minimal side effects of immobility. **Rationale:** Aggressive, consistent nursing care prevents or limits the complications of immobility and decreases length of stay.

3. Verbalization of comfort. **Rationale:** Analgesics and non-pharmacologic interventions decrease anxiety and promote relaxation.

Unexpected Outcomes

1. Motor/sensory function deteriorates. **Rationale:** Overdistraction or stretching of the spinal cord results in motor weakness, numbness, tingling, or other sensory changes. Motor and sensory function also can deteriorate as a result of evolution (edema and neural disruption) of the spinal cord injury. Radiographs must be obtained to identify any orthopedic malposition of the vertebrae. *Notify the physician immediately in the event of motor/sensory changes.*

2. Dislodged pins/tongs. **Rationale:** May result in further neurologic damage as a result of disruption of traction, alignment, and cervical stability. See Skill 15–3 for interventions required for pin/tong dislodgment. *Notify the physician immediately if this occurs.*

3. Malposition or disruption of weights on pulley device/rope. **Rationale:** May result in additional motor weakness and/or sensory abnormalities. *Notify the physician immediately if this occurs.*

4. Intolerance to repositioning. **Rationale:** If the patient is on a Stryker frame, he or she may experience a variety of responses to pronating, from dizziness and discomfort to cardiovascular compromise and rhythm disturbances. If these responses interfere with turning the patient, then the patient must be placed on another type of bed to achieve mobility and avoid skin breakdown. If the patient is on a rotating kinetic table, he or she may not tolerate continuous rotation because of discomfort, dizziness, and nausea. The bed may be turned and locked manually to help the patient build up a tolerance to rotation.

5. Pulmonary compromise. **Rationale:** Both immobility and spinal cord injury may result in poor pulmonary function. The patient may require elective or emergency intubation with ventilatory assistance.

6. Skin breakdown. **Rationale:** Both immobility and spinal cord injury predispose the patient to skin disruption associated with pressure and poor skin perfusion.

Documentation

Documentation in the patient record should include date, time, and frequency of pin/tong assessment; traction setup and amount of weight applied; type of tongs/pins inserted; any changes in traction; serial motor/sensory function assessments; pulmonary, cardiovascular, integumentary, neurologic, and nutritional status and nursing interventions performed on the patient to optimize status; tolerance to repositioning; effectiveness of bowel and bladder elimination; joint mobility; pain; patient's body position/alignment; type of bed utilized; and the development of any unexpected outcomes. **Rationale:** Provides a record of nursing interventions and expected and unexpected outcomes and serves as a legal document of the events.

Patient/Family Education

1. Review with the patient and family the pathology of the disease or injury, such as displaced vertebra, spinal instability, and effects of spinal cord injury. **Rationale:** Provides a knowledge base for further education.
2. Discuss with the patient and family the immediate goals of traction, such as to support and align the spine and ensure immobilization. **Rationale:** Enhances understanding of treatment and mobility restrictions.
3. Describe the type of bed the patient will be on in order to maintain traction and immobility, the process of inserting tongs/pins, and the importance of cooperation with serial motor/sensory examinations. **Rationale:** Decreases anxiety and ensures cooperation with serial testing.
4. Review the following restrictions:
   a. Nothing should be placed under the patient's head or shoulders *unless* it is approved by the physician. **Rationale:** Pillows and towel rolls placed under the patient's head or shoulders interfere with spinal alignment and cervical flexion/extension. *However*, in some instances, orthopedic alignment is enhanced by placement of a towel roll or other device to achieve a specific position. This must be evaluated by radiograph, and care must be taken not to disturb devices placed to achieve improved vertebral alignment.
   b. The patient may not turn independently while affixed to cervical traction. **Rationale:** Physically repositioning the patient may be contraindicated because of spinal instability. Specialty beds, such as a rotating kinetic table or Stryker frame, negate the need to reposition the patient. Log-rolling techniques are indicated when manual repositioning is needed to ensure neutrality and provide support to the spine.
5. Discuss with the patient and family the body's multisystem response to immobility and spinal cord injury, and explain nursing interventions aimed at minimizing complications. **Rationale:** This information comprises the initiation of the rehabilitative process in the intensive care unit. The patient and family will ultimately learn to manage these problems independently; this basic information is needed to provide a groundwork upon which to build rehabilitative skills and concepts.

Performance Checklist
Skill 15–2: Maintenance of the Desired Traction

Critical Behaviors	Complies yes	no
1. Wash hands.		
2. Perform pin care.		
3. Reposition the patient.		
4. Perform pulmonary toilet.		
5. Perform range-of-motion exercises to extremities.		
6. Appropriately apply orthotic devices.		
7. Maintain the patient's proper body alignment.		
8. Wash hands.		
9. Document care in patient record.		

SKILL 15–3

Tong and Pin Care

Once the pins are inserted under aseptic conditions, external fixation devices require local care to prevent or assess for local infection. Since the pins are inserted through the skin into the bone, local infections can become devastating and may result in cranial osteomyelitis.

Tong and pin care is essentially the same for all devices. The areas are assessed for signs and symptoms of infection. Definitive skin care at pin sites remains controversial. It is generally recommended that the sites be cleansed with a peroxide-saline solution. The use of an iodine or Povidone-iodine preparation is not recommended (Rutecki and Seligson, 1980). Usually, pin sites do not require a dressing unless there is excessive drainage.

Occasionally, the pin or tong becomes disengaged from the skull. If the skin is tented beneath the pin or the pin is not attached to the skull, the patient should be placed supine with the weights and the neck stabilized. The physician should be notified *immediately* for pin or tong disengagement as well as any redness, swelling, or exudate at the pin site.

Purpose

The nurse performs tong or pin care to

1. Assess pin sites for signs and symptoms of infection, loosening, or displacement.
2. Remove exudate at pin sites.

Prerequisite Knowledge and Skills

Prior to tong or pin site care, the nurse should understand

1. Normal tong or pin site placement.
2. Muscle control of chewing and eyelid closure.
3. Specific system involvement related to cervical lesions.
4. Principles of infection control.
5. Universal precautions.

The nurse should be able to perform

1. Proper handwashing technique (see Skill 35–5).
2. Universal precautions (see Skill 35–1).
3. Wound assessment.
4. Assessment of chewing function.
5. Assessment of eyelid closure.

Assessment

1. Assess tong and pin sites for integrity or skin tenting. **Rationale:** Determines that pins have not slipped or loosened.
2. Assess tong and pin sites for signs and symptoms of infection. **Rationale:** Identifies pins and tongs that demonstrate drainage, redness, or swelling.
3. Assess mastication and eyelid closure. **Rationale:** Bitemporal tong placement may interfere with mastication; anterior halo pin placement may result in incomplete eyelid closure.

Nursing Diagnoses

1. Potential for infection related to pin/tong placement. **Rationale:** Pins and tongs penetrate the skin and interrupt the first barrier to infection.
2. Altered nutrition related to impaired mastication. **Rationale:** Masseter muscles are pierced during bitemporal pin placement.
3. Potential for injury related to incomplete eyelid closure. **Rationale:** Anterior halo pin may impair normal eyelid closure and interfere with protection and lubrication of the cornea.

Planning

1. Individualize the following goals for tong and pin care:
   a. Prevent infection or skin breakdown of pin/tong sites. **Rationale:** Pins/tongs are placed through the skin and penetrate the bone. Infection may necessitate relocating pin sites, administering systemic antibiotics, or discontinuing therapy earlier than expected.
   b. Clean pin sites free of exudate. **Rationale:** Excessive exudate provides a culture medium for bacterial growth. Exudate may be sent for culture and sensitivity analysis.
2. Prepare all necessary equipment and supplies. **Rationale:** Facilitates quick and efficient tong and pin care.
   a. Hydrogen peroxide (1 oz).
   b. Razor/clipper.
   c. Sterile normal saline solution (2 oz).
   d. Sterile cotton tip applicators (eight).
   e. Sterile specimen containers (two).
3. Prepare the patient.
   a. Explain the procedure to the patient. **Rationale:** To decrease anxiety, gain patient cooperation, and provide baseline information for long-term pin care.
   b. Position patient. **Rationale:** To adequately view pin insertion sites and to gain access for local care.

Implementation

Steps	Rationale	Special Considerations
1. Wash hands.	Reduces transmission of microorganisms.	
2. Mix 1 oz peroxide with 1 oz normal saline in sterile container.	Makes half-strength solution.	Solutions may be kept in covered sterile container for 24 hours. Label, date, and time solution containers.
3. Place 1 oz normal saline in a second sterile container.	Prepares a solution for rinsing.	

Table continues on following page

Steps	Rationale	Special Considerations
4. Cleanse the area around each pin and tong with a cotton-tip swab and half-strength H_2O_2/normal saline solution. Use a separate swab for each site to decrease the chance of cross-contamination.	Removes crusty drainage and prevents excessive exudate.	Some serous drainage may occur in the first 2 to 3 days.
5. Rinse site with saline-soaked swab.	Removes H_2O_2 and any further exudate.	
6. Wash hands.	Reduces transmission of microorganisms.	

Evaluation

Perform pin-tong site care every 8 hours and p.r.n. **Rationale:** Detects any loosening, redness, or infection at early stages so appropriate measures may be taken.

Expected Outcomes

1. Pin/tong sites will remain intact. **Rationale:** Validates stability of pins and traction and site integrity.
2. Site will be free of infection. **Rationale:** Clean, dry pin site decreases the incidence of skin breakdown and infection.
3. Effective eye closure. **Rationale:** Ensures that pins do not interfere with eyelid closure (halo ring only).

Unexpected Outcomes

1. Pin/tong displacement. **Rationale:** If pin/tong is not in proper place, tenting of skin or total displacement can occur. This interferes with proper traction and may result in further neurologic injury. If tongs/pins are displaced, maintain patient in a flat position with head in a neutral position, and *notify the physician immediately*.
2. Infection at site of pin/tong. **Rationale:** Local infection may lead to skull osteomyelitis. Systemic antibiotics may be used to treat pin-site infection (Glaser et al., 1986). The pin site may need to be changed if the patient does not respond to antibiotics.
3. Inadequate/limited nutritional intake. **Rationale:** Mastication is impaired, and patient cannot meet nutritional requirements. Nutritional supplements, soft diet, or enteral feedings may be needed.
4. Eye injury occurs. **Rationale:** Eyelids do not close, and cornea is injured. Alternative anterior pin sites should be identified. This may be avoided by having the patient close his or her eyes during insertion (Nazaroff et al., 1989).

Documentation

Documentation in the patient record should include date and time of pin/tong care; assessment data, including motor/sensory/cranial nerve function and condition of the skin and pin/tong insertion sites; any unexpected outcomes and interventions taken; and if a physician is consulted, the date, time, reason, and name of the physician notified. **Rationale:** Documents nursing care provided and expected and unexpected outcomes and serves as a legal document of the events.

Patient/Family Education

1. Discuss with the patient and family the basic concepts regarding pin and tong care, such as the need for cervical immobilization, the principles of handwashing, the principles of clean technique, the possible complications of pins/tongs, and that pin sites should not be touched by patient or family except to deliver site care. **Rationale:** Provides baseline information.
2. Assess the readiness of the patient and family to assume the responsibility of pin care. **Rationale:** Provides an opportunity to evaluate and educate the family about the long-term plan of care.
3. Teach the patient to notify the nurse about any increase in pain, tenderness, or swelling at the pin sites. **Rationale:** Allows patient to understand the importance of pin-site assessment to prevent infection and maintain traction.

Performance Checklist
Skill 15–3: Tong and Pin Care

Critical Behaviors	Complies yes	no
1. Wash hands.		
2. Mix 1 oz peroxide with 1 oz normal saline.		
3. Place 1 oz normal saline in sterile container.		

Table continues on following page

Critical Behaviors	Complies	
	yes	no
4. Cleanse areas with half-strength peroxide and saline solution.		
5. Rinse site with saline-soaked swab.		
6. Wash hands.		
7. Document in patient record.		

SKILL 15–4

Halo Traction Care

Patients having an unstable cervical spine injury will require long-term cervical traction and immobilization with halo traction. Halo traction may be applied preoperatively or postoperatively according to the physician's preference. Halo traction also may be applied as definitive treatment for certain spinal fractures. The patient may wear halo-vest traction for up to 10 to 12 weeks, the length of time required for bony healing.

The halo vest allows for patient mobility while still maintaining cervical traction. The apparatus consists of a halo ring with four skull pins, four vertical struts (two anterior and two posterior), and a hard plastic vest with anterior and posterior portions lined with sheepskin (Fig. 15–7). Two pins are placed anteriorly above the eyes in the frontal area and two posterolaterally in the temporo-occipital area. The anterior and posterior portions of the vest are attached with two shoulder and two side straps. It is important that the vest fit snuggly, that it is tight enough to prevent slippage but loose enough to prevent pressure sores or restrict breathing (Ohman and Spaniol, 1990).

Emergency access to the thoracic area is dependent on the specific halo-vest device used. Some vests are manufactured with breakaway struts that can collapse (when necessary) to facilitate access for CPR. Other vests are designed so that the anterior plastic vest can be deliberately broken for access to the thoracic area. Check the manufacturers' guidelines for emergency features of specific vests.

The newer models of halo rings and struts are made of graphite with titanium pins that are MRI compatible. The trend now is to immobilize the patient, realign the vertebrae, and reduce the fracture initially, and then place the patient in a halo-vest device prior to surgical stabilization to facilitate mobility for such diagnostic studies as CT scans, MRIs, tomograms, and myelograms.

Purpose

The nurse provides care for a patient in halo-vest traction to

1. Maintain cervical traction.
2. Mobilize the patient.
3. Maintain skin integrity.
4. Gain access to the patient for pulmonary care.

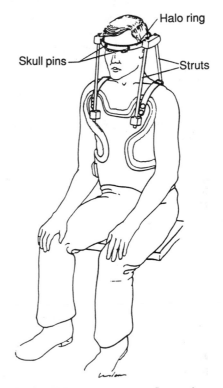

FIGURE 15–7. Halo-vest apparatus. Supportive struts and ring are attached to plastic vest, thereby applying cervical traction while allowing for patient mobility. (Reprinted with permission from M. F. Colbert and S. L. Kincade, Halo immobilization device. In S. L. Kincade and J. Lohrman (Eds.), *Critical Care Nursing Procedures.* Philadelphia: B. C. Decker, 1990, p. 286. Jim Wilson, illustrator.)

Prerequisite Knowledge and Skills

Prior to caring for the patient in halo-vest traction, the nurse should understand

1. Vertebral and spinal cord anatomy.
2. System-specific sequelae related to spinal cord injury (see Table 15–1).
3. The parts and mechanics of the halo-vest device, including how to access the anterior chest in case of cardiac arrest.
4. Proper body mechanics.
5. Principles of chest physiotherapy (see Skill 3–1).
6. Anatomy and reflexes associated with swallowing.

The nurse should be able to perform:

1. Proper handwashing technique (see Skill 35–5).
2. Pulmonary assessment.

3. Pulmonary toilet, including chest physiotherapy and quad-assist coughing.
4. Skin assessment.
5. Motor/sensory assessment.
6. Pain/discomfort assessment.
7. Assessment of halo vest stability.
8. Dysphagia assessment.
9. Technique for anterior chest access.

Assessment

1. Assess the stability of the pins within the skull and the halo ring. **Rationale:** Ensures that pins have not slipped or loosened. Torquing the pins ensures stability of the ring in the skull with equal pressure applied to all pin sites. Normal torque is 4 to 8 inch pounds. The physician will adjust the torque pressure after the halo ring has been positioned correctly and then within 48 hours and p.r.n. for loosening (Botte et al., 1989; Hummelgard and Martin, 1982).
2. Assess integrity of struts and halo-vest system by asking patient to nod head. Patient should have no cervical mobility while in halo-vest device. **Rationale:** Validates that system is intact and cervical traction is maintained.
3. Assess pulmonary function. **Rationale:** Halo vest may decrease vital capacity (Lind et al., 1987). Spinal cord injury patients may have decreased innervation to respiratory accessory muscles.
4. Assess motor/sensory function. **Rationale:** To follow trends and identify effectiveness of cervical traction.
5. Assess body position in halo vest. **Rationale:** Ensures that body vest fits correctly and cervical traction is maintained. The physician will adjust the torque of the superstructure of the halo vest. Normal torque for the superstructure is 24 inch pounds.
6. Assess patient's pain/discomfort. **Rationale:** Identifies potential complications related to halo-vest device specifically after torquing of pins.
7. Assess for dysphagia. **Rationale:** Hyperextension required for cervical alignment may impair swallowing, leaving patient at increased risk for airway obstruction or aspiration.
8. Assess skin integrity. **Rationale:** The halo vest should fit snugly, sometimes resulting in pressure areas, specifically at the scapulae, sternum, and rib areas.

Nursing Diagnoses

1. Potential impaired skin integrity related to immobility and vest placement. **Rationale:** Insensate patients are more prone to skin breakdown because they are unable to feel pressure and reposition themselves.
2. Impaired physical mobility related to immobilization device or spinal cord injury. **Rationale:** Device limits mobility because the patient must turn head/body as unit and device weight changes the patient's center of gravity. The patient may be clumsy when device is first placed. Assistance and physical therapy may help patient improve coordination. The limitations imposed by the halo-vest device also may be coupled with sensory/motor deficits.
3. Dressing/grooming self-care deficit related to limited neck and shoulder movement. **Rationale:** The patient is unable to turn his or her head and neck unless the entire body turns; shoulder movement is limited by vest placement.
4. Potential for impaired gas exchange related to decreased vital capacity or decreased innervation to respiratory accessory muscles (Lind et al., 1987). **Rationale:** Predisposes the patient to retained secretions and subsequently diminished gas exchange.

Planning

1. Individualize the following goals for performing halo-vest care:
    a. Maintain skin integrity. **Rationale:** Prevents decubiti and infection.
    b. Utilize care as a teaching opportunity for patient and family. **Rationale:** Interactions with nursing staff should facilitate explanations and questions.
2. Prepare all necessary equipment and supplies. **Rationale:** Facilitates quick and efficient halo-vest care.
    a. Towels and wash cloths.
    b. Soap, water, and basin.
    c. Stethoscope.
    d. Clean anterior and/or posterior sheepskin.
    e. Cornstarch or powder.
    f. Lotion.
3. Use proper body mechanics. Obtain sufficient assistance to turn, lift, transfer, and position patient. *Do not* lift, turn, or pull patient by struts. Move halo vest and patient as an intact unit. **Rationale:** Maintains cervical traction without placing undue pressure on halo-vest device (Nazaroff et al., 1989).
4. Prepare the patient.
    a. Explain the procedure to the patient. **Rationale:** Decreases anxiety and increases patient cooperation.
    b. Position patient with head of bed flat, and turn patient to side. Assistance may be needed if patient is paralyzed or has motor deficits. **Rationale:** Maintains proper alignment.
5. Identify emergency equipment in case of airway obstruction or cardiac arrest. A wrench for removing the anterior portion of the vest should be taped to the vest. Newer models may have a hinge that facilitates immediate removal for CPR. If an airway obstruction occurs, the jaw-thrust method must be used to open the airway. If intubation is required, a blind nasal intubation is recommended. **Rationale:** Know the limitations of mobility with the patient in a halo vest, and anticipate needs before emergencies arise.

Implementation

Steps	Rationale	Special Considerations
1. Wash hands.	Reduces transmission of microorganisms.	
2. Unbuckle one side of halo vest while maintaining spinal alignment.	Gains access to underlying skin.	Inadvertent rotation of shoulders or hips may result in torsion of spinal cord.
3. Perform skin assessment.	Identifies potential or actual alterations in skin integrity.	Insensate patients may be more vulnerable to skin breakdown. The halo should fit snugly but not cause pain over pressure areas. For insensate patients, it is the nurse who assesses the fit of the halo on a daily basis. Sternum, ribs, scapulae, and clavicle areas are especially high risk for breakdown.
4. Bathe skin with soap and water.	To cleanse and protect.	Dry skin thoroughly, and avoid excessive lotion or powder, since these agents tend to mat the sheepskin.
5. Auscultate breath sounds.	To identify adventitious breath sounds.	Anticipate decreased breath sounds at bases in patients with poor diaphragm and intercostal function.
6. Perform pulmonary toilet, including anterior and posterior chest physiotherapy.	Enhances secretion maintenance and facilitates airway clearance.	There may be a slight decrease in vital capacity related to vest placement; assess in light of baseline pulmonary status.
7. Rebuckle vest.	Maintains cervical traction.	Be sure strap is secured to ensure proper fit.
8. Turn patient to opposite side, keep head flat, and repeat steps 2 to 8.	For assessment of opposite side of body.	
9. Change anterior sheepskin as needed: a. Place patient supine with head of bed flat. b. Unbuckle both side straps of vest. c. Remove soiled anterior sheepskin liner. d. Match clean liner to Velcro guides on anterior vest, and press into place. e. Buckle both sides of vest.	Provides comfort and cleanliness and protects skin. Provides support and alignment. To assess anterior portion of chest. Secures liner in place. Maintains cervical traction.	Anterior portion of sheepskin liner may require frequent changes because of secretions or drainage from tracheostomy or spills while eating. *Note:* The halo vest side panels may be opened simultaneously only when the patient is flat and supine.
10. Change posterior sheepskin: a. Position patient with head of bed flat and patient turned to side-lying position. b. Unbuckle one side of halo vest. c. Roll soiled liner from edge to center of vest. d. Match half the clean liner to corresponding portion of posterior vest, and roll remainder to center of vest. e. Buckle side strap.	Provides comfort and protects skin. To provide support and maintain alignment. Simplifies liner change. Provides comfort and protects skin. Maintains cervical tractions.	

Table continues on following page

Steps	Rationale	Special Considerations
f. Roll patient to opposite side.	Accesses liner.	
g. Unbuckle side strap, and remove remainder of soiled liner.		
h. Unroll clean liner, and match to corresponding Velcro strips on vest.	Secures liner in place.	
i. Buckle side strap.	Maintains cervical traction.	
11. Wash hands.	Reduces transmission of microorganisms.	

Evaluation

1. Evaluate skin integrity every 8 hours and p.r.n. **Rationale:** Identifies areas of irritation and breakdown.

2. Monitor integrity and fit of halo-vest device every 8 hours. Evaluate pin sites, struts, and vest shell. **Rationale:** Loosening of pins may alter dynamics of halo vest and cervical traction, resulting in neurologic deterioration. Loosening of strut rods interferes with cervical traction stability. Vest shell maintains stability of struts and halo ring.

3. Evaluate motor/sensory function every 4 hours. **Rationale:** Ensures that manipulation of halo-vest device has not resulted in further neurologic deterioration.

4. Evaluate pulmonary status every 8 hours and p.r.n. **Rationale:** Ensures that halo-vest therapy has not caused atelectasis or decreased respiratory function.

5. Evaluate pain/discomfort every 4 hours and p.r.n., especially after torque adjustment. **Rationale:** Indicates whether pain is normal discomfort after torque adjustment.

Expected Outcomes

1. Cervical traction is maintained. **Rationale:** Ensures stability to cervical area while allowing for patient mobility.

2. The underlying skin remains intact. **Rationale:** Provides barrier to infection.

3. Mobility is maintained. **Rationale:** Ensures that no further motor/sensory deficits occur secondary to halo-vest treatment. Early mobilization prevents multisystem complications.

Unexpected Outcomes

1. Perforation of the dura. **Rationale:** If the patient falls while wearing a halo vest, direct pressure to one of the four stabilizing pins may cause it to perforate the inner table of the skull, dura, and underlying cortical structures. If this occurs, maintain patient in a flat position, and *notify the physician immediately.* This can predispose the patient to CSF leak or infection.

2. Traction is not maintained because of pin loosening; i.e., patient is able to nod. **Rationale:** Loose pins causing structural instability may cause cervical mal-

alignment, damage to cervical grafts, and further neurologic injury.

3. Difficulty swallowing. **Rationale:** Hyperextension required for cervical alignment may result in dysphagia. The physician should be notified if this occurs, since further evaluation may be necessary. It is possible to perform the Heimlich maneuver on a patient in a halo vest.

Documentation

Documentation in the patient record should include date, time, and name of physician applying halo vest; skin assessment; pin assessment; pin-site care; integrity of the halo vest; pulmonary assessment; date and time chest physiotherapy is performed; motor/sensory assessment; patient's response to the procedure; and any unexpected outcomes and interventions taken. **Rationale:** Documents nursing care given and provides ongoing documentation of patient response to halo-vest therapy.

Patient/Family Education

1. Assess the patient and family for readiness to learn and ability to perform halo-vest care. Specific criteria affecting readiness to learn and ability to perform include physical or emotional limitations that may impede independent living, requirements for ongoing PT, OT, or extensive rehabilitation, availability of individual(s) to assist with patient's care, and cognitive/educational level of the patient and family. **Rationale:** Readiness to learn has an impact on compliance with care.

2. Discuss and demonstrate the following aspects of halo care: pin-site assessment, pin-site care, halo care, skin inspection, and care of sheepskin liners. **Rationale:** Encourages cooperation and understanding. Enables the patient and family to ask questions throughout skill.

3. Observe return demonstration by individual(s) who will be providing care at home. **Rationale:** Facilitates questions in safe environment; identifies concerns in individual's technique, understanding, and ability to learn.

4. Explain the signs and symptoms of complications

related to halo-vest care, such as localized infection, halo-vest instability, potential for falls, temperature elevations greater than 101°F, and additional motor/sensory deficits. **Rationale:** Enables the patient and family to recognize when further evaluation by the physician is indicated.

5. Evaluate the patient and family for their readiness for long-term maintenance of the halo vest. Most patients will remain in the halo vest for 8 to 12 weeks. Family should be able to perform pin-site assessment and care,

identify potential complications and the interventions needed when these occur, identify when the physician should be notified, understand the self-care deficits associated with this immobilization device, and understand what to do if the device becomes unstable. **Rationale:** Allows the nurse to anticipate needs for patient's discharge home with the halo vest.

6. Identify resources in the community for the patient and family. **Rationale:** Facilitates transition to the community.

Performance Checklist
Skill 15–4: Halo Traction Care

Critical Behaviors	Complies yes	no
1. Wash hands.		
2. Unbuckle one side of halo vest while maintaining spinal alignment.		
3. Perform skin assessment.		
4. Bathe skin under halo vest.		
5. Auscultate breath sounds.		
6. Perform pulmonary toilet and chest PT.		
7. Rebuckle vest.		
8. Turn patient to opposite side, and repeat steps 2 to 8.		
9. Change anterior liner:		
a. Place patient supine with HOB flat.		
b. Unbuckle both side straps of vest.		
c. Remove soiled anterior liner.		
d. Replace with clean liner.		
e. Rebuckle both sides of vest.		
10. Change posterior liner:		
a. Position patient on side with HOB flat.		
b. Unbuckle one side of vest.		
c. Roll soiled liner to center.		
d. Match clean liner to posterior vest, and roll remainder to center of vest.		
e. Buckle side strap.		
f. Roll patient to opposite side.		
g. Unbuckle side strap.		
h. Unroll clean liner, and match to vest.		
i. Buckle side strap.		
11. Wash hands.		
12. Document procedure in patient record.		

REFERENCES

Botte, M. J., Garfin, S. R., Byrne, T. P., et al. (1989). The halo skeletal fixator: Principles of application and maintenance. *Clin. Orthop.* 239:12–17.

Garfin, S. R., Botte, M. J., Waters, R. L., and Nickel, V. L. (1986). Complications in the use of the halo fixation device. *J. Bone Joint Surg.* 68A(3):320–325.

Glaser, J. A., Whitehall, R., Stamp, W. G., and Jane, J. A. (1986). Complications associated with the halo vest. *J. Neurosurg.* 65:762–769.

Hickey, J. V. (1986). *The Clinical Practice of Neurological and Neurosurgical Nursing*, 2d Ed. Philadelphia: Lippincott.

Hummelgard, A., and Martin, E. (1982). Management of the patient in a halo brace. *J. Neurosurg. Nurs.* 14(3):113–118.

Lind, B., Bake, B., Lindquist, C., and Nordwall, A. (1987). Influence of halo vest on vital capacity. *Spine* 12(5):449–452.

Nazaroff, K. S., Stanton, J. H., Magana, K. R., and Kaufman, R. L. (1989). Halo-body jacket immobilization in rheumatoid arthritis patients with cervical myelopathy. *Nurs. Clin. North Am.* 32(1):209–223.

Ohman, K., and Spaniol, D. (1990). Halo immobilization: Discharge planning and patient education. *J. Neurosci. Nurs.* 22(6):351–357.

Rutecki, B., and Seligson, D. (1980). Caring for the patient in a halo apparatus. *Nursing 80* 10(10):73–77.

BIBLIOGRAPHY

Adelstein, W. (1989). C1–C2 fractures and dislocations. *J. Neurosci. Nurs.* 21(3):149–159.

Botte, M. J., Byrne, T. P., and Garfin, S. R. (1987). Application of the halo device for immobilization of the cervical spine utilizing an increased torque pressure. *J. Bone Joint Surg.* 69(5):750–752.

Browner, C. M., Hadley, M. N., Sonntag, V. K., and Mattingly, L. G. (1987). Halo immobilization brace care: An innovative approach. *J. Neurosci. Nurs.* 19(1):25–29.

Kinkade, S., and Lohrman, J. (1990). *Critical Care Nursing Procedures.* Philadelphia: B. C. Decker.

Lind, B., Sihlbom, H., and Nordwell, A. (1988). Halo-vest treatment of unstable traumatic cervical spine injuries. *Spine* 13(4):425–432.

McRae, R. (1989). *Practical Fracture Treatment*, 2d Ed. Edinburgh: Churchill-Livingstone.

Millar, S., Sampson, L., and Soukup, M. (1985). *AACN Procedure Manual for Critical Care.* Philadelphia: Saunders.

Nickel, V. L., Perry, J., Garrett, A., and Heppenstall, M. (1989). The halo: A spinal skeletal traction fixation device. *Clin. Orthop.* 239:4–11.

Olson, B., and Ustanko, L. (1990). Self-care needs of patients in the halo brace. *Orthop. Nurs.* 9(1):27–33.

Rudy, E. B. (1984). *Advanced Neurological and Neurosurgical Nursing.* St. Louis: Mosby.

Snyder, M. (1991). *A Guide to Neurological and Neurosurgical Nursing*, 2d Ed. Albany, N.Y.: Delmar.

INTRACRANIAL PRESSURE MONITORING

After completing this chapter, the nurse will be able to

- Define the key terms.
- Describe the methods for monitoring intracranial pressure.
- Identify patient's requiring intracranial pressure monitoring.
- Discuss and describe the safe application and maintenance of intracranial pressure monitoring.
- Identify and discuss the clinical significance of increased intracranial pressure and pressure waveforms.
- Identify potential complications of intracranial pressure monitoring.
- Discuss methods for troubleshooting intracranial pressure monitoring devices.

Intracranial pressure (ICP) reflects the dynamic pressure relationship between the brain, cerebrospinal fluid (CSF), and the cerebral circulation. Since the cranium is essentially a closed system, any change in the volume of one of these critical elements causes a change in cerebral dynamics. Normal ICP is 0 to 15 mmHg (50 to 200 cmH$_2$O), as measured at the level of the foramen of Monro (measured at the level of the outer canthus of the eye) in the supine patient. In the unimpaired brain, increases in ICP result in automatic protective responses in an effort to maintain this dynamic equilibrium.

One protective mechanism of the brain is the ability to shunt CSF to the subarachnoid space surrounding the spinal cord, thereby effectively decreasing CSF volume in the cranium. Another protective mechanism is autoregulation, a property by which the brain ensures optimal blood flow by vasoconstricting or vasodilating cerebral arterioles in response to systemic pressure and chemical stimuli (PCO$_2$, PO$_2$, lactic acid, pyruvic acid). When ICP continues to rise despite the brain's attempt to alleviate it, autoregulatory responses are lost, resulting in intracranial hypertension (Fig. 16–1).

Intracranial hypertension is defined as sustained ICP of 15 mmHg or greater. Intracranial hypertension can be caused by a variety of conditions that affect intracranial content volume (Table 16–1). Increases in intracranial pressure also can be precipitated by pharmacologic, chemical, emotional, and physical activity (Table 16–2). Malignant (intracranial) hypertension is used by some to describe a sustained (greater than 20 minutes) ICP of 20 mmHg or greater (Hickey, 1986). Uncontrolled intracranial hypertension results in secondary cerebral ischemia, brain herniation, and ultimately, the death of neural cells.

Specific clinical signs and symptoms may indicate increased ICP (Fig. 16–2). Herniation syndromes occur as a result of the forcing of semisolid brain matter against inelastic structures such as bone and dura. This pressure causes dysfunction of the neural structures involved and correlates directly with the clinical signs and symptoms identified (Table 16–3). Central or transtentorial herniation results from downward displacement of the cerebral hemispheres and central structures of the brain (basal ganglia and diencephalon) resulting in midbrain compression against the tentorium cerebelli. Uncal herniation results when the lateral edge of the temporal lobe is forced through the tentorial notch. Infratentorial herniation occurs with compression on the brainstem or cerebellum, either upward against the tentorium cerebelli or downward through the foramen magnum.

Measurement of intracranial pressure is of paramount importance to the critically ill neurologic patient because changes or dramatic increases in ICP cannot be deduced consistently from signs and symptoms. The ultimate goal of caring for the brain-injured patient is the prevention or minimization of secondary ischemic injury. Advances in ICP monitoring technology have facilitated early, aggressive treatment of intracranial hypertension. The primary goals of intracranial monitoring are identification of pressure trends and evaluation of therapeutic interventions.

In order to obtain accurate intracranial pressures, a pressure monitoring device must be placed within the cranium. The three monitoring devices most commonly used are (1) fiberoptic, (2) hydraulic (fluid-filled), and (3) sensor. Anatomic positions for the monitoring device include the subarachnoid space, the epidural space, the intraventricular space, and the intraparenchymal space. Each system and anatomic location has specific advantages and disadvantages and risks and benefits.

The ICP waveform results from the transmission of arterial and venous pressure waves through the CSF and brain parenchyma. A normal ICP waveform resembles a somewhat dampened arterial waveform (Fig. 16–3). The ICP waveform normally has three or more defined peaks (Fig. 16–4) identified as P$_1$, P$_2$, and P$_3$. The first

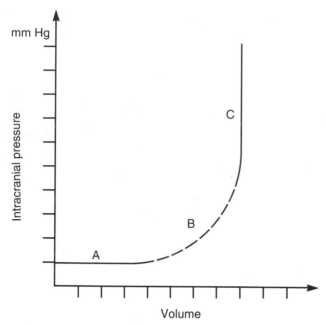

FIGURE 16–1. Intracranial pressure volume curve. Areas *A*, *B*, and *C* correspond to minimal, moderate, and severe increases in intracranial pressure.

peak on the ICP configuration is P_1, also called the *percussion wave*; it has a sharp peak and a consistent amplitude. P_2 is called the *tidal wave*. It has a variable amplitude and shape and ends on the dicrotic notch. P_3, the *dicrotic wave*, is located immediately after the dicrotic notch and slopes into the diastolic baseline position. Intracranial compliance can be observed by comparing P_1 and P_2.

Germon (1988) defines *intracranial compliance* as "an expression of the relationship between the change in ICP as a result of a change in the intracranial volume." When autoregulatory mechanisms are intact, increases in intracranial contents should cause reciprocal decreases in another intracranial element in order to maintain a steady dynamic equilibrium. However, when increases in intracranial volume precipitate a significant increase in ICP, there is a failure of normal intracranial compensatory mechanisms, and a state of decreased compliance exists.

This is noted on the ICP tracing when P_2 is of equal or greater amplitude than P_1 (Fig. 16–5). Other indicators of decreased compliance are (1) a sustained increase in ICP (greater than 10 mmHg for greater than 3 minutes) in response to a given nursing procedure and (2) the patient's rapid neurologic deterioration (Germon, 1988; Mitchell et al., 1988).

Continuous ICP monitoring reflects intracranial pressure trends (also called *waves*) over a period of time. Three types of ICP waves are identified: A waves, B waves, and C waves (Figs. 16–6, 16–7, and 16–8). A waves, also known as pressure or plateau waves, are an ominous sign and indicate severe intracranial decompensation. A waves are characterized by sudden steep increases in ICP to 50 to 100 mmHg, are of 5 to 20 minutes duration, occur spontaneously or with physiologic alterations, are frequently accompanied by neurologic deterioration, occur at varying intervals, and indicate impending herniation. Of all the pressure waves, plateau waves are the most clinically significant.

B waves are sharp, rhythmic oscillations that occur every ½ to 2 minutes. ICP increases to 20 to 50 mmHg during this trend. B waves may be seen prior to the onset of plateau waves.

C waves reflect elevations in ICP up to 20 mmHg. These waves occur every 4 to 8 minutes and are not thought to be clinically significant (Hickey, 1986). See Table 16–4 for comparisons of pressure trends.

More important than the direct measurement of ICP is the indirect or calculated cerebral perfusion pressure (CPP). CPP considers both the mean arterial pressure (MAP), that is, the ability of the body to deliver blood to the brain, and the intracranial pressure, that is, the resistance the systemic pressure must overcome to perfuse the brain. Normal range for CPP is 60 to 150 mmHg; CPP is calculated by subtracting the ICP from the MAP. Clinical situations resulting in severe hypertension, hypotension, cardiopulmonary collapse, and increased intracranial pressure may impair the brain's autoregulatory ability by pushing the CPP above or below the preferred range (less than 50 mmHg or greater than 150 mmHg). Once the brain loses the ability to control its blood supply, the CPP becomes reactive to subsequent changes in systemic pressure and intracranial pressure. Net decreases in CPP indicate diminished cerebral perfusion

TABLE 16–1 CONDITIONS RESULTING IN INTRACRANIAL HYPERTENSION

Increased brain volume	Space-occupying lesions such as epidural and subdural hematomas, tumors, abscesses, or aneurysms
	Cerebral edema related to head injuries, cardiopulmonary arrest, and metabolic encephalopathies (cytotoxic and vasogenic edema)
Increased blood volume	Obstruction of venous outflow
	Hyperemia
	Hypercapnia
	Disease states associated with increased blood volume, such as Reye's syndrome
Increased cerebrospinal fluid (CSF)	Increased production of CSF
	Decreased absorption of CSF
	Obstruction to CSF flow

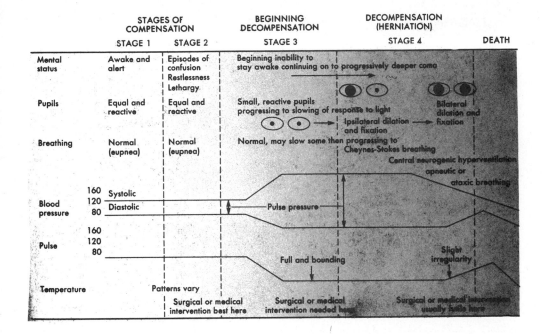

FIGURE 16–2. Clinical correlates of increased intracranial pressure. (Reprinted with permission from P. Beare and J. Myers, *Principles and Practice of Adult Health Nursing*. St. Louis: Mosby, 1990.)

TABLE 16–2 CONTRIBUTING FACTORS FOR ELEVATIONS IN INTRACRANIAL PRESSURE

Factors	Possible Causes
Hypercapnia (PCO_2 > 45 mmHg)	Sleep, sedation, shallow respirations, coma, neuromuscular impairment, improper mechanical ventilator settings
Hypoxemia (PO_2 < 50 mmHg)	Insufficient oxygen concentration in supplemental oxygen therapy, inadequate lung ventilation, inadequate lung perfusion
Drug-induced cerebral vasodilation	Administration of nicotinic acid, cyclandelate, histamine, nylidrin hydrochloride, and anesthetic agents such as halothane, enflurance, isoflurane, and nitrous oxide
Valsalva maneuver	Straining at stool; moving or turning in bed
Body positioning	Any position that obstructs venous return from the brain, such as Trendelenburg, prone position, extreme flexion of hips, and neck flexion
Isometric muscle contractions	Isometric exercises, such as pushing against resistance, shivering, and decerebration
Coughing/sneezing	Allergies, colds, normal postoperative cough
REM sleep	Rapid eye movements are associated with cerebral activity; arousal from sleep also increases ICP
Emotional upset	Unpleasant or stimulating conversation
Noxious stimuli	Visceral discomfort, painful nursing procedures or stimuli associated with assessment, loud noises, jarring of the bed
Clustering of activities	Cumulative effect of closely spaced care-related activities

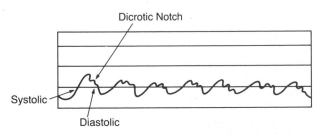

FIGURE 16–3. Normal intracranial pressure waveform.

FIGURE 16–4. Components of the intracranial pressure waveform: P_1, P_2, and P_3.

TABLE 16–3   SIGNS AND SYMPTOMS OF HERNIATION SYNDROMES

	Central		Uncal		Infratentorial	
	Early	**Late**	**Early**	**Late**	**Early**	**Late**
Pupils	Small reactive	Bilateral fixed, dilated	Ipsilateral dilated pupil; sluggish nonreactive	Midposition and fixed	Midposition or small and nonreactive	Bilateral fixed
Level of arousal	Difficulty with concentration; agitated/drowsy	Stupor leads to coma	Normal to restless	Stupor may rapidly become coma	Stupor	Coma
Motor	Contralateral hemiparesis	Bilateral decortication/ decerebration/ flaccidity	Contralateral hemiparesis	Decortication/ decerebration/ flaccidity	Hemiparesis, hemiplegia	Decortication/ decerebration/ flaccidity
Respiration	Yawning, deep sighs, pauses, central neurogenic hyperventilation	Cheyne-Stokes, ataxic	Normal	Cheyne-Stokes, ataxic	Variable depending on level of lesion	Respiratory arrest
Extraocular signs	Normal; roving	Dysconjugate gaze	Ipsilateral ptosis	Extraocular paralysis	Ophthalmoplegias; early loss of upward gaze	Extraocular paralysis

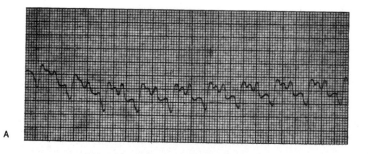

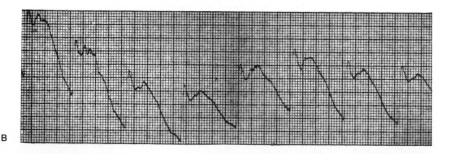

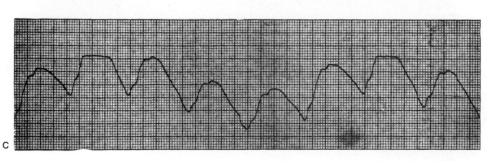

FIGURE 16–5.   Example of intracranial pressure waveform with P$_2$ elevation indicating decreased cerebral compliance.

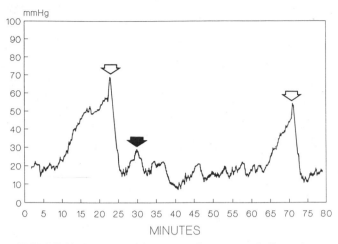

FIGURE 16–6. A or plateau waves. Open arrows indicate plateau elevations in intracranial pressure. Note that when intracranial pressure falls, it does not return to baseline preceding the first wave (*closed arrow*). (Reprinted with permission from S. B. Marshall, L. F. Marshall, H. R. Vos, and R. M. Chesnut, *Neuroscience Critical Care: Pathophysiology and Patient Management.* Philadelphia: Saunders, 1990.)

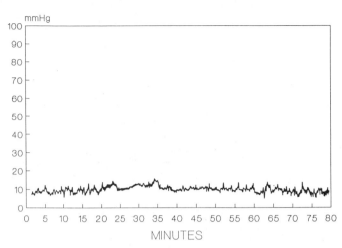

FIGURE 16–8. Lundberg or C waves. The intracranial pressure changes are much less impressive than in A or B waves and reflect changes in arterial blood pressure. (Reprinted with permission from S. B. Marshall, L. F. Marshall, H. R. Vos, and R. M. Chesnut, *Neuroscience Critical Care: Pathophysiology and Patient Management*, Philadelphia: Saunders, 1990.)

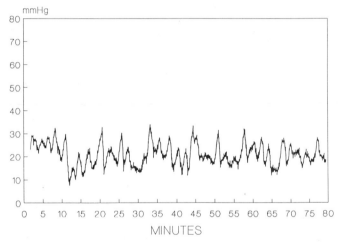

FIGURE 16–7. Elevations in intracranial pressure represent B waves. The intracranial pressure rise is steep and rapid, but to heights less than those observed with A waves and much briefer. (Reprinted with permission from S. B. Marshall, L. F. Marshall, H. R. Vos, and R. M. Chesnut, *Neuroscience Critical Care: Pathophysiology and Patient Management*, Philadelphia: Saunders, 1990.)

and may result in dysfunction of neural tissue at the cellular level, thereby jeopardizing ultimate cerebral function. Hypoxia and irreversible neurologic dysfunction are associated with CPPs less than 30 mmHg.

This chapter focuses on those procedures necessary to establish and monitor intracranial pressure.

KEY TERMS

autoregulation	foramen of Monro
burr hole	herniation
cerebral metabolic rate	intracranial pressure
cerebral perfusion	intracranial pressure
cerebral perfusion pressure	monitoring
cranium	intracranial hypertension
diencephalon	intraventricular
dura mater	meninges
epidural space	plateau waves
epidural catheter	subarachnoid space
foramen magnum	uncus

TABLE 16–4 COMPARISON OF ICP PRESSURE TRENDS

Description	Pressure, mmHg	Clinical Signs and Symptoms
A waves	50–100	Abnormal changes in respiratory patterns, abnormal pupillary responses, altered motor function, dysphagia, symptoms related to cerebral dysfunction, changes in vital signs, headache, vomiting
B waves	20–50	Fluctuating respiratory pattern, decreased level of consciousness, agitation, drowsiness
C waves	4–20	No accepted clinical significance
Normal	4–15	Normal

SKILLS

GUIDELINES

The following assessment guidelines assist the nurse in formulating nursing diagnoses and an individualized plan of care for the patient with an intracranial pressure monitor.

1. Know the patient's baseline neurologic assessment.
2. Know the patient's baseline vital signs.
3. Know the patient's past medical history, including allergies, previous neurologic assessment, previous cognitive level, previous surgeries (especially eye surgery), cardiac history, lung disease, chronic illnesses, and psychosocial support systems.
4. Identify associated injuries that may modify the plan of care for intracranial hypertension, such as shock, burns, pulmonary compromise, abdominal injury, bone fractures, or spinal cord injury.
5. Know the current goals of intracranial pressure monitoring.
6. Determine appropriate interventions for neurologic deterioration.
7. Become adept with the equipment required to initiate and maintain intracranial pressure monitoring.

SKILL 16–1

Assisting with Insertion of an Intracranial Pressure Monitoring Device

Intracranial pressure monitoring involves the placement of a pressure-sensing device into the cranium. Regions for anatomic placement of the monitoring device include the subarachnoid or epidural space, intraventricularly, or intraparenchymally (Figs. 16–9 and 16–10). Each system and anatomic location has distinct advantages, disadvantages, risks, and benefits (see Tables 16–5 and 16–6).

The most recent advance in intracranial pressure management is the use of fiberoptic monitoring. This technique has proven to be accurate and dependable for measuring and reporting ICP data. The fiberoptic catheter is extremely versatile; it can be placed in virtually any intracranial location because the transducer is located at the tip of the catheter. The fiberoptic catheter can be incorporated within a subarachnoid bolt, within a ventriculostomy, or directly into cortical tissue. The system requires no fluid flush and is calibrated only once immediately prior to insertion.

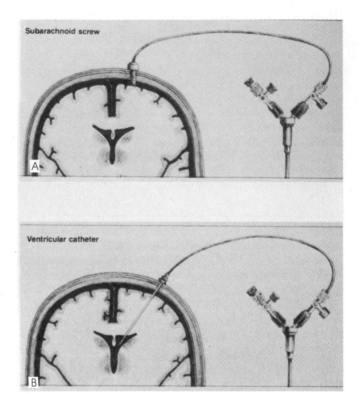

FIGURE 16–9. Anatomic placement of intraventricular monitoring devices. (*A*) Intraventricular catheter. (*B*) Subarachnoid bolt. (Reprinted with permission from Cordona, Hurn, and Basnajel et al. *Trauma Nursing from Resuscitation through Rehabilitation.* Philadelphia: Saunders, 1988.)

Malfunctions with the fiberoptic catheter reflect the state of fiberoptic technology. Fragile filaments are easily damaged as a result of tension or catheter crimping. Unfortunately, once the fibers are damaged, the device is rendered inoperative. Another disadvantage of this system is that specialized equipment is required to establish, monitor, and record ICP.

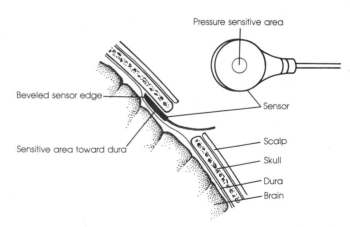

FIGURE 16–10. Anatomic placement of an epidural sensor. (Reprinted with permission from E. Rudy, *Advanced Neurological and Neurosurgical Nursing,* St. Louis: Mosby, 1984.)

TABLE 16–5 COMPARISON OF ICP MONITORING SITES

System	Advantages	Disadvantages
Intraventricular catheter	Considered the gold standard for ICP monitoring Allows treatment of increased ICP through drainage of CSF Access for determination of volume-pressure curve	May have difficulty in locating ventricles Increased risk of infection from penetration of catheter into center of brain Invasive procedure with risk of intracerebral bleeding in cannula track
Subarachnoid/ subdural	No penetration of brain necessary for insertion Easier placement than intraventricular catheter Decreased risk of infection over intraventricular catheter	Unable to drain CSF Unreliable at high ICP when brain tissue herniates up into monitoring device
Epidural	Easy to insert No penetration of dura Minimal risk of infection	Question of accuracy of ICP reflected through dura Separate dedicated monitoring system required Unable to drain CSF
Intraparenchymal	Allows for measurement of ICP selectively in brain parenchyma Easy to place Decreased risk of infection	Unable to drain CSF Separate monitoring system required

Source: Reprinted with permission from S. B. Marshall, L. F. Marshall, H. R. Vos, and R. M. Chesnut, *Neuroscience Critical Care: Pathophysiology and Patient Management.* Philadelphia: Saunders, 1990, page 371.

TABLE 16–6 COMPARISON OF ICP MONITORING SYSTEMS

	Fluid-Filled	Epidural	Fiberoptic Transducer Catheter
Placement	Intraventricular or subarachnoid	Epidural only	Intraventricular, subarachnoid, or intraparenchymal
CSF drainage	Able to drain with ventricular catheter; no continuous ICP recording while draining	No drainage capability	Able to drain with ventricular catheter while continuously recording ICP
Infection risk	Static fluid column with stopcocks, tubing, etc. may increase risk of infection	Lack of static fluid column and intact dura minimize risk of infection	Lack of static fluid column may reduce risk of infection
Waveform	Uses bedside monitoring equipment to display waveform and generate alarm system	Requires dedicated equipment; does not interface with bedside monitor; displays mean pressure trend only	Requires dedicated equipment that displays waveform or interfaces with bedside monitor for display and alarm system
Artifact	May be present with movement of system or patient; also present with air or kinks in tubing	Minimal to none	Minimal to none
Zero reference	Repeated zero adjustment necessary; done at bedside while system connected to patient	Factory set, cannot be checked after insertion	Zero adjustment done at time of insertion, cannot be checked after insertion
Transducer calibration	Required before patient use; able to check during patient use	Factory set, no calibration required	Factory set, no calibration required; may be calibrated to bedside monitor

Source: Reprinted with permission from S. B. Marshall, L. F. Marshall, H. R. Vos, and R. M. Chesnut, *Neuroscience Critical Care: Pathophysiology and Patient Management.* Philadelphia: Saunders, 1990, page 371.

Purpose

The nurse assists with intracranial pressure monitor insertion to

1. Assess intracranial dynamics.
2. Establish a system in which CSF can be collected.
3. Document the intracranial pressure and waveform.
4. Establish a system for introducing dye or a chemotherapeutic agent.

Prerequisite Knowledge and Skills

Prior to assisting the physician with insertion of an intracranial pressure monitor, the nurse should understand

1. Principles of neuroanatomy and physiology.
2. Principles of intracranial pressure dynamics.
3. Principles of intracranial pressure monitoring.
4. Indications for each type of intracranial pressure monitoring device.
5. Principles of asepsis.
6. Differences between hydraulic, fiberoptic, and sensor systems.

The nurse should be able to perform

1. Proper handwashing technique (see Skill 35–5).
2. Aseptic technique.
3. Neurologic assessment.
4. Vital signs assessment.
5. Universal precautions (see Skill 35–1).

Assessment

1. Observe for *early* signs and symptoms of increased intracranial pressure, such as altered or decreased level of consciousness, restlessness, agitation, irritability, anxiety, lethargy or drowsiness, confusion, apathy, motor weakness (i.e., hemiparesis), headaches, pupillary dysfunction, or seizures (see Fig. 16–2). **Rationale:** Pressure on cortical structures results in an alteration in level of consciousness, but metabolic offenders such as ETOH, sedation, ketoacidosis, hepatic coma, renal failure, and recreational drug use must be ruled out because they produce similar effects.
2. Identify *late* signs of increased intracranial pressure, such as continuing alteration in level of consciousness progressing to coma, alteration in motor/sensory assessment (i.e., hemiparesis, decortication, decerebration), alteration in pupillary response and extraocular movements, alteration in respiratory pattern or rate (Cheyne-Stokes, central neurogenic hyperventilation, apneustic, ataxic patterns), elevation in blood pressure, widened pulse pressure, and bradycardia (Cushing's reflex), alterations in brainstem reflexes, and possibly vomiting (see Fig. 16–2). **Rationale:** Alterations result from increasing pressure exerted on brainstem structures, specifically the midbrain, pons, and medulla. The cranial nerves governing extraocular movements have nuclei

originating in the midbrain and pons. Respiratory centers are found throughout the brainstem and may result in abnormal breathing patterns associated with specific structures involved.
3. Signs of increased intracranial pressure in the infant include tense or bulging anterior fontanel, separation of suture lines or increased head circumference, irritability, projectile vomiting, drowsiness, high-pitched cry, "sunset eyes" (i.e., eyeball deviated downward so only upper portion of pupil is visible), and "cracked pot" sound on percussion of skull (Germon and Grant, 1989).

Nursing Diagnoses

1. Potential for infection related to entry into the skin, cranium, meninges, CSF circulation, and cortical parenchyma. **Rationale:** Interruption of normal protective barriers increases the risk of infection.
2. Potential for injury related to placement of device. **Rationale:** A subarachnoid device or a ventriculostomy may cause hemorrhage or hemotoma by disrupting cortical veins. Underlying structures of the cerebral cortex may be further damaged by the passage of the ventriculostomy into the lateral ventricle.
3. Discomfort related to invasive procedure. **Rationale:** Depending on the patient's level of consciousness, discomfort may be perceived when the skin and dura are entered.
4. Knowledge deficit related to need for intracranial monitoring. **Rationale:** The need for intracranial monitoring implies a serious patient condition. Any information given to the patient and family may help to alleviate anxiety. This will serve as a groundwork to build further information if more aggressive interventions become necessary.

Planning

1. Individualize goals for insertion of intracranial pressure monitoring device. Identify intracranial pressure trends and assess the effectiveness of therapeutic interventions. **Rationale:** Abnormal or sustained elevations in intracranial pressure predispose the patient to neurologic decompensation.
2. Collect all necessary equipment and supplies for device placement. **Rationale:** Assembly of all the necessary equipment ensures that insertion of an intracranial pressure monitoring device will be completed quickly and efficiently. Individual institutional policy may dictate many aspects of this procedure; for example, some institutions require that this be performed in the operating room to decrease the risk of infection. The following items should be available either individually or as part of a prepackaged insertion tray.
   a. Razor.
   b. Povidone-iodine scrub solution or swabs.
   c. Sterile gloves.
   d. Surgical caps, masks, sterile gowns.

e. Sterile towels and/or drapes (2 each).
f. Local anesthetic with epinephrine (lidocaine 1% or 2%).
g. Luer-lok syringes and needles for anesthetic administration, 18-gauge needle and 5-cc syringe for drawing up lidocaine, 23-gauge needles for local anesthetic administration.
h. Twist drill and bits.
i. Suture material, 2-0 nylon, 3-0 silk.
j. Scalpel with no. 11 knife blade (1).
k. Scalp retractor.
l. Forceps.
m. Sterile scissors.
n. Needle holder.
o. Suction and sterile suction catheter setup.
p. Bone wax or Gelfoam.
q. Light source.
r. Occlusive dressing or 4 × 4 gauze pads (12 to 15).
s. Tape (1-in rolls).
t. Two 4-in Kling or Kerlex rolls.
u. Subarachnoid bolt or Silastic ventricular catheter.

3. Prepare all necessary equipment and supplies to establish monitoring system. **Rationale:** While intracranial pressure monitoring systems may vary, the principles in caring for the patient are essentially the same. Each system will require specific equipment. See package inserts or instruction manuals for specific manufacturer's recommendations.

HYDRAULIC SYSTEM

a. Monitoring equipment, including ECG, arterial pressure monitor, respiratory monitor, and ICP modules.
b. Transducer cable.
c. Sterile transducer.
d. Pressure tubing.
e. Three-way stopcocks and sterile "dead end" ports or 40-μm filters.
f. Luer-lok syringe, 10 cc (1).
g. Sterile gloves.
h. Sterile towels or barriers (2).
i. Saline without preservative (may use IV solution of 0.9% sodium chloride).
j. Sterile drainage collection bag and tubing (for ventriculostomy only).

k. Carpenter's level.

FIBEROPTIC SYSTEM

a. Monitoring equipment, including ECG, arterial pressure monitor, respiratory monitor, and ICP modules, in addition to microprocessor, preamp connector, bedside monitoring cable to primary monitoring system.
b. Kit containing fiberoptic catheter, bolt, or ventricular catheter, insertion and calibration tools.
c. Sterile gloves.
d. Sterile towels or barriers (2).

SENSOR SYSTEM

a. Monitoring equipment, including ECG, arterial pressure monitor, and respiratory modules.
b. Epidural monitoring module and sensor.
c. Ronguers, Cushing type, Kerrison, angle and straight.

4. Prepare the patient and family.
a. Explain the procedure to the patient and family. **Rationale:** The nurse reinforces the need for intracranial monitoring and identifies misconceptions the patient and family may have regarding the procedure. Provides for cooperation.
b. Position the patient in a semi-Fowler's position at 30–45 degrees with head in neutral position. **Rationale:** Facilitates venous outflow.
c. Administer prescribed sedation as needed. **Rationale:** The patient must remain still throughout procedure to minimize the risk of further injury. The restless or agitated patient may require additional sedation during procedure. Any pharmacologic agent used must have a short half-life or be reversible so as not to inhibit the neurologic examination.
d. Ensure a patent airway. **Rationale:** Prevents hypoxia during the procedure. The patient should be suctioned if needed prior to the procedure.
e. Discuss the steps involved in placement of the device. **Rationale:** Allays anxiety and reviews comfort measures.
f. Determine any patient allergies to local anesthetic agents. **Rationale:** Decreases the incidence of allergic reactions.

Implementation

Steps	Rationale	Special Considerations
1. Wash hands.	Reduces transmission of microorganisms.	

Table continues on following page

Steps	Rationale	Special Considerations
2. Assemble hydraulic system:	Facilitates procedure.	
a. Set up sterile field and sterile equipment.	For easy access to equipment.	
b. Don sterile gloves.	Universal precautions.	
c. Assemble equipment per institutional procedure.	Ensures proper setup.	See institution for specific guidelines regarding setup of the device used. Generally, the system consists of pressure tubing that attaches to the device at the proximal end and the transducer at the distal end. Stopcocks and syringes may be added to the system for access and flushing according to policy.
d. Flush system with additive-free sterile saline. Remove all air bubbles.	Bubbles dampen waveform. Alcohol preservative in saline may cause cortical necrosis.	
e. Wrap system in sterile towel.	Maintains system sterility until device insertion.	Minimizes risk of infection; a closed system must be maintained at all times.
3. Turn on monitor.	Ensures monitor is working and allows for appropriate warm-up time.	Monitor should be plugged in when not in use to keep battery charged.
4. Check function of suction.	Ensures that suction is functional for insertion.	Facilitates the removal of blood and bone fragments from the insertion site.
5. Assist physician in identifying area for device placement.	Identifies access site.	Care should be taken to place the device in patient's nondominant side. The presence of skull fractures, localized infection, or tissue injury from penetrating trauma may limit site placement.
6. Shave and prepare insertion site with povidone-iodine solution.	Visualizes surface of insertion site. Reduces microorganisms and minimizes risk of infection.	Preparation protocols vary from institution to institution. A surgical prep is usually performed.
7. Drape head in sterile fashion.	Protects insertion site from contamination.	
8. Open sterile trays, and obtain system setup wrapped in the sterile towel.	Facilitates easy access to equipment.	Nurse may assist in pouring solutions into sterile containers.
9. Remove sterile towels and hand system to physician.	Allows tubing setup and transaction to be connected.	System is now ready for zero balance and calibration.
10. Monitor patient throughout placement of device for neurologic and vital signs changes.	Identifies any acute change and indicates the need for sedation.	
11. Calibrate transducer. Fiberoptic and sensor catheters must be calibrated *before* insertion. Sensor systems are internally calibrated during the manufacturing process. Hydraulic systems are calibrated *after* insertion.	Provides baseline for ongoing monitoring.	Fiberoptic and sensor catheters can only be calibrated once before insertion. Studies show that the calibration is accurate up to 5 days (Hollingsworth-Friedlund et al., 1988). Hydraulic systems may be recalibrated whenever necessary.
a. When the fiberoptic catheter kit is opened, the sterile transducer connection from the catheter is attached to the microprocessor connector.	Zero balances to atmospheric pressure.	

Table continues on following page

Steps	Rationale	Special Considerations
b. Press the zero button on the microprocessor.	Starts zero balancing.	If it does not read zero, the tool from the catheter kit is used to adjust the setting to zero.
12. Zero balance fiberoptic system with bedside monitoring system:	Allows waveform to be viewed with ECG and other pressure tracings.	
a. Depress the zero control until the number 0 appears.	Provides accurate digital readout on both systems.	
b. Continue to press zero control while pressing zero on bedside ICP monitor.	Calibrates bedside monitor to microprocessor.	
c. When the number 0 appears on the bedside monitor, release the zero control on the microprocessor.	System is now zeroed and calibrated.	
13. Recheck system connections.	Identifies any loose connections or potential sites for contamination.	Flush to remove any air bubbles in system that have occurred as a result of device placement.
14. *For ventriculostomies only*, attach drainage system distal to transducer (see Skill 16–4 regarding care of ventriculostomies).	Ensures accurate pressure readings.	
15. For *hydraulic system*, position transducer at level of the foramen of Monro reference point, and zero, balance, and calibrate transducer.	Provides accurate pressure readings.	The transducer is placed at either the outer canthus of the eye or the external auditory canal. A domed transducer system must be placed with the transducer level to one of these reference points (Fig. 16–11).
16. Apply antibacterial ointment and occlusive dressing to insertion site. In addition, head dressing may be applied.	Protects site from microorganisms.	Institutional policy may dictate specific care of site.
17. Obtain recording of waveform.	Documents baseline waveform and pressure.	The sensor will not have a waveform, since it does not have direct contact with CSF. Pressures should be monitored in the "mean" mode to reflect average pressure.
18. Discard supplies.	Universal precautions.	
19. Wash hands.	Reduces transmission of microorganisms.	

Evaluation

1. Perform a postprocedure neurologic assessment and compare with preprocedure assessment. **Rationale:** Identifies any changes that occurred during insertion and the need for intervention.

2. Evaluate the functioning of the monitoring system. **Rationale:** Ensures accurate waveform and/or pressure readings.

3. Monitor vital signs. **Rationale:** Identifies complications; may identify the need for further sedation.

4. Note trends in pressure waves and intracranial dynamics. **Rationale:** Identifies early pressure trends and patient's response to stimuli and nursing/medical interventions.

Expected Outcomes

1. The monitoring system will provide reliable data. **Rationale:** Provides data for appropriate, planned interventions.

2. The device will be placed in an anatomically correct position, as demonstrated by waveform analysis and pressure reading. **Rationale:** Correct placement of the device is necessary for accurate pressure reading and to identify changes associated with therapeutic modalities.

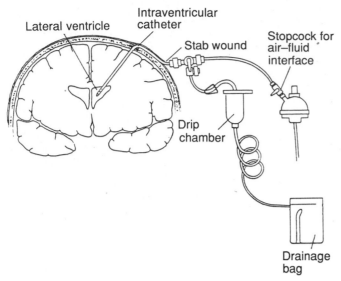

FIGURE 16–11. Intraventricular catheter drainage setup. (Illustration by Jim Wilson. Reprinted with permission from S. Kinkade and J. Lohrman, *Critical Care Nursing Procedures: A Team Approach*, Philadelphia: Decker, 1990.)

Unexpected Outcomes

1. Device cannot be placed. **Rationale:** Structural damage related to trauma and/or edema may obscure normal anatomy and prevents device placement.

2. Waveform and pressures do not correlate with neurologic assessment. **Rationale:** Other causes of neurologic deterioration and/or coma not associated with increases in intracranial pressure must be ruled out.

3. Dampened pressure waveform or obstruction of bolt. **Rationale:** Reflect unreliable data. Troubleshooting of the device is required.

Documentation

Documentation in the patient record should include the date and time of insertion, a baseline neurologic assessment, the insertion site, the device used, the patient's response to the procedure, including any changes that occurred, intracranial pressure, pressure wave recordings, cerebral perfusion pressure, and patient's response to therapeutic measures. **Rationale:** Documents nursing care given, expected and unexpected outcomes, and the interventions taken.

Patient/Family Education

1. Assess the cognitive level and readiness and ability to process information of patient and family. **Rationale:** The ability to learn and process information may be impaired as a result of high level stress and anxiety.

2. Reinforce the need for device placement to both patient and family. **Rationale:** Information regarding the need for device placement, such as to monitor intracranial pressure and evaluate therapeutic modalities, must be reinforced by the nurse. Identify and discuss risks and benefits of monitoring. Provides opportunity to ask questions.

3. Although patients are not discharged with intracranial monitoring devices, implications of potential brain injury and the need for long-term rehabilitation should be discussed with the patient and family. **Rationale:** Brain injury predisposes the patient to a wide array of cognitive and social impairments. Quality of life, functional rehabilitation, social interaction, and identification of resources are all issues affecting the patient's return to activities of daily living.

Performance Checklist
Skill 16–1: Assisting with Insertion of an Intracranial Pressure Monitoring Device

Critical Behaviors	Complies yes	no
1. Wash hands.		
2. Assemble hydraulic system:		
a. Set up sterile field.		
b. Don sterile gloves.		
c. Assemble equipment.		
d. Flush system with additive-free sterile saline.		
e. Wrap system in a sterile towel.		
3. Turn on monitor.		
4. Check suction equipment.		
5. Assist physician with identifying placement site.		

Table continues on following page

Critical Behaviors	Complies yes	no
6. Prepare site.		
7. Drape head in sterile fashion.		
8. Open sterile trays, and obtain system setup.		
9. Remove sterile towels, hand system to physician.		
10. Monitor patient throughout placement for neurologic and vital signs changes.		
11. Calibrate transducer.		
12. For fiberoptic system, zero with bedside monitor.		
13. Recheck system connections.		
14. For ventriculostomies, attach drainage system distal to transducer.		
15. For hydraulic system, position transducer at level of the foramen of Monro, and zero, balance, and recalibrate transducer.		
16. Apply antibacterial ointment and occlusive dressing to site. Apply head dressing if desired.		
17. Obtain recording of pressure waveform.		
18. Discard supplies.		
19. Wash hands.		
20. Document procedure in patient record.		

SKILL 16–2

Care of Intracranial Pressure Monitoring Device and System

Nursing care for patients with an intracranial pressure monitoring device focuses on maintaining the monitoring system, assessing the dressing/insertion site, evaluating waveforms, and obtaining pressure measurements. Interventions will vary with the type of device used as well as with institutional policy. The duration of monitoring generally ranges from 1 to 5 days (average 72 hours) with a single monitoring device. The patient requiring long-term monitoring (greater than 5 days) will require discontinuation and replacement of the original device and system. If the device is replaced, it should be inserted in the opposite hemisphere (if possible) to avoid the potential for contamination from the previous site. Duration of monitoring and the necessity of additional intracranial monitors increase the risk of infection-related complications.

When properly cared for, the intracranial pressure device provides reliable data to guide the therapy of the neurologically impaired patient.

Purpose

The nurse maintains the intracranial pressure monitoring device to

1. Ensure the accuracy of waveforms and pressure readings.
2. Maintain system and device integrity.
3. Minimize the risk of infection.

Prerequisite Knowledge and Skills

Prior to caring for the patient with an intracranial pressure monitoring device, the nurse should understand

1. Principles of hemodynamic monitoring.
2. Principles of asepsis.
3. Neuroanatomy and physiology.
4. Pathophysiology of increased intracranial pressure.

The nurse should be able to perform

1. Neurologic assessment.
2. Proper handwashing technique (see Skill 35–5).
3. Vital signs and hemodynamic assessments.
4. Calculation of cerebral perfusion pressure.
5. Universal precautions (see Skill 35–1).

Assessment

1. Assess the trends in intracranial pressure and the waveform tracing every hour and p.r.n. (note institutional policies). **Rationale:** Drastic changes or trends to-

ward undesirable pressure readings and waveform tracings indicate either an acute pathophysiologic event or mechanical malfunction.

2. Assess the system and device integrity, stability, loose/leaking connections, covered stopcock ports, and drainage on head dressing. **Rationale:** Decreases the risk of infection and invasion of microorganisms.

3. Assess the temperature; white blood cell count; cerebrospinal fluid cultures; device cultures (if obtained); and insertion site for signs and symptoms of inflammation and infection and observe for signs and symptoms of meningitis such as photophobia and neck stiffness. **Rationale:** Abnormalities in these indicators suggest central nervous system or local infection. Other indicators, such as headache, decreasing level of consciousness, seizures, cranial nerve dysfunction, and, uncommonly, endocrine disorders (such as SIADH), are symptoms of meningitis in the older child and adult. Symptoms of meningitis in young children include fever, refusal to eat, vomiting, diarrhea, listlessness, shrill cry, and bulging fontanels (Hickey, 1986).

Nursing Diagnoses

1. Potential for impaired cerebral tissue perfusion. **Rationale:** Cerebral perfusion pressure is determined by mean arterial pressure and related to increased intracranial pressure.

2. Potential for infection related to invasive device placement. **Rationale:** Normal defense mechanisms are interrupted (scalp, cranium, and dura), exposing the CNS to microorganisms, and placing the patient at increased risk for infection-related complications and subsequent potentially permanent neurological impairment.

Planning

1. Individualize the following goals for the patient undergoing intracranial pressure monitoring:
   a. Maintain intracranial pressure within normal limits. **Rationale:** Preserves neurological function or preserves neural tissue.
   b. Maintain system integrity. **Rationale:** Supports accurate intracranial pressure waveforms and pressure readouts; reduces potential for infection.
   c. Prevent infection. **Rationale:** CNS or local infection increases the patient's morbidity, extends the length of hospital stay, and may be associated with further neurologic injury.

2. Prepare the patient and family.
   a. Simplistically explain the meaning of intracranial pressure and its relationship to the treatment plans. **Rationale:** Intracranial pressure monitoring can be a source of confusion for the patient's family. Frequently, the family will learn to observe the intracranial pressure on the monitor independently and demonstrate anxiety when it is perceived that the numbers are "bad" or project an optimistic outcome if the numbers are "good." The patient and family must receive consistent reassurance and information regarding the patient's clinical status and understand therapies instituted to decrease intracranial pressure. They should be encouraged to ask questions and state their concerns.
   b. Position the patient in high semi-Fowler's position with head in neutral position. **Rationale:** Facilitates venous drainage from the cranium and prevents or minimizes an increase in intrathoracic pressure, which in turn will minimize intracranial pressure.

Implementation

Steps	Rationale	Special Considerations
Maintaining the Monitoring System		
1. Validate the accuracy of the system setup.	Unexpected changes in ICP or changes in waveform configuration require assessing device placement and stability and/or troubleshooting the system (Skill 16–3).	
2. Assess the system and connections for leaks.	Loose or leaking connections suggest that the integrity of the system has been disrupted, thus the potential for microorganism invasion.	Changing the setup or even replacing the device may be indicated. Discuss your findings with the physician.
3. Assess the stability of device.	The device must be intact and seated in the skull to provide accurate data.	Care should be taken while repositioning the patient to avoid dislodging the device.

Table continues on following page

Steps	Rationale	Special Considerations
4. Change the head dressing and assess the device insertion site per institutional protocol or physician's order using aseptic technique.	Assesses device stability and allows for direct visualization of insertion site.	Practices regarding changing the head dressing and providing local care to the insertion site are extremely variable. Some authors advocate a dressing change and site care every 24 hours Pollack-Latham, 1987a and b; Sphritz, 1983). Wisinger and Mest-Beck (1990) advocate that the dressing be changed only when wet, contaminated, or loose. It is agreed by all that an occlusive dressing should be applied to the insertion site. Responsibility for changing the head dressing and providing site care is institutional specific. Check your institution's policy. For dressings that are not changed, observe for drainage.

Pressure Measurements and Recalibration

Steps	Rationale	Special Considerations
1. Obtain and record ICP every hour and p.r.n. ICP pressure should be read on the "mean" standard.	Intracranial pressure is a component of overall neurological assessment.	Pressure trends over a period of time are most significant. Trends allow for the identification of pressure waves and evaluation of therapeutic modalities.
2. Confirm the position of the transducer at the foramen of Monro. (Reference point for hydraulic systems only.) Tape or secure disposable transducers to the dressing. A Velcro strap may also be used.	Ensures accurate pressure and waveform data.	Anatomically, the reference point is equivalent to the level of the ear or the outer canthus of the eye. Fiberoptic catheters and sensor transducers are located at the tip of the catheter; the zero reference point is *not* utilized.
3. Calculate and record CPP every hour and p.r.n.	Evaluates critical blood flow to the brain.	Preferred range for CPP is 60 to 150 mmHg. CPP = MAP − ICP, MAP = [2 (diastolic) + systolic]/3. Check your institutional policies or physician's orders for frequency of recordings.
4. Balance and recalibrate the system by turning the system off to the patient and opening the transducer to air/atmospheric pressure (for hydraulic systems only).	Ensures accuracy of readings.	The presence of an air filter on the transducer or stopcock will help prevent contamination of system. Zeroing and recalibration are recommended every 2 to 4 hours and p.r.n. (Pollack-Latham, 1987a and b). See package inserts for manufacturers' recommendations.

Changing the System Setup

Steps	Rationale	Special Considerations
1. Change the system setup per institutional protocol (for hydraulic systems only) using aseptic technique.	Complies with infection control guidelines and/or to maintain system integrity.	There is limited research about the frequency of changing the system setup. Earlier works suggest changing the pressure tubing/system setup every 24 hours (Sphritz, 1983). Recent publications suggest that the setup should *not* be changed at arbitrary intervals.

Discontinuing Intracranial Pressure Monitoring

Steps	Rationale	Special Considerations
1. Secure suture material, sterile hemostat, scissors, and clamp or twist drill.	Facilitates removal of the device.	Have a sterile palm-sized twist drill handle available to facilitate removal.

Table continues on following page

Steps	Rationale	Special Considerations
2. Wash hands.	Reduces transmission of microorganisms.	
3. Once device is removed, apply povidone-iodine ointment to site. Apply an occlusive dressing over site.	Decreases risk of infection.	Occlusive dressing folded 4 × 4 with overlying tape or a translucent type of dressing.
4. Discard supplies in appropriate receptacle.	Universal precautions.	
5. Wash hands.	Reduces transmission of microorganisms.	

Evaluation

Compare the patient's intracranial pressure and pressure waves and identify intracranial pressure trends on an ongoing basis. **Rationale:** Evaluates the patient's response to interventions.

Expected Outcomes

1. ICP is maintained within normal limits. **Rationale:** Therapeutic interventions have been effective.
2. Absence of infection. **Rationale:** System integrity and appropriate infection control measures have been maintained.

Unexpected Outcomes

1. CNS or local infection. **Rationale:** The presence of an intracranial pressure monitoring device increases the risk of infection-related complications. The risk increases if the device penetrates the dura.
2. Device becomes dislodged. **Rationale:** Device may become inadvertently dislodged during routine turning of the patient *or* if the patient is extremely restless or agitated.
3. Pressure readings and waveforms inconsistent with neurologic assessment. **Rationale:** May occur with device malfunction or when unilateral intracranial pressure monitored by a device is not consistent with overall or central intracranial pressure.
4. CSF leakage and/or infection. **Rationale:** May indicate dislodgment of device or breaks in the system.

Documentation

Documentation in the patient record should include date and time of system and device checks, baseline neurologic assessment, ICP, CPP, therapies instituted to decrease ICP and optimize CPP and patient's response to these therapies, signs and symptoms of CNS or local infection, identification of loose, cracked, or leaking connections or catheters and related interventions, any manipulation of the system, significant changes in ICP resulting from transducer recalibration, dampened or altered waveforms, and significant changes in pressure trends. **Rationale:** Documents nursing care given, expected and unexpected outcomes, and interventions taken.

Patient/Family Education

1. Assess the readiness of the patient and family to process information. **Rationale:** Situational anxiety and stress may reduce the ability of the patient and family to process information and demonstrate/verbalize learning.
2. Review the goals of intracranial pressure monitoring. **Rationale:** The patient and family should understand the short- and long-term goals of intracranial monitoring to decrease anxiety and to facilitate understanding of additional therapies.

Performance Checklist
Skill 16–2: Care of Intracranial Pressure Monitoring Device and System

Critical Behaviors	Complies yes	no
MAINTAINING THE MONITORING SYSTEM 1. Observe and review the system setup.		
2. Assess the system and connections for leaks.		
3. Assess the stability of the device.		
4. Change the head dressing and assess the device insertion site per institutional protocol.		

Table continues on following page

Critical Behaviors	Complies	
	yes	no
OBTAINING PRESSURE MEASUREMENTS AND RECALIBRATING THE MONITORING SYSTEM		
1. Obtain and record the intracranial pressure every hour and p.r.n.		
2. Confirm the position of the transducer.		
3. Calculate and record CPP every hour and p.r.n.		
4. Balance and recalibrate the system.		
CHANGING THE SYSTEM SETUP		
1. Change the system setup per institutional protocol.		
DISCONTINUING ICP MONITORING		
1. Secure suture material, sterile hemostat, scissors, and twist drill to remove device.		
2. Wash hands.		
3. Apply povidone-iodine ointment to site after removal, and apply dressing over site.		
4. Discard supplies.		
5. Wash hands.		
6. Document procedure in patient record.		

SKILL 16–3

Troubleshooting an Intracranial Pressure Monitoring Device

The implications for accurate ICP monitoring cannot be underestimated. Therapeutic modalities used to treat elevations in ICP and maintain adequate cerebral perfusion will affect the long-term outcome of the patient. Each intervention must be carefully evaluated for effectiveness. Since herniation is always a concern in the patient with increased ICP, any acute change must be evaluated for system failure versus changes in cerebral hemodynamics.

Each type of device has specific concerns associated with its use (see Table 16–6). The fiberoptic catheter will work only if the fiberoptics have not been damaged. The hydraulic system may develop a leak, air bubbles may become trapped in the system, or the tubing or device can become occluded with brain tissue or blood, resulting in a dampened waveform (Fig. 16–12). The sensor system can easily become displaced or wedged against the skull. Troubleshooting the system will require a working knowledge of the equipment and policies specific to the institution and the manufacturer's guidelines for its use.

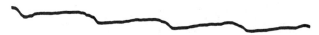

FIGURE 16–12. Dampened intracranial pressure waveform.

Purpose

The nurse troubleshoots the ICP monitoring device and system to

1. Determine if changes in waveforms or pressure are a result of mechanical failure.
2. Prevent the unnecessary replacement of the ICP monitoring device.
3. Ensure accurate readings.
4. Assess the insertion site for infection.
5. Assess for system integrity.

Prerequisite Knowledge and Skills

Prior to troubleshooting the ICP monitoring system, the nurse should understand

1. Principles of ICP.
2. Significance of ICP pressure and the various waveforms.
3. Factors that affect intracranial pressure.
4. Operation of specific ICP devices.

The nurse should be able to perform

1. Patient positioning.
2. Recalibration of the system.
3. Correct transducer placement.
4. Interpretation of waveforms and analysis of trends.
5. Proper handwashing techniques (see Skill 35–5).
6. Universal precautions (see Skill 35–1).

Assessment

1. Observe for signs and symptoms of increased ICP, including changes in level of consciousness, changes in respiratory pattern, and abnormal waveforms (see Fig. 16–2). **Rationale:** Identifies early signs of increased ICP and possible impending herniation.

2. Identify changes in stimuli that could account for the changes in ICP (i.e., suctioning, repositioning, coughing, pain, straining, or clustered activities. **Rationale:** Identifies the need for change in interventions, sedation, positioning, or stimulation.

3. Assess for mechanical difficulties specific to the monitoring system. **Rationale:** Identifies the need for interventions specific to the system.

Nursing Diagnoses

1. Potential alteration in cerebral tissue perfusion related to increased intracranial pressure. **Rationale:** Accuracy of intracranial monitoring must be ensured when implementing therapeutic interventions to minimize the risk of herniation.

2. Potential for injury related to system malfunction. **Rationale:** Inaccurate pressure readings, dampened waveforms, broken fiberoptics, and wedged sensors may lead to a delay in treating intracranial hypertension or may cause treatment to be initiated in the presence of normal ICP.

Planning

1. Individualize the following goals when troubleshooting:

   a. Maintain system integrity. **Rationale:** Promotes proper functioning and accurate measurements.

   b. Prevent infection at site or in CSF. **Rationale:** System disrupts normal protective barriers.

2. Prepare all necessary equipment and supplies. **Rationale:** Facilitates prompt and efficient intervention.

   a. Replacement system available in case of failure or breakage.

   b. Equipment needed to flush hydraulic system:
     (1) Sterile gloves, 1 pair.
     (2) Preservative-free sterile saline solution, 1 vial.
     (3) Luer-lok 10-cc syringe.
     (4) 18-gauge needle.
     (5) Sterile stopcocks × 2.
     (6) Sterile drape × 2.
     (7) Alcohol swabs × 3.

   c. Equipment needed to flush ventricular catheter or subarachnoid bolt:
     (1) Sterile gloves, 1 pair.
     (2) Preservative-free sterile saline solution, 1 vial.
     (3) Tuberculin 1-cc syringe.
     (4) 18-gauge needle.
     (5) Sterile stopcocks × 2.
     (6) Sterile drape × 2.
     (7) Alcohol swabs × 3.

   d. Sedation, self-inflating resuscitation bag connected to oxygen source, mannitol, readily available in case of intracranial hypertension or herniation. **Rationale:** Facilitates immediate intervention.

   e. Establish IV access. **Rationale:** Facilitates medication administration.

Implementation

Steps	Rationale	Special Considerations
Fiberoptic System		
1. Loss of waveform:		
a. Check cable connections; reconnect as needed.	Cable may have become loose or disconnected. Reconnection preamplifies cable.	
b. Increase gain or range.	Elevated or plateau waves may be higher than normal pressure range.	
c. Physician may need to reposition catheter tip.	Catheter tip near drain or non-intact skull.	Catheter should be placed away from drain sites, evacuated areas, or non-intact skull.
d. Replace fiberoptic catheter.	Fiberoptic catheter may break if catheter is kinked, coiled, or bent.	Loosely coil catheter with no sharp angles or tension on cable. Secure preamplifier cable to head dressing.
2. Falsely elevated ICP reading:		
Physician may need to reposition catheter.	Catheter tip occluded with tissue.	Avoid by flushing bolt immediately before catheter insertion.
3. Negative ICP readings:		
Digital number less than zero. Notify physician.	Catheter near open drain or non-intact skull.	Avoid these areas when placing catheter.

Table continues on following page

Steps	Rationale	Special Considerations
4. Monitor reads >350 mmHg or −99:		
Fiberoptic catheter must be replaced.	Fiberoptic fibers are damaged.	Avoid kinking catheter.
5. Monitor reads 888:		
Fiberoptic catheter must be replaced.	Fiberoptic fibers are damaged.	Replace fiberoptic preamplifier cable.
6. Microprocessor reading and bedside monitor do not correlate:		
a. Check zero and calibration on fiberoptic microprocessor and bedside monitor by depressing the zero control on the microprocessor. Continue to press zero control, while pressing zero on bedside monitor. When zero appears on bedside monitor, release the zero control on the microprocessor.	Recalibrates bedside monitor to microprocessor.	
b. Check connections.	Cable may be loose or disconnected.	
Hydraulic System		
1. Loss of waveform:		
a. Check stopcock connections and tighten as needed.	Connections may be loose.	
b. Don sterile gloves.	Universal precautions.	
c. Turn stopcock off to patient, and flush system with preservative-free sterile saline.	Protects patient from mechanical injury. Eliminates air bubbles.	
d. Close system.	Reduces transmission of microorganisms.	
e. Turn stopcock on to patient.	Allows for transmission of pressure and waveform.	
f. Check monitor cable.	Monitor may be disconnected.	
g. Increase gain or range.	Elevated or plateau waves may be higher than normal pressure range.	
h. Flush intraventricular catheter or screw as per physician order; 0.25 cc sterile saline may be used.	Device may be occluded with blood or tissue. Limit amount of fluid injected into subarachnoid or ventricular system because this will increase ICP.	
2. Falsely high reading:		
a. Zero balance and recalibrate the system.	Calibrates monitor to atmospheric pressure.	This may need to be repeated every 2 to 4 hours.
b. Position transducer at the external auditory canal or the outer canthus of the eye.	Provides accurate, consistent data (see Fig. 16–11).	
c. Check system for air bubbles.	Air may falsify readings by attenuating or amplifying pressure signal.	Air will displace CSF. If air bubbles are found, system must be flushed to remove them.
d. Flush system as above in 1b to 1e.	Establishes accurate pressure and waveform readouts.	
3. Falsely low reading:		
a. Check connections.	Loose connections will falsify readings.	Also increases the risk of infection.

Table continues on following page

Steps	Rationale	Special Considerations
b. Flush system as above in 1b to 1e.	Bolt or catheter may be occluded with blood or tissue.	
c. Check transducer level. Transducer should be placed at the level of the foramen of Monro (see Fig. 16–11).	Provides accurate, consistent data.	
4. Low ICP pressure:		
a. Check patient for otorrhea/ rhinorrhea (see Skill 17–3).	May be secondary to decompression.	Otorrhea/rhinorrhea indicates a CSF leak.
b. For ventriculostomy, refer to Skill 16–4.	Ventricles may collapse due to overdrainage.	Always remove CSF against a pressure gradient.
Sensor System		
1. Loss of waveform:		
Check connections.	Cable may be loose or disconnected.	
2. Sensor becomes dislodged:		
a. Apply sterile dressing to site.	Reduces risk of infection.	Notify physician. Reinsertion may be necessary.
b. Observe for CSF leak.	Dura may be torn.	
3. Elevated readings:		
a. High pressure trend: Assess neurologic status, and notify physician of any changes.	Before intervening, correlate ICP with total neurological assessment.	High pressure readings with sensors may be inaccurate.
b. Falsely elevated pressures: Assess neurologic status and system integrity, and notify physician of any changes.	Correlates ICP with total neurological assessment. Wedging of sensor between dura and table of skull may cause this.	Notify physician for possible reinsertion.

Evaluation

Evaluate patient's response to interventions throughout procedure, and perform neurologic assessment and compare with previous assessment levels. **Rationale:** Determine if troubleshooting interventions have caused any undesirable effects. Correlate neurological assessment with trended ICP and waveforms.

Expected Outcomes

1. Reliable, accurate, trended data. **Rationale:** Properly functioning system provides reliable data on which interventions will be based.
2. Acute changes in ICP or waveform will be identified and promptly treated. **Rationale:** Preserves neural tissue and thus neurological function.

Unexpected Outcomes

1. Inaccurate data. **Rationale:** Identifies need for troubleshooting and neurologic assessment.
2. Inoperable fiberoptic catheter. **Rationale:** The fiberoptics must not be kinked or damaged.
3. Displacement or "wedged" sensor catheter. **Rationale:** Wedging of the sensor against the dura and inner table of the skull results in inaccurate data.
4. Occluded hydraulic system. **Rationale:** Intracranial pressure elevations may cause blood or tissue to be pushed into device.

Documentation

Documentation in the patient record should include the patient's neurologic status before and after troubleshooting, the assessed problem, and the necessary intervention. **Rationale:** Provides evidence of nursing care given, expected or unexpected outcomes, and interventions taken.

Patient/Family Education

Reinforce the need for and purpose of ICP monitoring with both patient and family. **Rationale:** Decreases anxiety and provides an opportunity to ask questions.

Performance Checklist
Skill 16–3: Troubleshooting an Intracranial Pressure Monitoring Device

Critical Behaviors	Complies	
	yes	no
FIBEROPTIC SYSTEM		
1. Loss of waveform:		
a. Check cable connections; reconnect as needed.		
b. Increase gain or range.		
c. Assist physician in repositioning or replacing catheter.		
2. Falsely elevated ICP reading: assist physician in repositioning catheter.		
3. Negative ICP readings: notify physician.		
4. Monitor reads >350 mmHg or −99: assist physician in replacing fiberoptic catheter.		
5. Monitor reads 888: assist physician in replacing fiberoptic catheter.		
6. Microprocessor reading and bedside monitor do not correlate:		
a. Rezero and calibrate.		
b. Check connections.		
HYDRAULIC SYSTEM		
1. Loss of waveform:		
a. Check stopcock connections.		
b. Don sterile gloves.		
c. Turn stopcock off to patient, and flush system.		
d. Close system.		
e. Turn system on to patient.		
f. Check monitor cable.		
g. Increase gain or range.		
h. Flush intraventricular catheter or screw as directed by physician.		
2. Falsely high reading:		
a. Rezero and calibrate.		
b. Reposition transducer.		
c. Check system for air bubbles.		
d. Flush system (see steps 1b to 1e).		
3. Falsely low reading:		
a. Check connections.		
b. Flush system (see steps 1b to 1e).		
c. Check transducer level.		
4. Low ICP pressure:		
a. Check patient for otorrhea/rhinorrhea.		
b. For ventriculostomy, refer to Skill 16–4.		
SENSOR SYSTEM		
1. Loss of waveform:		
a. Check connections.		

Table continues on following page

Critical Behaviors	Complies	
	yes	no
2. Sensor becomes dislodged:		
a. Apply sterile dressing to site.		
b. Observe for CSF leak.		
3. Elevated readings. High pressure trend and/or falsely elevated pressures:		
a. Assess neurologic status.		
b. Notify physician.		
4. Document any troubleshooting interventions in the patient record.		

SKILL 16–4

Care of Intraventricular Devices

A ventriculostomy is beneficial in the management of neurologically impaired patients for ICP monitoring, drainage of cerebrospinal fluid (CSF) or blood in the subarachnoid space, collection of CSF samples, injection of intrathecal medications, and evaluation of therapy aimed at reducing ICP (Wisinger and Mest-Beck, 1990). Associated with the highest risk of infection, ventriculostomy is considered the most accurate mode of ICP monitoring. The ventriculostomy can be incorporated into a hydraulic, fluid-filled, or fiberoptic monitoring system.

Indications for intraventricular catheter use vary; Robinet (1985) describes its use in a select group of head-injured patients only, but other authors indicate that the ventricular catheter is the preferred method of any intracranial monitoring (Wisinger and Mest-Beck, 1990).

Clinical situations benefiting from ventriculostomy placement include (1) acute-onset hydrocephalus, (2) meningitis/encephalitis resulting in malabsorption of CSF, (3) tumor growth occluding CSF pathway, (4) selected postcraniotomy monitoring, (5) head injury requiring close ICP monitoring, and (6) subarachnoid/intracerebral hemorrhage.

Certain situations preclude the placement of an intraventricular device. They are (1) intracranial abscess/infection, (2) scalp infection, (3) anticoagulation abnormalities, including heparin therapy, (4) severe midline shift resulting in ventricular displacement, and (5) cerebral edema resulting in ventricular collapse (slit ventricles).

The greatest risk to ventriculostomy placement is infection. Other risks include development of hemorrhage due to puncture of the brain, CSF leakage, air in ventricles, or sudden decompression of ventricles (from overdraining) precipitating or accentuating midline shift or upward herniation (Pollack-Latham, 1987a and b).

The ventricular catheter may be utilized in two ways: It can be primarily a pressure monitoring device with intermittent drainage capabilities or it can be a continuous drainage device with intermittent pressure sensing. This skill should be performed as an adjunct to Skill 16–2.

Purpose

The nurse maintains intraventricular devices to:

1. Monitor intracranial pressure.
2. Provide a mechanism for drainage of CSF.
3. Obtain CSF cultures.
4. Instill intrathecal chemotherapy.

Prerequisite Knowledge and Skills

Prior to working with intravascular devices the nurse should understand

1. Neuroanatomy and physiology.
2. Intracranial pressure dynamics.
3. CSF production and pathway.
4. Principles of asepsis.
5. Principles of pressure monitoring.
6. Implications of positioning the neurologically impaired patient.
7. Universal precautions.

The nurse should be able to perform

1. Proper handwashing technique (see Skill 35–5).
2. Neurologic assessment.
3. Vital signs assessment.
4. Universal precautions (see Skill 35–1).

Assessment

See Skills 16–1 and 16–2 for assessment of the patient with an intracranial monitoring device. Once the ventriculostomy system is in place, the nurse should also assess:

1. Observe for *early* signs and symptoms of increased intracranial pressure, such as altered or decreased level of consciousness, restlessness, agitation, irritability, anxiety, lethargy or drowsiness, confusion, apathy, motor weakness (i.e., hemiparesis), headaches, pupillary dysfunction, or seizures (see Fig. 16–2). **Rationale:** Pressure on cortical structures causes an alteration in level of consciousness, but metabolic offenders such as ETOH, sedation, ketoacidosis, hepatic coma, renal failure, and

recreational drug use must be ruled out because they produce similar effects.

2. Identify *late* signs of increased intracranial pressure, such as continuing alteration in level of consciousness progressing to coma, alteration in motor/sensory assessment (i.e., hemiparesis, decortication, decerebration), alteration in pupillary response and extraocular movements, alteration in respiratory pattern or rate (Cheyne-Stokes, central neurogenic hyperventilation, apneustic, ataxic patterns), elevation in blood pressure, widened pulse pressure, and bradycardia (Cushing's reflex), alterations in brainstem reflexes, and possibly vomiting (see Fig. 16–2). **Rationale:** Alterations result from increasing pressure exerted on brainstem structures, specifically the midbrain, pons, and medulla. The cranial nerves governing extraocular movements have nuclei originating in the midbrain and pons. Respiratory centers are found throughout the brainstem and may result in abnormal breathing patterns associated with specific structures involved.

3. Signs of increased intracranial pressure in the infant include tense or bulging anterior fontanel, separation of suture lines or increased head circumference, irritability, projectile vomiting, drowsiness, high-pitched cry, "sunset eyes" (i.e., eyeball deviated downward so only upper portion of pupil is visible), and "cracked pot" sound on percussion of skull (Germon and Grant, 1989).

4. Assess the trends in intracranial pressure and the waveform tracing every hour and p.r.n. (note institutional policies). **Rationale:** Drastic changes or trends toward undesirable pressure readings and waveform tracings indicate either an acute pathophysiologic event or mechanical malfunction.

5. Assess the system and device integrity, stability, loose/leaking connections, covered stopcock ports, and drainage on head dressing. **Rationale:** Decreases the risk of infection and invasion of microorganisms.

6. Assess the temperature; white blood cell count; cerebrospinal fluid cultures; device cultures (if obtained); and insertion site for signs and symptoms of inflammation and infection and observe for signs and symptoms of meningitis such as photophobia and neck stiffness. **Rationale:** Abnormalities in these indicators suggest central nervous system or local infection. Other indicators, such as headache, decreasing level of consciousness, seizures, cranial nerve dysfunction, and, uncommonly, endocrine disorders (such as SIADH), are symptoms of meningitis in the older child and adult. Symptoms of meningitis in young children include fever, refusal to eat, vomiting, diarrhea, listlessness, shrill cry, and bulging fontanels (Hickey, 1986).

7. Patency of the ventriculostomy. **Rationale:** Patent system allows for accurate monitoring, fluid drainage, and/or medication injection.

8. Amount, color, and character of CSF that has drained. **Rationale:** Abnormal characters are indicative of pathologic conditions.

Nursing Diagnoses

1. Potential for neurologic injury related to overdrainage and upward herniation. **Rationale:** Fluid drain off may result in ventricular displacement.

2. Potential for infection related to device penetration of the dura and the cerebral cortex. **Rationale:** Disruption of anatomical protective barriers increases the risk of infection.

Planning

1. Individualize the following goals for the patient with a ventriculostomy:
   a. Maintain patent system. **Rationale:** Facilitates drainage of CSF and ensures an accurate ICP measurements.
   b. Minimize risk of infection. **Rationale:** Infection-related complications may jeopardize the patient's long-term functional outcome.

2. Prepare the patient.
   a. Explain the procedure. **Rationale:** Reduces anxiety, and encourages cooperation and questions.
   b. Explain the importance of the patient remaining still during the procedure. **Rationale:** Decreases risk of contaminating monitoring system.

3. Assemble closed monitoring/drainage system. Setup for drainage will vary among institutions. Some drainage systems will be prepackaged as a set from the manufacturer. If the nurse must construct the drainage system, sterile technique must be utilized, and care must be taken to avoid multiple connections and open ports, which increase the risk of infection.

Implementation

Steps	Rationale	Special Considerations
Drainage System Setup		
1. Wash hands.	Reduces transmission of microorganisms.	
2. Attach assembled drainage system to device per institutional protocol using aseptic technique.	Allows for CSF drainage.	The drainage system is usually attached to the system via a stopcock port. The drainage system should be placed distal to the transducer (if a hydraulic system is utilized) or can be attached to any stopcock in the fiberoptic system.

Table continues on following page

Steps	Rationale	Special Considerations
Instituting Continuous Pressure Monitoring with Intermittent Drainage		
1. Position the patient, with the head of the bed at a consistent level (usually 30 to 60 degrees) and level transducer with reference point—hydraulic system only (see Skill 16–2).	Maintains ICP within normal parameters and prevents overdrainage of CSF.	The patient's head and neck should be maintained in a neutral position. This can be accomplished with small pillows or towel rolls for support. Care should be taken to avoid flexion and hyperextension of neck. Avoid Trendelenburg position, which can exacerbate intracranial pressure by interfering with venous jugular drainage.
2. Monitor ICP until a drainage parameter has been identified or as prescribed.	Allows for identification of ICP trends.	Fluid-filled systems may require that the stopcock be turned on to the transducer and off to the drainage system. Fiberoptic systems require closure or clamping of the drainage system only.
3. Hydraulic system: Open system to drain by turning stopcock off to transducer and on to drainage system. Fiberoptic system: Unclamp or open drainage system.	Allows for drainage of CSF.	Only small amounts of CSF should be drained at any one time. Robinet (1985) suggests 2 cc of CSF. Rapid cerebral decompression by overdrainage of CSF may result in neurologic deterioration due to upward herniation.
4. Monitor patency of system when system is open for drainage.	Ensures adequate CSF flow to relieve increased ICP.	Blood, tissue, or kinks in the tubing may occlude CSF flow and impede CSF drainage. See Skill 16–3 to identify other variables that impair the system.
5. Close drainage system when prescribed parameters are met. Hydraulic system: Turn the stopcock off to the drainage system and on to the transducer. Fiberoptic system: Close or clamp the drainage system.	Avoids overdrainage and decreases potential for herniation.	
Continuous Drainage System with Intermittent Pressure Monitoring		
1. Identify drainage parameters as prescribed by the physician. These should include: a. Amount of CSF to be drained over a period of time. b. Intervals at which ICP should be measured.	Facilitates drainage for patients requiring frequent or continuous CSF drainage as a result of persistently increased ICP. Maintains ICP within normal limits.	These parameters may vary institutionally or within specific protocols.
2. Place the ventricular drainage system at appropriate height for drainage as prescribed by the physician.	The height of the system will control the pressure at which CSF will drain.	The drainage system should be placed at a specific level, prescribed by the physician or protocol, above the zero reference point (foramen of Monro). For example, if the system is to be drained at a pressure of 15 mmHg, place the drainage bag 15 cm above the reference point.
3. Open drainage system by opening stopcock or clamp to drainage tubing and bag.	Allows for continuous flow of CSF at the prescribed pressure.	See Skill 16–3 for problems with flow of CSF. Normally, patency is demonstrated by fluctuation of CSF in the tubing and collection chamber.

Table continues on following page

Steps	Rationale	Special Considerations
a. Hydraulic system: Close the drainage system to assess and record ICP per institutional protocol or as prescribed by the physician.	Monitors ICP pressure.	The fiberoptic system allows for continuous drainage as well as pressure monitoring.
b. Turn the stopcock off to the transducer and on to the drainage system.	Reestablishes continuous drainage.	

Changing the Drainage System

Steps	Rationale	Special Considerations
1. Obtain equipment to establish new drainage system and assemble (if necessary) on sterile field.	Equipment readiness avoids prolonged system exposure to atmosphere.	Equipment needed: system specific tubing and drainage bag; sterile specimen container; sterile mask, gloves and cap; sterile capped needles.
2. Don cap, mask, and sterile gloves.	Universal precautions.	
3. Close the system off to the drainage collection tubing and bag.	Prevents leakage of CSF when tubing is disconnected.	
4. Disconnect old tubing from stopcock connection.	Allows for connection of new drainage tubing and bag.	
5. Place a sterile needle and cap on the end of the tubing to be discarded.	Prevents leakage of CSF from discarded tubing.	One way to obtain a CSF sample is by using CSF in the discarded tubing. See obtaining CSF sample below.
6. Insert new tubing and drainage bag at connection.	Reestablishes drainage system.	
7. Place drainage system at height prescribed by physician or protocol.	Maintains CSF drainage against prescribed pressure gradient.	
8. Discard used supplies and old drainage system in appropriate receptacle.	Universal precautions.	

Obtaining CSF Sample

Steps	Rationale	Special Considerations
1. If using CSF in tubing to be discarded:		Several methods are described to obtain a CSF sample. Operationalizing this procedure depends on institutional policy. Two methods will be described, one involves withdrawing CSF from the intact system; the other describes CSF collection from the discarded system. System sampling for culture and analysis is usually performed once a day.
a. Gather sterile gloves and sterile specimen container.	Maintains sterile technique.	
b. Open container and don sterile gloves.	Avoids contamination of CSF sample.	
c. Obtain discarded drainage bag/ tubing and release clamp.	CSF in tubing is released for analysis.	
d. Direct flow of CSF from tubing into opened sterile container.	Provides sample for analysis.	This method allows for the most recent CSF drained in tubing to be sent for analysis.
e. Close sterile container.	Prevents contamination of specimen.	
f. Discard supplies in appropriate receptacle.	Universal precautions.	

Table continues on following page

Steps	Rationale	Special Considerations
g. Send CSF for appropriate studies as prescribed by the physician or by unit protocol.	Identification of microorganism growth.	See Table 16–7 for normal characteristics of CSF. CSF is typically sent for culture and sensitivity, glucose, white blood cell count, and protein.
2. If obtaining CSF sample by invasive method:		
a. Obtain mask, cap, sterile gloves, 23-gauge needle, 5-cc syringe, sterile container, and povidone-iodine solution or alcohol.	In order to perform procedure in aseptic manner.	
b. Don mask, cap, and sterile gloves.	Reduces transmission of microorganisms.	
c. Locate dead-end port/connection from which to obtain CSF sample.	Identifies the port for preparation.	
d. Swab port with povidone-iodine or alcohol solution.	Reduces transmission of microorganisms.	Specific preparation will vary institutionally. Refer to your institutional guidelines and protocols.
e. Attach 23-gauge needle to 5-cc syringe.	Provides method to withdraw CSF.	
f. Insert needle into prepared dead-end port and slowly withdraw 2 cc of CSF.	Obtains CSF sample.	Care should be taken to avoid rapid withdrawal of CSF to avoid sudden cerebral decompression and upward herniation.
g. Withdraw needle from dead-end port.	Disengages needle from drainage system.	
h. Place specimen into opened sterile container. Avoid contamination of sample.	Provides sample for analysis.	
i. Close sterile container.	Prevents contamination of specimen.	
j. Swab dead-end port with Betadine or alcohol.	Reduces transmission of microorganisms.	
k. Discard supplies in appropriate receptacle.	Universal precautions.	
l. Send CSF for appropriate studies as prescribed.	For identification of microorganism growth.	
Administering Intrathecal Medications		
1. Gather equipment: povidone-iodine solution/swabs, 23-gauge needle and 25-gauge butterfly set, 3-cc syringe, and sterile gloves, mask, and cap to be used for administration of intrathecal medication.	Facilitates efficiency of procedure.	
2. Locate appropriate port for medication injection.	Identifies the port for injection.	Medication may be injected through a prepared dead-end self-sealing port on the stopcock. Institutions have varying guidelines regarding the nurse's role in administering intrathecal medication. *Refer to institutional policies and guidelines prior to administering intrathecal medication.* Also note the type of medication to be administered to determine if the patient requires preparation prior to administration (such as with amphotericin).

Table continues on following page

Steps	Rationale	Special Considerations
3. Close system off to pressure and drainage pathways.	Ensures that the medication will be injected into the ventricle, not into the system.	
4. Don mask, cap, and sterile gloves.	Reduces transmission of microorganisms.	The smallest gauge needle should be used to inject medication to minimize disruption of the self-sealing stopcock cap.
5. Prepare syringe with medication. Cap with 25-gauge needle.	Needed to inject medication.	
6. Insert needle of medication syringe into the diaphragm on dead-end cap.	Accesses system for instillation of medication.	
7. Instill medication *slowly* into prepared port.	Minimizes risk of increasing ICP with additional volume.	In some patients, it may be appropriate to withdraw CSF equal to the amount to be injected to minimize potential for increased ICP and neurologic deterioration. Because of the risks of volume infusion, the medication should be prepared in as *little* solute as safely possible. Generally, intrathecal medications are of a lesser dose than systemic medications.
8. Observe patient for signs and symptoms of increased ICP or reaction to administered medication.	Prevents neurological deterioration or adverse problems.	Observe for nausea, vomiting, rash, chills, fever, headache, anaphylaxis, or behavior changes.
9. Withdraw needle and dispose of in appropriate receptacle.	Reestablishes a closed system. Universal precautions.	
10. Swab dead-end port with povidone-iodine or alcohol.	Reduces transmission of microorganisms.	
11. Reestablish pressure monitoring or drainage system.	For continuous pressure monitoring or CSF drainage.	

Evaluation

1. Evaluate neurological status secondary to manipulation of the ventriculostomy. **Rationale:** Identifies neurologic changes resulting from interventions.

2. Ensure patency of system. **Rationale:** Continued drainage, particularly of bloody CSF (such as seen in subarachnoid hemorrhage) and particulates, impedes CSF flow through drainage system.

3. Verify system integrity. **Rationale:** Manipulating the system in any way may loosen system connections resulting in leaks.

4. Evaluate ICP trends and waveforms. **Rationale:** Manipulation of the system may cause dampening of waveform (if air bubbles have been introduced inadvertently) and may necessitate recalibration or zeroing of the system.

5. Evaluate the patient for signs and symptoms of CNS infection. **Rationale:** Ventriculostomy is associated with the highest risk of infection when compared to other intracranial monitoring systems.

6. Evaluate effects specific to intrathecal medication administration (if applicable). **Rationale:** Identifies neurologic changes related to intrathecal administration.

Expected Outcomes

1. Absence of infection. **Rationale:** The occurrence of infection lengthens hospital stay and jeopardizes long-term patient outcomes.

2. Device remains stable and provides accurate ICP trends, waveforms, and drainage. **Rationale:** Optimizes patient outcome.

Unexpected Outcomes

1. Overdrainage of CSF. **Rationale:** Overdrainage can occur if the system is drained for too long a period of time, if the system is inadvertently left open, if the CSF pressure is inordinately high and drains excessively,

TABLE 16–7 CHARACTERISTICS OF CSF

Volume

The volume of CSF increases with hydrocephalus and decreases with space-occupying lesions. The normal range is 135 to 150 ml.

Specific Gravity

The normal value is 1.007.

Color

Xanthochromia is the term used to describe discoloration of the CSF. It is most often due to blood in the CSF. This discoloration may be yellow, orange, or brown, and is due to the red blood cell (RBC) breakdown and the liberation of bilirubin.

Turbidity or Cloudiness of the CSF

Turbidity usually indicates an increased number of white blood cells (WBCs) in the CSF. A high protein content or microorganisms in the CSF can cause clouding. An infection process would increase the WBC and microorganism counts. Elevated protein levels occur with brain tumors.

Cell Count

Blood can appear in the CSF as soon as 3 hours after the blood enters the CSF from a subarachnoid hemorrhage. The discoloration of the CSF can continue for up to 28 days after the initial bleeding. There are no RBCs normally present in CSF.

White Blood Cells (WBCs)

The range of 0 to 5 cells/mm^3 is considered normal as long as these cells are agranulocytes. If there are 5 to 10 cells/mm^3, it is highly suspicious of abnormality. More than 10 cells/mm^3 indicates disease of the central nervous system. Leukocytosis in the CSF can result from an inflammatory process within the ventricular system of the brain or the meninges. The most common cause of such an inflammatory process is meningitis. Inadequately treated open head injuries, brain abscess, sinusitis, or mastoiditis can be the underlying cause by which invading microorganisms enter the meninges, thereby causing inflammation. Intracranial tumors, spinal tumors, and multiple sclerosis also elevate the whole blood count of the CSF.

Protein Content

The protein count is elevated with tumors, infections, and hemorrhages. The normal range is 15 to 45 mg/100 ml.

Glucose

Normally 60 to 80 mg/100 ml (approximately 80%) of the blood glucose level is found. An elevated CSF glucose level has no specific significance; however, a decreased glucose level indicates the presence of glycolytic substances such as bacteria in the CSF.

Electrolytes in CSF

The following is a list of values for four electrolytes:
- Sodium: 141 mEq/liter (= to blood: 135–145)
- Potassium: 3.3 mEq/liter (< than in blood: 3.5–5.0)
- Chloride: 118 to 132 mEq/liter (> than in blood: 96–105)
- Calcium: 2.5 mEq/liter (< than in blood: 5.0)

Colloidal Gold Curve

The colloidal gold curve is a test that indicates alterations in the albumin–globulin ratio in CSF. Reactions in this test are sometimes seen in neurosyphilis, multiple sclerosis, and purulent meningitis. This is an unreliable test with many false positives and false negatives; therefore, a diagnosis is never made solely on the basis of this test.

Culture and Sensitivity

CSF can be cultured to identify the invading organism within the fluid. Sensitivity can also be determined to identify what drug therapy will be the most effective.

Smears

Smears for Gram stain are essential in diagnosing specific meningitis, such as tubercular meningitis.

Serology

Serology testing of CSF can be performed to diagnose neurosyphilis.

Source: Reprinted with permission from J. Hickey, *The Clinical Practice of Neurological and Neurosurgical Nursing*, 2d Ed. Philadelphia: Lippincott, 1986, p.97.

---

or if the patient is maintained at a higher level than the reference point on the system, thereby decreasing the pressure gradient over which the CSF must overcome to drain.

2. Infection. **Rationale:** Nosocomial infection may occur as a result of intracranial device placement. See Skill 16–1 for other unexpected outcomes and rationales related to intracranial monitoring devices.

Documentation

Documentation in the patient record should include the date and time of setup, system change, CSF sample obtained, and medication instillation; the color, amount, and character of CSF drainage; the frequency and duration of drainage; cultures sent; and test results.

Patient/Family Education

1. Explain the rationale for ICP monitoring and CSF drainage. **Rationale:** Reduces patient and family anxiety.

2. Reinforce risks and benefits of ventricular drainage. **Rationale:** Improves understanding and cooperation with further therapies.

3. Explain the signs and symptoms of increased ICP and CNS infection. **Rationale:** This enables the patient and family to recognize neurologic deterioration and the need for intervention.

Performance Checklist
Skill 16–4: Care of Intraventricular Devices

Critical Behaviors	Complies yes	no
DRAINAGE SYSTEM SETUP 1. Wash hands.		
2. Attach closed drainage system to appropriate port using aseptic technique.		
INSTITUTING CONTINUOUS PRESSURE MONITORING WITH INTERMITTENT DRAINAGE 1. Position the patient and level transducer (hydraulic system only).		
2. Monitor ICP.		
3. Open drainage system to allow CSF flow.		
4. Monitor patency of system.		
5. Close drainage system as prescribed.		
ESTABLISHING CONTINUOUS DRAINAGE SYSTEM WITH INTERMITTENT PRESSURE MONITORING 1. Identify level at which to maintain system.		
2. Place system at specific height.		
3. Open drainage system to allow for continuous drainage.		
4. Close drainage system to intermittently observe and assess intracranial waveforms and pressure trends.		
5. Reestablish continuous drainage.		
CHANGING THE DRAINAGE SYSTEM 1. Obtain appropriate equipment.		
2. Don appropriate attire.		
3. Close system off to drainage bag.		
4. Disconnect old tubing and drainage bag.		
5. Place sterile cap on end of tubing to be discarded.		
6. Insert new tubing and drainage bag at connection.		
7. Place new drainage system at appropriate height.		
8. Reserve discarded CSF for sampling (if applicable), and discard used supplies and old drainage system.		
OBTAINING CSF SAMPLE		
ADMINISTERING INTRATHECAL MEDICATIONS 1. Gather equipment.		
2. Locate port for injection.		
3. Close system to pressure and drainage pathways.		
4. Don mask, cap, and sterile gloves.		
5. Obtain syringe and needle with medication, and puncture diaphragm on dead-end cap.		
6. Inject medication slowly.		
7. Assess the patient thoroughly after injection.		
8. Withdraw needle and syringe, and dispose of appropriately.		
9. Swab dead-end port with Betadine or alcohol.		
10. Reestablish pressure monitoring or drainage system.		

Table continues on following page

Critical Behaviors	Complies	
	yes	**no**
HEAD DRESSING, SITE CARE, AND REMOVAL OF DEVICE 1. See Skill 16–2.		
2. Document all procedures in the patient record.		

REFERENCES

Beare, P. and Myers, J. (1990). *Principles and Practice of Adult Health Nursing.* St. Louis: Mosby.

Cardona, V., Hurn, P., Bastnagel, P. et al. (1988). *Trauma Nursing: from Resuscitation through Rehabilitation.* Philadelphia: Saunders.

Germon, C. (1988). Interpretation of ICP pulse waves to determine intracerebral compliance. *J. Neurosci. Nurs.* 20:344–349.

Germon, C., and Grant, M. (1989). Increased Intracranial Pressure. In *Core Curriculum of Neuroscience Nursing.* Chicago: Am. Assoc. Neurosci. Nurses.

Hickey, J. (1986). *The Clinical Practice of Neurological and Neurosurgical Nursing,* 2d Ed. Philadelphia: Lippincott.

Hollingsworth-Friedlund, P., Vos, H., and Daily, E. (1988). Use of fiberoptic pressure transducer for intracranial pressure measurements: A preliminary report. *Heart Lung* 17:111–120.

Lundgren, J. (1986). *Acute Neuroscience Nursing: Concepts of Care.* Boston: Jones and Bartlett.

Marshall, S. B., Marshall, L., Vos, H., and Chesnut, R. (1990). *Neuroscience Critical Care: Pathophysiology and Patient Management.* Philadelphia: Saunders.

Mitchell, P., Hodges, L., Muwaswes, M., and Walleck, C. (1988). *AACN's Neuroscience Nursing: Phenomena and Practice.* Norwalk, Conn.: Appleton & Lange.

Pollack-Latham, C. (1987a). Intracranial pressure monitoring: Part I. *Crit. Care Nurs.* 7(4):40–51.

Pollack-Latham, C. (1987b). Intracranial pressure monitoring: II. Patient care. *Crit. Care Nurs.* 7(6):53–72.

Robinet, K. (1985). Increased intracranial pressure: Management with an intraventricular catheter. *J. Neurosurg. Nurs.* 17(2):95–104.

Shpritz, D. (1983). Craniocerebral trauma. *Crit. Care Nurs.* 3(2):49–61.

Spielman-McGinnis, G. (1988). Central Nervous System I: Head Injuries. In V. Cardona et al. (Eds.), *Trauma Nursing from Resuscitation through Rehabilitation.* Philadelphia: Saunders.

Walleck, C. (1989). Controversies in the management of the head-injured patient. *Crit. Care Clin. North Am.* 1(1):67–74.

Wisinger, D., and Mest-Beck, L. (1990). Ventriculostomy: A guide to nursing management. *J. Neurosci. Nurs.* 22:365–369.

BIBLIOGRAPHY

Boortz-Marx, R. (1985). Factors affecting intracranial pressure: A descriptive study. *J. Neurosurg. Nurs.* 17(2): 89–94.

Bruya, M. (1981). Planned periods of rest in the intensive care unit: Nursing care activities and intracranial pressure. *J. Neurosurg. Nurs.* 13(4): 184–194.

Chambers, L., Mendelow, A., Sinar, E., and Modha, P. (1990). A clinical evaluation of the Camino subdural screw and ventricular monitoring kits. *Neurosurgery* 26: 421–423.

Crutchfield, J.S., Narayan, R., Robertson, C., and Micheal, L. (1990). Evaluation of a fiberoptic intracranial pressure monitor. *J. Neurosurg.* 72: 482–487.

Gilliam, E. (1990). Intracranial hypertension: Advances in intracranial pressure monitoring. *Crit. Care Nurs. Clin. North Am.* 2: 21–27.

Hickman, K., Mayer, B., and Muwaswes, M. (1990). Intracranial pressure monitoring: A review of risk factors associated with infection. *Heart Lung* 19(1): 84–90.

March, K., Mitchell, P., Grady, S., and Winn, R. (1990). Effect of backrest position on intracranial and cerebral perfusion pressures. *J. Neurosci. Nurs.* 22: 375–381.

Millar, S., Sampson, L.K., and Soukup, M. (1985). *AACN Procedure Manual for Critical Care,* (2d Ed.) Philadelphia: Saunders.

BEHAVIORAL OBJECTIVES

After completing this chapter, the nurse will be able to

- Define the key terms.
- Describe the methods of specific neurologic procedures.
- Discuss techniques used to support the patient during the procedure.
- Demonstrate the skills involved in assisting with special neurologic procedures.
- State the significance of the test results.

Special neurologic procedures are essential for evaluating, planning, and treating patient needs in individualized situations. The nurse is responsible for giving or reinforcing information concerning these tests to the patient and family. The nurse is also responsible for correlating the patient's clinical status with the test results, planning patient care, and identifying specific teaching needs.

The procedures in this chapter are diagnostic in nature, and most involve the nurse as an assistant and patient care provider through the testing process.

KEY TERMS

coma	extraocular movements
conjugate	nuchal rigidity
doll's eyes	nystagmus
dysconjugate	tentorium cerebri

SKILLS

17–1 Assisting with Lumbar and Cisternal Punctures
17–2 Assisting with Ice-Water Caloric Testing for Vestibular Function
17–3 Assessment Technique for Cerebrospinal Fluid Drainage

GUIDELINES

The following assessment guidelines assist the nurse in formulating a nursing diagnosis and developing an individualized plan of care for the patient undergoing special neurological procedures.

1. Know the patient's baseline neurologic assessment.
2. Know the patient's baseline vital signs.
3. Know the patient's medical history.
4. Know the patient's current medical treatment.
5. Assess the ability of the patient and family to learn and comprehend.

SKILL 17–1

Assisting with Lumbar and Cisternal Punctures

A lumbar or cisternal puncture accesses the subarachnoid space to support a diagnosis of subarachnoid hemorrhage, central nervous system (CNS) tumor, infection, or an autoimmune disorder. Absolute contraindication to lumbar or cisternal puncture exists if the patient has a known or suspected intracranial mass or greatly increased intracranial pressure (ICP). Patients with mass lesions and/or significant cerebral edema with a shifting of the intracranial contents develop a large pressure gradient between cerebral and lumbar subarachnoid spaces. A sudden release of pressure below the intracranial contents may precipitate cerebral herniation through the tentorial notch or brainstem or cerebellar herniation through the foramen magnum.

Using strict aseptic technique, a needle with a stylet is inserted either at the level of L3–4 or L4–5 (Fig. 17–1) or in the cisterna magna (Fig. 17–2) to access small reservoirs of cerebrospinal fluid (CSF).

A lumbar puncture is the usual procedure to obtain CSF, but a cisternal (C1–2) puncture is done when the lumbar area is not accessible, when the contrast material cannot circulate freely in the subarachnoid space due to a complete block at a specific vertebral level, if the patient's spinal positioning is restricted (such as in spinal cord injury), or if the patient cannot tolerate or assume the position needed to undergo lumbar puncture.

Once the needle is inserted in the correct location, initial CSF (opening) pressures are obtained; then CSF samples are collected for analysis. The CSF is placed in three sterile test tubes and is sent to the laboratory for analysis of color, turbidity, cell count (RBCs), WBCs, protein, glucose, and culture and sensitivity. The physician also may ask the nurse to assist in performing the Queckenstedt test. This may be done during the lumbar puncture if an obstruction in the spinal subarachnoid space is suspected. Complete or partial obstruction of the spinal subarachnoid space may be caused by a herniated intervertebral disk or a spinal tumor. This test is performed by compressing *both* jugular veins for 10 seconds; serial pressure readings are recorded from the CVP

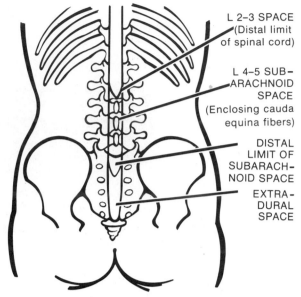

FIGURE 17–1. The body of the spinal cord ends at L2–3. The region below, L4–5, encloses the cauda equina (a bundle of lumbar and sacral nerve roots) within the subarachnoid space. It is this area that is appropriate for lumbar puncture.

manometer at 5 and 10 seconds. After 10 seconds, the jugular veins are released and the CSF pressure is read and recorded every 5 seconds for 30 seconds or until the pressure returns to baseline. In patients who *do not* have a spinal subarachnoid blockage, this maneuver will cause a sudden, sharp increase in CSF pressure. Patients with a partial subarachnoid block may experience a small or slight rise in CSF pressure, and compete blockage of CSF circulation will result in *no* increase in CSF pressure. This maneuver is *contraindicated* in patient's with increased intracranial pressure or subarachnoid hemorrhage because herniation or rebleeding may occur as a result of the imposed increase in ICP. A lumbar puncture is considered an invasive, traumatic, and somewhat painful

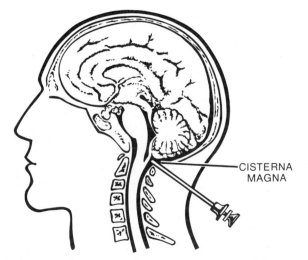

FIGURE 17–2. The cisterna magna, located at the base of the skull between the second cervical vertebrae and under the posterior rim of the foramen magnum.

test. The physician should explain the procedure and its risks and benefits, and the patient should sign an informed consent prior to initiation of the procedure.

Purpose

A lumbar or cisternal puncture is performed to:
1. Measure the pressure of the CSF.
2. Examine CSF for the presence of blood.
3. Collect CSF for laboratory studies.
4. Evaluate spinal dynamics for signs of CSF flow obstruction.
5. Inject air, oxygen, or contrast media to visualize CNS structures radiographically.
6. Remove CSF to alleviate increased ICP.
7. Provide access for intrathecal injection of chemotherapeutic or antibacterial agents.
8. Introduce spinal anesthesia for surgical/obstetrical procedures.

Prerequisite Knowledge and Skills

Prior to assisting with lumbar or cisternal puncture, the nurse should understand
1. Anatomy and physiology of the spinal column and CSF circulation.
2. The anticipated dynamic response following CSF removal.
3. Potential risks and benefits of this procedure.
4. Principles of asepsis.

The nurse should be able to perform
1. Neurologic assessment.
2. Vital signs assessment.
3. Handwashing technique (see Skill 35–5).
4. Aseptic technique.
5. Proper patient positioning techniques.
6. Universal precautions (see Skill 35–1).

Assessment

1. Identify symptomatology that indicates the need for lumbar or cisternal puncture, including changing levels of consciousness, photophobia, nuchal rigidity, or temperature elevations. **Rationale:** Symptoms are indicative of an infectious process in the central nervous system.
2. Identify any developmental or anatomic abnormalities or changes in the lumbar region or at the foramen magnum level. **Rationale:** Abnormal lumbar anatomy, such as severe scoliosis or anatomic changes from previous lumbar surgery/fusion, may preclude the use of the lumbar area for puncture to decrease risk to the patient and to optimize correct placement of lumbar needle. Abnormalities at the foramen magnum or cervical regions may preclude the use of these areas for puncture; the patient may be unable to achieve the required position

of flexing the neck with chin to the chest, or a specific anomoly may interfere with accurate needle placement.

3. Identify patients who are at risk for complication and those in which a lumbar or cisternal puncture is contraindicated, including patients with an intracranial mass or cerebral edema causing a shift of the intracranial contents, those with local infection at the lumbar or cisternal site, patient's who are anticoagulated, or patients with medication or contrast material allergies. **Rationale:** A lumbar or cisternal puncture increases the risk for brainstem herniation, infection, hematoma, or allergic reaction.

4. Assess patient's degree of cooperativeness. **Rationale:** It is imperative that the patient be able to cooperate with instructions and positioning required for proper needle placement. *Inadvertent patient movement may result in injury by displacing the spinal needle.*

Nursing Diagnoses

1. Anxiety related to invasive procedure. **Rationale:** Invasive procedures may result in anxiety and fear.

2. Potential for injury related to procedure. **Rationale:** The patient is at risk for hematoma with resultant neurologic decompensation when undergoing lumbar or cisternal puncture.

3. Potential for infection. **Rationale:** Needle entry through the dura increases the risk of procedure-related infection.

4. Pain related to invasive procedure. **Rationale:** Even when using local anesthetic, the patient may feel or perceive pain and discomfort during needle placement, especially when puncturing the dura.

5. Potential for altered pattern in urine elimination. **Rationale:** Irritation of spinal nerve roots at the region of lumbar puncture (specifically the sacral nerve roots) may cause temporary urine retention. If this occurs, the physician should be notified, because the patient may require intermittent catheterization until the irritation resolves.

Planning

1. Individualize the following goals for the patient undergoing lumbar or cisternal puncture:
   a. Patient cooperation and comprehension of the procedure. **Rationale:** Prior to the procedure ascertain whether explanation to patient and family regarding the need for the test, the steps of the procedure, and the restrictions enforced after the procedure have supported their compliance and cooperation, and reduced their anxiety. Since patients are often fearful of paralysis, the nurse should stress that the needle is not placed directly in the spinal cord but in the space *surrounding* the spinal cord. Discuss the specific positions the patient will need to assume. It is beneficial to discuss specific ways comfort can be maintained, such as the use of local anesthesia and practicing breathing/relaxation techniques.
   b. Patient safety will be ensured. **Rationale:** Proper positioning reduces risk of patient injury.
   c. Patient comfort will be ensured. **Rationale:** Puncture-site discomfort and/or postprocedural headache may be relieved by bed rest and analgesics. The degree of discomfort the patient perceives is dependent on individual pain tolerance and the degree of technical difficulty present during the lumbar or cisternal puncture.

2. Prepare all necessary equipment and supplies. **Rationale:** Facilitates initiation and progression of procedure.
   a. Sterile gloves.
   b. Spinal needle with stylet (20 gauge, 3 to 3½ in).
   c. Sterile gauze pads (4 × 4s).
   d. Povidone-iodine solution.
   e. Three-way stopcock.
   f. Manometer.
   g. Sterile fenestrated drape.
   h. Three or four small sterile specimen containers (test tubes).
   i. Needles (no. 18 to draw up anesthetic; no. 22 to inject local anesthetic).
   j. Syringe, 5 cc.
   k. Band-Aid or sterile dressing.
   l. Disposable razor (for cisternal puncture).
   m. Lidocaine 1% to 2% (without epinephrine).
   n. Adequate light source.
   o. Two overbed tables (one for sterile field, one to position patient if necessary).
   p. Rolled towels or small pillows to support patient during positioning.
   q. Cardiopulmonary resuscitation equipment.
   Note: Check institution for availability of prepackaged lumbar puncture kit.

3. Prepare the patient.
   a. Have patient empty bladder (if necessary). **Rationale:** The patient will not be able to interrupt the procedure in progress.
   b. For *lumbar puncture*, position patient in lateral decubitus (fetal) position with head and neck flexed and knees up toward chest (Fig. 17–3). **Rationale:** This position widens the interspinous process space (space between the vertebrae) and facilitates entry of the spinal needle into the subarachnoid space.
   c. For *cisternal puncture*, assist the patient to flex the chin to the chest. **Rationale:** This position brings the brainstem and spinal cord forward in the canal, making the site accessible for puncture.

4. Administer light sedative as prescribed by physician. **Rationale:** Reduces anxiety and facilitates cooperativeness. A light sedative (such as diazepam 5 mg) may be administered prior to procedure.

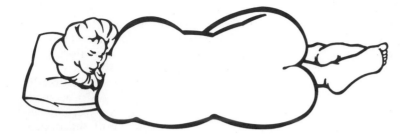

FIGURE 17–3.   The lateral decubitus (fetal) position appropriate for lumbar puncture. The patient's knees are drawn tightly up to the chest, and the patient flexes the chin down to the chest. This increases the intraspinous space to facilitate needle insertion.

Implementation

Steps	Rationale	Special Considerations
1. Wash hands.	Reduces transmission of microorganisms.	
2. Close patient's door or draw curtain around bed.	Provides privacy.	
3. Ensure correct position of the patient.	Provides for spinal alignment and allows physician access to the area.	The patient should be able to tolerate a side-lying position with head flat. If the patient is obese or cannot tolerate a flat position, this test (both lumbar and cisternal) may be done with the patient sitting upright and leaning over a bedside table. For *lumbar punctures*, to help the patient maintain this position, the nurse should place one arm behind the patient's head and the other arm around the knees. Provide stability to the patient's shoulder by standing in front of him or her. For *cisternal punctures*, to maintain this position, support the crown of the head and the patient's jaw.
4. Prepare the skin with povidone-iodine solution.	Reduces microorganisms and prevents infection.	For cisternal puncture, the physician will shave the nape of the neck.
5. Assist in draping area.	Decreases risk of contamination and provides a sterile field for procedure.	The physician may wish to defer draping during the cisternal puncture so as not to obscure anatomic landmarks.
6. Assist the physician in identifying the appropriate anatomic site for puncture.	*Lumbar* punctures: *below* the level of L2 to prevent damage to the spinal cord. (In the *adult*, the body of the spinal cord ends at L1 or L2.) *Cisternal* punctures: the skull base is used to select for puncture.	The physician draws an imaginary line vertically between the two iliac crests, and a second line is imagined horizontally across the spinous processes. These lines should intersect the L3–4 area, and the puncture can be performed here or one level below at L4–5. The second cervical vertebrae is the *first* palpable spinous process. The needle is inserted slightly above this level.
7. Assist with administration of local anesthesia.	Prevents or decreases pain from needle insertion.	The skin is injected initially; then a deeper injection of anesthetic is administered to the interspinous ligament.

Table continues on following page

Steps	Rationale	Special Considerations
8. Monitor the patient's neurologic, respiratory, and cardiovascular status during procedure.	Placement of spinal needle can result in neurologic symptoms or decompensation.	During lumbar procedures, the patient may experience pain or abnormal sensation radiating down the legs as a result of spinal nerve irritation. This may necessitate a change in patient or needle position. During cisternal punctures, the patient is observed carefully for signs of respiratory depression or an altered level of consciousness due to needle proximity to medulla (Rudy, 1984).
9. Once the needle is in place, instruct patient to relax, breath normally, and avoid holding his/her breath.	Increased muscle tension or intrathoracic pressure may falsely elevate CSF pressure.	Patients undergoing lumbar puncture also may straighten legs, since severe leg flexion can increase intrathoracic pressure.
10. Using aseptic technique, assist in attaching manometer to spinal needle via a three-way stopcock.	Obtains CSF pressure measurement while maintaining needle and field sterility.	Readings taken at the cisternal area or with the patient in a sitting position are of little value due to altered pressure mechanics. Normal CSF pressure readings taken at the lumbar area range from 110 to 150 mmHg (Rudy, 1984).
11. If an obstruction in the spinal subarachnoid space is suspected, assist in performing Queckenstedt test by simultaneously compressing the jugular veins for 10 seconds.	A normal response indicates the pathway between the skull and lumbar needle is patent.	Normally, there is a rapid increase in CSF pressure with resultant decrease when compression is released. If there is a complete or partial spinal block, the pressure will *not* rise or will rise slowly and remain at the increased level when jugulars are released. Also, if the CSF pressure does not rise with the Queckenstedt maneuver, the cause may be improper needle placement. The Queckenstedt test is *contraindicated* in patients with increased ICP or subarachnoid hemorrhage.
12. Assist with the collection of CSF specimens in sterile tubes.	The physician must stabilize the manometer system with one hand and turn stopcock with the other.	Care should be taken to use aseptic technique and to avoid rapid loss of CSF. Place 1 cc of fluid in each tube.
13. Label each tube with type of specimen, patient name, and order in which the specimen was collected.	The order in which the specimen was collected is needed for accurate laboratory interpretation.	The laboratory may differentiate between blood in the CSF or traumatic tap by evaluating each numbered specimen. Red blood cell (RBC) dissipation through consecutive samples is indicative of traumatic tap; consistent RBC presence is indicative of subarachnoid hemorrhage.
14. Apply antiseptic and dressing to puncture site after physician removes needle.	Provides sterile dressing at access site.	
15. Instruct patient to remain flat in bed for 6 to 24 hours after the procedure unless otherwise prescribed by the physician. Patient *may* log-roll.	Allows punctured dura to seal.	Postprocedure positioning restrictions remain controversial, but the flat position is helpful in relieving headache associated with CSF withdrawal and leakage of CSF at puncture site.
16. Discard supplies in appropriate receptacle.	Universal precautions.	
17. Wash hands.	Decreases transmission of microorganisms.	

Table continues on following page

Steps	Rationale	Special Considerations
18. Send specimens to laboratory for evaluation.	For diagnostic processing.	See Table 16–7 on p. 502 for normal components of CSF.

Evaluation

1. Evaluate the patient's neurologic and respiratory status every 15 minutes for the first hour, every hour for the next 4 hours, then every 4 hours for the following 24 hours. Evaluation should include motor and sensory status, level of consciousness, respiratory rate, and breathing pattern. **Rationale:** Neurologic and respiratory status should be consistent.
2. Monitor needle puncture site. **Rationale:** Identifies any complications such as bleeding or CSF leak at puncture site.
3. Evaluate the patient for pain or discomfort. **Rationale:** The patient may experience pain or discomfort at the puncture site, which can be relieved with mild analgesia.

Expected Outcomes

1. Test findings of CSF are diagnostic. **Rationale:** Xanthochromia may indicate the presence of RBCs; turbidity may indicate the presence of bacteria.
2. Patient's vital signs and level of consciousness remain stable before, during, and after the procedure. **Rationale:** No extreme changes in CSF pressure result in neurologic decompensation.
3. Absence of headache, neck stiffness, local pain at puncture site, leg spasms, or slight elevation in temperature. **Rationale:** Any of these symptoms may be related to meningeal irritation resulting from entry into the subarachnoid space. These symptoms are transient and can be relieved with analgesics and position changes. Administration of fluids (if appropriate) may enhance CSF replenishment and decrease headache symptoms.

Unexpected Outcomes

1. Significant change in level of consciousness and/or vital signs. **Rationale:** Overdrainage of CSF can result in herniation of the cerebellar tonsils through the foramen magnum. Maintain patient in a flat position, notify physician immediately, and begin emergency procedures as needed.
2. Inability to void spontaneously. **Rationale:** Difficulty in voiding may result from nerve irritation related to lumbar needle entry, since lumbar nerve roots govern bowel and bladder control. The patient also may have difficulty voiding because of position restrictions. This

symptom should be transient and resolve when the patient is allowed to sit upright or when nerve irritation resolves. Persistent inability to void may indicate hematoma formation or nerve damage at the lumbar site. If the patient cannot void for greater than 6 hours and the bladder is palpable, notify the physician immediately for further evaluation, and prepare to catheterize the patient.
3. CSF is not obtained. **Rationale:** This may occur because of difficulty in puncturing the dura, patient's intolerance of procedure, or poor needle placement.
4. Prolonged headache, stiff neck, photophobia, and acute rise in temperature. **Rationale:** Symptoms indicate CNS infection, possibly resulting from puncture.
5. Excessive drainage at puncture site. **Rationale:** Indicates subcutaneous tract leakage of CSF or blood.
6. Persistent complaints of pain and/or tingling in lower extremities. **Rationale:** Needle trauma to the spinal nerves may result in nerve injury.

Documentation

Documentation in the patient record should include the date, time of the procedure, the status of the puncture site, and amount of CSF collected; the character of the CSF, neurologic and respiratory assessment before and after the procedure, complaints of pain, unexpected outcomes, and interventions needed. **Rationale:** Provides documentation regarding the procedure and the patient's response to the procedure.

Patient/Family Education

1. Assess patient and family understanding of positioning restrictions after the procedure and the common occurrence of selected symptoms. **Rationale:** Reinforcement of information may be necessary to reduce patient's anxiety related to restrictions and symptoms.
2. Teach patient and family about the signs and symptoms of CNS infection, specifically meningeal signs, such as neck stiffness, increased temperature, photophobia, nausea, vomiting, and change in level of consciousness. **Rationale:** The risk for CNS infection occurs whenever the dura is disrupted.

Performance Checklist
Skill 17–1 Assisting with Lumbar and Cisternal Punctures

Critical Behaviors	Complies yes	no
1. Wash hands.		

Table continues on following page

Critical Behaviors	Complies	
	yes	no
2. Close patient's door or draw curtain around bed.		
3. Position the patient properly.		
4. Prepare skin with antimicrobial solution.		
5. Assist in draping area.		
6. Assist in identifying appropriate site.		
7. Assist with administration of local anesthetic.		
8. Monitor patient's neurologic status during procedure.		
9. Provide relaxation measures.		
10. Assist in obtaining CSF pressures.		
11. Perform Queckenstedt test as requested.		
12. Assist in collection of CSF samples.		
13. Label tubes with appropriate information.		
14. Apply antiseptic and dressing to puncture site.		
15. Instruct the patient regarding positioning restrictions.		
16. Discard supplies.		
17. Wash hands.		
18. Send specimens to laboratory.		
19. Document procedure in patient record.		

SKILL 17–2

Assisting with Ice-Water Caloric Testing for Vestibular Function

Caloric testing for vestibular function (oculovestibular testing) is a diagnostic procedure to test the vestibular portion of the eighth (acoustic) cranial nerve. Oculovestibular testing is also performed to assess brainstem function in the comatose patient. Assessment of the oculovestibular response can be one component of the evaluation for brain death.

The oculovestibular reflex can be elicited by introducing cold or warm water into the external auditory canal for 30 seconds to 3 minutes. This stimulates the semicircular canals and generates an impulse in the vestibular nerve. This impulse is relayed via the brainstem to the third (oculomotor) and sixth (abducens) cranial nerves, both of which govern extraocular movement (see Fig. 17–4). Normal responses depend on whether the patient is awake or unconscious. The awake patient should demonstrate a two-component response. Unilateral cold water (86°F or 30°C) irrigation results in a slow initial nystagmic eye movement *toward* the irrigated ear and then a fast component of nystagmus *away* from the irrigated ear. Unilateral warm water irrigation (110°F or 44°C) results in rapid nystagmus toward the irrigated ear. The mnemonic *COWS* (cold, opposite; warm, same) re-

fers only to the expected eye direction of the fast nystagmic component. The unconscious patient may have diminished reflex response to the fast (nystagmic) component; therefore, a normal response in the comatose patient is reflex conjugate eye movement toward the cold water–irrigated ear. An abnormal (dysconjugate) or absent response to cold water testing in the unconscious patient may indicate brainstem dysfunction and a poor prognosis (Fig. 17–5).

Hallpike caloric testing involves irrigating the ear (with intact tympanic membrane) for 40 seconds with 250 to 500 cc warm or cold water. The patient is observed for tonic and nystagmic eye movements (Hickey, 1986).

Caution should be used when interpreting the patient's eye movements during this procedure. The presence of a normal response implies intact brainstem function, but an abnormal response does not definitively indicate brainstem dysfunction. Agents or conditions that potentially interfere with the oculovestibular reflex include

1. Ototoxic drugs.
2. Neurosuppressant drugs such as barbiturates, phenytoin, sedatives, and tricyclic antidepressants.
3. Neuromuscular blockers.
4. Preexisting vestibular disease.
5. Preexisting cranial nerve disorders involving the abducens nerve (cranial nerve VI).

Frontal cortex

Medial longitudinal fasciculus

Decreased firing of vestibular nerve

Relative increased firing of vestibular nerve

Slow

Slow

Fast

Fast

Ice water

III Medial rectus subnucleus of oculomotor complex

—— Fast phase (corrective, cortical) pathway

– – – Slow phase (active, vestibular) pathway

Vestibular nuclei

VI Pontine gaze center and abducens nucleus innervating lateral rectus muscle

FIGURE 17–4. Physiology of the oculovestibular reflex. Cold water irrigation of a patient will elicit this reflex if both the cerebral hemisphere and the brainstem are intact. The signal passes through the pathways from the medulla to the midbrain, resulting in a slow movement of the eyes toward the irrigated ear. Then, as the impulse travels to the intact ipsilateral hemisphere, a rapid corrective movement of the eyes (nystagmus away from the irrigated ear) can be observed. (Reprinted with permission from Patient Care Magazine, page 29, Medical Economics Publishing, 1981.)

Patient response with intact brainstem

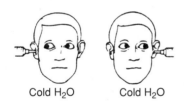

Cold H₂O Cold H₂O

Abnormal or absent patient response

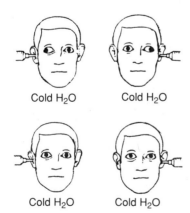

Cold H₂O Cold H₂O

Cold H₂O Cold H₂O

FIGURE 17–5. Cold water caloric responses in the comatose patient. If the patient's brainstem is intact, the normal response to cold water irrigation is slow movement *toward* the irrigated ear. When the brainstem is not intact, an abnormal (dysconjugate) or absent response may be observed. (Adapted with permission from F. Plum and J. Posner, *The Diagnosis of Stupor and Coma*, 3d Ed. Philadelphia: F. A. Davis, 1980.)

The physician performs this test *only* after it has been determined that the patient's tympanic membrane is intact. Caloric testing is also contraindicated in patients with active labyrinth diseases, such as Meniere's disease.

Purpose

The nurse assists with oculovestibular testing to

1. Evaluate brainstem function.
2. Evaluate the vestibular portion of the eighth cranial nerve.

Prerequisite Knowledge and Skills

Prior to assisting with oculovestibular testing, the nurse should understand

1. Neurologic anatomy and physiology.
2. The normal and abnormal responses associated with stimulating the oculovestibular reflex.
3. The significance of the patient's response to testing.

The nurse should be able to perform

1. Neurologic assessment.
2. Cranial nerve assessment.
3. Vital signs assessment.
4. Proper handwashing technique (see Skill 35–5).
5. Universal precautions (see Skill 35–1).

Assessment

1. Identify the awake patient's need for oculovestibular testing (may arise to assess cranial nerve function). **Rationale:** Patients with acoustic neuroma or Meniere's disease may exhibit a diminished or absent response to oculovestibular testing.

2. Identify the comatose patient's need for oculovestibular testing (may be performed to determine the integrity of the brainstem). **Rationale:** A normal response in the comatose patient indicates that brainstem pathways between the third, sixth, and eighth cranial nerves (whose nuclei are found in the midbrain and pons, respectively) are intact. An absent or abnormal response may indicate brainstem dysfunction or brain death.

Nursing Diagnoses

1. Pain related to stimulation of the semicircular canal (in the awake patient). **Rationale:** Water irrigation of the ear may elicit the following systemic responses: nausea, vomiting, vertigo, or dizziness in the awake patient.

2. Anxiety related to uncertainty of patient's diagnosis and prognosis (family response). **Rationale:** The need to perform oculovestibular testing on the unconscious patient may be a situationally anxiety-producing experience for the patient's family.

Planning

1. Individualize goals for the patient and family related to oculovestibular testing.

a. Determine brainstem function. **Rationale:** Necessary to determine coma and/or brain death.
b. Determine the response of cranial nerve VIII (vestibular portion). **Rationale:** Determines brainstem function of the awake and comatose patient.

2. Prepare all necessary equipment and supplies: 50-cc irrigating syringe, receptacle for water (emesis basin), tap water at appropriate temperature, towels/protective bedding.

3. Prepare the patient.
a. Explain the procedure to the patient. **Rationale:** Reduces anxiety and facilitates cooperation. The comatose patient's family should receive education and emotional support related to the need for oculovestibular testing.
b. Keep awake patient NPO 6 to 8 hours prior to procedure. **Rationale:** Nausea, vomiting, and dizziness may occur as a side effect of testing.
c. Position the patient in supine position, and tilt patient's head as directed by physician. **Rationale:** The patient's head may be tilted forward 30 degrees to test the vertical canals and backward 60 degrees to test the horizontal canals. This maneuver may need to be modified depending on the patient's tolerance to positioning. Head tilting may be deferred if the patient has an actual or suspected cervical spine injury.
d. Instruct the awake patient to keep his or her eyes open and focused forward. The comatose patient will require intervention to keep eyes open. **Rationale:** This allows for visualization of eye movements.

Implementation

Steps	Rationale	Special Considerations
1. Wash hands.	Reduces transmission of microorganisms.	
2. Verify that the integrity of the tympanic membrane has been assessed.	This test is contraindicated for patient's with punctured tympanic membrane.	
3. Maintain patient's head position depending on whether horizontal or vertical testing is performed.	The patient's head may be tilted backward and forward throughout procedure to test vertical and horizontal canals.	This technique may be contraindicated for a patient with actual or suspected cervical spine injury.
4. Observe patient's eye movements during instillation of water. Note the time interval between instillation and response. If cold water irrigant is used for the awake patient, it should be utilized in very small amounts (1 cc) to minimize untoward effects that the patient may experience. Larger amounts of cold water irrigant may be required for the unconscious patient to maintain stimulation adequate to effect a response.	Provides information regarding the oculovestibular reflex.	The comatose patient will require the nurse to keep the eyes open to visualize movement. Test each ear separately in order to stimulate both cranial nerves. A 5-minute wait between irrigations is suggested to allow patient relief from untoward symptoms so as not to confound reflex responses.

Table continues on following page

Steps	Rationale	Special Considerations
5. Assess patient's tolerance to procedure.	The external meatus is irrigated for 30 seconds to 3 minutes. Irrigations are discontinued when untoward effects, such as nausea, vomiting, or dizziness occur.	
6. Discard supplies in appropriate receptacles.	Universal precautions.	
7. Wash hands.	Reduces transmission of microorganisms.	

Evaluation

1. Evaluate occurrence of untoward effects of testing, such as nausea, vomiting, dizziness, and vertigo. **Rationale:** Caloric testing can precipitate these effects.
2. Monitor vital signs, pupillary response, and motor response of the lethargic or comatose patient. **Rationale:** Ensures that these indicators remain at baseline values.
3. Evaluate the patient's response to caloric testing. **Rationale:** Indicates the status of the brainstem and VIII cranial nerve (oculovestibular portion).

Expected Outcomes

1. Successful assessment of the awake patient's cranial nerve and brainstem function. **Rationale:** Determines if there is an abnormality in neural function.
2. Assessment of the comatose patient's brainstem and cranial nerve integrity. **Rationale:** Demonstration of the expected or normal comatose response (nystagmus toward the cold water–irrigated ear) indicates neural function at a very basic level. Additional brain death criteria, such as assessing for spontaneous respirations, doll's eyes (oculocephalic) reflex, cerebral blood flow studies, and calculations of cerebral perfusion pressure supports the diagnosis of brain death.

Unexpected Outcomes

1. Diagnostic testing is unable to be completed. **Rationale:** The awake patient must be able to keep his or her eyes open and comply with focusing ahead in order to accurately assess response.
2. Patient develops nausea, vomiting, dizziness, or vertigo. **Rationale:** Stimulation of the vestibular nerve can cause these untoward effects.

Documentation

Documentation in the patient record should include date and time procedure performed, identification of intact tympanic membrane, temperature and amount of solution instilled, the time interval between the beginning of instillation and the patient's response, a description of the patient's eye movements or untoward responses, the patient's general tolerance to the procedure, and a postprocedure vital signs, pupillary responses, and motor function before and after the procedure. **Rationale:** Provides documentation regarding the procedure and the patient's response to the procedure.

Patient/Family Education

Reinforce what diagnostic information caloric testing can provide. **Rationale:** Caloric testing is but one component of brain-death testing.

Performance Checklist
Skill 17–2: Assisting with Ice-Water Caloric Testing for Vestibular Function

Critical Behaviors	Complies	
	yes	no
1. Wash hands.		
2. Verify the integrity of tympanic membrane with the physician.		
3. Position patient and hold patient's head as requested.		
4. Observe patient's eye movements following instillation of cold or warm water. Note time interval between instillation and response.		
5. Assess patient's tolerance to procedure.		
6. Discard supplies according to institutional policy.		
7. Wash hands.		
8. Document procedure in patient record.		

SKILL 17–3

Assessment Technique for Cerebrospinal Fluid Drainage

The integrity of the dura, the outermost meningeal membrane found directly beneath the cranium, is jeopardized whenever damage occurs to the skull. Any type of open or closed cranial injury may cause compromise to the dura by stretching, tearing, or penetrating the membrane. Most often associated with basilar skull fractures, this loss of integrity can result in a cerebrospinal fluid (CSF) leak (Fig. 17–6). The dura entered for neurosurgical procedures is also at risk for leak.

Although any skull fracture can cause a break in the protective covering of the brain, those associated with dural tears predispose the patient to an even higher risk of infection because a tear in the dura permits CNS exposure to the environment.

The patient with a CSF leak may experience otorrhea (leakage of CSF from the ear), rhinorrhea (leakage of CSF from the nares), leaking of CSF into the nasopharynx, or CSF fluid collection or drainage at an operative site. CSF drainage can sometimes be identified by a characteristic "halo" sign, a yellowish ring surrounding the drainage on dressings or linens.

Most CSF leaks spontaneously resolve within 7 to 10 days. The patient is usually placed on bed rest and may be given antibiotics prophylactically to reduce the risk of CNS infection. If the CSF leak persists, it may be treated by intermittent drainage of CSF by lumbar puncture or continuous drainage via a lumbar subarachnoid drain. Dural repair may be required if other methods of treatment are not successful.

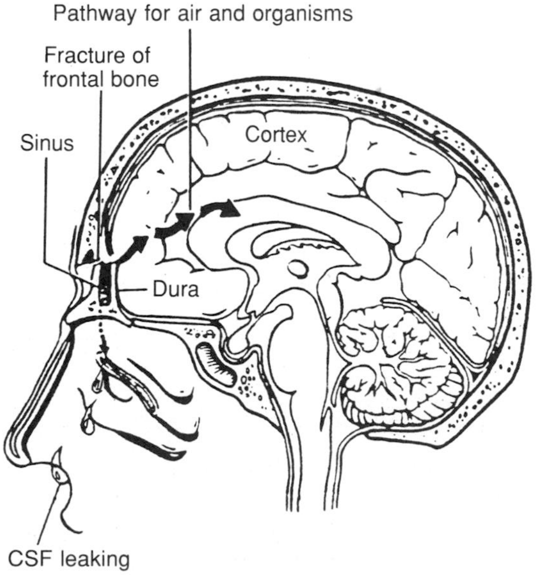

FIGURE 17–6. Cerebrospinal fluid leak resulting from skull fracture. This diagram depicts a CSF leak from the nose (rhinorrhea), but CSF drainage also may be experienced from the ear (otorrhea), nasopharyngeally (described as postnasal drip), and rarely, in tears. (Reprinted with permission from M. Snyder and M. Jackie, *Neurologic Problems: A Critical Care Nursing Focus*, Englewood Cliffs, N. J.: R. J. Brady, 1981.)

Purpose

The nurse identifies CSF drainage to decrease the risk of CNS infection.

Prerequisite Knowledge and Skills

Prior to assessing for CSF, the nurse should understand

1. Neuroanatomy.
2. Conditions placing the patient at risk for CSF leak.
3. The relationship between CSF leak and CNS infection.

The nurse should be able to perform

1. A "halo" test.
2. Neurologic assessment.
3. Proper handwashing technique (see Skill 35–5).
4. Universal precautions (see Skill 35–1).

Assessment

1. Assess the high risk patient for nasal and/or aural drainage or new onset postnasal drip. **Rationale:** When CSF drains from the paranasal sinuses, it is often sensed as a postnasal drip or increased frequency of swallowing. The nurse *should not attempt* to pack or irrigate any of the areas suspected of CSF leak.

2. Assess postoperative neurosurgical patients for clear or serous fluid from operative site or surgically placed drains. **Rationale:** A CSF leak will most likely be noted at the operative site as drainage or a "boggy" area around the incision, or persistent serous drainage from a surgical drain.

Nursing Diagnosis

Potential for infection related to disruption of the brain's protective barrier. **Rationale:** Increases the risk of infection.

Planning

1. Individualize the following goals for identification of CSF leak:
   a. Identification of patients at high risk for CSF leak. **Rationale:** A CSF leak is suspected on all patients presenting with open or closed head trauma.
   b. Prompt determination of drainage as CSF. **Rationale:** Facilitates interventions for CSF leak and for decreasing risk of infection.

2. Prepare all necessary equipment and supplies:
   a. Sterile dressing.
   b. Glucose dip sticks.
   c. Small test tube (if there is enough drainage to collect).
   d. Clean linen.

e. Nonsterile examination gloves.
3. Prepare the patient.
   a. Explain the technique of CSF identification to the patient. **Rationale:** If CSF drainage is identified, it is likely to lengthen the patient's stay and direct his or her course of treatment.

b. Assist patient to a comfortable position that makes the drainage site visible. **Rationale:** Observation of the leakage site and application of new dressing may necessitate a change in patient positioning (particularly if leakage is noted at the posterior aspect of the skull.)

Implementation

Steps	Rationale	Special Considerations
1. Wash hands.	Reduces transmission of microorganisms.	
2. Identify area of CSF drainage.	Prepares for collection and assessment of fluid.	The nurse may need to reposition the patient onto side if the area to be assessed is a posterior surgical wound.
3. Don examination gloves.	Universal precautions.	
4. Obtain moist dressing or linen with fresh drainage evident, or collect drainage in small tube (if possible).	Provides for testing or the examination for the presence of glucose or "halo" sign.	Collecting drainage in a tube, although sometimes difficult, allows for better evaluation of the drainage. If a nasal leak is present, the tube may be held at the naris to collect fluid. Postoperative drainage may be collected from the drain.
5. Assess drainage for "halo" sign, a combination of blood encircled by a yellowish stain.	A yellowish ring around the drainage perimeter is indicative of CSF.	This sign is difficult to see on some dressings and is perhaps best observed on linen (pillowcase).
6. Evaluate test tube sample with glucose stick.	The presence of glucose is indicative of CSF, since glucose is a component of normal CSF.	If the drainage is particularly sanguinous, this test may not be accurate.
7. Discard soiled dressing/linen in appropriate receptacle.	Universal precautions.	
8. Replace sterile dressing at site.	Minimizes the risk of infection.	Dressings may need frequent replacement. The nose or ear should not be packed in any way with these dressings. Drainage should be allowed to freely flow into the loose fitting dressing.
9. Wash hands.	Reduces transmission of microorganisms.	
10. Notify physician if testing indicates presence of CSF.	If CSF is identified, the patient will need a course of prophylactic antibiotic therapy.	A lumbar drain may need to be inserted if leak is excessive.

Evaluation

Evalute the patient for signs and symptoms of CNS infection, such as photophobia, neck stiffness, nausea, and elevated temperature. **Rationale:** CSF leak predisposes the patient to CNS infection.

Expected Outcome

Prompt identification of CSF leak. **Rationale:** Patient will need to be evaluated by a physician and will probably be placed on prophylactic antibiotics.

Unexpected Outcome

Development of a CNS infection. **Rationale:** Increased exposure to the environment will increase the patient's risk of infection. This may be insidious if the patient has no symptoms of CSF leak or does not report symptoms such as a postnasal drip or the need to swallow frequently.

Documentation

Documentation in the patient record should include the date and time drainage was noted, color and character of the drainage, the site from which drainage was collected, and observations made (such as "halo" sign or positive glucose test). If pads or sponges are used to absorb drainage, record the number of dressing changes required within a specific time frame (1 hour intervals).

Patient/Family Education

1. Reinforce that the patient with a CSF leak should not blow the nose, sneeze, or cough. **Rationale:** Increased pressure at the leak site will inhibit healing.

2. Prior to discharge, the signs and symptoms of CSF leak should be reviewed again with the patient and family. If signs and symptoms of leak occur, have the patient notify the physician immediately. **Rationale:** The patient should be able to recognize and report the occurrence of drainage.

3. Prior to discharge, the patient and family should be knowledgeable regarding the presence and significance of meningeal signs, such as neck stiffness, high temperature, photophobia, nausea, vomiting, and change in mental status. **Rationale:** Signs and symptoms of CNS infection may not occur until after the patient has been discharged to home.

Performance Checklist
Skill 17–3: Assessment Technique for Cerebrospinal Fluid Drainage

Critical Behaviors	Complies	
	yes	no
1. Wash hands.		
2. Identify area of CSF drainage.		
3. Don examination gloves.		
4. Obtain dressing/linen for evaluation.		
5. Evaluate dressing/linen for "halo" sign.		
6. Test drainage for glucose (when appropriate).		
7. Discard gloves, dressings, and supplies.		
8. Replace sterile dressing at site (if possible).		
9. Wash hands.		
10. Notify physician if CSF is present.		
11. Document procedure in patient record.		

REFERENCES

Hickey, J. (1986). *The Clinical Practice of Neurological and Neurosurgical Nursing*, 2d Ed. Philadelphia: Lippincott.

Millar, S., Sampson, L. K., and Soukup, M. (1985). *AACN Procedure Manual for Critical Care*. Philadelphia: Saunders.

Plum, F. and Posner, J. (1980). *The Diagnosis of Stupor and Coma*. Philadelphia: F. A. Davis.

Ricci, M. (1985). Lumbar and cisternal punctures (assisting with). In S. Millar, L. K. Sampson, and S. M. Soukup (Eds.), *AACN Procedure Manual for Critical Care*, 2d Ed. (pp 341–345). Philadelphia: Saunders.

Rudy, E. (1984). *Advanced Neurological and Neurosurgical Nursing*. St. Louis: Mosby.

Synder, M. and Jackie, M. (1981). *Neurologic Problems: A Critical Care Nursing Focus*. Englewood Cliffs, NJ: R. J. Brady.

BIBLIOGRAPHY

Lower, J. (1986). Maxillofacial trauma. *Nurs. Clin. North Am.*, 21(4):611–625.

McGruder, J. Cooke, J. Conroy, J. and Baker, J. (1988). Headache after lumbar puncture: review of the epidural blood patch. *South. Med. J.*, 81(10):1249–1252.

Rupp, S. and Wilson, C. (1989). Treatment of spontaneous cerebrospinal fluid leak with epidural blood patch: Case report. *J. Neurosurg.*, 70(5):808–810.

Snyder, M., and Jackie, M. (1981). *Neurologic Problems: A Critical Care Nursing Focus*, Englewood Cliffs, NJ: R. J. Brady.

Zegeer, L. (1989). Oculocephalic and vestibulo-ocular responses: significance for nursing care. *J. Neurosci. Nurs.*, 21 (1):46–55.

UNIT IV

THE GASTROINTESTINAL SYSTEM

18

MANAGEMENT OF GASTROINTESTINAL DISORDERS

BEHAVIORAL OBJECTIVES

After completing this chapter, the nurse will be able to

- Define the key terms.
- Describe methods for managing gastrointestinal disorders.
- Discuss indications for specific interventions to manage gastrointestinal disorders.
- Demonstrate the skills involved in managing gastrointestinal disorders.

This chapter focuses on procedures utilized in the diagnosis and treatment of gastrointestinal disorders. The nurse needs to collect specimens for laboratory analysis, test specimens at the bedside, and implement and manage therapies designed to treat certain conditions.

18–4 Esophagogastric Tamponade Tube
18–5 Scleral Endoscopic Therapy
18–6 Vasopressin Infusion

GUIDELINES

The following assessment guidelines assist the nurse in formulating a nursing diagnosis and an individualized plan of care in the management of gastrointestinal disorders:

1. Know the patient's medical history and presenting symptoms.
2. Identify the patient's baseline vital signs, cardiac rhythm, and respiratory status.
3. Review the patient's laboratory test results.
4. Perform an abdominal assessment.
5. Select the appropriate intervention for the assessment findings.
6. Become proficient with the equipment used to manage gastrointestinal disorders.

KEY TERMS

Edlich tube
endoscope
endoscopic sclerotherapy
Ewald tube
gastric distension
gastric lavage

Levin tube
nasogastric tube
oropharynx
Salem sump
varix (varices)

SKILLS

18–1 Nasogastric Tube Insertion
18–2 Gastric Lavage in Hemorrhage
18–3 Gastric Lavage in Overdose

SKILL 18–1

Nasogastric Tube Insertion

Nasogastric intubation is used for both diagnostic and therapeutic purposes. The most frequent indication for nasogastric tube insertion is for decompression of the stomach and evacuation of gastric contents in the presence of an ileus, hemorrhage, or overdose. Feedings and medications may be instilled for therapeutic reasons. Samples of gastric contents also may be removed for diagnostic testing.

Nasogastric intubation is performed by passing a small- or large-bore tube into a nostril and advancing it through the oropharynx and esophagus into the stomach. Gastric intubation also may be accomplished by inserting the tube into the oral cavity and advancing it through the oropharynx and esophagus into the stomach (orogastric intubation).

Nasogastric tubes are available with weighted and non-weighted tips and with single or double lumens (Fig. 18–1). The Levin tube, a nonweighted single-lumen tube, is unsuitable for use with suction because it does not have an air vent. An air venting system prevents a nasogastric tube from adhering to the mucosal surface when the tube is attached to suction. The Salem sump, a nonweighted double-lumen tube, is suitable for use with suction because the secondary lumen functions as the air vent. Both tubes are unsuitable for long-term management because they stiffen with prolonged use, increasing the risk of mucosal erosion.

Small-bore single-lumen weighted tubes are preferred for enteral feedings. These tubes do not allow for aspiration of large amounts of gastric contents nor can they be attached to suction (see Chap. 32).

Purpose

The nurse inserts a nasogastric tube to

1. Decompress the stomach and proximal small intestine.
2. Evacuate blood or secretions.
3. Evacuate ingested drugs or toxins.
4. Instill medications and feedings.

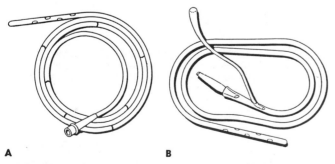

FIGURE 18–1. (*A*) Nonvented single-lumen (Levin) tube. (*B*) Vented double-lumen (Salem sump) tube. (Reprinted with permission from B. A. Norton and A. M. Miller, *Skills for Professional Nursing Practice.* Norwalk, Conn.: Appleton-Century-Crofts, 1986).

5. Obtain samples of gastric contents for analysis.
6. Administer warm lavage fluid to correct hypothermia.

Prerequisite Knowledge and Skills

Prior to inserting a nasogastric tube, the nurse should understand

1. Principles of universal precautions (see Skill 35–1).
2. Anatomy and physiology of the nasopharynx, esophagus, and stomach.
3. Anatomy of the upper respiratory tract.
4. Principles of fluid and electrolyte balance.

The nurse should be able to perform

1. Proper handwashing technique (see Skill 35–5).
2. Universal precautions (see Skill 35–1).
3. Respiratory system assessment.
4. Vital signs assessment.
5. Abdominal assessment.

Assessment

1. Identify patient history of nasal deformity, surgery, or trauma. **Rationale:** Provides information about the patency of the nares.
2. Assess the patient for a history of varices or recent esophageal or gastric surgery. **Rationale:** May increase the risk of developing complications during tube insertion.
3. Assess the patient for signs of gastric distension or irritation (i.e., nausea, vomiting, and absence of or hypoactive bowel sounds). **Rationale:** Accumulation of secretions and air in the stomach increases the risk or vomiting and aspiration.
4. Determine the need for analysis of gastric contents. **Rationale:** Provides data to assist in the diagnosis and treatment of selected disorders (i.e., peptic ulcer disease, esophageal varices).
5. Assess history for ingestion of drugs or toxins. **Rationale:** Immediate evacuation or neutralization of gastric contents is necessary to prevent absorption and/or tissue damage.
6. Assess ability of patient to take medications and feedings by mouth. **Rationale:** Prescribed medication(s) and nutritional support form a component of the therapeutic plan of care.
7. Assess the patient for profound hypothermia. **Rationale:** Administration of warm fluid lavage is a method to correct profound hypothermia.

Nursing Diagnoses

1. Potential for aspiration related to accumulation of intestinal secretions. **Rationale:** Distension caused by accumulated secretions increases the risk of vomiting and thus aspiration.

2.   Potential for aspiration related to impaired gag reflex. **Rationale:** Ineffective gag reflex may lead to aspiration of food and fluids.

3.   Potential for poisoning related to ingestion of drugs or toxins. **Rationale:** Intestinal absorption of drugs or toxins may lead to local and systemic complications.

4.   Altered nutrition: less than body requirements related to inability to take sufficient nutrition by mouth. **Rationale:** May lead to nutritional deficiencies.

5.   Hypothermia related to (specify mechanism). **Rationale:** Profound hypothermia interferes with normal cell metabolism and normal clotting mechanism.

6.   Potential fluid volume deficit related to accumulated blood and intestinal secretions. **Rationale:** Fluids and electrolytes sequestered within the gastrointestinal tract are lost to circulating volume and cellular utilization.

Planning

1.   Individualize the following goals for nasogastric tube insertion based on patient indications:
    a.   Decompression of stomach and small intestine. **Rationale:** Minimizes the risk of aspiration and allows for quantifying gastric fluid loss.
    b.   Evacuation of drugs and/or toxins. **Rationale:** Prevents poisoning and local tissue injury.
    c.   Administration of medications and/or nutritional support. **Rationale:** Contributes to the overall therapeutic plan for the patient.
    d.   Gastric sampling for analysis. **Rationale:** Contributes to the diagnosis and response to treatment.
    e.   Warming of core temperature. **Rationale:** Restores normal cell metabolism and normal clotting mechanism.

2.   Assemble and prepare all necessary equipment and supplies. **Rationale:** Facilitates efficient and effective nasogastric tube insertion.
    a.   Nasogastric tube: Levin tube or Salem sump (nos. 12 to 18 French for an adult, nos. 8 to 14 French for a child).
    b.   Water-soluble lubricant.
    c.   Irrigation kit with 50- to 60-cc irrigating syringe and normal saline solution for irrigation.
    d.   Two emesis basins.
    e.   Ice.
    f.   Cup of water with straw or ice chips.
    g.   Suction source with connecting tube (if tube is to be connected to suction).
    h.   Nonsterile gloves.
    i.   Stethoscope.
    j.   Rubber band.
    k.   Safety pin.
    l.   Paper tape or suction tube attachment device.
    m.   pH test paper (if appropriate).
    n.   Gastroccult slide (if appropriate).

3.   Prepare the patient.
    a.   Explain procedure and reason for tube insertion. **Rationale:** Decreases patient anxiety.
    b.   Explain patient's role in assisting with passage of the tube. **Rationale:** Elicits patient cooperation and facilitates insertion.
    c.   Assist the patient to assume a high Fowler's, semi-Fowler's, or left lateral position. **Rationale:** Facilitates passage of the tube into the stomach and prevents aspiration.

4.   Estimate length of tube to be passed.
    a.   Measure total length from bridge of nose to earlobe to tip of xiphoid process (Fig. 18–2). **Rationale:** Determines length of tube to be passed.
    b.   Mark this length on tube with tape. **Rationale:** Estimates distance from nasal orifice to stomach.

5.   Place tube on ice. **Rationale:** Stiffens tube to prevent coiling during insertion.

6.   Assess patency of nostrils: Occlude one nostril at a time; ask patient to breathe through nose; select nostril with better airflow. **Rationale:** Nostril with better airflow and patency eases insertion and improves patient's tolerance of the tube.

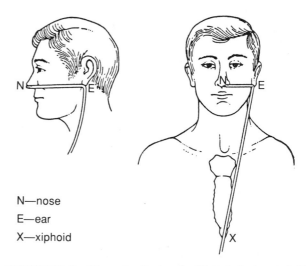

N—nose
E—ear
X—xiphoid

FIGURE 18–2.   Measuring the length of tube to be inserted. (Reprinted with permission from L. S. Brunner and D. S. Suddarth, *Textbook of Medical-Surgical Nursing*, 6th Ed. Philadelphia: Lippincott, 1988, p. 754.)

Implementation

Steps	Rationale	Special Considerations
1. Wash hands.	Reduces transmission of microorganisms.	

Table continues on following page

Steps	Rationale	Special Considerations
2. Lubricate 6 to 10 cm of distal end of tube with water-soluble lubricant.	Minimizes mucosal injury and irritation during insertion.	
3. Don nonsterile gloves.	Universal precautions.	
4. Insert tube into opening of selected nostril.	Directs tube toward correct placement.	
5. Position curved edge of tube downward, and direct tube along base of nostril.	Minimizes injury to the nasal turbinates.	If resistance is met, *do not force insertion* since this could damage nasal turbinates/mucosa and cause severe bleeding.
6. When tube reaches posterior nasopharynx, flex patient's neck forward.	Facilitates passage of tube into esophagus rather than into trachea.	Especially helpful in the intubated patient.
7. Ask patient (if appropriate) to swallow sips of water through a straw or to suck on ice chips to initiate the swallowing maneuver, or ask the patient to simulate the swallowing maneuver.	Causes epiglottis to close off trachea and directs tube toward esophagus.	
8. Continue to pass tube until marked position is at the rim of the nostril.	Advances tube into the stomach.	
9. Confirm position of tube in stomach:		
a. Aspirate contents from primary lumen into 50- to 60-cc irrigating syringe. Discard drainage in appropriate receptacle. Rinse out irrigating syringe with normal saline.	Indicates correct placement of tube in stomach.	Test specimen for pH and blood before discarding.
b. Inject 15 to 20 cc of air into primary lumen while auscultating with stethoscope placed over gastric bulb (left upper quadrant, just below rib cage) (Fig. 18–3).	Rapid bolus of air can be auscultated because stomach is a hollow organ.	

Table continues on following page

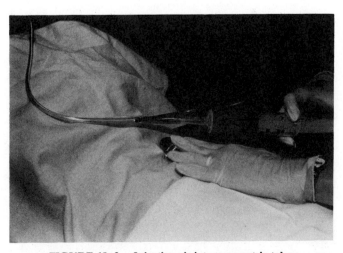

FIGURE 18–3.   Injecting air into nasogastric tube.

Steps	Rationale	Special Considerations
10. Secure tube in position:		
a. Wrap tape around tube, securing tape to bridge of nose, mustache area, or cheek (Fig. 18–4).	Maintains tube in correct position and prevents inadvertent dislodgment.	Avoid exerting pressure against rim of nostril with tube because it may cause ulceration.
b. Or apply adhesive area of suction tube attachment device to bridge and side of nose, and close clamp around the nasogastric tube (Fig. 18–5).		
11. Attach primary lumen to suction, gravity drainage, or tube feeding, or clamp off primary lumen to prevent leakage of gastric contents.	Initiates therapy as prescribed.	Salem sump: continuous or intermittent suction <80 mmHg. With Salem sump, keep air vent above level of stomach; a "rushing" sound should be heard at air vent (indicates airflow through vent). *Do not clamp air vent.* If gastric secretions accumulate in air vent, flush with 30 to 60 cc of air, reposition tube, and irrigate primary lumen.
12. Secure tube to patient's gown or robe 10 to 12 in from nose. Loop rubber band around tube, and pin rubber band to desired clothing.	Prevents tube from pulling and putting pressure against rim of nostril. Provides another protection against tube dislodgment.	Unpin rubber band from clothing before removal.
13. Reassess position of tube as per unit routine/patient condition and before instillation of any medication, irrigant, or feeding.	Incorrect position of tube increases risk of aspiration.	
14. Irrigate tube as per unit routine/ patient condition and p.r.n. with 20 to 30 cc normal saline.	Ensures patency of tube.	
15. Wash hands.	Reduces transmission of microorganisms.	

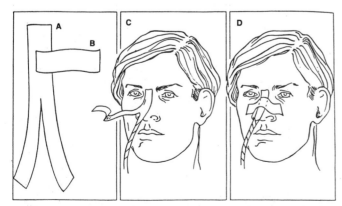

FIGURE 18–4. Securing the tube to the bridge of the nose. (Reprinted with permission from J. R. Ellis, E. A. Nowlis, and P. M. Bentz, *Modules for Basic Nursing Skills*, 4th Ed. Boston: Houghton-Mifflin, 1988, p. 45.)

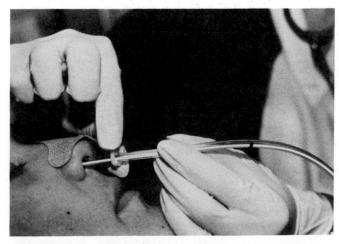

FIGURE 18–5. Securing the nasogastric tube attachment device.

Evaluation

1. Monitor intake and output through tube every hour or as determined by unit routine or patient condition. **Rationale:** Provides data for fluid balance.

2. Evaluate tube position and function every hour or as determined by unit routine or patient condition. **Rationale:** Adequate evacuation of secretions and proper administration of feedings or medications are dependent on proper tube placement and function.

3. Monitor patient tolerance of tube placement. **Rationale:** Tube placement may cause mild discomfort, bleeding, respiratory aggravation, or cardiac dysrhythmias.

Expected Outcomes

1. Accurate placement of nasogastric tube in the stomach. **Rationale:** Accurate tube placement is necessary for proper tube function and use.

2. Decompression of stomach and proximal small intestine. **Rationale:** Tube provides conduit for evacuation of secretions, blood, air, drugs, and/or toxins.

Unexpected Outcomes

1. Incorrect placement of tube in trachea, bronchus, or esophagus. **Rationale:** Tube may pass into respiratory tree during insertion or may be incompletely passed into the stomach.

2. Bleeding during or after tube insertion. **Rationale:** Injury to nasal mucosa or nasal turbinates may occur as a result of inadequate lubrication or forceful insertion. Injury to varices may occur as tube passes through esophagus.

3. Bradycardia during insertion. **Rationale:** Vagal stimulation may occur during insertion.

Documentation

Documentation in the patient record should include the date, time, and the reason for nasogastric tube insertion, size and type of tube inserted, orifice that was cannulated, assessment of tube placement, patient assessment during and after tube insertion, patient tolerance of procedure, occurrence of any unexpected outcomes, and amount and characteristics of gastric contents. **Rationale:** Documents nursing actions, status of gastrointestinal drainage, and any unexpected outcomes and interventions taken.

Patient/Family Education

1. Explain indications and procedure for tube insertion and maintenance to both patient and family. **Rationale:** Decreases patient's and family's anxiety. Encourages patient cooperation and understanding of procedure and therapeutic plan of care.

2. Evaluate the patient's need for long-term enteral feeding via nasogastric/nasointestinal tube. **Rationale:** Allows nurse to plan patient and family discharge teaching and to coordinate services needed for home enteral feeding (see Chap. 32).

Performance Checklist
Skill 18–1:   Nasogastric Tube Insertion

Critical Behaviors	Complies	
	yes	no
1. Wash hands.		
2. Lubricate distal end of tube.		
3. Don nonsterile gloves.		
4. Insert tube into selected nostril.		
5. Position curved edge of tube downward, and direct tube along nostril base.		
6. When tube reaches posterior nasopharynx, flex patient's neck forward.		
7. Ask patient to swallow or simulate swallowing.		
8. Stop passing the tube at the taped marker.		
9. Confirm correct position of tube.		
10. Secure tube in position.		
11. Manage primary lumen of tube as indicated.		
12. Secure tube to patient's clothes.		
13. Reassess correct tube placement.		

Table continues on following page

Critical Behaviors	Complies	
	yes	no
14. Irrigate tube.		
15. Wash hands.		
16. Document procedure in patient record.		

SKILL 18–2

Gastric Lavage in Hemorrhage

Major upper gastrointestinal hemorrhage leads to a severe volume loss and a profound decrease in the oxygen-carrying capacity of the blood, causing life-threatening complications. In the presence of hemorrhage, gastric lavage provides a mechanism to stop bleeding, to prepare the patient for further diagnostic evaluation, and to evacuate the blood before absorption of a high nitrogen load.

Lavage may be performed with iced or room-temperature solution. Iced solutions cause vasoconstriction, which decreases bleeding. However, it has been demonstrated that iced solutions interfere with platelet function and may not be efficient in maintaining clot formation at the bleeding site. Additionally, iced solutions may predispose the patient to hypothermia, which interferes with the normal clotting mechanism. Room-temperature solutions have been shown to be effective in clearing the stomach of blood and clots, in promoting hemostasis, and in preventing hypothermia.

Purpose

The nurse performs gastric lavage in hemorrhage to
1. Stop or control upper gastrointestinal bleeding.
2. Quantify volume loss from upper gastrointestinal bleeding.
3. Decrease or prevent absorption of a high nitrogen load.
4. Cleanse the stomach of blood and clots in preparation for endoscopy or scleral therapy.
5. Prevent the aspiration of blood.

Prerequisite Knowledge and Skills

Prior to performing gastric lavage in hemorrhage, the nurse should understand
1. Principles of universal precautions (see Skill 35–1).
2. Anatomy and physiology of the upper gastrointestinal tract.
3. Anatomy and physiology of the upper respiratory tract.
4. Major causes of upper gastrointestinal bleeding.

5. Cardiac effects of vagal stimulation.

The nurse should be able to perform
1. Proper infection-control measures (see Chap. 35).
2. Assessment of gastric tube placement (see Skill 18–1).
3. Assessment of respiratory status.
4. Interpretation of cardiac dysrhythmias.
5. Insertion of oral airway and bite block (see Skill 1–1).

Assessment

1. Assess patient history for varices or recent esophageal or gastric surgery. **Rationale:** Varices or recent surgery may predispose the patient to complications during tube insertion.
2. Observe the patient for signs and symptoms of major blood volume loss, including tachycardia, hypotension, decreased urine output, and decreased filling pressures, hematocrit, hemoglobin, and coagulation studies. **Rationale:** Physical signs and symptoms result from major blood volume loss.
3. Assess the patient's baseline cardiac rhythm. **Rationale:** Passage of a large-bore tube increases the risk of developing cardiac dysrhythmias.
4. Assess the patient's respiratory status (i.e., rate, depth, pattern, and characteristics of secretions). **Rationale:** Topical anesthesia in the oropharynx may diminish the gag reflex, increasing the risk of aspiration. Large-bore tube also may interfere with breathing status. Accumulation of a large amount of blood in the stomach increases risk of vomiting with aspiration.

Nursing Diagnoses

1. Fluid volume deficit related to major upper gastrointestinal hemorrhage. **Rationale:** Blood loss into the gastrointestinal tract decreases intravascular volume.
2. Potential for aspiration related to accumulation of blood and clots in stomach. **Rationale:** Gastric distension and stimulation of gag reflex during insertion of lavage tube increase the risk of vomiting and aspiration.
3. Potential altered body temperature related to instillation of large amounts of fluids less than normal body temperature. **Rationale:** Body heat transfers to lavage fluid.

Planning

1. Individualize the following patient goals for gastric lavage:
   a. Maintain fluid volume. **Rationale:** Adequate intravascular volume is necessary for tissue perfusion.
   b. Quantify blood volume loss into gastrointestinal tract. **Rationale:** Provides basis for adequate volume replacement.
   c. Prevent absorption of high nitrogen load. **Rationale:** May lead to changes in neurologic status secondary to nitrogen conversion and encephalopathy.
   d. Remove blood and clots from upper gastrointestinal tract prior to diagnostic and therapeutic interventions. **Rationale:** Interferes with visualization of esophageal and gastric tissue and structures.
   e. Prevent aspiration of blood. **Rationale:** Gastric distension increases the risk of aspiration.

2. Assemble and prepare all necessary equipment and supplies. **Rationale:** Ensures that gastric lavage will be conducted quickly and efficiently.
   a. Lavage tube, no. 32 to 36 French gastric tube (Ewald or Edlich) or no. 16 to 18 French Levin tube or Salem sump.
   b. Irrigating kit with 50- to 60-cc irrigating syringe.
   c. Water-soluble lubricant.
   d. Lavage fluid (normal saline or tap water, iced or at room temperature).
   e. Disposable basin for aspirate (large).
   f. Suction source and connecting tube (optional).
   g. Topical anesthetic agent.
   h. Bite block or oral airway (optional).
   i. Continuous lavage kit (if available), or assemble
      (1) Y connector
      (2) Infusion tubing
      (3) Tapered connector
      (4) Connecting tubing
      (5) Drainage container
      (6) Two rubber-shod clamps.
   j. Stethoscope.
   k. Emergency intubation equipment.
   l. Endotracheal suction equipment.
   m. Cardiac monitor.
   n. Nonsterile gloves.

3. Prepare the patient.
   a. Explain the indications and the procedure for gastric lavage in hemorrhage. **Rationale:** Decreases patient anxiety.
   b. Explain the patient's role in assisting with passage of the tube and lavage of the stomach. **Rationale:** Elicits patient cooperation.
   c. Place patient on cardiac monitor. **Rationale:** Cardiac dysrhythmias may occur as a result of vagal stimulation during passage of a large-bore tube.
   d. Position patient in left lateral or semi-Fowler's position. After tube is inserted, position patient in left lateral position with head of the bed at a 20-degree angle. **Rationale:** Facilitates passage of tube into stomach and prevents aspiration.

Implementation

Steps	Rationale	Special Considerations
1. Wash hands.	Reduces transmission of microorganisms.	
2. Don nonsterile gloves.	Universal precautions.	
3. Coat 6 to 10 cm of distal end of the lavage tube with water-soluble lubricant.	Minimizes mucosal injury and irritation during insertion of tube.	
4. Insert Ewald or Edlich tube (Fig. 18–6):	Large bore (no. 32 to 36 French) is preferred for the evacuation of blood and clots.	*Do not pass nasally because severe nasal trauma will occur.*
a. Anesthetize posterior oropharynx with topical agent.	Decreases discomfort caused by passing tube.	*Caution:* Gag reflex may be compromised by topical anesthesia, increasing the risk of aspiration. Have emergency intubation equipment available.
b. Insert oral airway or bite block.	Prevents patient from biting on tube or inserter's fingers.	Remove dentures if appropriate.
c. Position tube toward posterior pharynx over tongue.		Heart rate may decrease as a result of vagal stimulation. Administer atropine as necessary.

Table continues on following page

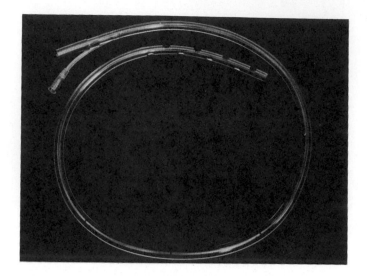

FIGURE 18–6. Ewald tube. (Reprinted with permission from K. D. DeGroot and M. B. Damato, *Critical Care Skills*. Norwalk, Conn.: Appleton & Lange, 1987, p. 252.)

Steps	Rationale	Special Considerations
d. Pass tube slowly into stomach (approximately 20 in). Encourage patient to attempt to swallow while passing tube.	Rapid passage may stimulate vomiting and increase risk of aspiration. Swallowing maneuver causes epiglottis to close trachea and directs tube into esophagus.	
5. *Or* insert Levin tube or Salem sump (see Skill 18–1).	Larger-lumen tube (no. 16 to 18 French) helps to prevent drainage ports from becoming blocked with clots.	
6. Aspirate gastric contents through lavage tube using irrigating syringe, *or* allow gastric contents to drain by gravity into large collection container.	Removes gastric contents (blood and clots) from stomach.	
7. Intermittent lavage: a. Instill 50 to 200 cc lavage fluid into lavage tube using irrigating syringe.	Aids in breaking up clots and rinsing out the stomach of blood.	Lavage fluid may be drained immediately or retained in stomach for about 30 minutes before draining to facilitate dissolving clots.
b. Aspirate gastric contents through lavage tube using irrigating syringe.	Evacuates gastric contents from stomach.	
c. *Or* allow gastric contents to drain by gravity into large collection container.		
d. *Or* connect lavage tube to suction (<80 mmHg).		
e. Continue intermittent lavage until returns are clear and free of clots.		
8. Continuous lavage: a. Assemble equipment:	Aids in breaking up of clots and rinsing stomach of blood.	
(1) Connect infusion tubing to lavage fluid container.	Prepares system for continuous lavage.	

Table continues on following page

Steps	Rationale	Special Considerations
(2) Connect distal end of infusion tubing to stem end of Y connector.		
(3) Connect tapered connector to one limb of Y connector, and attach to lavage tube (Ewald, Edlich, or nasogastric tube).		
(4) Attach connecting tubing to other limb of Y connector.		
(5) Attach distal end of connecting tubing to drainage container (Fig. 18–7).		
b. Instill lavage fluid:	Directs fluid into the stomach.	Lavage fluid may be retained in stomach for 30 minutes before draining to facilitate dissolving clots.
(1) Clamp connecting tubing just distal to Y connector with rubber-shod clamp.		
(2) Open clamp on infusion tubing and instill desired amount of fluid into stomach (usually 150 to 200 cc).		
(3) Close clamp on infusion tubing.		
c. Remove clamp on connecting tubing.	Allows fluid to siphon from stomach into drainage container.	Speed and amount siphoned depend on height of siphon column. To increase speed and amount, raise height of patient in reference to drainage container.
d. Allow gastric contents to drain by gravity into drainage container.		
e. Repeat steps 8b through d until returns are clear and free of clots.		
9. Remove Ewald or Edlich tube, if used:	Prevents tissue injury.	
a. Clamp tube with rubber-shod clamp.	Prevents leakage of contents remaining within lumen and possible aspiration of contents during removal.	
b. Pull tube out slowly and steadily.	Minimizes risk of vomiting.	
10. Insert nasogastric tube, if needed (see Skill 18–1).	Provides access to gastric contents.	
11. Dispose of equipment in appropriate receptacle.	Universal precautions.	
12. Wash hands.	Reduces transmission of microorganisms.	

Evaluation

1. Measure blood volume loss. **Rationale:** Contributes to fluid balance assessment and fluid resuscitation requirements.

2. Monitor for recurrence of bleeding. **Rationale:** Cessation of bleeding with lavage may be a temporary measure.

3. Evaluate blood ammonia levels. **Rationale:** Provides an estimate of the nitrogen load that has been absorbed systemically.

Expected Outcomes

1. Cessation or control of upper gastrointestinal bleeding. **Rationale:** Lavage contributes to cessation of bleeding through vasoconstriction and removal of clots.

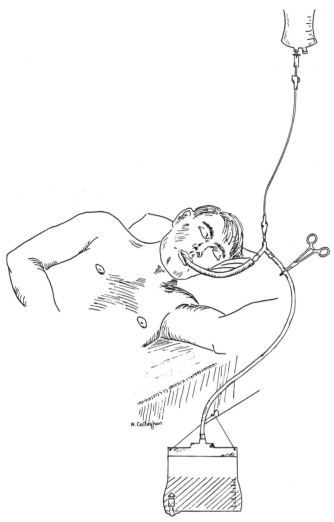

FIGURE 18–7. Continuous lavage system.

2. Evacuation of blood and clots from the stomach. **Rationale:** Provides for adequate visualization of tissues and structures during diagnostic and therapeutic procedures.

3. Prevention of absorption of high nitrogen load. **Rationale:** Blood is protein, and absorption of a large amount of protein (nitrogen) can contribute to encephalopathy.

Unexpected Outcomes

1. Impaired airway. **Rationale:** Inappropriate placement of tube into trachea or bronchus.

2. Bradydysrhythmias. **Rationale:** Passage of a large-bore tube may cause vagal stimulation.

3. Aspiration of gastric contents. **Rationale:** Protective gag reflex may be impaired secondary to topical anesthesia in oropharynx; passage of a large-bore tube may stimulate vomiting reflex.

Documentation

Documentation in the patient record should include the date, time, and reason for performing gastric lavage, size and type of lavage tube inserted, assessment of tube placement, patient tolerance of tube placement and lavage procedure, occurrence of any unexpected outcomes and actions taken, amount and characteristics of aspirate, assessment of gastric drainage after lavage, and amount of fluid used to lavage. **Rationale:** Documents nursing process, status of gastrointestinal bleeding, and any unexpected outcomes and interventions taken.

Patient/Family Education

Explain the indications and procedure for gastric lavage to both patient and family. **Rationale:** Encourages patient and family cooperation and understanding of procedure.

Performance Checklist
Skill 18–2: Gastric Lavage in Hemorrhage

Critical Behaviors	Complies	
	yes	no
1. Wash hands.		
2. Don nonsterile gloves.		
3. Lubricate tube.		
4. Insert Ewald or Edlich tube (or insert Levin tube or Salem sump):		
a. Anesthetize posterior oropharynx.		
b. Insert oral airway or bite block.		
c. Position tube toward posterior pharynx over tongue.		
d. Slowly pass tube into stomach.		
5. Aspirate gastric contents, *or* allow gastric contents to drain by gravity.		

Table continues on following page

Critical Behaviors	Complies	
	yes	no
6. Perform intermittent or continuous lavage:		
a. Instill gastric lavage fluid.		
b. Aspirate gastric contents, *or* allow gastric contents to drain by gravity, *or* connect lavage tube to suction.		
7. Continue lavage until returns are clear and free of clots.		
8. Remove Ewald or Edlich tube, if used.		
9. Insert nasogastric tube, if appropriate.		
10. Dispose of soiled equipment appropriately.		
11. Wash hands.		
12. Document procedure in patient record.		

SKILL 18–3

Gastric Lavage in Overdose

Ingestion of large amounts of drugs or toxins into the gastrointestinal tract presents potentially lethal consequences. In order to prevent or minimize serious sequelae, drugs and toxins must be evacuated from the stomach before significant systemic absorption occurs.

Removal of harmful substances may be accomplished by induced vomiting, unless contraindicated, or by lavage. Lavage or cleansing of the stomach is accomplished by instilling a large amount of neutral fluid into the stomach and then draining the contents and lavage fluid out of the stomach. Repeated lavages are performed until all potentially harmful material is removed.

Purpose

The nurse performs gastric lavage in overdose to

1. Prevent or minimize the serious consequences of systemic absorption of drugs or toxins.
2. Prevent or minimize damage to gastrointestinal tissue.

Prerequisite Knowledge and Skills

Prior to performing gastric lavage in overdose, the nurse should understand

1. Principles of universal precautions (see Skill 35–1).
2. Anatomy and physiology of the upper gastrointestinal tract.
3. Anatomy and physiology of the upper respiratory tract.
4. Harmful effects of the ingestion of drugs and toxic agents.
5. Cardiac effects of vagal stimulation.

The nurse should be able to perform

1. Proper infection-control measures (see Chap. 35).
2. Assessment of gastric tube placement (see Skill 18–1).
3. Interpretation of cardiac dysrhythmias.
4. Insertion of oral airway and bite block (see Skill 1–1).

Assessment

1. Assess the patient's history for ingestion of drugs or toxic agents. **Rationale:** History may show contraindication to vomiting and/or need for gastric lavage.
2. Determine the patient's level of consciousness and adequacy of gag reflex. **Rationale:** Induced vomiting may be the treatment of choice if the patient is alert and awake with an intact gag reflex, making lavage unnecessary.
3. Determine specific or suspected agents ingested. Contact Poison Control Center if unsure that lavage is indicated. **Rationale:** Certain agents may require neutralization before attempting tube evacuation. Specific side effects can be anticipated with the ingestion of particular drugs and toxic agents.
4. Assess the patient's baseline cardiac rhythm. **Rationale:** Passage of a large-bore tube and side effects of selected toxic agents increase the risk of cardiac dysrhythmias.
5. Assess the patient's baseline respiratory status (i.e., rate, depth, pattern, and characteristics of secretions). **Rationale:** Topical anesthesia in the oropharynx may alter the gag reflex and increase the risk of aspiration. Passage of a large-bore tube may compromise the airway. Instillation of large amounts of lavage fluid increases the risk of aspiration. Central nervous system depression and respiratory depression are side effects of certain drugs and toxic agents.

Nursing Diagnoses

1. Potential for poisoning related to ingestion of (specify actual or suspected agent). **Rationale:** Toxic side effects occur with ingestion of excessive amounts of certain agents.

2. Potential for injury related to ingestion of (specify actual or suspected agent). **Rationale:** Certain agents injure tissue upon contact.

3. Potential for aspiration related to drug or toxin effect. **Rationale:** Certain drugs or toxins cause central nervous system depression, increasing the risk of aspiration.

Planning

1. Individualize the following patient goals for gastric lavage:
   a. Prevent or minimize absorption of drugs or toxic agents. **Rationale:** Drugs or toxic agents may cause severe systemic effects if absorbed.
   b. Prevent or minimize local tissue damage. **Rationale:** Contact with certain toxic agents causes injury to gastrointestinal tissue.

2. Assemble and prepare all necessary equipment and supplies. **Rationale:** Ensures that gastric lavage in overdose will be completed efficiently.
   a. No. 16 or 18 French Levin tube or Salem sump or a no. 32 to 36 French gastric tube (Ewald or Edlich).
   b. Irrigating kit with 50- to 60-cc irrigating syringe.
   c. Water-soluble lubricant.
   d. Lavage fluid: normal saline or tap water.
   e. Disposable basin for aspirate.
   f. Topical anesthetic agent.
   g. Bite block or oral airway.
   h. Specimen container for aspirate.
   i. Continuous lavage kit (if available) or
      (1) Y connector
      (2) Infusion tubing
      (3) Tapered connector
      (4) Connecting tubing (4 ft)
      (5) Drainage container
      (6) Two rubber-shod clamps.
   j. Stethoscope.
   k. No. 16 or 18 French Levin tube or Salem sump (if not used for lavage tube).
   l. Absorptive agent for instillation (as prescribed).
   m. Peristaltic agent for instillation (as prescribed).
   n. Emergency intubation equipment.
   o. Endotracheal suction equipment.
   p. Cardiac monitor.
   q. Nonsterile gloves.

3. Prepare the patient.
   a. Explain the indications and the procedure for gastric lavage in overdose. **Rationale:** Decreases patient anxiety.
   b. Explain the patient's role in assisting with passage of the tube and lavage of stomach. **Rationale:** Elicits patient's cooperation during the procedure.
   c. Place patient on cardiac monitor. **Rationale:** Cardiac dysrhythmias may result from passage of a large-bore tube or as an effect of ingested drugs or toxins.
   d. Assist the patient to assume a left lateral or semi-Fowler's position. **Rationale:** Facilitates passage of the tube into the stomach and prevents aspiration.

Implementation

Steps	Rationale	Special Considerations
1. Wash hands.	Reduces transmission of microorganisms.	
2. Don nonsterile gloves.	Universal precautions.	
3. Coat 6 to 10 cm of distal end of lavage tube with water-soluble lubricant.	Minimizes mucosal injury and irritation during insertion of tube.	
4. Insert Ewald or Edlich tube (see Fig. 18-6):	Large-bore tube is preferred to evacuate undigested pills and capsules. Smaller-lumen tubes may become blocked with solid material.	*Do not pass this tube nasally because severe nasal trauma will occur.*
a. Anesthetize posterior oropharynx with topical agent.	Decreases discomfort caused by passage of tube.	*Caution:* Patient's gag reflex may be compromised by topical anesthesia and increase the risk of aspiration. Keep emergency intubation equipment available.
b. Insert oral airway or bite block.	Prevents patient from biting on tube or inserter's fingers.	Remove dentures if appropriate.

Table continues on following page

Steps	Rationale	Special Considerations
c. Position tube toward posterior pharynx over tongue.		
d. Pass tube slowly into stomach (approximately 20 in), and encourage patient to simulate swallowing while passing tube.	Rapid passage may stimulate vomiting and increase risk of aspiration. Swallowing maneuver causes epiglottis to close trachea and directs tube into esophagus.	Heart rate may decrease as a result of vagal stimulation. Administer atropine as needed.
5. *Or* insert Levin tube or Salem sump (see Skill 18–1).	Smaller-lumen tube may be used with ingestion of liquid agents or with liquified tablets or capsules.	
6. Aspirate gastric contents through lavage tube using irrigating syringe, and save specimen for analysis.	Withdraws gastric contents and toxic agents out of stomach. Confirms position of lavage tube in stomach.	Send aspirate to laboratory for toxicology screen, if appropriate.
7. Intermittent lavage:	Aids in diluting toxic agents and removing them from the stomach before absorption.	May use normal saline or tap water.
a. Instill 150 to 200 cc lavage fluid into stomach using irrigating syringe.	Distends rugae to allow lavage of all areas of stomach.	
b. Aspirate gastric contents through lavage tube using irrigating syringe.	Evacuates gastric contents and ingested toxic agents.	
c. *Or* allow gastric contents to drain by gravity into large collection container.		
d. Continue lavage until returns are clear and free of particulate matter.	Removes toxic agents and prevents systemic absorption of toxic agents.	
8. Continuous lavage (see Fig. 18–7):	Aids in diluting toxic agents and removing them from the stomach before absorption.	May use normal saline or tap water.
a. Assemble all equipment:		
(1) Connect infusion tubing to lavage fluid container.		
(2) Connect distal end of infusion tubing to stem end of Y connector.		
(3) Connect tapered connector to one limb of Y connector, and attach to lavage tube (Ewald, Edlich, or nasogastric tube).		
(4) Attach connecting tubing to other limb of Y connector.		
(5) Attach distal end of connecting tubing to drainage container.		
b. Instill lavage fluid:	Distends rugae to allow lavage of all areas of stomach.	
(1) Clamp connecting tubing just distal to Y connector with rubber-shod clamp.		
(2) Open clamp on infusion tubing and instill desired amount of fluid into stomach (usually 150 to 200 cc).		

Table continues on following page

Steps	Rationale	Special Considerations
(3) Close clamp on infusion tubing.		
c. Remove clamp on connecting tubing.		
d. Allow gastric contents to drain by gravity into drainage container.		
e. Continue lavage, until returns are clear and free of particulate matter.		
9. Remove Ewald or Edlich tube, if used:	Prevents tissue injury.	Ensure complete lavage before tube removal.
a. Clamp tube with rubber-shod clamp.	Prevents leakage of contents remaining within lumen and possible aspiration of contents during removal.	
b. Pull tube out slowly and steadily.	Minimizes risk of vomiting.	
10. Insert nasogastric tube, if needed (see Skill 18–1).	Provides access for administration of medications and may be used in event of nausea and vomiting.	
11. Administer prescribed agents into stomach via nasogastric tube, and clamp tube to prevent inadvertent leaking of gastric drainage or prescribed agents.	Agents that absorb toxic substances may be used to prevent systemic absorption. Peristaltic agents may be used to increase rate of excretion and therefore decrease absorption of toxic agents.	Liquified activated charcoal is most commonly used absorptive agent. Magnesium citrate is the most commonly used peristaltic agent.
12. Discard equipment in appropriate receptacle.	Universal precautions.	
13. Wash hands.	Reduces transmission of microorganisms.	

Evaluation

1. Evaluate the amount and characteristics of the lavage returns. **Rationale:** Ensures adequate clearance of toxic agents.

2. Monitor patient for signs and symptoms of the side effects of toxic agents. **Rationale:** Absorption of the toxic agent may have occurred prior to lavage.

Expected Outcomes

1. Prevention or minimization of systemic complications secondary to the absorption of drugs or toxic agents. **Rationale:** Certain drugs and toxic agents will depress the respiratory and central nervous systems and/or cause cardiac dysrhythmias.

2. Minimization of tissue damage by toxic agents. **Rationale:** Neutralization and evacuation of toxic agents may prevent or minimize injury to gastrointestinal tissue.

Unexpected Outcomes

1. Impaired airway. **Rationale:** Inappropriate placement of lavage tube in trachea or bronchus.

2. Bradydysrhythmias. **Rationale:** Passage of a large-bore tube may cause vagal stimulation.

3. Aspiration of gastric contents. **Rationale:** Protective gag reflex may be altered because of topical anesthesia in the oropharynx. Passage of a large-bore tube may stimulate vomiting reflex.

Documentation

Documentation in the patient record should include the date, time, size, and type of lavage tube inserted, assessment of tube placement, patient tolerance of tube placement and lavage procedure, occurrence of any unexpected outcomes, amount and characteristics of aspirate, assessment of gastric drainage after lavage, instillation of type and amounts of agents after lavage, and aspirated specimens sent to laboratory for analysis. **Rationale:** Documents nursing interventions, evacuation of the stomach, and any unexpected outcomes and interventions taken.

Patient/Family Education

1. Explain the indications and the procedure for gas-

tric lavage to both patient (if possible) and family. **Rationale:** Encourages patient and family cooperation and understanding of procedure.

2. Evaluate patient and family need for information on prevention of accidental ingestion of drugs or toxic agents. **Rationale:** Patient and family may have been unaware or uninformed that the agent or drug is (potentially) toxic.

3. Evaluate patient and family need for information on emergency treatments for accidental ingestion of drugs or toxic agents. **Rationale:** Emergency first-aid measures may decrease potential toxicity/systemic absorption.

4. Evaluate the patient's need for follow-up psychiatric support for suicide ideation. **Rationale:** Overdose may reflect suicidal intent.

Performance Checklist
Skill 18–3:   Gastric Lavage in Overdose

Critical Behaviors	Complies	
	yes	no
1. Wash hands.		
2. Don nonsterile gloves.		
3. Lubricate distal portion of tube.		
4. Insert Ewald or Edlich tube:		
a. Anesthetize posterior oropharynx.		
b. Insert oral airway or bite block.		
c. Position tube toward posterior pharynx over tongue.		
d. Pass tube slowly into stomach.		
5. *Or* insert Levin tube or Salem sump.		
6. Aspirate gastric contents, and send aspirate to appropriate laboratory for toxicology screen.		
7. Perform intermittent lavage.		
8. *Or* perform continuous lavage.		
9. Remove Ewald or Edlich tube, if used.		
10. Insert nasogastric tube, if needed.		
11. Administer prescribed agents into nasogastric tube, and clamp tube.		
12. Dispose of equipment appropriately.		
13. Wash hands.		
14. Document procedure in patient record.		

SKILL 18–4

Esophagogastric Tamponade Tube

Esophagogastric tamponade therapy is indicated to control bleeding from gastric and esophageal varices that are unresponsive to medical therapy. Tamponade therapy provides direct pressure against bleeding vessels in the esophagus and upper portion of the stomach. This pressure is created by the inflation of balloon(s) that is (are) attached to a large-bore nasogastric or orogastric tube.

Tamponade therapy is a short-term intervention because of the potential complications caused by the inflated balloon(s): airway obstruction with the movement of an inflated balloon upward into the oropharynx, isch-emia and necrosis to esophageal and gastric mucosa precipitated by the inflated balloon constricting capillary blood flow to the esophagus, and esophageal rupture caused by overinflation of the balloon and/or weakening of the esophageal musculature.

A variety of tamponade tubes are available for patient use. A three-lumen tube, the Linton tube, has a gastric balloon and lumens for esophageal and gastric suction. This tube is not widely used today because of its limited features. Another three-lumen tube, the Sengstaken-Blakemore tube, has gastric and esophageal balloons and a lumen for gastric drainage. A four-lumen tube, the Minnesota tube, has two balloons (one gastric and one esophageal) and two drainage lumens (one gastric and one esophageal). The Sengstaken-Blakemore and Minnesota tubes are the standard for tamponade therapy (Figures 18–8 and 18–9).

Purpose

The nurse utilizes esophagogastric tamponade therapy to control bleeding from gastric and esophageal varices.

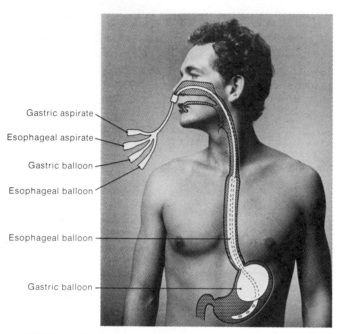

Gastric aspirate
Esophageal aspirate
Gastric balloon
Esophageal balloon
Esophageal balloon
Gastric balloon

FIGURE 18–8. Minnesota four-lumen tube. (Reprinted with permission from P. L. Swearingen, *Photo Atlas of Nursing Procedures.* Reading, Mass.: Addison-Wesley, 1991, p. 229.)

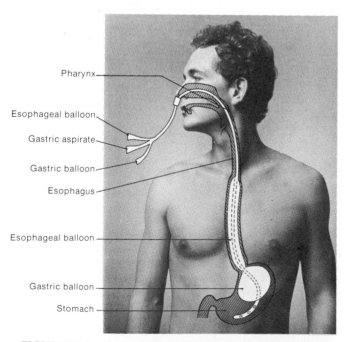

Pharynx
Esophageal balloon
Gastric aspirate
Gastric balloon
Esophagus
Esophageal balloon
Gastric balloon
Stomach

FIGURE 18–9. Sengstaken-Blakemore tube. (Reprinted with permission from P. L. Swearingen, *Photo Atlas of Nursing Procedures.* Reading, Mass.: Addison-Wesley, 1991, p. 228.)

Prerequisite Knowledge and Skills

Prior to performing esophagogastric tamponade therapy, the nurse should understand

1. Principles of universal precautions (see Skill 35–1).
2. Anatomy and physiology of the upper gastrointestinal tract.
3. Pathophysiology of gastric and esophageal varices.
4. Anatomy and physiology of the respiratory tract.
5. Cardiac effects of vagal stimulation.
6. Physiology of tissue perfusion.
7. Principles of balanced suspension traction.

The nurse should be able to perform

1. Proper handwashing technique (see Skill 35–5).
2. Assessment of gastric tube placement (see Skill 18–1).
3. Assessment of respiratory status.
4. Interpretation of cardiac dysrhythmias.
5. Insertion of oral airway and bite block (see Skill 1–1).
6. Irrigation of gastric tube (see Skill 18–1).
7. Management of balanced suspension traction.

Assessment

1. Observe the patient for signs and symptoms of major blood volume loss, including tachycardia; hypotension; decreased urine output; decreased filling pressures (PAP, PCWP, CVP); decreased platelets, hematocrit, and hemoglobin; and elevated PT and PTT. **Rationale:** Significant blood loss can be experienced with esophageal/gastric varices.
2. Assess patient history for varices. **Rationale:** Varices result from portal hypertension, which may be caused by prolonged alcohol abuse, portal venous thrombosis, and/or chronic liver disease.
3. Assess the patient's response to medical therapy to control bleeding. **Rationale:** Failure to respond to gastric lavage, correction of coagulation disorders, and vasopressin administration indicates the need for balloon tamponade.
4. Assess the patient's baseline cardiac rhythm. **Rationale:** Passage of a large-bore tube causes vagal stimulation and bradydysrhythmias.
5. Assess the patient's baseline respiratory status (i.e., rate, depth, pattern, and characteristics of secretions). **Rationale:** Topical anesthesia in the oropharynx alters the gag reflex and increases the risk of aspiration. Passage of a large-bore tube may impair airway. Accumulation of large amounts of blood in the stomach predisposes one to aspiration.

Nursing Diagnoses

1. Fluid volume deficit related to major variceal bleeding. **Rationale:** Blood loss into the gastrointestinal tract decreases intravascular volume.

2. Potential for aspiration related to accumulation of blood and clots in stomach. **Rationale:** Gastric distension and stimulation of the gag reflex increase the risk of vomiting and aspiration.

3. Potential for injury related to presence of large-bore tamponade tube and inflated balloons. **Rationale:** Nasal insertion increases the risk of pressure necrosis of nasal mucosa. Inflated balloon under traction increases risk of pressure necrosis of the esophageal and gastric mucosa. •

Planning

1. Develop individualized patient goals for esophago-gastric tamponade to maintain the intravascular volume necessary for adequate tissue perfusion. **Rationale:** Significant loss of blood into gastrointestinal tract depletes circulating volume.

2. Assemble and prepare all necessary equipment and supplies. **Rationale:** Access to all necessary equipment and supplies ensures that therapy will be completed efficiently.
   a. Tamponade tube, Linton, Sengstaken-Blakemore, or Minnesota tube.
   b. Nasogastric tube, no. 16 to 18 French (if Sengstaken-Blakemore tube is used).
   c. Irrigating kit with two 50- to 60-cc irrigating syringes.
   d. Normal saline for irrigation.
   e. Water-soluble lubricant.
   f. Topical anesthetic agent.
   g. Bite block or oral airway.
   h. Sponge-rubber cube (used with nasal insertion).
   i. Weight (1 to 2 lb) with balanced suspension traction apparatus or football helmet.
   j. Stethoscope.
   k. Sphygmomanometer.
   l. Y-shaped rubber tubing (supplied with tamponade tube).
   m. Y connector.
   n. Four rubber-shod clamps.
   o. Scissors (to be kept at bedside).
   p. Suture material (if Sengstaken-Blakemore tube is used).
   q. Adhesive tape.
   r. Two suction setups with connecting tubing.
   s. Emergency intubation equipment.
   t. Endotracheal suction equipment.
   u. Cardiac monitor.

3. Prepare the patient.
   a. Explain the indications and the procedure for esophagogastric tamponade therapy. **Rationale:** Decreases patient anxiety.
   b. Explain the patient's role in assisting with passage of the tube and maintenance of tamponade pressure. **Rationale:** Elicits patient cooperation during the procedure and therapy.
   c. Place patient on cardiac monitor. **Rationale:** Cardiac dysrhythmias may occur during passage of a large bore tube.

4. Position patient: high Fowler's, semi-Fowler's, or left lateral. **Rationale:** Facilitates passage of tube into stomach and prevents aspiration.

5. Test function of tamponade tube:
   a. Inflate balloon(s) with small amount of air. **Rationale:** Ensures proper function of balloon(s) prior to insertion.
   b. Hold air-filled balloon(s) under water to test for leaks. **Rationale:** Intact balloon(s) produces no air bubbles.

Implementation

Steps	Rationale	Special Considerations
1. Wash hands.	Reduces transmission of microorganisms.	
2. Don nonsterile gloves.	Universal precautions.	
3. Empty stomach and esophagus of large quantities of blood and clots (see Skill 18–2).	Prevents vomiting and aspiration during tube insertion and minimizes risk of blocking tube with clots.	
4. Coat the tamponade tube with water-soluble lubricant:	Minimizes mucosal injury and irritation during insertion.	
a. Lubricate balloon(s).		
b. Lubricate the distal 15 cm of tube.		
5. With Sengstaken-Blakemore tube, affix no. 18 French nasogastric tube aside tamponade tube with suture material. Position distal tip of nasogastric tube just above esophageal balloon on Sengstaken-Blakemore.	Provides for evacuation of secretions that accumulate in esophagus above inflated balloon.	Not necessary with the Minnesota and Linton tubes because they have a lumen for esophageal drainage and suction.

Table continues on following page

Steps	Rationale	Special Considerations
6. Estimate length of tube to be passed:	Estimates distance to stomach.	
a. Measure total length from bridge of nose to earlobe to tip of xiphoid process (see Fig. 18–2).		
b. Mark this point on tube with tape.		
7. Anesthetize the posterior oropharynx (and nostril, if tube is to be passed nasally) with topical agent.	Decreases discomfort caused by insertion.	*Caution:* Gag reflex and cough reflex may be compromised by topical anesthesia, increasing the risk of aspiration. *Keep emergency intubation equipment available.* Patient may be intubated prophylactically to prevent airway compromise.
8. Insert oral airway or bite block if tube is to be passed orally (see Skill 1–1).	Prevents patient from biting on tube or inserter's fingers.	Remove dentures if appropriate.
9. Insert tamponade tube into mouth or selected nostril:	Eases passage of tube.	Heart rate may decrease as a result of vagal stimulation. Administer atropine if necessary.
a. Ensure that balloons are completely deflated before insertion.		
b. Pass tube into stomach to at least 50-cm mark or 10 cm beyond estimated length to reach stomach (see Figs. 18–8 and 18–9).	Ensures that entire gastric balloon is placed within stomach.	
10. Confirm tube placement:	Outline of partially inflated gastric balloon can be visualized on x-ray. Ensures placement of entire gastric balloon within the stomach.	If gastric balloon is partially located in the esophagus, complete inflation of gastric balloon could cause esophageal rupture.
a. Aspirate drainage from gastric suction port.		
b. Inject about 15 to 20 cc air into gastric suction lumen of tube while auscultating with a stethoscope over gastric bulb (left upper quadrant, just below rib cage).		
c. Inject 20 cc air into gastric balloon lumen, double clamp gastric balloon lumen with rubber-shod clamps, and obtain abdominal x-ray.		
11. Inflate gastric balloon with 200 to 350 cc air after confirmation of position by x-ray, and double clamp balloon lumen with rubber-shod clamps.	Inflated balloon fills stomach. Clamps prevent air leak from gastric balloon.	
12. Withdraw tamponade tube until resistance is met.	Positions gastric balloon at gastroesophageal junction.	
13. Maintain gentle tension on tube:	Fixes position of gastric balloon and exerts pressure on vessels.	
a. Apply gentle traction with 1 to 2 lb of weight attached to the tamponade tube with balanced suspension traction (Fig. 18–10).		

Table continues on following page

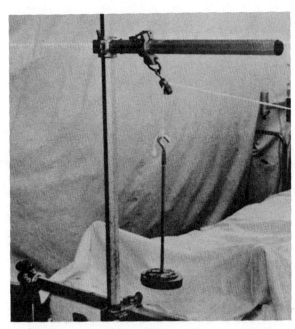

FIGURE 18–10. Balanced suspension traction securing tampon-ade tube placement. (Reprinted with permission from K. D. DeGroot and M. Damato, *Critical Care Skills.* Norwalk, Conn.: Appleton & Lange, 1987, p. 257.)

Steps	Rationale	Special Considerations
b. *Or* tape tube to sponge cube as it exits nostril and tape sponge cube to nose if tube is passed *nasally* (Fig. 18–11), or tape tube securely to cheek if tube is passed *orally*.		
c. *Or* apply football helmet to patient, and tape tube to mouth guard on helmet (Fig. 18–12).		If helmet used, pad inside of helmet to prevent pressure ulcer formation on back of head.
14. Mark tube with piece of tape as it exits mouth or nose.	Reference point to assess tube migration outward.	
15. Lavage stomach via gastric suction lumen.	Ensures patency and prevents blood clots from blocking the tube.	
16. Connect gastric suction lumen to continuous or intermittent suction <80 mmHg.	Provides for evacuation of gastric contents and for assessment of continuation of bleeding.	
17. Connect esophageal suction lumen or primary lumen of nasogastric tube to continuous or intermittent suction <80 mmHg.	Provides for evacuation of secretions that accumulate above inflated balloon.	
18. Inflate esophageal balloon if bleeding is not controlled by gastric tamponade (Fig. 18–13): a. Connect one limb of Y rubber tubing to esophageal balloon lumen. b. Connect one limb of Y rubber tubing to bulb of sphygmomanometer.	Produces direct pressure on esophageal vessels.	Maintain esophageal balloon pressures as prescribed. Monitor pressures every 2 to 4 hours while esophageal balloon is inflated. Reinflate to prescribed pressure as needed.

Table continues on following page

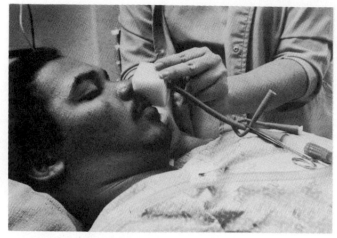

FIGURE 18–11. Tamponade tube secured in position with nasal insertion. (Reprinted with permission from K. D. DeGroot and M. Damato, *Critical Care Skills*. Norwalk, Conn.: Appleton & Lange, 1987, p. 258.)

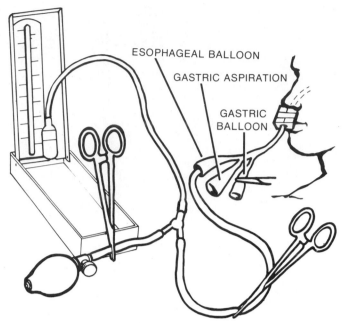

FIGURE 18–13. Inflation of esophageal balloon. (Courtesy of Davol, Inc.)

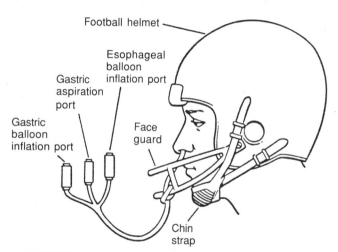

FIGURE 18–12. Tamponade tube secured in position with helmet. (Reprinted with permission from C. B. Persons, *Critical Care Procedures and Protocols: A Nursing Process Approach*. Philadelphia: Lippincott, 1987, p. 204.)

Steps	Rationale	Special Considerations
c. Connect one limb of Y rubber tubing to sphygmomanometer tubing.		
d. Pump bulb of sphygmomanometer to inflate esophageal balloon to prescribed pressure (safe inflation range is 25 to 45 mmHg).	Higher pressures may cause necrosis of esophageal mucosa.	
e. Read esophageal balloon inflation pressure on sphygmomanometer.	Pressure within esophageal balloon is transmitted to mercury column in sphygmomanometer.	
f. Double clamp esophageal balloon lumen.	Prevents air leaks from esophageal balloon.	

Table continues on following page

Steps	Rationale	Special Considerations
19. Maintain tamponade therapy as needed: maximum of 24 to 36 hours for esophageal balloon, 48 to 72 hours for gastric balloon.	Longer inflation time may cause necrosis or ulceration of tissue.	
20. Provide nares care every 2 hours when tube is inserted nasally.	Prevents drying and ulceration of mucosa.	Remove dried blood/secretions from nasal orifice and proximal nares. Apply lubricating ointment or gel to keep mucosa moist.
21. Provide oral care every 2 hours.	Prevents drying and ulceration of mucosa.	Swab mouth with cleansing and moisturizing agents.
22. Discontinue tamponade therapy in stages:	Provides for gradual reduction in tamponade in order to assess successful discontinuance of bleeding.	*Never deflate gastric balloon while esophageal balloon remains inflated.* The inflated esophageal balloon will migrate upward into oropharynx and cause airway obstruction. If airway obstruction occurs, *cut tamponade tube to deflate balloons and remove immediately.*
a. Deflate esophageal balloon by unclamping esophageal balloon lumen, and aspirate lumen with irrigating syringe to ensure complete deflation.		
b. Observe for recurrence of bleeding over 12 to 24 hours. If bleeding recurs, reinflate esophageal balloon.	Bleeding may recur with release of pressure on esophageal vessels.	
c. Deflate gastric balloon by unclamping gastric balloon lumen, and aspirate lumen with irrigating syringe to ensure complete deflation.		
d. Observe for recurrence of bleeding over 12 to 24 hours. If bleeding recurs, reinflate gastric balloon.	Bleeding may recur with release of pressure on gastric vessels.	
23. Cut tube with scissors, and remove tamponade tube slowly.	Ensures complete balloon deflation prior to removal.	
24. Dispose of equipment in appropriate receptacle.	Universal precautions.	
25. Wash hands.	Reduces transmission of microorganisms.	

Evaluation

1. Evaluate the patient for recurrence of variceal bleeding. **Rationale:** Bleeding may recur with removal of or despite esophagogastric tamponade therapy.
2. Monitor the patency of the airway and respiratory status. **Rationale:** Presence or movement of a large-bore tube may impair the upper airway.
3. Monitor output accurately. Irrigate gastric lumen with 20 to 30 cc normal saline every 2 to 4 hours or as needed to keep patent.
4. Monitor output accurately. Irrigate esophageal lumen with 10 to 15 cc normal saline every 2 to 4 hours or as needed to keep patent.

Expected Outcomes

1. Cessation of variceal bleeding. **Rationale:** Tamponade therapy applies direct pressure on bleeding vessels to stop bleeding.

2. Gastric decompression. **Rationale:** Decreases risk of aspiration and absorption of nitrogen load (blood).

Unexpected Outcomes

1. Inappropriate placement of tamponade tube. **Rationale:** May cause airway obstruction or rupture of esophagus when balloon(s) is (are) inflated.
2. Gastric or esophageal necrosis. **Rationale:** High balloon pressures for extended periods of time against mucosal tissue may lead to tissue damage.
3. Esophageal rupture. **Rationale:** Esophageal rupture may occur as a consequence of extensive tissue necrosis caused by high balloon pressures or by inadvertent inflation of gastric balloon within the esophagus.
4. Airway obstruction. **Rationale:** Obstruction of airway occurs if tube migrates upward into oropharynx.
5. Cardiac dysrhythmias during insertion or removal of tube. **Rationale:** Passage of a large-bore tube may cause vagal stimulation and bradydysrhythmias.

6. Aspiration of gastric or oropharyngeal contents into respiratory tract. **Rationale:** Protective gag reflex may be impaired secondary to topical anesthesia in oropharynx. Passage of a large-bore tube may initiate vomiting with resultant aspiration. Accumulated oropharyngeal secretions above inflated gastric and esophageal balloons may be aspirated into the respiratory tract.

Documentation

Documentation in the patient record should include date and time of the procedure, reason for insertion, route of insertion (oral or nasal), assessment of tube placement, x-ray confirmation of placement, patient tolerance of procedure, inflation status of each balloon (inflated or deflated), volume in gastric balloon, pressure of esophageal balloon, provision of suction on gastric and esophageal lumens, time of measurements of esoph-

ageal balloon pressures and pressure readings, need to add pressure to esophageal balloon to maintain ordered pressure, amount and characteristics of gastric and esophageal drainage, performance and amount of irrigation of drainage lumens, occurrence of any unexpected outcomes, and method of traction and maintenance of traction. **Rationale:** Documents nursing care given, provides baseline to compare/trend patient assessments, and documents any unexpected outcomes and interventions taken.

Patient/Family Education

Explain the indications and the procedure for insertion and maintenance of esophagogastric tamponade tube to both patient and family. **Rationale:** Encourages patient and family cooperation and understanding of procedure and ongoing care.

Performance Checklist
Skill 18–4: Esophagogastric Tamponade Tube

Critical Behaviors	Complies yes	no
1. Wash hands.		
2. Don nonsterile gloves.		
3. Evacuate patient's stomach.		
4. Lubricate tamponade tube.		
5. If using a Sengstaken-Blakemore tube, secure no. 16 to 18 French nasogastric tube.		
6. Estimate length of tube to be passed.		
7. Anesthetize oropharynx and nostril if appropriate.		
8. For oral insertion, remove dentures and insert oral airway or bite block.		
9. Insert tamponade tube.		
10. Confirm tube placement.		
11. Inflate gastric balloon with 200 to 350 cc air, and double clamp lumen.		
12. Withdraw tube until resistance is met.		
13. Maintain gentle tension on tube.		
14. Mark tube at exit from mouth or nose.		
15. Lavage stomach via gastric suction lumen.		
16. Connect gastric suction lumen to suction.		
17. Connect esophageal suction or primary lumen of nasogastric tube to suction.		
18. Inflate esophageal balloon as needed to control bleeding.		
19. Maintain tamponade therapy as needed.		
20. Provide nares care every 2 hours.		
21. Provide oral care every 2 hours.		
22. Discontinue tamponade therapy in stages:		

Table continues on following page

Critical Behaviors	Complies	
	yes	no
a. Deflate esophageal balloon.		
b. Observe for recurrence of bleeding.		
c. Deflate gastric balloon.		
d. Observe for recurrence of bleeding.		
e. Reinflate balloon(s) as needed to control bleeding.		
23. Cut tamponade tube and withdraw slowly.		
24. Dispose of equipment appropriately.		
25. Wash hands.		
26. Document procedure in patient record.		

SKILL 18–5

Scleral Endoscopic Therapy

Increased portal venous pressure caused by obstruction to blood flow through the liver leads to the development of collateral channels for drainage of portal blood. These channels redirect portal blood flow to low-resistance venous beds, most commonly within the esophagus. As these low-pressure veins become distended with blood, varices develop. These varices are under high pressure and are friable, and they are predisposed to bleeding. Blood loss can be profound.

Scleral endoscopic therapy can be an acute, chronic, or preventive intervention used to control bleeding from esophageal varices. A fiberoptic endoscope is passed through the esophagus into the stomach. Through an opening in the scope, a sclerosing agent is introduced into the varices that causes thrombosis and ultimately prevention of or cessation of bleeding.

Purpose

The purpose of scleral endoscopic therapy is to prevent or control bleeding from esophageal varices.

Prerequisite Knowledge and Skills

Prior to assisting with scleral endoscopic therapy, the nurse should understand

1. Principles of universal precautions.
2. Anatomy and physiology of the gastrointestinal tract.
3. Pathophysiology of gastric and esophageal varices.
4. Anatomy and physiology of the respiratory system.
5. Actions and side effects of sclerosing agents.
6. Cardiac effects of vagal stimulation.

The nurse should be able to perform

1. Proper handwashing technique (see Skill 35–5).
2. Universal precautions (see Skill 35–1).
3. Assessment of respiratory status.
4. Interpretation of cardiac dysrhythmias.
5. Insertion of oral airway and bite block (see Skill 1–1).

Assessment

1. Assess the patient for a history of esophageal or gastric varices. **Rationale:** Sclerotherapy is used for acute, chronic, and preventive treatment for varices.
2. Assess the patient's PT, PTT, and platelet counts. **Rationale:** Grossly abnormal coagulation factors should be corrected prior to sclerosing.
3. Assess the patient's baseline cardiac rhythm. **Rationale:** Passage of a large-bore tube may cause vagal stimulation and bradydysrhythmias.
4. Assess the patient's baseline respiratory status (i.e., rate, depth, pattern, characteristics of secretions, and breath sounds). **Rationale:** Gag reflex may be diminished with application of topical anesthesia. Passage of a large-bore tube may cause airway obstruction. Risk of aspiration is increased with large amounts of blood in the stomach. Analgesics and sedatives may cause respiratory depression.

Nursing Diagnoses

1. Potential for injury related to injection or spraying of sclerosing agent. **Rationale:** Injection of sclerosing agent too deeply into the esophageal muscle can cause tissue necrosis. Accidental spraying of sclerosing agent in the eye can cause damage to eye structures.
2. Potential for aspiration related to the passage of large-bore tube. **Rationale:** Gag reflex may be diminished with topical anesthesia application.

3. Potential ineffective breathing pattern related to dosage and ability to metabolize analgesics and sedatives. **Rationale:** Esophageal varices are associated with liver impairment. Patients may have limited ability to metabolize these drugs.

4. Potential fluid volume deficit related to variceal bleeding. **Rationale:** Significant loss of circulating volume occurs with bleeding varices.

Planning

1. Individualize the following patient goals for scleral endoscopic therapy:
   a. Treatment or prevention of variceal bleeding. **Rationale:** Bleeding from gastric and esophageal varices may lead to massive blood volume loss.
   b. Maintenance of adequate circulating volume for tissue perfusion. **Rationale:** Vascular volume can fall precipitously with uncontrolled variceal bleeding.
2. Ensure that a completed informed consent form is present in the medical record prior to initiating the procedure. **Rationale:** Legal requirement for performing an invasive procedure.
3. Assemble and prepare all necessary equipment and supplies. **Rationale:** Ensures that bleeding will be controlled quickly and efficiently.
   a. Endoscope (flexible or rigid, physician preference).
   b. Endoscopic injector needle (usually 23 gauge, 4-mm needle).
   c. Three 10-cc syringes filled with sclerosing agent.
   d. Suction setup with connecting tubing.
   e. Safety goggles for each assistant and patient.
   f. Waterproof covering for patient (optional).
   g. Nonsterile gloves.
   h. Water-soluble lubricant.
   i. Gastric lavage equipment (if needed).
   j. Topical anesthesia.
   k. Two 30- to 50-cc syringes.
   l. Normal saline or tap water for irrigation.
   m. Oral airway or bite block.
   n. Pulse oximeter (optional) (see Skill 6–1).
   o. Automatic blood pressure device (optional).
   p. Premedications as prescribed.
   q. Emergency intubation equipment.
   r. Endotracheal suction equipment.
   s. Nasogastric tube or esophagogastric tamponade tube (as requested).

4. Prepare the patient.
   a. Explain the indications and the procedure for scleral endoscopic therapy. **Rationale:** Decreases anxiety.
   b. Explain the patient's role in assisting with the procedure and postprocedure care. **Rationale:** Elicits cooperation during and after procedure.
   c. Place patient on cardiac monitor. **Rationale:** Vagal stimulation may result in cardiac dysrhythmias.
   d. Place pulse oximeter and automatic blood pressure device on the patient (if an arterial pressure line is not in place). **Rationale:** Allows for continuous assessment of respiratory status and blood pressure throughout the procedure.
   e. Ensure venous access. **Rationale:** For administration of premedications as ordered.
   f. Allow only clear liquids 8 to 12 hours prior to procedure. **Rationale:** Undigested material in the stomach increases the risk of aspiration and decreases visualization of varices and mucosa.
   g. Position the patient as requested by the physician, usually left lateral with the head of the bed elevated 30 degrees. **Rationale:** Facilitates passage of the endoscope and decreases the risk of aspiration.
   h. Premedicate patient as requested by physician. Common sedatives: diazepam, midazolam, meperidine; vagal lytic agent: atropine. **Rationale:** Light sedation decreases patient anxiety and encourages cooperation during procedure. Vagal lytic agent protects against profound bradycardia during insertion of endoscope.
   i. Remove dentures if present. **Rationale:** Dentures interfere with safe passing of endoscope.
   j. Protect patient's eyes with goggles or waterproof covering. **Rationale:** Provides protection against accidental spraying with sclerosing agent.
5. Determine the patient's PT, PTT, and platelet counts. **Rationale:** Abnormal coagulation factors increase risk of bleeding from varices after needle injection.
6. Obtain the patient's baseline vital signs (i.e., blood pressure, heart rate and rhythm, respiratory rate and pattern, and SaO_2). **Rationale:** Untoward changes in vital signs may reflect intolerance to procedure or complications related to bleeding or to respiratory compromise.

Implementation

Steps	Rationale	Special Considerations
1. Wash hands.	Reduces transmission of microorganisms.	
2. Don nonsterile gloves.	Universal precautions.	

Table continues on following page

Steps	Rationale	Special Considerations
3. Perform or assist the physician with gastric lavage if needed (see Skill 18–2).	Large amounts of blood or clots in stomach or esophagus obstruct visualization of varices and increase the risk of aspiration during the procedure.	Monitor heart rate/rhythm and respiratory status during lavage.
4. Don protective goggles.	Provides protection against accidental spraying with sclerosing agent.	
5. Assist physician with insertion of endoscope:	Endoscope allows for visualization of esophagus and stomach to locate varices.	*Caution:* Gag reflex and cough reflex may be compromised by topical anesthetic, increasing the risk of aspiration. *Keep emergency intubation equipment available.* Monitor heart rate/rhythm and respiratory status during endoscopy.
a. Anesthetize the posterior oropharynx with topical agent.	Decreases discomfort caused by passage of endoscope.	
b. Insert oral airway or bite block (see Skill 1–1).	Prevents patient from biting on endoscope or inserter's fingers.	
c. Lubricate 10 to 15 cm of distal end of endoscope with water-soluble lubricant.	Minimizes mucosal injury and irritation during insertion of endoscope.	
d. Encourage patient to simulate swallowing while tube is being passed.	Swallowing maneuver causes epiglottis to close trachea and directs endoscope into esophagus.	
6. Inject air or irrigant via endoscope as requested by physician.	Expands tissue folds and cleanses area to increase visualization of tissue.	Patient may have gastric distension or belching after procedure due to air insertion.
7. Apply suction via endoscope as requested by physician.	Evacuates secretions and irrigant as needed to increase visualization of tissue.	
8. Manipulate sclerosing needle as requested by physician (Fig. 18–14).	Ensures that sclerosing needle is in proper position for injection and does not injure tissue during movement of endoscope.	Needle must be retracted before manipulation of endoscope.
9. Inject sclerosing agent as requested by physician.		Most common sclerosing agents are sodium morrhuate and ethanolamine oleate 5%.

Table continues on following page

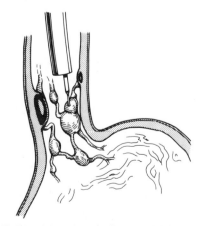

FIGURE 18–14. Sclerosing needle placed into varix. (Reprinted with permission from M. V. Sivak, *Endoscopic Sclerotherapy of Esophageal Varices* (Gastroenterology Series Vol. 1). New York: Praeger, 1984, p. 131.)

Steps	Rationale	Special Considerations
10. Insert nasogastric tube or esophagogastric tamponade tube after removal of endoscope as requested by physician (see Skills 18–1 and 18–4).	Nasogastric tube provides for assessment of recurrent bleeding; esophagogastric tamponade tube may be used to apply pressure to oozing varices.	*Caution:* Insertion of nasogastric tube may disrupt fragile varices and initiate bleeding. Chest x-ray is usually performed to rule out aspiration or esophageal perforation.
11. Dispose of equipment in appropriate receptacle.	Universal precautions.	
12. Wash hands.	Reduces transmission of microorganisms.	

Evaluation

1.   Monitor vital signs (i.e., blood pressure, respiratory rate, SaO$_2$, and heart rate/rhythm) every ½ to 1 hour for 2 to 4 hours after procedure. **Rationale:** Unusual pain and/or changes in vital signs may indicate complications related to the procedure.

2.   Monitor for signs of recurrent bleeding; note hematocrit, hemoglobin, intake and output, nasogastric drainage, and vomitus. **Rationale:** Bleeding may occur from untreated varices or injection sites of treated varices.

3.   Assess for return of normal pharyngeal function. Keep patient on side with head of bed elevated to prevent aspiration until gag, swallowing, and cough reflexes are intact. **Rationale:** Pharyngeal function may be compromised after topical anesthesia or passage of a large-bore tube.

4.   Provide cool clear liquids with return of pharyngeal function. Progress diet slowly, avoiding solid food for 16 to 24 hours. **Rationale:** Prevent aspiration. Food may act as an irritant to newly sclerosed varices.

5.   Administer antacids, histamine blockers, and sucralfate as prescribed by the physician. **Rationale:** Provides protection to fragile varices from gastric acids.

Expected Outcome

Thrombosis of bleeding varice(s). **Rationale:** Aim of therapy is to prevent recurrent bleeding.

Unexpected Outcomes

1.   Continued bleeding from injected varices. **Rationale:** Bleeding may continue secondary to high venous pressure and altered coagulation factors.

2.   Esophageal sloughing or ulceration. **Rationale:** Leakage of sclerosing agent out of varices will necrose esophageal tissue.

3.   Esophageal perforation. **Rationale:** May occur with use of rigid endoscope, injection of sclerosing agent too deep into esophageal tissue or outside of varices, or extension of mucosal ulceration.

4.   Substernal chest pain. **Rationale:** Chest pain (noncardiac in nature) is a side effect of irritating sclerosing agent.

5.   Fever. **Rationale:** Contaminants in sclerosing agents may cause fever, and inflammation secondary to sclerosing may cause fever.

6.   Allergic response to sclerosing agent. Allergic response may be as simple as rash or hives or full anaphylaxis. **Rationale:** Foreign agents may initiate antigen-antibody reaction.

7.   Aspiration pneumonia. **Rationale:** Altered breathing pattern and accumulation of blood may cause aspiration of gastric or oropharyngeal secretions into the lungs.

Documentation

Documentation in the patient record should include date and time of procedure, baseline vital signs, premedications administered, gastric lavage (if performed), patient tolerance of procedure, occurrence of any unexpected outcomes, insertion of nasogastric or tamponade tube (if inserted), postprocedure vital signs, position of patient after procedure, assessment of gag/cough reflex, return of normal gag/cough reflex, any postprocedure medications administered, and any untoward events during the procedure or unexpected outcomes and interventions taken. **Rationale:** Documents nursing care given, provides baseline to compare patient assessments, and documents any unexpected outcomes and interventions taken.

Patient/Family Education

1.   Explain the indications and the procedure for endoscopic sclerotherapy to both patient and family. **Rationale:** Encourages patient and family cooperation and understanding of procedure and participation during procedure.

2.   Explain signs and symptoms to report (i.e., fever, late chest pain, difficulty swallowing, or bleeding). **Rationale:** Unexpected outcomes may occur days or weeks after completion of procedure.

3.   Explain progression of diet after procedure. **Rationale:** Decreases risk of aspiration until the full return of gag reflex.

4.   Explain medication therapy for gastric acid control. **Rationale:** Reflux of gastric acid may irritate friable varices and initiate bleeding.

Performance Checklist
Skill 18–5: Scleral Endoscopic Therapy

Critical Behaviors	Complies	
	yes	no
1. Wash hands.		
2. Don nonsterile gloves.		
3. Perform or assist with gastric lavage.		
4. Don protective goggles.		
5. Assist physician with endoscopy as requested.		
6. Inject air or irrigant via endoscope as requested.		
7. Apply suction via endoscope as requested.		
8. Manipulate sclerosing needle as requested.		
9. Inject sclerosing agent as requested.		
10. Insert nasogastric tube as requested.		
11. Dispose of equipment appropriately.		
12. Wash hands.		
13. Document procedure in patient record.		

SKILL 18–6

Vasopressin Infusion

Vasopressin is a peptide hormone secreted by the posterior pituitary gland. Vasopressin acts as a smooth-muscle constrictor. Since the vessel walls of the gastrointestinal tract are composed of smooth muscle, vasopressin is a useful adjunct in the treatment of gastrointestinal bleeding. Constriction of vessel walls leads to decreased blood flow, which contributes to the formation of a thrombus at the bleeding site.

Vasopressin may be infused *selectively*, directly into the bleeding vessels, or *nonselectively*, into the general venous circulation. For selective infusion, an angiogram is performed to locate the specific bleeding vessel. The catheter is then advanced to the site of bleeding. For nonselective infusion, a simple venipuncture is performed to initiate infusion. It was believed that selective infusion would minimize the systemic side effects of vasopressin, but this has not been confirmed in clinical practice. Since nonselective infusion demonstrates a satisfactory reduction in bleeding, is less invasive, avoids the potential complications of an angiogram, and has shown no increase in systemic side effects, it has become the route of choice for vasopressin infusion.

The most common side effects of vasopressin are reflected in the cardiovascular system: dysrhythmias, hypertension, peripheral cyanosis, decreased renal blood flow, and pulmonary edema. Nitroglycerin (infusion or paste) is often used concomitantly to counteract these effects. Continuous monitoring of the cardiac rhythm is absolutely essential during infusion.

Purpose

The nurse initiates vasopressin infusion therapy to stop or control gastrointestinal bleeding.

Prerequisite Knowledge and Skills

Prior to performing vasopressin infusion, the nurse should understand

1. Principles of universal precautions.
2. Actions, indications for use, dosages, adverse effects, and contraindications of vasopressin.
3. Principles of management of arterial and venous infusion catheters.

The nurse should be able to perform

1. Proper handwashing technique (see Skill 35–5).
2. Aseptic technique.
3. Universal precautions (see Skill 35–1).
4. Assessment of arterial and venous infusion catheter systems (see Skills 9–1 and 10–2).
5. Calculation of drug dosage infusion rate.
6. Preparation of solutions for infusion.
7. Interpretation of cardiac dysrhythmias.
8. Setup and management of a controlled infusion device (see Skills 33–3 and 33–4).

Assessment

1. Observe the patient for signs and symptoms of

major blood volume loss, including tachycardia, hypotension, decreased urine output, decreased filling pressures (PAP, PCWP, CVP) hematocrit, hemoglobin and clotting factors (PT, PTT, platelets), frank blood per rectum, and/or nasogastric aspirate. **Rationale:** Gastrointestinal bleeding can result in significant volume loss and corresponding changes in vital signs.

2. Validate patency of arterial or venous infusion access site. **Rationale:** Extravasation of vasopressin may cause tissue necrosis.

3. Assess the patient's history for cardiac and cardiovascular disease. **Rationale:** Side effects of vasopressin may exacerbate cardiac and cardiovascular deficits.

4. Assess the patient's baseline cardiac rate and rhythm, and cardiac enzymes. **Rationale:** Side effects of vasopressin may alter cardiac status.

Nursing Diagnoses

1. Fluid volume deficit related to major gastrointestinal bleeding. **Rationale:** Blood loss into the gastrointestinal tract decreases circulating/intravascular volume.

2. Altered tissue perfusion (renal, cerebral, cardiopulmonary, and peripheral) related to vasopressin infusion. **Rationale:** Vasoconstrictive action of vasopressin decreases blood flow to major organs.

3. Potential for injury related to vasopressin infusion. **Rationale:** Extravasation of vasopressin causes localized tissue necrosis.

Planning

1. Individualize the following patient goals for vasopressin infusion:

a. Control of intravascular volume loss into the gastrointestinal tract. **Rationale:** Maintenance of intravascular volume is necessary for adequate tissue perfusion.

b. Prevention of extravasation of vasopressin into the tissue. **Rationale:** Extravasation of vasopressin causes localized tissue necrosis.

2. Assemble and prepare all necessary equipment and supplies. **Rationale:** Ensures that vasopressin infusion will be accomplished quickly and efficiently.

a. Vasopressin (Pitressin), 20 units per vial.

b. 250 to 500 ml normal saline or D_5W for intravenous administration.

c. Controlled infusion device (if intraarterial infusion is being administered, *must* use infuser that will pump against arterial pressure).

d. IV administration tubing for use with infusion device.

e. Cardiac monitor.

3. Prepare the patient.

a. Explain the indications and the procedure for vasopressin infusion therapy. **Rationale:** Decreases patient anxiety.

b. Explain the patient's role in assisting with management of the vascular access used for infusion of vasopressin. **Rationale:** Elicits patient cooperation with the maintenance of access.

c. Place patient on cardiac monitor **Rationale:** To detect dysrhythmias.

4. Establish the patient's baseline cardiovascular function (i.e., rate/rhythm, blood pressure, peripheral pulses, breath sounds, and urine output). **Rationale:** Establishes baseline for comparison during therapy.

5. Obtain a 12-lead electrocardiogram. **Rationale:** Provides a baseline should ECG changes be observed.

Implementation

Steps	Rationale	Special Considerations
1. Wash hands.	Reduces transmission of microorganisms.	
2. Assess patency of intravascular access.	Extravasation of vasopressin can cause tissue necrosis.	Venous or arterial access may be used. Arterial access is inserted via femoral artery and advanced under fluoroscopy to a mesenteric artery branch near the bleeding vessel.
3. Prepare and administer a bolus infusion of vasopressin as prescribed by the physician.	Bolus infusion raises blood levels of drug rapidly.	Normal bolus infusion: 20 units in 20 to 50 cc D_5W or normal saline infused over 5 to 30 minutes.
4. Prepare continuous vasopressin infusion: a. Add 100 units vasopressin to 250 to 500 cc D_5W or normal saline (0.2 to 0.4 unit/cc). b. Label infusion.	To control bleeding with a continuous infusion.	Vasopressin is compatible with both D_5W and normal saline. Concentrate infusion as necessary to control fluid intake.

Table continues on following page

Steps	Rationale	Special Considerations
5. Connect vasopressin infusion to controlled infusion device.	Necessary to provide a constant and accurate flow rate. Arterial infusion requires an infusion pump that overcomes arterial pressure.	
6. Infuse vasopressin at prescribed dose in units per minute.	Concentrations of infusions may vary affecting dose per cc.	Dose range: 0.1 to 0.6 units/min (up to 0.9 units/min has been infused safely).
7. Keep cannulated extremity immobilized.	Dislodgment of arterial access may result in arterial bleeding or infusion of vasopressin into an inappropriate area. Dislodgment of venous access may lead to subcutaneous infiltration and localized tissue necrosis.	
8. Wean and discontinue vasopressin infusion as prescribed by physician.	Abrupt discontinuation may precipitate acute recurrence of bleeding.	Wean infusion over 12 to 24 hours. Assess patient during weaning for recurrence of bleeding.
9. Maintain patency of access after discontinuance of infusion.	Provides ready access should therapy need to be reinitiated.	
10. Dispose of equipment in appropriate receptacles.	Universal precautions.	
11. Wash hands.	Reduces transmission of microorganisms.	

Evaluation

1. Monitor the patient for the presence or absence of active bleeding, vital signs, hematocrit, hemoglobin, and coagulation factors. **Rationale:** Provides data to determine effectiveness of vasopressin infusion.

2. Evaluate the patient for ischemic changes on the ECG, angina, or myocardial infarction. **Rationale:** Vasoconstrictive action decreases coronary artery perfusion and may increase blood pressure. *Note:* Patient may be placed on a nitroglycerin infusion or paste to counteract cardiovascular complications of vasopressin. Bradycardia is most common cardiovascular effect of vasopressin.

3. Assess the patient for abdominal cramps. **Rationale:** Vasopressin causes abdominal muscles (smooth muscles) to contract.

4. Monitor the patient's urine output. **Rationale:** Vasopressin is a synthetic form of antidiuretic hormone, which causes increased reabsorption of water by the kidneys.

5. Monitor placement and function of intravascular device, including patency and extravasation, every hour. **Rationale:** Extravasation can cause tissue necrosis.

6. Monitor pulse, color, and temperature of extremity distal to the infusion site. **Rationale:** Presence of arterial access may compromise distal circulation.

Expected Outcomes

1. Cessation of gastrointestinal bleeding. **Rationale:** Vasopressin slows or stops bleeding by vasoconstrictive action on bleeding vessels.

2. Maintenance of vascular access integrity. **Rationale:** Prevents tissue necrosis secondary to vasopressin extravasation.

Unexpected Outcomes

1. Continued bleeding despite vasopressin infusion. **Rationale:** Bleeding may not respond to vasopressin therapy.

2. Extravasation of vasopressin into the tissue. **Rationale:** Failure to maintain vascular access integrity.

3. Occurrence of major cardiovascular complications, such as bradydysrhythmias, ischemic cardiac rhythms, hypertension, angina, myocardial infarction, peripheral mottling or cyanosis, decreased renal blood flow with decreased urine output, or pulmonary edema. **Rationale:** Possible adverse effects of vasopressin.

Documentation

Documentation in the patient record should include the date, time, and indications for initiating vasopressin infusion, location and size of vascular access, condition of access site, solution used and concentration of vasopressin infusion, and dose of infusion in units per minute (bolus and continuous). Also *include* changes made with titration, use of continuous cardiac monitoring, and cardiovascular and abdominal assessment findings. **Rationale:** Documents nursing interventions, patient response to therapy, and patient status.

Patient/Family Education

Explain the indications, the procedure for initiation, and the maintenance of vasopressin infusion to both pa-

tient and family. **Rationale:** Encourages patient and family cooperation and understanding of procedure.

Performance Checklist
Skill 18–6:   Vasopressin Infusion

Critical Behaviors	Complies yes	no
1. Wash hands.		
2. Assess patency of intravascular access.		
3. Prepare and administer bolus infusion as prescribed.		
4. Prepare continuous infusion.		
5. Connect vasopressin infusion to controlled infusion device.		
6. Infuse vasopressin at prescribed dose.		
7. Immobilize cannulated extremity.		
8. Wean and discontinue vasopressin infusion as prescribed by physician.		
9. Maintain patency of vascular access after discontinuing infusion.		
10. Dispose of equipment appropriately.		
11. Wash hands.		
12. Document infusion and patient assessment in patient record.		

BIBLIOGRAPHY

DeGroot, K. D., and Damato, M. B. (1987). *Critical Care Skills*. Norwalk, Conn.: Appleton & Lange.

Drossman, D. A. (Ed.) (1987). *Manual of Gastroenterologic Procedures*, 2d Ed. New York: Raven Press.

Gruber, M. (1985). Endoscopic injection sclerotherapy: Nursing responsibilities. *Crit. Care Q.* March 73–80.

Jenkins, J. L., and Loscaizo, J. (1986). *Manual of Emergency Medicine*. Boston: Little, Brown.

Millar, S., Sampson, L. K., and Soukoup, M. (1985). *AACN Procedures Manual for Critical Care*. Philadelphia: Saunders.

Persons, C. B. (1987). *Critical Care Procedures and Protocols: A Nursing Process Approach*. Philadelphia: Lippincott.

Siegel, B. (1986). *Diagnostic Patient Studies in Surgery*. Philadelphia: Lea & Febiger.

Sivak, M. V. (Ed.) (1987). *Gastroenterologic Endoscopy*. Philadelphia: Saunders.

White, J. V., Milazza, J. V., and Comerota, A. J. (1985). Management of massive hemorrhage from esophageal varices. *Crit. Care Q.* September 69–79.

Zschoche, D. A. (Ed.) (1986). *Mosby's Comprehensive Review of Critical Care*, 3d Ed. St. Louis: Mosby.

SPECIAL PROCEDURES USED IN THE DIAGNOSIS AND TREATMENT OF GASTROINTESTINAL PROBLEMS

BEHAVIORAL OBJECTIVES

After completing this chapter, the nurse will be able to

- Define the key terms.
- Describe the procedures used to diagnose and treat gastrointestinal problems.
- Discuss the indications for procedures used to diagnose and treat gastrointestinal problems.
- Assist with procedures used to diagnose and treat gastrointestinal problems.
- Care for the patient undergoing special procedures for gastrointestinal problems.
- Demonstrate skills involved in special procedures for gastrointestinal problems.

Selected procedures that provide direct access to the gastrointestinal tract and abdominal cavity are performed by the physician for the diagnosis and treatment of particular gastrointestinal disorders. This access allows for the examination of tissue and fluid samples and for performing interventions designed to correct or alleviate the problem.

KEY TERMS

abdominal girth   peritoneal lavage
ascites   sigmoid colon
paracentesis

SKILLS

19–1 Assisting with Paracentesis
19–2 Assisting with Peritoneal Lavage
19–3 Assisting with Bedside Upper Gastrointestinal Endoscopy
19–4 Assisting with Bedside Sigmoidoscopy

GUIDELINES

The following assessment guidelines assist the nurse in formulating a nursing diagnosis and an individualized plan of care for the patient undergoing special procedures for gastrointestinal problems:

1. Review the patient's history and physical symptoms.
2. Perform an abdominal girth measurement.
3. Review laboratory results.
4. Determine the desired outcome of the procedure.
5. Review the function of the equipment used to perform special procedures.
6. Determine the special needs and preparation of the patient undergoing the procedure.

SKILL 19–1

Assisting with Paracentesis

Paracentesis is a procedure in which fluid is removed from the peritoneal cavity for diagnostic and therapeutic purposes. A needle, trocar, or soft, flexible tubing is used to remove peritoneal fluid for laboratory analysis to support a diagnosis of ascites or other acute abdominal conditions. Paracentesis is also performed in the evaluation of blunt or penetrating trauma to the abdomen.

The accumulation of large amounts of ascitic fluid within the peritoneal cavity exerts pressure on the diaphragm and abdominal organs and vasculature, leading to respiratory compromise and increased work of breathing. Paracentesis relieves intraabdominal and diaphragmatic pressures, diminishing the work of breathing.

Purpose

Paracentesis is utilized to

1. Obtain fluid samples from the peritoneal space for diagnostic examination.
2. Evacuate fluid (ascites) from the peritoneal space.
3. Alleviate respiratory compromise related to pressure on the diaphragm caused by ascitic fluid.

Prerequisite Knowledge and Skills

Prior to assisting with paracentesis, the nurse should understand

1. Principles of universal precautions.
2. Anatomy and physiology of the lower quadrants of the abdomen.
3. Formation of ascitic fluid.
4. Normal and abnormal composition of peritoneal fluid.

The nurse should be able to perform

1. Proper handwashing technique (see Skill 35–5).

2. Universal precautions (see Skill 35–1).
3. Abdominal assessment.
4. Urinary catheterization.
5. Bladder percussion.

Assessment

1. Assess the patient's history and symptoms for abdominal injury, major gastrointestinal pathology, liver disease, and portal hypertension. **Rationale:** Certain conditions of the gastrointestinal tract may be diagnosed and treated with paracentesis.

2. Assess the patient's respiratory status (i.e., rate, depth, excursion, gas exchange, and use of accessory muscles). **Rationale:** Paracentesis may be indicated to decrease work of breathing.

3. Assess the patient's baseline fluid and electrolyte status. **Rationale:** Removal of peritoneal fluid may cause compartment shifting of intravascular volume, electrolytes, and proteins, leading to a decreased circulating volume.

4. Assess the patient for bladder distension. **Rationale:** Bladder distension increases the risk of bladder perforation during the procedure.

5. Measure the patient's abdominal girth. **Rationale:** Abdominal girth measurement provides information on changes in fluid accumulation within the peritoneal cavity.

6. Assess the patient's coagulation studies (i.e., PT, PTT, and platelets). **Rationale:** Abnormal clotting studies may increase the risk of bleeding during and after the procedure. Therapy may be necessary to correct clotting studies before paracentesis.

Nursing Diagnoses

1. Potential fluid volume deficit related to intravascular fluid shifts into peritoneal space. **Rationale:** Evacuation of peritoneal fluid may cause compartment shifting of intravascular volume, serum electrolytes, and proteins, decreasing the circulating volume.

2. (Potential) Ineffective breathing pattern related to accumulation of peritoneal fluid exerting pressure on the diaphragm. **Rationale:** Large amount of fluid accumulated in the peritoneal space interferes with diaphragm movement and increases the work of breathing.

3. Potential for injury (perforation of bowel/bladder) related to insertion of needle into peritoneal space. **Rationale:** Intestines and bladder lie underneath the abdominal surface where needle access to peritoneal space is performed.

4. Potential for infection related to invasive procedure. **Rationale:** Direct access into the peritoneal cavity provides a mechanism for entry of microorganisms into the peritoneal space.

Planning

1. Individualize the following patient goals for paracentesis:

a. Obtain fluid samples needed for diagnostic examination. **Rationale:** Analysis of fluid samples provides diagnostic information.

b. Evacuate ascitic fluid from peritoneal space. **Rationale:** Removal of fluid relieves intraabdominal pressure.

c. Relieve respiratory compromise created by accumulated peritoneal fluid. **Rationale:** Evacuation of fluid accumulation within the peritoneal space will relieve respiratory difficulties.

2. Assemble and prepare all necessary equipment and supplies. **Rationale:** Ensures that paracentesis will be completed efficiently.

a. Sterile gloves.
b. Povidone-iodine solution.
c. Sterile towels or sterile drape.
d. Local anesthetic for injection.
e. 5-cc syringe with 21- or 25-gauge needle.
f. Trocar with stylet or needle (16, 18, or 20 gauge).
g. Polyethylene tubing, 16 gauge, 12 to 18 cm long (optional).
h. Two 10-cc syringes.
i. Two 50-cc syringes.
j. Sterile tubes for specimens.
k. Knife blade, no. 11.
l. Three-way stopcock.
m. Sterile 1-L collection bottle with connecting tubing.
n. Suture material with needle.
o. Hemostat.
p. 4 to 6 sterile gauze pads 4 × 4 in.
q. Sterile gauze dressing with tape or Band-Aid.

3. Prepare the patient.

a. Explain the indications and the procedure for paracentesis to the patient. **Rationale:** Decreases patient anxiety.

b. Explain the patient's role in assisting with the procedure and postprocedure care. **Rationale:** Elicits patient cooperation during and after the procedure.

c. Decompress the bladder. Palpate bladder to ensure decompression if patient is not catheterized. **Rationale:** A distended bladder increases the risk of bladder perforation during the procedure.

4. Ascertain that an informed consent form has been signed. **Rationale:** Paracentesis is an invasive procedure requiring a signed consent.

5. Obtain PT, PTT, and platelet counts before beginning the procedure. **Rationale:** Abnormal coagulation factors increase the risk of bleeding during invasive procedure. Report abnormal findings to physician immediately.

6. Position patient as requested by physician. Usual position is supine with head of bed elevated 45 to 90 degrees or sitting over the side of the bed. **Rationale:** Fluid accumulates in dependent areas.

Implementation

Steps	Rationale	Special Considerations
1. Wash hands.	Reduces transmission of microorganisms.	
2. Assist physician with preparing equipment and sterile field.	Facilitates easy access to needed equipment.	Maintain aseptic technique.
3. Prepare the insertion site with povidone-iodine solution.	Reduces risk of infection.	Use sterile technique.
4. Assist physician with injection of local anesthesia.	Local anesthesia minimizes pain and discomfort.	Assess for anesthesia of area.
5. Assist physician with insertion of trocar or needle.	Provides access to peritoneal fluid for evacuation.	Inserted through small stab wound at midline below umbilicus.
6. Assist physician with attaching syringe(s) or stopcock and tubing to withdraw peritoneal fluid (Figs. 19–1 and 19–2).	Fluid may be gently aspirated or siphoned by gravity or vacuum into collection device.	Retain fluid for laboratory analysis. Monitor amount of fluid removed. Removal of large amount of fluid (>1 L) may cause hypotension.
7. Record amount and characteristics of fluid withdrawn.	Provides information on fluid balance and patient diagnosis.	
8. Assess patient for signs and symptoms of pain, hypovolemia, hemorrhage, bowel perforation, and bladder perforation.	Unusual pain or changes in vital signs may indicate complications related to the procedure.	

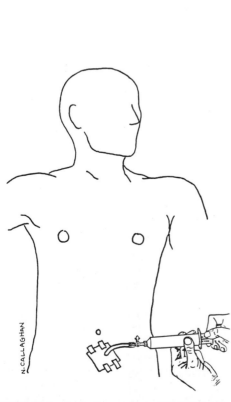

FIGURE 19–1 Aspirating peritoneal fluid into a syringe.

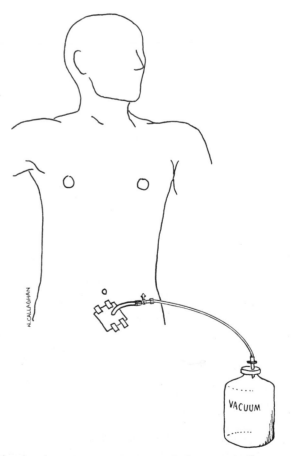

FIGURE 19–2 Peritoneal trocar attached to a gravity flow vacuum container.

Steps	Rationale	Special Considerations
9. Prepare and send fluid specimens for laboratory analysis.	Provides information about patient status.	Routine laboratory tests include specific gravity, total protein and albumin, RBC and WBC counts, amylase, culture, and cytology.
10. Apply sterile dressing to wound site after removal of trocar and wound closure.	Provides a barrier to infection and collects fluid that may leak from wound site.	
11. Dispose of equipment and soiled material in appropriate receptacle.	Universal precautions.	
12. Wash hands.	Reduces transmission of microorganisms.	

Evaluation

1.   Evaluate changes in abdominal girth. **Rationale:** Provides evidence of fluid reaccumulation.

2.   Monitor for changes in respiratory status (i.e., rate, depth, and pattern). **Rationale:** Removal of ascitic fluid will relieve pressure on the diaphragm and the resulting respiratory distress.

3.   Monitor for potential complications, including bowel/bladder perforation, bleeding, and intravascular volume loss. **Rationale:** Paracentesis interrupts the integrity of the skin and underlying peritoneum.

4.   Monitor vital signs, temperature, insertion site for drainage and/or evidence of infection, and laboratory data. **Rationale:** Infection is a complication of paracentesis.

5.   Monitor intake and output. **Rationale:** Provides data for evaluation of fluid-balance status.

Expected Outcomes

1.   Evacuation of peritoneal fluid for laboratory analysis. **Rationale:** Assists in establishing a diagnosis and provides a direction for treatment.

2.   Decompression of peritoneal cavity. **Rationale:** Accumulated ascitic fluid within peritoneal space causes compression of abdominal and respiratory structures.

3.   Relief of respiratory compromise. **Rationale:** Accumulated ascitic fluid can cause respiratory compromise.

Unexpected Outcomes

1.   Perforation of bowel or bladder. **Rationale:** Intestines and bladder underlie the abdominal surface where needle access to the peritoneal cavity is performed.

2.   Local or systemic infection. **Rationale:** Invasive procedure into the peritoneal space provides portal of entry for microorganisms.

3.   Hypovolemia, hypotension. **Rationale:** Large amount of fluid shifting from intravascular space after procedure may lead to hypovolemia and significant decrease in blood pressure.

4.   Bleeding from paracentesis site. **Rationale:** Uncorrected clotting abnormalities or inadequate surgical hemostasis contributes to continued bleeding.

5.   Ascitic leak from paracentesis site. **Rationale:** Intraabdominal pressure may contribute to leakage of fluid out of the surgical wound.

Documentation

Documentation in the patient record should include date and time of procedure, patient tolerance of procedure, assessment of insertion site, occurrence of any unexpected outcomes, amount and characteristics of fluid removed, specimens sent for laboratory analysis, and postprocedure vital signs, respiratory status, and abdominal girth. **Rationale:** Documents nursing actions, patient response, and patient status.

Patient/Family Education

1.   Explain the indications and the procedure for paracentesis to both patient and family. **Rationale:** Encourages patient and family cooperation and understanding of procedure and participation during procedure.

2.   Explain the signs and symptoms to report to caregiver, such as fever, abdominal pain, decreased urine output, bleeding, and leakage of fluid from surgical wound site. **Rationale:** Unexpected outcomes may not manifest themselves for a period of time following the procedure.

Performance Checklist
Skill 19–1: Assisting with Paracentesis

Critical Behaviors	Complies yes	Complies no
1. Wash hands.		
2. Assist with preparation of equipment.		
3. Prepare insertion site.		
4. Assist with injection of local anesthetic.		
5. Assist with insertion of trocar.		
6. Assist with withdrawal of ascitic fluid.		
7. Record amount and characteristics of fluid.		
8. Monitor patient during procedure.		
9. Prepare and send fluid samples for laboratory analysis.		
10. Apply sterile dressing to insertion site.		
11. Dispose of equipment appropriately.		
12. Wash hands.		
13. Document procedure in patient record.		

SKILL 19–2

Assisting with Peritoneal Lavage

Peritoneal lavage is a procedure in which the peritoneal space is washed or cleansed with sterile fluid for diagnostic and therapeutic purposes. The peritoneal space is accessed using a needle, trocar, or soft, flexible tubing inserted into the lower abdomen.

Peritoneal lavage is performed most frequently in the evaluation and diagnosis of injuries following blunt trauma to the abdomen. The presence of blood, intestinal enzymes, or microorganisms in lavage returns assists in the diagnosis of organ injuries and in determining further treatment.

Peritoneal lavage also may be used for irrigation and cleansing of purulent exudate in peritonitis or intraabdominal abscess. Normal saline, dilute povidone-iodine, or antibacterial solutions are frequently used for therapeutic lavage.

Purpose

Peritoneal lavage is utilized to

1. Diagnose intraabdominal bleeding and organ injury through analysis of lavage returns.
2. Cleanse the peritoneum of purulent exudate for the treatment of peritonitis and abscess.

Prerequisite Knowledge and Skills

Prior to assisting with peritoneal lavage, the nurse should understand

1. Principles of universal precautions.
2. Anatomy and physiology of the lower quadrants of the abdomen.
3. Normal and abnormal composition of peritoneal fluid.

The nurse should be able to perform

1. Proper handwashing technique (see Skill 35–5).
2. Universal precautions (see Skill 35–1).
3. Abdominal assessment.
4. Urinary catheterization.
5. Bladder percussion.

Assessment

1. Assess the patient's history and symptoms for abdominal injury, peritonitis, or intraabdominal abscess. **Rationale:** Diagnosis and treatment of certain abdominal conditions may be accomplished with peritoneal lavage.
2. Assess the patient's baseline fluid status and serum electrolytes and proteins. **Rationale:** Lavage fluid may cause shifting of fluid out of the intravascular space, leading to the loss of fluid, electrolytes, and proteins from the vascular space.
3. Assess the patient for bladder distension. **Rationale:** Bladder distension increases the risk of bladder perforation during insertion of the trocar.
4. Assess the patient's PT, PTT, and platelet counts. **Rationale:** Abnormal clotting studies may increase the risk of bleeding during and after the procedure. Therapy may be necessary to correct clotting studies before initiation of procedure.

Nursing Diagnoses

1. Potential for infection related to invasive procedure. **Rationale:** Direct access into peritoneal cavity pro-

vides a mechanism for entry of microorganisms into the peritoneal space.

2. Potential for injury (bowel/bladder perforation) related to insertion of needle or trocar into the peritoneal space. **Rationale:** Intestines and bladder underlie abdominal surface where needle/trocar access is performed.

3. Potential fluid volume deficit related to intravascular fluid shifts into peritoneal space. **Rationale:** Fluid evacuation may cause compartment shifting of intravascular volume, essential serum electrolytes, and proteins, leading to intravascular depletion.

4. (Potential) Fluid volume excess related to inadequate drainage of lavage fluid. **Rationale:** Undrained lavage fluid may be absorbed into intravascular space.

5. (Potential) Ineffective breathing pattern related to indwelling lavage fluid. **Rationale:** Indwelling lavage fluid places pressure on diaphragm and intraabdominal organs, resulting in difficulty breathing.

Planning

1. Individualize the following patient goals for peritoneal lavage:
   a. Confirm diagnosis of internal abdominal injury. **Rationale:** Characteristics of lavage returns are used to diagnose certain abdominal injuries.
   b. Cleanse the peritoneum of purulent exudate. **Rationale:** Purulent fluid in the intraabdominal cavity is washed out with lavage fluid.

2. Assemble and prepare all necessary equipment and supplies. **Rationale:** Ensures that peritoneal lavage will be completed efficiently.
   a. Sterile gloves.
   b. Povidone-iodine solution.
   c. Sterile towels or sterile drape.
   d. Local anesthetic for injection.
   e. 5-cc syringe with 21- or 25-gauge needle.
   f. Trocar with stylet.
   g. Polyethylene tubing, 16 gauge, 12 to 18 cm long (optional).
   h. Two 10-cc syringes.
   i. Sterile tubes for specimens.
   j. Knife blade, no. 11.
   k. Three-way stopcock.
   l. Suture material with needle.
   m. Hemostat.
   n. 4 to 6 sterile gauze pads 4 × 4 in.
   o. Sterile gauze dressing with tape.
   p. Lavage fluid:
      (1) Diagnostic fluid: normal saline or Ringer's lactate
      (2) Therapeutic fluid: physician prescribed.
   q. Intravenous tubing.
   r. Drainage collector.

3. Prepare the patient.
   a. Explain the indications and the procedure for peritoneal lavage. **Rationale:** Decreases patient anxiety.
   b. Explain the patient's role in assisting with the procedure and postprocedure care. **Rationale:** Elicits patient cooperation during and after procedure.
   c. Have patient void or catheterize patient before procedure. **Rationale:** Distended bladder increases risk of nicking bladder during procedure. Palpate bladder to ensure decompression.
   d. Position patient as requested by physician. **Rationale:** Fluid accumulates in dependent areas. Usual position is supine, either flat or with head of bed elevated 30 degrees.

Implementation

Steps	Rationale	Special Considerations
1. Wash hands.	Reduces transmission of microorganisms.	
2. Assist physician with setup of sterile field and equipment.	Maintains aseptic technique.	
3. Set up lavage equipment: a. Attach IV tubing to lavage fluid, and clear tubing of air. b. Attach IV tubing to one port of three-way stopcock. c. Attach drainage collector to second port of three-way stopcock.	Provides closed system for instillation and drainage of lavage fluid.	
4. Prepare insertion site, and assist physician with insertion of trocar.	Trocar provides access to peritoneal cavity.	Inserted through small stab wound at midline, below umbilicus. Physician may withdraw fluid sample through trocar prior to lavage.

Table continues on following page

Steps	Rationale	Special Considerations
5. Attach trocar to remaining port of three-way stopcock (Fig. 19–3).	Completes closed lavage system.	
6. Instill lavage fluid: a. Turn stopcock off to drainage collector. b. Open clamp on IV tubing. c. Instill amount of fluid as requested by physician. d. Close clamp on IV tubing when infusion is completed.	Directs lavage fluid into peritoneal space.	Usual lavage fluid is 1 L normal saline or Ringer's lactate infused over 10 to 15 minutes.
7. Rotate patient side to side (if not contraindicated).	Facilitates sampling of fluid that may accumulate in pockets on either side.	
8. Drain lavage fluid: a. Turn stopcock off to IV tubing. b. Allow fluid to drain into drainage collector.	Directs lavage fluid from peritoneal space to drainage collector.	In therapeutic peritoneal lavage, the physician may order "dwell time," the amount of time the fluid remains within the cavity before draining.
9. Rotate patient side to side (if not contraindicated).	Facilitates drainage of fluid that may accumulate in pockets on either side.	
10. Repeat steps 6 to 9 as specified by physician.	Physician may request continued lavage to cleanse peritoneal space.	If repeat cycles are used, a soft peritoneal catheter is usually inserted.

Table continues on following page

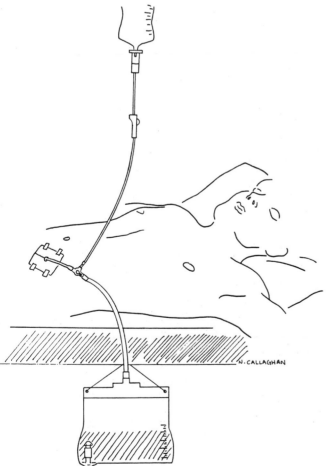

FIGURE 19–3 Continuous lavage system.

Steps	Rationale	Special Considerations
11. Calculate "true" drainage: Total drainage minus lavage fluid input.	Monitors fluid balance.	
12. Prepare and send fluid for laboratory analysis as requested by physician.	Laboratory analysis of fluid specimen provides information about patient status.	Routine laboratory tests include RBC and WBC counts, amylase, lipase, and culture and sensitivity.
13. Apply sterile dressing to insertion site after removal of trocar and wound closure.	Provides barrier to infection and collects fluid that may leak from wound site.	
14. Dispose of equipment in appropriate receptacle.	Universal precautions.	
15. Wash hands.	Reduces transmission of microorganisms.	

Evaluation

1. Evaluate visual and laboratory characteristics of lavage return. **Rationale:** Characteristics of lavage returns are used to diagnose patient conditions and to evaluate the effectiveness of the lavage procedure.
2. Monitor for changes in respiratory status (i.e., rate, depth, and pattern). **Rationale:** Indwelling lavage fluid places pressure on the diaphragm and intraabdominal organs, resulting in difficulty breathing.
3. Monitor for potential complications, including bowel/bladder perforation, bleeding, and intravascular volume loss. **Rationale:** Potential complications of insertion of trocar.
4. Monitor vital signs, temperature, and insertion site for drainage and/or evidence of infection. **Rationale:** Provides information on hemodynamic status and development of infection.

Expected Outcomes

1. Obtain lavage fluid returns for diagnostic evaluation. **Rationale:** Visual and laboratory analyses of lavage returns assist with diagnosis.
2. Cleanse peritoneum of purulent exudate and microorganisms. **Rationale:** Repeated lavaging of the peritoneum removes exudate and eliminates microorganisms.

Unexpected Outcomes

1. Perforation of bowel or bladder. **Rationale:** Intestines and bladder underlie the abdominal surface where access to the peritoneal space is performed.
2. Local or systemic infection. **Rationale:** Invasive procedure provides portal of entry for microorganisms.
3. Hypovolemia, hypotension. **Rationale:** Large fluid shifts into the peritoneal space may lead to hypovolemia and a significant decrease in blood pressure.

4. Hypervolemia. **Rationale:** Large fluid shifts into the intravascular space may lead to hypervolemia.
5. Inadequate drainage of lavage fluid. **Rationale:** Technical problems in lavage system or sequestering of fluid in dependent areas may lead to incomplete drainage of irrigant.
6. Bleeding from trocar insertion site. **Rationale:** Uncorrected clotting abnormalities or inadequate surgical hemostasis contributes to continued bleeding.
7. Respiratory compromise. **Rationale:** Instillation of large amount of lavage fluid increases intraabdominal pressure, leading to decreased diaphragmatic excursion.

Documentation

Documentation in the patient record should include date and time of procedure, patient tolerance of procedure, assessment of insertion site, occurrence of any unexpected outcomes, type and amount of lavage fluid instilled, amount and characteristics of lavage returns, specimens sent for laboratory analysis, and postprocedure vital signs. **Rationale:** Documents nursing interventions, patient response status, and expected/unexpected outcomes.

Patient/Family Education

1. Explain the indications and the procedure for peritoneal lavage to both patient and family. **Rationale:** Encourages patient and family cooperation and understanding of procedure and participation during procedure.
2. Explain signs and symptoms to report to caregiver, such as fever, abdominal pain, bleeding, leakage of fluid from wound site, and difficulty breathing. **Rationale:** Encourages patient and family participation in ongoing monitoring of procedure.

Performance Checklist
Skill 19–2:   Assisting with Peritoneal Lavage

Critical Behaviors	Complies	
	yes	no
1. Wash hands.		
2. Assist with equipment and sterile field setup.		
3. Set up lavage equipment.		
4. Prepare incision/puncture site, and assist with insertion of trocar.		
5. Attach trocar to stopcock.		
6. Instill lavage fluid.		
7. Rotate patient from side to side.		
8. Drain lavage fluid.		
9. Rotate patient from side to side.		
10. Repeat lavage sequence as requested.		
11. Calculate true drainage.		
12. Prepare and send fluid for laboratory analysis.		
13. Apply sterile dressing to wound site.		
14. Dispose of equipment appropriately.		
15. Wash hands.		
16. Document procedure in patient record.		

SKILL 19–3

Assisting with Bedside Upper Gastrointestinal Endoscopy

Endoscopy provides direct access to and visualization of the upper gastrointestinal tract. Endoscopy consists of passing a tube through the mouth, esophagus, and stomach into the proximal small intestine. A wide variety of rigid and flexible endoscopes, varying in size and length, are available for clinical use.

Once the upper gastrointestinal tract is accessed via the endoscope, numerous diagnostic and therapeutic procedures can be performed. Direct visual inspection of esophageal, stomach, and duodenal tissue can be accomplished. Removal of tissue samples for diagnostic evaluation through biopsy and washings may be performed.

Purpose

Bedside endoscopy is utilized to provide access to the upper gastrointestinal tract to

1.   Visualize structures and tissues of the upper gastrointestinal tract.
2.   Obtain tissue samples for laboratory analysis.
3.   Treat certain conditions of the upper gastrointestinal tract.

Prerequisite Knowledge and Skills

Prior to assisting with bedside endoscopy, the nurse should understand

1.   Principles of universal precautions.
2.   Anatomy and physiology of the upper gastrointestinal tract.
3.   Anatomy and physiology of the respiratory tract.
4.   Cardiac effects of vagal stimulation.

The nurse should be able to perform

1.   Proper handwashing technique (see Skill 35–5).
2.   Universal precautions (see Skill 35–1).
3.   Assessment of respiratory status.
4.   Interpretation of cardiac dysrhythmias.
5.   Insertion of an oral airway or bite block (see Skill 1–1).

Assessment

1.   Assess the patient's history and symptoms for factors indicating the need for direct access to the upper gastrointestinal tract, such as history of peptic ulceration, esophageal varices, upper gastrointestinal bleeding, carcinoma of upper gastrointestinal tract, esophageal stricture, vomiting, hiatus hernia, or pyloric obstruction. **Rationale:** Diagnosis and treatment of certain abnormalities may be accomplished with endoscopy.

2. Assess the patient's PT, PTT, and platelet count. **Rationale:** Abnormal clotting studies may increase the risk of bleeding during and after the procedure. It may be necessary to correct clotting studies before beginning the procedure.

3. Assess the patient's baseline cardiac rhythm. **Rationale:** Passage of a large-bore tube causes vagal stimulation with resultant cardiac dysrhythmias.

4. Assess the patient's baseline respiratory status (i.e., rate, depth, pattern, characteristics of secretion, and breath sounds). **Rationale:** Topical anesthesia in oropharynx may alter the gag reflex, thus increasing the risk of aspiration. Passage of a large-bore tube interferes with airway. Analgesics and sedatives may cause respiratory depression.

5. Assess the patient's stomach for accumulation of secretions or blood. **Rationale:** Accumulation of large amounts of secretions or blood decreases the ability to visualize tissue and structures and increases the risk of aspiration during the procedure.

Nursing Diagnoses

1. Potential for aspiration related to the passage of a large-bore tube through oropharynx. **Rationale:** Topical anesthesia applied to the oropharynx prior to passage of the tube may diminish the gag reflex and thus increase the risk of aspiration.

2. (Potential) Ineffective breathing pattern related to administration of analgesics and sedatives. **Rationale:** Patient requires a moderate degree of sedation prior to gastroscopy to facilitate cooperation.

3. Potential for injury related to insertion of a large-bore tube. **Rationale:** Passage and manipulation of the tube may injure tissues and structures of the upper gastrointestinal tract.

Planning

1. Individualize the following patient goals for bedside gastrointestinal endoscopy:
   a. Visualization of tissue and structures. **Rationale:** Endoscopy provides direct access to upper gastrointestinal tract.
   b. Tissue sampling. **Rationale:** Provides for diagnostic evaluation through biopsy and washings.
   c. Treatment of certain abnormalities. **Rationale:** The most common therapeutic procedures are removal of foreign bodies, scleral injection therapy, esophageal dilatation, pyloric dilatation, laser therapy, electrocoagulation and injection for bleeding lesions, and placement of tubes into the esophagus, stomach, and duodenum.

2. Ensure that a completed informed consent form is present in the patient record prior to initiating the procedure. **Rationale:** Requirement for performing an invasive procedure.

3. Assemble and prepare all necessary equipment and supplies. **Rationale:** Ensures that bedside endoscopy will be completed efficiently.
   a. Endoscope and accessories as requested by physician.
   b. Suction setup with connecting tubing.
   c. Nonsterile gloves.
   d. Water-soluble lubricant.
   e. Topical anesthesia.
   f. Oral airway or bite block.
   g. Two 30- to 50-cc syringes.
   h. Normal saline or tap water for irrigation.
   i. Pulse oximeter (optional).
   j. Automatic blood pressure device (optional).
   k. Gastric lavage equipment (if needed).
   l. Premedication as prescribed by physician.
   m. Emergency intubation equipment.
   n. Endotracheal suction equipment.

4. Prepare the patient.
   a. Explain the indications and the procedure for bedside endoscopy. **Rationale:** Decreases patient's anxiety.
   b. Explain the patient's role in assisting with the procedure and postprocedure care. **Rationale:** Elicits patient cooperation during and after procedure.
   c. Place the patient on a cardiac monitor and evaluate rhythm. **Rationale:** Cardiac dysrhythmias may occur during passage of a large-bore tube secondary to vagal stimulation.
   d. Place a pulse oximeter and automatic blood pressure device on the patient (if an arterial line is not in place). **Rationale:** Allows for continuous assessment of respiratory status and blood pressure throughout the procedure.
   e. Ensure a venous access. **Rationale:** Venous access is required for administration of premedication and in case of emergency.
   f. Keep patient NPO or allow *only* clear liquids 8 to 12 hours prior to procedure. **Rationale:** Undigested material in stomach increases the risk of aspiration and decreases visualization of tissue.
   g. Position patient as requested. Usual position: left lateral with head of bed elevated 30 degrees. **Rationale:** Positioning patient appropriately facilitates passage of endoscope into stomach and prevents aspiration.
   h. Premedicate patient as prescribed by physician. Common sedatives: diazepam, midazolam, meperidine. Vagal lytic: atropine. **Rationale:** Light sedation decreases patient anxiety and provides cooperation during procedure. Vagal lytic agent protects against profound bradycardia during insertion of endoscope.

Implementation

Steps	Rationale	Special Considerations
1. Wash hands.	Prevents transmission of microorganisms.	
2. Don nonsterile gloves.	Universal precautions.	
3. Remove dentures, if appropriate.	Dentures may interfere with safe passage of the endoscope.	
4. Perform or assist physician with gastric lavage, if necessary (see Skill 18–2).	Large amounts of blood or clots will obstruct visualization of tissue and increase risk of aspiration.	Monitor heart rate and respiratory status during lavage.
5. Assist physician with insertion of endoscope:	Endoscope provides visualization of esophagus, stomach, and duodenum.	*Caution*: Patient's gag and cough reflexes may be compromised by topical anesthesia, increasing the risk of aspiration. *Keep emergency intubation equipment available.*
a. Anesthetize posterior oropharynx with topical agent.	Decreases discomfort caused by passage of scope.	
b. Insert oral airway or bite block.	Prevents patient from biting on endoscope or inserter's fingers.	
c. Lubricate 10 to 15 cm distal end of scope.	Minimizes mucosal injury and irritation during insertion.	
d. Encourage patient to simulate swallowing while endoscope is being passed.	Swallowing maneuver causes epiglottis to close trachea and directs endoscope into esophagus.	
6. Inject air or irrigant via endoscope as requested.	Expands tissue folds and cleanses area to increase visualization of tissue.	Patient may have gastric distension or belching after procedure due to air insertion.
7. Apply suction via endoscope as requested.	Evacuates secretions and irrigant as needed to improve visualization of tissue.	
8. Assist with obtaining tissue sample(s) as requested.	Analysis of tissue samples aids in diagnostic evaluation of patient.	Specimens may be obtained by direct biopsy, brush techniques, or tissue washing techniques.
9. Prepare and send tissue samples for laboratory analysis as requested.	Laboratory analysis provides information about patient status.	
10. Dispose of equipment in appropriate receptacle.	Universal precautions.	
11. Wash hands.	Reduces transmission of microorganisms.	

Evaluation

1. Evaluate blood pressure, heart rate/rhythm, and respiratory rate and SaO$_2$ in light of patient's baseline vital signs. **Rationale:** Gastrointestinal bleeding may occur after procedure.

2. Monitor for signs of gastrointestinal bleeding. **Rationale:** Gastrointestinal bleeding may occur after procedure.

3. Assess pharyngeal function, and keep patient NPO until return of normal pharyngeal function. **Rationale:** Pharyngeal function may be compromised after topical anesthesia.

Expected Outcomes

1. Visualization and sampling of tissue and structures of upper gastrointestinal tract. **Rationale:** For confirmation of medical diagnosis.

2. Successful institution of therapeutic modalities. **Rationale:** A variety of therapeutic procedures can be performed via endoscopy.

Unexpected Outcomes

1. Bleeding from upper gastrointestinal tract. **Rationale:** Injury to tissue during procedure may cause bleeding.

2. Inadequate visualization of tissue and structures. **Rationale:** Accumulated secretions or bleeding may interfere with visualization of tissue. Patient's intolerance of procedure may necessitate premature discontinuance.

3. Esophageal perforation. **Rationale:** Perforation is more likely to occur with use of a rigid endoscope, extension of ulceration, patient agitation, or passage of the endoscope through weakened tissue.

4. Aspiration. **Rationale:** Compromised pharyngeal function with an accumulation of blood and secretions in the stomach predisposes the patient to aspiration.

Documentation

Documentation in the patient record should include date and time of procedure, baseline vital signs, premedications administered, patient tolerance of procedure, specimens obtained during the procedure, specific therapeutic procedures performed during the endoscopy, occurrence of any unexpected outcomes and interventions instituted, postprocedure vital signs, assessments of gag and cough reflexes after the procedure, and re-

sumption of oral intake and patient's tolerance. **Rationale:** Provides documentation, nursing care given, expected and unexpected outcomes, and interventions taken.

Patient/Family Education

1. Explain the indications and the procedure for endoscopy to both patient and family. **Rationale:** Encourages patient and family cooperation and understanding and participation during procedure.

2. Explain the indications and any specific therapeutic modalities to be performed. **Rationale:** Increases patient and family understanding of treatment.

3. Explain the signs and symptoms to report to caregiver, such as fever, chest pain, difficulty swallowing, or bleeding. **Rationale:** Some unexpected outcomes may present a considerable amount of time after the procedure.

4. Explain the progression of diet after procedure. **Rationale:** Decreases risk of aspiration until full return of the gag reflex.

Performance Checklist
Skill 19–3: Assisting with Bedside Upper Gastrointestinal Endoscopy

Critical Behaviors	Complies	
	yes	no
1. Wash hands.		
2. Don nonsterile gloves.		
3. Remove denture (if appropriate).		
4. Perform or assist with gastric lavage, if needed.		
5. Assist with insertion of endoscope.		
6. Inject air and irrigant as requested.		
7. Apply suction as requested.		
8. Assist with obtaining tissue sample(s).		
9. Process tissue samples.		
10. Dispose of equipment appropriately.		
11. Wash hands.		
12. Document procedure in patient record.		

SKILL 19–4

Assisting with Bedside Sigmoidoscopy

Sigmoidoscopy provides direct access to the distal portion of the lower gastrointestinal tract. Sigmoidoscopy consists of passing a tube through the anus and rectum into the sigmoid colon. A wide variety of rigid or flexible sigmoidoscopes, varying in size and length, are available for clinical use.

Once the distal portion of the lower gastrointestinal

tract is accessed via the sigmoidoscope, direct visual inspection of rectal and sigmoid tissue is possible. Removal of tissue samples for diagnostic evaluation through biopsy and tissue washings may be performed.

Purpose

Sigmoidoscopy is utilized to access the distal portion of the lower gastrointestinal tract to

1. Diagnose and treat abnormalities.
2. Obtain tissue samples for laboratory analysis.

Prerequisite Knowledge and Skills

Prior to assisting with sigmoidoscopy, the nurse should understand

1. Principles of universal precautions.
2. Anatomy and physiology of the lower gastrointestinal tract.
3. Cardiac effects of vagal stimulation.

The nurse should be able to perform

1. Proper handwashing technique (see Skill 35–5).
2. Universal precautions.
3. Interpretation of cardiac dysrhythmias.

Assessment

1. Assess the patient's history and symptoms for factors indicating the need for direct access to lower gastrointestinal tract, such as lower gastrointestinal bleeding, changes in bowel routine, abdominal distension, and abdominal pain. **Rationale**: Diagnosis and treatment of certain conditions of the lower gastrointestinal tract may be accomplished through sigmoidoscopy.
2. Assess the patient's PT, PTT, and platelet count. **Rationale:** Abnormal coagulation studies may increase the risk of bleeding during or after the procedure. Therapy may be necessary to correct clotting studies before initiation of the procedure.
3. Identify the patient's baseline cardiac rhythm. **Rationale:** Passage of a large-bore tube via the rectum causes vagal stimulation, possibly resulting in cardiac dysrhythmias.
4. Assess the patient's rectum and distal colon for the presence of stool. **Rationale:** The presence of stool in the rectum or sigmoid colon interferes with direct visualization of tissues and structures. Enemas may be needed to cleanse the bowel of stool prior to initiating the procedure.

Nursing Diagnosis

Potential for injury related to passage of a tube into the rectum and sigmoid colon. **Rationale:** Passage and manipulation of tube may injure tissue and structures of the lower gastrointestinal tract.

Planning

1. Individualize the following patient goals for sigmoidoscopy:
   a. Visualization of tissue and structures of the rec-

tum and sigmoid colon. **Rationale:** Provides direct access to lower gastrointestinal tract.
   b. Tissue sampling. **Rationale:** For laboratory analysis and diagnostic evaluation.
   c. Treatment of selected abnormalities of rectum and sigmoid colon. **Rationale:** The most common therapeutic procedures performed via the sigmoidoscope include removal of polyps, coagulation of bleeding lesions, reduction of volvulus, removal of foreign bodies, decompression of an atonically distended colon, and dilatation of strictures.
2. Ensure that a completed informed consent form is present in the patient record prior to initiating the procedure. **Rationale:** Requirement for performing an invasive procedure.
3. Assemble and prepare all necessary equipment and supplies. **Rationale:** Ensures that sigmoidoscopy will be completed efficiently.
   a. Sigmoidoscope and accessories as requested.
   b. Suction setup with connecting tubing.
   c. Nonsterile gloves.
   d. Water-soluble lubricant.
   e. Two 30- to 50-cc syringes.
   f. Normal saline or tap water for irrigation.
   g. Pulse oximeter (optional).
   h. Automatic blood pressure device (optional).
   i. Premedication as requested.
4. Prepare the patient.
   a. Explain the indications and the procedure for sigmoidoscopy. **Rationale:** Decreases patient and family anxiety.
   b. Explain the patient's role in assisting with the procedure. **Rationale:** Elicits patient cooperation during the procedure.
   c. Cleanse the patient's rectum and sigmoid colon prior to examination (usual prep: Fleets enema or soapsuds enema). **Rationale:** Presence of stool decreases visualization of tissues and structures.
   d. Place the patient on a cardiac monitor. **Rationale:** Cardiac dysrhythmias may occur during passage of a large-bore tube via the rectum.
   e. Place a pulse oximeter and automatic blood pressure device on the patient (if an arterial line is not in place). **Rationale:** Allows for continuous assessment of respiratory status and blood pressure throughout the procedure.
   f. Premedicate patient as prescribed (common sedatives: diazepam, midazolam, meperidine). **Rationale:** Some patients require light sedation to relax and cooperate during the procedure.
   g. Position patient as requested. Usual position: left lateral, flat. **Rationale:** Facilitates passage of sigmoidoscope.
   h. Support patient during digital rectal examination. **Rationale:** Provides initial examination of rectum and evaluation of bowel cleansing.

Implementation

Steps	Rationale	Special Considerations
1. Wash hands.	Prevents transmission of microorganisms.	
2. Don nonsterile gloves.	Universal precautions.	
3. Lubricate distal 10 to 15 cm of sigmoidoscope (Fig. 19–4).	Minimizes mucosal injury and irritation during insertion of sigmoidoscope.	Use water-soluble lubricant.
4. Assist physician with insertion of sigmoidoscope.	For direct visualization.	Physician may request assistance with advancing sigmoidoscope.
5. Inject air or irrigant via sigmoidoscope as requested.	Expands tissue folds and cleanses area to improve visualization.	
6. Apply suction via sigmoidoscope as requested.	Evacuates secretions and irrigant as needed to improve visualization.	
7. Assist with obtaining tissue samples as requested.	Analysis of tissue samples aids in diagnostic evaluation.	
8. Prepare and send tissue samples for laboratory analysis.	Laboratory analysis provides information about patient status.	
9. Comfort patient during manipulation of scope.	Mild to moderate abdominal discomfort occurs with manipulation of sigmoidoscope.	Encourage patient to relax abdominal muscles and take deep breaths.
10. Dispose of equipment in appropriate receptacle.	Universal precautions.	
11. Wash hands.	Reduces transmission of microorganisms.	

Evaluation

1. Evaluate the patient's blood pressure, heart rate/rhythm, respiratory rate, SaO_2, temperature, abdominal/rectal pain, and rectal bleeding in light of baseline values. **Rationale:** Evaluates patient's tolerance of procedure and postprocedure status.

2. Monitor for complications of procedure, such as rectal bleeding and bowel perforation. **Rationale:** Instrumentation of the gastrointestinal tract may result in tissue injury.

3. Monitor for abdominal distension secondary to instillation of air during the procedure. **Rationale:** Disten-

sion may cause significant patient discomfort, which may be relieved with a flatus tube or bag.

Expected Outcomes

1. Visualization and sampling of tissues and structures. **Rationale:** Supports diagnostic evaluation of distal lower portion of gastrointestinal tract.

2. Successful institution of therapeutic modality(s). **Rationale:** A variety of therapeutic procedures may be conducted with sigmoidoscopy.

Unexpected Outcomes

1. Bleeding from rectum or sigmoid colon. **Rationale:** Sigmoidoscope may tear or otherwise injure weakened, ulcerated tissue.

2. Inadequate visualization of tissues and structures. **Rationale:** Retained stool, bleeding, or obstruction may interfere with visualization of tissue. Patient intolerance to procedure may necessitate premature discontinuance.

3. Perforation of rectum or sigmoid colon. **Rationale:** Perforation may occur with use of a rigid sigmoidoscope, extension of tissue lesion, patient agitation, or passage of the sigmoidoscope through weakened tissue.

Documentation

Documentation in the patient record should include date and time of procedure, baseline and postprocedure

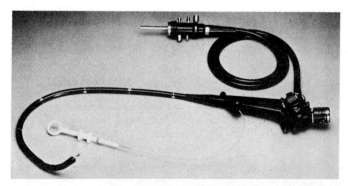

FIGURE 19–4 Flexible sigmoidoscope. (Reprinted with permission from R. M. Katon, E. B. Keefe, and C. S. Melnyk, *Flexible Sigmoidoscopy*. New York: Grune & Stratton, 1985, p. 64.)

vital signs, premedications administered, patient tolerance of procedure, occurrence of any unexpected outcomes and interventions taken, specimens obtained and processed during procedure, and specific therapeutic procedures performed during sigmoidoscopy. **Rationale:** Documents nursing care given, expected and unexpected outcomes, and interventions taken.

Patient/Family Education

1. Explain the indications and the procedure for sigmoidoscopy to both patient and family. **Rationale:** Encourages patient and family cooperation and understanding and participation during procedure.

2. Explain the indications and any specific interventions to be performed during the procedure. **Rationale:** Increases patient and family understanding of treatment.

3. Explain the signs and symptoms to report to caregiver, such as fever, rectal pain, difficulty passing stool, and bleeding. **Rationale:** Some unexpected outcomes may manifest at a considerable period of time after completion of the procedure.

Performance Checklist
Skill 19–4   Assisting with Bedside Sigmoidoscopy

Critical Behaviors	Complies yes	no
1. Wash hands.		
2. Don nonsterile gloves.		
3. Lubricate sigmoidoscope.		
4. Assist with insertion of scope.		
5. Inject air or irrigant via scope.		
6. Apply suction as requested.		
7. Assist with obtaining tissue samples.		
8. Prepare and send tissue samples for laboratory analysis.		
9. Comfort patient during scope manipulation.		
10. Dispose of equipment appropriately.		
11. Wash hands.		
12. Document procedure in patient record.		

BIBLIOGRAPHY

Dent, T. L., Strodel, W. E., and Turcotte, J. B. (1985). *Surgical Endoscopy*. Chicago: Year Book Medical Publishers.

Drossman, D. A. (Ed.) (1987). *Manual of Gastroenterologic Procedures*, 2d Ed. New York: Raven Press.

Knezevich, B. A. (1986). *Trauma Nursing: Principles and Practices*. Norwalk, Conn.: Appleton-Century-Crofts.

Millar, S., Sampson, L. K., and Soukup, M. (1985). *AACN Procedure Manual for Critical Care*, 2d Ed. Philadelphia: Saunders.

Persons, C. B. (1987). *Critical Care Procedures and Protocols: A Nursing Process Approach*. Philadelphia: Lippincott.

Schapiro, M., and Lehman, G. B. (Eds.) (1990). *Flexible Sigmoidoscopy: Techniques and Utilization*. Baltimore: Williams & Wilkins.

Siegal, B. (1986). *Diagnostic Patient Studies in Surgery*. Philadelphia: Lea & Febiger.

Sivak, M. V. (1987). *Gastroenterologic Endoscopy*. Philadelphia: Saunders.

20

STOMA/FISTULA MANAGEMENT

BEHAVIORAL OBJECTIVES

After completing this chapter, the nurse will be able to

- Define the key terms.
- Describe methods of stoma/fistula discharge containment.
- Describe the principles of peristomal skin protection.
- Demonstrate the skills involved in stoma/fistula management.
- Develop a nursing care plan for stoma/fistula management.

The focus of stoma/fistula management is the collection of discharge while protecting surrounding tissue. A *stoma* or *ostomy* is a surgically created opening in the large bowel (colostomy), small bowel (ileostomy), or urinary system (a urostomy). Each requires specific stomal and peristomal care, pouches, and barriers.

Effective and consistent discharge containment will control odor, protect peristomal skin, facilitate volume and electrolyte replacement when indicated, and provide patient comfort. Stoma and fistula care is a clean procedure requiring only examination gloves to comply with universal precautions.

This chapter will address containment of stoma/fistula discharge and the attendant peristomal skin care and irrigation of a colostomy. Examples of commercial products to be discussed in this chapter include barriers (also called wafers or flanges), pouches, adhesives, skin sealants, powders, and paste or caulk.

KEY TERMS

colostomy	*mucocutaneous junction*
denuded	*peristomal/perifistula skin*
fistula	*stoma*
hyperkeratosis	*stoma necrosis*
ileal/colon conduit	*transverse colostomy*
Koch pouch (continent	*urostomy*
stoma)	

SKILLS

20–1   Stoma Pouching
20–2   Fistula/Draining-Wound Pouching
20–3   Colostomy Irrigation

GUIDELINES

The following assessment guidelines assist the nurse in formulating a nursing diagnosis and an individualized plan of care for a patient with a stoma and/or a fistula:

1. Know the type of stoma or the reason for the fistula.
2. Know the patient's prior stoma management for the previously created stoma.
3. Assess stoma viability and peristomal/fistula skin condition.
4. Assess the nature and volume of output.
5. Become familiar with available pouching equipment within your institution.
6. Determine appropriate intervals for pouch emptying and change.

SKILL 20–1

Stoma Pouching

Stoma discharge is contained by applying a collecting pouch with a protective skin barrier or wafer (Fig. 20–1*A* to *C*). Colostomy/ileostomy discharge is contained in an open-end pouch with a clamp for ease in emptying. For the bedridden or supine patient, the pouch may be angled to the side to facilitate emptying. The opening in the protective skin barrier or flange is sized to fit ⅛-in (0.5-cm) around the base of the stoma. The ⅛-in (0.5-cm) sizing adjustment allows for the peristaltic movement that occurs in the stoma. Paste is used to caulk this small area so that no peristomal skin is exposed.

Urine from a urostomy is collected in a pouch with a drain spigot (Fig. 20–1*D*), preferably one with an antireflux membrane. The urinary drain pouch is always connected to drainage when the patient is in bed. The urinary stoma may be pouched with either a barrier that is highly resistant to urine or a pouch with only an adhesive backing. When using an adhesive-backed urinary pouch, the opening may be cut wider than the stoma because urine flowing freely over the skin does not cause skin irritation. Skin is only irritated by urine when it is allowed to pool around the stoma, leading to hyperkeratosis from the continual maceration of the peristomal area. If urine is highly alkaline, usually a result of insufficient water intake, alkaline crystals may form on the stoma. Any condition causing a change in the balance of normal skin flora combined with the continual moisture places the

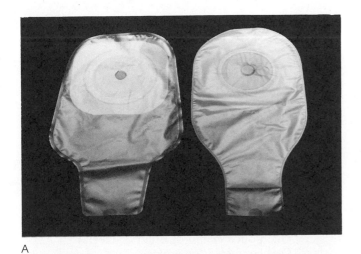

A

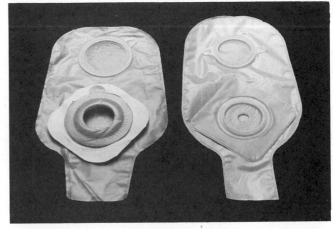

C

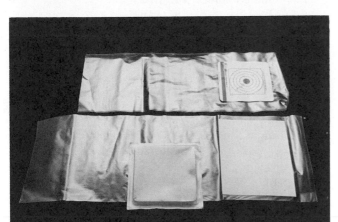

B

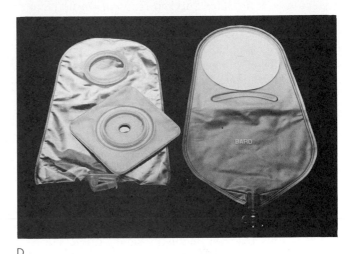

D

FIGURE 20–1. Colostomy pouches. (*A*) One-piece precut or cut-to-fit open-end pouches with an attached skin barrier (Hollister and ConvaTec). (*B*) Two-piece open-end pouches with a barrier and flange (Hollister and ConvaTec). (*C*) Pouches that may be custom cut (United and Bard) and added to a skin barrier (United). (*D*) Urostomy pouches with a drain spout (ConvaTec and Bard).

person with a urinary stoma at increased risk to develop a peristomal fungal infection. A fungal infection requires specific treatment with an antifungal powder because it will spread rapidly, denude the skin, and make pouch adhesion difficult, as well as cause patient discomfort.

When properly applied, a pouch should provide 3 to 5 days' wear. The pouch is routinely emptied whenever it is one-half to one-third full.

Purpose

The nurse performs the stoma pouching to

1. Contain bowel/bladder discharge.
2. Protect the peristomal skin.
3. Control odor,
4. Maintain patient comfort.

Prerequisite Knowledge and Skills

Prior to applying a stoma pouch, the nurse should understand

1. Anatomy and physiology of altered bowel/bladder elimination.
2. Anatomy and physiology of the skin.
3. Universal precautions.
4. Common concerns related to altered body image.

The nurse should be able to perform

1. Proper handwashing technique (see Skill 35–5).
2. Universal precautions (see Skill 35–1).
3. Correct selection and sizing of pouch.

Assessment

1. Observe for indications of pouch leakage, including odor, patient complaint or evidence of itching, and burning or wetness around stoma or pouch. **Rationale:** Physical signs resulting from leakage under faceplate or pouch barrier necessitate an immediate change.
2. Note quantity and nature of discharge. **Rationale:** Provides data to assess and monitor gastrointestinal/genitourinary function.
3. Observe the condition of the stoma, such as size

(in centimeters), height (in centimeters), color, and presence or absence of edema. **Rationale:** Physical signs reflect stoma viability; determines proper pouch size.

4.   Observe the condition of the peristomal skin. **Rationale:** Detects any irritation.

5.   Assess the patient's attitude toward the stoma and its care. **Rationale:** Provides information regarding the patient's coping mechanisms with a body image disturbance.

Nursing Diagnoses

1.   Bowel incontinence related to ostomy surgery. **Rationale:** Surgical revision of bowel/bladder system alters elimination pattern.

2.   Altered patterns of urinary elimination related to cystectomy. **Rationale:** Surgical removal of the bladder alters elimination pattern.

3.   Potential for impaired skin integrity related to bowel/bladder/fistula discharge. **Rationale:** Feces/urine/fistula drainage will irritate peristomal/perifistula skin.

4.   Knowledge deficit related to stoma management. **Rationale:** Creation of a stoma requires learning new skills for self-care.

5.   Body image disturbance related to alteration in bowel/bladder elimination and feelings of loss of control. **Rationale:** Physical changes caused by surgery and loss of continence usually result in altered perception of body image.

6.   Potential for sexual dysfunction related to damage of parasympathetic/sympathetic nerves. **Rationale:** Wide bowel resection or cystectomy may damage nerves, resulting in impotence for men and vaginal dryness or contour for women.

Planning

1.   Develop individualized goals for stoma pouching to maintain an intact pouching system. **Rationale:** Con-

tained stoma discharge maintains skin integrity, eliminates odor, increases patient comfort, and provides a sense of security.

2.   Select and prepare all necessary supplies. **Rationale:** Assembly of all necessary supplies ensures pouch change will be completed quickly and efficiently.
a.   Appropriate pouch and barrier.
b.   Paste.
c.   Skin sealant.
d.   Powder (if appropriate).
e.   One set clean scissors.
f.   Deodorant/ostomy cleaner.
g.   Two to three wet wash cloths.
h.   One dry cloth or towel.
i.   One pair exam gloves.
j.   One pouch clamp or drain connector.
k.   One container for drainage.
l.   One disposable underpad.
m.   One roll of 2-in nonallergic paper tape.
n.   One plastic bag for disposal of pouch.
o.   4 x 4 gauze pads (for urinary stoma).

3.   Prepare the patient and family.
a.   Explain the procedure to the patient and family. **Rationale:** Patient and family will begin to learn steps in pouch change.
b.   Explain the degree of participation expected from the patient. **Rationale:** Patient and family become involved with physical/emotional adaptation.
c.   Place the patient in the position to best empty, remove, and reapply the pouch. **Rationale:** Slightly turning patient to the affected side enhances gravity flow for pouch emptying and may provide the best body contour for application of the pouch.

Implementation

Steps	Rationale	Special Considerations
1. Wash hands.	Reduces transmission of microorganisms.	
2. Don exam gloves.	Universal precautions.	
3. Remove old clamp and set aside (if urinary, save bedside drain bag connector).	Can be reused when new pouch is applied.	
4. Empty contents from old pouch.	Prevents spillage during removal.	Fold back cuff of pouch before emptying to keep from soiling bottom edges of pouch.
5. Gently remove pouch by supporting skin while pulling pouch up and away.	Prevents adhesive from denuding the skin.	To facilitate removal, use warm water. To control odor, spray a small amount of deodorant in the room prior to opening or removing the pouch.

Table continues on following page

Steps	Rationale	Special Considerations
6. Dispose of old pouch in plastic bag, and place in appropriate receptacle.	Pouches cannot go into sewer systems. Plastic bag contains odor and leakage of body fluids.	
7. Gently wash the stoma and surrounding peristomal skin with warm water and pat dry. Do *not* use soap because it leaves a residue and is drying to the skin.	Removes feces or urine.	Stoma may bleed slightly. This is normal. If stoma is new, observe for intact sutures, color, and absence or presence of stents.
8. When pouching a urinary stoma, take 4 x 4's and make a roll, and apply the gauze rolls as a wick on the stoma to keep the skin clean and dry.	Urinary stomas discharge continuously.	Best time to change is in the early morning if no fluid was consumed overnight. If patient is on IV hydration only, this will not apply. *Exception*: A continent urostomy (Koch pouch) does not empty spontaneously. It must be catheterized and drained.
9. Measure stoma: Make a pattern by placing a clear piece of plastic over the stoma and drawing the outline of stoma.	Opening must be made ⅛-in (0.5-cm) larger than stoma.	If stoma is oval, the opening must be made oval-shaped. Be careful not to reverse the pattern if stoma is not round.
10. Select and prepare appropriate skin barrier and pouch (Table 20–1):	Improves "wearing time" of the pouch.	
a. Trace stoma pattern onto the paper back of the pouch barrier or flange, and cut out opening in the barrier.	Provides a custom fit for the stoma (Fig. 20–2).	Adjust pattern accordingly if pouch will be applied sideways for the patient who is primarily supine.
b. If using a Karaya pouch, select the appropriate size.	Karaya ring or precut pouches also must have ⅛-in (0.5-cm) allowance.	Karaya does not hold up well to urine. Karaya pouches may require a belt if there is no surrounding collar of paper tape.
11. Remove protective paper backing from barrier, and set barrier aside.	In order to adhere to the skin.	Do not touch adhesive back.
12. Check that the peristomal skin is still clean and dry.	Discharge may be expelled at any time.	This is an important step. Barriers will not stick to wet skin. Rewash and dry if necessary.
13. Apply the protective skin sealant around the stoma where barrier and tape will be applied.	Protects the skin from denuding when pouch is removed.	If skin is denuded, first apply a light dusting of stoma powder and *then* skin sealant.

Table continues on following page

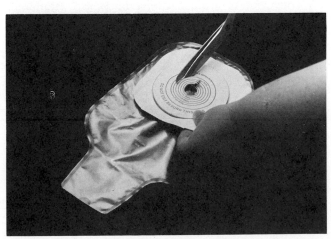

FIGURE 20–2. The adhesive barrier backing of the pouch is cut ⅛ in (0.5 cm) larger than the stoma.

Steps	Rationale	Special Considerations
14. Apply a ring of stoma paste around the base of the stoma *or* around the cutout opening on the adhesive side of barrier.	Fills in or caulks the ⅛-in (0.5-cm) opening and protects peristomal skin.	Do *not* use with urinary stoma. Urine will wash paste away.
15. Fit barrier around stoma, and seal in place with gentle pressure:	Eliminate cracks or channels for the urine or stool to flow through.	Adhesive-backed pouches without a barrier may be slightly more difficult to apply. Carefully slit the paper backing into four sections, peeling off one section at a time as it is applied to the skin.
a. Attach pouch to barrier if two-piece system is used, and apply as one-piece unit.	For easier application.	
b. Apply pouch sideways if patient is primarily supine.	Facilitates emptying when patient is supine.	
16. Apply clamp to bottom of pouch, folding over *only* once.	Prevents stretching plastic clamps.	When unclasping pouch for emptying, fold a cuff back to prevent soiling entire pouch with stool. A very small amount of ostomy soap (Peri-wash) or deodorant may be sprayed into the bottom of the pouch after emptying to help neutralize odor and keep feces from sticking to the pouch.
17. For urinary pouch, attach to bedside drainage bag.	Provides continuous drainage and prevents pooling of urine around stoma.	
18. Place soiled equipment and refuse in appropriate receptacles.	Universal precautions.	
19. Wash hands.	Reduces transmission of microorganisms.	

Evaluation

1. Evaluate the patient for odor, complaints or evidence of itching and burning, and wetness around the stoma or pouch. **Rationale:** Indicates that pouching system is not intact and will need to be reapplied.
2. Evaluate integrity of peristomal skin. **Rationale:** Signs and symptoms of denuded skin indicate that the seal around the stoma is not intact.
3. Evaluate the amount and nature of the discharge. **Rationale:** Evidence of how colostomy/ileostomy/urostomy is functioning.

Expected Outcomes

1. Pouch remains secure. **Rationale:** Discharge is contained.
2. Peristomal skin remains intact. **Rationale:** Prevents secondary infections and patient discomfort.

Unexpected Outcomes

1. Peristomal skin is damaged or denuded. **Rationale:** Previous pouches did not have an intact seal, resulting in leakage of discharge on peristomal skin with subsequent breakdown.
2. Odor, complaint or evidence of itching and burning, or wetness around stoma or pouch. **Rationale:** Pouching system is not intact. A new pouch will need to be applied.
3. Absence of discharge. **Rationale:** May signal surgical emergency because colostomy/ileostomy/urostomy is malfunctioning. *Exception:* A continent ileostomy/urostomy (Koch pouch) will not discharge spontaneously. Such a pouch must be catheterized.

Documentation

Documentation in the patient record should include date and time of procedure, the condition of the stoma, mucocutaneous junction, and peristomal skin; the amount and nature of discharge; type of pouch applied; and the patient's response to the procedure (i.e., ability to look at stoma, assist with the procedure). **Rationale:** Documents nursing care given, the condition of the stoma

TABLE 20–1 Product Selection Guide for Stoma Pouching

Product	Use	Examples
Drainable pouches: 1. One-piece vs. two-piece 2. Starter opening vs. precut opening 3. With or without skin barrier attached	For fecal ostomies that need frequent emptying.	Hollister Convatec United Bard NuHope
Urinary pouches: 1. One-piece vs. two-piece 2. Starter opening vs. precut opening 3. With or without skin barrier attached 4. With or without antireflux valve	To collect urine and provide an easy spout for emptying and connecting to bedside drainage.	Bard United Cymed Hollister Convatec NuHope
Closed-end pouches: 1. One-piece vs. two-piece 2. With or without skin barrier attached	To collect any unexpected discharge between colostomy irrigations.	Hollister Convatec
Skin barriers: 1. Pectin based 2. Karaya based 3. Preattached to pouch 4. Separate wafer	To protect the skin from stomal discharge and provide support for pouch.	Stomahesive Premium Barrier Reliaseal United Barrier
Pastes: 1. Pectin based 2. Karaya based	To protect the inner-pouch seal around the stoma, increasing pouch wearing time.	Stomahesive Paste Premium Paste Karaya Paste

and peristomal area, patient's adaptation to an altered body image, and expected and unexpected outcomes.

Patient/Family Education

1. Assess the ability and readiness of the patient and family to begin participation in stoma care. **Rationale:** Psychomotor and/or cognitive impairment may necessitate delaying patient and family teaching.
2. Discuss and demonstrate preparation of pouch and supplies for pouch change with both patient and family. **Rationale:** Encourages acceptance and understanding and enables the patient and family to ask questions.
3. Explain the need for regular emptying of pouch. **Rationale:** Scheduled emptying prevents leakage.
4. Explain to the patient and family the need for home care follow-up, and initiate an enterostomal therapy nurse referral if available. **Rationale:** Adjustment and learning of new skills for ostomy care take place over time and are facilitated by a nurse trained in this specialty.

Performance Checklist
Skill 20–1:   Stoma Pouching

Critical Behaviors	Complies yes	no
1. Wash hands.		
2. Don exam gloves.		
3. Remove and set aside pouch clamp or drain connector.		
4. Empty contents from pouch without soiling patient.		
5. Remove old pouch.		
6. Dispose of old pouch correctly.		
7. Gently wash the peristomal skin and stoma, and pat dry.		
8. For a urinary stoma, apply gauze rolls as a wick to keep skin clean and dry.		
9. Measure stoma.		

Table continues on following page

Critical Behaviors	Complies	
	yes	no
10. Select and prepare appropriate skin barrier and pouch.		
11. Remove protective backing from barrier, and set barrier aside.		
12. Check that peristomal skin is still clean and dry.		
13. Apply protective skin sealant around stoma.		
14. Apply a ring of stoma paste around stomal base or cutout opening on adhesive side of barrier.		
15. Fit barrier around stoma, and seal with gentle pressure.		
16. Apply clamp to bottom of pouch.		
17. For urinary pouch, attach to bedside drainage bag.		
18. Discard soiled equipment and refuse properly.		
19. Wash hands.		
20. Document procedure in patient record.		

SKILL 20–2

Fistula/Draining-Wound Pouching

The discharge from a fistula or draining wound can have wide variations in both amount and type. The opening of a fistula may be irregularly shaped and located almost anywhere in the body. There are preassembled wound-management pouches with an attached barrier and access door that work well for draining incisional wounds or drain sites requiring frequent access for packing, irrigation, or manipulation of the drain. A custom pouch made of barrier, adhesive, and a drainage-collection bag works best for irregular shapes or difficult locations. The principles and purpose of fistula or draining-wound management are the same as for pouching a stoma.

Purpose

The nurse performs fistula/draining-wound pouching to

1. Contain fistula/draining-wound discharge.
2. Protect perifistula skin.
3. Control odor.
4. Maintain patient comfort.

Prerequisite Knowledge and Skills

Prior to applying a fistula or draining-wound pouch, the nurse should understand

1. Universal precautions.
2. Quantity and quality of discharge.

TABLE 20–2 Assessment Guide for Fistulas or Draining Wounds

Assessment Variable	Characteristics	Significance for Pouch Selection
Location of fistula or draining wound	Fistula within an incision	Include incision in pouch
	Retention sutures	Cut opening around sutures
	Irregular skin surface	Use flexible skin barrier or adhesive; build up irregular surface or crevices with paste
	In fold or near bony prominence	Avoid rigid flanges
Nature of discharge	Volume >500 ml per 24 hours or thick, pasty discharge	Requires open-end pouch
	Watery/thin discharge	May connect to drainage
	Corrosive, i.e., alkaline, bile, pancreatic, small bowel	Requires maximum skin protection, i.e., barrier, sealant, paste, possibly cement
Integrity of perifistula or wound skin	Smooth and intact	Wide selection of pouches
	Denuded, weeping blistered, painful	No alcohol-based products; use powder to absorb exudate; may require cement

3. Anatomy and pathophysiology of fistula and/or draining wound.

The nurse should be able to perform

1. Proper handwashing technique (see Skill 35–5).
2. Correct selection and construction of pouching system.
3. Universal precautions (see Skill 35–1).

Assessment

1. Observe for indications of pouch leakage, including odor, patient complaint of burning or itching, or wetness. **Rationale:** Physical signs resulting from leakage that necessitate an immediate change.
2. Note quantity and nature of discharge. **Rationale:** Monitors fluid and electrolyte balance.
3. Evaluate the fistula or draining wound (Table 20–2). **Rationale:** Characteristics will determine pouching system selected.

Nursing Diagnoses

1. Potential for impaired skin integrity related to fistula or wound drainage. **Rationale:** Discharge may be highly caustic.

2. Potential fluid and electrolyte imbalance related to fistula or wound drainage. **Rationale:** Fistulas and draining wounds may be a source of significant fluid and electrolyte losses.

Planning

1. Develop individualized goals for fistula/draining-wound pouching to maintain an intact pouching system. **Rationale:** Contained discharge maintains skin integrity and increases patient comfort.
2. Select and prepare all necessary supplies (Table 20–3). **Rationale:** Assembly of all supplies and equipment ensures that pouch change will be completed quickly and efficiently.
   a. Appropriate pouch(s) and barrier(s).
   b. Paste.
   c. Skin adhesive.
   d. Powder (if appropriate).
   e. Sealant (if appropriate).
   f. Skin adhesive (if appropriate).
   g. One set of scissors.
   h. Two to three wet wash cloths.
   i. One dry cloth or towel.
   j. One pair exam gloves.

TABLE 20–3 Product Selection Guide for Fistulas or Draining Wounds

Product	Use	Examples

Pouches:
  1. Preattached adhesive only*
  2. Preattached solid skin barrier
  3. Odor-proof vs. non-odor-proof
  4. With or without access door
  5. Various sizes
  6. With or without drain connector
	To contain the discharge, protect the perifistula/wound skin, and facilitate the measurement of discharge†	Fistula pouches:
		  United
		  Bard
		  Coloplast
		  Greer
		Wound manager with access door:
		  Convatec
		  Hollister

Solid skin barriers	To protect the skin from discharge, provide a base for pouch attachment, and provide suitable environment for healing denuded tissue	United Skin Barrier Stomahesive Premium Comfeel 4 x 4, 6 x 6, 8 x 8
Skin sealants	To protect the top layer of the epidermis from stripping when adhesives/barriers are removed; apply to intact skin and allow to dry	United Skin Prep Bard Protective Barrier Hollister Skin Gel
Adhesives	To attach two surfaces, enhance the seal of the pouching system, and provide some protection against discharge	United Skin Bond Cement Marlen Cement Hollister Medical Adhesive Spray
Pastes	A semisolid form of skin barrier used to caulk the edges of a solid barrier; also used to level irregular skin surfaces	Stomahesive Paste Karaya Paste
Powders	Applied to moist, denuded skin only to absorb serous secretions; dust off excess or it will interfere with effectiveness of adhesives	Stomahesive Powder Karaya Powder

*Double faced adhesive discs can be added to the adhesive already on a pouch to extend the size of the opening.
†Commercial drain/tube exit ports or baby nipples may be attached to a pouch for the exit of drain/tubes.

k. One pouch clamp or drain connector.
l. One drain-tube holder (if catheters or drains need to exit pouch).
m. One disposable underpad.
n. One roll 2-in nonallergic paper tape.
o. Deodorant.
p. One bottle sterile normal saline for irrigation.
q. One plastic bag for disposal of pouch.

3. Prepare the patient and family.
    a. Explain the procedure to the patient and family. **Rationale:** To allay anxiety.
    b. Position the patient so that fistula/wound is clearly visible and as flat as possible. **Rationale:** Correct positioning provides best body contour to apply the pouch.

Implementation

Steps	Rationale	Special Considerations
1. Wash hands.	Reduces transmission of microorganisms.	
2. Don exam gloves.	Universal precautions.	
3. Remove old clamps or bedside drain-bag connector, and set aside.	Can be reused when new pouch applied.	
4. Empty contents from old pouch.	Prevents spillage during removal.	
5. Gently remove pouch by supporting skin while pulling pouch up and away.	Prevents adhesive from denuding the skin.	To facilitate removal, use warm water. Cement or paste can be rolled away.
6. Dispose of old pouch in plastic bag, and place in appropriate receptacle.	Universal precautions.	
7. Gently clean any residue from the old pouch off the surrounding skin with warm water or solvent remover; then rinse off solvent remover.	Provides a clean base for the next application.	Do *not* use soap because it leaves a residue and is drying to the skin.
8. Irrigate the fistula/wound and surrounding skin with normal saline until clear return; then dry surrounding skin gently with sterile 4 x 4 gauze.	Clean discharge from area.	For copious drainage, place a sterile 4 x 4 gauze sponge into the wound or fistula to temporarily absorb drainage while preparing surrounding skin.
9. Measure fistula or wound: a. Make a pattern by placing a clear piece of plastic over area to be pouched and draw the outline (Fig. 20–3A). b. Cut out the center of the pattern.	Irregular shape/size must be followed as closely as possible.	Clear plastic pouch wrapper may be used to trace pattern. Place clean side over wound.
10. Select and prepare appropriate skin barrier and pouch or wound manager (see Table 20–3): a. Trace fistula or wound pattern (from 9a and b) onto the paper back of the pouch barrier, and cut opening in the barrier. b. Cut an opening into collecting pouch (if not using preattached system) slightly larger than the opening cut into the barrier.	Opening is cut to fit as close to wound edges as possible. Provides a custom fit.	Barrier will not adhere to denuded skin.
11. Remove protective paper backing from the barrier, and set barrier/pouch aside.	In order to adhere to the skin.	Do *not* touch adhesive back.

Table continues on following page

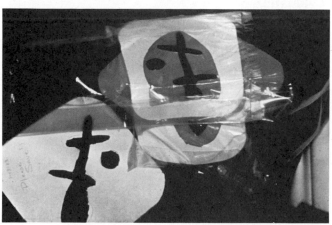
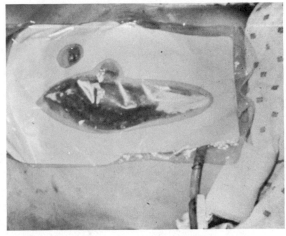

A B

FIGURE 20–3. Fistula/draining-wound pouch patterns. (*A*) Pattern cut out of barrier and pouch applied to fit over an open incision wound (note cutouts for retention sutures and fistula opening). (*B*) Open draining wound with an adjacent open drain site pouched with a large custom-fit pouch.

Steps	Rationale	Special Considerations
12. Prepare the skin around the wound or fistula by	Prevents epidermal denuding with pouch removal.	
a. Protecting with skin sealant.		
b. Dusting with light coat of powder prior to skin sealant if the area is denuded.		
13. Apply skin adhesive.	Provides additional tack and smooth surface for solid skin barrier.	Where wound edge is uneven or there are creases or folds, place wedges of solid skin barrier to provide level surface.
14. Apply prepared solid skin barrier (opening cut to previously made pattern; Fig. 20–3*B*) around wound or fistula:	Protects skin and provides base for pouch.	If preattached barrier and pouch, apply as one piece.
a. Caulk the edges of the solid barrier proximal to the fistula or wound with paste (Fig. 20–4).	Fills crevices and extends life of pouch.	May be applied via access door in wound manager.
b. Start by applying the pouch at the lower margin of the site, removing the gauze pads as you seal the pouch in place.	Contains the discharge.	
15. If a drain tube is to be connected to a suction source, pull drain tube through an opening made in front of pouch as you apply pouch.	May use commercially available exit port or tape over opening cut in pouch (Fig. 20–5*A* and 5*B*).	
16. Close the pouch with a clamp, rubber band, or drain connection to bedside bag.	Contains discharge.	
17. Connect drainage or catheters exiting pouch to suction or separate drainage receptacle.	Allows drainage to be contained and collected.	
18. Place soiled equipment and refuse in appropriate receptacles.	Universal precautions.	Place items soiled with body fluids in an impervious bag.
19. Wash hands.	Prevents transmission of microorganisms.	

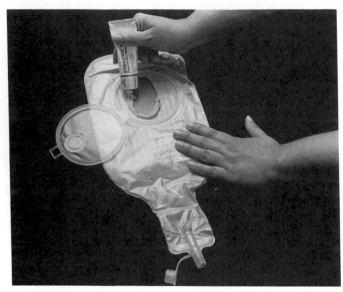

FIGURE 20–4. Adherence is increased by caulking the edges of the barrier with paste.

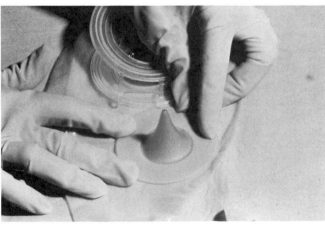

A

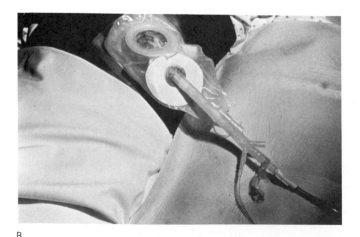

B

FIGURE 20–5. Drain exit ports. (*A*) A commercially made exit port is applied to the front of the pouch (NuHope). (*B*) A sump drain is drawn through the exit port and connected to suction.

Evaluation

1. Evaluate complaints or evidence of itching and burning, odor, or wetness around fistula or wound. **Rationale:** Signs that pouching system is not intact and will need to be reapplied.

2. Evaluate the integrity of the perifistula or wound skin. **Rationale:** Signs and symptoms of irritation indicate that the seal around the barrier is not intact.

3. Evaluate the patient's daily weights and electrolyte profile. **Rationale:** Voluminous fistula or wound drainage may cause fluid and electrolyte derangements.

4. Monitor patient's temperature for elevations and drainage for purulence, foul smell, and the culture, and sensitivity. **Rationale:** Indications of an infectious process.

Expected Outcomes

1. Pouch will remain intact a minimum of 24 hours. **Rationale:** Frequent manipulation of the skin surrounding the wound or fistula is prone to irritation and breakdown. Pouching a draining wound or fistula initially requires more time than a dressing change. Cost/benefit/comfort ratio is achieved only if dressing changes are decreased and perifistula or wound skin is protected.

2. Perifistula or wound skin remains intact or shows evidence of healing. **Rationale:** Prevents secondary infection and patient discomfort.

Unexpected Outcomes

1. Fistula or wound pouch leaks. **Rationale:** Opening in barrier may have been cut too large. Caulking has not filled crevices. Incorrect selection of pouch for fistula/wound drainage.

2. Perifistula or periwound skin is damaged or denuded. **Rationale:** Previous pouch did not have an intact seal, resulting in leakage of discharge with subsequent breakdown.

Documentation

Documentation in the patient record should include the date and time of pouching, the condition of the perifistula/wound skin, amount and nature of the discharge, type of pouch applied, and the effectiveness and/or modifications made in the pouching system. **Rationale:** Documents nursing care given, the condition of the perifistula/wound area, and the quantity and nature of the discharge.

Patient/Family Education

1. Explain the rationale for pouching fistulas or draining wounds to both patient and family. **Rationale:** To allay anxiety.

2. Provide an opportunity for the patient and family to ask questions. **Rationale:** Encourages patient and family understanding of and participation in the treatment plan.

Performance Checklist
Skill 20–2: Fistula/Draining-Wound Pouching

Critical Behaviors	Complies	
	yes	no
1. Wash hands.		
2. Don exam gloves.		
3. Remove and set aside pouch clamp or drain connector.		
4. Empty contents from pouch without soiling patient.		
5. Remove old pouch.		
6. Dispose of old pouch correctly.		
7. Gently clean perifistula or wound skin.		
8. Irrigate wound (if appropriate).		
9. Measure fistula or wound.		
10. Prepare skin barrier and pouch according to pattern.		
11. Remove protective backing from barrier, and set barrier aside.		
12. Prepare skin around the wound or fistula.		
13. Apply skin adhesive.		
14. Apply prepared skin barrier.		
15. Caulk the edges of the skin barrier.		
16. Apply pouch.		
17. If appropriate, pull drain tube through opening in pouch.		
18. Apply clamp or drain connector.		
19. Connect drainage or catheters exiting pouch to suction or separate drainage.		
20. Discard soiled equipment and refuse appropriately.		
21. Wash hands.		
22. Document procedure in patient record.		

SKILL 20–3

Colostomy Irrigation

Routine colostomy irrigation is no longer recommended, but colostomy irrigation may be done to prepare the patient for radiologic studies, relieve constipation, or stimulate peristalsis. A physician order is usually required. An ileostomy or urostomy is *never* irrigated.

Purpose

The nurse irrigates a colostomy to

1. Empty the colon.
2. Prepare the lower bowel for radiologic or other studies.

3. Stimulate peristalsis.

Prerequisite Knowledge and Skills

Prior to irrigating a colostomy, the nurse should understand

1. Anatomy and physiology of altered bowel elimination.
2. Universal precautions.
3. The location of proximal and distal stomas if there is a double-barrel or loop colostomy.

The nurse should be able to perform

1. Proper handwashing technique (see Skill 35–5).
2. Removal and application of stoma pouch.
3. Universal precautions (see Skill 35–1).

Assessment

1. Observe the patient for signs and symptoms of abdominal distension (i.e., increased girth and firmness). **Rationale:** May indicate a full colon.

2. Determine the angle of the bowel by digital examination of stoma opening if not noted in the patient record. **Rationale:** Irrigation cone is inserted toward open angle of bowel.

3. Determine the time of the last stoma discharge, the consistency, and the amount. **Rationale:** Recent large amount of discharge may indicate an evacuated bowel.

Nursing Diagnosis

Constipation. **Rationale:** Failure to evacuate the large bowel results in constipation.

Planning

1. Develop individualized goals for irrigating a colostomy to promote bowel evacuation. **Rationale:** Relieves constipation and cleanses the bowel for radiographic or other studies.

2. Prepare all necessary equipment and supplies. **Rationale:** Assembly of all supplies and equipment ensures that irrigation will be completed efficiently.
   a. Equipment for pouching a stoma (see Skill 20–1).
   b. One irrigation bag, tubing, and stoma cone (Fig. 20–6A).
   c. Irrigant (physician order).
   d. Irrigation sleeve.
   e. One package of lubricating gel.
   f. One bedpan, bedside commode, or drainage container.
   g. One disposable underpad.
   h. One pair of exam gloves.
   i. Room deodorant.
   j. Mild liquid soap.

3. Prepare the patient.
   a. Explain the procedure. **Rationale:** To allay anxiety.
   b. Place the patient on bedside commode or chair. Bedridden patient should be placed in semi-Fowler's position if possible. **Rationale:** Facilitates return of irrigation fluid.

Implementation

Steps	Rationale	Special Considerations
1. Verify physician's order.	Reduces risk of error.	The physician's order should include type, amount of irrigant, and frequency of irrigation.
2. Wash hands.	Reduces transmission of microorganisms.	
3. Don exam gloves.	Universal precautions.	
4. Remove the patient's pouch.	Gains access to the stoma.	Spray a small amount of room deodorant to neutralize odor during irrigation.
5. Attach an irrigation sleeve: a. To flange of two-piece pouching system. b. To peristomal skin with adhesive back if one-piece pouching system is in use.	Prevents irrigation return from soiling patient and surrounding area.	The sleeve has a top opening for administration of fluid through stoma and is long enough to reach into the commode or drainage receptacle with the patient in an upright or semi-Fowler's position. A small amount of liquid soap placed in the sleeve prevents feces from sticking to the sides of sleeve and helps in cleaning it after irrigation.
6. Fill irrigation bag with ordered amount and type of irrigant; temperature should be lukewarm.	Amount of irrigant will be prescribed by the physician based on the patient's condition.	500 to 1000 cc is average. Common irrigants are room-temperature plain tap water or normal saline.
7. Attach the irrigation cone tip to the end of irrigation bag tubing and lubricate to allow easy insertion.	Prevents perforation of bowel lumen.	Never use the semirigid tubing of an irrigation or enema bag because of its potential to perforate the bowel wall.

Table continues on following page

Steps	Rationale	Special Considerations
8. Gently insert the irrigation cone tip into the opening of the stoma, directing the tip toward the proximal bowel, and hold cone tip snugly against stoma.	Cone tip will prevent backflow of irrigation fluid during procedure. This enhances colon distension and effectiveness of irrigation (Fig. 20–6B).	Irrigation bag is hung at patient's shoulder height.
9. Adjust clamp on irrigation set to allow irrigant to flow slowly into bowel.	A rapid flow rate or fluid that is too cold may cause cramping. The irrigant entering slowly will gradually open the bowel behind the stoma.	If cramping occurs, slow flow rate and instruct patient to breathe slowly in and out through the mouth. Irrigation can stimulate the vagal response; monitor patient's heart rate and rhythm.
10. Remove cone tip after prescribed amount of fluid has been administered, and close top of irrigation sleeve.	Peristalsis will evacuate the bowel contents.	If there is no or minimal return of irrigant, this may indicate that the patient is dehydrated and the fluid has been absorbed in the bowel.
11. Allow 20 to 60 minutes for the bowel to evacuate. The abdomen may be gently massaged to stimulate peristalsis.	The return is individual and dependent primarily on peristalsis.	If there is minimal or no return of irrigant, an additional amount of fluid may need to be instilled. Obtain physician order.
12. Reapply the patient's pouch (see Skill 20–1).	After complete evacuation, leakage may still occur, pouch will contain discharge.	
13. Place soiled equipment and refuse in appropriate receptacle.	Universal precautions.	Irrigation bag, tubing, and cone are reusable, as are some sleeves.
14. Wash hands.	Reduces transmission of microorganisms.	

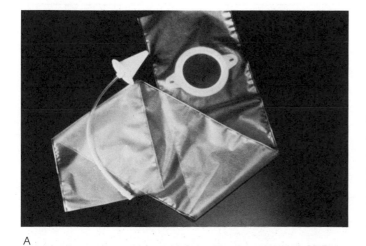
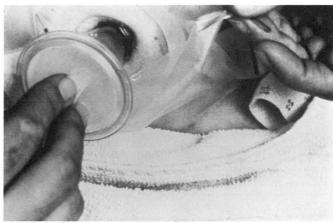

A   B

FIGURE 20–6. (*A*) An irrigation sleeve and cone tip (Hollister). (*B*) The cone tip is gently inserted into the stoma through the top of the irrigation sleeve.

Evaluation

1. Return should be equal to or greater than the amount of irrigant administered. **Rationale:** Evidence of fluid and electrolyte balance and success of irrigation procedure.
2. Evaluate the patient's bowel sounds every 1 to 2 hours. **Rationale:** Provides evidence of peristalsis.
3. Monitor the frequency and amount of colostomy discharge following irrigation procedure. **Rationale:** Provides evidence of colostomy function.

Expected Outcome

Bowel evacuation. **Rationale:** Irrigation stimulates peristalsis.

Unexpected Outcomes

1. Minimal or complete absence of return of irrigant.

Rationale: Patient is most likely dehydrated and fluid has been reabsorbed.

2. Bowel perforation. **Rationale:** Irrigation cone (or an inappropriate irrigating device) has punctured the bowel. Notify the physician immediately should this be suspected. Patient may experience sharp abdominal pain and/or bleeding without return of irrigant.

3. Slight bleeding from stoma. **Rationale:** Stoma is a mucous membrane that may bleed easily with friction from cone; this should cease spontaneously.

4. Bradycardia and/or syncope. **Rationale:** Vagus nerve pathway may be stimulated with bowel stimulation.

Documentation

Documentation in the patient record should include the date and time of the irrigation; amount of irrigant administered; the amount, color, and consistency of the return; the patient's tolerance of the procedure; and any unexpected outcomes and interventions taken. **Rationale:** Documents nursing care given, the effectiveness of irrigation, and expected outcomes and unexpected outcomes.

Patient/Family Education

1. Explain the reason for irrigation (i.e., diagnostic test, surgery preparation, stimulation of peristalsis, release of impaction) to both patient and family. **Rationale:** Encourages acceptance and understanding and enables the patient and family to ask questions.

2. If it is a newly created sigmoid colostomy and the patient is a candidate for irrigation as management, initiate an enterostomal therapy nurse referral to assist the patient and family in learning colostomy irrigation prior to discharge from the hospital. **Rationale:** Colostomy irrigation is an option only for the patients with a sigmoid colostomy or lower descending colostomy.

Performance Checklist
Skill 20–3: Colostomy Irrigation

Critical Behaviors	Complies yes	Complies no
1. Verify physician order for irrigation.		
2. Wash hands.		
3. Don exam gloves.		
4. Remove pouch.		
5. Attach an irrigation sleeve.		
6. Fill irrigation bag with ordered irrigant.		
7. Attach and lubricate cone tip.		
8. Insert cone, holding firmly in place.		
9. Adjust clamp and instill irrigation fluid slowly.		
10. Remove cone, closing irrigation sleeve.		
11. Allow 20 to 60 minutes for bowel to evacuate.		
12. Apply new colostomy pouch.		
13. Discard soiled equipment and refuse appropriately.		
14. Wash hands.		
15. Document procedure in patient record.		

BIBLIOGRAPHY

Broadwell, D. C. (1986). Gastrointestinal System. In J. M. Thompson and G. K. McFarland (Eds.), *Clinical Nursing.* St. Louis: Mosby.

Broadwell, D. C., and Jackson, B. S. (1982). *Principles of Ostomy Care.* St. Louis: Mosby.

Cheney, T. (1985). Nursing implications in the care of the ostomy patient receiving radiation and chemotherapy. *J. Enterostomal Ther.* 12:175–181.

Dobkin, K., and Broadwell, D. C. (1986). Nursing considerations for the patient undergoing colostomy surgery. *Semin. Oncol. Nurs.* 2(4):249–255.

Irrang, S., and Bryant, R. (1984). Management of the enterocutaneous fistula. *J. Enterostomal Ther.* 11(6):211–225.

Pettengill, C. (1989). Treatment of extraordinary wounds: Ingenuity and cooperation. *J. Enterostomal Ther.* 16(1):29–33.

Smith, D. B., and Johnson, D. E. (1986). *Ostomy Care and the Cancer Patient: Surgical and Clinical Considerations.* New York: Grune & Stratton.

Watt, R. C. (1986). Nursing management of a patient with a urinary diversion. *Semin. Oncol. Nurs.* 2(4):265–269.

UNIT V

THE RENAL SYSTEM

21

ACUTE HEMODIALYSIS

BEHAVIORAL OBJECTIVES

After completing this chapter, the nurse will be able to

- Define the key terms.
- Identify the components of the hemodialysis system.
- Describe the various types of vascular accesses used for hemodialysis.
- Demonstrate the skills involved in acute hemodialysis.
- Develop a plan of care for the patient receiving hemodialysis.

The basic goal of dialysis is volume regulation, acid–base balance, and electrolyte and azotemia control. Dialysis or continuous renal replacement therapy (CRRT) may be prescribed as acute support therapies for electrolyte imbalances (i.e., hyperkalemia), acidosis, and pericarditis, with isolated ultrafiltration for fluid management. Hemodialysis and hemoperfusion are therapies of choice in the majority of drug overdoses and chemical poisonings. Finally, dialysis is a maintenance therapy for patients with end-stage renal disease or those in whom conservative management (diet, medications) is insufficient. Basic knowledge of the principles of diffusion, osmosis, hydrostatic pressure, and the components of the dialysis system is essential for understanding hemodialysis.

KEY TERMS

bruit	hemodialysis
cannulation	steal syndrome
dialysate	thrill
dialyzer	transmembrane (negative)
diffusion	pressure
dry weight	ultrafiltration
extracorporeal	vascular access

SKILLS

21–1 Hemodialysis: Subclavian Catheter Coupling/Uncoupling
21–2 Hemodialysis: Cannulation of the Arteriovenous Vascular Access Fistula/Graft
21–3 Hemodialysis: Maintenance of Vascular Access
21–4 Hemodialysis: Initiation and Termination
21–5 Continuous Renal Replacement Therapy: Slow Continuous Ultrafiltration (SCUF) and Continuous Arteriovenous Hemofiltration (CAVH)

GUIDELINES

The following assessment guidelines assist the nurse in formulating a nursing diagnosis and an individualized plan of care for the patient receiving hemodialysis:

1. Know the patient's baseline vital signs.
2. Know the patient's fluid status by analyzing weight (current versus dry), skin turgor, mucous membranes, edema, and intake and output.
3. Know the patient's serum electrolyte levels.
4. Know the patient's underlying medical condition and its dynamic effect on renal functioning.
5. Know the patient's current medical treatment.
6. Perform systematic cardiovascular, respiratory, neurologic, and renal assessments.

7. Perform assessment of vascular access.
8. Determine appropriate interventions for assessment findings.
9. Become adept with equipment used for hemodialysis.

SKILL 21–1

Hemodialysis: Subclavian Catheter Coupling/Uncoupling

Temporary external access devices such as the subclavian, jugular, or femoral vein catheter are used for acute intervention until dialysis is no longer needed or a permanent access can be placed for chronic therapy. Cannulation is accomplished with a specially designed semirigid or rigid, single- or double-lumen Teflon catheter. The catheter may be used immediately for dialysis after placement has been verified by x-ray.

Purpose

The nurse performs the coupling/uncoupling procedure to initiate or terminate hemodialysis.

Prerequisite Knowledge and Skills

Prior to performing subclavian coupling/uncoupling, the nurse should understand

1. Anatomy of the subclavicular/femoral area.
2. Dynamics of blood circulation.
3. Principles of aseptic technique.
4. Universal precautions.

The nurse should be able to perform

1. Proper handwashing technique (see Skill 35–5).
2. Universal precautions (see Skill 35–1).
3. Setup of a sterile field.
4. Flushing and heparinization of a catheter lumen.

Assessment

1. Assess the patient for maintenance of a closed system, including secured limb caps and occlusive dressing. **Rationale:** Open system may result in infection or air embolism or impair catheter functioning.
2. Assess the catheter insertion site for signs and symptoms of infection, including redness, swelling, drainage/crusting, or odor. **Rationale:** Catheter exit-site infections may result in septicemia or subacute bacterial endocarditis. Signs and symptoms of exit-site infections may warrant a change in the catheter site or further interventions, such as culture of the drainage and antibiotic therapy.
3. Assess catheter patency, including signs of catheter kinking, and ability to aspirate blood from the catheter. **Rationale:** Optimal blood flow while on dialysis is dependent on a patent lumen.

Nursing Diagnosis

Potential for infection related to break in aseptic technique with possible transmission of microorganisms. **Rationale:** The open system provides a direct portal of entry for microorganisms that can be transported throughout the body via the circulation.

Planning

1. Develop individualized goals for performing coupling/uncoupling of the subclavian/femoral catheter for hemodialysis to prevent infection. **Rationale:** Maintenance of aseptic technique reduces the transmission of microorganisms.
2. Prepare all necessary equipment and supplies. **Rationale:** Assembly of all the necessary equipment at the bedside decreases the risk of environmental contamination.

COUPLING EQUIPMENT

a. Two masks and head coverings (to be worn by patient and nurse).
b. Sharps container.
c. Goggles.
d. One pair sterile gloves.
e. Four 10-cc syringes.
f. One 20- to 30-cc syringe (if serum lab is required).
g. Two 19-gauge needles.
h. Sterile normal saline (for infusion, at least 20 cc).
i. One subclavian tray, which includes
   (1) Sterile barriers
   (2) Six 4 × 4 gauze pads
   (3) Two 2 × 2 gauze pads
   (4) One transparent dressing
   (5) One roll of 1-in Micropore tape.
j. Povidone-iodine solution.
k. One vial heparin (1000 U/1 cc) (amount prescribed per unit policy).
l. Sterile solution container.

UNCOUPLING EQUIPMENT

a. Two masks and head coverings (to be worn by patient and nurse).
b. Two sterile catheter caps.
c. One vial heparin (1000 U/1 cc).
d. One sterile 3- or 5-cc syringe, depending on amount of heparin.
e. Two sterile 10-cc syringes.
f. Two sterile 19-gauge needles.
g. Three packages sterile 2 × 2 gauze pads.
h. Sterile barrier.

3. Prepare the patient.
   a. Explain the procedure to the patient. **Rationale:** Reduces anxiety.
   b. Provide the patient with a mask and cap. **Ratio-**

nale: Decreases the risk of airborne pathogens.

c. Assist the patient to a comfortable position, generally supine or Trendelenburg. Based on the patient's respiratory status, a low semi-Fowler's position may be used. **Rationale:** Promotes comfort.

Implementation

Steps	Rationale	Special Considerations
Coupling		
1. Wash hands.	Reduces transmission of microorganisms.	
2. Don mask and cap.	Infection control precautions.	
3. Open subclavian tray, removing sterile barriers, 2 × 2's, 4 × 4's, and transparent dressing from tray, and place onto sterile field.	Prepares material and maintains aseptic technique.	
4. Open sterile needles and syringes. Place on sterile field.	Readies equipment and maintains aseptic technique to prevent transmission of microorganisms.	
5. Attach 19-gauge needles to 10-cc syringes and draw up normal saline. If planning to give a loading dose of heparin, draw heparin up in syringe first, then fill remaining portion of syringe with normal saline.	Prepares syringe for catheter flushing.	*Recommend* 9 cc of normal saline and 1 cc (1000 units) of heparin or as per unit policy.
6. Fill one-quarter of the sterile basin with povidone-iodine solution.	Prepares solution used to cleanse catheter.	
7. Remove dressing from subclavian exit site, taking care not to contaminate or dislodge cannula.	Allows access to exit site.	Inspect for signs and symptoms of exit-site infection: drainage, crusting, swelling, redness, exudate, or complaints of pain at the site.
8. Discard soiled dressing in appropriate disposal container.	Universal precautions.	
9. Wash hands.	Reduces transmission of microorganisms.	
10. Don sterile gloves.	To maintain aseptic technique.	
11. Place sterile barrier beneath subclavian catheter.	Sets up sterile field.	Do not touch catheter with gloves. Should gloves accidently touch the catheter, a change is necessary to maintain aseptic technique.
12. Saturate four of the 4 × 4's in povidone-iodine solution. Partially wring out a soaked 4 × 4, and perform a 1-minute scrub of the arterial limb of the catheter.	Povidone-iodine serves as a bactericidal agent.	Scrub catheter in vertical direction, being careful not to create tension. Use enough friction to remove any crust or drainage.
13. Wrap second povidone-iodine soaked 4 × 4 around arterial limb and leave in place for approximately 3 to 5 minutes.	Reduces transmission of microorganisms.	
14. After 3 to 5 minutes, remove povidone-iodine soaked 4 × 4, and discard in appropriate receptacle.	Universal precautions.	
15. Remove cap from arterial limb of catheter and discard appropriately.	Provides access to arterial side of catheter. Universal precautions.	Be sure slide clamp is closed before removing arterial limb catheter cap.

Table continues on following page

Steps	Rationale	Special Considerations
16. Attach an empty 10-cc syringe to the arterial limb, open the slide clamp, and gently aspirate 10 cc of blood. Then close the slide clamp, remove syringe, and discard in appropriate receptacle.	Verifies patency of catheter limb.	If you have difficulty aspirating blood, notify physician. If serum laboratory work is required, attach another empty syringe to the arterial limb and aspirate required amount of blood.
17. Repeat steps 12 through 16 on the venous limb.	To verify patency of venous limb.	Observe for clots.
18. Attach heparinized normal saline flush syringe to arterial limb, open slide clamp and gently aspirate 2 to 3 cc of blood, and then slowly flush catheter with heparin. Then, close slide clamp.	Positive pressure prevents backup of blood into the catheter after flushing.	Syringe should be left attached to catheter limb until replaced with dialyzer tubing connector.
19. Repeat step 18 on venous limb.	Prevents clotting of blood until dialysis is initiated.	Syringe should be left attached to catheter limb until replaced with dialyzer tubing connector.
20. Soak two 2 × 2's in povidone-iodine solution, and cleanse connection site.	Cleanses connection site.	
21. Remove 10-cc normal saline flush syringe from arterial limb, and attach arterial line securely to the catheter limb.	Connects to dialysis machine.	
22. Tape connections securely.	Prevents accidental separation of lines.	
23. Open slide clamp on the arterial limb and turn on blood pump.	Primes the blood lines with blood.	
24. When the venous drip chamber located on the hemodialysis machine is pink, turn off the blood pump and clamp the venous line. Then remove 10-cc normal saline flush syringe from the venous limb, and securely attach to the venous tubing.	Indicates blood has circulated through dialyzer to the venous line.	The venous limb should be left in clamped position.
25. Tape connections securely.	Prevents accidental separation on lines.	
26. Remove gloves, and discard soiled material in appropriate receptacle.	Universal precautions.	
27. Wash hands.	Reduces transmission of microorganisms.	
Uncoupling		
1. Wash hands.	Reduces transmission of microorganisms.	
2. Don mask and cap.	Infection control precautions.	
3. Open syringes, caps, needles, and 2 × 2's, and place on sterile field.	Maintains aseptic technique.	
4. Fill two syringes with desired amount of heparin, depending on type of catheter used.	Heparin is used to maintain patency of access.	
5. Remove tape from the arterial and venous limbs; and wrap both limbs with povidone-iodine soaked 2 × 2's and scrub for 1 minute.	Povidone-iodine acts as a bactericidal agent.	Scrub catheter in vertical direction, being careful not to create tension. Use enough friction to remove any crust or drainage.

Table continues on following page

Steps	Rationale	Special Considerations
6. Place sterile barrier under catheter limbs.	Sets up a sterile field.	
7. Don sterile gloves.	Maintains aseptic technique.	
8. Clamp arterial and venous limbs.	Prevents blood loss from catheter.	
9. Using the same povidone-iodine soaked 2 × 2 to handle the dialysis tubing, disconnect arterial line from the limb and attach a 10-cc syringe with normal saline.	Povidone-iodine acts as a bactericidal agent.	
10. Unclamp slide clamp, and inject 10 cc of normal saline into arterial limb. Then reclamp and remove syringe.	Prevents blood from entering the tip of the catheter.	
11. Attach a 3- or 5-cc syringe with heparin, unclamp slide clamp, and inject prescribed amount of heparin.	Maintains catheter patency by preventing clotting of blood.	Heparin dosage will vary depending on type of catheter utilized and unit policy.
12. Clamp, disconnect syringe, and cap the arterial limb.	Prevents loss of blood.	
13. Repeat steps 9 through 12 on venous limb.	Maintains patency by preventing clotting of blood.	
14. Apply transparent occlusive dressing to subclavian catheter site per established policy.	Prevents contamination of catheter exit site.	Occlusive dressing should be maintained and changed at least weekly.
15. Discard soiled material in appropriate receptacle.	Universal precautions.	
16. Wash hands.	Reduces transmission of microorganisms.	

Evaluation

Assess the condition of catheter, exit site, and dressing, and compare with preprocedure assessments. **Rationale:** Monitors for signs and symptoms of infection, and catheter patency.

Expected Outcomes

1. Exit site is free of drainage, redness, swelling, and crusting. **Rationale:** Absence of signs and symptoms of infection.
2. Blood is easily aspirated. **Rationale:** Patency of catheter is maintained.

Unexpected Outcomes

1. Blood flow problems and/or decreased catheter patency. **Rationale:** Catheter handling during coupling/uncoupling procedure may cause kinking, hematoma formation, or catheter dislodgment.
2. Drainage, redness, swelling, pain and/or crusting at exit site. **Rationale:** Indicates signs and symptoms of infection.
3. Catheter dislodgment. **Rationale:** Loss of access for dialysis procedure.
4. Environmental contamination with blood. **Rationale:** Break in universal precautions.

Documentation

Documentation in the patient record should include date and time of coupling/uncoupling, condition of catheter exit site, patency of catheter lumens, quality of blood flow, date and time of dressing application, and any unexpected outcomes encountered and interventions taken. **Rationale:** Documents nursing care given and patient response to expected and unexpected outcomes.

Patient/Family Education

1. Discuss the need to maintain subclavian catheter placement and strict aseptic technique during coupling and uncoupling procedure with both patient and family. Instruct that this catheter is a temporary vascular access. **Rationale:** Promotes an understanding of the treatment plan and encourages the patient and family to ask questions.
2. Evaluate the patient's need for long-term permanent access. **Rationale:** Allows for planning of chronic vascular access and attendant patient and family education.

Performance Checklist
Skill 21–1: Hemodialysis: Subclavian Catheter Coupling/Uncoupling

Critical Behaviors	Complies	
	yes	no
COUPLING		
1. Wash hands.		
2. Don mask and cap.		
3. Open subclavian tray, and place barriers, gauze pads, and dressings on sterile field.		
4. Open sterile needles and syringes, and place on sterile field.		
5. Attach 19-gauge needles to 10-cc syringes, and draw up normal saline, with heparin (if appropriate).		
6. Fill sterile basin one-quarter full with povidone-iodine.		
7. Remove dressing from subclavian exit site.		
8. Discard soiled dressing appropriately.		
9. Wash hands.		
10. Don sterile gloves.		
11. Place sterile barrier underneath catheter using aseptic technique.		
12. Perform 1-minute scrub of subclavian catheter.		
13. Wrap arterial and venous limbs with povidone-iodine soaked 4 × 4.		
14. After 3 to 5 minutes, remove 4 × 4 and discard appropriately.		
15. Remove cap from arterial limb of catheter and discard.		
16. Aspirate blood from arterial limb to verify patency.		
17. Repeat steps 12 to 16 on venous limb.		
18. Gently flush arterial limb with normal saline and close with slide clamp.		
19. Repeat step 18 on venous limb.		
20. Soak two 2 × 2's in povidone-iodine and cleanse connection site.		
21. Remove 10-cc normal saline flush syringes from arterial limb, and attach arterial line to catheter limb.		
22. Tape catheter and tubing connections securely.		
23. Prime dialysis line with arterial blood.		
24. Clamp venous line when venous drip chamber becomes pink.		
25. Remove 10-cc normal saline flush syringe and attach to venous tubing.		
26. Tape connections.		
27. Discard soiled materials appropriately.		
28. Wash hands.		
UNCOUPLING		
1. Wash hands.		
2. Don mask and cap.		
3. Place syringes, caps, needles, and 2 × 2's on sterile field.		
4. Fill syringes with appropriate amount of heparin.		

Table continues on following page

Critical Behaviors	Complies	
	yes	no
5. Remove tape and wrap arterial and venous limbs with povidone-soaked 2 × 2. Scrub for one minute.		
6. Place sterile barrier under catheter.		
7. Don sterile gloves.		
8. Clamp both limbs.		
9. Disconnect arterial line and flush with normal saline. Reclamp.		
10. Flush with prescribed amount of heparin and reclamp.		
11. Cap the arterial limb.		
12. Repeat Steps 9 through 11 on venous limb.		
13. Apply occlusive dressing to catheter site.		
14. Discard soiled materials appropriately.		
15. Wash hands.		
16. Document procedure in patient record.		

SKILL 21–2

Hemodialysis: Cannulation of the Arteriovenous Vascular Access Fistula/Graft

The arteriovenous (A-V) fistula (Fig. 21–1) and graft are vascular access devices used in patients requiring maintenance hemodialysis. The A-V fistula is a surgically created anastomosis of an artery to a vein. Blood is redirected from the artery to the vein, causing the vein to dilate with increased blood flow. The A-V fistula matures in 4 to 6 weeks, and cannulation should not be attempted prior to that time. A bruit over the A-V fistula indicates patency of the vascular access.

The A-V graft is an internal access in which an artery is anastomosed to a vein by use of synthetic material called polytetrafluoroethylene (PTFE). One end of the graft is sutured to the artery, tunneled under the skin through subcutaneous tissue, and sutured into a vein. As with the A-V fistula, arterial blood is redirected through the graft material. Although a 2- to 3-week maturation period is optimal, these grafts can be cannulated when swelling in the limb has decreased (approximately 7 to 10 days). A bruit in the A-V graft indicates patency of the access.

Purpose

The nurse performs cannulation of the A-V fistula or graft to access the vascular circulation for hemodialysis.

Prerequisite Knowledge and Skills

Prior to performing cannulation, the nurse should understand

1. Anatomy and physiology of the vascular system.
2. Principles of intravenous therapy.
3. Principles of aseptic technique.
4. Universal precautions.

The nurse should be able to perform

1. Proper handwashing technique (see Skill 35–5).
2. Universal precautions (see Skill 35–1).
3. Venipuncture techniques (see Skill 9–1).
4. Assessment of vascular access patency.
5. Doppler use.

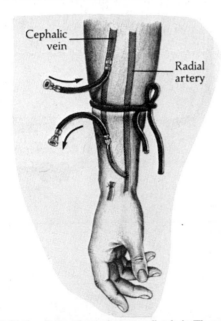

FIGURE 21–1. Internal arteriovenous fistula in Thompson, J. M., McFarland, G. K., Hirsch, J. E., Tucker, S. M., and Bowers, A. C. (eds.) *Mosby's Manual of Clinical Nursing*. St. Louis, C.V. Mosby Co., 1989, with permission.

Assessment

1. Assess the access site for the presence of bruit, edema, inflammation, suppuration, and quality of blood flow in underlying vessel. **Rationale:** Physical signs and symptoms indicate vascular access patency and presence of infection.
2. Assess the circulatory status of the vascular access limb (i.e., capillary refill, color, pulse, bruit/thrill, and skin temperature). **Rationale:** Physical signs and symptoms indicate circulatory status of limb.
3. Palpate vascular access to determine area for cannulation (i.e., blood vessel filling, thrill). If unable to palpate a thrill, use a Doppler to assess presence of blood flow. **Rationale:** Findings indicate a mature vessel for cannulation.

Nursing Diagnoses

1. Pain related to venipuncture. **Rationale:** Venipuncture is a noxious stimulus.
2. Potential alteration in tissue perfusion related to trauma of the vascular access. **Rationale:** Poor vessel entry during cannulation may cause blood to leak out of the access, resulting in hematoma formation and sluggish blood flow during dialysis. Incorrect needle placement within the vessel also may obstruct blood flow during dialysis.

Planning

1. Individualize the following goals for performing cannulation:
   a. Maintain patency of vascular access. **Rationale:** Without patency of access, hemodialysis cannot be performed.

b. Maintain needle alignment within access. **Rationale:** To provide optimal blood flow for hemodialysis.
2. Prepare all necessary equipment and supplies. **Rationale:** Assembly of all necessary equipment ensures that cannulation will be completed quickly and efficiently.
   a. Two 10-cc syringes.
   b. Two 19-gauge needles.
   c. One vial heparin (1000 U/ml).
   d. One vial normal saline (for injection).
   e. Two fistula needles (generally 14 to 16 gauge in an adult).
   f. Two povidone-iodine swabs (or 2 × 2 gauze pads, soaked).
   g. Two TB syringes (if lidocaine is used).
   h. One tourniquet (A-V fistula only).
   i. Antiseptic soap.
   j. Two 4 × 4 gauze pads.
   k. Adhesive tape, 1-in roll.
   l. Two bulldog clamps.
   m. One sterile barrier.
   n. Goggles.
   o. One set examination gloves.
   p. One vial lidocaine 1%.
3. Prepare the patient.
   a. Explain the procedure to the patient. **Rationale:** Reduces anxiety and encourages cooperation.
   b. Assist the patient to a comfortable position while exposing site of vascular access. **Rationale:** Promotes comfort and reduces strain to vascular access limb.
   c. Palpate the vascular access site to determine the area to be cannulated. **Rationale:** Validates patency of the vessel.
   d. Ascertain if patient prefers cannulation site to be anesthetized. **Rationale:** Reduces anxiety and promotes patient comfort.

Implementation

Steps	Rationale	Special Considerations
1. Wash hands.	Reduces transmission of microorganisms.	
2. Wash access arm for 1 full minute with antiseptic soap and a 4 × 4, and rinse off with water.	Reduces the number and transmission of microorganisms.	
3. Place arm on sterile barrier.	Maintains aseptic technique.	
4. Starting at the site for insertion, moving out in concentric circles for 2 to 3 in, wash access area with povidone-iodine swabs or soaked 2 × 2 for 1 full minute.	Povidone-iodine solution serves as a bactericidal agent.	
5. Repeat step 4 with second, new swab or 2 × 2.		

Table continues on following page

Steps	Rationale	Special Considerations
6. Using two 10-cc syringes and two 19-gauge needles, draw up prescribed amount of heparin and normal saline in each syringe.	Prepares syringes for flushing fistula/graft.	
7. Attach heparinized saline-filled syringes to fistula needle tubing, and prime fistula needles.	Prevents clotting of blood in fistula needles.	
8. Place a bulldog clamp on each catheter.	Prevents loss of heparinized solution and backflow of blood.	
9. Apply tourniquet to upper portion of access limb for *A-V fistula cannulation only*.	Facilitates site determination for cannulation.	
10. Don examination gloves and goggles.	Universal precautions.	
11. Select site to be used.	Decreases recirculation of dialyzed blood.	Arterial site should be at least 3 in from arterial anastomosis. Venous needle must be in the direction of venous flow and, if possible, 3 in or more from the arterial needle.
12. Grasp butterfly wings or hub of fistula needle between thumb and index finger of dominant hand with needle tip bevel up.	Provides secure grasp of needle upon cannulation.	Optional: Prior to insertion of fistula needle, lidocaine may be injected intradermally to make a small wheal as per patient preference.
13. Remove needle guard.	Exposes fistula needle.	
14. Hold skin taut with nondominant hand.	Prevents rolling of vessel.	Avoid contamination of area to be punctured.
15. With dominant hand, insert needle at a 45-degree angle to the skin (if lidocaine was used, use same puncture site for needle).	Prevents shearing of graft material.	
a. *A-V Fistula*: Advance bevel up to hub of the needle.	Accesses arterial vascular system.	
b. *A-V Graft*: As soon as tip is through the graft, rotate needle 180 degrees, and advance needle to hub, bevel down.	Accesses arterial vascular system.	Bevel down position prevents shearing of graft.
16. Remove tourniquet before infusing normal saline or heparin (if A-V fistula).	Prevents clotting.	
17. Remove bulldog clamp from needle limb, and aspirate blood.	Verifies correct placement and patency of access.	
18. Infuse heparinized saline, and reclamp catheter with bulldog clamp.	Prevents clotting and backflow of blood.	
19. Secure needle with adhesive tape over insertion site.	Maintains angle of needle so that it floats freely in the vessel/graft.	
20. Repeat steps 12 through 18 for insertion of second needle.	Cannulation of venous site.	Hemodialysis can now be initiated.
21. Discard soiled material in appropriate receptacle.	Universal precautions.	
22. Wash hands.	Reduces transmission of microorganisms.	

Evaluation

1. Evaluate the vascular access for edema, swelling, redness, pain, hematoma formation, and bleeding. **Rationale:** Injury and inflammation of the intima and medial layer of a vessel may cause phlebitis and clot formation.
2. Monitor for alignment of needles and force of blood flow during dialysis (i.e., good blood flow without sucking of air, arterial pressure on dialysis machine between 0 and 20 mmHg). **Rationale:** Incorrect placement of needles within the vessel can hinder or obstruct blood flow during dialysis.
3. Monitor circulatory status of vascular access limb. **Rationale:** Ischemia of digits distal to cannulation site is indicative of inadequate blood flow. Notify the physician.

Expected Outcomes

1. Pulsating blood flow in the dialysis tubing set. **Rationale:** Indicates proper cannulation of A-V fistula or A-V graft.
2. Vascular access limb has pulses distal to access site. **Rationale:** Evidence of adequate circulation.

Unexpected Outcomes

1. Hematoma formation. **Rationale:** Penetration of both vessel walls by the fistula needles results in leakage of blood into tissue layers under the skin.
2. Poor blood flow. **Rationale:** Incorrect needle gauge or needle placement within the vessel may obstruct blood flow.

Documentation

Documentation in the patient record should include date and time of cannulation, quality of blood flow, presence of bruit, appearance of site before and after cannulation, circulatory assessment of vascular access limb, needle gauge used for cannulation, and any unexpected outcomes encountered and the interventions taken. **Rationale:** Documents cannulation, status of graft/fistula and vascular access limb, and expected and unexpected outcomes and interventions taken.

Patient/Family Education

1. Assess the readiness and ability of the patient and family to perform maintenance access care. **Rationale:** Cognitive and/or psychomotor impairments may necessitate delay and/or alterations in the teaching plan.
2. Demonstrate how to assess for circulatory patency of the vascular access to both patient and family. **Rationale:** Fosters an understanding and encourages participation in treatment plan.
3. Discuss the signs and symptoms of an infected and/or clotted vascular access. **Rationale:** Enables the patient and family to recognize problems and seek prompt attention.
4. Evaluate the patient's and family's understanding of maintenance access care. **Rationale:** Allows anticipation of discharge needs and discharge instruction (see Skill 21–3).

Performance Checklist
Skill 21–2: Hemodialysis: Cannulation of the Arteriovenous Vascular Access Fistula/Graft

Critical Behaviors	Complies	
	yes	no
1. Wash hands.		
2. Perform antiseptic scrub of access limb.		
3. Place access limb on sterile barrier.		
4. Cleanse access site with povidone-iodine solution.		
5. Repeat step 4 with a second soaked 4 × 4.		
6. Fill two 10-cc syringes with prescribed amount of heparin and normal saline.		
7. Prime fistula needles with heparinized saline.		
8. Clamp catheter with bulldog clamps.		
9. Apply tourniquet (only with A-V fistula access).		
10. Don examination gloves and goggles.		
11. Select site to be used.		
12. Grasp butterfly wings or hub of fistula needles and hold needle tip bevel up.		
13. Remove needle guard.		
14. Hold skin taut with nondominant hand.		
15. Insert needle at 45-degree angle, bevel up.		

Table continues on following page

Critical Behaviors	Complies yes	no
a. With A-V graft access, insert needle, rotate 180-degrees, and then advance to the hub with bevel down.		
b. With A-V fistula access, advance needle to hub, bevel up.		
16. Remove tourniquet from arm if using A-V fistula for cannulation.		
17. Remove bulldog clamp, and aspirate for blood return.		
18. Heparinize the fistula needle, and reclamp.		
19. Secure needle to maintain a fully floating angle.		
20. Repeat steps 12 to 18 for second needle.		
21. Discard soiled dressings and materials in appropriate disposal receptacle.		
22. Wash hands.		
23. Document procedure in patient record.		

SKILL 21–3

Hemodialysis: Maintenance of Vascular Access

Patency of the vascular access is of paramount importance in the dialysis patient. The quality of blood flow through the vascular access is monitored by evaluating the bruit and thrill. The extremity with the vascular access is also examined for circulatory changes and indicators of a potential infectious process.

Purpose

The nurse maintains the vascular access to
1. Provide direct vascular access.
2. Prevent graft/fistula loss.

Prerequisite Knowledge and Skills

Prior to maintaining a vascular access, the nurse should understand

1. Principles of aseptic technique.
2. Principles of universal precautions.
3. Principles of vascular access.
4. Principles of clotting mechanism.

The nurse should be able to perform

1. Proper handwashing technique (see Skill 35–5).
2. Universal precautions (see Skill 35–1).
3. Palpation of vascular access.
4. Doppler use.

Assessment

1. Observe the patient for signs and symptoms of adequate circulation of vascular access limb. **Rationale:** To detect circulatory deficits in the limb secondary to vascular access placement.

2. Assess the access site for erythema, swelling, tenderness, and drainage. **Rationale:** To identify infectious process.

Nursing Diagnoses

1. Potential for infection related to break in skin from venipuncture. **Rationale:** The skin provides the first line of defense, so a break or opening in the skin (surgical or trauma) increases the risk of infection.
2. Potential alteration in tissue perfusion related to trauma of the vascular access. **Rationale:** Incorrect needle gauge or placement during cannulation may cause blood to leak out of the access, resulting in hematoma formation.

Planning

1. Individualize the following goals for vascular access care:
   a. Maintain patency. **Rationale:** Without a patent access, hemodialysis cannot be performed.
   b. Prevent infection. **Rationale:** Maintenance of aseptic technique reduces transmission of microorganisms.
2. Prepare all necessary equipment and supplies. **Rationale:** Assembly of all necessary equipment ensures efficient completion of procedure.
   a. Stethoscope.
   b. Doppler (optional).
3. Prepare the patient.
   a. Explain the procedure to the patient. **Rationale:** Reduces anxiety and encourages cooperation.
   b. Assist the patient to a comfortable position that facilitates exposure of the vascular access site. **Rationale:** Promotes comfort and reduces strain to vascular access limb.

Implementation

Steps	Rationale	Special Considerations
1. Wash hands.	Reduces transmission of microorganisms.	
2. Evaluate the patency of the vascular access every 8 hours: a. Gently palpate along entire length of the graft or over the access for a thrill. b. Auscultate with the stethoscope for the presence of a bruit.	Indicates patency of vascular access. Indicates patency of vascular access. Auscultation is helpful if extremity is edematous and thrill is difficult to palpate.	*Thrill*: Feel of vibrations or purring beneath your fingers. *Bruit*: Sounds like rushing water. Absence of a bruit does not confirm occlusion. Auscultate with a Doppler if unable to hear bruit with a stethoscope and/or palpate a thrill.
3. Evaluate the circulation of the vascular limb: a. Palpate pulses distal to the vascular access. b. Observe for bleeding or signs of hematoma formation. c. Check capillary refill. d. Compare color and temperature of both extremities.	Indicates circulatory status of vascular access limb and patency of vascular access. Validates circulation May impair circulation in extremity. Quantifies circulation. To detect ischemic changes in digits distal to access site.	
4. Identify changes in sensation distal to vascular access.	May indicate the "steal" syndrome.	Numbness and tingling may be expected within the first 24 hours.
5. Assess for erythema, swelling, tenderness, or drainage.	Indicates possible signs and symptoms of infection.	
6. Place sign above patient's bed indicating which limb contains the vascular access.	Alerts personnel not to use affected extremity for blood pressure, venipuncture, tourniquet, or blood draw, which may traumatize vessel.	Refrain from placing restraints, gauze, and tape circumferentially around the vascular access limb.
7. Wash hands.	Reduces transmission of microorganisms.	

Evaluation

Compare assessment findings with previous findings of vascular access. **Rationale:** Alerts caregiver to changes that may indicate clot formation, impending graft/fistula loss, inadequate limb circulation, and/or infection.

Expected Outcomes

1. Positive bruit and thrill. **Rationale:** Indicates patent vascular access for hemodialysis.
2. Absence of erythema, swelling, drainage, or tenderness. **Rationale:** These are physical signs of infection of the access.

Unexpected Outcomes

1. Thrombosis. **Rationale:** Injury and inflammation of the intima and medial layer of a vessel may cause clot formation.
2. Hematoma. **Rationale:** Indicates injury to vessel wall that allows escape of blood into tissue layers.

3. Infection. **Rationale:** The skin provides the first line of defense, so a break or opening potentiates invasion by microorganisms.
4. Steal syndrome. **Rationale:** Vascular access limb is deprived of retrograde blood flow resulting in ischemia.

Documentation

Documentation in the patient record should include date and time of assessment, the presence or absence of a thrill and/or a bruit, character of bruit's sound, condition of skin of vascular access limb, any variations between extremities, pulses distal to the access, general appearance of the site, subjective sensations at or distal to the site, and any unexpected outcomes and interventions taken. **Rationale:** Documents assessment findings for future comparisons, expected and unexpected outcomes, and interventions taken.

Patient/Family Education

1. Assess the patient's and family's readiness and ability to perform maintenance access care. **Rationale:** Cognitive and/or psychomotor impairments may necessitate delay and/or alteration in the teaching plan.

2. Discuss the discharge instructions with the patient and family, including check for the presence of a thrill three times a day, especially upon awakening, cleanse access extremity at least daily with a deodorant soap, avoid constrictive clothing or jewelry on access limb, avoid sleeping in a posture that exerts pressure directly on access, avoid venipuncture, blood pressure, and blood draws to access extremity, and inform medical personnel of decreased circulation in extremity, decreased access patency, or signs of infection. **Rationale:** Enables the patient and family to ask questions and gain an active role in self-care.

Performance Checklist
Skill 21-3: Hemodialysis: Maintenance of Vascular Access

Critical Behaviors	Complies	
	yes	no
1. Wash hands.		
2. Evaluate the patency of the vascular access:		
a. Palpate for a thrill above the A-V fistula or along the entire length of the graft.		
b. Auscultate with a stethoscope/Doppler for a bruit.		
3. Evaluate the circulation of the vascular access:		
a. Palpate pulses distal to the access.		
b. Observe for bleeding or hematoma/clot formation.		
c. Check for capillary refill.		
d. Compare temperature and color of extremities.		
4. Inquire about altered sensation distal to vascular access.		
5. Assess for signs of infection.		
6. Place sign above bed indicating limb with vascular access.		
7. Wash hands.		
8. Document procedure in patient record.		

SKILL 21–4

Hemodialysis: Initiation and Termination

Hemodialysis requires a closed extracorporeal circuit that provides a conduit to propel blood between the body and the dialyzer (artificial kidney) (Fig. 21–2). The dialyzer removes accumulated uremic toxins and corrects fluid and electrolyte imbalances. The essential component of the dialyzer is a semipermeable membrane that interfaces with both blood and dialysate and allows passage of select molecules through small pores. The dialysate passes through the dialyzer on the outside of the semipermeable membrane, while blood flows in a countercurrent direction on the inside of the membrane. After substances are exchanged, the dialysate admixture is discarded via an outflow port and the blood is returned to the patient. Dialyzers currently in use are categorized as hollow fiber, parallel plate, or hemoperfusion devices.

Hollow fiber: Composed of 10,000 to 20,000 cuprammonium rayon or regenerated cellulose fibers that have an internal diameter of approximately 200 μm. Blood flows through the fibers, while dialysate flows countercurrent or crosscurrent on the outside of the fibers (Fig. 21–3).

Parallel plate: Composed of cuprophan sheets layered between grooved rigid supports. Dialyzing fluid flows outside the cellophane membrane countercurrent to the flow of blood in the cellophane layers (Fig. 21–4).

Hemoperfusion cartridge: Utilizes a cartridge containing biocompatible activated carbon that has the capacity to efficiently remove drugs with fat-soluble or protein-bound drugs. Dialysate is not required; however, heparin is necessary to prevent extracorporeal clotting of the blood.

The dialysate bath is a concentrated electrolyte mixture of water, sodium chloride, potassium chloride, calcium chloride, and magnesium chloride with glucose

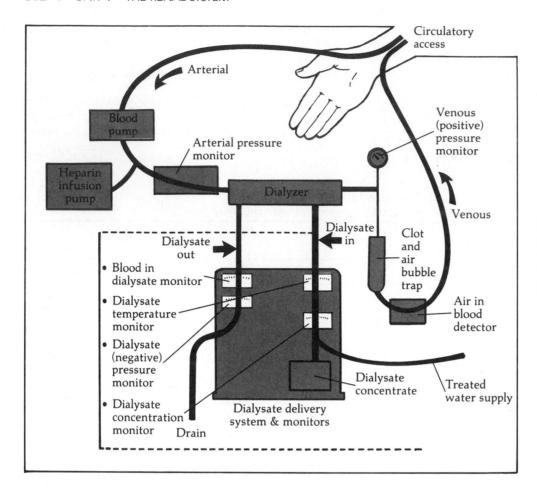

FIGURE 21–2. Components of a typical hemodialysis system in Thompson, J. M., McFarland, G. K., Hirsch, J. E., Tucker, S. M., and Bowers, A. C. (eds.) *Mosby's Manual of Clinical Nursing.* St. Louis, C.V. Mosby Co., 1989, with permission.

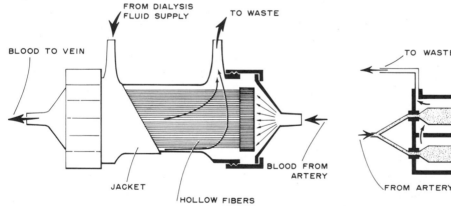

FIGURE 21–3. Hollow fiber or capillary dialyzer in Price, S. and Wilson, L. (eds.) *Pathophysiology–Clinical Concepts of Disease Processes.* New York, McGraw-Hill, 1982, with permission.

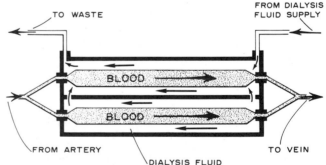

FIGURE 21–4. Parallel plate dialyzer in Price, S. and Wilson, L. (eds.) *Pathophysiology–Clinical Concepts of Disease Processes.* New York, McGraw-Hill, 1982, with permission.

added to achieve a desired osmolality. A base of acetate or bicarbonate is used to help replenish body buffer stores and provide additional buffer reserves. Bicarbonate is the preferred buffer because problems with cramping, hypotension, nausea, and vomiting are reported less frequently. Dialysate prescriptions may be individualized by altering additives of calcium, potassium, and glucose based on the patient's biochemical parameters.

The major function of the fluid delivery system is to combine the concentrated electrolyte mixture with water and then transport this dialysate fluid to the hemodialyzer. Figure 21–2 represents a typical hemodialysis system. Three systems currently used are the proportioning, batch, and sorbent regenerating systems.

Proportioning system: Uses a metering pump to automatically mix processed tap water and liquid concentrate. It is delivered to the dialyzer and then discarded. Water processing methods available include filtration, softening, distillation, deionization, and reverse osmosis.

Batch system: Water and concentrated solution are manually mixed in a 100-L tank to achieve the correct composition of dialysate, and the mixture is pulled up from a holding tank to the dialyzer, which sits in a small reservoir on top of the machine. Dialysate is pulled by a flowmeter at a rate of 400 to 600 ml/min and circulates through the dialyzer and is then discarded.

Sorbent regenerating system: Less than 6 L of water is used. Dialysate is converted through ion exchange and absorption into reusable water through a multilayered sorbent cartridge. No additional water processing or plumbing is required as the dialysate recirculates in the system.

Purpose

The nurse performs hemodialysis to maintain volume regulation, acid–base balance, electrolyte and azotemia control.

Prerequisite Knowledge and Skills

Prior to performing hemodialysis, the nurse should understand

1. Universal precautions.
2. Principles of aseptic technique.
3. Principles of renal physiology and dynamics of renal disease.
4. Principles of fluid, electrolyte, and acid–base balance.
5. Vascular access.
6. Principles of hemodialysis.
7. Components of the dialysis system, including dialyzer, fluid delivery system, and water treatments.

The nurse should be able to perform

1. Proper handwashing techniques (see Skill 35–5).
2. Universal precautions (see Skill 35–1).
3. Systematic patient assessment.
4. Cannulation of vascular access (see Skill 21–2).

Assessment

1. Observe for the quality of blood flow in the vascular access (i.e., bruit, thrill, arterial pressure gauge readings on the hemodialysis machine—varies greatly with a fistula subclavian catheter or graft—usually between -50 and -150 mmHg). **Rationale:** Validates patency of vascular access.
2. Monitor the patient's vital signs (i.e., temperature, pulse, respiration, and blood pressure). **Rationale:** Alterations in vital signs may indicate a decreased cardiovascular response as fluid volume is removed.
3. Assess the patient's fluid, electrolyte, and acid–base status (i.e., edema, lung and heart sounds, current weight versus dry weight, neck vein distension, dysrhythmias, weakness, nausea, vomiting, and diarrhea). **Rationale:** The dialysis prescription may vary in terms of ul-

trafiltration required, concentration of dialysate bath, and/or dialyzer selection when fluid, electrolyte, and acid–base imbalances occur.
4. Monitor the hemodialysis circuit (i.e., arterial and venous pressures, temperature, conductivity, and dialyzer membrane and blood lines for leaks). **Rationale:** These symptoms must be monitored to prevent technical problems of the delivery system and untoward patient complications.

Nursing Diagnoses

1. Fluid volume excess related to intravascular volume overload, hypertension, and edema. **Rationale:** In renal disease, a decreased glomerular filtration rate (GFR) and a decreased renal excretion of waste products result in an excess intravascular volume.
2. Potential for decreased cardiac output related to rapid intravascular volume removal. **Rationale:** Hypovolemia can be potentiated with excessive fluid removal.
3. Anxiety related to loss of kidney function and hemodialysis therapy. **Rationale:** Renal disease and dialysis treatment regimen create many stresses for the patient, causing loss of control over environment and self.
4. Potential for injury related to susceptibility to bleeding. **Rationale:** Decreased clotting factors, increased nitrogenous waste products, platelet defects, and anticoagulation therapy potentiate this complication during dialysis.
5. Pain related to muscle cramping, nausea, or vomiting. **Rationale:** Fluid and electrolyte shifts potentiate symptoms.
6. Potential for infection related to repeated venipunctures. **Rationale:** Portal of entry for transmission of microorganisms occurs with cannulation of vascular access.

Planning

1. Develop individualized goals for patients on hemodialysis to maintain euvolemic status, acid–base balance, electrolyte balance, and azotemia control. **Rationale:** Dialysis removes accumulated waste products to restore fluid, electrolyte, and acid–base balance.
2. Prepare all necessary equipment and supplies. **Rationale:** Assembly of all necessary equipment ensures that the procedure will be completed efficiently.

INITIATION

   a. Single-patient system machine, tubes, dialyzer, and dialysate.
   b. Tape, 1 in.
   c. Two bulldog clamps.
   d. One set exam gloves.
   e. Goggles.
   f. One vial heparin (if loading dose ordered by physician).

g. One 30-cc syringe.
h. One 18-gauge needle.
i. One sterile 4 × 4 gauze pad.
j. Antiseptic soap.
k. One sterile barrier.

TERMINATION

a. Single-patient system machine.
b. Four bulldog clamps.
c. Four 2 × 2 gauze pads.
d. Normal saline, 1000 ml.
e. One set exam gloves.
f. Goggles.
g. Four bandages.
h. Sharps container.

3. Prepare the patient.
   a. Explain the procedure. **Rationale:** Reduces anxiety and enhances cooperation of the patient.
   b. Position patient in a prone position with the head elevated at 45 degrees or as tolerated (varies with individualized hemodynamic parameters). **Rationale:** Promotes easy breathing, comfort and ease of hemodialysis initiation.
4. Verify physician order for dialysis. Physician order should include type of dialyzer, number of hours for dialysis run, heparinization required, ultrafiltration, lab work, dialysate bath. **Rationale:** Reduces possibility of error.
5. Set up single-patient system machine according to manufacturer's directions. **Rationale:** Ensures safe and proper assembly.

Implementation

Steps	Rationale	Special Considerations
Initiation		
1. Wash hands.	Reduces transmission of microorganisms.	
2. Don exam gloves and goggles.	Universal precautions.	
3. Wash access arm for 1 full minute with antiseptic soap and a sterile 4 × 4, and place arm on sterile barrier.	Reduces transmission of microorganisms and establishes a sterile field.	
4. Cannulate vascular access (see Skills 21–1 and 21–2).	Provides access to vascular system.	
5. Connect arterial access to arterial patient line.	Provides a circuit between the patient and the dialyzer.	
6. Place the venous dialyzer tubing line into the retaining clamps of the fluid catch-all on the side of the dialysis machine.	Prevents contamination of venous tubing.	Be careful not to immerse the end of the venous line below the fluid level.
7. Tape arterial cannula connections securely.	Prevents accidental disconnection.	
8. Remove bulldog clamp from arterial line.	Permits flow of blood.	
9. Adjust blood pump to 100 ml/min until blood reaches the venous drip chamber.	Slow rate prevents symptoms of rapid blood loss and allows for assessment of blood flow from the arterial limb.	Heparin loading dose may be given via bolus in arterial line, if ordered.
10. Turn off blood pump.	Prevents blood loss from dialyzer and cannula.	
11. Clamp the end of the venous tubing below the drip chamber with a bulldog clamp.	Prevents introduction of air.	
12. Remove venous line tubing from fluid catch-all and connect to the venous patient cannula.	Completes pathway circuit for return of blood from the dialyzer to the patient.	
13. Tape venous connections securely.	Prevents accidental separation.	
14. Remove bulldog clamp from venous tubing.	Permits flow of blood.	

Table continues on following page

Steps	Rationale	Special Considerations
15. Turn on blood pump, and adjust flow to 100 ml/min.	Initiates flow of blood from patient to the dialyzer.	
16. Immediately move foam detector switch from bypass to alarm position.	Sets the foam detector alarm monitor to on.	The air/foam monitor detects minute air leaks.
17. Adjust the blood level in the arterial and venous drip chambers to three-quarters full.	Prevents accumulation of air in tubing and dialyzer.	
18. Turn dialyzer over so that arterial (red) port is at the top.	Establishes countercurrent flow.	
19. If patient is receiving systemic heparinization, set parameters on heparin infusion pump as prescribed.	Provides anticoagulation.	A 30-cc syringe containing heparinized saline (dose dependent on prescription of physician and number of hours on dialysis) is placed in the heparin infusion pump. The rate of infusion can be set from 0.5 to 5.5 cc/hr.
20. Secure cannula connections and blood tubing to patient's extremity/gown.	Additional precaution against accidental disconnection.	
21. Slowly increase blood pump speed to prescribed rate while continuing to assess patient (level of consciousness, complaints of chest pain, dysrhythmias, and changes in hemodynamic variables).	Prevents complications from rapid removal of blood.	Identify on your dialysis machine the indicators for *actual* pressure vs. the high and low pressure alarm limits.
22. Set alarm limit indicators for both arterial and venous pressures 50 mmHg above and below actual pressure gauge indicator.	Sets the safety alarm system.	Ascertain whether your dialysis machine requires a manual setting of the dialysate pressure alarm. This alarm may be a built-in feature on newer dialysis machines.
23. Calculate patient's transmembrane pressure (TMP).	To remove desired ultrafiltrate.	Formula: Weight to be removed × 500 ml − KUF = TMP. (KUF is the coefficient of ultrafiltration of the dialyzer. Each type/size of dialyzer has a different KUF, which can be obtained from the package insert.)
24. Set TMP or negative pressure.	Allows for ultrafiltration.	
25. Wash hands.	Reduces transmission of microorganisms.	
26. Continuously monitor patient status and machine function throughout treatment.	Prevents complications and minimizes effects of fluid and electrolyte shifts.	Patient assessment should include vital signs and symptoms related to fluid and electrolyte shifts (such as cramping, hypotension, nausea, and vomiting). Monitor the machine for blood flow rate, arterial and venous pressure readings, dialysate pressure, and blood circuit for clotting or air.

Termination

Steps	Rationale	Special Considerations
1. Wash hands.	Reduces transmission of microorganisms.	
2. Don clean examination gloves and goggles.	Universal precautions.	
3. Move the arterial, venous, and dialysate pressure alarms to the maximum low/high limits.	Prevents machine from alarming when terminating as pressures drop.	

Table continues on following page

Steps	Rationale	Special Considerations
4. Turn TMP or negative pressure off.	Removes negative pressure, thereby stopping ultrafiltration.	
5. Turn off the heparin infusion pump.	Discontinues heparinization prior to the end of dialysis, thus allowing clotting times to return to normal shortly after treatment.	
6. Decrease the blood pump flow to 100 cc/min.	Reduces blood flow.	
7. Check amount of normal saline, and hang a new bag if necessary.	Minimizes the danger of air embolism on return of blood to patient.	Normal saline (100 cc) or air rinse is used to return blood to patient.
8. Maintain the blood level in the arterial and venous drip chambers at three-quarters full.	Prevents air in tubing and dialyzer.	
9. Turn off the blood pump.	Stops blood flow.	
10. Clamp the arterial tubing with a bulldog clamp between patient and blood pump.	Prevents loss of blood if the tubing becomes separated.	
11. Disconnect tubing from vascular access device.	Terminates dialysis.	
12. Turn on blood pump to rate of 100 cc/min, and simultaneously unclamp the patient end connector of the arterial tubing.	Promotes slow return of blood in tubing back to patient.	
13. When blood level is just above the arterial chamber, clamp the tubing above the arterial chamber with a bulldog clamp.	Minimizes the danger of air embolism on return of blood to the patient.	
14. Unclamp the normal saline IV line.	Flushes the tubing.	
15. Maintain blood pump at 100 cc/min, and clear the blood tubing and dialyzer with saline until satisfactory rinse-back is achieved.	Promotes rinse-back of blood to patient.	Satisfactory rinse-back is achieved when venous chamber has pink-tinged normal saline return.
16. Turn off blood pump.	Terminates flow of blood.	
17. Clamp venous access with a bulldog clamp.	Prevents backflow of blood.	
18. If using a subclavian catheter, complete uncoupling (see Skill 21–1).	Discontinues vascular access.	Maintain aseptic technique.
19. A-V fistula/A-V graft: When fistula needles are used, remove both cannulas from patient's access site, one at a time. Using sterile 2 × 2 gauze pad, apply moderate pressure to access site until bleeding has stopped.	Discontinues vascular access.	Maintain aseptic technique.
20. Dress access site(s) with remaining sterile 2 × 2 gauze pad and bandages.	Provides protective barrier.	
21. Dispose of soiled material/equipment in appropriate disposal receptacle.	Universal precautions.	

Table continues on following page

Steps	Rationale	Special Considerations
22. Sanitize single-patient machine according to established procedure.	Reduces transmission of microorganisms and readies it for future use.	
23. Wash hands.	Reduces transmission of microorganisms.	

Evaluation

1. Evaluate any complications related to the vascular access (i.e., bleeding, clotting, poor flow), physical/metabolic patient problems (i.e., dysrhythmia, chest pain, acid–base imbalance), and technical problems (i.e., blood leak, clotted dialyzer) during, and after dialysis. **Rationale:** Continuous evaluation during, and after dialysis assists in prompt identification and management of complications and any untoward effects to the patient when identifying the effectiveness of the hemodialysis treatment.

2. Assess the patient's vital signs (i.e., blood pressure, pulse, temperature, weight, respirations, and PAP/PCWP) and laboratory values (i.e., sodium, potassium, CO_2, chloride, blood urea nitrogen, creatinine, hemoglobin, and hematocrit) before and after dialysis. **Rationale:** Evaluates the patient's response to therapy and effectiveness of hemodialysis treatment.

Expected Outcomes

1. Removal of accumulated waste products and restoration of acid–base/electrolyte/fluid balance. **Rationale:** The process of hemodialysis removes excess nitrogenous waste products, fluid, and electrolytes, but since the dialysis bath has higher concentrations of electrolytes depleted by renal failure, those needed by the patient are replaced or maintained.

2. Weight at or near dry weight, BUN and creatinine decreased from predialysis value, and electrolytes within normal limits. **Rationale:** Decrease in uremic manifestations and complications thereof promotes homeostasis.

Unexpected Outcomes

1. Complications related to vascular access (i.e., hematoma, vascular spasm, clotting, or poor blood flow). **Rationale:** Without patency of access, hemodialysis cannot be performed.

2. Physiologic complications (i.e., dysrhythmias, chest pain, acid–base imbalance, hypotension, nausea and vomiting, seizures, headaches, muscle cramping, or dyspnea). **Rationale:** Rapid removal of fluid and waste products and shifts in electrolytes may potentiate adverse outcomes.

3. Technical problems (i.e., blood leak, clotted di-

alyzer, air leak, disconnection of lines, or hemolysis). **Rationale:** These problems may alert staff to dialysis equipment/machine malfunctions or problems.

Documentation

Documentation in the patient record should include the date, time, and length of hemodialysis; assessments of access site, respiratory, cardiovascular, and neurologic status; vital signs; weight before and after dialysis; and any complications. **Rationale:** Documents nursing care given and provides data to trend the effectiveness of dialytic therapy.

Patient/Family Education

1. Assess the patient's and family's level of knowledge related to the disease process and treatment plan. **Rationale:** Enables patient and family members to ask questions and the nurse to give feedback.

2. Discuss with the patient and family the treatment modality in terms of process, access required, risks, and benefits. **Rationale:** This enables the patient and family to participate in decision making and to take part in the treatment plan.

3. Instruct the patient and family in the signs and symptoms of possible complications of dialysis (i.e., chest pain, bleeding, muscle cramps, and nausea and vomiting). **Rationale:** Assists the patient and family in recognizing complications to properly notify the staff when symptoms occur or develop. Enables the patient and family to take an active part in the treatment plan.

4. Evaluate the patient's need for long-term dialysis intervention. **Rationale:** Since long-term dialysis therapy is located in outpatient facilities, early discharge planning facilitates patient placement.

5. Implement instructions regarding diet and fluid restrictions, medications, access care, and follow-up appointments. **Rationale:** Enables patient to make decisions and become an active member of the treatment plan.

6. Assess the patient's need for home health care and durable medical equipment. **Rationale:** Promotes continuity of care for the discharged patient.

Performance Checklist
Skill 21–4:   Hemodialysis: Initiation and Termination

Critical Behaviors	Complies yes	no
INITIATION		
1. Wash hands.		
2. Don gloves and goggles.		
3. Wash access arm for 1 minute with antiseptic soap.		
4. Cannulate vascular access.		
5. Connect arterial access to arterial patient line.		
6. Appropriately place venous patient line in retaining clamps of fluid catch-all.		
7. Tape arterial connections securely.		
8. Remove bulldog clamp from arterial line.		
9. Slowly adjust blood pump to 100 ml/min.		
10. When blood reaches venous drip chamber, turn off blood pump.		
11. Clamp off venous tubing below drip chamber.		
12. Remove venous line tubing from fluid catch-all and connect to venous cannula.		
13. Tape venous connection securely.		
14. Remove bulldog clamp from venous tubing.		
15. Turn on blood pump and adjust blood flow to 100 ml/min.		
16. Set foam detector switch to alarm position.		
17. Adjust blood level in drip chambers to three-quarters full.		
18. Change position of dialyzer to establish countercurrent flow.		
19. Set correct parameters on heparin pump, if appropriate.		
20. Secure needles and tubes.		
21. Slowly increase blood pump speed to prescribed rate.		
22. Set alarm limits for arterial and venous pressures.		
23. Calculate TMP.		
24. Set TMP or negative pressure.		
25. Wash hands.		
26. Monitor patient throughout treatment.		
27. Document procedure in patient record.		
TERMINATION		
1. Wash hands.		
2. Don clean gloves and goggles.		
3. Spread alarm limits.		
4. Turn TMP or negative pressure off.		
5. Turn heparin infusion pump off.		
6. Decrease blood flow to 100 cc/min.		

Table continues on following page

Critical Behaviors	Complies	
	yes	no
7. Check amount of normal saline, and hang replacement bag if necessary.		
8. Maintain appropriate blood levels in arterial and venous drip chambers.		
9. Turn off blood pump.		
10. Clamp arterial tubing with bulldog clamp.		
11. Disconnect tubing from vascular access.		
12. Simultaneously turn on blood pump and unclamp the patient end connector of arterial tubing.		
13. Clamp arterial line when air reaches chamber.		
14. Unclamp IV normal saline line to promote rinse-back of blood.		
15. Maintain blood pump speed to clear tubing and dialyzer of blood.		
16. Turn blood pump off.		
17. Clamp venous access.		
18. Complete uncoupling from subclavian catheter.		
19. *Or* decannulate A-V fistula/graft.		
20. Dress access sites.		
21. Dispose of soiled material/equipment in appropriate receptacles.		
22. Sanitize machine according to established procedure.		
23. Wash hands.		
24. Document procedure in patient record.		

SKILL 21–5

Continuous Renal Replacement Therapy: Slow Continuous Ultrafiltration (SCUF) and Continuous Arteriovenous Hemofiltration (CAVH)

Continuous renal replacement therapy is a process whereby fluid and solutes are removed in patients who do not require or tolerate conventional methods of hemodialysis. Two methods commonly used are slow continuous ultrafiltration (SCUF) and continuous arteriovenous hemofiltration (CAVH). Both are relatively simple procedures requiring minimal volumes of priming fluid.

Both methods use a hemofilter connected to arterial and venous access lines (Fig. 21–5). Blood flows from the arterial line through the hemofilter, where the removal of plasma water and all unbound substances with molecular weights between 500 and 10,000 daltons (ultrafiltrate) is regulated via a volumetric pump, slide clamp, or suction. The ultrafiltrate exits through a side port, and blood is returned to the patient via the venous access limb. Heparin is continuously infused to prevent clotting of the hemofilter.

The force of the arterial blood pressure propels the blood through the circuit. For successful performance, the mean arterial pressure must be 60 mmHg. The hemofilter has a large surface area, high sieving coefficient, and low resistance, so patients with low mean arterial pressures can tolerate the procedure. Arterial and venous access is required. The femoral artery is a common site for percutaneous cannulation. An arteriovenous shunt may also be used but is less desired.

With CAVH, there is a slow, continuous removal of fluid and solutes (400–800 cc/hr). Usually, one-half to three-fourths of the ultrafiltrate removed is replaced in the next hour's infusion of intravenous fluid. Thus the patient's intravascular volume and electrolyte values are gradually changed causing fewer problems than with conventional hemodialysis. It is particularly useful in hemodynamically unstable patients with fluid overload and azotemia. CAVH can be alternated with hemodialysis thus decreasing the number of hemodialysis treatments needed. Contraindications to CAVH include a hypercatabolic state, hyperkalemia, poisoning, low blood pressure (MAP<60 mmHg), shock or low colloid oncotic pressure, congestive heart failure, and severe atherosclerosis. CAVH should not be used in situations when the rapid removal of unwanted substances is necessary.

While CAVH provides a greater exchange of solutes through hemodilution, SCUF primarily removes plasma water in much smaller volumes (150–300 cc/hr). The replacement fluid will consist of the patient's usual hourly intravenous infusion (maintenance IV, vasoactive phar-

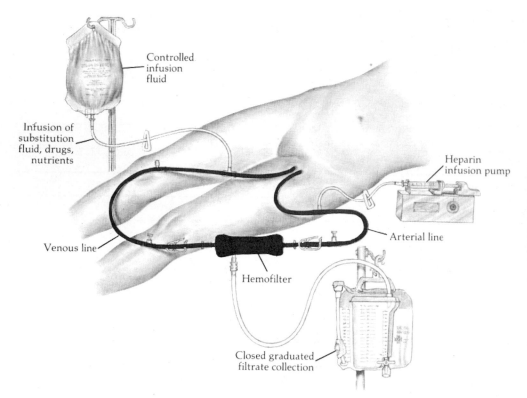

Controlled infusion fluid

Infusion of substitution fluid, drugs, nutrients

Venous line

Heparin infusion pump

Arterial line

Hemofilter

Closed graduated filtrate collection

FIGURE 21–5. Continuous arteriovenous hemofiltration with femoral cannulations in Thompson, J. M., McFarland, G. K., Hirsch, J. E., Tucker, S. M., and Bowers, A. C. (eds.) *Mosby's Manual of Clinical Nursing.* St. Louis, C.V. Mosby Co., 1989, with permission.

macotherapeutics, total parenteral nutrition, etc). SCUF is commonly used to control fluid balance between hemodialysis treatments and fluid volume overload in patients with congestive heart failure unresponsive to diuretic therapy.

Purpose

The nurse performs continuous ultrafiltration to remove fluid and/or solute from patients with uncomplicated acute oliguric renal failure, especially those who are hemodynamically unstable on conventional methods of dialysis.

Prerequisite Knowledge and Skills

Prior to performing CAVH/SCUF, the nurse should understand

1. Universal precautions.
2. Principles of aseptic technique.
3. Principles of vascular access cannulation and venipuncture.
4. Principles of fluid, electrolyte, and acid–base balance.
5. The theoretical and technical aspects of the hemofiltration membrane.

The nurse should be able to perform

1. Proper handwashing technique (see Skill 35–5).
2. Systematic patient assessment.
3. Cannulation of vascular access (see Skill 21–1 or 21–2).

4. Preparation and priming of hemofiltration equipment.
5. Determination of activated clotting time (ACT).

Assessment

1. Assess the vascular access for patency and infection (i.e., bruit, thrill, clotting, bleeding, purulent drainage, erythema, pain, or warmth around site). **Rationale:** Validates patent access and the presence of infection.
2. Assess the patient's vital signs (i.e., temperature, pulse, respiration, blood pressure—mean arterial pressure above 60 mmHg—and CVP/PAP/PCWP). **Rationale:** Alterations in vital signs may indicate a decreased cardiovascular response as fluid volume is removed.
3. Assess the patient's fluid, electrolyte, and acid–base balance (i.e., edema, lung and heart sounds, current weight versus dry weight, weakness, dysrhythmias, nausea, vomiting, or diarrhea). **Rationale:** Untoward effects may indicate that the patient is not tolerating the hemofiltration.
4. Assess the patient's anticoagulation status (i.e., prothrombin time (PT), partial thromboplastin time (PTT) and platelet count). **Rationale:** Maintains patency in system for continued hemofiltration.
5. Determine the patient's hematocrit. **Rationale:** With hematocrits greater than 40%, the blood may sludge and clot in the hemofilter.

Nursing Diagnoses

1. Fluid volume excess related to too-rapid infusion of replacement fluid. **Rationale:** CAVH utilizes an IV

system to infuse fluid, drugs, and nutrients into the venous circuit.

2. Potential for fluid volume deficit related to decreased cardiac output. **Rationale:** Too-rapid fluid removal or bleeding decreases the circulating volume, thus decreasing the cardiac output.

3. Potential for infection related to vascular access. **Rationale:** Portal of entry for transmission of microorganisms on cannulation of vascular access or venipuncture.

Planning

1. Individualize the following goals for performing continuous ultrafiltration:
   a. Maintain fluid/acid–base/electrolyte/balance. **Rationale:** Increased removal of fluid and shifts in electrolytes may potentiate adverse outcomes.
   b. Maintain patency of vascular access. **Rationale:** Without patency of access, hemofiltration cannot be maintained.
   c. Maintain prescribed anticoagulation ranges. **Rationale:** Monitoring of the Lee White or ACT helps to prevent inadequate or excessive anticoagulation and, therefore, a decreased likelihood of bleeding tendencies or membrane clotting.
2. Assemble all necessary equipment and supplies. **Rationale:** Preparation of all equipment and supplies will ensure that the procedure is initiated efficiently.

a. Hemofilter system.
b. Two infusion pumps (per hospital use).
c. Eight sterile 4 × 4's.
d. Two sterile barriers.
e. Tape, 1 in wide.
f. Two sterile bulldog clamps (nonserrated cannulated clamps).
g. Replacement fluid as ordered (IV or peritoneal solutions).
h. Sterile gloves.
i. Six to eight povidone-iodine swabs.
j. Four alcohol wipes.
k. One prefilled 20-cc syringe with 10 ml heparinized saline (10 U/ml), or according to established policy.
l. One 3-cc syringe containing 1 cc of heparin (5000 U/ml).
m. 2 L of 0.9% normal saline for IV infusion.
n. Blood tubes for anticoagulation specimens.
o. Drainage bag (peritoneal dialysis solution 5-L bag).
p. Goggles.
q. One set exam gloves.

3. Prepare the patient.
   a. Explain the purpose and procedure of hemofiltration. **Rationale:** Minimizes anxiety and facilitates cooperation.
   b. Explain the necessity for bed rest. **Rationale:** Patient will need to remain in bed throughout the procedure.

Implementation

Steps	Rationale	Special Considerations
Preparation		
1. Wash hands.	Reduces transmission of microorganisms.	
2. Remove hemofilter and lines from package, and check that protective caps are properly placed at the end of the arterial and venous blood lines.	Maintains a closed system for sterility.	Review the hemofilter and observe the minimal distance between the priming solution and the hemofilter and the collection/measuring device. By raising the priming solution higher than the rest of the system, the amount of time required to prime the system is decreased.
3. Maintain and check that blood line connections to hemofilter are secure.	To avoid accidental leaks or disconnections.	
4. Place the hemofilter with arterial end down (blood inlet) in the holder, and lock the holder.	Positions hemofilter for priming procedure.	
5. Connect 1000 cc of 0.9% normal saline to the end of the venous line (blood outlet), and position bag at the level of the hemofilter.	Used as a flushing solution.	

Table continues on following page

Steps	Rationale	Special Considerations
6. Attach the ultrafiltration (UF) line to the uncapped port on the hemofilter (across from arterial inlet port).	Provides a closed system for collection of ultrafiltrate.	Maintain aseptic technique.
7. Connect the UF line to the closed collection/measuring device.	Completes assembly of system and facilitates measurement of the priming solution.	
8. Hang the collection system approximately 20 in (no less than 16 in) below the level of the hemofilter.	Priming position enhances movement of the priming solution across the membrane of the hemofilter.	
9. Check that all lines are securely connected.	Prevents leaks or disconnections.	Check that the cap on the dialysate inlet port (across from the venous line) is secure.
10. Close clamp on arterial blood line, and keep venous line, UF line, and rinsing bag clamps open.	Primes the system.	Bulldog clamps can be used if roller clamps are lost. These are nonserrated cannulated clamps that prevent cutting of tubing.
11. Prepare 2 L of heparinized 0.9% normal saline: Instill 5000 U heparin per 1000 cc of 0.9% normal saline.	Priming solution.	Heparin may vary. Check the unit protocol or the physician's order.
12. Hang the heparinized normal saline solution at least 48 in above the level of the hemofilter.	Facilitates priming of the hemofilter by gravity.	
13. Connect infusion pump to arterial line.	Prevents clotting of hemofilter.	

Priming

Steps	Rationale	Special Considerations
1. Wash hands.	Reduces transmission of microorganisms.	
2. Unclamp the arterial line, and flush all connecting lines with the heparinized 0.9% normal saline solution.	Initiates priming of the system.	Make sure that whenever there is fluid, either priming solution or blood, moving through the blood compartment of the hemofilter, the ultrafiltrate line remains unclamped. If the UF line is clamped during the priming procedure, you may have inadequate removal of air or cause some of or all the layers of the hemofilter to collapse, rendering it nonfunctional.
3. Intermittently clamp and unclamp the venous line for 3 to 5 seconds.	Enhances removal of air from the blood compartment.	Some normal saline may appear in the UF line; this is normal.
4. When 1000 ml of priming solution has flowed into system, clamp the venous line, and rotate the hemofilter so that the arterial line is up.	Initiates thorough priming of the ultrafiltrate compartment.	Hemofilter must be rinsed to remove glycerin coating, ethylene oxide (from sterilization), and all air bubbles.
5. Hang another 1000 ml of heparinized 0.9% normal saline.	For priming ultrafiltrate compartment.	
6. Continue priming with heparinized 0.9% normal saline until 400 ml of normal saline has collected in the ultrafiltrate collection/measuring device.	Ensures that ultrafiltrate compartment is thoroughly primed.	

Table continues on following page

Steps	Rationale	Special Considerations
7. Rotate the hemofilter so that the arterial line end is down.	To complete priming of the hemofilter.	
8. Unclamp the venous line.	Allows drainage of fluid from the hemofilter.	
9. Infuse 500 ml to flow through the venous blood side, and intermittently clamp and unclamp the venous line.	Promotes purging of air bubbles from the hemofilter.	
10. When 100 ml of the heparinized 0.9% normal saline remains in the IV bag, clamp the arterial line.	Prevents introduction of air into the system.	If air bubbles persist, continue flushing the system with heparinized 0.9% normal saline.
11. Clamp the venous and UF lines.	Prevents loss of priming solution from system and potential for air accumulation.	
12. Drain and discard the normal saline in UF collection device. The system is now ready for patient use.	Excludes normal saline priming solution from ultrafiltrate volume.	

Initiation

Steps	Rationale	Special Considerations
1. Wash hands.	Reduces transmission of microorganisms.	
2. Establish vascular access (see Skills 9–1, 21–1, or 21–2).	Provides route for hemofiltration.	Subclavian and venipuncture access may be initiated depending on established protocols. Ensure that patient has an arterial access and a venous access.
3. Position hemofilter parallel to the patient's access.	Allows for flow of ultrafiltrate by gravity.	
4. Don goggles and gloves.	Universal precautions.	
5. Administer initial heparin dose, if ordered, per established policy.	Provides anticoagulation to prevent clotting of hemofilter.	
6. Connect setup lines to access.	Establishes closed system for hemofiltration.	Secure access sites and filter for safety.
7. Position the UF collection/measuring device below the level of the patient.	Encourages flow of ultrafiltration by gravity.	Level of collection device determines rate of ultrafiltration. Raising the level decreases the negative pressure and rate of ultrafiltration; lowering the collection devices increases the negative pressure and rate of ultrafiltration.
8. Securely tape all connections.	Prevents leaks or disconnections.	
9. Ensure that system is flowing well.	Validates effectiveness of hemofiltration.	
10. Dispose of soiled material in appropriate receptacle.	Universal precautions.	
11. Wash hands.	Prevents transmission of microorganisms.	

Monitoring

Steps	Rationale	Special Considerations
1. Administer maintenance heparin as prescribed or per unit protocol.	Prevents decrease in UF formation and clotting.	Heparin dose varies according to patient condition.

Table continues on following page

Steps	Rationale	Special Considerations
2. Initiate replacement fluids as per established policy or as ordered.	Prevents hypotensive episodes.	Replacement fluids are dependent on the patient's baseline assessment (electrolyte status, volume status). Normal saline or Ringer's lactate solutions are preferred. Total parenteral nutrition solutions can be infused with replacement fluid without fluid overload. Formula: Amount of previous hour's ultrafiltrate plus previous hour's total output minus previous hour's IV fluids plus desired net hourly fluid loss equals amount of replacement fluid $(UF + TO) - (IV + FL) = RF$.
3. Monitor for occlusion or kinks in ultrafiltrate line, blood lines, and vascular access.	Prevents decrease in UF formation.	
4. Monitor security of all connections.	Prevents accidental disconnection.	
5. Monitor UF for		
a. Rate: Should be 200 cc/h or less.	Prevents excessive fluid removal and decreases potential for hypotensive episodes.	If UF volume decreases sharply (greater than 20%), assess system for clotting. If you want to decrease UF rate during therapy, raise the ultrafiltrate collection/measuring device.
b. Clarity of filtrate: If blood-tinged, clamp UF tubing and notify physician immediately.	Pink or red-tinged color indicates filter leak or rupture.	
c. Position of hemofilter.	Maintains adequate UF rate.	
d. Level of collection/measuring device: Should be approximately 20 in (no less than 16 in) below the level of the filter.	Allows for gravity drainage.	
e. Presence of air bubbles.	Air is entering the system, negative pressure is too high; disconnected lines, leaks, cracks, or clotting in filter.	
6. Monitor vital signs. If the patient becomes acutely hypotensive:	Fluid can be ultrafiltrated faster than it can be equilibrated into the vasculature, causing hypotension.	Continuously monitor intake and output, hemodynamic variables, and heart rate and rhythm.
a. Clamp UF tubing. Blood will continue to flow through the filter, but no UF will be formed.	Prevents further ultrafiltration.	
b. Increase rate of replacement fluids as prescribed by physician.	Increases volume status, thus decreasing hypotensive state.	
7. Monitor clotting times as per unit protocol.	Prevents clotting of system.	Clotting time generally monitored every hour or as ordered.
8. Monitor rate of fluid replacement (see step 2 under Monitoring).	Prevents excessive infusion/depletion.	$(UF + TO) - (IV + FL) = RF$.

Table continues on following page

Steps	Rationale	Special Considerations
9. Monitor laboratory data per established protocol (i.e., BUN, electrolytes, CBC, creatinine, and coagulation studies).	Evaluates hydration and effects of solute removal.	
10. Monitor the patient's access site and all lines for		
a. Uniform color of blood in filter.	Indicates no clotting.	
b. Lack of separation or appearance of white flecks in tubing.	Indicates clotting of blood.	
Termination		
1. Wash hands.	Reduces transmission of microorganisms.	
2. Don gloves and goggles.	Universal precautions.	
3. Clamp fluid replacement line.	Prevents further administration of fluid.	
4. Clamp the arterial and venous lines.	Prevents the loss of blood if tubing becomes separated.	
5. Bulldog-clamp the arterial access line, and remove tape.	Prevents further flow of blood.	
6. Clean connection site with alcohol wipe × 2.	Reduces transmission of microorganisms.	
7. Disconnect arterial access line from arterial system line.	Breaks system to terminate from the arterial side.	
8. Repeat steps 6 and 7 for venous system line.	Breaks system to terminate from the venous side.	
9. Prepare for the disconnection/ decannulation (see Skill 21–1).	Discontinues vascular access.	Maintain aseptic technique.
10. Dispose of soiled material in disposal receptacle.	Universal precautions.	
11. Wash hands.	Reduces transmission of organisms.	

Evaluation

1.   Evaluate during and following hemofiltration any complications related to physical/metabolic patient problems (i.e., dysrhythmias, chest pain, acid–base imbalance), vascular access (i.e., poor flow, clotting), and technical problems (i.e., clotted hemofilter). **Rationale:** Continuous evaluation assists in prompt identification and management of complications and untoward effects to the patient.

2.   Assess vital signs (i.e., blood pressure, pulse, temperature, weight, respiration, PAP, PCWP,CVP, JVD) and weight before, during, and after CAVH/SCUF. **Rationale:** Evaluates the patient's response to therapy and monitors for any patient complications.

Expected Outcomes

1.   Removal of prescribed amount of fluids and solutes slowly over 24 to 72 hours. **Rationale:** Slow removal helps to prevent hemodynamic alterations.

2.   Weight at or near dry weight, electrolytes within normal limits, absence of peripheral edema, absence or decrease in respiratory distress, and adequate filling pressures. **Rationale:** Reduces cardiac workload.

Unexpected Outcomes

1.   Physiologic complications (i.e., dysrhythmias, chest pain, acid–base imbalance, hypotension, nausea and vomiting, headaches, or dehydration). **Rationale:** Excessive removal of fluid without adequate fluid re-

placement and shift in electrolytes may potentiate adverse outcomes.

2. Complications with vascular access (i.e., clotting or poor blood flow). **Rationale:** Without patency of access, hemofiltration process cannot be performed.

3. Technical problems (i.e., clotted hemofilter, disconnection of lines, air leak, or blood leak). **Rationale:** When one of these technical problems occurs, a new hemofilter system must be instituted.

Documentation

Documentation in the patient record should include date, time, and length of procedure, continuous assessments of the patient's intake and output, weight, vital signs, coagulation profile, and serial clotting times, laboratory data (i.e., electrolytes, CBC, BUN, and creatinine as ordered) and assessment of the ultrafiltrate for clarity, filtration rate, and UF fluid changes, also medications administered, and any unexpected outcomes and interventions taken. **Rationale:** Documents nursing care given and effectiveness of therapy.

Patient/Family Education

1. Assess the patient's and family's level of knowledge of the disease process, the related treatment regimen and its role in life support. **Rationale:** Enables the patient and family to ask questions, give feedback, and reduce anxiety.

2. Instruct the patient and family in the signs and symptoms of the possible complications of CAVH/SCUF (i.e., volume depletion, hemorrhage, hypotension). **Rationale:** Supports the informed consent process.

Performance Checklist
Skill 21–5: Continuous Renal Replacement Therapy: Slow Continuous Ultrafiltration (SCUF) and Continuous Arteriovenous Hemofiltration (CAVH)

Critical Behaviors	Complies	
	yes	no
PREPARATION 1. Wash hands.		
2. Ensure that protective caps are placed securely on arterial and venous lines of filter.		
3. Ensure that blood lines to hemofilter are secure and taped.		
4. Lock hemofilter in holder, arterial end down.		
5. Connect rinsing bag to venous blood outlet.		
6. Attach UF line to arterial blood line.		
7. Assemble collection system and connect to UF line.		
8. Hang collection system 20 in below level of hemofilter.		
9. Check all line connections.		
10. Clamp arterial blood line, leaving venous, UF, and rinsing bag lines open.		
11. Prepare heparinized normal saline solution (priming solution).		
12. Hang heparinized normal saline 48 in above hemofilter.		
13. Connect heparinized normal saline to arterial line.		
PRIMING 1. Wash hands.		
2. Unclamp arterial line, and flush all lines.		
3. Intermittently clamp and unclamp venous line.		
4. Clamp venous line and rotate filter, arterial end up, when filter has been primed with 1000 ml.		
5. Hang another 1000 ml of normal saline.		
6. Continue priming until 400 ml of normal saline collects in the ultrafiltrate collection/measuring device.		
7. Rotate the filter with the arterial end down.		

Table continues on following page

Critical Behaviors	Complies	
	yes	no
8. Unclamp venous line.		
9. Flush blood side with 500 ml solution.		
10. Clamp arterial line when 100 ml remains of the flush priming solution.		
11. Clamp the venous and UF lines.		
12. Drain and discard saline in the UF collection device.		
13. Wash hands.		
INITIATION		
1. Wash hands.		
2. Establish vascular access.		
3. Position filter parallel to patient's access.		
4. Don goggles and gloves.		
5. Administer initial heparin dose.		
6. Connect setup lines to access.		
7. Position UF collection device below level of patient.		
8. Secure all connections with tape.		
9. Ensure that system is flowing well.		
10. Dispose of soiled material in appropriate receptacle.		
11. Wash hands.		
MONITORING		
1. Administer maintenance heparin as prescribed.		
2. Initiate replacement fluids as prescribed.		
3. Monitor vascular access, blood, and ultrafiltrate lines for occlusion or kinks.		
4. Monitor security of all connections.		
5. Monitor rate, clarity, and position of UF.		
6. Monitor vital signs.		
7. Monitor clotting times.		
8. Monitor rate of fluid replacement.		
9. Monitor laboratory profile.		
10. Monitor access site.		
11. Document in the patient record.		
TERMINATION		
1. Wash hands.		
2. Don goggles and gloves.		
3. Clamp fluid replacement line.		
4. Clamp arterial and venous lines.		
5. Clamp arterial access line, and remove tape.		
6. Clean connection site twice.		

Table continues on following page

Critical Behaviors	Complies	
	yes	no
7. Disconnect arterial access line from arterial system line.		
8. Repeat steps 6 and 7 for venous access line.		
9. Prepare access for uncoupling/decannulation according to established policy.		
10. Dispose of soiled material in appropriate receptacle.		
11. Wash hands.		
12. Document in the patient record.		

BIBLIOGRAPHY

Daugirdas, J. T. and Ing, T. S. (Eds.) (1988). *Handbook of Dialysis.* Boston: Little, Brown.

Dirkes, S. (1989). Making a critical difference with CAVH. *Nursing 89* 19(11):57–60.

Gutch, C. F., and Stoner, M. H. (1975) *Review of Hemodialysis for Nurses and Dialysis Personnel*, (2d Ed.) St. Louis: Mosby.

Henderson, L. (1987). Hemofiltration. *Kidney* 20(6):25–30.

Jackle, M. and Rasmussen, C. (1980). *Renal Problems: A Critical Care Nursing Focus.* Bowie, MD.: Robert J. Brady Company.

Kiely, M. (1984). Continuous arteriovenous hemofiltration. *Crit. Care Nurs.* 4(4):39–49.

Lancaster, L. E. (Ed.) (1989). *Core Curriculum for Nephrology Nursing.* Pitman, N.J.: Anthony J. Jannetti.

Larson, E., Lindbloom, L., and Davis, K. (Eds.) (1982). *Development of the Clinical Nephrology Practitioner: A Focus on Independent Learning.* St. Louis: Mosby.

Lawyer, L. A., and Velasco, A. (1989). Continuous arteriovenous hemodialysis in the ICU. *Crit. Care Nurs.* 9(1): 29.

Locke, S., Groth, N., and Lees, P. (1985). Continuous arteriovenous hemofiltration: An alternative to standard hemodialysis in unstable patients. *Am. Nephrol. Nurses Assoc. J.* 12(2):127–131.

Paganini, E. P. (Ed.) (1986). *Acute Continuous Renal Replacement Therapy.* Boston: Martinus Nijhoff.

Price, C. A. (1989). Continuous arteriovenous ultrafiltration: A monitoring guide for ICU nurses. *Crit. Care Nurs.* 9(1): 12.

Ulrich, B. T. (1989). *Nephrology Nursing Concepts and Strategies.* Norwalk, Conn.: Appleton & Lange.

Whittaker, A., Brown, C., Grabenbauer, K., and Cauble, L. (1986). Preventing complications in continuous arteriovenous hemofiltration. *Dimens. Crit. Care Nurs.* 5(2):72–79.

Williams, V., and Perkins, L. (1984). Continuous ultrafiltration: A new ICU procedure for ten treatment of fluid overload. *Crit. Care Nurs.* 4(4):44–49.

PERITONEAL DIALYSIS

BEHAVIORAL OBJECTIVES

After completing this chapter, the nurse will be able to

- Define the key terms.
- Differentiate between the three modes of peritoneal dialysis.
- Identify the three phases of the peritoneal dialysis exchange.
- Discuss the techniques of catheter care.
- Demonstrate the skills involved in peritoneal dialysis.

Peritoneal dialysis removes metabolic waste products and fluid from the body via osmosis and diffusion through the peritoneal membrane. The technique involves the infusion of a dialyzing fluid into the peritoneal cavity through a flexible Silastic catheter (Fig. 22–1). Substances in the blood and dialysate chemically and osmotically equilibrate across the peritoneal membrane, which acts as a semipermeable membrane. Toxins and catabolites can be removed and electrolyte imbalances can be corrected when a solution with ionic concentrations similar to plasma is used. Fluid removal can be enhanced by the addition of dextrose to the dialysate, thereby increasing the osmotic gradient.

The average adult patient can tolerate up to 2 L of dialysate at a time. The process of peritoneal dialysis involves several exchanges or cycles, each involving three phases. The *inflow*, or *infusion, phase* is the time required to infuse the prescribed volume of dialysate. Factors influencing inflow by gravity include catheter diameter, length of tubing, height of solution, intraabdominal pressure, fibrin formation, or kinked tubing. Infusion by gravity takes approximately 10 minutes for 2 L.

The *dwell*, or *diffusion, phase* is the length of time that the dialysate remains in the peritoneal cavity and provides the time for osmosis and diffusion to take place. Dwell time varies with the clinical condition and type of peritoneal dialysis method utilized.

The *drain*, or *outflow, phase* is the time required to drain the peritoneal cavity of infused dialysate plus excess extracellular fluid. By gravity, outflow time may be altered by external or internal obstructions: tubing kinks, clamped tubing, fibrin formation, catheter position, or intraabdominal pressure.

KEY TERMS

cycler	*exchange*
dialysate	*inflow phase*
diffusion	*osmosis*
diffusion phase	*outflow phase*
dwell time	*peritoneal dialysis*
effluent	*semipermeable membrane*

SKILLS

22–1 Peritoneal Dialysis: Exit-Site and Catheter Care
22–2 Peritoneal Dialysis: Coupling/Uncoupling
22–3 Peritoneal Dialysis: Continuous Ambulatory Peritoneal Dialysis (CAPD)

GUIDELINES

The following assessment guidelines assist the nurse in formulating a nursing diagnosis and an individualized plan of care for the patient receiving peritoneal dialysis:

1. Know the patient's baseline vital signs.
2. Know the patient's fluid status by analyzing weight (current versus dry), skin turgor, mucous membranes, edema, and intake and output.
3. Know the patient's serum electrolyte levels.
4. Know how the patient's underlying medical condition affects renal function.
5. Know the patient's current medical treatment.
6. Perform systematic cardiovascular, respiratory, neurologic, and renal assessments.
7. Perform catheter insertion-site assessment and care.
8. Determine appropriate interventions for assessment findings.
9. Become adept with equipment used for peritoneal dialysis.

SKILL 22–1

Peritoneal Dialysis: Exit-Site and Catheter Care

Peritoneal dialysis requires access to the peritoneal cavity. Several commercially prepared types of peritoneal catheters are available (Fig. 22–2). The trocar and single-cuff Silastic catheter are most often used for temporary acute dialysis. The trocar is a rigid plastic catheter with multiple perforations at the peritoneal end for dispersion of peritoneal fluid. This trocar is inserted at the bedside via a stylet that is removed with entry into the peritoneal cavity. Once the stylet is removed, the trocar

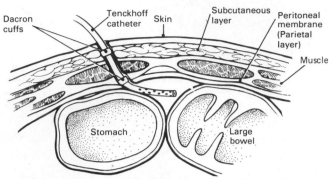

FIGURE 22–1 Tenckhoff catheter used in peritoneal dialysis in Lewis, S.M. and Collier, I.C.: *Medical-Surgical Nursing Assessment and Management of Clinical Problems,* **2nd ed. New York: McGraw-Hill Book Co. 1987, with permission.**

Prerequisite Knowledge and Skills

Prior to performing peritoneal dialysis exit-site and catheter care, the nurse should understand

1. Anatomy and physiology of the peritoneal cavity.
2. Principles of osmosis and diffusion.
3. Principles of aseptic technique.
4. Universal precautions.

The nurse should be able to perform

1. Proper handwashing technique (see Skill 35–5).
2. Setup of a sterile field.
3. Application of a sterile dressing.
4. Specimen taking for culture and sensitivity (see Skill 28–2).
5. Abdominal assessment.
6. Universal precautions (see Skill 35–1).

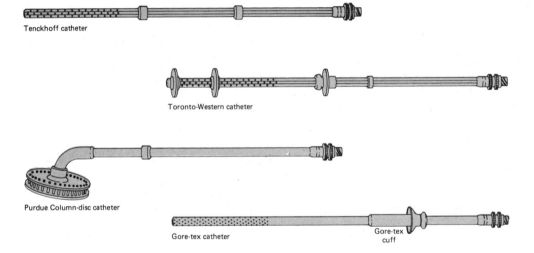

FIGURE 22–2 Peritoneal catheters used for peritoneal dialysis in Lewis, S.M. and Collier, I.C. *Medical-Surgical Nursing Assessment and Management of Clinical Problems,* **2nd ed. New York: McGraw-Hill Book Co. 1987, with permission.**

is advanced toward the pelvis. A protective metal disk may be placed around the catheter at the skin surface to prevent accidental removal. An alternative acute access device is a single-cuff Silastic catheter. The cuff is composed of Dacron felt bonded to the catheter, and the cuff provides a barrier against bacterial invasion.

Catheters for chronic use are similar to the acute single-cuff Silastic catheter, but they have a double Dacron cuff. One cuff is positioned in the subcutaneous tissue beneath the skin at the exit site, and the other is in the fascia outside the peritoneal cavity. Ingrowth of tissue around the Dacron cuffs closes the sinus tracts, providing an effective barrier against bacterial invasion. These catheters are surgically implanted through a percutaneous incision below the umbilicus, are tunneled through subcutaneous tissue, and exit through a stab wound on either side of the abdomen (Fig. 22–3).

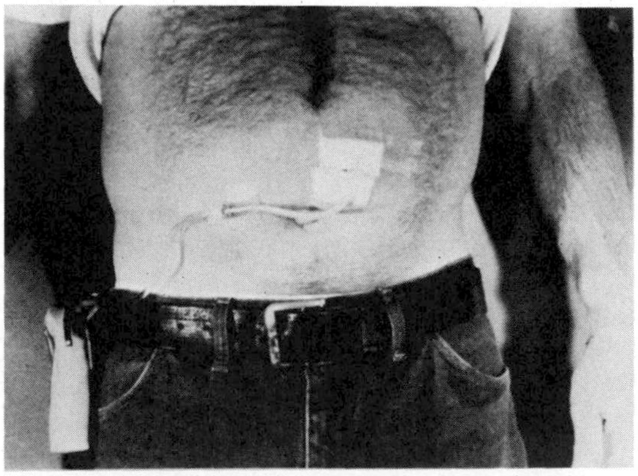

FIGURE 22–3 Placement of peritoneal catheter in Lewis, S.M. and Collier, I.C. *Medical-Surgical Nursing Assessment and Management of Clinical Problems,* **2nd ed. New York: McGraw-Hill Book Co. 1987, with permission.**

Purpose

The nurse performs exit-site and catheter care to:

1. Prevent local and systemic infection.
2. Assess skin integrity at the exit site.

Assessment

1. Auscultate the patient's abdomen for bowel sounds (i.e., location, quantity, duration), and measure

the patient's abdominal girth at the midpoint of the abdomen. **Rationale:** Assesses bowel activity and identifies signs and symptoms of abdominal distension, infection, or volume overload.

2. Assess the dressing and catheter site for leakage and/or drainage. **Rationale:** Any leak in the tubing or connection or drainage from the exit site signifies that the peritoneal cavity has been contaminated and the patient requires antibiotic coverage.

3. Assess the patient for signs and symptoms of peritonitis (i.e., cloudy effluent, abdominal pain, fever, and chills). **Rationale:** Effluent and/or wound drainage carries a high risk for transmission of pathogens.

4. Assess the peritoneal catheter for kinking, puncture sites, and loose connections. **Rationale:** Any alteration in catheter integrity may potentiate infection and necessitate removal of the catheter.

5. Assess the peritoneal exit site for crusting, drainage, redness, swelling, odor, and tenderness on palpation. **Rationale:** May be an indicator of peritonitis or local site infection.

6. Assess fluid status (i.e., skin turgor, edema, weight, intake and output, vital signs, and lung sounds). **Rationale:** Provides an indication of volume excess or deficit.

Nursing Diagnoses

1. Potential for infection related to catheter placement and disruption of skin integrity. **Rationale:** The skin is the first line of defense both anatomically and chemically. Aseptic technique prevents the growth and/or transmission of microorganisms.

2. Potential for fluid volume excess related to inadequate ultrafiltration. **Rationale:** Any alteration, either mechanical or physiologic, may inhibit fluid removal.

Planning

1. Individualize the following goals for performing peritoneal dialysis exit-site and catheter care:
   a. Prevent infection. **Rationale:** Effluent and/or wound drainage carries a high risk for transmission of pathogens.
   b. Maintain catheter integrity. **Rationale:** Peritoneal dialysis requires access to the peritoneal cavity. Any alteration in catheter integrity may potentiate infection and necessitate removal of the catheter.

2. Prepare all necessary equipment and supplies. **Rationale:** Efficient assembly of equipment decreases the risk for contaminating the patient's catheter during the procedure.
   a. Two masks (for nurse and patient).
   b. Goggles.
   c. Culturette for drainage.
   d. Five packages of sterile 4 × 4's.
   e. 60 cc hydrogen peroxide.
   f. 60 cc povidone-iodine solution.
   g. One roll adhesive tape (1-in size).
   h. Two 60-cc sterile containers (for the hydrogen peroxide and povidone-iodine solutions).
   i. Two pairs of sterile gloves.
   j. One suture removal kit.
   k. One sterile barrier.

3. Prepare the patient:
   a. Explain the procedure to the patient. **Rationale:** Reduces anxiety and increases cooperation.
   b. Assist the patient in applying the mask. **Rationale:** Decreases risk of contamination with airborne pathogens.
   c. Assist the patient to a comfortable position, commonly flat or low semi-Fowler's. **Rationale:** Position usually depends on patient's respiratory status.

Implementation

Steps	Rationale	Special Considerations
1. Wash hands.	Reduces transmission of microorganisms.	
2. Don mask and goggles.	Reduces transmission of microorganisms.	
3. Open sterile containers and place on flat surface.	Prevents contamination and spilling of cleansing solutions.	
4. Open 4 × 4's and suture removal kit onto sterile barrier.	Maintains aseptic technique.	
5. Pour approximately 60 cc of hydrogen peroxide into a sterile container.	Maintains aseptic technique.	
6. Pour approximately 60 cc of povidone-iodine solution into the second sterile container.	Maintains aseptic technique.	

Table continues on following page

Steps	Rationale	Special Considerations
7. Don sterile gloves.	Universal precautions.	
8. Remove tape and top layers of old dressing from catheter site.	Gains access to catheter site.	
9. Leave a 4 × 4 underneath the catheter.	Prevents contamination of catheter by skin flora.	
10. Discard dressing and gloves in appropriate receptacle.	Universal precautions.	Note odor, color, and amount of any drainage on dressing.
11. Don a new pair of sterile gloves.	Maintains aseptic technique.	
12. Using nondominent hand, pick up distal end of catheter with a sterile 4 × 4.	To maintain aseptic technique, the catheter should be considered sterile and handled with a dry sterile 4 × 4 to prevent contamination.	Avoid tugging on catheter.
13. Using forceps, remove remaining 4 × 4 under catheter and discard both appropriately.	Maintain sterility by using forceps to remove old dressing.	
14. Inspect catheter exit site, catheter tunnel, and surrounding area for leakage, infection, and/or trauma.	Provides assessment for possible complications.	Note evidence of pain, warmth, crusting, discharge, bleeding, redness, or unusual swelling, which may indicate infection.
15. Using a sterile 4 × 4, palpate the subcutaneous catheter segments and cuff.	Checks for pain or accumulated drainage.	There should be no pain when exit-site cuff is palpated gently. Obtain culture of drainage if present.
16. While still holding the catheter off the skin, soak a 4 × 4 in the hydrogen peroxide solution and gently cleanse the catheter from the cap to the exit site. Then cleanse the skin moving in concentric circles from the catheter exit site outward 2 to 4 in (5–10 cm).	Hydrogen peroxide dries RBCs and is helpful in removing old secretions.	Use enough friction and hydrogen peroxide to remove any crusting or drainage.
17. Soak remaining 4 × 4's in povidone-iodine solution. Squeezing out excess solution from 4 × 4's, cleanse the catheter and catheter exit site as in step 16, and repeat three times. Allow to air dry. Do *not* wipe off excess iodine solution or pat dry.	Acts as a bactericidal agent.	At least a 5-minute scrub.
18. Proceed with coupling and initiation of peritoneal dialysis, or apply occlusive dressing.	Facilitates initiation of dialysis. Maintains aseptic technique.	
19. Discard soiled gloves, materials, and equipment in appropriate receptacle.	Universal precautions.	
20. Wash hands.	Reduces transmission of microorganisms.	

Evaluation

Compare condition of peritoneal dialysis catheter, access, exit site, and dressing with previous assessment findings. **Rationale:** Alerts caregiver to changes that may indicate impaired catheter integrity and/or infection.

Expected Outcomes

1. Maintenance of catheter and exit-site integrity. **Rationale:** Provides patent access for dialysis.
2. Exit site is free of signs and symptoms of infection. **Rationale:** Exit site is a portal of entry for microorganisms.

Unexpected Outcomes

1. Leakage of effluent. **Rationale:** Implies contamination of peritoneal cavity and predisposes the patient to peritonitis.

2. Drainage from tunnel/exit site. **Rationale:** Sign of a tunnel infection of the subcutaneous tissue.

Documentation

Documentation in the patient record should include date and time of exit-site and catheter care, findings of the abdominal assessment (note in particular the location, quality, and duration of abdominal pain); the condition of the catheter and exit site; presence of drainage (note color, odor, and amount); any leakage of effluent (note color, clarity, consistency, and odor); any specimens sent; signs and symptoms of peritonitis; and patient's response to the procedure. **Rationale:** Documents nursing care and provides data regarding the effectiveness of therapy.

Patient/Family Education

1. Explain the rationale for aseptic technique with catheter and exit-site care to both patient and family. **Rationale:** Promotes understanding of procedure and cooperation and relieves anxiety.

2. Instruct the patient and family about the signs and symptoms of peritonitis and tunnel/exit-site infections. **Rationale:** Promotes an understanding of the treatment plan.

3. If peritoneal dialysis treatments are to become chronic, evaluate the patient's and family's understanding of and ability to perform aseptic technique and catheter care. **Rationale:** Allows for planning of instructional sessions and acquisition of necessary supplies for discharge.

Performance Checklist
Skill 22–1: Peritoneal Dialysis: Exit-Site and Catheter Care

Critical Behaviors	Complies yes	no
1. Wash hands.		
2. Don mask and goggles.		
3. Open sterile containers and place on flat surface.		
4. Open 4 × 4's and suture removal kit onto sterile barrier.		
5. Prepare 60 cc of hydrogen peroxide.		
6. Prepare 60 cc of povidone-iodine.		
7. Don sterile gloves.		
8. Remove tape and top layers of old dressing.		
9. Leave a 4 × 4 under catheter.		
10. Discard dressing and gloves appropriately.		
11. Don a new pair of sterile gloves.		
12. Use sterile 4 × 4 to pick up distal end of catheter.		
13. Use forceps to remove remaining dressing from catheter.		
14. Inspect catheter and exit site.		
15. Palpate subcutaneous catheter segments and cuff.		
16. Perform catheter and exit-site scrub with hydrogen peroxide.		
17. Perform catheter and exit-site scrub with povidone-iodine.		
18. Proceed with coupling and initiation of peritoneal dialysis or apply occlusive dressing.		
19. Discard soiled gloves, materials, and equipment in appropriate disposal receptacle.		
20. Wash hands.		
21. Document in the patient record.		

SKILL 22–2

Peritoneal Dialysis: Coupling/Uncoupling

Peritoneal dialysis requires an access to the peritoneal cavity with use of a temporary device. Acute devices such as the trocar or single-cuff Silastic catheter may be used for acute intervention until peritoneal dialysis is no longer required or a permanent Tenkhoff catheter can be placed for chronic therapy.

Purpose

The nurse performs peritoneal dialysis coupling/uncoupling to initiate/terminate peritoneal dialysis.

Prerequisite Knowledge and Skills

Prior to performing peritoneal dialysis coupling/uncoupling, the nurse should understand

1. Principles of aseptic technique.
2. Universal precautions.
3. Principles of peritoneal dialysis.

The nurse should be able to perform

1. Proper handwashing technique (see Skill 35–5).
2. Peritoneal dialysis catheter and exit-site care (see Skill 22–1).
3. Abdominal assessment.
4. Universal precautions (see Skill 35–1).

Assessment

1. Assess the patient for maintenance of a closed system, including an occlusive dressing. **Rationale:** Open system increases the likelihood for infection or impairment of catheter functioning.
2. Assess the patient for redness, swelling, tenderness on palpation, drainage/crusting, or odor from catheter exit site. **Rationale:** Physical signs and symptoms of infection.
3. Assess the patency of the peritoneal catheter, including signs of catheter kinking, puncture sites, and loose connections. **Rationale:** Peritoneal dialysis requires access to peritoneal cavity. Any alteration in catheter integrity may potentiate infection and necessitate removal of the catheter.
4. Assess the patient's baseline weight, vital signs, abdominal girth, and neurologic status. **Rationale:** Baseline data will assist in early recognition of potential complications.

Nursing Diagnosis

Potential for infection related to a break in aseptic technique. **Rationale:** Coupling or uncoupling provides a direct route for the transmission of microorganisms into the peritoneal cavity.

Planning

1. Develop individualized goals for performing peritoneal dialysis coupling/uncoupling to prevent infection. **Rationale:** Maintenance of aseptic technique reduces the transmission of microorganisms.
2. Prepare all necessary equipment and supplies. **Rationale:** Assembly of all the necessary equipment assists in completing the procedure efficiently.

COUPLING EQUIPMENT

   a. Two masks and/or goggles (for nurse and patient).
   b. One pair of sterile gloves.
   c. One sterile container.
   d. 60 cc povidone-iodine solution.
   e. Five packages of sterile 4 × 4's.
   f. One sterile barrier.
   g. One suture removal kit.

UNCOUPLING EQUIPMENT

   a. Two masks and/or goggles (for nurse and patient).
   b. One pair of sterile gloves.
   c. One sterile container.
   d. 60 cc povidone-iodine solution.
   e. Three packages of sterile 4 × 4's.
   f. One catheter cap (if needed).
   g. One suture removal kit.
   h. One sterile barrier.
   i. One roll of adhesive tape (1 in).
   j. Two hemostats.

3. Prepare the patient.
   a. Explain the procedure to the patient. **Rationale:** Reduces anxiety and increases cooperation.
   b. Assist patient to a comfortable position, commonly flat or low semi-Fowler's. Position will ultimately depend on patient's respiratory status. **Rationale:** Facilitates cooperation with aseptic technique.
   c. Assist the patient with application of the mask. **Rationale:** Prevents contamination with airborne pathogens.

Implementation

Steps	Rationale	Special Consideration
Coupling		
1. Wash hands.	Reduces transmission of microorganisms.	

Table continues on following page

Steps	Rationale	Special Considerations
2. Don mask and/or goggles.	Prevents contamination with airborne pathogens.	
3. Open sterile container and place on a flat surface.	Prevents contamination and spilling of cleansing solution.	
4. Pour approximately 60 cc of povidone-iodine solution into the sterile container.	Maintains aseptic technique.	
5. Open sterile 4 × 4's and suture removal kit onto sterile barrier.	Maintains aseptic technique.	
6. Don sterile gloves.	Universal precautions.	
7. If present, remove tape and top layers of old dressing from catheter site.	Gains access to catheter site.	Note odor, color, and amount of any drainage on dressing.
8. Leave a 4 × 4 underneath the catheter (if Silastic catheter is used).	Prevents contamination of catheter by skin flora.	
9. Discard gloves and dressing in appropriate receptacle.	Universal precautions.	
10. Don a new pair of sterile gloves.	Maintains aseptic technique.	
11. Using nondominant hand, pick up peritoneal dialysis line with sterile 4 × 4, and remove the protective cap with the dominant hand (*not* the sterile 4 × 4).	To maintain aseptic technique, nonsterile equipment should be handled with sterile 4 × 4's to prevent contamination.	
12. Then, using the dominant hand, pick up distal end of catheter with a sterile 4 × 4 and connect to the peritoneal dialysis line.	To maintain aseptic technique, the catheter should be considered nonsterile and handled with a dry sterile 4 × 4 to prevent contamination.	Avoid tugging on the catheter. Check catheter/dialysis connection to ensure a tight connection.
13. Using sterile forceps, remove remaining 4 × 4 under the catheter and dispose of appropriately.	Maintains sterility.	
14. Remove the plastic clamp from the Silastic catheter (if catheter placement is surgically performed).	Provides open access of catheter and permits drainage for procedure.	Acute Silastic catheter will usually have a plastic clamp and cap after surgical placement in the operating room. Trocar will have a cap after bedside placement.
15. Soak a sterile 4 × 4 with povidone-iodine solution and wrap it around the connection site.	Prevents contamination with airborne organisms.	
16. Discard soiled gloves, materials, and equipment in appropriate receptacle.	Universal precautions.	
17. Wash hands.	Prevents transmission of microorganisms.	
Uncoupling		
1. Wash hands.	Prevents transmission of microorganisms.	
2. Don mask and/or goggles.	Prevents contamination with airborne organisms.	

Table continues on following page

Steps	Rationale	Special Considerations
3. Observe outflow of last peritoneal dialysis cycle, and make sure effluent is completely drained.	Patient's abdomen must be empty of dialysis fluid.	
4. Clamp catheter and peritoneal dialysis patient line with hemostats or the roller clamps secured to the lines.	Prevents leakage or drainage of effluent and prevents contamination with microorganisms.	
5. Don sterile gloves.	Universal precautions.	
6. Unwrap gauze dressing from around catheter connection and discard appropriately.	Permits access to connection for uncoupling procedure.	
7. Remove sterile gloves and discard appropriately.	Universal precautions.	
8. Open sterile container and place on a flat surface.	Prevents contamination and spilling of cleansing solution.	
9. Pour approximately 60 cc of povidone-iodine solution into the sterile container.	Maintains aseptic technique.	
10. Open catheter cap and place in the povidone-iodine solution container.	Acts as a bactericidal agent.	
11. Open sterile 4 × 4's and suture removal kit onto sterile barrier.	Maintains aseptic technique.	
12. Don sterile gloves.	Universal precautions.	
13. Lift the catheter cap with sterile forceps out of the povidone-iodine solution container and place on sterile barrier.	Maintains aseptic technique.	
14. Grasp both the patient's catheter and the peritoneal dialysis line with sterile 4 × 4's.	Maintains sterility and aseptic technique.	Keep patient's catheter in an upright position.
15. Discard the dialysis line, but continue to hold patient's catheter with the sterile 4 × 4.	Initiates uncoupling.	
16. Carefully pick up the catheter cap and screw it onto the patient's catheter.	Maintains aseptic technique.	Catheter caps are changed weekly.
17. Tape catheter to abdomen. Rotate direction of tubing to prevent irritation to one part of the exit site.	Prevents accidental pulling.	
18. Apply an occlusive dressing.	Maintains aseptic technique.	Dressing should be changed daily.
19. Discard soiled gloves, materials, and equipment in appropriate receptacle.	Universal precautions.	
20. Wash hands.	Prevents transmission of microorganisms.	

Evaluation

Evaluate the condition of the catheter and exit site and compare with previous assessments. **Rationale:** Assesses for signs of infection and/or technical complications.

Expected Outcomes

1. Exit site is free of crusting, drainage, pain, redness, and swelling. **Rationale:** Absence of signs and symptoms of infection.

2. Integrity and placement of catheter are maintained. **Rationale:** Provides patent access for peritoneal dialysis.

Unexpected Outcomes

1. Poor inflow/outflow. **Rationale:** Kinking or dislodgment of the catheter may have occurred during the coupling/uncoupling procedure.

2. Infected exit site. **Rationale:** Exit site is potential portal of entry for microorganisms.

3. Catheter dislodgment. **Rationale:** Implies improper handling or securing during peritoneal dialysis.

Documentation

Documentation in the patient record should include the date and time of coupling/uncoupling, condition and placement of catheter, patency of the catheter, direction catheter was taped, appearance of the exit site, patient's response to the procedure, and any unexpected outcomes encountered and actions taken. **Rationale:** Documents nursing care given and status of catheter/exit site.

Patient/Family Education

1. Explain the necessity for stringent aseptic technique, mode of pathogen transmission, and the procedure to both patient and family. **Rationale:** Promotes understanding by the patient and family and relieves anxiety.

2. If peritoneal dialysis treatments are to become chronic, evaluate the patient's and family's understanding of aseptic technique and catheter care in relation to coupling/uncoupling. **Rationale:** Allows for planning of instructional sessions prior to discharge.

Performance Checklist
Skill 22–2:   Peritoneal Dialysis: Coupling/Uncoupling

Critical Behaviors	Complies	
	yes	no
COUPLING		
1. Wash hands.		
2. Don mask and/or goggles.		
3. Open sterile container and place on flat surface.		
4. Prepare povidone-iodine solution.		
5. Open sterile 4 × 4's and suture removal kit onto sterile barrier.		
6. Don sterile gloves.		
7. Remove tape and top layers of old dressing.		
8. Leave a 4 × 4 under catheter.		
9. Discard gloves and dressing appropriately.		
10. Don a new pair of sterile gloves.		
11. Use a sterile 4 × 4 to remove protective cap from peritoneal dialysis line.		
12. Use a sterile 4 × 4 to pick up distal end of catheter and connect to peritoneal dialysis line.		
13. Use a sterile forceps to remove remaining 4 × 4 under catheter and discard.		
14. Remove the clamp from the catheter.		
15. Wrap the connection site with a 4 × 4 soaked with povidone-iodine solution.		
16. Discard soiled gloves, materials, and equipment in appropriate receptacle.		
17. Wash hands.		
18. Document procedure in the patient record.		
UNCOUPLING		
1. Wash hands.		
2. Don mask and/or goggles.		
3. Make sure effluent is completely drained.		

Table continues on following page

Critical Behaviors	Complies	
	yes	no
4. Clamp catheter and peritoneal dialysis patient line with hemostats.		
5. Don sterile gloves.		
6. Remove old soaked 4 × 4 from around connection and discard.		
7. Remove and discard gloves in appropriate container.		
8. Open sterile container and place on flat surface.		
9. Prepare povidone-iodine solution.		
10. Open catheter cap and place in povidone-iodine solution.		
11. Open sterile 4 × 4's and suture removal kit onto sterile barrier.		
12. Don sterile gloves.		
13. Remove catheter cap from povidone-iodine solution and place on sterile barrier.		
14. Use sterile 4 × 4 to grasp patient catheter and peritoneal dialysis line.		
15. Discard dialysis line, but continue to hold patient catheter.		
16. Using sterile forceps, lift catheter cap from povidone-iodine solution and screw on catheter, maintaining aseptic technique.		
17. Tape catheter to abdomen, rotating direction of tubing.		
18. Apply occlusive dressing.		
19. Discard soiled gloves, materials, and equipment in appropriate receptacle.		
20. Wash hands.		
21. Document in the patient record.		

SKILL 22–3

Peritoneal Dialysis: Continuous Ambulatory Peritoneal Dialysis (CAPD)

Three modes of peritoneal dialysis commonly used are intermittent peritoneal dialysis (IPD), continuous cyclic peritoneal dialysis (CCPD), or continuous ambulatory peritoneal dialysis (CAPD). IPD is generally performed for 8 to 10 hours per treatment, three times each week, utilizing an automated cycling machine (Fig. 22–4). In the critical care unit, this procedure may be done manually if a cycling machine is not available.

In CAPD, the patient performs three to four exchanges over a 24-hour period, 7 days a week. Each 2 L of dialysate dwells in the peritoneal cavity for approximately 4 hours. On the final exchange, the 2 L remains in the peritoneal cavity overnight. This dialysate is drained the following morning.

CCPD is a combination of the IPD and CAPD modes. The patient receives dialysis exchanges during the night via a cycler machine. On the final exchange, the last 2 L remains in the peritoneal cavity during the day. This dialysate is drained in the evening at initiation of the cycling mode.

Purpose

The nurse performs CAPD to
1. Remove metabolic waste products.
2. Maintain fluid, electrolyte, and acid–base balances.
3. Control azotemia.
4. Facilitate machine-free dialysis.

Prerequisite Knowledge and Skills

Prior to performing CAPD, the nurse should understand
1. Principles of aseptic technique.
2. Universal precautions.
3. Principles of fluid, electrolyte, and acid–base balances.
4. Anatomy and physiology of the peritoneum.
5. Principles of osmosis and diffusion.
6. Components of the peritoneal system: access and dialysate.

The nurse should be able to perform

1. Proper handwashing technique (see Skill 35–5).
2. Vital signs assessment.
3. Peritoneal catheter care (see Skill 22–1).
4. Abdominal assessment.
5. Universal precautions (see Skill 35–1).

Assessment

1. Assess the patient for maintenance of a closed system. **Rationale:** Leaks in the system predispose the patient to infection and peritonitis.

2. Assess the patient's vital signs (i.e., temperature, pulse, respirations, and blood pressure). **Rationale:** Provides baseline data to monitor effectiveness of dialytic therapy.

3. Assess fluid status (i.e., periorbital, sacral, or extremity edema; jugular vein distension; and weight). **Rationale:** Provides information on effectiveness of ultrafiltration.

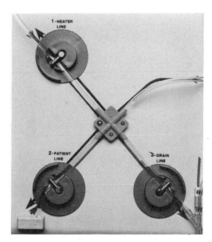
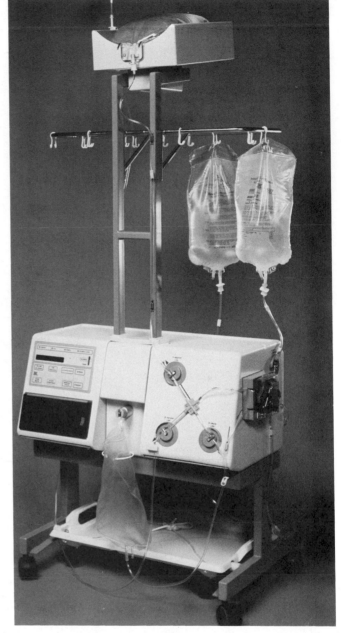

FIGURE 22–4 Automated cycling machine. The peritoneal automated cycler with X-connector set. (Travenol Laboratories, with permission.)

Nursing Diagnoses

1. Fluid volume excess related to an increased intravascular volume, hypertension, and peripheral edema. **Rationale:** In renal disease, a decreased glomerular filtration rate (GFR) and a decreased renal excretion of water result in an increased intravascular volume.

2. Potential for decreased cardiac output related to increased intravascular volume removal. **Rationale:** Hypovolemia can be potentiated with excessive intravascular fluid removal.

3. Anxiety related to loss of kidney function and initiation and termination of peritoneal dialysis therapy.

Rationale: Renal disease and the dialysis treatment regimen create many stresses for the patient, causing loss of control over environment and self.

4. Potential for infection related to coupling/uncoupling procedure. **Rationale:** Open catheter is a portal of entry for microorganisms.

Planning

1. Develop individualized goals for performing CAPD to maintain euvolemic status, acid–base and electro-

lyte balances, and azotemia control. **Rationale:** By the processes of osmosis and diffusion through the peritoneal membrane, accumulated waste products and excess fluid are removed.
2. Prepare all necessary equipment and supplies. **Rationale:** Assembly of all necessary equipment ensures that the procedure will be completed efficiently.
    a. Two masks (nurse and patient).
    b. One bottle of povidone-iodine.
    c. One sterile barrier.
    d. One roll of tape (1 in).
    e. One bag of dianeal solution.
    f. Two outlet port clamps.
    g. One cloth belted pouch.
3. Prepare the patient.
    a. Assist the patient in putting on the mask. **Rationale:** Prevents contamination with airborne pathogens and prevents transmission of microorganisms.
    b. Explain the procedure. **Rationale:** Promotes the patient's understanding and compliance with the procedure.
    c. Assist the patient to a comfortable position. **Rationale:** Facilitates cooperation during the procedure.

Implementation

Steps	Rationale	Special Considerations
Preparing for Outflow		
1. Wash hands.	Reduces transmission of microorganisms.	
2. Remove collapsed dianeal drainage bag from clothing, and place below the mid-abdominal area.	Enhances gravity outflow.	Be careful to avoid pulling on the catheter.
3. Open roller clamp and permit fluid from peritoneal cavity to drain.	Promotes drainage of effluent.	Allow 15 to 20 minutes for outflow.
4. When effluent has completely drained, close the roller clamp.	Prevents leakage of fluid and decreases incidence of site and environmental contamination.	
5. Wash hands.	Reduces transmission of microorganisms.	
Preparing New Bag		
1. Wash hands.	Reduces transmission of microorganisms.	
2. Don mask.	Prevents contamination with airborne pathogens.	
3. Remove a new dianeal solution bag from its protective overpouch wrapping.	Protects solution when in storage.	
4. Check dianeal bag for dialysate percent, expiration date, clarity, and/or leaks.	Prevents contamination of fluid entering the peritoneal cavity.	
5. Place drainage dianeal bag, filled with effluent, next to the new dianeal bag for instillation.	Proximity of bags promotes easy transfer of spikes.	
6. Extend ports of both containers over edge of work surface.	Provides accessibility to ports.	Ports are very similar to those found on intravenous bags.
7. Remove iodine shields from the ports of the effluent and drainage bags and discard.	Permits access to ports.	
8. Firmly clamp the outlet port of the drainage bag.	Prevents leakage of fluid and decreases incidence of site and environmental contamination.	The clamp should be flush with the cuff on the port.

Table continues on following page

Steps	Rationale	Special Considerations
Exchange		
1. Remove protective covering from port of new dianeal bag.	Provides access for spiking of dianeal bag.	Maintain aseptic technique.
2. Using a twisting motion, remove the spike from the effluent drainage bag.	Completes disconnection.	Do not touch the spike. Maintain aseptic technique.
3. Without interruption, immediately transfer spike to the new dianeal bag, twisting and pushing the spike until it is flush with the port on the dianeal bag.	Minimizes environmental exposure of the spike to prevent possible contamination.	
4. Remove outlet port clamp from newly spiked dianeal bag.	Allows for flow of dianeal fluid.	
5. Place iodine shield over spiked connection.	Provides bacteriostatic properties.	
Inflow		
1. Hang the dianeal bag above the level of the peritoneal cavity, and open the roller clamp.	Time for inflow cycle depends on height of dianeal bag.	Inflow will take approximately 10 minutes. For CAPD, inflow/outflow times are not specified.
2. When inflow is complete, close roller clamp.	Prevents backflow of effluent.	Leave a minute amount of dianeal fluid in collapsed container because it facilitates folding and drainage on next exchange.
Dwell		
1. Remove dianeal bag from the IV pole and fold so that spike connection is on the inside.	Provides stabilization for the connection and reduces risk of disconnection.	Dwell time is usually approximately 3 to 4 hours, depending on the number of exchanges per 24 hours.
2. Secure folded container on patient with cloth belted pouch.	Provides support and prevents catheter movement.	
3. Discard effluent into biohazardous waste receptacle, being careful to avoid splashing of effluent.	Universal precautions.	
4. Discard empty dianeal container into appropriate disposal receptacle.	Universal precautions.	
5. Wash outlet port clamps in soapy water, place on clean surface, and let air dry.	Clean technique promotes proper handling of equipment.	
6. Wash hands.	Reduces transmission of microorganisms.	

Evaluation

1. Evaluate effluent for amount, color, and clarity, and compare with previous exchanges. **Rationale:** Identifies effectiveness of CAPD exchanges and monitors for possible complications such as bowel perforation, bleeding, or peritonitis.

2. Evaluate catheter and connections for leaks and/or kinks. **Rationale:** Alterations in the catheter integrity potentiate infection.

3. Evaluate exit site for crusting, drainage, redness, swelling, odor, and tenderness or pain on palpation. **Rationale:** Physical signs and symptoms indicative of infection.

4. Monitor vital signs (i.e., blood pressure, pulse, respirations, temperature, and weight) and laboratory values of sodium, potassium, CO_2, chloride, blood urea nitrogen, and creatinine before and after dialysis. **Rationale:** Evaluates the patient's response to therapy.

Expected Outcomes

1. Removal of accumulated waste products, resto-

ration of acid–base balance, electrolyte balance, and fluid control. **Rationale:** The process of CAPD removes excess nitrogenous waste products, fluid, and electrolytes, but since the dialysis bath has higher concentrations of electrolytes depleted by renal failure, those needed by the patient are replaced or maintained.

2. Weight at or near dry weight, BUN, and creatinine decreased from predialysis values and electrolytes within normal limits. **Rationale:** Decrease in uremic manifestations and complications promotes homeostasis.

3. Maintenance of catheter and exit-site integrity. **Rationale:** Provides patent access for dialysis.

4. Exit site is free of signs and symptoms of infection. **Rationale:** Exit site is a portal of entry for microorganisms.

Unexpected Outcomes

1. Complications related to access (i.e., poor flow, infection, kinking, and leakage). **Rationale:** Without a patent access, peritoneal dialysis cannot be performed.

2. Physiologic complications (i.e., hypotension, nausea and vomiting, dysrhythmias, headache, and cramps). **Rationale:** Excessive removal of fluid and shifts in electrolytes may potentiate a condition of disequilibrium.

Documentation

Documentation in the patient record should include findings of catheter and exit-site assessment (i.e., leak-age, kinking, redness, drainage, odor, swelling, or crusting); procedure parameters (i.e., date and time of exchanges, percentage of dianeal fluid, and number of exchanges); characteristics of effluent (i.e., color, clarity, consistency, and odor); and patient's response to the procedure. **Rationale:** Documents nursing care and provides data regarding the effectiveness of the procedure.

Patient/Family Education

Note: Formal patient/family education for CAPD is performed by experienced dialysis personnel.

1. Assess the patient's and family's level of knowledge related to the disease process and treatment plan. **Rationale:** Enables patient and family to ask questions and the nurse to give feedback.

2. Explain to the patient and family the signs and symptoms of possible complications (i.e., infection, inadequate dialysis flow, and fluid overload). **Rationale:** Enables the patient and family to take an active part in the treatment plan and seek assistance when complications arise.

3. Assess patient and family understanding of the need to adhere with follow-up appointments. **Rationale:** CAPD is a self-care procedure. Follow-up with dialysis personnel will ensure that the patient is able to perform safe and effective CAPD, and that the patient has the necessary supplies and equipment for the procedure.

Performance Checklist
Skill 22–3: Peritoneal Dialysis: Continuous Ambulatory Peritoneal Dialysis (CAPD)

Critical Behaviors	Complies	
	yes	no
PREPARING FOR OUTFLOW 1. Wash hands.		
2. Remove collapsed dianeal drainage bag, and place in drainage position.		
3. Open roller clamp and drain peritoneal cavity.		
4. Close roller clamp when drainage is completed.		
5. Wash hands.		
PREPARING NEW BAG 1. Wash hands.		
2. Don mask.		
3. Remove new dianeal bag from wrapping.		
4. Check new dianeal bag.		
5. Place filled drainage bag next to new dianeal bag.		
6. Extend ports of both bags over edge of work surface.		
7. Remove iodine shield from ports of both dianeal and drainage bags and discard.		
8. Firmly clamp outlet port of drainage bag.		

Table continues on following page

Critical Behaviors	Complies yes	no
EXCHANGE		
1. Remove protective covering from port of new dianeal bag.		
2. Remove spike for effluent drainage bag.		
3. Spike new dianeal bag.		
4. Remove outlet port clamp from newly spiked dianeal bag.		
5. Place iodine shield over spiked connection.		
INFLOW		
1. Hang dianeal bag, and infuse dialysate.		
2. After infusion, close roller clamp.		
DWELL		
1. Remove dianeal bag from IV pole and fold with spiked connection inside.		
2. Secure folded bag on patient.		
3. Discard effluent without splashing.		
4. Discard used supplies and equipment in appropriate disposal receptacle.		
5. Wash outlet port clamps.		
6. Wash hands.		
7. Document procedure in patient record.		

BIBLIOGRAPHY

Daugirdas, J. T., and Ing, T. S. (Eds.) (1988). *Handbook of Dialysis.* Boston: Little, Brown.

Jackle, M., and Rasmussen, C. (1980). *Renal Problems: A Critical Care Nursing Focus.* Bowie, MD: Robert J. Brady Company.

Jensen, S., Pomeroy, M., Davidson, M., et al. (1989). Evaluation of dressing protocols that reduce peritoneal dialysis catheter exit site infections. *Am. Nephrol. Nurses Assoc. J.* 16(6):425–431.

Lancaster, L. E. (Ed.) (1987). *Core Curriculum for Nephrology Nursing.* Pitman, N.J.: Anthony J. Jannetti.

Larson, E., Lindbloom, L., and Davis, K. (Eds.) (1982). *Development of the Clinical Nephrology Practitioner: A Focus on Independent Learning.* St. Louis: Mosby.

Prowant, B., Schmidt, L., Twardowski, Z., et al. (1988). Peritoneal dialysis catheter exit site care. *Am. Nephrol. Nurses Assoc. J.* 15(4):219–221.

Ulrich, B. T. (1989). *Nephrology Nursing Concepts and Strategies.* Norwalk, Conn.: Appleton & Lange.

UNIT VI

THE MUSCULOSKELETAL SYSTEM

23

PRESSURE-RELIEVING AND PRESSURE-REDUCING DEVICES

BEHAVIORAL OBJECTIVES

After completing this chapter, the nurse will be able to

- Define the key terms.
- Identify devices for pressure reduction and pressure relief.
- List the indications for pressure-reducing and pressure-relieving devices.
- State the nursing responsibilities when using pressure-reducing and pressure-relieving devices.
- State the indications for discontinuing use of a pressure-reducing or pressure-relieving device.

The body weight of a patient on a relatively firm standard hospital mattress causes areas of high pressure (40 to 120 mmHg) on the skin and underlying tissues. High and/or prolonged pressures may close the capillaries in those areas, which prevents blood from reaching surrounding tissues to deliver oxygen and nutrients and remove waste products. Pressure necrosis may occur with high pressure in a short period of time or with low pressure over a long period of time.

The goal of any pressure-relieving device is to reduce the pressure over bony prominences to below capillary closing pressure (approximately 25–32 mmHg) to prevent tissue ischemia. Capillary closing pressure is the normal pressure exerted within the vessel that forces the capillary to remain patent. A *pressure-relieving* device is one that *consistently* maintains external skin pressure at below 32 mmHg, whereas a *pressure-reducing* device maintains external skin pressures at lower than a standard hospital mattress.

Devices may be classified as static or dynamic. *Static*

devices (pressure-reducing) are motionless, except in response to patient movement, and provide proper weight distribution and comfort. A static device is one that is nonpowered. Examples of static devices or mattress overlays include foam, gel, water, and some air mattresses. *Dynamic* devices (pressure-relieving) have moving parts and require energy or physical force for motion. Dynamic systems include air fluidized beds, low air loss beds, oscillating support beds, and alternating air pressure mattresses.

The decision to use a specific device is usually dictated by hospital policy. Many institutions have implemented scales (i.e., Braden, Bergstrom, Hemphill, Norton, and Gosnell) to determine the risk for pressure sore development and use these scales as a guide for the selection of pressure-reducing/pressure-relieving devices. Table 23–1 lists the major indications, advantages, disadvantages, and contraindications for these devices.

This chapter focuses on the purposes and procedures involved in the selection and use of pressure-relieving or

TABLE 23–1   Pressure-Relieving/Reducing Devices: Major Indications, Contraindications, Advantages, and Disadvantages

Device	Indications	Contraindications	Advantages	Disadvantages
Air fluidized therapy	Patients with large area burns, posterior flaps and grafts, deep and/or multiple pressure sores, intractable pain associated with pressure, contraindications for turning.	Patients with severe pulmonary problems, unstable spine, body weight greater than 250 lbs, height greater than 6 ft.	Relieves pressure, moisture, friction, and shear; permits positioning on donor sites or grafts; relieves pain associated with external pressure; drainage or incontinence is absorbed by beads in bed; some have built-in scales to ease in weighing patient.	Perceptual/sensory deprivation; potential systemic dehydration (i.e., evaporation of body fluids); potential for local dehydration (i.e., dries wound base); difficult to transfer patient; patients cannot be transported in bed; and a foam wedge is required to elevate head of bed.
Low air loss therapy	Patients with spinal cord/ multiple trauma, posterior flaps and grafts, deep and/or multiple pressure sores, contraindications for turning.	Patients with severe agitation, unstable spine, and uncontrolled claustrophobia.	Relieves pressure, moisture, friction, and shear; permits positioning on donor sites or grafts; adapts to all types of traction; patient transfers easily; some have built-in scales for ease in weighing patient; and patient can control head and foot of bed; nurses report ease of use.	Positioning difficult on low-friction surface; requires battery pack for patient transportation; potential for local dehydration (i.e., dries wound base).
Lateral rotation therapy tables	Patients with spinal cord injuries, trauma, continuous head/skeletal traction, severe pulmonary problems, and pulmonary, vascular, and urinary stasis.	Patients with increased intracranial pressure with agitation, large cranial defects, severe diarrhea, body weights greater than 500 lbs, hemodynamic instability.	Can be adapted to traction; can be used for patients with unstable spines; and reduces complications of immobility.	Skin shearing can occur on support surface; can cause agitation or motion sickness; rotation must be 20 of 24 hours; produces external pressure when rotation is stopped for more than 30 minutes; and potential sleep deprivation.
Lateral rotation therapy cushions	Patients with severe pulmonary problems, spinal cord injury, multiple trauma, deep and/or multiple pressure sores, pulmonary, vascular, and urinary stasis, and contraindications for turning.	Patients with cardiovascular instability, skeletal traction, unstable spine, who weigh more than 300 lbs, and who adjust rotation with fracture.	Relieves pressure, moisture, friction, and shear; only cushions rotate, not entire bed; some models provide low air loss with rotation and pulsation; patient can control head and foot of bed; some models have built-in scales.	Potential local dehydration; cannot rotate with traction; low-friction surface; requires battery pack for patient transportation.
Foam mattress	Patients with existing superficial pressure sores or moderate risk for pressure sores.	Patients with no two intact skin surfaces to be turned onto and who require pressure reduction rather than pressure relief.	Ease of use; can be sent home with patient; may be inexpensive for patient.	Potentially induces perspiration; easily soiled; disposal can be costly.
Air mattress	Patients with existing superficial pressure sores or moderate risk for pressure sores.	Patients with no two intact skin surfaces to be turned onto or who require pressure reduction rather than pressure relief.	Ease of use; can be sent home with patient, although some may require pump rental.	Potentially induces perspiration; easily punctured; some require reinflation with a pump; some may not be used for extended periods of time.

pressure-reducing devices. Techniques discussed include transfer, positioning, and cardiopulmonary resuscitation of patients maintained on these devices.

KEY TERMS

air fluidized therapy
capillary closing pressure
decubitus
dermal wound
dynamic device
ischemia
low air loss therapy

oscillating support therapy
pressure reduction
pressure relief
pressure-relieving devices
pressure sore
static device

SKILLS

23–1 Pressure-Relieving Devices: Air Fluidized Therapy
23–2 Pressure-Relieving Devices: Low Air Loss Therapy
23–3 Pressure-Relieving Devices: Oscillating Support Therapy
23–4 Pressure-Reducing Devices: Foam and Air Mattresses

GUIDELINES

The following assessment guidelines assist the nurse in formulating a nursing diagnosis and an individualized plan of care to maintain skin integrity:

1. Assess the patient's risk for pressure sores.
2. Know the patient's baseline skin/wound assessment.
3. Know the patient's medical history.
4. Know the patient's current medical treatment.
5. Know the patient's nutritional status/requirements.
6. Perform systematic wound and skin assessments (especially over bony prominences) in a timely fashion.
7. Determine appropriate intervention for assessed finding.
8. Become adept with devices used for pressure reduction/relief.

SKILL 23–1

Pressure-Relieving Devices: Air Fluidized Therapy

Air fluidized therapy beds are classified as dynamic pressure-relieving devices. These beds also may be known as high air loss, bead, or sand beds. Air fluidized therapy reduces pressure on the skin to approximately 5 to 16 mmHg, allowing existing pressure sores (decubitus, dermal wounds) to heal and preventing the development of new pressure sores.

The air fluidized therapy bed is a rectangular tank that contains millions of sandlike grains (microspheres) and

is covered loosely by a closely woven filter sheet. When an air compressor blows warm, filtered air through the microspheres from below, the fluidized bed has a soft gel consistency that supports the body equally with no areas of high pressure. The loose-fitting filter sheet yields to the contours of the body, preventing dermal shearing or friction.

Body fluids, such as urine or wound exudate, pass through the filter sheet and mix with the microspheres, forming dense clumps that sink to the bottom of the tank. The high pH of the microspheres, along with the warm air, desiccate the bead clusters. The contaminated microspheres are sieved (cleaned) and the filter sheet is changed between patients or every 2 weeks by the company.

Purpose

The nurse utilizes air fluidized therapy (AFT) to

1. Alleviate pressure on burned tissue.
2. Alleviate pressure on posterior skin flaps and grafts.
3. Provide pressure relief on deep or multiple pressure sores when conventional methods fail.
4. Reduce the risk of pressure sores when immobilization is expected to be lengthy.
5. Reduce intractable pain not alleviated by conventional methods.
6. Reduce friction, shearing, and moisture on the skin when conventional methods fail.
7. Reduce the risk of pathologic fractures.

Prerequisite Knowledge and Skills

Prior to placing a patient on AFT, the nurse should understand

1. Principles of preventing pressure-induced injury.
2. Pathophysiology of tissue ischemia.
3. Principles of wound healing.
4. Principles of AFT.
5. Clinical features of AFT bed, such as safety features, maintenance and repair, advantages and disadvantages, and nursing responsibilities.
6. Principles of fluid and electrolyte balance.
7. The necessity for turning and repositioning on AFT to reduce the hazards of immobility (i.e., circulatory, pulmonary, and urinary stasis).

The nurse should be able to perform

1. Proper handwashing technique (see Skill 35–5).
2. Universal precautions (see Skill 35–1).
3. Skin assessment.
4. Assessment of nutritional status.
5. Assessment of fluid and electrolyte balance.
6. Assessment of wound healing.
7. Pain assessment.
8. Pulmonary assessment.
9. Motor/sensory assessment.
10. Scheduled turning/repositioning techniques.

11. Pressure sore prevention and care techniques (see Chapter 29).

Assessment

1. Inspect the patient's bony prominences for evidence of pressure sore formation. **Rationale:** Pressure relief and airflow reduce factors that contribute to pressure sore formation. Bony prominences most often affected includes: sacrum, shoulders, elbows, heels, ankles and knees.

2. Assess the patient's fluid balance: weight change(s), blood pressure, heart rate, filling pressures, intake and output, electrolyte profile, hemoglobin and hematocrit, skin turgor, mucous membranes, and urine specific gravity. **Rationale:** Exposure of the skin to continuous warm, dry airflow causes evaporation of moisture on both the skin and mucous membranes.

3. Assess the patient's wound(s): type and amount of drainage, areas of necrosis, surrounding skin for maceration and inflammation, and any pain or palpation of surrounding area. **Rationale:** Absence of pressure, friction, and shearing of skin should allow wound(s) to heal.

4. Assess the patient's pain/comfort level (i.e., scale of 0–10). **Rationale:** Pressure relief can reduce intractable pain.

5. Assess the patient's pulmonary status: adventitious breath sounds, rate and depth, cough, cyanosis, dyspnea, use of accessory muscles, nasal flaring, arterial blood gases, decreased mental acuity, and restlessness. **Rationale:** Recumbent position and lack of firm back support cause difficulty in mobilizing secretions.

6. Perform motor/sensory assessment: changes in kinesthetic and vestibular senses and/or changes in perceptual characteristics. **Rationale:** Floating sensation alters perception in some patients.

Nursing Diagnoses

1. Potential/actual impaired tissue integrity related to high and/or prolonged external pressures. **Rationale:** High or prolonged external pressure decreases or prevents blood flow causing tissue ischemia.

2. Knowledge deficit related to effects of tissue compression and rationale for device. **Rationale:** Affects cooperation and acceptance of a therapy that is not usually a common experience for the patient and family.

3. Pain related to disease process or injury. **Rationale:** External pressure can intensify intractable pain.

4. Impaired physical mobility related to disease process and/or injury. **Rationale:** Limitation of physical movement can cause prolonged or elevated external pressure which decreases or prevents blood flow causing tissue ischemia.

Planning

1. Individualize the following goals on the basis of the assessment:
   a. Reduce the amount or duration of external pressure to the patient's skin. **Rationale:** High and/or prolonged external pressure exceeds closing capillary pressure causing tissue ischemia.
   b. Decrease effects of urinary/fecal incontinence or other bodily excretions on the patient's skin. **Rationale:** Excessive moisture causes maceration, increasing potential for skin breakdown or increasing severity of existing pressure sores.
   c. Manage intractable pain. **Rationale:** External pressure can intensify intractable pain.
   d. Promote wound healing. **Rationale:** Relief of external pressure supports wound healing.

2. Obtain physician's order, and initiate mechanism to procure bed. **Rationale:** A physician's order is generally required for reimbursement purposes. Some hospitals have specific approval criteria for placing a patient on AFT. Check with your institution's policy regarding AFT use and the mechanism by which this is ordered/obtained.

3. Prepare patient for transfer to AFT bed.
   a. Discuss rationale for AFT with patient. **Rationale:** Reduces anxiety.
   b. Explain the principles of AFT to patient. **Rationale:** Encourages cooperation.

4. Set up AFT bed.
   a. Check sign indicating the date and time the bed can be used. **Rationale:** Sign will be posted by the company.
   b. Check the temperature indicator to be certain the temperature of bed is at least 88°F (31.1°C). **Rationale:** Temperature less than 88°F (31.1°C) results in bed too cold for patient comfort.
   c. If the patient does *not* have a new flap or graft, turn bed off. **Rationale:** Eases transfer of patient onto bed.
   d. If patient has a new flap or graft *do not* turn bed off. **Rationale:** Keeping bed on eliminates even small amount of pressure to new flap or graft site.

5. Tape company representative's name and telephone number at the foot of the bed. **Rationale:** Facilitates contact should problems arise. Most companies have 24-hour per day consultation/troubleshooting service.

Implementation

Steps	Rationale	Special Considerations
Placing Patient on AFT Bed		
1. Wash hands.	Reduces transmission of microorganisms.	

Table continues on following page

Steps	Rationale	Special Considerations
2. Place one hospital flat sheet over polyester filter sheet.	Use of more than one sheet can result in blockage of airflow through the filter sheet.	
3. Lift patient onto bed.	Completes transfer.	
4. Turn bed on.	Initiates therapy.	Company initiates a warmup period that must be completed before patient is placed on the bed.
5. After transfer, remove all linen except flat sheet.	Plastic linen savers or multiple linens will impede airflow to patient's skin, diminishing efficacy of therapy.	
6. Gently pull filter sheet loose around patient's body, especially under feet.	Tightened filter sheet can produce pressure, especially in foot area. Prevents "hammocking" effect.	
7. Institute turning/repositioning schedule.	Reduces hazards of immobility and allows for skin assessment.	

Turning Patient on AFT Bed

1. Ensure loose fit of filter sheet around patient.	Tight filter sheet may cause pressure on the skin.	
2. Gather hospital sheet in close to the patient at shoulder and hip.	Provides support when moving patient.	
3. Pull patient to side of bed.	Eases turning.	
4. Pulling upward and over with the sheet, turn the patient away from you into a side-lying position.	Supports proper body mechanics and completes turning.	
5. Cross one leg in front of the other, with the upper leg slightly bent at the knee and hip.	Stabilizes the patient.	
6. If bony prominences come into contact with one another, separate with a pillow.	Relieves pressure.	
7. If turning to perform treatment, hold the patient in the desired position and turn bed off.*	Beads in the bed will hold the patient in fixed position.	

Cardiopulmonary Resuscitation on AFT Bed

1. Hyperextend patient's neck into the microspheres.	Opens airway.	
2. Turn bed off.	Immobilizes patient.	
3. Unplug bed from wall.	Prevents automatic refluidizing and promotes a hard surface for CPR.	
4. Initiate CPR.	*No* cardiac backboard is necessary.	
5. Position patient's arms, legs, and torso away from the metal rails before defibrillating (see Skill 8–1).	Maintains electrical safety.	

*See manufacturer's manual for other procedures: bedpan placement and removal, dressing changes, hypothermia, hyperthermia, proning patient, traction, x-rays.

Evaluation

1. Maintain turning/positioning schedule every 2 hours. **Rationale:** Prevents circulatory, pulmonary, and urinary stasis.

2. Evaluate skin (particularly areas over bony prom- inences) for evidence of pressure sore/necrosis. **Rationale:** Relief of external pressure prevents pressure sores.

3. Evaluate existing pressure sores, wounds, flaps, grafts, etc. for evidence of healing. **Rationale:** Relief of external pressure supports wound healing.

4. Evaluate skin for evidence of friction, shearing, or

moisture. **Rationale:** These factors may contribute to skin breakdown.

5. Evaluate pain level (on a scale of 0–10) if the patient was placed on the bed for comfort. **Rationale:** External pressure can intensify intractable pain.

6. Evaluate for the development of pathologic fractures. **Rationale:** Reduced external pressure and ease of movement reduce the risk of pathologic fractures.

7. Evaluate patient's acceptance of and adaptation to the device. **Rationale:** Increases cooperation and decreases anxiety.

8. Determine when therapy should be discontinued. **Rationale:** Pressure relief is no longer required.

Expected Outcomes

1. Absence of pressure sores. **Rationale:** Relief of external pressure reduces risk of pressure sores.

2. Evidence of wound healing. **Rationale:** Relief of external pressure supports wound healing.

3. Verbalization of decreased pain. **Rationale:** External pressure can intensify intractable pain.

4. Absence of friction, shearing, and moisture on skin. **Rationale:** Pressure relief and airflow reduce these factors that contribute to pressure sore formation.

5. Integrity of skeletal system is maintained. **Rationale:** Pressure relief reduces the risk of pathologic fractures.

Unexpected Outcomes

1. Dehydration. **Rationale:** The exposure of the skin to continuous warm, dry airflow can cause evaporation of moisture on both the skin and the mucous membranes and in the base of the wound.

2. Development of or deterioration of existing pressure sores. **Rationale:** Other factors contributing to pressure sores (i.e., nutrition, immobility, incontinence) remain uncontrolled.

4. Pulmonary congestion. **Rationale:** Recumbent position and lack of firm back support causes difficulty in mobilizing secretions.

5. Perceptual/sensory deprivation. **Rationale:** Floating sensation alters perception in many patients.

Documentation

Documentation in the patient record should include date and time AFT therapy is initiated, rationale for use of AFT, serial skin assessments; status of wound healing if applicable, degree of comfort achieved, development of pathologic fracture(s), patient's response to AFT, implementation of turning schedule, any unexpected outcomes and interventions taken, and phone number and name of company representative. **Rationale:** Documents nursing care delivered, status of patient's skin, and any expected or unexpected outcomes and interventions taken.

Patient/Family Education

1. Explain to patient and family the effects of tissue compression. **Rationale:** Encourages understanding and enables patient and family to ask questions.

2. Explain how AFT achieves pressure relief. **Rationale:** Increases cooperation.

3. Evaluate the patient's need for long-term pressure reduction (i.e., acute/chronic health problems remain uncontrolled and/or chronic pressure sores). **Rationale:** Allows the nurse to anticipate the need for patient discharge with pressure-relieving device.

Performance Checklist
Skill 23–1: Pressure-Relieving Devices: Air Fluidized Therapy

Critical Behaviors	Complies	
	yes	no
PLACING PATIENT ON AFT BED 1. Wash hands.		
2. Place one hospital flat sheet on bed.		
3. Lift patient onto bed.		
4. Turn bed on.		
5. Remove all linen except hospital flat sheet.		
6. Gently pull filter sheet loose around patient's body.		
7. Tape company representative's name and phone number at foot of bed.		
8. Institute turning/repositioning schedule.		
TURNING PATIENT ON AFT BED 1. Gently pull filter sheet loose around patient's body.		
2. Gather hospital sheet to patient at shoulder and hip.		
3. Pull patient to side of bed.		

Table continues on following page

Critical Behaviors	Complies	
	yes	no
4. Pulling upward and over, turn patient on side.		
5. Cross one of the patient's legs over the other, upper leg slightly bent.		
6. Separate bony prominences with pillows.		
CARDIOPULMONARY RESUSCITATION ON AFT BED 1. Hyperextend patient's neck.		
2. Turn bed off.		
3. Unplug bed.		
4. Initiate CPR.		
5. Position patient's arms, legs, and torso away from rails before defibrillating.		
6. Document procedure in patient record.		

SKILL 23–2

Pressure-Relieving Devices: Low Air Loss Therapy

Low air loss therapy beds are classified as dynamic pressure-relieving devices. These devices also may be known as a specialty/therapeutic beds (but do not include bead or sand beds) or as air-suspension therapy beds.

Low air loss beds relieve pressure well below 25–32 mmHg. Low air loss refers to the airflow system of the bed. The controlled low emission of air is designed to prevent dehydration (as can occur with high air loss therapy, i.e., air fluidized beds) while promoting dry skin. Maximum patient weight ranges from 300 to 500 pounds depending on the low air loss bed model.

Most units have 21 to 23 waterproof polyurethane-coated nylon sacs that are vapor permeable to allow for evaporation of perspiration and excessive moisture. A 0.1-μm filter continually removes particulate matter and most bacteria from the airflow. The multiple air-filled nylon sacs are inflated by an air compressor and are divided into four or five sections that are mounted on a regular hospital-type bed frame. Each section has separate controls that inflate or deflate the individual section to provide support as well as relieve pressure.

The entire bed can be raised or lowered, and the head and foot can be adjusted for patient comfort and transfer. In addition, cushions can be deflated to ease patient transfer to a sitting position or chair.

Several types of cushions can be substituted for the standard low air loss therapy mattress. Split or U-shape cushions enhance pressure relief for the head, sacral, and heel areas. Proning cushions provide extra comfort for patients maintained in the prone position. Extended-height cushions are available to prevent shorter patients from sliding down in bed. High air loss cushions can reduce moisture over extensive body areas, and heavy-duty cushions are available for use with external fixators, weight of casts, and/or obese patients. Draw sheets made of the same material as the air sacs also are available for the incontinent patient.

Purpose

The nurse utilizes low air loss therapy (LALT) to

1. Alleviate external pressure in spinal cord–injured or multiple-trauma patients.
2. Provide pressure relief with deep or multiple pressure sores when conventional methods fail.
3. Reduce the risk of pressure sores when immobilization will be lengthy.
4. Alleviate external pressure on burns, flaps, and grafts.
5. Reduce friction, shearing, and moisture on the skin when conventional methods fail.

Prerequisite Knowledge and Skills

Prior to placing a patient on LALT, the nurse should understand

1. Principles of preventing pressure-induced injury (see Skill 29–1).
2. Pathophysiology of tissue ischemia.
3. Principles of wound healing (see Chapters 28 and 29).
4. Principles of LALT.
5. Clinical features of the LALT bed, such as safety features, maintenance and repair, advantages and disadvantages, and nursing responsibilities.
6. Patient turning and repositioning.

The nurse should be able to perform

1. Proper handwashing technique (see Skill 35–5).
2. Universal precautions (see Skill 35–1).
3. Skin assessment.
4. Assessment of nutritional status.
5. Assessment of wound healing.
6. Scheduled turning/repositioning techniques.
7. Pressure sore prevention and care techniques (see Chapter 29).

Assessment

1. Inspect the patient's bony prominences for evidence of pressure sore formation. **Rationale:** Pressure relief and airflow reduce factors that contribute to the formation of pressure sores.

2. Assess the patient's wound(s): type and amount of drainage, areas of necrosis, surrounding skin for maceration and inflammation, and any pain on palpation of surrounding area. **Rationale:** Relief of external pressure facilitates wound healing.

Nursing Diagnoses

1. Potential/actual impaired tissue integrity related to high and/or prolonged external pressure. **Rationale:** Capillary pressure greater than 25–32 mmHg causes tissue ischemia.

2. Knowledge deficit related to the effects of tissue compression and rationale for the device. **Rationale:** Affects cooperation and acceptance of a therapy that is not usually a common experience for the patient and family.

3. Impaired physical mobility related to disease process or injury. **Rationale:** Limitation of physical movement can cause prolonged or elevated external pressure, which closes capillaries causing tissue ischemia.

Planning

1. Individualize the following goals on the basis of the assessment:
    a. Reduce the amount or duration of external pressure to the patient's skin. **Rationale:** Elevated and/or extended external pressure exceeds closing capillary pressure causing tissue ischemia.

b. Decrease the effects of incontinence or other bodily excretions on the patient's skin. **Rationale:** Excessive moisture on the skin causes maceration, increasing the potential for skin breakdown or the severity of existing pressure sores.

c. Promote wound healing. **Rationale:** Relief of external pressure allows wound healing.

2. Obtain physician's order and initiate mechanisms to procure the bed. **Rationale:** A physician's order is generally required for reimbursement purposes. Some hospitals have specific approval criteria for placing patients on LALT. Check your institution's policy regarding specialty bed use and the mechanism by which they are ordered/obtained.

3. Prepare the patient for transfer to the LALT bed.
    a. Discuss the rationale for LALT with patient. **Rationale:** Reduces anxiety.
    b. Explain the principles of LALT to patient. **Rationale:** Encourages cooperation.

4. Prepare the LALT bed.
    a. Adjust the height of the LALT bed to that of stretcher or regular bed. **Rationale:** Eases transfer of patient onto bed. There are widely diverse LALT units with specific guidelines for use. Always review manufacturer's instructions for the specific model you are using.
    b. Push the foot pedal to lock the wheels. **Rationale:** Ensures patient safety.
    c. Inflate air cushions to maximum (see manufacturer's manual). **Rationale:** Eases patient transfer.

5. Tape company representative's name and telephone number at the foot of bed. **Rationale:** Facilitates contact should problems arise. Most companies have 24-hour per day consultation/troubleshooting service.

Implementation

Steps	Rationale	Special Considerations
Placing a Patient on an LALT Bed		
1. Wash hands.	Reduces transmission of microorganisms.	
2. Place cover sheet provided by company on bed.	Cover sheet reduces friction.	
3. Slide patient onto bed.	Completes transfer.	
4. Position patient on bed; pressures are initially set by the company representative according to the patient's body-weight distribution.	Many manufacturers have specifications for patient positioning.	
5. Turn off maximum inflate switch.	Pressure cushions will adjust automatically to preset optimal levels.	
6. Use pads provided by the company for draining wounds or incontinence.	Permits air flow to reach patient.	The use of plastic linen savers or impervious sheets should be avoided to maximize air flow.

Table continues on following page

Steps	Rationale	Special Considerations
7. Institute turning/repositioning schedule.*	Reduces hazards of immobility.	
Repositioning a Patient on an LALT Bed		
1. Increase air cushions to maximum inflate.	Provides firm surface.	
2. Turn and reposition patient as on standard hospital bed.	No special procedures are required on LALT bed.	
3. Turn maximum inflate switch off.	Pressure cushions will adjust automatically to preset optimal levels.	
4. If bony prominences are in contact with one another, separate with a pillow.	Relieves pressure.	
5. For CPR: deflate air cushions according to manufacturer's guidelines.	Firm surface is necessary for effective cardiac compression.	
6. Wash hands.	Reduces transmission of microorganisms.	

*Consult manufacturer's manual for other procedures, such as bathing/daily hygiene, dressing changes, pressure sores, traction, bedpan placement/removal, hypo/hyperthermia, proning patient, transfer to wheelchair, charting, patient chair transfer, removal/replacement of air sacs, and x-rays.

Evaluation

1. Monitor turning/repositioning schedule every 2 hours. **Rationale:** Prevents circulatory, pulmonary, and urinary stasis.
2. Evaluate skin (particularly areas over bony prominences) for evidence of pressure sore/necrosis. **Rationale:** Relief of external pressure prevents pressure sores.
3. Evaluate existing pressure sores, wounds, flaps, grafts, etc. for evidence of healing. **Rationale:** Relief of external pressure supports healing.
4. Evaluate skin for evidence of friction, shearing, or moisture on skin. **Rationale:** These factors contribute to pressure sore formation.
5. Evaluate patient's acceptance of and adaptation to the device. **Rationale:** Increases cooperation and decreases anxiety.
6. Determine when the therapy should be discontinued. **Rationale:** Pressure relief is no longer required.

Expected Outcomes

1. Absence of pressure sores. **Rationale:** Relief of external pressure reduces risk of pressure sores.
2. Evidence of wound healing. **Rationale:** Relief of external pressure facilitates wound healing.
3. Absence of friction, shearing, and moisture on skin. **Rationale:** Pressure relief and continuous airflow reduce these factors that contribute to pressure sore formation.

Unexpected Outcomes

1. Local dehydration of open wounds. **Rationale:** Constant warm, dry airflow can dry out the moisture in the base of the wound.

2. Pressure sores or further deterioration of existing pressure sores. **Rationale:** Other factors contributing to pressure sores (i.e., nutrition, immobility, incontinence, etc.) remain uncontrolled.

Documentation

Documentation in the patient record should include the date and time LALT therapy is initiated, rationale for use of LALT, serial skin assessments, status of wound healing if applicable, patient's response to LALT, implementation of turning schedule, any unexpected outcomes and interventions taken, and the phone number and name of the company representative. **Rationale:** Documents nursing care delivered, status of patient's skin, and any unexpected outcomes and interventions taken.

Patient/Family Education

1. Explain to the patient and family the effects of tissue compression. **Rationale:** Encourages understanding and enables the patient and family to ask questions.
2. Explain how LALT achieves pressure relief. **Rationale:** Increases cooperation.
3. Evaluate the patient's need for long-term pressure reduction (i.e., acute/chronic health problems remain uncontrolled and/or chronic pressure sores). **Rationale:** Allows the nurse to anticipate the need for patient discharge with pressure-reducing device.

Performance Checklist
Skill 23–2: Pressure-Relieving Devices: Low Air Loss Therapy

Critical Behaviors	Complies yes	no
PLACING A PATIENT ON AN **LALT** BED		
1. Wash hands.		
2. Place cover sheet on low air loss bed.		
3. Slide patient onto bed.		
4. Turn off maximum inflate switch.		
5. Use pads provided by company for draining wounds/incontinence.		
6. Tape company representative's name and phone number at foot of bed.		
7. Institute turning/repositioning schedule.		
REPOSITION A PATIENT ON AN **LALT** BED		
1. Increase air cushions to maximum inflate.		
2. Turn and position patient as on standard hospital bed.		
3. Turn maximum inflate switch off.		
4. Use pillows to separate bony prominences.		
5. For CPR: deflate cushions as per manufacturer's guidelines.		
6. Wash hands.		
7. Document in the patient record.		

SKILL 23–3

Pressure-Relieving Devices: Oscillating Support Therapy

Lateral rotation therapy tables are classified as dynamic pressure-relieving devices, also known as rotating or mechanical tables or oscillating support therapy (OST). They consist of a flat surface with adjustable foam support packs that function as a mattress and also maintain body alignment. They provide continuous, slow, side-to-side turning of the patient by rotating the bed frame. The motion assists in preventing secondary complications of immobility by providing constant postural drainage and repositioning that stimulates body systems.

The bed turns to a maximum of 62 degrees on each side, either intermittently or constantly, every 4 to 4.5 minutes, with a turning frequency of 200 to 300 times per day. The bed should remain in motion for 20 hours of each 24-hour period.

Head and shoulder packs provide cervical stability, and lateral arm and leg hatches facilitate range of motion. Some beds have special features such as variable settings for turning frequency and a flotation mattress.

Hatches underneath the bed located in the cervical, thoracic, and rectal areas provide access for skin care, catheter maintenance, and bladder and bowel management.

Lateral rotation therapy *cushions* are classified as dy-namic pressure-reducing devices, and these provide low air loss technology in addition to lateral rotation. The rotation assists in preventing/treating pulmonary complications by promoting drainage of lung secretions. These cushions also enhance venous return from lower extremities and facilitate urine flow. Some lateral rotation therapy cushions provide pulsation, which enhances patient comfort.

Purpose

The nurse utilizes oscillating support therapy to

1. Provide a special support surface for unstable trauma patients, unstable spinal cord injury/surgery patients, and patients requiring continuous head and skeletal traction.
2. Alleviate severe pulmonary problems.
3. Prevent stasis of pulmonary secretions.
4. Prevent complications of venous stasis and thrombosis.
5. Prevent urinary stasis.
6. Reduce the risk of pressure sores.
7. Provide pressure relief for patients with deep or multiple pressure sores when conventional methods fail.
8. Reduce pressure, friction, and shearing.

Prerequisite Knowledge and Skills

Prior to placing a patient on oscillating support therapy, the nurse should understand

1. Principles of preventing pressure-induced injury (see Skill 29–1).
2. Pathophysiology of tissue ischemia.
3. Principles of wound healing (see Chapters 28 and 29).
4. Principles of oscillating support therapy.
5. Clinical features of oscillating support therapy, such as safety features, maintenance and repair, advantages and disadvantages, and nursing responsibilities.
6. Effects of immobility on body systems, including factors contributing to impaired circulation, including venous stasis and thrombosis, pulmonary and urinary stasis.

The nurse should be able to perform

1. Proper handwashing technique (see Skill 35–5).
2. Universal precautions (see Skill 35–1).
3. Skin assessment.
4. Assessment of nutritional status.
5. Assessment of wound healing.
6. Peripheral vascular system assessment.
7. Pulmonary system assessment.
8. Bladder palpation.
9. Motor/sensory assessment.
10. Pressure sore prevention and care techniques (see Chapter 29).

Assessment

1. Inspect the patient's bony prominences for evidence of pressure sore formation. **Rationale:** Pressure relief reduces the risk for pressure sores. For lateral rotation therapy table, also assess for the presence of friction and shearing, which can occur with movement of the table.
2. Assess the patient's wounds: type and amount of drainage, area of necrosis, surrounding skin for maceration and inflammation, and any pain on palpation of surrounding skin. **Rationale:** Relief of external pressure facilitates wound healing.
3. Assess the patient's vascular system: ischemic rest pain, arterial pulses, condition of the skin and hair of lower extremities, and presence of atrophic nails. **Rationale:** Lateral movement discourages venous stasis.
4. Assess the patient's pulmonary status: adventitious breath sounds, rate and depth of respirations, cough, cyanosis, dyspnea, nasal flaring, arterial blood gases, decreased mental acuity, and restlessness. **Rationale:** Lateral movement provides postural drainage and mobilizes secretions.
5. Assess the patient's bladder: distended bladder, feelings of incomplete bladder emptying, and/or urinary infrequency. **Rationale:** Lateral movement decreases urinary stasis.

Nursing Diagnoses

1. Potential or actual impaired tissue integrity related to high and/or prolonged external pressure. **Rationale:** High or prolonged external pressure closes capillaries causing tissue ischemia.
2. Knowledge deficit related to the effects of tissue compression and the rationale for therapy. **Rationale:** Affects cooperation and acceptance of a therapy that is not usually a common experience for the patient and family.
3. Impaired physical mobility related to disease process or injury. **Rationale:** Limitation of physical movement can cause prolonged or elevated external pressure that closes capillaries causing tissue ischemia.
4. Alteration in peripheral tissue perfusion related to immobility. **Rationale:** External pressure causes a decrease in capillary blood flow.
5. Ineffective airway clearance related to immobility. **Rationale:** Inability to turn or ambulate contributes to adventitious breath sounds and diminished respiratory depth.
6. Urinary retention related to immobility. **Rationale:** Limited mobility and recumbent position may cause urinary stasis.

Planning

1. Individualize the following goals on the basis of assessment:
   a. Decrease the effects of immobility:
      (1) Reduce the amount or duration of external pressure to the patient's skin. **Rationale:** Elevated and/or extended external pressure exceeds closing capillary pressure causing tissue ischemia.
      (2) Implement measures to increase circulation. **Rationale:** Prolonged or elevated external pressure decreases capillary blood flow.
      (3) Implement measures to improve respiratory function. **Rationale:** Inability to turn or ambulate results in pulmonary stasis.
      (4) Implement measures to decrease urinary retention. **Rationale:** Immobility results in urinary stasis, which can cause urinary calculi and infection.
   b. Decrease the effects of incontinence or exudate on the patient's skin. **Rationale:** Excessive moisture on the skin causes maceration, increasing the potential for skin breakdown or the severity of existing pressure sores.
   c. Promote wound healing. **Rationale:** Relief of external pressure supports wound healing.
2. Obtain physician's order and initiate the mechanisms to procure the device. **Rationale:** A physician's order is generally required for reimbursement purposes. Some hospitals have specific approval criteria for use of lateral rotation therapy. Check your institution's

policy regarding specialty bed use and the mechanism by which they are ordered/obtained. The representative assembles the bed to fit the patient and makes later adjustments.
3. Prepare the patient for transfer to oscillating support therapy.

a. Discuss the rationale for use with patient. **Rationale:** Reduces anxiety.
b. Explain the principles of therapy to patient. **Rationale:** Encourages cooperation.

Implementation

Steps	Rationale	Special Considerations
Placing a Patient on a Lateral Rotation Therapy Table		
1. Wash hands.	Reduces transmission of microorganisms.	
2. Be sure bed is locked in horizontal position and drive is disengaged.	Ensures patient safety.	The holes in the frame that the side supports fit are near the surface of the base packs.
3. Check all hatches to be certain they are properly latched, and be sure castors are locked.	Prevents unplanned movement of bed.	
4. Slide the patient gently to center of bed.*	Bouncing patient can result in skin abrasions.	May cover pillar bars with a towel or folded paper sheet to avoid possibility of abrasion.
Positioning a Patient on a Lateral Rotation Therapy Table		
1. Center patient on the bed by aligning nose, umbilicus, and pubis with center posts.	Facilitates proper balance. Rotating to one side indicates that patient is not centered.	To initiate CPR, return bed to horizontal position and lock in place.
2. Place thoracic side supports in appropriate holes provided in the frame, and be sure they are tightened securely.	These are the main supporting apparatus.	Packs and supports are labeled for patient's right and left sides.
3. Adjust knee assembly to a position slightly above the patient's knee.	Provides support.	
4. Place disposable leg support in a position under the thigh and calf so that it fits under the ankle and knee but not beneath the heel.	Decreases external pressure on the heels.	Leg supports should be changed periodically when soiled.
5. Place foot supports in foot bracket assembly. Assembly should be positioned so that the foot rests in anatomic position. Tighten the foot assembly.	Maintains the foot in proper anatomic position.	The foot supports should not be left in place longer than 2 hours at a time. A schedule of 2 hours on and 2 hours off should be maintained continuously. Side-to-side motion does not relieve pressure on the soles of the feet.
6. Install abductor packs into preset metal brackets.	Provides support.	
7. Place side leg supports snugly against the patient's hips, and tighten securely.	Provides support.	
8. Install knee packs in a position such that your hand just fits between the knee and the pack.	Prevents pressure on the knee.	Knee packs can be adjusted to allow for variation in abduction and flexion of patient's legs. They maintain proper posture of the lower limbs in the spastic patient, discouraging contracture formation.
9. Adjust the head and shoulder support assembly.	Provides further support.	

Table continues on following page

Steps	Rationale	Special Considerations
10. Place a hand on the patient's shoulder, and adjust the shoulder pack to lightly touch your hand.	Prevents pressure sores.	Should always be 1 in (2.54 cm) clearance between patient's shoulder and the shoulder pack. If cervical traction causes the patient to slide up on the bed during rotation, place patient in reverse Trendelenburg position.
11. Adjust head pack so that it does not touch the patient's ears or come in contact with the tongs of cervical traction, tighten head and shoulder assemblies securely.	Provides support.	To remove the head and shoulder packs, loosen the handle of the shoulder pack and slide to the side or lift entire assembly.
12. Tighten clamps on crossbar to secure assemblies in correct lateral position.	Provides support.	
13. Install disposable foam arm supports.	To ensure that the hand is in a position of function and the ulnar nerve and elbow are protected.	
14. Secure arm supports in holes provided on frame.	Provides support.	
15. Safety straps are to be in place whenever a confused or restless patient is on the bed. One safety strap is used to hold down the shoulder assembly. Place the other strap in proper position.	Prevents falls and patient injury.	
16. Maintain bed in motion for 20 hours of every 24-hour period.	Provides proper rotation.	
17. Wash hands.	Reduces transmission of microorganisms.	

Placing a Patient on Lateral Rotation Therapy Cushions

Steps	Rationale	Special Considerations
1. Wash hands.	Reduces transmission of microorganisms.	There are widely diverse units with specific guidelines for use. Always review specific manufacturer's guidelines.
2. Adjust height of bed to that of stretcher or bed.	Eases transfer of patient onto bed.	
3. Push foot pedal to lock wheels.	Ensures patient safety.	
4. Inflate air cushions to maximum.	Decreases distance to which patient has to be lowered.	
5. Place cover sheet provided by company on bed.	Cover sheet decreases friction on skin.	
6. Slide patient onto bed.	Completes transfer.	
7. Position patient on bed. Pressures are initially set by the representative according to the patient's body weight distribution.	Many manufacturers have specifications for patient positioning.	To initiate CPR, deflate air cushions by pushing deflate switch.
8. Turn off maximum inflate switch.	Pressure cushions will adjust automatically to preset optimal levels.	
9. For draining wounds or incontinence, use pads provided by the company.	Company's pads permit airflow to reach patient.	The use of plastic linen savers or impervious sheets is to be avoided to maximize airflow.

Table continues on following page

Steps	Rationale	Special Considerations
10. Tape company representative's name and telephone number at the foot of the bed.	Facilitates contact should problems arise.	Most companies have 24-hour per day troubleshooting service.

Repositioning a Patient on Lateral Rotation Therapy Cushions

Steps	Rationale	Special Considerations
1. Increase air cushions to maximum inflate.	Provides firm surface for moving the patient.	
2. Turn and reposition patient as on standard hospital bed.	No special procedures are required to reposition patients on this bed.	
3. Turn maximum inflate switch off.	Pressure cushions will adjust automatically to preset optimal levels.	
4. If bony prominences are in contact with one another, separate with a pillow.	Relieves pressure.	
5. Wash hands.	Reduces transmission of microorganisms.	

*Consult manufacturer's manual for other procedures, such as bathing, bowel/bladder care, chest tubes, cleaning of bed, controlling patient's temperature, IV therapy, physical therapy, placement of bedpan, placement of amputee on bed, pulmonary care, skin care, sleep deprivation, traction, vomiting, and x-rays.

Evaluation

1. Evaluate the patient's skin (particularly areas over bony prominences) for evidence of pressure necrosis. **Rationale:** Relief of external pressure prevents pressure sores.

2. Evaluate the patient's existing pressure sores, wounds, flaps, grafts, etc. for evidence of healing. **Rationale:** Relief of external pressure facilitates healing.

3. Evaluate the skin for evidence of friction, shearing, or moisture. **Rationale:** These factors contribute to pressure sore formation.

4. Evaluate the patient's peripheral vascular circulation. **Rationale:** Lateral movement discourages venous stasis.

5. Evaluate the patient's pulmonary function. **Rationale:** Lateral movement provides continuous postural drainage and mobilization of secretions.

6. Evaluate the patient for urinary retention. **Rationale:** Lateral movement decreases urinary stasis.

7. Evaluate the patient's acceptance of and adaptation to the device. **Rationale:** Increases cooperation and decreases anxiety.

8. Determine when therapy should be discontinued. **Rationale:** Oscillating support therapy is no longer required.

Expected Outcomes

1. Intact skin integrity. **Rationale:** Decreased external pressure reduces risk of pressure sores.

2. Wound healing. **Rationale:** Relief of external pressure supports wound healing.

3. Absence of friction, shearing, and moisture on skin. **Rationale:** Pressure relief and continuous airflow reduce these factors contributing to pressure sores.

4. Improved peripheral circulation. **Rationale:** Lateral movement improves blood flow.

5. Improved urinary elimination. **Rationale:** Lateral movement decreases urinary stasis.

6. Maximum pulmonary function is achieved. **Rationale:** Lateral movement provides postural drainage and mobilizes secretions.

Unexpected Outcomes

1. Lateral movement of table may cause friction and shearing, motion sickness, agitation and disorientation, and falls if patient is not strapped in properly. **Rationale:** Table is in continuous motion.

2. Pressure sore formation or further deterioration of existing pressure sores. **Rationale:** Other factors contributing to pressure sores (i.e., incontinence, nutrition, etc.) remain uncontrolled.

Documentation

Documentation in the patient record should include the date and time the therapy is instituted, rationale for use of oscillating support therapy, number of hours patient is in rotation mode, serial skin assessments, status of wound healing if applicable, patient's response to therapy, any unexpected outcomes and interventions taken, and the phone number and name of the company representative. **Rationale:** Documents nursing care delivered, status of patient's skin, and any unexpected outcomes.

Patient/Family Education

1. Explain to the patient and family the effects of tissue compression. **Rationale:** Encourages understanding and enables patient and family to ask questions.

2. Explain how therapy achieves pressure relief. **Rationale:** Increases cooperation.

3. Evaluate the patient's need for long-term pressure reduction (i.e., acute/chronic health problems remain un-controlled and/or chronic pressure sores). **Rationale:** Allows the nurse to anticipate the need for patient discharge with pressure-reducing device.

Performance Checklist
Skill 23–3:   Pressure-Relieving Devices: Oscillating Support Therapy

Critical Behaviors	Complies	
	yes	no
PLACING PATIENT ON A LATERAL ROTATION THERAPY TABLE 1. Wash hands.		
2. Lock bed in horizontal position and disengage drive.		
3. Lock all hatches and castors.		
4. Slide patient gently to center of bed.		
POSITIONING A PATIENT ON A LATERAL ROTATION THERAPY TABLE 1. Align patient with center posts.		
2. Place and tighten thoracic side supports.		
3. Adjust knee assembly just above patient's knee.		
4. Place leg supports under thigh and calf, avoiding patient's heel.		
5. Assemble and tighten foot assembly.		
6. Install abductor packs.		
7. Place and tighten side leg supports snugly against patient's hips.		
8. Position knee packs so that hand can fit between pack and knee.		
9. Adjust head and shoulder support assembly.		
10. Adjust the shoulder pack so that pack and shoulder are 1 in (2.5 cm) apart.		
11. Adjust head pack to avoid contact with patient's ears or tongs of cervical traction and tighten.		
12. Tighten clamps on crossbar.		
13. Install foam arm supports.		
14. Secure arm supports in holes on frame.		
15. Use safety straps when appropriate.		
16. Maintain bed in motion for 20 hours of every 24-hour period.		
17. Wash hands.		
18. Document in patient record.		
PLACING A PATIENT ON LATERAL ROTATION THERAPY CUSHIONS 1. Wash hands.		
2. Adjust height of bed to stretcher or bed.		
3. Push foot pedal to lock wheels of bed.		
4. Inflate air cushions to maximum inflation.		
5. Place cover sheet on bed.		
6. Slide patient gently onto bed.		
7. Position patient on bed according to manufacturer's guidelines.		
8. Turn off maximum inflate switch.		

Table continues on following page

Critical Behaviors	Complies	
	yes	no
9. Use pads provided by company for draining wounds/incontinence.		
10. Tape company representative's name and phone number at foot of bed.		
REPOSITIONING A PATIENT ON LATERAL ROTATION THERAPY CUSHIONS 1. Increase air cushions to maximum inflate.		
2. Turn and reposition patient as on standard hospital bed.		
3. Turn maximum inflate switch off.		
4. Use pillows to separate bony prominences.		
5. Wash hands.		
6. Document in patient record.		

SKILL 23–4

Pressure-Reducing Devices: Foam and Air Mattresses

The 4-in (10 cm) dense foam overlay is classified as a static pressure-reducing device. The overlay has head, trunk, and foot sections with varying degrees of foam density and contours that reduce pressure in these areas. Most overlays have an optional film sleeve protective cover that is vapor-permeable to help decrease heat and moisture buildup as well as protect the foam from soiling by incontinence and/or perspiration. The foam overlay is used for the prevention of pressure sores or for those patients with existing pressure sores who can be turned and repositioned onto at least two intact skin surfaces.

Polyurethane 2-in (5 cm) convoluted foam pads have pyramid-shaped peaks and are placed on top of the standard hospital mattress. Although very popular and inexpensive, they are not classified as either a pressure-relieving or a pressure-reducing device but are predominately used for patient comfort. *Note*: This skill refers specifically to the 4-in (10 cm) dense foam overlay.

Air mattresses are classified as static pressure-reducing devices and provide pressure reduction over bony prominences to prevent impairment in tissue integrity. The static air mattress is an inflatable vinyl mattress with interconnecting air compartments (cells). The mattress is inflated with an air pump to the level where the sacrum is not palpable beneath the air compartments. There are a great many static air mattresses with varying shapes and numbers of air cells. Daily reinflation may be required.

With the dynamic alternating air mattress, a bedside pump alternately inflates and deflates interconnecting cells to reduce the tissue interface pressures and stimulate capillary action. The cells inflate and deflate on a preset, timed schedule, which varies according to manufacturer's model. Such air mattresses may have options such as constant airflow or alternating airflow, and some may be a combination of alternating air mattress with a thin foam pad.

The air mattress is placed on top of the standard hospital mattress underneath the bed linen and is used to prevent pressure sores or for patients with existing pressure sores who can be turned and repositioned onto at least two intact skin surfaces.

Purpose

The nurse utilizes a foam overlay to

1. Reduce the risk of pressure sores.
2. Provide pressure reduction for patients with existing superficial pressure sores *if* the patient can be turned and positioned off the pressure sores.

Prerequisite Knowledge and Skills

Prior to placing a patient on a foam overlay/air mattress, the nurse should understand

1. Principles of preventing pressure-induced injury (see Skill 29–1).
2. Pathophysiology of tissue ischemia.
3. Principles of wound healing (see Chapters 28 and 29).
4. Principles of the pressure-distributing properties or foam or alternating air mattress.
5. Repositioning to promote circulation.

The nurse should be able to perform

1. Proper handwashing technique (see Skill 35–5).
2. Universal precautions (see Skill 35–1).
3. Skin assessment.
4. Assessment of nutritional status.
5. Assessment of wound healing.
6. Scheduled turning/repositioning techniques.
7. Pressure sore prevention and care techniques (see Chapter 29).

Assessment

1. Assess the patient's bony prominences (i.e., trochanters, sacrum, heels) for evidence of effects of ex-

ternal pressure. **Rationale:** Effect of tissue compression is first seen over bony prominences; pressure relief rather than pressure reduction may be required for patient.

2. Assess the patient's wound(s): type and amount of drainage, areas of necrosis, surrounding skin for maceration and inflammation, and any pain on palpation of surrounding skin. **Rationale:** Reduction of external pressure facilitates wound healing.

Nursing Diagnoses

1. Potential or actual impaired skin integrity related to high and/or prolonged external pressure. **Rationale:** High or prolonged external pressure closes capillaries causing tissue ischemia.

2. Knowledge deficit related to the effects of tissue compression and the rationale for use of the device. **Rationale:** Affects cooperation and acceptance of a therapy that is not usually a common experience for patient and family.

3. Impaired physical mobility related to disease process or injury. **Rationale:** Limitation of physical movement can cause prolonged or elevated external pressure

that exceeds capillary-closing pressure causing tissue ischemia.

Planning

1. Develop individualized goals on the basis of the assessment to reduce the amount or duration of external pressure on the skin. **Rationale:** High and/or prolonged external pressure exceeds capillary closing pressure causing tissue ischemia.

2. Initiate mechanism to procure the foam overlay or air mattress. Check to see if a physician's order is required for reimbursement purposes, and order as per hospital procedure. **Rationale:** Your hospital may have specific guidelines for ordering and procuring foam overlays or air mattresses.

3. Prepare the patient for transfer to a foam overlay.
   a. Discuss the rationale for pressure-reducing device use with patient. **Rationale:** Reduces anxiety.
   b. Explain the principles of pressure-reducing device use to patient. **Rationale:** Encourages cooperation.

Implementation

Steps	Rationale	Special Considerations
Foam Overlay		
1. Wash hands.	Reduces transmission of microorganisms.	
2. Remove linen from bed.	For optimal pressure reduction.	
3. Remove foam from package and allow to swell.	Foam is compressed in transit.	
4. Ensure that the head and foot of the foam are in the proper position on the bed.	Head and foot areas have increased density to disperse higher pressures.	To initiate CPR, place backboard between patient and foam.
5. If required, place protective cover over foam loosely. Sleeve should not compress foam.	Sleeve protects foam from soiling.	
6. Replace linens on bed, being careful not to pull too tight.	Compression of foam reduces pressure reduction.	
7. Place patient on bed.	Initiates pressure reduction.	
8. If bony prominences are in contact with one another, separate with a pillow.	Relieves pressure.	
9. Institute turning/repositioning schedule.	Reduces hazards of immobility.	
10. Wash hands.	Reduces transmission of microorganisms.	
Air Mattress		
1. Wash hands.	Reduces transmission of microorganisms.	
2. Place air mattress in correct direction on the bed.	Mattress may have specific areas with increased pressure-reducing capabilities.	Head and foot areas are marked on the air mattress.

Table continues on following page

Steps	Rationale	Special Considerations
3. Inflate mattress with air pump provided by company as per manufacturer's guidelines.	Initiates pressure reduction.	Can be inflated under patient if necessary.
4. Position straps around corners of standard mattress.	Holds mattress in place.	
5. Cover with one hospital flat sheet.	Too many sheets under patient can cause pressure and reduce the effects of the air mattress.	
6. Place patient on air mattress.	Completes transfer.	Mattress must be deflated before initiating CPR. Most units have instant deflate mechanisms.
7. Institute turning/repositioning schedule.	Reduces hazard of immobility and risk of pressure sore formation.	
8. Perform hand check once every 8 hours when patient is on the air mattress:	To maintain mattress at proper pressures.	
a. Slide hand *beneath* the air mattress under patient's bony prominences.	Areas most susceptible to air mattress "bottoming out."	
b. Hand should be palm up, fingers flat.	If the fingers are flexed, the hand check will be misleading.	
c. If bony prominences are felt, reinflation is required.	Identifies the need for air installation.	No air is added if bony prominences are not detected.
9. Wash hands.	Reduces transmission of microorganisms.	

Evaluation

1. Monitor the turning/repositioning schedule every 2 hours. **Rationale:** Prevents circulatory, pulmonary, and urinary stasis and other effects of immobility.
2. Evaluate the patient's skin (particularly areas over bony prominences) for evidence of pressure sore formation/necrosis. **Rationale:** Reduction of external pressure prevents pressure sores.
3. Evaluate the patient's existing pressure sores for evidence of healing. **Rationale:** Reduction of amount or duration of external pressure supports wound healing.
4. Monitor skin for evidence of friction, shearing, or moisture. **Rationale:** These factors contribute to pressure sore formation.
5. Evaluate the patient's acceptance of and adaptation to the device. **Rationale:** Increases cooperation and decreases anxiety.
6. Determine when therapy should be discontinued. **Rationale:** Pressure reduction no longer required.

Expected Outcomes

1. Intact skin integrity. **Rationale:** Reduction of external pressure reduces risk of pressure sore formation.
2. Evidence of wound healing. **Rationale:** Reduction of external pressure supports wound healing.

Unexpected Outcomes

1. Patient complains of feeling overheated with foam overlay. **Rationale:** Polyurethane may decrease evaporation and cause perspiration.
2. Pressure sore formation or deterioration of existing pressure sores. **Rationale:** Patient may require pressure relief rather than pressure reduction. Other factors contributing to impaired tissue integrity (i.e., immobility, nutrition, incontinence, etc.) remain uncontrolled.

Documentation

Documentation in the patient record should include the date and time the patient was placed on the pressure reducing device and its rationale for use, serial skin assessments, status of wound healing if applicable, patient's response to foam overlay or air mattress, implementation of turning schedule, and any unexpected outcomes and interventions taken. **Rationale:** Documents nursing care delivered, status of patient's skin, and any expected and unexpected outcomes and interventions taken.

Patient/Family Education

1. Explain to both patient and family the effects of tissue compression. **Rationale:** Encourages understanding and enables patient and family to ask questions.
2. Explain how foam overlay/air mattress achieves pressure reduction. **Rationale:** Increases cooperation.

3. Evaluate the patient's need for long-term pressure reduction (i.e., acute/chronic health problems remain uncontrolled and/or chronic pressure sores). **Rationale:** Allows the nurse to anticipate the need for patient discharge with pressure-reducing device.

Performance Checklist
Skill 23–4:   Pressure-Reducing Devices: Foam and Air Mattresses

Critical Behaviors	Complies	
	yes	no
FOAM OVERLAY		
1. Wash hands.		
2. Remove linen from bed.		
3. Remove foam from package and allow to swell.		
4. Properly position foam at head and foot of bed.		
5. If required, place protective sleeve loosely over foam.		
6. Replace linens loosely over foam overlay.		
7. Place patient on bed.		
8. Pad any prominences in contact with each other.		
9. Institute turning/repositioning schedule.		
10. Wash hands.		
11. Document in patient record.		
AIR MATTRESS		
1. Wash hands.		
2. Position mattress on bed appropriately.		
3. Inflate mattress according to manufacturer's directions.		
4. Position straps around corners of standard mattress.		
5. Place one sheet over mattress.		
6. Position patient as on standard hospital mattress.		
7. Initiate turning/repositioning schedule.		
8. Perform hand check once every 8 hours.		
9. Wash hands.		
10. Document in patient record.		

BIBLIOGRAPHY

Allman, R. M. (1989). Pressure ulcers among the elderly. *N. Engl. J. Med.* 320(13):850–853.

Andrews, J., and Balai, R. (1988). The prevention and treatment of pressure sores by use of pressure distributing mattresses. *Decubitus* 1(4):14–15, 18–21.

Arnell, I. (1988). Aggressive and successful prevention of skin breakdown. *Today's OR Nurse* 10(10):10–14.

Beaver, M. J. (1986). Mediscus low air loss beds and the prevention of decubitus ulcers. *Crit. Care Nurs.* 6(5):32–33.

Becker, D. M., Gonzalez, M., Gentili, A., et al. (1987). Prevention of deep venous thrombosis in patients with acute spinal cord injuries: Use of rotating treatment tables. *Neurosurgery* 20(5):675–677.

Ceccio, C. M. (1990). Understanding therapeutic beds. *Orthop. Nurs.* 9(3):57–70.

Fink, M. P., Helsmoortel, C. M., Stein, K. L., et al. (1990). The efficacy of an oscillating bed in the prevention of lower respiratory tract infection in critically ill victims of blunt trauma: A prospective study. *Chest* 97(1):132–137.

Gentilello, L., Thompson, D. A., Tonnesen, A. S., et al. (1988). Effect of a rotating bed on the incidence of pulmonary complications in critically ill patient. *Crit. Care Med.* 16(8):783–786.

Greer, D. M., Morris, J. E., Walsh, N. E., et al. (1988). Cost-effectiveness and efficacy of air-fluidized therapy in the treatment of pressure ulcers. *J. Enterostomal Ther.* 15(6):247–251.

International Association for Enterostomal Therapy (1987). *Standards of Care: Dermal Wounds; Pressure Sores.* Irvine, Calif.: IAET.

Jackson, B.S., Chagares, R., Nee, N., and Freeman, K. (1988). The effects of a therapeutic bed on pressure ulcers: An experimental study. *J. Enterostomal Ther.* 15(6):220.

Jester, J., and Weaver, V. (1990). A report of clinical investigation of various tissue support surfaces used for the prevention, early intervention, and management of pressure ulcers. *Ostomy/Wound Management* 26:39–45.

Kelley, R. E., Vibulsresth, S., Bell, L., and Duncan, R. C. (1987). Evaluation of kinetic therapy on the prevention of complications of prolonged bed rest secondary to stroke. *Stroke* 18(3):638–642.

Klein, L., and Gilroy, K. (1989). Evaluating mattress overlays and pressure-relieving systems: A question of perception or reality? *J. Enterostomal Ther.* 16:58–60.

Krouskop, T. A., Noble, P. S., Brown, J., and Marburger, R. (1986). Factors affecting the pressure-distributing properties of foam mattress overlays. *J. Rehabil. Res. Dev.* 23(3):33–39.

Lovell, H. W., and Anderson, C. L. (1990). Put your patient on the right bed. *RN* 53(5):66–72.

Scheulen, J. J., and Munster, A. (1986). Improved surgical care of posterior burns and donor sites using air-fluidized support. *J. Burn Care Rehabil.* 7(1):40–41.

Willey, T. (1989). High-tech beds and mattress overlays: A decision guide. *Am. J. Nurs.* 89(9):1142–1145.

University Hospital Consortium Technology Advancement Center (1990). Guidelines for the Use of Pressure Relief Devices in the Treatment and Prevention of Pressure Ulcers. Chicago: University Hospital Consortium.

24

IMMOBILIZATION CASTS

BEHAVIORAL OBJECTIVES

After completing this chapter, the nurse will be able to

- Define the key terms.
- Discuss the various types of casts and their indications.
- Recognize potential complications of a patient in a cast.
- Demonstrate the skills involved in cast immobilization.

The anatomic structure of the musculoskeletal system includes bones, muscles, tendons, ligaments, cartilage, blood vessels, and nerves. These structures function to support the body, protect underlying organs, provide movement, act as a vehicle for storage of mineral salts and fats, and produce blood cells.

Immobilization is most often associated with injuries to the musculoskeletal system. The purpose of immobilization is to support, protect, and maintain the position of realigned bones after a fracture or dislocation or to prevent or correct deformities.

This chapter addresses the purpose, recognition, assessment, and intervention of musculoskeletal injuries requiring immobilization with a cast. Techniques discussed include assisting with cast application and removal and care of the patient with a cast.

KEY WORDS

bivalve	malunion
body cast	moleskin
cast	open reduction
cast cutter	petaling
cast syndrome	plaster of paris
compartment syndrome	setting time
computerized axial	spica cast
tomography (CAT scan)	stabilization
"green" cast	stockinette
magnetic resonance	webril
imaging (MRI)	windowing

SKILLS

24–1   Assisting with Cast Application
24–2   Cast Care
24–3   Cast Removal

GUIDELINES

The following assessment guidelines assist the nurse in formulating an individualized plan of care based on the nursing diagnoses to maintain immobilization of the musculoskeletal system with the use of a cast.

1.   Ascertain the mechanism and type of the injury, acute versus chronic nature of the injury, congenital versus acquired cause of the deformity, and any previous history of immobilization or casting.

2.   Identify the patient's nutritional status for its impact on wound healing.

3.   Know the results of the physical examination of the affected area before and after casting.

4.   Identify the results of diagnostic tests (i.e., x-ray, CAT scan, MRI, coagulation studies, CBC, UA, and ABGs, if chest spica cast).

5.   Determine the appropriate nursing interventions based on the assessment findings.

6.   Become familiar with the supplies and instrumentation required for cast application and removal.

SKILL 24–1 _____

Assisting with Cast Application

Casting is an immobilization technique in which a rigid external structure is molded to the contour of the affected body part. Applied correctly, a cast will promote proper stabilization and subsequent bone healing. Although other methods of immobilization (traction or internal or external fixation) are available, casts have the advantage of being easy to apply and care for, less expensive, and less restrictive to patient activities. The cast is applied to a wide area encompassing the affected bone, joint, or tissue, as well as to the joint directly above and/or below the injured site (Table 24–1). Temporary stabilization with posterior plaster splints is often used for several days following an injury to an extremity to allow for maximum swelling prior to immobilization with a cast.

Casts can be made of layers of plaster bandages or synthetic materials. The cast material chosen depends on the type of fracture or deformity, the amount of stabilization required, physician preference, the availability of materials, and patient comfort and expected activity level.

TABLE 24–1 Types of Casts

Type	Area Included	Indications
Short arm (Fig. 24–1)	Proximal palmar crease to elbow	Stable fracture of carpal bones and radius
Long arm (Fig. 24–2)	Proximal palmar crease to axillary fold; elbow at 90-degree angle	Unstable fracture of wrist; stable fracture of distal humerus; fracture of radius, ulna, or both
Hanging arm (Fig. 24–3)	Long-arm cast with loop close to wrist; strap around patient's neck	Displaced fracture of humerus
Short leg (Fig. 24–4)	Base of toes to knee	Stable fracture of ankle/metatarsals; fractures of calcaneous and talus
Long leg (Fig. 24–5)	Base of toes to middle or upper thigh	Fracture of tibia, fibula, and ankle
Long-leg cylinder (Fig. 24–6)	Long-leg cast with foot and ankle free	Stable injuries of distal femur, proximal tibia, and knee joint
Spica: Thumb (Fig. 24–7)	Short-arm cast with spical bandage between hand and affected thumb	Fractures of navicular and thumb metacarpal
Shoulder (Fig. 24–8)	Body jacket plus long-arm cast with spical bandage between trunk and affected arm	Unstable fracture of shoulder girdle or humerus
Hip (Fig. 24–9)	Nipple line down entire length of affected leg; unaffected leg may be fully, partially, or not included; spical bandage from trunk or unaffected leg to affected leg	Fracture of femur
Body (Fig. 24–10)	Encloses the trunk; may extend from neck to the groin	Injury to vertebrae

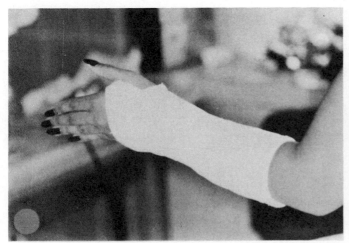

FIGURE 24–1. Short-arm cast. (From K. K. Wu, *Techniques in Surgical Casting and Splinting*. Lea & Febiger, Philadelphia, 1987, p. 58, with permission.)

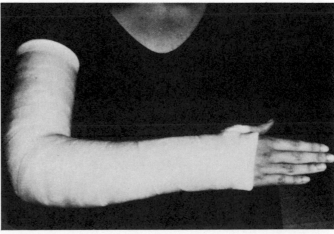

FIGURE 24–2. Long-arm cast. (From K. K. Wu, *Techniques in Surgical Casting and Splinting*. Lea & Febiger, Philadelphia, 1987, p. 89, with permission.)

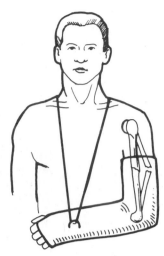

FIGURE 24–3. Hanging arm cast. (From K. K. Wu, *Techniques in Surgical Casting and Splinting*. Lea & Febiger, Philadelphia, 1987, p. 97, Fig. 6–11, with permission.)

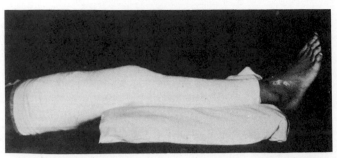

FIGURE 24–6. Long-leg cylinder cast. (From F. Freuler, W. Wiedmer, and D. Bianchini, *Cast Manual for Adults and Children*, Heidelberg, Springer-Verlag, 1979, p. 54, with permission.)

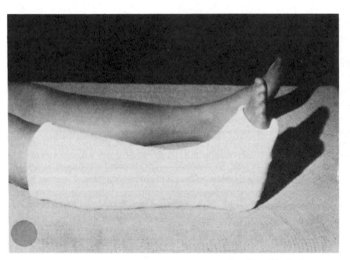

FIGURE 24–4. Short-leg cast. (From K. K. Wu, *Techniques in Surgical Casting and Splinting*. Lea & Febiger, Philadelphia, 1987, p. 124, with permission.)

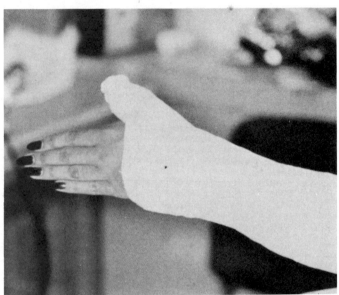

FIGURE 24–7. Thumb spica cast. (From K. K. Wu, *Techniques in Surgical Casting and Splinting*. Lea & Febiger, Philadelphia, 1987, p. 62, with permission.)

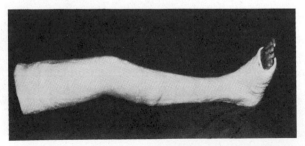

FIGURE 24–5. Long-leg cast. (From F. Freuler, W. Wiedmer, and D. Bianchini, *Cast Manual for Adults and Children*, Heidelberg, Springer-Verlag, 1979, p. 62, with permission.)

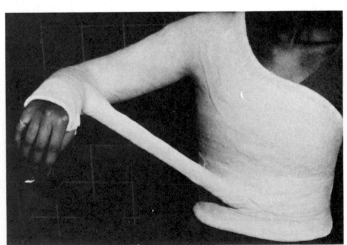

FIGURE 24–8. Shoulder spica cast. (From K. K. Wu, *Techniques in Surgical Casting and Splinting*. Lea & Febiger, Philadelphia, 1987, p. 109, with permission.)

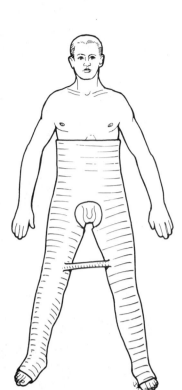

FIGURE 24–9. Hip spica cast. (From K. K. Wu, *Techniques in Surgical Casting and Splinting.* Lea & Febiger, Philadelphia, 1987, p. 198, Fig. 10–1, with permission.)

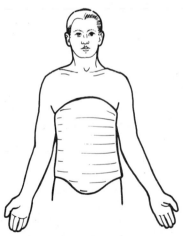

FIGURE 24–10. Body cast. (From K. K. Wu, *Techniques in Surgical Casting and Splinting.* Lea & Febiger, Philadelphia, 1987, p. 223, Fig. 11–1*B*, with permission.)

Purpose

The nurse assists with application of a cast to

1. Provide for the patient's physical care, safety, and comfort during the procedure.
2. Maintain proper body alignment of the affected area during the procedure.

Prerequisite Knowledge and Skills

Prior to assisting with the application of a cast, the nurse should understand

1. Anatomy and physiology of the affected body part.
2. Physiology of bone healing.
3. Proper body mechanics to avoid injury to the patient or self during the application.
4. Properties of cast setting and drying (Table 24–2).

The nurse should be able to perform

1. Proper handwashing technique (see Skill 35–5).
2. Neurovascular assessment.
3. Proper positioning of limb to be casted.
4. Proper handling of plaster or synthetic rolls.
5. Proper handling of plaster splints.

Assessment

1. Perform neurovascular checks on the affected body part, noting color, temperature, capillary filling time, pulses, sensation, motion, presence or absence of edema. Assessment findings should be compared with the findings on the unaffected side or body part. **Rationale:** Provides baseline data for prevention of compartment syndrome.
2. Assess alignment of the affected area. **Rationale:** To prevent contracture formation.
3. Assess skin integrity of the area to be casted for scars, open lacerations, bruises, or rashes. **Rationale:** To prevent complications and provide baseline data.
4. Assess nutritional status, including 24-hour dietary intake; protein; vitamins A, D, and C; calcium; phosphorus; and magnesium. **Rationale:** Intake of adequate nutrients optimizes the anabolic process necessary for repair and growth of bone and soft tissue to prevent delayed and/or nonunion of fractures.
5. Assess blood loss from fracture: hemoglobin less than 8 g/dl, hematocrit less than 25 percent, heart rate above 120 beats/min, and blood pressure below 80/60 mmHg. **Rationale:** An extremity fracture can result in a loss of 1 to 3 units of blood.

Nursing Diagnoses

1. Fear related to cast application. **Rationale:** Uncertainty of outcome of procedure may produce feeling of dread.
2. Impaired physical mobility related to musculoskeletal injury and/or cast. **Rationale:** Immobilization to maintain alignment of bone fragments is required for proper healing in cast.
3. Pain related to musculoskeletal injury. **Rationale:** Injury to soft tissue surrounding fracture results in muscle spasm, which produces pain.
4. Potential decrease in peripheral tissue perfusion related to edema formation and/or hemorrhage. **Ratio-**

TABLE 24–2 Cast Materials

Material	Characteristics	Drying Time
Plaster of paris	Inexpensive Durable Easily molded Heavy Porous Translucent for x-rays "Messy" application	24 hours for arm/leg cast; up to 48 hours for weight-bearing cast; up to 72 hours for body cast
Synthetic	Expensive Light weight Easy to clean Not easily molded Difficult to "petal"	Fiberglass: dry in 10 to 15 minutes; weight-bearing in 30 minutes Polyurethane: dry in 7 minutes; weight-bearing in 20 minutes

nale: Swelling occludes the arterial blood supply and venous return in the affected extremity, resulting in ischemia and/or necrosis.

5. Potential for injury related to neurovascular compromise. **Rationale:** Posttraumatic edema, hemorrhage, and/or excessively restrictive dressings may cause compression of the neurovascular structures of the extremity, leading to development of compartment syndrome.

6. Potential for impaired skin integrity related to mechanism of injury or pressure beneath cast. **Rationale:** Adequate precasting skin care of the affected extremity decreases the risk of skin breakdown.

Planning

1. Individualize the following goals for immobilization of the affected extremity with a cast:
    a. Maintain proper alignment. **Rationale:** Prevents contracture formation.
    b. Promote stabilization and bone healing. **Rationale:** Prevents malunion.
2. Determine the type of cast and casting materials to be used. **Rationale:** The needed amount of supplies must be available before the casting procedure is initiated.
3. Prepare all necessary equipment and supplies. **Rationale:** Time and motion efficiency is critical once application is initiated.
    a. Precasting x-rays
    b. Positioning equipment:
        (1) Finger traps and weights (Fig. 24–11), if applicable.
        (2) Spica table (Fig. 24–12), if applicable.
        (3) Supports (pillows, stools, foam padding).
    c. Plastering equipment:
        (1) Cast cart if available.
        (2) Pail for water.
        (3) Appropriate size and quantity of cast material; width of plaster of paris varies from

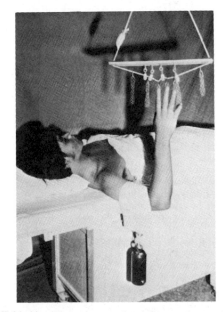

FIGURE 24–11. Finger traps and weights may be required in order to reduce a fracture of the wrist prior to immobilization in a cast. From J. F. Burke, R. J. Boyd, and C. J. McCabe, *Trauma Management*, Chicago: Yearbook Medical Publishers, 1988, p. 340.

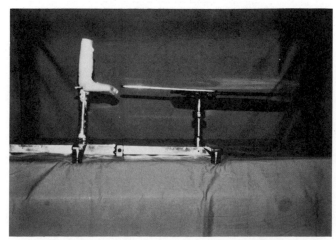

FIGURE 24–12. Patients will be suspended on a spica table for application of hip spica or body casts.

2 to 6 in; width of fiberglass varies from 2 to 5 in to suit different body parts.

(4) Knife or scissors to trim cast.

(5) Appropriate size and quantity of cast padding, webril, or stockinette.

(6) Plastic drapes to protect patient and equipment.

(7) Disposable exam gloves.

(8) Specific adjuncts required for the cast to be applied (e.g., walking heel for short-leg cast).

4. Clean the parts of the body to be casted with soap and water prior to application when possible. Dry thoroughly. Do *not* apply lotions and creams. **Rationale:** Maintains skin integrity and prevents irritation and/or infection of skin. Creams and lotions may soften skin and cause the cast to stick.

5. Assess the patient's level of pain on a scale of 0 to 10, and medicate as prescribed prior to casting. **Rationale:** Decreases pain from extensive manipulation of affected area.

6. Prepare the patient.

   a. Discuss the nature and purpose of the cast. **Rationale:** Enlists patient cooperation during the casting procedure.

   b. Discuss the sensations the patient will experience during application of cast, especially heat and weight. **Rationale:** Facilitates the patient's understanding and decreases fear of the unknown.

7. Warm room, if possible. **Rationale:** Patient may have large body surface area exposed during cast application. In a cold room, a limb in plaster becomes very cold, increasing the patient's thermoregulatory demands.

8. Fill the bucket with water at the temperature appropriate for the type of cast to be applied. **Rationale:** Temperature of water affects setting time; the warmer the water, the more rapid the setting. Average temperature for plaster of paris is 25 to 30°C; for synthetic materials it is 21 to 27°C. If water is too warm, a weak cast will result. Hot water could burn the patient's skin. Cold or warm water may be used for very large casts to prevent them from setting before cast application is complete.

Implementation

Steps	Rationale	Special Considerations
1. Wash hands.	Reduces transmission of microorganisms.	
2. Supply cast padding or stockinette as requested.	When swelling is anticipated, padding is required to permit expansion within cast without constriction of the limb's blood supply.	Extra padding is needed over bony prominences or in thin patients.
3. Don disposable exam gloves.	Plaster is abrasive to the skin.	
4. Remove rolls of plaster or synthetic bandages from packaging wrapper with dry hands. Place rolls away from water to prevent premature wetting of plaster.	Consistency of plaster of paris will be altered if premature or uneven wetting occurs.	
5. Unroll edge of bandage a few inches, and hold the distal end in the nondominant hand and the roll in the dominant hand (Fig. 24–13).	Facilitates finding end after immersion.	
6. If using splints, immerse splint, holding one end in each hand, push together accordian style to remove excess water, and smooth out remaining wrinkles by running between two fingers.	Prepares material for use.	
7. Immerse one roll of plaster at a time immediately before use, holding plaster under water.	Plaster roll must be wet for proper molding.	If bandage is dropped to bottom of bucket, crystallized plaster will adhere to it and make hard areas on bandage.
8. Remove plaster from water when bubbling stops.	Oversoaking will adversely affect setting time.	

Table continues on following page

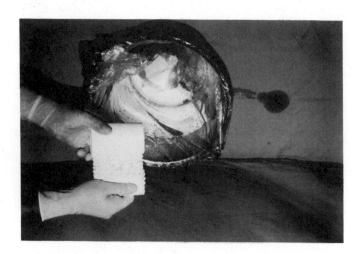

FIGURE 24–13. Prior to immersion in water, the roll of plaster of paris is unrolled a few inches.

Steps	Rationale	Special Considerations
9. Squeeze gently to remove excess water from plaster of paris. Remove excess water without wringing out plaster; it should remain "sloppy."	Eliminates undue soiling of personnel and environment.	Do *not* squeeze synthetic material because the cooling effect is lost.
10. Continue to supply plaster in the same manner until casting is complete.	On the adult patient, more than one roll of plaster is usually needed for a proper cast.	The number of rolls depends on the extremity or body surface and the desired strength of the cast.
11. Wash excess plaster from patient's skin with warm water.	Plaster is abrasive to skin.	
12. Strain water used for casting procedure through piece of cloth material prior to discarding.	Residue in water from plaster of paris can clog plumbing system.	
13. Wash hands.	Reduces transmission of microorganisms.	
14. Move the casted extremity using the palms of your hands to prevent indentations from your fingers.	Indentations on a wet cast may cause pressure areas to develop.	
15. Elevate the extremity on plastic pillow.	Elevation facilitates venous return, decreasing edema.	Rubber pillow does not allow heat to dissipate.

Evaluation

1. Perform neurovascular assessment every hour for 24 hours and every 4 hours thereafter and compare with precasting and previous assessments. **Rationale:** Early detection of compromised tissue perfusion prevents complications, especially development of compartment syndrome, which can occur up to 6 days after initial trauma. Emphasis is placed on the five P's of assessment (Fig. 24–14).
   a. *Pain.* Note location, pattern, duration, and intensity out of proportion to injury.
   b. *Pallor.* Note presence of absence of cyanosis, mottling, and erythema.
   c. *Paresthesia.* Note and report tingling, numbness, and lack of sensation.
   d. *Pulse.* Note decreased quality of pulses distal to injury compared with unaffected extremity.
   e. *Paralysis.* Note absence of mobility of distal joints.
2. Monitor skin integrity of areas around edges of the cast, and note patient complaints of pressure and/or burning sensation. **Rationale:** Skin breakdown predisposes the patient to infection.
3. For patients in a spica cast, monitor gastrointestinal, genitourinary, and respiratory function and compare

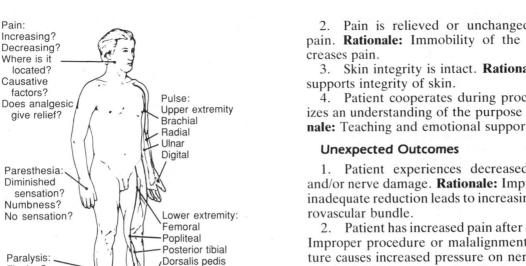

Pain:
Increasing?
Decreasing?
Where is it
   located?
Causative
   factors?
Does analgesic
   give relief?

Pulse:
Upper extremity
Brachial
Radial
Ulnar
Digital

Paresthesia:
Diminished
   sensation?
Numbness?
No sensation?

Lower extremity:
Femoral
Popliteal
Posterior tibial
Dorsalis pedis

Paralysis:
Flexion?
Extension?
Abduction?
Adduction?
Rotation?

Pallor:
Capillary filling after pressure?
Skin cool or warm to touch?

FIGURE 24–14. The five P's of neurovascular assessment (from K. J. Webb, Early assessment of orthopedic injuries. *Am. J. Nurs.* 74:1048, 1974, with permission.)

2. Pain is relieved or unchanged from precasting pain. **Rationale:** Immobility of the affected area decreases pain.

3. Skin integrity is intact. **Rationale:** Proper casting supports integrity of skin.

4. Patient cooperates during procedure and verbalizes an understanding of the purpose of the cast. **Rationale:** Teaching and emotional support decrease fear.

Unexpected Outcomes

1. Patient experiences decreased tissue perfusion and/or nerve damage. **Rationale:** Improper technique or inadequate reduction leads to increasing pressure on neurovascular bundle.

2. Patient has increased pain after casting. **Rationale:** Improper procedure or malalignment of affected structure causes increased pressure on nerve fibers.

3. Malalignment is visualized on postcasting x-ray films. **Rationale:** Improper reduction may require repeat of casting procedure.

4. Patient develops compartment syndrome. **Rationale:** Postinjury edema, hemorrhage, or restrictive cast may cause compromise of neurovascular structures.

with precasting baseline. **Rationale:** Cast syndrome can occur in patients with body cast.

4. Obtain postcasting x-ray. **Rationale:** Documents the proper alignment of the bone.

5. Observe for signs and symptoms of cast syndrome, which is a series of events leading to small bowel obstruction. It occurs most commonly in patients with body or spica casts but also can occur with an extremity cast. Signs and symptoms include anxiety; vague abdominal distension; dyspnea; increases in blood pressure, pulse, and respirations; and low-grade temperature. **Rationale:** Cast syndrome results from the compression of the superior mesenteric artery by the patient's cast.

Expected Outcomes

1. Neurovascular assessment is improved or unchanged from precasting assessment. **Rationale:** Proper casting procedure reduces or eliminates pressure on neurovascular structure.

Documentation

Documentation in the patient record should include the date and time of procedure, type of cast material, the area of body involved, name of physician applying cast, patient's tolerance of the procedure, level of pain, medication and dose administered, degree of comfort achieved, serial neurovascular assessments, integrity of the skin, and for those patients in a spica cast, the status of the gastrointestinal and genitourinary functions (i.e., bowel sounds, presence of bowel or bladder distension, abdominal tenderness, nausea and/or vomiting, and elimination pattern or lack thereof); and any unexpected outcomes and the medical and nursing interventions taken. **Rationale:** Documents baseline nursing assessment and care as well as medical interventions taken.

Patient/Family Education

Emphasize the need to report immediately the signs and symptoms of neurovascular compromise. **Rationale:** Essential to recognize early warning signs of complications for prompt intervention.

Performance Checklist
Skill 24–1: Assisting with Cast Application

Critical Behaviors	Complies	
	yes	no
1. Wash hands.		
2. Supply cast padding or stockinette as requested.		
3. Don gloves.		

Table continues on following page

Critical Behaviors	Complies	
	yes	no
4. Remove rolls of plaster or synthetic bandages from packaging wrapper with dry hands.		
5. Unroll edge of bandage a few inches and hold ends in hands.		
6. If using splints, immerse, holding one end in each hand.		
7. Immerse one roll of plaster at a time immediately before use, holding plaster under water.		
8. Remove plaster from water when bubbling stops.		
9. Squeeze gently to remove excess water from plaster of paris.		
10. Continue to support plaster in the same manner until casting is complete.		
11. Wash excess plaster from patient's skin with warm water.		
12. Strain water used for casting procedure through piece of cloth material prior to discarding.		
13. Wash hands.		
14. Move casted extremity with palms of hands, *not* fingers.		
15. Elevate extremity on plastic pillow.		
16. Document in patient record.		

SKILL 24–2

Cast Care

Care of a patient in a cast begins with procedures for drying and finishing the cast. A dry cast becomes a rigid structure that exerts external pressure on the body part(s) it encases. The focus in cast care is to prevent limb-threatening complications and systemic infections while striking a balance between a clean, functional cast and patient comfort.

Patient and family teaching is important from the onset, since many patients, especially those with large body casts, will be discharged prior to removal of the cast.

Purpose

The nurse performs cast care to

1. Maintain proper alignment of fracture fragments or deformity.
2. Prevent complications related to improper immobilization.
3. Provide for patient safety and comfort.

Prerequisite Knowledge and Skills

Prior to caring for the patient in a cast, the nurse should understand

1. Anatomy and physiology of the affected body part(s).
2. Principles of bone healing.
3. Principles of compartment pressure.
4. Properties of cast setting.
5. Principles of drying by evaporation.
6. Principles of body mechanics to avoid injury to patient or self.

The nurse should be able to perform

1. Neurovascular assessment specific for casted area (Table 24–3).
2. Proper handwashing technique (see Skill 35–5).
3. Proper techniques of lifting and turning.

Assessment

1. Assess the patient's neurovascular status (the five P's) every 4 hours after setting occurs. Assess color, temperature, capillary refill, quality of pulses distal to the cast, presence or absence of sensation, presence of pain with passive motion, ability to actively move joints or digits distal to fracture/cast, and presence or absence of edema. **Rationale:** Compartment syndrome may develop after casting.
2. Observe for signs and symptoms of bleeding under cast. Note the presence and amount of drainage or frank blood or changes in vital signs and/or decreasing hemoglobin and hematocrit, indicative of blood loss. **Rationale:** Bleeding may occur under cast from fracture or operative site and may not be visible externally.
3. Assess for signs and symptoms of infection, including elevated temperature, increasing white blood cell count, foul-smelling drainage, or positive culture results. **Rationale:** Traumatic injuries or suture line may become infected under cast, leading to osteomyelitis.
4. Observe for signs and symptoms of fat emboli, including changing level of consciousness with potential

TABLE 24–3 Guide for Assessment of Peripheral Nerves

Nerve	Sensory Test	Motor Test
Axillary	Ask patient to abduct shoulder.	Prick areas of insertion of deltoid.
Radial	Ask patient to extend wrist and fingers.	Prick area between thumb and forefinger on dorsum.
Median	Ask patient to abduct thumb.	Prick tip of thumb and index and middle fingers on palmar side.
Ulnar	Ask patient to abduct index finger toward thumb.	Prick tip of fifth finger on palmar side of hand.
Peroneal	Ask patient to dorsiflex ankle and extend toes.	Prick lateral surface of great toe and medial surface of second toe.
Tibial	Ask patient to plantar flex ankle and flex toes.	Prick medial and lateral surfaces of sole of foot.

progression to unresponsiveness and comatose state, increased heart rate, tachypnea, increased temperature (usually greater than 100°F [37.8°C]), and petecheae over upper trunk. **Rationale:** Fat emboli are most commonly associated with fractures of long bones, occurring 12 to 36 hours after fracture.

5. Assess for development of pressure sore(s) underneath cast, demonstrated by persistent or intermittent burning (early) deteriorating to markedly decreased or an absence of pain (late). **Rationale:** Pressure sore(s) with the destruction of nerve endings may result from indentations in the cast.

6. Observe for signs and symptoms of cast syndrome, including hypoactive or absent bowel sounds, intake exceeding output, nausea and vomiting, and diminished breath sounds. **Rationale:** Cast syndrome may result from compression of superior mesenteric artery. Respiratory compromise may result from restriction of thoracic cavity in patients with a body cast.

7. Assess nutritional status, including daily caloric intake and nitrogen balance, as evidenced by serum total protein and albumin levels and dietary intake. **Rationale:** Patients with the metabolic stress of bone healing requires additional energy sources.

8. Assess for history of hypo/hyperthyroidism and/or renal calculi. **Rationale:** Preexisting calcium imbalance can affect bone healing.

Nursing Diagnoses

1. Impaired physical mobility related to rigid structure of the cast and consequent limitations. **Rationale:** Immobilization is required for proper bone healing.

2. Knowledge deficit related to self-care of cast. **Rationale:** Unfamiliarity with cast or cognitive limitation from the injury may impair ability to participate in cast care.

3. Potential decreased tissue perfusion of limb related to edema formation and hemorrhage. **Rationale:** Hemorrhage and/or swelling may disrupt arterial blood supply. Edema may impede venous return.

4. Potential for injury related to neurovascular com-

promise. **Rationale:** Undetected neurovascular compromise may be limb-threatening.

5. Potential for impaired skin integrity related to pressure points underneath cast. **Rationale:** Uneven distribution of pressure under cast may lead to tissue necrosis.

6. Potential for infection related to contaminated wounds, sutured limb, or soiled casts. **Rationale:** Warm, moist, dark environment under cast provides medium for microorganisms.

7. Potential decreased gastrointestinal tissue perfusion related to compression of the superior mesenteric artery associated with cast syndrome. **Rationale:** Bending of the superior mesenteric artery may be caused by improper casting.

8. Potential for ineffective breathing patterns related to restricted chest movement. **Rationale:** Patients in a body cast may have feelings of claustrophobia.

9. Potential for impaired gas exchange related to fat emboli. **Rationale:** Hypoxia results from pulmonary insufficiency following fat emboli.

10. Potential for altered nutritional status less than body requirements for bone healing. **Rationale:** Energy requirements are increased during periods of metabolic stress.

Planning

1. Individualize the following goals for the care of the cast:
   a. Maintain tissue perfusion. **Rationale:** Excessive edema formation and/or hemorrhaging may result in neurovascular compromise.
   b. Prevent infection. **Rationale:** Dark, warm environment underneath the cast is conducive to bacterial proliferation.

2. Prepare all necessary positioning equipment for drying the cast. **Rationale:** Decreases unnecessary and potentially painful movements for the patient.
   a. Plastic pillow
   b. Woolen blanket or absorbent towel
   c. For large body casts, circulating fan or hair dryer

3. Prepare all necessary equipment to finish and maintain the cast. **Rationale:** Rough edges of cast encourage skin breakdown.
   a. Stockinette (will be pulled over edges if used under cast for padding)
   b. "Petal" material (tape or moleskin) (Fig. 24–15)
   c. For spica cast or long-leg cast, waterproof material

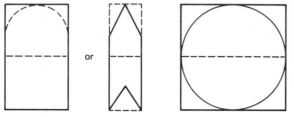

FIGURE 24–15. "Petals" to finish a cast can be made of adhesive tape or moleskin.

d. Cleanser
e. One cast saw

4. Place cast saw at bedside. **Rationale:** Anticipate development of complications. Spica casts need to be removed to perform CPR. Circumferential casts of the extremity may need to be removed rapidly in light of a declining neurovascular status.
5. Prepare the patient.
   a. Explain the procedure and equipment to be used. **Rationale:** Reduces fear.
   b. Explain the desired level of patient's participation and anticipated movements for repositioning and/or manipulation. **Rationale:** Encourages cooperation.
6. Provide pain medication as prescribed in anticipation of repositioning and/or manipulation. **Rationale:** Promotes comfort and facilitates cooperation with the procedure.

Implementation

Steps	Rationale	Special Considerations
Drying The Cast		
1. Elevate casted area on plastic pillow covered with woolen blanket or absorbent towel.	Blanket or towel absorbs moisture. Elevation reduces tissue swelling and prevents cast indentation.	Avoid rubber pillows or rubber sheeting on pillow. Airtight rubber covering on pillow may combine with heat produced with drying, which may cause chemical injury.
2. Always move casted extremity with palms until completely dry.	Fingertips may cause indentations in a wet cast.	
3. Expose cast to room air.	Circulating warm room air is the best method to dry a cast.	
4. Provide adequate warmth for areas of patient not casted.	Casts dry by evaporation, causing the patient to feel cold.	
5. Avoid use of external dryers if possible.	Cast should be allowed to dry from inside out.	Rapid drying may cause cast to crack.
6. Facilitate drying of large body casts, if required. Use any of the following as permitted in hospital:	The drying process may need to be accelerated if patient becomes hypothermic.	
a. Fan to circulate air. Do not blow fan directly on cast.		
b. Hair dryer. Use on low setting only.		
7. Reposition patient or extremity every 2 to 3 hours during drying process.	Facilitates even drying.	
Finishing the Cast		
1. When cast is dry, pull edges of stockinette out over cast, if applicable.	Covers rough edges that may irritate skin.	
2. If edges are not covered with stockinette at time of application, make "petals" to cover rough edges (see Fig. 24–15).	Prevents irritation and abrasion of skin.	Adhesive tape or moleskin may be used. Point of petal is directed toward inside of cast (Fig. 24–16). Wrinkled petals will provide irritation and defeat purpose of finishing.

Table continues on following page

Steps	Rationale	Special Considerations
3. Assist with windowing cast if necessary to observe drainage or suture line or to relieve pressure (Fig. 24–17).	A portion of the cast is removed to observe underlying area.	If window is to be replaced, pad area with equal depth of dressing prior to retaping window.
4. For hip spica cast, protect groin area with waterproof material.	Eliminates possible source of contamination.	

Basic Cast Care

Steps	Rationale	Special Considerations
1. Apply ice to casted area for 48 hours after cast is dry.	Initial application of ice will help decrease edema.	Ensure that ice is placed in waterproof plastic bag to prevent cast from becoming wet.
2. Keep extremity elevated above heart level.	Reduces swelling by increasing venous return.	If compartment syndrome is suspected, do not elevate above heart (see Chap. 26).
3. Label and initial drainage from wounds and/or suture line, if applicable.	Provides baseline for subsequent assessments.	Small amounts of drainage will diffuse through porous material.
4. Provide skin care for exposed areas around cast. Alcohol or small amounts of soap and water may be used as cleansing agent.	Alcohol evaporates while excess water will soften cast.	Alcohol may have a drying effect on skin. Apply lotion as needed.
5. Perform or assist with passive or active ROM exercises to joints distal and proximal to cast every 2 to 4 hours.	Decreases muscle atrophy.	Perform passive ROM if patient is unable to actively exercise.
6. Perform or assist with passive or active ROM exercises in uncasted extremities.	Maintains muscle strength and increases circulation.	Quadricep muscles begin to atrophy within 1 week.
7. Elevate head of bed when placing patient in a spica cast on bedpan.	Minimizes contamination of cast in perineal area.	A fracture bedpan facilitates the procedure.
8. Initiate a referral for nutritional support to ensure adequate dietary intake.	Bone healing may require intake of additional calories, proteins, and vitamins.	
9. Monitor blood calcium levels frequently if patient is on bed rest.	High calcium levels and immobility predispose to renal calculi.	Maintain blood calcium level within normal range (8.5 to 10.5 mg/dl).

Table continues on following page

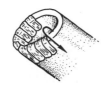

FIGURE 24–16. "Petals" are applied with the point directed into cast. (From S. M. Lewis and I. C. Collier, *Medical-Surgical Nursing*, 3rd. Ed., St. Louis, Mosby Year Book, 1992, p. 1681.)

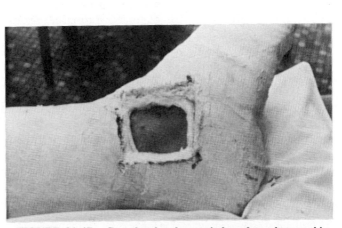

FIGURE 24–17. Cast that has been windowed to observe skin, wound, or incision below. (From J. Farrell, *Illustrated Guide to Orthopedic Nursing*, 3d Ed. Philadelphia: Lippincott, 1986, p. 62, with permission.)

Steps	Rationale	Special Considerations
10. Promote fluid intake up to 3000 ml per day.	Oral or intravenous fluid prevents dehydration and renal complications.	Patients with cast syndrome may have copious nasogastric secretions.
11. Clean plaster cast when soiled with household cleanser (e.g., Comet, Ajax) and damp cloth. Do *not* "waterproof" cast.	Oversaturation may soften cast. A soaked cast may predispose to infection. Covering cast prevents evaporation and may cause excoriation of skin.	A double thickness of plaster of the exact size may be added over soiled area. Fiberglass casts are impervious to water and may be immersed with physician permission. Cast should be dried following immersion to prevent skin excoriation.
12. Refer patient to physical and/or occupational therapist as appropriate.	Working with other health care professionals assists in meeting the patient's rehabilitation needs.	

Evaluation

1. Evaluate the patient's response to the cast. **Rationale:** Occasionally, a patient will experience claustrophobia from encasement in a cast.

2. Evaluate serial neurovascular assessments every hour for 24 hours and every 4 hours thereafter. **Rationale:** Sequential evaluations alert the nurse to progressive compromise, which can occur up to 6 days following the initial trauma.

3. Monitor the patient's skin integrity in areas around the cast. **Rationale:** Meticulous attention to skin care is essential during the entire time the patient is casted to maintain integrity.

4. Report signs and symptoms of fat emboli immediately to the physician. **Rationale:** Fat emboli to the lungs or other vital organs may result in a life-threatening crisis.

5. For patients in a body cast, report signs and symptoms indicative of developing cast syndrome. **Rationale:** Undetected, cast syndrome will progress to a medical emergency.

Expected Outcomes

1. Optimal muscle strength, limited loss of muscle mass, and positive nitrogen balance. **Rationale:** Adequate nutrition and exercise will promote muscle strength.

2. Patient verbalizes comfort with minimal or no complaints of pain. **Rationale:** Pain should decrease as healing takes place.

3. Integrity of cast is maintained. **Rationale:** Proper bone union is dependent on a clean, dry, intact cast.

4. Wounds or surgical incision achieve closure by primary intention. **Rationale:** Aseptic technique and wound care prevent infectious complications.

5. If the patient is primarily bedridden, maintain normal bowel and bladder elimination patterns. **Rationale:** Adequate fluid intake, nutrition, and exercise promote normal patterns.

6. Maintenance of effective breathing patterns (when patient is in a body cast). **Rationale:** A properly applied body cast does not restrict respiratory excursion.

Unexpected Outcomes

1. Nonunion or malunion of affected area. **Rationale:** Inadequate initial reduction and casting, disruption of cast continuity, or presence of infection may lead to malunion of fragments.

2. Osteomyelitis. **Rationale:** Direct infection from a penetrating wound, bacteremia, or infection of wound and/or suture line below cast can lead to osteomyelitis. Indirect seeding can occur from urinary tract infection, dental abscess, etc.

3. Pressure sore(s) under the cast. **Rationale:** Undetected pressure points are present within cast and/or padding is not adequate to protect skin over bony prominences.

4. Cast syndrome. **Rationale:** Most commonly, abdominal portion of spica cast is constrictive.

Documentation

Documentation in the patient record should include date and time of serial neurovascular assessment(s); evaluation of skin integrity, bowel sounds, and presence or absence of bowel movements; respiratory rate; depth and complaints of difficulty breathing; analysis of CBC, which suggests infectious processes or hemorrhaging; evaluation of electrolytes (calcium) or a negative nitrogen balance (total protein and albumin); patient's tolerance of the cast; patient's verbalization of signs and symptoms of neurovascular compromise; and referrals to physical therapy, occupational therapy, or nutritionist. A flow sheet may facilitate comparisons and trending of data. **Rationale:** Documentation provides a basis for communication with other members of health care team and a basis of comparison for future assessment findings.

Patient/Family Education

1. Instruct the patient and family to report immediately the signs and symptoms of neurovascular compromise. **Rationale:** Essential to recognize and report early signs to prevent future complications.

2. Assess the patient's and family's understanding of the nature, purpose, and care of the cast. **Rationale:** Provides the basis for an individualized patient and family education plan.

3. Have the patient and family perform active ROM exercises to unaffected body parts and passive ROM exercises to affected body parts as tolerated. **Rationale:** Helps in maintaining muscle strength and limiting muscle atrophy.

4. Evaluate the anticipated length of confinement with a cast. **Rationale:** Enables the nurse to initiate appropriate referrals should the patient be discharged home with the cast.

Performance Checklist
Skill 24–2: Cast Care

Critical Behaviors	Complies yes	Complies no
DRYING THE CAST		
1. Place casted area on pillow covered with woolen blankets or absorbent towel.		
2. Move cast with palms of hands, *not* fingers.		
3. Expose cast to room air to dry.		
4. Adequately cover body area of patient not involved in cast.		
5. Avoid use of external dryers, if possible.		
6. Facilitate drying of large body casts through the use of a fan or a hair dryer.		
7. Reposition patient or extremity every 2 to 3 hours until cast is completely dry.		
FINISHING THE CAST		
1. Pull stockinette over edges of cast.		
2. Make adhesive or moleskin "petals" if stockinette is not used.		
3. Assist in windowing of cast, if necessary.		
4. Apply waterproof material to groin areas of spica cast.		
BASIC CAST CARE		
1. Apply ice to casted area for 48 hours.		
2. Keep extremity elevated above level of heart.		
3. Correctly label and initial any drainage on cast.		
4. Provide skin care to exposed areas around cast.		
5. Perform passive or active ROM exercises to joints above and below cast.		
6. Perform active or passive ROM exercises to unaffected areas.		
7. Elevate head of bed when placing patient in spica cast on bedpan.		
8. Provide proper nutritional support.		
9. Monitor blood calcium levels.		
10. Promote fluid intake up to 3000 ml per day.		
11. Clean cast if soiled.		
12. Refer patient to physical or occupational therapy.		
13. Document all interventions in patient record.		

SKILL 24–3

Cast Removal

Cast removal is performed when proper healing of the affected part has been achieved, as evidenced by x-ray, when complications arise (i.e., foul-smelling odor arising from cast), or in the event that further treatments are necessary (i.e., open reduction with internal fixation). It is a safe and simple procedure, since it is the vibration of the blade that bivalves the cast, not the cutting action.

Once the cast has been removed, patient and family education is necessary to prevent potential refracture or dislocation of the affected part.

Purpose

The nurse assists with cast removal to

1. Facilitate removal of the cast.
2. Provide emotional support to the patient.

Prerequisite Knowledge and Skills

Prior to assisting with cast removal, the nurse should understand

1. Anatomy and physiology of the affected body part.
2. Physiology of bone healing.
3. Complications of casting.
4. Proper body mechanics to avoid injury to patient or self during cast removal.

The nurse should be able to perform

1. Neurovascular assessment.
2. Proper handwashing technique (see Skill 35–5).
3. Proper waste disposal of items in contact with bodily fluids or secretions.

Assessment

1. Assess the patient's neurovascular status, including color, temperature, capillary refill, pulse(s), movement of body part(s) distal to site of fracture or deformity, sensation(s), and presence or absence of edema. **Rationale:** Provides baseline data for evaluation after removal.
2 Verify adequate bone union, as evidenced by radiographic films. **Rationale:** Bone union takes approximately 6 to 12 weeks.

Nursing Diagnoses

1. Fear related to use of cast cutter for removal of cast. **Rationale:** Patients are often fearful of being lacerated by cast cutter.
2. Knowledge deficit related to equipment and procedure for cast removal. **Rationale:** Lack of patient education about procedure and equipment prior to removal of cast results in deficit.
3. Potential for injury related to decreased muscle strength, atrophy, instability of the joint in the affected part, and/or lack of knowledge of activity restrictions. **Rationale:** Proper and adequate education aids in physical activities within the patient's tolerance and endurance.
4. Impaired physical mobility related to decreased muscle strength and potential instability of the joint(s) in the affected body part. **Rationale:** Patient may be reluctant to resume motion of the extremity for fear of reinjury.

5. Potential body-image disturbance related to muscle atrophy of the affected body part. **Rationale:** Muscle atrophy may make affected body part appear smaller than unaffected part(s).

Planning

1. Individualize the following goals for cast removal:
   a. Patient's fears regarding cast removal will be alleviated. **Rationale:** This is a new and unfamiliar experience for most patients.
   b. Prevent refracture or dislocation. **Rationale:** Decreased muscle mass results in diminished support to the bony union and/or joint.
2. Prepare all necessary equipment and supplies. **Rationale:** Ensures that procedure will be completed efficiently.
   a. X-ray film taken immediately prior to cast removal.
   b. One cast cutter (Fig. 24–18).
   c. One cast spreader (Fig. 24–19).
   d. One pair of bandage scissors.
   e. Appropriate supportive device(s), such as a brace, splint, elastic stocking, or Ace bandage (Fig. 24–20).
   f. Skin emollient, such as skin oil, creams, or lotions.
   g. Cast cart, if available.
3. Prepare the patient.
   a. Explain the procedure and the equipment to the patient. **Rationale:** Reduces apprehension and enlists the patient's cooperation, which will facilitate the process.
   b. Assist the patient in assuming a position that is comfortable yet facilitates the procedure for the patient, nurse, and physician. **Rationale:** Provides for patient's comfort and efficient cast removal.
4. Ensure that cast cutter has been approved for use by biomedical engineering department. **Rationale:** Proper seeding of blade on cast ensures patient safety.

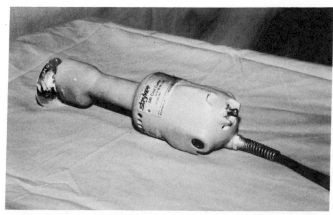

FIGURE 24–18. Electric cast cutter used for removal of plaster cast.

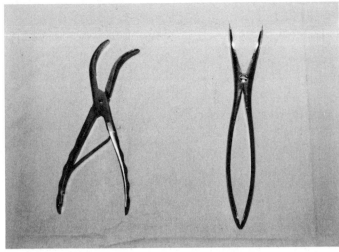

FIGURE 24–19. Two types of cast spreaders for ease of cast removal.

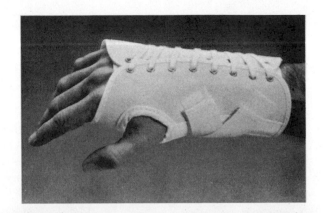

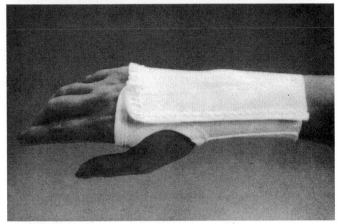

FIGURE 24–20. Two types of splints may be applied to the upper extremity after cast removal for support. Ace bandages are commonly used following removal of lower extremity cast. (Courtesy of Smith & Nephew Rolyan Inc.)

Implementation

Steps	Rationale	Special Considerations
1. Wash hands.	Reduces transmission of microorganisms.	
2. Assist in bivalving the cast with the saw cutter by stabilizing the cutter with one thumb resting on the cast. Support the patient's position while the cast is bivalved with the cast cutter.	Stabilizing the cutter provides even pressure and prevents undue injury to the patient.	Ensure that the cutter does not touch skin after the cutter cuts through the cast.
3. Separate the cast edges with a cast spreader.	Facilitates easy removal of cast.	
4. Cut the padding using scissors.	Facilitates easy removal of padding.	
5. Gently remove the cast, removing the anterior portion, followed by the posterior portion. Ensure that the joints of the extremity are well supported.	Facilitates removal of the cast without damaging the affected part. Prevents undue pain and muscle spasm.	Muscles of the affected part may be weak and unstable.
6. Assess the condition of the affected part. Note the skin integrity, the color of the skin, and degree of muscle strength and atrophy.	For early detection and prevention of complications, as well as baseline data.	

Table continues on following page

Steps	Rationale	Special Considerations
7. Clean the skin carefully with soap without removing the dead skin. Gently pat dry the casted area. Do *not* rub with towel.	Provides comfort and prevents abrasion from forceful removal of dead skin.	
8. Apply skin emollients following cleansing prior to application of supportive devices.	Provides comfort and prevents irritation from supportive devices.	
9. Assist in the application of supportive devices as prescribed.	For support of weak muscles and unstable joints in the affected part.	
10. Wash hands.	Reduces transmission of microorganisms.	

Evaluation

1. Monitor the patient's neurovascular status every 8 hours following removal of the cast. **Rationale:** Supportive devices can compromise tissue perfusion. Neurovascular deficit also may indicate reinjury.

2. Monitor the skin integrity of the casted area. **Rationale:** Establishes a baseline for early detection and prevention of complications.

3. Monitor the stability of the joints and muscle strength of the affected part. **Rationale:** Prevents potential injury as well as anticipates the need for a supportive device.

Expected Outcomes

1. Neurovascular assessment of the affected part with supportive device remains consistent with the baseline established upon cast removal. **Rationale:** Improperly applied device may cause pressure on the neurovascular structure. Neurovascular deficits also may indicate reinjury.

2. Skin integrity in the casted area is intact. **Rationale:** It is possible for the skin to be lacerated with the cast cutter upon cast removal.

3. Union of the affected bone is maintained after removal of the cast. **Rationale:** Patient and family education is necessary with regard to activity restrictions, proper exercise, and use of supportive device(s) to prevent reinjury.

4. Successful coping with the appearance of the affected extremity. **Rationale:** Muscle strength and appearance of the affected part will return to preinjury status with proper exercise.

5. Full range of motion of the affected part. **Rationale:** Correct alignment and successful union of the affected part in conjunction with an aggressive exercise program will result in full range of motion.

Unexpected Outcomes

1. Compromised tissue perfusion of the affected part. **Rationale:** Most commonly associated with improper application of the supportive devices that causes pressure on neurovascular bundle.

2. Decreasing physical mobility associated with increasing edema formation and complaints of pain. **Rationale:** Increasing edema and complaints of pain are suggestive of malalignment or nonunion of the affected part.

Documentation

Documentation in the patient record should include date and time of the procedure, name of the individual removing the cast, patient's tolerance of procedure, baseline neurovascular assessment, condition of the casted area's skin, baseline assessment of joint stability, muscle strength and degree of muscle atrophy, response to patient and family education, and any unexpected outcomes and interventions taken. **Rationale:** Documents nursing care given, expected and unexpected outcomes, and interventions taken.

Patient/Family Education

1. Discuss the expected outcomes after cast removal with the patient and family, including mild dependent edema, fragility and brittleness of the bone in the affected part(s), scaly, soft, slightly discolored skin in the casted area with sloughing of the epidermis, decreased muscle strength and presence of muscle atrophy, and instability of joints. **Rationale:** To prevent potential refracture or dislocation of the affected part, to decrease anxiety and patient's fear, and to support successful coping with an altered body image.

2. Instruct the patient to notify the health care professional immediately with the onset of severe pain and/or extensive swelling of the affected part. **Rationale:** May indicate early signs of complications, refracture, or dislocation.

3. Emphasize the importance of maintaining the exercise program. **Rationale:** Builds muscle strength and mass and contributes to the prevention of reinjury.

Performance Checklist
Skill 24–3: Cast Removal

Critical Behaviors	Complies	
	yes	no
1. Wash hands.		
2. Maintain patient position while assisting in bivalving of cast.		
3. Separate the cast edges with a cast spreader.		
4. Cut the padding using scissors.		
5. Gently remove the cast.		
6. Assess the condition of the affected part.		
7. Clean the skin carefully.		
8. Apply lotions, creams, or emollients to skin.		
9. Assist with the application of the supportive device(s) as needed.		
10. Wash hands.		
11. Document in the patient record.		

BIBLIOGRAPHY

Caine, R. M., and Bufalino, P. M. (1987). *Nursing Care Planning Guide for Adults*. Baltimore: Williams & Wilkins.

Cardona, V. D., Hurn, P. D., Bastnagel-Mason, P. J., et al. (1988). *Trauma Nursing from Resuscitation through Rehabilitation*. Philadelphia: Saunders.

Corkery, E. (1989). Discharge planning and home health care: What every staff nurse should know. *Orthop. Nurs.* 8(6):18–26.

Duncan, H. A. (1989). *Duncan's Dictionary for Nurses*, 2d Ed. New York: Springer.

Farrell, J. (1986). *Illustrated Guide to Orthopedic Nursing*, 3d Ed. Philadelphia: Lippincott.

Gates, S. J., and Mooar, P. A. (1989). *Orthopaedics and Sports Medicine for Nurses*. Baltimore: Williams & Wilkins.

Mourad, L. A. (1988). *The Nursing Process in the Care of the Adult with Orthopaedic Conditions*, 2d Ed. New York: Wiley.

Pellino, T. A., Mooney, N. E., Salmond, S. W., and Verdisco, L. A. (1986). *Core Curriculum for Orthopaedic Nursing*. Pittman, N.J.: Janetti.

Perry, A. G., and Potter, P. A. (1986). *Clinical Nursing Skills and Techniques: Basic, Intermediate, Advanced*. St. Louis: Mosby.

Riley, M. K., and Beltran, M. J. (1986). *Clinical Nursing Interventions with Critical Elements*. New York: Wiley.

Schoen, D. C. (1986). *The Nursing Process in Orthopedics*. Norwalk, Conn.: Appleton-Century-Crofts.

Stewart, J. D. M., and Hallett, J. P. (1988). *Traction and Orthopaedic Appliances*, 2d Ed. New York: Churchill-Livingstone.

25

TRACTION

BEHAVIORAL OBJECTIVES

After completing this chapter, the nurse will be able to

- Define the key terms.
- Discuss the mechanics of traction.
- Describe the types and indications of tractions frequently used.
- Identify the complications of traction.
- Demonstrate the skills involved in the use of traction.

Traction exerts a pulling force on a body part by overcoming the effects of muscle tone and gravity or the mechanical forces that caused the fracture. The constant pulling or drawing can be achieved manually or with a mechanical device to reduce a fracture and realign bone fragments until calcification occurs, reduce and treat a dislocation of a joint or pelvis, prevent the development of contractures or lessen the deformity, relieve and reduce pain and muscle spasm, immobilize and rest a limb in its optimal functional position, preventing further nerve and tissue damage, and promote bone and soft-tissue healing.

Traction may be applied to an upper or lower limb by means of skeletal traction and skin traction or to other body parts, such as the spine or pelvis. The kind of traction used depends on the type and location of the fracture or disorder and the physician's preference. With skin traction, force is applied through the skin, whereas in skeletal traction, force is applied via the bones.

KEY TERMS

alignment
arthrodesis
blister
Buck's traction
callus
cancellous bone
claustrophobia
contraction
countertraction
embolism
fat embolism
femoral condyles
femur
fracture

humerus
immobilize
Kirschner wire
malleoli
neurovascular check
osteomyelitis
osteotomy
reduce/reduction
spasm
stabilization
Steinmann pin
threaded pin(s)
traction
union

SKILLS

25–1   Skin Traction
25–2   Balanced Suspension Skeletal Traction
25–3   External Fixation Traction

GUIDELINES

The following assessment guidelines assist the nurse in formulating nursing diagnoses and an individualized plan of care for a patient in traction.

1.   Know the patient's medical history, the mechanism and type of injury, and the purpose and indication for traction.
2.   Know the patient's nutritional status for its impact on wound healing.
3.   Know the patient's neurovascular status and current range of motion in the joints proximal and distal to the affected body part.
4.   Know the results of the physical examination and diagnostic tests performed before and after application of traction.
5.   Determine appropriate nursing interventions based on assessment findings.
6.   Become adept with supplies and equipment utilized in traction.

SKILL 25–1

Skin Traction

Skin traction is the application of any commercial skin traction strips/tape or other skin traction devices such as a pelvic belt, boot, or halter directly to the patient's skin. Skin traction is applied intermittently over a period of time to relieve muscle spasm and pain caused by pressure on the nerves surrounding an injury. In the event of a fracture, skin traction is used for immobilization of the affected body part prior to definitive management of the injury.

Certain considerations should be kept in mind when applying skin traction. Skin traction is never applied over an open wound. The patient should be observed for potential allergic reaction to the commercial skin traction strips/tape. Pressure on the bony prominence of the affected body part must be avoided, especially over the iliac crests with pelvic traction. Different types of skin traction are discussed in Table 25–1, and shown in Figs. 25–1 and 25–2.

TABLE 25–1 Skin Traction

Type of Traction	Description	Indications	Special Considerations
Buck's extension traction (see Fig. 25–1)	The patient is supine. Traction is affixed to the affected extremity/limb and is attached to weights and pulleys, allowing force to be in one direction.	Used preoperatively to maintain immobility for a hip fracture or subtrochanteric fracture of the femur.	May be removed for neurovascular and skin assessment. Soap and water are used for skin care. Patient may be turned to unaffected side, keeping affected extremity in abduction.
Pelvic traction (see Fig. 25–2)	Pelvic belt is applied around the pelvis and is hooked to a wide spreader bar. The belt has long straps attached to the foot of the bed with ropes, pulleys, and weights. Both knees and hips should be flexed to minimize pressure on the lumbar spine, which can cause a considerable increase in pain.	Used most often to relieve muscle spasms of the lower back and to reduce pressure on spinal nerve roots after a herniated or ruptured disk and with pelvic fractures.	For maximum effectiveness, the patient lies quietly in bed to stabilize the pelvis, decreasing irritation of the injured nerves or muscles and relieving pain and inflammation. Patient may be log-rolled with bed flattened if traction must be continuous. A fracture bedpan should be used if lifting is difficult. The area over the iliac crest may be the first to experience irritation, since the belt is applied directly over the skin. Constipation will add to the discomfort of the patient in pelvic traction for low back pain; measures should be taken to prevent constipation.

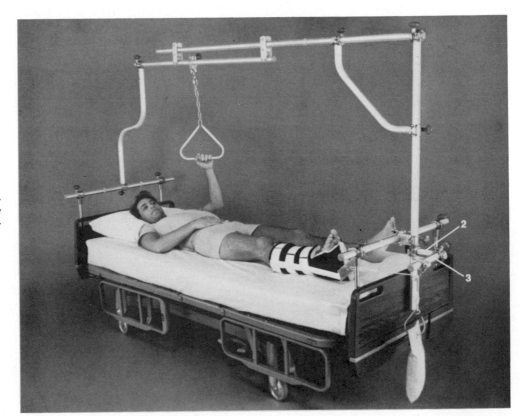

FIGURE 25–1. Buck's extension traction. (With permission, *The Traction Handbook,* **6th Ed. Warsaw, Ind.: Zimmer, 1989, p. 27.)**

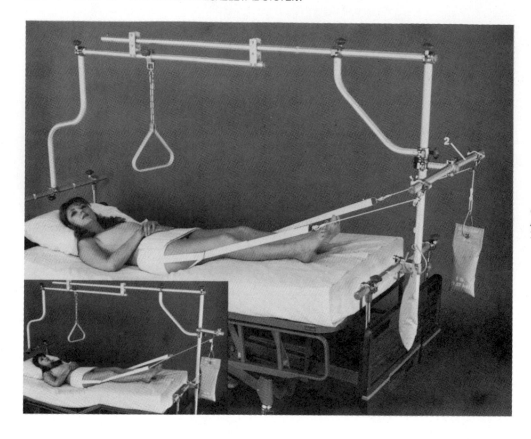

FIGURE 25–2. Pelvic traction. (With permission, *The Traction Handbook*, 6th Ed. Warsaw, Ind.: Zimmer, 1989, p. 25.)

Purpose

The nurse assists with the establishment and maintenance of skin traction to

1. Maintain proper alignment of body part(s).
2. Immobilize the extremity.
3. Relieve muscle spasm and reduce pain.
4. Prevent joint contractures.
5. Maintain skin integrity while in traction.

Prerequisite Knowledge and Skills

Prior to the application of skin traction, the nurse should understand

1. Anatomy and physiology of the affected body part.
2. Proper alignment of affected body part.
3. Physiology of bone healing.
4. Principles of skin traction.
5. Proper body mechanics.
6. Effects of immobilization on the patient.

The nurse should be able to perform

1. Proper handwashing technique (see Skill 35–5).
2. Neurovascular assessment.
3. Range-of-motion exercises.
4. Proper skin care with soap and water.
5. Proper body mechanics.

Assessment

1. Assess the skin integrity of the area to be placed in skin traction. **Rationale:** Provides baseline data and determines the ability of the skin to tolerate traction.
2. Review the patient's radiographic studies to assess the alignment of the bone fragments. **Rationale:** Verifies fracture prior to reduction.
3. Assess neurovascular status of the affected body part(s), including pain (note location, pattern, and duration), pallor (note presence or absence of cyanosis, mottling, and erythema), paresthesia (note any reports of numbness, tingling, or lack of sensation), pulselessness (i.e., decrease in the quality of the pulse distal to the injury), and paralysis (i.e., absence of mobility of joints distal to the injury). Assessment findings should be compared with the findings on the unaffected side or body part. **Rationale:** Provides baseline data for detection of complications, including redness, numbness, tingling sensation, increased pain, muscle spasm, or compartment syndrome (see Chap. 26).
4. Assess the patient for signs and symptoms of pulmonary/fat emboli (i.e., rate and depth of respiration, presence or absence of cough, sputum production, changes in sensorium, presence of petechial rash over chest and neck, tachycardia, and decreased blood pressure. **Rationale:** Fat emboli are most commonly associated with fractures of the long bones. Transient petechial rash occurs in 5–10% of patients with fat emboli.
5. Assess the severity of the patient's pain. **Rationale:** Provides baseline data and determines the effectiveness of traction to relieve muscle spasm.
6. Assess the patient's nutritional status, including caloric intake, protein balance, vitamins A, D, and C, calcium, phosphorus, and magnesium. **Rationale:** Sup-

plying adequate nutrients optimizes the anabolism necessary for repair and growth of bone and soft tissue in order to prevent delayed union or nonunion of the fracture.

7. Assess the patient's ability to do active or passive ROM exercises on the unaffected extremity. **Rationale:** Maintains muscle tone and strength in the unaffected extremities.

Nursing Diagnoses

1. Impaired physical mobility related to musculoskeletal injury and/or skin traction. **Rationale:** Continuous immobilization and maintenance of proper alignment of bone fragments are required with skin traction.

2. Pain related to muscle spasm or musculoskeletal injury. **Rationale:** Traction helps restore function, thus relieving muscle spasm/contraction. Pain also may be an indication of impending neurovascular compromise.

3. Fear related to unfamiliarity with skin traction. **Rationale:** Most patients have not seen or had experience with traction equipment and setup.

4. Potential for injury related to neurovascular compromise. **Rationale:** Malalignment of bones and/or skin traction that is too tight may lead to occlusion of the arterial blood supply and impairment of venous return, leading to compartmental syndrome.

5. Potential for impaired skin integrity related to pressure points and blister formation. **Rationale:** Skin attachment requires adhesive application to the skin to provide traction.

Planning

1. Individualize the following goals for using skin traction:
   a. Immobilize and maintain realignment of the af-

fected body part(s). **Rationale:** Continuous immobilization and maintenance of proper alignment of bone fragments are required for adequate bone healing.
   b. Maintain skin integrity. **Rationale:** Intact skin prevents potential for infection.
   c. Maintain neurovascular integrity. **Rationale:** Prevents pressure on neurovascular bundle.
   d. Promote patient comfort. **Rationale:** Fear, injury to soft tissues surrounding the fractured bone, and impending neurovascular compromise contribute to a patient's pain.

2. Prepare the patient.
   a. Explain the procedure to the patient. **Rationale:** Reduces anxiety and encourages cooperation.
   b. Explain the patient's participation. **Rationale:** Refocuses patient's attention, reduces fear, and encourages compliance with activity restrictions.
   c. Discuss the patient's positioning during and after the application of skin traction. **Rationale:** Eliminates or decreases fear.

3. Prepare and assemble all the necessary equipment and supplies for skin traction. **Rationale:** Ensures that application of skin traction will be completed quickly and efficiently.
   a. Velcro boots/straps for Buck's traction.
   b. Pelvic strap/belt for pelvic traction.
   c. Bed frame for attachment of traction.
   d. Ropes, weights, pulleys, and weight holder.
   e. Heel protectors.
   f. Spreader bars.
   g. Foot support.
   h. Padding (i.e., sheepskin, of appropriate size).

4. Measure patient's girth at the crest of the ilium. **Rationale:** Ensures correct size of pelvic belt. Prevents skin irritation caused by friction.

Implementation

Steps	Rationale	Special Considerations
1. Wash hands.	Reduces transmission of microorganisms.	
2. Assist with positioning the affected body part as requested by the physician while the pelvic belts (pelvic traction), adhesive strips, padding over the bony prominences, elastic bandages, and foot support are applied.	Provides stability to prevent movement that could result in additional trauma.	Velcro boots can serve as foot support in preventing peroneal palsy (foot drop). For the patient who is unable to do active ROM, high-top sneakers may be used. Lower portion of pelvic belt should be at or slightly below the greater trochanter (see Fig. 25–2).
3. Assist as requested with attachment of spreader bar, ropes, pulleys, and weights as prescribed.	Ensures proper alignment of the bone fragments/body part(s).	Trapeze facilitates care, helps patient help himself or herself, and enables the patient to be more active. Spreader bar is used to maintain a steady pull of the affected body part and to ensure distribution of traction weight.
4. Wash hands.	Reduces transmission of microorganisms.	

Evaluation

1. Monitor the patient's neurovascular status (the 5 P's) every 1 to 2 hours until stabilized and then every 4 hours. **Rationale:** Early detection of neurovascular compromise prevents complications.

2. Monitor the entire setup and functioning of skin traction every 8 hours. Check that the prescribed weights are hanging freely, knots are secured, ropes are in pulleys, and position of affected body part is correct. **Rationale:** Prevents potential injury and ensures that traction and countertraction are maintained.

3. Evaluate the patient for skin irritation and/or development of blisters every 4 hours. **Rationale:** Prevents complications of impaired skin integrity.

4. Evaluate the patient's comfort level. **Rationale:** Pain may be a symptom of skin irritation, friction from the skin apparatus, and/or improper functioning of traction.

5. Perform passive ROM exercise to joints distal and proximal to affected extremity or body part. Ensure that a patient consultation is initiated with a physical therapist. **Rationale:** Exercise promotes circulation and maintains muscle strength of the affected extremity, thus preventing contracture formation.

6. Evaluate nutritional status for adequate intake to promote bone healing (i.e., vitamins A, D, and C, calcium, phosphorus, magnesium, and proteins). **Rationale:** Supplying adequate nutrients optimizes the anabolism necessary for repair and growth of bone and soft tissues to prevent delayed union and/or nonunion of fractures and to minimize catabolism secondary to trauma.

Expected Outcomes

1. Proper alignment of body part. **Rationale:** Supports union of fractured bone.

2. Relief of muscle spasm/pain. **Rationale:** Functioning traction maintains alignment of bone fragments by countertraction, thus relieving muscle spasm/pain until definitive treatment can be instituted.

3. Patient comfort with minimal or no complaints of pain. **Rationale:** Proper alignment of bone fragments and a functioning traction relieve muscle spasm.

4. Maintenance of skin integrity. **Rationale:** Skin attachment requires adhesion to the skin to provide traction, putting the patient at high risk for skin breakdown.

5. Maintenance of normal bowel elimination pattern. **Rationale:** Immobilization decreases peristalsis.

6. Full range of motion in distal and proximal joints. **Rationale:** Prevents formation of contractures.

7. Adequate tissue perfusion. **Rationale:** Proper application of skin traction decreases or prevents injury to the neurovascular bundle.

Unexpected Outcomes

1. Neurovascular compromise. **Rationale:** Most commonly associated with improper application of traction that causes pressure on the neurovascular bundle. Deep vein thrombosis occurs with prolonged immobilization.

2. Progressive edema formation with complaints of pain. **Rationale:** Edema and increasing pain are suggestive of malalignment or nonunion of the affected part.

3. Pressure sores/blister formation. **Rationale:** Improper application of adhesive strips or elastic bandages or poor skin care may cause impaired skin integrity.

4. Fat embolism. **Rationale:** Risk of fat embolism 24 to 72 hours following long-bone fracture can be minimized by immobilization of the fracture site.

5. Joint contracture. **Rationale:** Lack of ROM exercises and malpositioning of the affected extremity contribute to joint contracture formation.

Documentation

Documentation in the patient record should include the date and time of the procedure, the type of traction, the name and title of the person applying the traction, the amount of weight used, alignment of the extremity involved, the patient's response to the procedure, serial neurovascular assessments, skin integrity of the affected extremity, evaluation of traction setup, ROM exercises performed and patient's tolerance thereof, bowel and bladder patterns, patient's comfort/pain level, the severity and frequency of pain manifested by the patient, the patient's response to narcotic and muscle relaxants, and any unexpected outcomes encountered and actions taken. **Rationale:** Documents patient's status, effectiveness of traction, and nursing care given.

Patient/Family Education

1. Discuss the nature of the equipment and the purpose of skin traction with both patient and family. **Rationale:** Eases anxiety.

2. Patient's family should not release weights from the skin traction to the affected extremity unless otherwise instructed. **Rationale:** Releasing the weights from the traction causes muscle contraction, which in turn can malalign the fracture and damage the surrounding nerves and vessels.

3. Instruct the patient and family to report signs and symptoms of increased pain, muscle spasm, numbness, tingling sensation, and/or change in temperature of extremity. **Rationale:** May herald the need for immediate intervention.

4. Have the patient and family perform active ROM exercises to the unaffected extremity and passive ROM exercises to the affected body part(s) as tolerated. **Rationale:** Maintains muscle strength and discourages muscle atrophy.

5. Instruct the patient and family to maintain activities of daily living as appropriate, and provide diversional activities while the patient is in traction. **Rationale:** Immobilization in skin traction for a period of time may cause the patient to experience a sense of claustrophobia and boredom.

Performance Checklist
Skill 25–1:   Skin Traction

Critical Behaviors	Complies yes	no
1. Wash hands.		
2. Ensure proper alignment of affected extremity during application of skin traction.		
3. Assist with attachment of the ropes, pulleys, prescribed weights, and weight holder.		
4. Wash hands.		
5. Document the procedure in the patient record.		

SKILL 25–2

Balanced Suspension Skeletal Traction

Skeletal traction is a common treatment for fractures of the long bones or for correction of orthopedic abnormalities. It is applied to immobilize and maintain alignment of a fractured bone, reduce the fracture, and overcome muscle spasm, thus promoting bone healing. Skeletal traction's pulling force is exerted directly to the bone using pins (Steinmann), wires (Kirschner), and screws. The sites chosen for pin or wire insertion are usually areas of strong cancellous bone.

Once initiated, traction must be continuously maintained. Lifting or releasing the weights can cause muscle contraction, which in turn can disrupt the fracture alignment, damaging the surrounding nerves and vasculature. Skeletal traction remains in place over a period of time, depending on the severity of the defect and factors that influence bone healing, such as type of bone, patient's age, nutritional status, inadequate fixation, infection, disturbance of blood supply, and metabolic disease.

Examples of skeletal traction seen in the critical-care setting, their descriptions, and their indications are listed in Table 25–2, and shown in Figs. 25–3 to 25–6.

Purpose

The nurse assists with the establishment and maintenance of skeletal traction to

1. Maintain proper bone alignment until calcification occurs.
2. Prevent joint contractures.
3. Immobilize the affected extremity to prevent further injury to the surrounding nerves, tissue, and vasculature.
4. Ensure the comfort and safety of the patient while in skeletal traction.

Prerequisite Knowledge and Skills

Prior to assisting with the establishment of the balanced suspension skeletal traction, the nurse should understand

1. Anatomy and physiology of the affected extremity.
2. Physiology of bone healing.
3. Principles of balanced suspension skeletal traction.
4. Proper alignment of the affected extremity.
5. Principles of aseptic technique.
6. Principles of body mechanics.
7. Effects of immobilization on the patient.

The nurse should be able to perform

1. Proper handwashing technique (see Skill 35–5).
2. Proper body mechanics.
3. Neurovascular assessment.
4. Sterile field setup.
5. Passive ROM exercises on joints distal to the affected area.

Assessment

1. Perform a neurovascular assessment (the 5 P's) of the affected extremity, including pain (note location, pattern, and duration), pallor (note presence or absence of cyanosis, mottling, and erythema), paresthesia (note any reports of numbness, tingling, or lack of sensation), pulselessness (i.e., decrease in the quality of the pulse distal to the injury), and paralysis (i.e., absence of mobility of joints distal to the injury). Compare assessment findings with those of the unaffected side. **Rationale:** Provides baseline data necessary to trend ongoing assessment findings.

2. Assess the integrity of skin surrounding the body part to be placed in skeletal traction. **Rationale:** Skin and/or soft-tissue damage around pin insertion site are a portal of entry for microorganisms into the bone, leading to osteomyelitis.

3. Assess the patient's nutritional status, including caloric intake, protein, vitamins A, D, and C, calcium, phosphorus, and magnesium. **Rationale:** Supplying adequate nutrients optimizes the anabolism necessary for repair and growth of bone and soft tissue to prevent delayed union and/or nonunion of fractures.

4. Assess the patient's ability to do active ROM exercises on the unaffected extremity and passive ROM exercises on joints distal to the site of injury. **Rationale:** Provide baseline data for prevention of contracture formation.

TABLE 25–2 Skeletal Traction

Type of Traction	Description	Indications	Special Considerations
Balanced suspension skeletal traction to the femur (see Fig. 25–3).	Foot of the bed elevated with patient flat on his or her back. Steinmann pins are used to achieve the skeletal traction. A Thomas splint (see Fig. 25–4) is usually used, with a Pearson attachment (see Fig. 25–5) to convert the splint to balanced suspension.	Used in the treatment of fractures of the femoral shaft, hip, and lower leg.	Countertraction is achieved by using the patient's body weight. Position patient supine with the affected leg in sling abduction and no rotation, toes straight up toward the ceiling. Ensure that hip flexion between the bed and the thigh does not exceed 20 degrees, except for meals and activities of daily living, to prevent the possibility of developing hip flexion contracture and pressure sores.
Dunlop's skeletal traction (see Fig. 25–6)	The upper arm is abducted 45 degrees, and the elbow is flexed 45 degrees. Position of the forearm is maintained by using a Buck's extension, a type of skin traction to prevent muscle spasm. Humeral counterweight is achieved by inserting a Kirschner wire through the distal humerus with spreader bow and weights attached.	Used in the treatment of fractures of the distal humerus.	Buck's extension (skin traction) is used to forearm, which helps maintain the position of the forearm while the Steinmann pin/ Kirschner wire is being inserted.

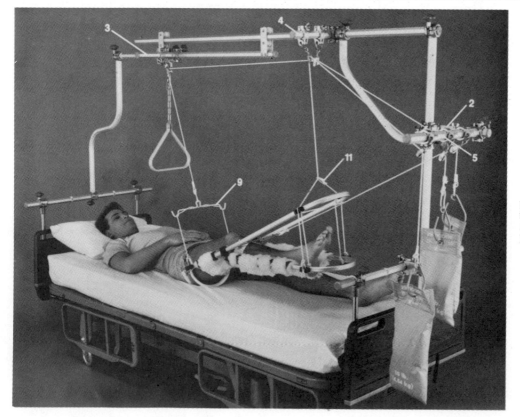

FIGURE 25–3. Balanced suspension skeletal traction to the femur. (With permission, *The Traction Handbook*, 6th Ed. Warsaw, Ind.: Zimmer, 1989, p. 37.)

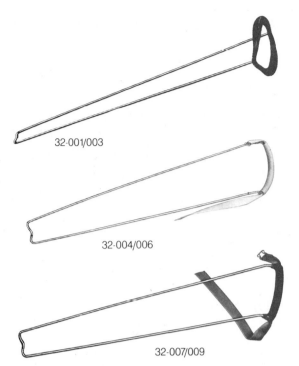

32-001/003

32-004/006

32-007/009

FIGURE 25–4. Thomas leg splint. (With permission, *The Traction Handbook*, 6th Ed. Warsaw, Ind.: Zimmer, 1989, p. 50.)

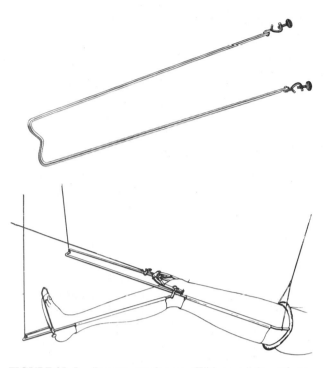

FIGURE 25–5. Pearson attachment. (With permission, *The Traction Handbook*, 6th Ed. Warsaw, Ind.: Zimmer, 1989, p. 51.)

FIGURE 25–6. Dunlop's skeletal traction. (With permission, *The Traction Handbook*, 6th Ed. Warsaw, Ind.: Zimmer, 1989, p. 21.)

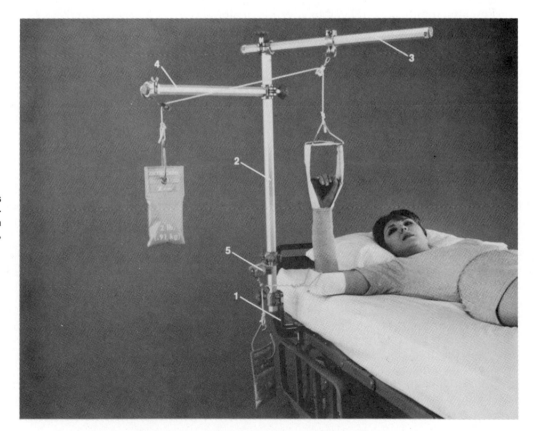

Nursing Diagnoses

1. Impaired physical mobility related to application of balanced suspension skeletal traction to the affected extremity. **Rationale:** Proper alignment and reduction of fracture fragments are dependent on continuous application of traction.

2. Fear related to unfamiliarity with balanced suspension skeletal traction. **Rationale:** Most patients have not seen or had experience with traction equipment and setup.

3. Pain related to musculoskeletal injury, muscle spasm, and/or tension from skeletal traction. **Rationale:** Injury to soft tissues surrounding the fractured bone results in muscle contraction, which can be very painful; pain also may be an indication of impending neurovascular compromise.

4. Impaired skin integrity related to insertion of Steinmann or threaded pins directly into the bone or mechanism of injury, i.e., open fracture. **Rationale:** Pin insertion or an open fracture disrupts the skin integrity and provides a portal of entry for microorganisms, which may lead to osteomyelitis.

5. Potential for injury related to neurovascular compromise. **Rationale:** Disruption of skeletal traction or improper alignment or reduction of fractured bone may cause occlusion of the arterial blood supply and impair venous return.

6. Potential for decreased tissue perfusion of the limb related to neurovascular compromise. **Rationale:** Malalignment of bone fragments may lead to occlusion of the arterial blood supply and/or impairment of venous return, leading to compartment syndrome.

7. Potential for infection related to insertion of Steinmann or threaded pins or Kirschner wires directly into the bone. **Rationale:** The pins and/or wires disrupt skin integrity and provide a portal of entry for microorganisms, which may lead to osteomyelitis.

Planning

1. Individualize the following goals for using balanced suspension skeletal traction:
   a. Maintain proper alignment of bone fragments. **Rationale:** Overcomes muscle spasms, reduces the fracture, and promotes bone healing.
   b. Maintain neurovascular integrity. **Rationale:** Malalignment, disruption of traction, and edema formation may cause neurovascular compromise.
   c. Prevent infection in the presence of impaired skin integrity. **Rationale:** The development of osteomyelitis is a serious complication with potentially long-term sequelae.
   d. Maintain range of motion in the joints proximal and distal to the injury site. **Rationale:** Active/passive range of motion maintains muscle tone and strength, thus decreasing the possibility of joint contractures.

e. Promote patient comfort. **Rationale:** Fear, soft-tissue injury, and/or impending neurovascular compromise contribute to patient's pain.

2. Administer pain medication as prescribed 20 to 30 minutes prior to establishing skeletal traction to the affected extremity. **Rationale:** Extensive manipulation of the affected limb can be quite painful.

3. Prepare and assemble all the necessary equipment and supplies for setting up the skeletal traction. **Rationale:** Ensures that application of traction to the affected extremity will be completed quickly and efficiently.
   a. Equipment for insertion of a Steinmann pin or Kirschner wire:
      (1) Hand drill.
      (2) One Kirschner spreader bar.
      (3) One scalpel with no 11 or no 15 blade.
      (4) Four sterile towels/drapes.
      (5) Two povidone-iodine prep sticks.
      (6) Lidocaine 1% solution, 30-cc vial.
      (7) One 10-cc syringe and one 22-gauge 1½-in needle and one 25-gauge ⅝-in needle.
      (8) One pair of sterile gloves.
      (9) Two packs of 4 × 4 sterile gauze pads.
      (10) One small packet of povidone-iodine ointment.
      Note: All these items may be found in a prepackaged sterile Steinmann pin/Kirschner wire tray.
   b. Equipment for skeletal traction:
      (1) Overhead frame for attachment of traction.
      (2) Ropes, weights, pulleys, and weight holder (weights vary from 1 to 5 lbs).
      (3) Heel protectors.
      (4) One or two 4-in elastic bandages.
      (5) Pearson attachment, padded.
      (6) Thomas splint.
      (7) Foot support.

4. Prepare the patient.
   a. Explain the procedure to the patient. **Rationale:** Reduces anxiety and encourages cooperation.
   b. Explain the patient's participation. **Rationale:** Refocuses patient's attention, reduces fear, and encourages compliance with activity restrictions.
   c. Discuss with the patient positioning of the affected extremity (depends on the type of skeletal traction and the extremity involved; see Table 25–2).

5. Assist with attachment of the ropes, pulleys, weights, and weight holders. Make sure the ropes are tied securely in knots and are passed through the pulleys to the weights. Knots should not be in contact with the pulleys on the foot of the bed. **Rationale:** Ropes and pulleys are used to hold the weights to provide traction to the affected extremity and provide the patient a certain amount of freedom of movement. The patient's body weight serves as a countertraction. Proper setup of traction equipment prior to pin/wire insertion facilitates rapid application of traction.

Implementation

Steps	Rationale	Special Considerations
1. Wash hands.	Reduces transmission of microorganisms.	
2. Clean the affected extremity to be placed in skeletal traction with povidone-iodine solution.	Reduces the potential for infection.	
3. Open pin/wire tray using aseptic technique.	Reduces the potential for infection.	
4. Maintain the position of the injured extremity as requested by the physician during injection of local anesthesia and insertion of pin/wire.	Ensures stability of the affected limb to prevent undue movement that could cause further trauma.	Positioning of the affected extremity depends on the type of skeletal traction to be used and extremity involved.
5. Assist with insertion of the pin or wire through the bone as requested.	Ensures stability of the affected limb to prevent undue movement that could cause further trauma.	
6. Assist as requested with application of the Thomas splint, Pearson attachment, spreader bar, foot support, and elastic bandage as needed.	Ensures proper alignment of the bone fragments placed under traction.	Spreader bar is used to achieve abduction of the affected part. Thomas splint comes in full- or half-ring styles and is used for fractures of the femoral shaft, hip, or lower leg. Pearson attachment converts Thomas splint to balanced suspension and allows passive motion of the knee without malalignment of the affected extremity. Foot support prevents peroneal paralysis (foot drop) and prevents the patient from sliding down to the end of the bed.
7. Assist as requested with the positioning of the affected extremity in suspension and in applying the ropes, pulleys, and prescribed weights.	Helps realign bone fragments and prevent muscle spasm.	Countertraction is the assistance, or back-pull, made to extension on a limb.
8. Position the patient's body in proper alignment.	Provides for patient safety and comfort and optimal traction.	Proper body positioning/alignment optimizes the repair and growth of bone and soft tissue in order to prevent delayed union and/or nonunion of fractures.
9. Wash hands.	Reduces transmission of microorganisms.	

Evaluation

1. Monitor the patient's neurovascular status every 1 to 2 hours for 4 hours or until stabilized and then every 4 hours. **Rationale:** Early detection prevents complications from neurovascular compromise.

2. Monitor skeletal traction every 4 hours. Check that the prescribed weights are hanging freely, knots are secured, ropes are in pulleys, and affected limb is in proper alignment with total body. **Rationale:** Prevents potential injury and ensures that traction and countertraction are maintained.

3. Ensure proper wound and pin/wire care with povidone-iodine solution every shift. Evaluate pin/wire insertion site for purulent drainage, redness, pain, swelling, and warmth. **Rationale:** Pin insertion disrupts skin integrity and provides a portal of entry for microorganisms that can cause infection, leading to osteomyelitis.

4. Evaluate the patient's comfort level. **Rationale:** Tell the patient that medications are given IM/IV initially but will quickly become PO or whatever is appropriate. Discuss how long the patient requires pain medications and whether muscle relaxants are used.

5. Evaluate mobility of distal/proximal joints. Ensure

that a patient consultation with physical therapy is initiated. **Rationale:** Exercise promotes circulation to the affected extremity and prevents potential for contracture formation.

6. Monitor the patient's nutritional intake and output for adequate bone healing (i.e., vitamins A, D, and C, calcium, phosphorus, magnesium, and proteins). **Rationale:** Supplying adequate nutrients optimizes the anabolism necessary for repair and growth of bone and soft tissue in order to prevent delayed union and/or nonunion of fractures.

Expected Outcomes

1. Adequate tissue perfusion. **Rationale:** Proper application of skeletal traction decreases or prevents the potential for injury to the neurovascular bundle.
2. Patient comfort. **Rationale:** Proper alignment of bone fragments and traction relieve muscle spasm.
3. Absence of infection with skin integrity. **Rationale:** Prevents osteomyelitis.
4. Maintenance of normal bowel and bladder elimination patterns. **Rationale:** Prevents bladder and bowel complications such as constipation and cystitis.
5. Satisfactory alignment of bone fragments on x-ray studies with evidence of beginning callous formation within 6 weeks. **Rationale:** Functioning traction realigns bone fragments, establishes countertraction, and thus promotes bone healing.
6. Optimal range of motion in distal and proximal joints. **Rationale:** Prevents contracture formation.

Unexpected Outcomes

1. Neurovascular compromise. **Rationale:** Most commonly associated with improper application/maintenance of traction that causes pressure on the neurovascular bundle.
2. Increasing edema formation and complaints of pain. **Rationale:** Edema and increasing pain are suggestive of malalignment of the affected part.
3. Osteomyelitis. **Rationale:** Improper pin and/or wound care or a break in aseptic technique during pin or wire insertion in a closed fracture may cause development of osteomyelitis.
4. Fat embolism. **Rationale:** Occurs most frequently within 24 to 72 hours of a long-bone fracture.
5. Contractures of joints distal and proximal to the injury site. **Rationale:** May be due to improper positioning of the affected extremity, lack of ROM exercises, or improper application of traction.
6. Skin irritation and/or pressure sores. **Rationale:**

Prolonged immobility without good skin care and/or changes of position predispose the patient to the development of pressure sores.

Documentation

Documentation in the patient record should include the date and time of the procedure, the extremity involved, the type of traction and amount of weight used, the name and title of the person applying the traction, the alignment of involved extremity, the patient's response to the procedure, consecutive neurovascular assessments, evaluation of the traction setup, skin integrity of the affected extremity, pin/wire care and assessment of insertion sites, wound care if applicable, ROM exercises to distal/proximal joints, evaluation of patient's nutritional status and oral intake, bowel and bladder patterns, and any unexpected outcomes encountered and actions taken. **Rationale:** Documents nursing care given.

Patient/Family Education

1. Discuss the nature of the equipment and the purpose of traction with both patient and family. **Rationale:** Helps ease patient's fear and anxiety.
2. Patient's family should be instructed not to release weights from the skeletal traction attached to the affected extremity. **Rationale:** Releasing the weights from the traction causes muscle contraction, which in turn can malalign the fracture and damage the surrounding nerves and vessels.
3. Instruct the patient and family to report increased pain, muscle spasm, numbness, change in temperature, or cold and/or tingling sensation in the affected extremity. **Rationale:** May herald the need for immediate intervention.
4. Have the patient and family perform active ROM exercises to the unaffected extremity and passive ROM exercises to the affected body parts as tolerated. **Rationale:** Helps in maintaining muscle strength, limiting muscle atrophy.
5. Instruct the patient and family to maintain activities of daily living as appropriate, and provide diversional activities while the patient is in traction. **Rationale:** Immobilization with skeletal traction for an extended period of time may cause the patient to experience a sense of claustrophobia and boredom.

Performance Checklist
Skill 25–2: Balanced Suspension Skeletal Traction

Critical Behaviors	Complies	
	yes	no
1. Wash hands.		
2. Clean the affected extremity to be placed in a balanced suspension skeletal traction with povidone-iodine solution.		

Table continues on following page

Critical Behaviors	Complies	
	yes	no
3. Open pin/wire tray using aseptic technique.		
4. Position the injured extremity as requested during injection of local anesthetic.		
5. Assist with insertion of pin or wire through the bone as requested.		
6. Assist as requested with application of the Thomas splint, Pearson attachment, spreader bar, foot support, and elastic bandage as needed.		
7. Assist as requested with attachment of the ropes, pulleys, weights, and weight holders, making sure the ropes are tied securely to the ends of the Thomas splint.		
8. Maintain proper body alignment.		
9. Wash hands.		
10. Document in the patient record.		

SKILL 25–3

External Fixation Traction

External fixation traction is a form of skeletal traction. It holds fragments in position while allowing for a wide variety of configurations (Fig. 25–7A and B).

External fixation traction, such as the Hoffman or Ibizarov devices, utilizes metal pins that are drilled into the bone and fixed to a rigid external frame or bar. These devices may be used for limb fractures associated with significant skin and tissue damage, extensive comminuted fracture, burns, delayed union, nonunion, and infected nonunion. Other indications include infected fractures, osteotomy, pelvic fracture, lengthening of a limb, and/or arthrodesis. The device will be inserted in the operating room or trauma admission area.

Purpose

The nurse cares for the patient in external fixation traction to

1. Maintain proper bone alignment until calcification occurs.
2. Immobilize and stabilize the affected body part to prevent further injury to the surrounding tissues, nerves, and vasculature.
3. Ensure safety and comfort while the patient is in the external fixator.
4. Prevent contractures in joints proximal and distal to the injury.

Prerequisite Knowledge and Skills

Prior to caring for the patient in external fixation traction, the nurse should understand

1. Anatomy and physiology of the affected body part.
2. Proper alignment of the affected body part.
3. Physiology of bone healing.
4. Principles of external fixation.

5. Principles of body mechanics.
6. Proper technique for using assistive supports (walker or crutches).
7. Principles of aseptic technique.

The nurse should be able to perform

1. Proper handwashing technique (see Skill 35–5).
2. Proper body mechanics.
3. Neurovascular assessment.
4. Range-of-motion exercises.

Assessment

1. Perform an initial neurovascular assessment (the 5 P's) of the affected extremity, including pain (note location, pattern, and duration), pallor (note presence or absence of cyanosis, mottling, and erythema), paresthesia (note any reports of numbness, tingling, or lack of sensation), pulselessness (i.e., decrease in the quality of the pulse distal to injury), and paralysis (i.e., absence of mobility of joints distal to injury). Compare the findings with those on the unaffected side. **Rationale:** Provides baseline data to monitor development of complications in the affected extremity.
2. Assess the skin integrity of the pin entrance and exit sites and areas contiguous to pin sites. **Rationale:** Pin sites provide a portal of entry for microorganisms.
3. Determine the amount, location, and severity of pain and/or muscle spasm. **Rationale:** Increase in pain may be from malposition of injured extremity or impending vascular compromise.
4. Review radiology studies to assess alignment of the bone fragments. **Rationale:** Knowledge of the amount of reduction achieved by the physician allows for the development of an individualized plan of care.
5. Assess the general condition of affected body part, including existing soft-tissue trauma, open areas, edema, bruises, rash, bleeding sites, and presence/risk of infection. **Rationale:** Provide baseline data for sequential evaluations.
6. Assess the patient for signs and symptoms of pul-

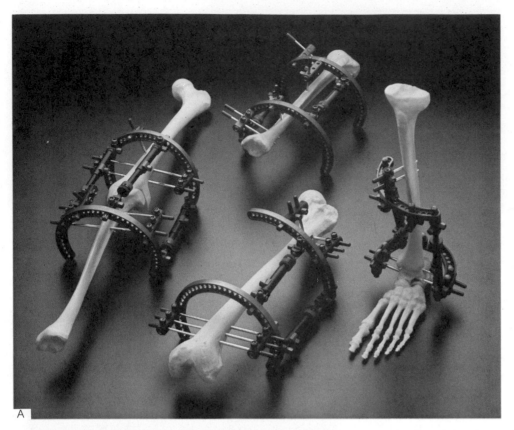

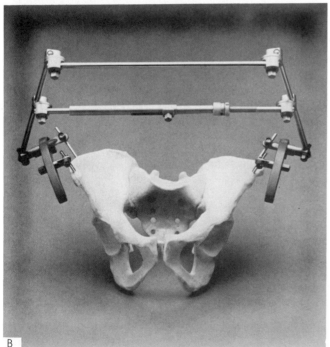

FIGURE 25–7. *(A)* External fixation devices for both upper and lower extremities. (Courtesy of Ace Medical, Los Angeles, Calif.) *(B)* External fixator for stabilization of pelvic fractures. (Courtesy of Ace Medical, Los Angeles, Calif.)

monary/fat emboli, including rate and depth of respiration, presence or absence of cough, sputum production, changes in sensorium, presence of petechial rash over chest and neck, tachycardia, and decreased blood pressure. **Rationale:** Fat emboli may occur following longbone trauma. Transient petechial rash occurs in 5–10% of patients with fat emboli.

7. Assess the patient's nutritional status, including caloric intake, protein balance, intake of vitamins A, D, and C, calcium, phosphorus, and magnesium. **Rationale:** Adequate nutritional intake optimizes the anabolism necessary for repair of bone and soft tissue in order to minimize delayed union or nonunion of the fracture.

8. Assess the mobility in uninvolved joints of the affected extremity. **Rationale:** Provides baseline data for assessment of contracture formation.

Nursing Diagnoses

1. Pain related to muscle spasm, musculoskeletal injury, open wounds, and/or tension from external fixation traction. **Rationale:** Injury to soft tissues surrounding the fractured bone results in muscle contraction, which can be very painful; pain also may be an indication of impending vascular compromise.

2. Fear related to unfamiliarity with external fixation traction. **Rationale:** Most patients have not seen or had experience with traction equipment and setup.

3. Potential for injury related to neurovascular compromise. **Rationale:** Disruption of traction or improper alignment/reduction of fractured bone may cause occlusion of the arterial blood supply and impair venous return.

4. Potential for infection related to traction pins directly inserted into the bone. **Rationale:** External fixators

are the treatment of choice for many unstable fractures with associated soft-tissue deficits. Hand drills should be used for pin insertion, since bone cells may be damaged by heat caused by process of drilling traction pins through bone if power drills are used.

5. Potential for decreased tissue perfusion of the affected limb related to edema formation. **Rationale:** Significant edema formation can occlude the arterial blood supply and venous return, resulting in ischemia and necrosis and potential loss of the limb.

6. Potential for infection related to initial injury and/or presence of skeletal pins. **Rationale:** Loss of skin at the site of injury predisposes patient to infection.

7. Potential for impaired gas exchange related to pulmonary and/or fat emboli. **Rationale:** Injury to long bones or immobility of lower extremity predisposes patient to pulmonary complications by obstructing blood flow in the pulmonary circulation.

8. Potential knowledge deficit related to treatment method and rehabilitation process. **Rationale:** Most patients and families are unfamiliar with external fixation devices.

Planning

1. Individualize the following goals for using the external fixation traction device:
   a. Maintain proper alignment of bone fragments. **Rationale:** Overcomes muscle spasms and aligns the fracture fragments.
   b. Immobilize the affected extremity to promote bone healing. **Rationale:** Micromotion at fracture ends predisposes to delayed union or nonunion.
   c. Maintain patient mobility and greater independence. **Rationale:** The injured extremity is exercise competent; therefore, partial use of limb is both possible and beneficial. Ambulation is possible with pelvic fixators if the acetabulum is not involved.
   d. Prevent infection in the presence of impaired skin integrity. **Rationale:** The development of osteomyelitis is a serious complication with potentially long-term sequelae.
   e. Maintain neurovascular integrity. **Rationale:** Malalignment, disruption of traction, and/or edema formation may cause neurovascular compromise.
   f. Maintain range of motion in the joints proximal and distal to the injury site. **Rationale:** Patients generally fear movement of affected area, predisposing to joint contractures in unaffected joints.
   g. Promote patient comfort. **Rationale:** Fear, soft-tissue injury, and/or impending neurovascular compromise contribute to patient's pain.
2. Assemble all the necessary equipment for traction maintenance. **Rationale:** External fixator care includes maintenance of the integrity of the device.

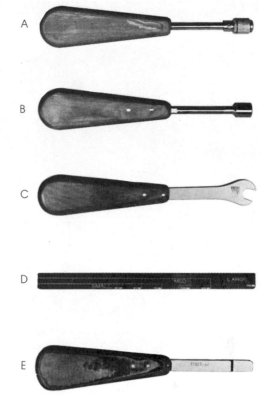

FIGURE 25–8. Assortment of wrenches for external fixation devices: (*A*) pin inserter, (*B*) socket wrench, (*C*) open-ended wrench, (*D*) tommy bar, (*E*) universal joint positioner. (Courtesy of Ace Medical, Los Angeles, Calif.)

   a. Appropriate tightening wrenches at bedside (Fig. 25–8).
   b. Box of alcohol wipes.
   c. One overhead frame and rope if lower extremity device is used (Fig. 25–9).
   d. Rubber caps (sufficient quantity to cover both ends of all pins).
   e. Two or three pillows to support frame.
3. Prepare all necessary equipment for pin-site care, according to institutional policy. **Rationale:** Prevents infection.
   a. One bottle of alcohol or one bottle hydrogen peroxide and normal saline (for half-strength mixture).
   b. Five to ten packets of sterile cotton applicators.
   c. One 10-cc syringe with 18-gauge angiocatheter for irrigation.
   d. 2 × 2 or 4 × 4 gauze pads (number depends on number of pin sites).
   e. 0.01% neomycin or povidone-iodine solution.
4. Prepare the patient.
   a. Explain the procedure to the patient. **Rationale:** Reduces anxiety and encourages cooperation.
   b. Explain the patient's participation. **Rationale:** Refocuses patient's attention, reduces fear, and encourages compliance with activity and/or restrictions.

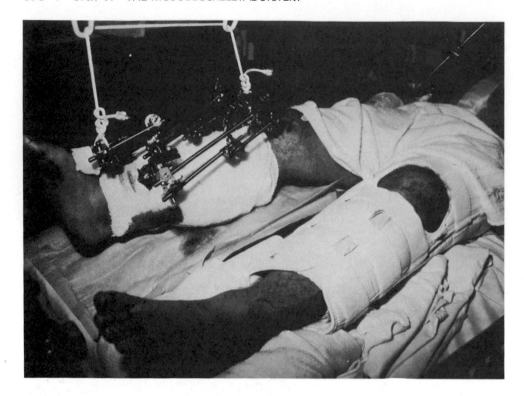

FIGURE 25–9. External fixator for lower extremity fracture suspended from overhead frame. (Used with permission from V. D. Cardonna et al., *Trauma Nursing: From Resuscitation Through Rehabilitation*. Philadelphia: Saunders, 1988, p. 552.)

Implementation

Steps	Rationale	Special Considerations
1. Perform pin care two to three times per day or according to physician orders:	Decreases entrance of skin flora into pin sites.	
a. Wash hands.	Reduces transmission of microorganisms.	
b. Don exam gloves. Remove initial dressing and discard in appropriate receptacle.	Allows visualization of pin sites. Universal precautions.	Initial dressing usually remains in place for 24 hours.
c. Wash hands.	Prevents transmission of microorganisms.	
d. Don sterile gloves.	Maintains aseptic technique.	
e. Cleanse skin opening around pin sites with sterile applicators soaked in alcohol.	Alcohol removes dried blood.	*Do not* remove scabs, which are part of healing process.
f. Apply small amount of antiseptic ointment to skin *around* pin. *Do not* place ointment into pin-site opening.	Occlusion of pin site will prevent drainage from pin site.	
g. Follow hospital protocol for type of dressing to be used, common options include: open to air, dry sterile dressings, wet to dry dressings.	Specific type of dressing depends on patient needs, physician preference, and/or institutional policy.	Kerlix bandage wraps may be used to prevent movement of skin on pins.
h. Perform wound irrigation if required for draining.	Cleanses wounds.	
i. Wash hands.	Reduces transmission of microorganisms.	

Table continues on following page

Steps	Rationale	Special Considerations
2. Cover exposed ends of fixation pins with rubber caps.	Prevents injury to patient and/or staff handling apparatus.	
3. Assist with ROM exercises on unaffected joints of injured limb, as well as in unaffected extremity, every 2 to 4 hours.	Improves venous return and prevents formation of thromboemboli and/or contractures.	
4. Elevate extremity to prevent complications:		
a. Use pillows to support external fixator frame.	Direct pressure on muscle groups may lead to compartment syndrome.	
b. Suspend from bed frame with traction rope.	Prevents development of pressure sores and decreases edema.	For patient comfort, make sure knee is flexed if lower extremity apparatus is used.
5. Reposition limb by moving apparatus, not limb itself.	Prevents malalignment of fractured bones.	
6. Turn patient in pelvic fixator to limitations of apparatus. *Do not use pelvic apparatus to turn patient.*	Pelvic fracture fragments do not have the stability of extremity fracture fragments.	The half pins used for pelvic fixator dislodge more easily than transfixation pins (Fig. 25–10).
7. Inspect apparatus every 8 hours for integrity.	Acceptable bone alignment may be lost if apparatus loosens.	Report loose pins to physician.
8. Wipe articulations and rods of external fixator with alcohol every 24 hours.	Reduces potential for transmission of microorganisms.	
9. Apply ice bags to lateral surface of injured extremity.	Decreases swelling and edema without compromising vascular flow.	Avoid placing pressure of bag over arterial areas.
10. Wash hands.	Reduces transmission of microorganisms.	

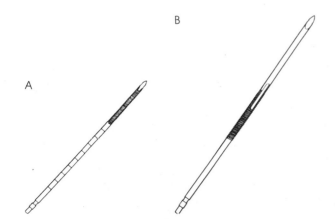

FIGURE 25–10. (*A*) Half pins are used for unilateral frames and pelvic fixators. (*B*) Transfixion pins have center threads and are used for double frames. (Courtesy of Howmedica, Inc., Rutherford, N.J.)

Evaluation

1. Evaluate the patient's neurovascular status every 1 to 2 hours for 24 hours or until stabilized and then every 4 hours. **Rationale:** Early detection prevents complications from pressure or compromised tissue perfusion.

2. Evaluate the alignment of the affected extremity. **Rationale:** Loose pins and/or loss of integrity of apparatus may cause malalignment of fracture fragments and/or drainage.

3. Monitor the patient's skin around the pin sites for evidence of inflammation and/or infection. **Rationale:** Pin insertion disrupts skin integrity and provides a portal of entry for microorganisms; infection may lead to osteomyelitis.

4. Evaluate the patient's comfort level. **Rationale:** Tell the patient that medications are given IM/IV initially but will quickly become PO or whatever is appropriate, and explain how long a patient usually requires pain medications.

5. Evaluate mobility of distal/proximal joints. Ensure that a physical therapy consult is initiated. **Rationale:** Exercise promotes circulation of the affected extremity, thus minimizing potential for contracture formation.

6. Monitor the patient's nutritional intake and output for adequate bone healing (i.e., vitamins A, D, and C, calcium, phosphorus, magnesium, and proteins). **Rationale:** Supplying adequate nutrients optimizes the ana-

bolism necessary for repair and growth of bone and soft tissue in order to prevent delayed union and/or nonunion of fracture.

Expected Outcomes

1. Neurovascular integrity. **Rationale:** Neurovascular checks evaluate for potential complications.
2. Patient comfort. **Rationale:** Proper alignment of bone fragments relieves pain and muscle spasm.
3. Absence of infection. **Rationale:** Reduces risk of osteomyelitis.
4. Alignment of bone fragments on x-ray studies with evidence of beginning callous formation. **Rationale:** Integrity of external fixator has been maintained.
5. Ambulation. **Rationale:** Use of external fixator devices permits early ambulation.

Unexpected Outcomes

1. Neurovascular compromise. **Rationale:** Improperly applied external fixation traction may cause pressure on the neurovascular bundles.
2. Increasing edema formation and complaints of pain. **Rationale:** Edema and increasing pain are suggestive of malalignment or nonunion of the affected part.
3. Osteomyelitis. **Rationale:** Improper pin and/or wound care or a break in aseptic technique during pin insertion.
4. Fat embolism. **Rationale:** Occurs most frequently within 24 to 72 hours after long-bone fracture.

Documentation

Documentation in the patient record should include the date and time of the procedure, the initial assessment of the extremity involved, serial neurovascular assessments, skin integrity of the affected extremity, pin care and assessment of the insertion sites, wound care (if applicable), the patient's response to the procedure, the patient's ability to weight-bear/ambulate, assessment(s) of nutritional status/oral intake, and any unexpected outcomes encountered and actions taken. **Rationale:** Documents baseline nursing assessments and care given.

Patient/Family Education

1. Discuss the nature, indications, and purpose of the external fixator with both patient and family. **Rationale:** Reduces anxiety.
2. Instruct the patient and family to report any signs and symptoms of neurovascular compromise. **Rationale:** May herald the need for immediate intervention.
3. Have the patient and family perform active ROM exercises on the affected extremity and passive ROM exercises on the unaffected body part within prescribed limitations. **Rationale:** Exercise prevents joint stiffness and muscle weakness as well as promoting blood circulation to the affected body part until ambulation is permitted.
4. The patient and family should be clearly informed of the amount of weight-bearing allowed with pelvic and/or lower extremity fractures if applicable. **Rationale:** Prevents confusion and/or additional trauma to the affected body part.
5. The patient and family should be taught the techniques for using crutches or a walker if applicable. Have the patient perform a return demonstration. **Rationale:** Prevents additional trauma to the affected body part.
6. Instruct the patient and family in proper pin care. Have the patient and family perform a return demonstration. **Rationale:** Reduces the risk of osteomyelitis, promotes independence, and enhances self-control.

Performance Checklist
Skill 25–3:   External Fixation Traction

Critical Behaviors	Complies	
	yes	no
1. Wash hands.		
2. Perform pin care two to three times per day or according to physician's orders.		
3. Cover exposed ends of fixation pins with rubber caps.		
4. Assist with ROM exercises on unaffected joints of injured limb, as well as affected extremity, every 2 to 4 hours.		
5. Elevate extremity to prevent complications.		
6. Reposition limb by moving apparatus, not limb itself.		
7. Turn patient in pelvic fixator to limitation of apparatus. *Do not* use pelvic apparatus to turn patient.		
8. Inspect apparatus every 8 hours for integrity.		
9. Wipe articulations and rods of external fixator with alcohol every 24 hours.		
10. Apply ice bags to lateral surface of injured extremity.		

Table continues on following page

Critical Behaviors	Complies	
	yes	no
11. Wash hands.		
12. Document in the patient record.		

REFERENCES

Burke, J. F., Boyd, R. J., and McCabe, C. J. (1988). *Trauma Management: Early Management of Visceral, Nervous System, and Musculoskeletal Injuries*. Chicago: Year Book Medical Publishers.

Corkery, E. (1989). Discharge planning and home health care: What every staff nurse should know. *Orthop. Nurs.* 8(6):18–26.

Dandy, D. J. (1989). *Essential Orthopaedics and Trauma*. New York: Churchill-Livingstone.

Farrell, J. (1986). *Illustrated Guide to Orthopedic Nursing*, 3d Ed. Philadelphia: Lippincott.

Mourad, L. D., and Drorte, M. M. (1988). *The Nursing Process in the Care of Adults with Orthopaedic Conditions*, 2d Ed. New York: Wiley.

Pellino, T. A., Mooney, N. E., Salmond, S. W., and Verdisco, L. A. (1986). *NAON Core Curriculum for Orthopedic Nursing*. Pitman, N.J.: Anthony J. Jannetti.

Perry, A. G., and Potter, P. A. (1986). *Clinical Nursing Skills and Techniques: Basic, Intermediate, Advanced*. St. Louis: Mosby.

Roaf, R., and Hodkinson, L. J. (1988). *Textbook of Orthopaedic Nursing*, 3d Ed. London: Blackwell Scientific.

Schoen, D. C. (1986). *The Nursing Process in Orthopaedics*. Norwalk, Conn.: Appleton-Century-Crofts.

Stewart, J. D. M., and Hallett, J. P. (1988). *Traction and Orthopaedic Appliances*, 2d Ed. New York: Churchill-Livingstone.

Zimmer, Inc. (1989). *The Traction Handbook*, 6th Ed. Warsaw, Ind.: Zimmer, Inc.

26

INTERCOMPARTMENTAL PRESSURE MONITORING

BEHAVIORAL OBJECTIVES

After completing this chapter, the nurse will be able to

- Define the key terms.
- Describe the indications for intracompartmental pressure monitoring.
- Describe two methods of continuous intracompartmental pressure monitoring.
- Identify the signs and symptoms of compartment syndrome.

Compartment syndrome is a potentially limb-threatening complication that often occurs after trauma to the skeletal or vascular systems. The detrimental effect of compartment syndrome is necrosis of muscle tissue caused by inadequate circulation at the capillary level. The patient may lose function of the affected muscles, progressing to loss of function of the entire extremity. Cosmetic defects may result, or amputation of the limb may be necessary. Serious systemic complications also may result from muscle necrosis. Infection within the compartment may result if treatment is delayed. Muscle necrosis also leads to the release of myoglobin and potassium into the circulation. Myoglobin blocks the renal tubules, leading to renal failure. Lethal cardiac dysrhythmias can result from the hyperkalemia associated with renal failure and/or the excess potassium released from the necrotic muscle. Finally, lactic acid released from the muscle can predispose the patient to metabolic acidosis.

Osteofascial compartments of the extremities represent an anatomic space with rigid boundaries. When interstitial pressure increases in the compartment or arteriolar pressure falls, blood flow to the area is compromised. The most common areas affected are the forearm and lower leg. See Table 26–1 for compartments in each extremity.

The critical closing pressure of arterioles in a compartment is a function of the difference in transmural pressure on either side of the vessel wall. Normal compartment pressure is 0 to −2 mmHg. When compartment pressure rises above the arteriolar pressure, the critical pressure point is reached and blood flow ceases (Fig. 26–1). Irreversible changes in muscle fiber occur when the compartment pressure reaches 30 mmHg. Left untreated, damage in the upper extremity can progress to the classic Volkmann's contracture (Fig. 26–2).

If the patient is awake and alert, a neurovascular assessment may be sufficient to diagnose compartment syndrome. In less reliable patients, such as those with an altered level of consciousness, the critically ill, or children, intracompartmental pressure monitoring may be indicated to confirm the clinical suspicion of compartment syndrome.

KEY TERMS

compartment	slit catheter
compartment syndrome	Volkmann's contracture
critical closing pressure	wick catheter

SKILLS

26–1 Assisting with Insertion of a Wick or Slit Catheter
26–2 Wick or Slit Catheter Care

GUIDELINES

The following assessment guidelines assist the nurse in formulating a nursing diagnosis and an individualized plan of care to monitor the intracompartmental pressure of an extremity.

1. Know the patient's baseline blood pressure.
2. Know the patient's baseline neurovascular assessment.
3. Know the mechanism of injury to the extremity.
4. Know the signs and symptoms of compartment syndrome.

SKILL 26–1 _____

Assisting with Insertion of a Wick or Slit Catheter

The goal when caring for a patient at risk for compartment syndrome is early diagnosis. Equivocal signs and symptoms make a definitive clinical diagnosis difficult. The development of techniques for measuring tissue pressures has provided an objective means for evaluating a compartment.

Three basic techniques exist for monitoring tissue pressure in the compartments of an extremity. A one-time measurement may be accomplished with a commercially prepared battery-operated kit. This technique may be

TABLE 26–1 Extremity Compartments

Compartment	Contents	Signs and Symptoms of Compartment Syndrome
Anterior compartment of leg	Tibialis anterior muscle (TA) Extensor hallucis longus (EHL) Extensor digitorum longus (EDL) Deep peroneal nerve (DPN)	Weak toe extension Weak foot dorsiflexion Pain on passive toe and foot flexion Hyperesthesia of first web space
Deep posterior compartment of leg	Tibialis posterior muscle (TP) Flexor hallucis longus (FHL) Flexor digitorum longus (FDL) Posterior tibial nerve (PTN)	Weak toe flexion Weak foot incision Pain on passive toe and foot extension Hyperesthesia of plantar surface Tenderness between tibia and Achilles tendon
Volar compartment of forearm	Flexor muscles of digits (FDL, FDP, FDS) Flexor muscles of forearm (PL, FCR, FCU) Median nerve (MN) Ulnar nerve (UN)	Weak finger and wrist flexion Pain on finger and wrist extension Hyperesthesia of volar aspect of fingers

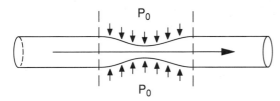

FIGURE 26–1. Increased tissue pressure causing collapse of an arteriole and cessation of blood flow. (Used with permission from F. A. Matsen, *Compartment Syndromes*. New York: Grune & Stratton, 1980, p. 11.)

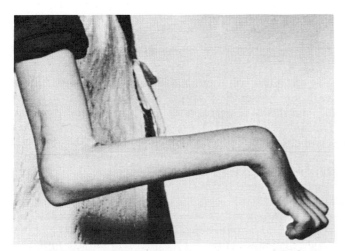

FIGURE 26–2. Volkmann's ischemic contracture of the forearm. (Used with permission from L. A. Mourad and M. M. Droste, *The Nursing Process in the Care of Adults with Orthopedic Conditions*, 2d Ed. New York: Wiley, 1988, p. 363.)

useful in the multisystem-injured patient when continuous monitoring is not practical. However, two techniques

are available for continuous monitoring of tissue pressure. Indirect measurements, with the aid of a manometer, monitor total tissue pressure (solid-tissue pressure plus interstitial-fluid pressure). Direct measurement of interstitial-fluid pressure can be determined by use of a wick (Fig. 26–3) or slit (Fig. 26–4) catheter.

Both the wick and slit catheters are simple to use and provide accurate, objective data when determining the need for surgical intervention in the treatment of compartment syndrome.

Choice of one catheter over the other depends on physician preference and availability and staff familiarity with each. The wick catheter has several advantages: The wick fibers maximize the area of contact with tissue fluid, patency can be maintained without a continuous infusion, equilibrium tissue-fluid pressure can be rapidly achieved, intracompartmental pressure can be measured even during exercise or muscle contraction, and small amounts of fluid can be collected for diagnosis. Prolonged use of a wick catheter can result in hydrolysis of the absorbable suture material used to make the wick. Catheter patency may be compromised by coagulation of blood around the tip, which requires flushing.

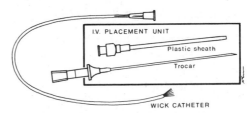

FIGURE 26–3. A wick catheter for intracompartmental pressure monitoring. (Used with permission from S. J. Mubarak and A. R. Hargens, *Compartment Syndromes and Volkmann's Contracture*. Philadelphia: Saunders, 1981, p. 114.)

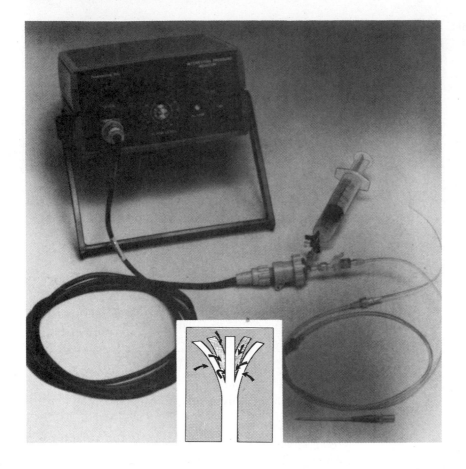

FIGURE 26–4. Slit catheter setup. Slit tip on catheter consists of 5 petals that allow a patent fluid path and prevent occlusion with material or tissue. (Photo courtesy of Howmedica, Inc.)

The design of the slit catheter decreases the problem of catheter patency. Therefore, good responses can be illicited on the monitor without excessive flushing of fluid into the compartment, which is already compromised.

Purpose

The nurse assists with insertion of a wick or slit catheter to

1. Monitor intracompartmental pressure.
2. Confirm clinical symptoms of compartment syndrome.
3. Clarify the pathologic process in patients unable to communicate symptoms.

Prerequisite Knowledge and Skills

Prior to assisting with insertion of a wick or slit catheter, the nurse should understand

1. Principles of aseptic technique.
2. Universal precautions.
3. Anatomy and physiology of the involved extremity.
4. Principles of transducer monitoring.

The nurse should be able to perform

1. Proper handwashing technique (see Skill 35–5).
2. Sterile technique.
3. Universal precautions (see Skill 35–1).
4. Proper skin preparation technique.
5. Neurovascular assessment.
6. Transducer system setup (see Skill 10–1).
7. Zeroing, leveling, and calibrating of the monitoring system (see Skill 10–1).

Assessment

1. Identify risk factors associated with compartment syndrome, including fractures with edema or hematoma formation, vascular and/or orthopedic procedures of the extremities, prolonged use of external pressure (i.e., pneumatic antishock garment), and decreased systemic (arteriolar) pressure below the compartment pressure. **Rationale:** Identification of patients at risk alerts the nurse to the need for intracompartmental pressure monitoring.
2. Compare affected extremity to unaffected extremity every 1 to 2 hours. **Rationale:** Serial assessments may indicate need for intracompartmental pressure monitoring. Pathologic changes are rarely bilateral.
3. Assess for throbbing pain in affected compartment, pain on passive stretching, firmness of compartment, and paresthesia distal to distribution of involved nerve (Fig. 26–5). **Rationale:** These symptoms, when they occur together, indicate the need for immediate intervention.
4. Determine the type of intracompartmental pres-

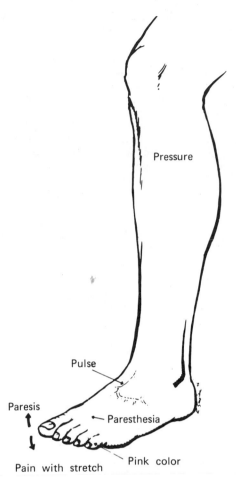

FIGURE 26–5. Early signs and symptoms of compartment syndrome of the lower extremity. (Used with permission from S. J. Mubarak, and A. R. Hargens, *Compartment Syndromes and Volkmann's Contracture.* Philadelphia: Saunders, 1981, p. 99.)

sure monitoring equipment to be used. Emphasis should be placed on one-time versus continuous monitoring, physician preference, and type of equipment available. **Rationale:** Type of monitor and setup required depend on resources available.

Nursing Diagnoses

1. Potential for impaired tissue integrity related to decreased perfusion. **Rationale:** Compartment syndrome often occurs following disruption of arterial flow.

2. Potential for injury related to increased tissue pressure. **Rationale:** Irreversible damage can occur within 5 to 6 hours of untreated increased compartment pressure.

3. Potential for injury related to neurovascular compromise. **Rationale:** Volkmann's contracture is a complication of compartment syndrome.

4. Potential for injury related to catheter insertion. **Rationale:** Improper insertion can result in further damage.

5. Potential for infection related to catheter insertion. **Rationale:** Invasive procedure provides a portal of entry for pathogens.

Planning

1. Individualize the following goals for monitoring compartmental syndrome:
    a. Maintain aseptic technique. **Rationale:** Monitoring setup is in direct communication with the compartment.
    b. Maintain functioning equipment. **Rationale:** Malfunctioning equipment may lead to incorrect measurements of tissue pressure and thus an inappropriate diagnosis.
    c. Maintain viability of extremity. **Rationale:** Confirmation of clinical findings with intracompartmental pressure monitoring provides early detection of potentially devastating complications.

2. Prepare all necessary supplies and equipment. **Rationale:** Assembly of all supplies and equipment allows for insertion to be performed quickly and efficiently.
    a. One monitor and amplifier.
    b. One monitoring kit, *or*
    c. One transducer, two three-way stopcocks, one high-pressure monitoring tube that is 48 in long or less.
    d. One 30-cc syringe.
    e. One heparin flush syringe, 100 units/cc.
    f. 20 to 25 cc normal saline solution for irrigation.
    g. One razor.
    h. Two or three povidone-iodine prep sticks.
    i. Local anesthetic (1% lidocaine), if prescribed.
    j. Wick or slit catheter (as per physician order).
    k. One roll of 1-in waterproof tape.
    l. One 3-0 atraumatic nylon suture with needle (or as per physician preference).
    m. Two packages sterile 4 × 4 gauze pads.

3. Prepare the patient.
    a. Assess the patient's ability to understand the procedure. **Rationale:** Associated trauma or age may affect cognitive ability.
    b. Explain the nature and purpose of the procedure. **Rationale:** Decreases anxiety and promotes patient cooperation.
    c. Describe the position of the extremity the patient will need to assume and maintain to prevent the compartment from having contact with the bed. **Rationale:** Promotes patient cooperation.
    d. Describe the sensations the patient will experience with catheter insertion. **Rationale:** Decreases anxiety and promotes cooperation.

Implementation

Steps	Rationale	Special Considerations
1. Turn monitor on (see Fig. 26–4).	Prevents calibration drift.	
2. Wash hands.	Reduces transmission of microorganisms.	
3. a. Obtain a 25-ml bag of 0.9% normal saline solution for injection.	Normal saline is preferred over Ringer's lactate.	A 30-cc syringe filled with 0.9% normal saline solution also may be used.
b. Assemble and prepare transducer-monitoring system (see Skill 10–1).	For continuous monitoring of compartment pressure.	
4. Position extremity so that compartment to be measured is not in contact with patient's bed.	Eliminates external pressure on compartment to be measured.	
5. Prepare insertion site with povidone-iodine.	Catheter must be inserted under aseptic technique.	Shave area first if excess hair will interfere with insertion or dressings.
a. Don sterile gloves.	Reduces transmission of microorganisms.	
b. Apply povidone-iodine solution beginning at insertion site and moving in concentric circles to periphery of extremity.	Reduces number of skin flora and transmission of microorganisms.	
c. Repeat with a clean prep stick.	Reduces transmission of microorganisms.	
d. Remove and discard gloves.	Prepares for handwashing.	
e. Wash hands.	Reduces transmission of microorganisms.	
6. Prepare local anesthetic agent if desired.	Injury may cause anesthesia to area.	
7. Attach wick or slit catheter to transducer setup, and check monitor:	Prepares system for monitoring compartment pressure.	Maintain aseptic technique.
a. First hold wick/slit catheter at level of transducer. Monitor should read 0.	Monitor automatically adjusts itself to zero. Zeroing negates the effect of atmospheric pressure.	Transducer should be at level of compartment.
b. Raise wick/slit catheter to eye level of nurse. Pressure should rise to 30 to 50 mmHg.	Validates response of system. False high or low pressure readings occur with improper setup, balancing, and calibration.	If slow response, suspect air bubbles; if pressure falls, suspect leak.
c. Lower wick/slit catheter to level of compartment (Fig. 26–6).	Pressure should return to 0.	
8. Assist physician as required with insertion of Jelco catheter (Fig. 26–7).	Catheter is inserted at 45-degree angle to the skin and is advanced into compartment.	Inner metal trocar is withdrawn, leaving plastic sheath in place.
9. Assist as required with insertion of wick/slit catheter through trocar (Fig. 26–8).	Allows measurements of intracompartmental pressure.	Plastic sheath of Jelco catheter is removed, leaving wick or slit catheter in place.
10. Secure wick/slit catheter in place with waterproof tape (Fig. 26–9).	Prevents inadvertent dislodgment of catheter.	Physician may suture in place.
11. Attach catheter to monitoring setup. Transducer must be at level of compartment for accurate measurement (Fig. 26–6).	Improper placement can result in inaccurate measurements.	Error of 2 mmHg will occur for every inch of discrepancy between transducer and compartment levels due to the hydrostatic pressure effect.

Table continues on following page

Steps	Rationale	Special Considerations
12. Check accuracy of monitoring system by palpating area over catheter tip or by having the patient flex-extend appropriate distal joint (Fig. 26–10). Large pressure deflection should occur.	Normal pressure response consists of a rapid rise with compression/contraction and a rapid fall to normal. Patients with compartment syndrome demonstrate a rapid rise in pressure with slow return to baseline.	Patient with compartment syndrome will complain of pain at pressures of 15–20 mmHg.
13. Obtain initial pressure measurement.	Provides baseline reading.	
14. Wash hands.	Prevents transmission of microorganisms.	

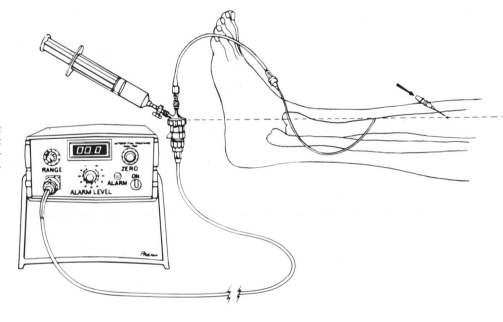

FIGURE 26–6. The open part of the venting stopcock is placed at the level of the tip of the intracompartmental catheter (*arrow*). Dashes show this level.

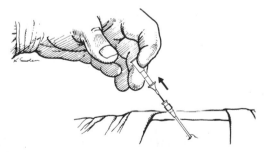

FIGURE 26–7. Jelco catheter used for insertion of wick catheter. (Used with permission from S. J. Mubarak and A. R. Hargens, *Compartment Syndromes and Volkmann's Contracture*. Philadelphia: Saunders, 1981, p. 114.)

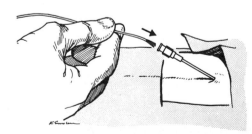

FIGURE 26–8. Threading wick catheter through Jelco catheter and into compartment to be measured. (Used with permission from S. J. Mubarak and A. R. Hargens, *Compartment Syndromes and Volkmann's Contracture*. Philadelphia: Saunders, 1981, p. 115.)

Evaluation

1. Recalibrate monitor every 4 to 8 hours or as per unit policy. **Rationale:** Improper calibration may lead to false high or low readings.

2. Monitor transducer setup for air bubbles. **Rationale:** Presence of air may cause abnormal readings.

3. Compare pre- and postinsertion neurovascular assessments. **Rationale:** Improper insertion of catheter can further compromise compartment and produces erroneous readings.

4. Evaluate initial pressure reading. **Rationale:** Decompression often occurs with a single reading of 40 mmHg in the presence of clinical symptoms.

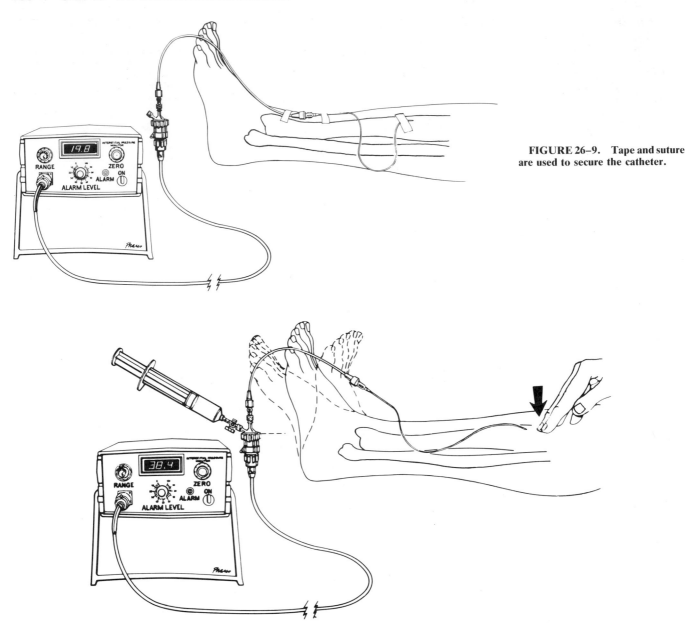

FIGURE 26–9. Tape and suture are used to secure the catheter.

FIGURE 26–10. The system's response can be checked either by palpating the area over the catheter tip (*arrow*) or by having the patient flex-extend the appropriate distal joint; observe the scope for small, temporary elevations in the pressure pattern.

Expected Outcomes

1. Monitoring setup is ready and available when required to monitor intracompartment pressure. **Rationale:** Determining compartment pressure is usually an acute event necessitating a prepared, functional monitoring setup.

2. Catheter is inserted without complication. **Rationale:** Decreases the incidence of tissue trauma and discomfort.

3. Accurate pressure readings are obtained. **Rationale:** Transducer is free from air and placed at level of the tip of intracompartmental catheter.

4. Viability of extremity is maintained. **Rationale:** Intracompartmental pressure monitoring provides for early recognition of intracompartmental pressure increases and prompt intervention.

Unexpected Outcomes

1. Inaccurate pressure readings. **Rationale:** Improper setup, leveling, or calibration produces erroneous pressure readings for which therapy may be instituted.

2. Bleeding into compartment following insertion. **Rationale:** Inadvertent vascular damage may contribute to sequelae of compartment syndrome.

3. Monitoring setup malfunctions. **Rationale:** Provides erroneous data for which therapies may be instituted.

4. Infection. **Rationale:** Invasive procedures, breaks

in aseptic techniques, or breaks in skin from initial injury provide a portal of entry for microorganisms.

Documentation

Documentation in the patient record should include the date and time of setup, composition of the flush solution, name and dose of medications added to the flush solution, name and title of person adding the medication, name of person preparing setup, date and time of procedure, pre- and postinsertion neurovascular assessments, type and location of catheter inserted, type and amount of local anesthesia used, name of physician inserting catheter, initial pressure reading, patient's tolerance of the procedure, and unexpected outcomes and interventions taken. **Rationale:** Documents nursing care given and baseline data for future trends.

Patient/Family Education

Discuss the importance of maintaining extremity position with both patient and family. **Rationale:** External pressure from movement on catheter may contribute to false readings.

Performance Checklist
Skill 26–1: Assisting with Insertion of a Wick or Slit Catheter

Critical Behaviors	Complies	
	yes	no
1. Turn monitor on.		
2. Wash hands.		
3. Obtain 20 to 25 cc normal saline solution for injection.		
4. Position involved extremity appropriately.		
5. Prepare insertion site.		
6. Prepare local anesthetic agent.		
7. Attach wick or slit catheter to transducer setup, and check monitor by raising catheter to eye level and observing for rise in pressure.		
8. Assist physician with insertion of Jelco catheter.		
9. Assist physician with insertion of wick or slit catheter.		
10. Secure wick or slit catheter in place with waterproof tape.		
11. Attach catheter to monitoring setup, and ensure that transducer is at level of compartment to be measured.		
12. Check accuracy of monitoring by palpating area over catheter tip or by having patient flex-extend distal joint.		
13. Obtain and record initial pressure measurement.		
14. Wash hands.		
15. Document procedure in the patient record.		

SKILL 26–2

Wick or Slit Catheter Care

Care of the patient with a wick or slit catheter focuses on local site care, troubleshooting the monitoring equipment, and assessment of trends in intracompartmental tissue pressure measurements. The goals are detection of developing compartment syndrome and prevention of devastating complications.

Purpose

The nurse performs wick or slit catheter care to

1. Prevent infection.
2. Provide accurate intracompartmental pressure readings.
3. Establish the clinical diagnosis of compartment syndrome.
4. Identify the need for decompression.

Prerequisite Knowledge and Skills

Prior to caring for the patient with a wick or slit catheter, the nurse should understand

1. Principles of aseptic technique.
2. Anatomy and physiology of involved extremity.

3. Principles of transducer monitoring.
4. Pathophysiology of compartment syndrome.

The nurse should be able to perform

1. Proper handwashing technique (see Skill 35–5).
2. Sterile dressing change.
3. Zeroing, leveling, and calibrating the transducer system (see Skill 10–1).
4. Neurovascular assessment.

Assessment

1. Assess the patient's skin integrity at the site of catheter insertion. **Rationale:** Catheter insertion provides a portal of entry for microorganisms.
2. Assess the patient for the symptoms of compartment syndrome (see Fig. 26–5 and Table 26–1) every 1 to 2 hours:
   a. Burning or searing pain. **Rationale:** Ischemic process results in this type of pain.
   b. Type and amount of narcotics required. **Rationale:** Pain of compartment syndrome may be disproportionate to injury.
   c. Edema and swelling of compartment. **Rationale:** The compartment will feel taut at pressure above 30 mmHg.
   d. Development of skin blisters. **Rationale:** May develop as compartment expands and/or treatment is delayed.
   e. Altered sensation. **Rationale:** Pressure on nerves within osteofascial compartment.
3. Assess accuracy of monitor readings every 4 to 8 hours or as per unit policy. **Rationale:** Inaccurate readings and misdiagnosis can occur with poorly calibrated monitors.
4. Assess blood and urine for myoglobin usually during the first 24 hours after injury. **Rationale:** Destruction of muscle tissue occurs during compartment syndrome and is not visibly apparent.

Nursing Diagnoses

1. Potential for infection related to presence of intracompartmental pressure monitoring catheter. **Rationale:** Catheter insertion provides a portal of entry for microorganisms.
2. Decreased tissue perfusion related to internal or external pressure on neurovascular structures. **Rationale:** Compartment syndrome occurs when the pressure within a space confined by bone and fascia increases to a point which decreases the perfusion of the muscle and nerves within that compartment.

Planning

1. Individualize the following goals for performing wick or slit catheter care:
   a. Maintain catheter patency. **Rationale:** Essential for accurate readings.
   b. Maintain aseptic technique. **Rationale:** Prevents infection.
   c. Maintain proper position of the extremity. **Rationale:** External pressure may cause falsely high readings.
2. Prepare the patient.
   a. Assess the patient's ability to cooperate with procedure. **Rationale:** Cognitive ability may be impaired by associated injuries or age.
   b. Explain the nature and purpose of the monitoring procedure. **Rationale:** Decreases anxiety and promotes cooperation.

Implementation

Steps	Rationale	Special Considerations
1. Wash hands.	Reduces transmission of microorganisms.	
2. Maintain extremity so that the catheter insertion site is free from external compression.	Prevents falsely elevated readings.	
3. Maintain the position of the transducer at the level of the catheter tip within the compartment (see Fig. 26–6).	Necessary for accurate readings.	
4. Calibrate the transducer by opening venting stopcock to air.	Necessary for accurate readings.	
5. Close venting stopcock and open monitoring stopcock.	Obtains intracompartmental pressure reading.	
6. Record pressure from monitor.	Provides written documentation of pressure readings.	

Table continues on following page

Steps	Rationale	Special Considerations
7. If reading shows borderline elevation, obtain serial measurements.	Trends may be important if readings are equivocal.	
8. Notify physician of pressure increases.	Decompression is usually performed for pressures above 30 mmHg for more than 4 hours.	
9. Assist with removal of catheter 48 hours after insertion.	Decreases risk of infection.	
10. Apply sterile dressing over insertion site.	Reduces transmission of microorganisms.	
11. Check removed catheter for presence of wick.	Avoids leaving a foreign body in compartment.	If wick detaches from catheter, pull the monofilament safety line attached to it for removal.
12. Wash hands.	Reduces transmission of microorganisms.	

Evaluation

1. Monitor compartment pressure every 2 hours or as ordered by physician. **Rationale:** Trends demonstrating an increasing pressure support the diagnosis of compartment syndrome.

2. Monitor insertion site for signs and symptoms of infection or inflammation. **Rationale:** May indicate the need for removal of catheter.

3. Monitor degree of pain and edema formation between readings. **Rationale:** Pain disproportionate to injury may indicate swelling/ischemia within the compartment.

4. Evaluate blood and urine samples daily for the presence of myoglobin. **Rationale:** Presence of myoglobin indicates necrosis of muscle tissue in the compartment.

Expected Outcomes

1. Adequate tissue perfusion to extremity is maintained. **Rationale:** Increasing compartment pressure supports a diagnosis of compartment syndrome and may indicate the need for immediate fasciotomy.

2. Catheter insertion site is without signs and symptoms of infection. **Rationale:** Infection of compartment may result in limb-threatening complications.

Unexpected Outcomes

1. Infection at catheter insertion site. **Rationale:** Breaks in aseptic technique or mechanism of initial injury contribute to infection.

2. Diminished tissue perfusion in extremity. **Rationale:** Continued swelling of the compartment results in decreased perfusion with limb-threatening consequences.

Documentation

Documentation in the patient record should include the position of the extremity, the date and times the equipment was calibrated, the date and times of compartment pressure readings, assessment of insertion site, the presence or absence of pain and edema formation, the date and time of dressing changes, the presence or absence of drainage, the date and time catheter was removed, a description of both catheter and insertion site after removal, any unexpected outcomes, and the interventions taken. **Rationale:** Documents nursing care given, expected and unexpected outcomes, and status of the compartment.

Patient/Family Education

1. Explain to the patient and family that compartment pressure monitoring will continue for approximately 48 hours after catheter insertion. **Rationale:** Inflammatory response (resulting in edema formation and decreased tissue perfusion) begins to subside within 48 hours.

2. Explain to the patient and family that a persistent rise in compartment pressure will necessitate surgical intervention (fasciotomy). **Rationale:** Encourages questions and eliminates fear of the unknown.

3. Discuss with the patient and family the need to report signs and symptoms of compartment syndrome after catheter removal. **Rationale:** For immediate assessment and intervention by a health care professional.

Performance Checklist
Skill 26–2: Wick or Slit Catheter Care

Critical Behaviors	Complies	
	yes	no
1. Wash hands.		
2. Position extremity so that involved compartment is off patient's bed.		
3. Position transducer at level of catheter tip.		
4. Calibrate transducer.		
5. Close venting stopcock, and open monitoring stopcock.		
6. Record pressure reading from monitor.		
7. Obtain serial measurements if reading shows borderline elevation.		
8. Notify physician of pressure increases.		
9. Assist with catheter removal 48 hours after insertion.		
10. Apply sterile dressing over insertion site.		
11. Check removed catheter for presence of wick.		
12. Wash hands.		
13. Document procedure in the patient record.		

BIBLIOGRAPHY

Allen, M. J., Stirling, A. J., Crawshaw, C. V., and Barnes, M. R. (1985). Intracompartmental pressure monitoring of leg injuries. *J. Bone Joint Surg.* 67B(1):53–57.

Cardona, V. D., Hurn, P. D., Bastnajel-Mason, P. J., et al. (1988). *Trauma Nursing from Resuscitation Through Rehabilitation*. Philadelphia: Saunders.

Gamron, R. B. (1988). Taking the pressure out of compartment syndrome. *Am. J. Nurs.* 88(8):1076–1080.

Matsen, F. A. (1975). Compartmental syndrome. *Clin. Orthop.* 113:8–14.

Mubarak, S. J., and Hargens, A. R. (1981). *Compartment Syndromes and Volkmann's Contracture*. Philadelphia: Saunders.

Proel, J. A. (1988). Compartment syndrome. *J. Emerg. Nurs.* 14(5):283–290.

UNIT VII

THE HEMATOLOGIC SYSTEM

27

HEMATOLOGIC MANAGEMENT

BEHAVIORAL OBJECTIVES

After completing this chapter, the nurse will be able to

- Define the key terms.
- Describe each constituent blood component.
- Discuss the indications for blood/blood component administration and autotransfusion.
- Demonstrate the skills involved in hematologic management.

Blood provides the vehicle for oxygen transport to the cells for aerobic metabolism and the production of adenosine triphosphate (ATP). With the advent of modern technology, blood may now be separated into its constituent components, allowing for specificity in transfusion therapy. The choice of which blood product to transfuse is based on the patient's clinical picture, complete blood count, coagulation studies, underlying pathophysiology, and hemodynamic status.

This chapter focuses on the procedures necessary for the management and care of a patient undergoing transfusion therapy.

KEY TERMS

albumin
autotransfusion
blood pump
cryoprecipitate
  antihemophilic factor
  (AHF)
fresh-frozen plasma
granulocytes
leukocyte-poor packed
  red blood cells
packed red blood cells
Plasmanate
platelet concentrate
transfusion reaction
type and crossmatch
whole blood

SKILLS

27–1 Blood and Blood Component Administration
27–2 Transfusion Reaction
27–3 Use of a Blood Pump
27–4 Determination of Microhematrocrit via Centrifuge
27–5 Autotransfusion (with Disposable Device)

GUIDELINES

The following assessment guidelines assist the nurse in formulating an individualized plan of care for the patient undergoing transfusion therapy:

1. Know the patient's medical history.
2. Know the patient's baseline complete blood count and, if appropriate, the results of coagulation studies.
3. Know the patient's baseline vital signs.
4. Know the patient's current medical treatment and its effect on the hematologic and immune systems.
5. Perform a systematic assessment of the hematologic and immune systems.
6. Determine appropriate interventions based on assessment findings.
7. Establish competency in the procedures used for blood and blood component administration.

SKILL 27–1

Blood and Blood Component Administration

Prior to administration of blood and blood components, the patient's blood must undergo a type and crossmatch with blood from a donor. This process involves testing the blood to avoid a possible transfusion reaction. Pretransfusion crossmatching ensures that the patient is issued the designated blood products, verifies that the blood products are ABO compatible, and detects most antibodies in the recipient's serum that react with the antigens in the donor's red blood cells.

Transfusion therapy is administered through a peripheral or central intravenous catheter.

Purpose

The nurse performs blood and blood component administration to

1. Provide volume replacement in the presence of massive hemorrhage.
2. Improve the blood's oxygen-carrying capacity by increasing the circulating volume of hemoglobin.
3. Replenish the blood with the constituents necessary for clotting to inhibit further bleeding.
4. Provide granulocytes for the neutropenic patient with an infection.

Prerequisite Knowledge and Skills

Prior to performing blood or blood component administration, the nurse should understand

1. Anatomy and physiology of the hematopoietic and immune systems, including knowledge of blood products (Table 27–1).
2. ABO and Rh compatibility (Table 27–2).
3. Principles of aseptic technique.
4. Universal precautions.
5. Principles of intravenous therapy administration.
6. Principles of hemodynamic pressures.
7. Principles of fluid and electrolyte balance.

The nurse should be able to perform

1. Proper handwashing technique (see Skill 35–5).
2. Universal precautions.
3. Vital signs assessment, including hemodynamic pressures.
4. Respiratory system assessment.
5. Assessment of fluid and electrolyte balance.
6. Assessment of the complete blood count and coagulation studies.
7. Assessment of the patient's previous transfusion history.
8. Administration of intravenous therapy.
9. Proper identification of client and donor type and crossmatch.

TABLE 27–1   SUMMARY OF BLOOD PRODUCTS AND ADMINISTRATION

Blood Component	Description	Actions	Indications	Administration	Complications
Whole blood	Red blood cells, plasma, and stable clotting factors	Restores oxygen-carrying capacity and intravascular volume	Symptomatic anemia with major circulating volume deficit Massive hemorrhaging with shock	Donor and recipient must be ABO compatible and Rh compatible Use microaggregate filter Rate of infusion: usually 2 to 4 hours but more rapid in cases of shock	Hemolytic reaction Allergic reaction Hypothermia Electrolyte disturbances Citrate intoxication Infectious diseases
Red blood cells	Red blood cells centrifuged from whole blood	Restores oxygen-carrying capacity and intravascular volume	Symptomatic anemia when patient is at risk for fluid overload Acute hemorrhaging	Donor and recipient must be ABO compatible and Rh compatible Use microaggregate filter Rate of infusion: 2 to 4 hours but more rapid in cases of shock	Infectious diseases Hemolytic reaction Allergic reaction Hypothermia Electrolyte disturbances Citrate intoxication

Table continues on following page

Blood Component	Description	Actions	Indications	Administration	Complications
Leukocyte-poor cells or washed red blood cells	Red blood cells from which leukocytes and plasma proteins have been reduced	Restores oxygen-carrying capacity and intravascular volume.	Symptomatic anemia when patient has history of repeated febrile nonhemolytic transfusion reactions Acute hemorrhaging	Donor and recipient must be ABO compatible and Rh compatible Use microaggregate filter Rate of infusion: 2 to 4 hours but more rapid in cases of shock	Allergic reaction Hemolytic reaction Hypothermia Electrolyte disturbances Citrate intoxication Infectious diseases
Fresh-frozen plasma	Plasma rich in clotting factors with platelets removed	Replaces clotting factors	Deficit of coagulation factors as in disseminated intravascular coagulopathy, liver disease, and coagulopathies from massive transfusions Major trauma victims with signs/symptoms of hemorrhage	Donor and recipient must be ABO compatible and Rh compatible Rate of infusion: 10 ml/min	Allergic reaction Febrile reactions Circulatory overload Infectious diseases
Platelets	Removed from whole blood	Increases platelet count and improves hemostasis	Thrombocytopenia Platelet dysfunction (prophylactically for platelet counts < 10,000 to 20,000/μl or evidence of bleeding with platelet count < 50,000/μl)	Do not use microaggregate filter; component filter obtained from blood bank ABO testing not necessary unless contaminated with RBCs but is usually done; usually give 6 units at one time	Infectious diseases Allergic reactions Febrile reactions
Cryoprecipitate antihemophilic factor (AHF)	Primarily coagulation Factor VIII with 250 mg of fibrinogen and 20 to 30 percent of Factor XIII	Used primarily with classic hemophilia A patients and patients with von Willebrand's disease, Factor XIII, and fibrinogen deficiencies	Hemophilia A, von Willebrand's disease Hypofibrinogenemia Factor XIII deficiency	Repeat doses may be necessary to attain satisfactory serum level Rate of infusion; approximately 10 ml of diluted component per minute	Allergic reactions Hepatitis
Albumin	Prepared from plasma	Intravascular volume expander by increasing osmotic pressure	Hypovolemic shock Liver failure	Special administration set with vial Rate of infusion over 30 to 60 minutes	Circulatory overload Febrile reaction
Granulocytes	Prepared by centrifugation or filtration leukopheresis, which removes granulocytes from whole blood	Increase the leukocyte level	Decreased WBC usually from chemotherapy or radiation	Must be ABO compatible and Rh compatible Rate of infusion: one unit over 2 to 4 hours; closely observe for reaction	Rash Febrile reaction Hepatitis
Plasma protein	Pooled from human plasma	Intravascular volume expander by increasing osmotic pressure	Hypovolemic shock	ABO compatability not necessary Rate of infusion; over 30 to 60 minutes	Circulatory overload Febile reaction

TABLE 27–2. ABO BLOOD SYSTEM WITH ABO AND Rh COMPATIBILITY

Blood Type	Antigens on Red Cell	Antibodies in Serum
A	A	Anti-B
B	B	Anti-A
AB	A, B	Neither Anti-A nor Anti-B
O	Neither A nor B	Anti-A and Anti-B

Whole Blood	Donor					
Recipient	A	B	O	AB	Rh Positive	Rh Negative
A	x					
B		x				
O			x			
AB				x		
Rh Positive					x	x
Rh Negative						x

Red Blood Cells	Donor					
Recipient	A	B	O	AB	Rh positive	Rh negative
A	x		x			
B		x	x			
O			x			
AB	x	x	x	x		
Rh Positive					x	x
Rh Negative						x

Plasma	Donor					
Recipient	A	B	O	AB	Rh Positive	Rh Negative
A	x			x		
B		x		x		
O	x	x	x	x		
AB				x		
Rh Positive					x	x
Rh Negative					x	x

Source: From *Transfusion Therapy Guidelines for Nurses*. Washington, D.C.: NIH Publication, 1990.

Assessment

1. Observe the patient for signs and symptoms of massive hemorrhage, including pale, clammy skin; hypotension (MAP < 60 mmHg); sinus tachycardia; tachypnea (RR > 30); dyspnea; overt blood loss (estimate amount in cc's); hemodynamic pressures (PAP < 2 mmHg, PCW < 2 mmHg, and CVP < 2 mmHg); decreased cardiac index (<2.0 L/min); and hourly urine output (<30 cc/h). **Rationale:** Significant loss of blood (hemoglobin < 8 g/dl) will require replacement with whole blood or packed red blood cells.

2. Evaluate patient's CBC for oxygen-carrying capacity deficit: hemoglobin < 8 g/dl and a hematocrit < 25 percent in relation to respiratory status and arterial blood gases. **Rationale:** Significant improvement may be seen in respiratory status by raising the patient's hemoglobin level to more than 10 g/dl. Hematocrit fluctuates with fluid and electrolyte status (i.e., a low hematocrit may reflect fluid volume excess).

3. Evaluate the patient's platelet count (< 20,000/μl) and coagulation studies, including prothrombin time and partial prothrombin time (1½ to 2 times greater than the control) and fibrinogen and fibrin split products (when assessing for DIC). **Rationale:** In addition to blood for volume replacement, patient may need clotting factors to prevent further bleeding and volume loss.

4. Observe the patient for signs and symptoms of coagulopathies and/or hematologic problems, including prolonged bleeding, ecchymotic areas, pallor, jaundice, epistaxis, bleeding gums, pain in the joints, back, or bone, dyspnea, angina, hemoptysis, hematuria, menorrhagia, amenorrhagia, lethargy, and cyanosis of skin, nailbeds, gums, and/or conjunctiva. **Rationale:** Administration of blood products may lead to serious side effects evidenced by these symptoms.

5. Assess the patient's transfusion history for the presence and severity of transfusion reaction(s). **Rationale:** A direct relationship exists between the number of transfusions a patient has had and the number of circulating antibodies and thus the likelihood of a transfusion reaction.

6. Assess the patient's pretransfusion vital signs, including temperature, heart rate/rhythm, blood pressure, respiratory rate, breath sounds, and if applicable, filling pressures (i.e., CVP, PAP, and PCWP). **Rationale:** Establishes baseline values when monitoring for fluid overload and/or transfusion reaction.

Nursing Diagnoses

1. Fluid volume deficit related to blood loss. **Rationale:** Hemorrhage will lead to a decreased circulating volume with inadequate tissue perfusion.

2. Decreased cardiac output related to hypovolemia. **Rationale:** Decreased circulating volume and decreased preload will impair stroke volume. Diminished oxygen-carrying capacity may lead to cardiac ischemia.

3. Potential for injury related to antigen-antibody complex formation. **Rationale:** Administration of blood or blood products may lead to a potentially life-threatening transfusion reaction.

Planning

1. Individualize the following goals for administering blood and/or blood components:
   a. Maintain adequate hemodynamic pressure. **Rationale:** Ensures adequate tissue perfusion.
   b. Enhance oxygen-carrying capacity. **Rationale:** Improves oxygenation status and cardiac output.
   c. Correct coagulation deficiencies. **Rationale:** Promotes hemostasis.

2. Ensure patency of the peripheral intravenous line (bore size minimum is 20 gauge; an 18-gauge is preferred) or subclavian catheter. **Rationale:** Flow at high pressure of blood through smaller-gauge

needles may damage red blood cells. For infusing whole blood or red blood cells, an 18- or 19-gauge needle gives an acceptable flow rate without discomfort to the patient.

3. Prepare all necessary equipment and supplies. **Rationale:** Assembly of all necessary equipment will facilitate prompt administration of blood and blood products.
   a. Appropriate administration set for blood/blood component to be transfused.
   b. 0.9% normal saline solution for intravenous administration (for whole blood and/or packed red blood cell administration).
   c. One alcohol prep.
   d. One 19-gauge needle.
   e. One set of examination gloves.
   f. Hemodynamic monitoring equipment (as applicable): blood pressure cuff/arterial line, central venous pressure manometer, and pulmonary artery catheter for measurement of PAP, PCW, and CVP.
   g. Stethoscope.
   h. Thermometer.
   i. Blood pump, if applicable.
   j. Blood warmer, if applicable.

4. Prepare the patient.
   a. Explain the procedure and the reason for administration to patient. **Rationale:** Reduces anxiety and provides opportunity for patient to ask questions.
   b. Explain the signs and symptoms of a transfusion reaction. **Rationale:** Patient may be the first to sense signs and symptoms of a transfusion reaction.

Implementation

Steps	Rationale	Special Considerations
Preparation		
1. Verify physician order for transfusion.	Required for transfusion therapy.	Physician order should include name of the specific blood component, amount, and duration of infusion.
2. Ascertain that a current type and crossmatch are available in the blood bank.	Type and crossmatch specimens are usually valid for 24 to 48 hours. Check your institution's policy for the number of days the type and crossmatch are valid.	
3. If type and crossmatch are not current or present, obtain a blood specimen for type and crossmatch and send to the blood bank.	Blood bank must have current specimen for processing.	Determine if the patient, family, or friends have donated blood/blood products for transfusion. If so, then alert the blood bank that a "directed unit" should be available.
4. Have patient sign consent form (if applicable).	Some institutions require this before administering transfusion.	
5. Obtain blood/blood component from blood bank.	Blood/blood products should be administered within 20 minutes of arrival on the unit unless stored in a special refrigerator where the temperature is maintained at 1 to 6° C.	
6. With another registered nurse, check blood/blood component record/label against the medical record/patient identification band, verifying the following data: a. Patient's name and hospital number. b. Type of blood component. c. Patient's blood group and Rh type. d. Donor's blood group and Rh type. e. Unit number.	Two registered nurses verifying the information reduces the risk of the patient receiving the wrong blood.	If there are any errors or inconsistencies, *do not administer the blood/blood product. Notify the blood bank immediately.* Patients receiving numerous transfusions over a period of time may need irradiated blood/blood products. Blood is irradiated so that lymphocytes will not proliferate and cause graft-versus-host disease.

Table continues on following page

Steps	Rationale	Special Considerations
f. Expiration date.		
g. Any abnormal color or appearance of the blood/blood component. *Note*: Check your institution's policy and procedure for checking blood/blood products prior to transfusion.		
7. Both registered nurses sign the transfusion forms.	Documents that proper verification was done.	A physician and registered nurse may verify blood/blood component product for administration. *Both* must sign the verification forms.
8. Wash hands.	Reduces transmission of microorganisms.	
9. Don gloves.	Universal precautions.	
10. Prepare administration set:		
a. For Y-tubing administration set:	Y-tubing is used with whole blood/packed red blood cell transfusions. Prevents spillage.	Y-set allows for easy switching to normal saline to flush the line after the transfusion.
(1) Turn roller clamps off.	Allows for filling of drip chamber.	
(2) Spike the 0.9% normal saline, open clamp between unit and drip chamber, fill drip chamber, covering filter, and prime the tubing.	Covering filter prevents hemolysis as blood drops from bag.	Y-tubing with filter can be used to administer a maximum of 2 units of whole blood or packed red blood cells.
(3) Close clamp to 0.9% normal saline.	Accesses contents.	You may fill the blood bag with 50 cc of 0.9% normal saline to decrease viscosity.
(4) Attach a 19-gauge needle to the distal end of the tubing.	For insertion into primary infusion.	
(5) Spike the unit of blood, keeping roller clamp closed.	Prevents spillage of blood.	
b. For single-tubing administration set:	Used for administration of fresh-frozen plasma.	Platelets, cryoprecipitate (AHF), albumin, granulocytes, and Plasmanate have specific infusion sets for administration that are supplied by either blood bank or pharmacy.
(1) Turn roller clamp off.	Prevents spillage.	
(2) Spike unit of blood.	Accesses unit.	
(3) Open clamp between unit and drip chamber, and fill drip chamber, covering filter.	Prevents damage to constituents.	
(4) Open roller clamp, and prime tubing.	Prevents air embolus.	
(5) Close roller clamp.	Prevents spillage.	
(6) Attach a 19-gauge needle to distal end of tubing.	For insertion into primary infusion.	

Table continues on following page

Steps	Rationale	Special Considerations
11. Cleanse Y-port of primary tubing proximal to the intravenous insertion site with an alcohol wipe.	Reduces transmission of microorganisms.	Y-port proximal to insertion site is selected to decrease the possibility of precipitation or hemolysis in primary tubing.
12. Insert needle into Y-port, and clamp off primary infusion.	Decreases potential for hemolysis or precipitation in tubing.	Maintain aseptic technique. Patient may continue intravenous therapy in other access sites.
13. Release roller clamp from blood bag.	Allows transfusion to proceed.	
14. Adjust clamp to infuse 10-15 gtts/minute for the first 15 minutes.	Ensures that patient will receive only a small amount of blood/blood product if reaction occurs.	
15. Monitor the patient continuously for the first 15 to 30 minutes of the transfusion.	Reactions usually occur within the first 15 to 30 minutes of infusion.	If signs and symptoms of a transfusion reaction occur (i.e., chills, flushing, rigor, itching, dyspnea, rash, urticaria, temperature spike), stop the infusion (see Skill 27–2).
16. Monitor the patient's vital signs every 15 minutes for the first hour then every half hour until the unit is infused.	Detects changes that suggest a transfusion reaction.	Monitor vital signs in this manner for each unit transfused.
17. Adjust the rate to infuse as prescribed. Transfusion should be completed within a maximum of 4 hours of initiating the infusion.	Blood begins to clot after 4 hours; likelihood of bacterial contamination markedly increases after 4 hours.	For patients on fluid restrictions, the blood bank can split units so that the chance of fluid volume excess is reduced.
18. For whole blood and packed red blood cell transfusions, at the completion of the infusion, flush the primary tubing with 0.9% normal saline.	Allows for infusion of blood in tubing.	
19. Clamp blood administration set, and adjust flow of primary infusion to prescribed rate.	Continues primary infusion.	

Evaluation

Evaluate the patient's response to transfusion, including hemoglobin and hematocrit levels; intravascular volume, reflected in increased blood pressure; filling pressures (CVP, PAP, PCWP), and cardiac index; decreased heart rate; increased urine output; and improved oxygenation/respiratory status. **Rationale:** Transfusion improves oxygen carrying capacity and provides fluid resuscitation in massive hemorrhage. One unit of packed red blood cells should raise the non-bleeding adult's hemoglobin level by 1 g/dL and the hematocrit by 3%.

Expected Outcomes

1. Hemoglobin and hematocrit improve. **Rationale:** Validates that transfusion has been adequate or that additional transfusions are necessary.
2. Stabilization of the hemodynamic status. **Rationale:** Reflects an adequate circulating volume.
3. Coagulopathies are corrected. **Rationale:** Bleeding will stop, since the blood product provides the necessary components to correct inadequacies in the coagulation cascade.
4. Absence of a transfusion reaction. **Rationale:** Patient has tolerated transfusion without adverse effects.

Unexpected Outcomes

1. Manifestation of signs and symptoms of a transfusion reaction. **Rationale:** Patient has reacted to transfusion as a foreign body.
2. Fluid volume excess. **Rationale:** Transfusion was either administered too quickly or patient's cardiovascular system was not able to handle the volume.
3. Development of a pyrogenic reaction. **Rationale:** Presence of bacterial contamination in the blood.
4. Hyperkalemia. **Rationale:** Stored blood develops a high potassium level due to red blood cell lysis.
5. Hypocalcemia. **Rationale:** The citrate ion in stored blood binds with calcium and is excreted from the body.

Documentation

Documentation in the patient record should include the pretransfusion assessment, date and time transfusion(s) was initiated and terminated, baseline and serial vital signs, transfusion record validated by two registered nurses, type and amount of blood/blood product administered, patient's response to transfusion (including laboratory data before and after transfusion), and any unexpected outcomes and interventions taken. **Rationale:** Documents nursing interventions, patient response, and expected and unexpected outcomes.

Patient/Family Education

1. Discuss the type of blood component administered, the rationale for its administration, and the signs and symptoms of a transfusion reaction to both patient and family. **Rationale:** Reaction to blood/blood products can occur hours after a transfusion.

2. Evaluate the patient's need for long-term blood/blood product administration. **Rationale:** Patient may need to carry a record of transfusions, history/severity of transfusion reactions, and requirement for irradiated blood/blood products to prevent a reaction.

Performance Checklist
Skill 27–1: Blood and Blood Component Administration

Critical Behaviors	Complies yes	no
PREPARATION		
1. Verify physician order for transfusion.		
2. Ascertain current type and crossmatch.		
3. If no type and crossmatch are available, obtain specimen for type and crossmatch.		
4. Have patient sign consent form, if applicable.		
5. Obtain blood/blood component from blood bank.		
6. Check blood/blood component with another registered nurse, verifying identification data: a. Patient's name and hospital number. b. Type of blood component. c. Patient's blood group and Rh type. d. Donor's blood group and Rh type. e. Unit number. f. Expiration date. g. Any abnormal color or appearance of the blood/blood component.		
7. Both nurses sign transfusion form.		
8. Wash hands.		
9. Don gloves.		

10. Prepare administration set:
a. For Y-tubing administration set:
  (1) Turn roller clamp off.
  (2) Spike the 0.9% normal saline, open clamp between unit and drip chamber, fill drip chamber, covering filter, and prime tubing.
  (3) Close clamp to 0.9% normal saline.
  (4) Attach a 19-gauge needle to the distal end of the tubing.
  (5) Spike the unit of blood, keeping roller clamp closed.
b. For single-tubing administration set:
  (1) Turn roller clamp off.
  (2) Spike unit of blood.
  (3) Open clamp between unit and drip chamber, and fill drip chamber, covering filter.
  (4) Open roller clamp, and prime tubing.
  (5) Close roller clamp.
  (6) Attach 19-gauge needle to distal end of tubing.		

11. Cleanse Y-port of primary tubing proximal to the intravenous insertion site.		
12. Insert needle into Y-port, and clamp off primary infusion.		
13. Release roller clamp from blood bag.		
14. Adjust rate to infuse 10 to 15 gtts/min for the first 15 to 30 minutes.		
15. Stay with patient and monitor for signs of reaction for first 15 to 30 minutes.		

Table continues on following page

Critical Behaviors	Complies	
	yes	no
16. Monitor vital signs every 15 minutes for the first hour and then every half hour until unit is infused.		
17. Adjust rate as prescribed but do not exceed 4 hours.		
18. At completion, flush tubing with 0.9% normal saline.		
19. Clamp line, and adjust flow of primary infusion.		
20. Remove and discard gloves.		
21. Wash hands.		
22. Document procedure in the patient record.		

SKILL 27–2

Transfusion Reaction

Transfusion of blood and blood products is generally a safe and effective method for correcting hematologic deficits, but adverse reactions can and do occur. An antigen-antibody reaction causes an acute hemolytic transfusion reaction and is mediated by neuroendocrine responses and by activating the complement and coagulation cascade. Clinically ominous events may include shock, disseminated intravascular coagulopathy (DIC), and acute tubular necrosis (ATN). The risks of granulocyte transfusions generally outweigh their benefits, so they are infused under very special circumstances, as in the bone marrow transplant patient whose white blood cell count remains severely depressed or nonexistent. Irradiating blood decreases the risk of a reaction by preventing the lymphocytes from proliferating and causing graft-versus-host disease.

Purpose

The nurse monitors the patient for a transfusion reaction to

1. Promptly identify early signs and symptoms of a reaction (see Tables 27–3 and 27–4).
2. Prevent life-threatening sequelae should a reaction occur.

Prerequisite Knowledge and Skills

Prior to intervening in the event of a transfusion reaction, the nurse should understand

1. Principles of ABO typing and Rh factor determination.
2. Principles of fluid and electrolyte balance.
3. Pharmacotherapy for a transfusion reaction.
4. Universal precautions.

The nurse should be able to perform

1. Vital signs assessment.
2. Respiratory system assessment.
3. Cardiovascular system assessment.
4. Oxygen administration (see Skills 2–1 and 2–2).
5. Administration of intravenous medications by bolus (IV push) (see Skill 33–2).
6. Cardiopulmonary resuscitation.
7. Universal precautions (see Skill 35–1).

Assessment

1. Observe the patient for life-threatening symptoms, including respiratory distress, hypotension, abdominal cramps, shock, and loss of consciousness. **Rationale:** Signs and symptoms of anaphylactic reaction usually occur immediately upon administration of only a few milliliters of blood. Patient remains afebrile.
2. Observe the patient for fever, chills, hypotension, lumbar pain, headache, palpitations, and malaise. **Rationale:** Indications of a nonhemolytic reaction, where fever is caused from patient's antibodies reacting with donor's antigens; also may be an indication of bacterial reaction, since bacteria can be transmitted through blood.
3. Observe the patient for hypothermia and cardiac dysrhythmias. **Rationale:** Occurs with the administration of large amounts of cold blood, which affects the conduction system of the heart.
4. Observe the patient for dyspnea, cyanosis, and elevated filling pressures. **Rationale:** Signs and symptoms of fluid volume excess leading to pump failure. Occurs in patients with congestive heart failure and elderly patients with limited cardiac reserve secondary to the oncotic force of the colloids. Diuretics may be necessary.
5. Assess the patient for local erythema, hives, and urticaria. **Rationale:** Signs and symptoms of an allergic reaction, since donor's blood contains antigens. Plasma may cause urticaria reactions. Diphenhydramine and acetaminophen may be given prior to the transfusion to counteract this effect.
6. Observe the patient for cardiac dysrhythmias, hypokalemia, alkalosis, circumoral tingling, and hypotension. **Rationale:** Signs and symptoms of citrate toxicity (citrate is used as an anticoagulant in whole blood and packed red blood cells). Occurs with rapid and massive transfusions of whole blood and packed red blood cells.

TABLE 27–3 SIGNS AND SYMPTOMS OF A TRANSFUSION REACTION FOR BOTH CONSCIOUS AND UNCONSCIOUS PATIENTS

Conscious Patients		*Unconscious Patient:*

General:
  Fever (rise of 1°C or 2°F)
  Chills
  Muscle aches, pain
  Back pain
  Chest pain
  Headache
  Heat at site of infusion or
    along vein
 	
Nervous system:
  Apprehension, impending
    sense of doom
  Tingling, numbness
 	
Respiratory system:
  Respiratory rate:
    Tachypnea
    Apnea
    Dyspnea
    Cough
    Wheezing
    Rales
 	
Gastrointestinal system:
  Nausea
  Vomiting
  Pain, abdominal cramping
  Diarrhea (may be bloody)
	Cardiovascular system:
	  Heart rate:
	    Brachycardia
	    Tachycardia
	  Blood pressure:
	    Hypotension, shock
	    Hypertension
	  Peripheral circulation:
	    Color cyanosis, facial
	      flushing
	    Temperature: cool/
	      clammy; hot/flushed/
	      dry
	    Edema
	  Bleeding:
	    Generalized DIC
	    Oozing at surgical site
	
	Renal System:
	  Changes in urine
	    volume:
	    Oliguria, anuria
	    Renal failure
	  Changes in urine color:
	    Dark, concentrated
	    Shades of red, brown,
	      amber
	    May indicate the
	      presence in urine of
	      RBCs (hematuria)
	      or of free
	      hemoglobin
	      (hemoglobinuria)
	
	Integumentary system:
	  Rashes, hives (urticaria),
	    swelling
	  Itching
	  Diaphoresis
		Weak Pulse
		Fever
		Hypotension
		Visible hemoglobinuria
		Increased operative
		  bleeding (oozing at
		  surgical site)
		Vasomotor instability
		  (tachycardia,
		  brachycardia,
		  or hypotension)
		Oliguria/anuria

Source: From *Transfusion Therapy Guidelines for Nurses*. Washington, D.C.: NIH, 1990.

Citrate combines with calcium and is excreted in the urine.

7. Continue to monitor the patient for fever and chills for 4 to 6 hours after the transfusion is completed. **Rationale:** Delayed hemolytic reaction (antibody reacts with antigen).

Nursing Diagnoses

1. Potential for injury related to antigen–antibody reaction. **Rationale:** Reactions almost always are due to ABO mismatch.

2. Potential for decreased cardiac output related to the antigen–antibody formation activating the neuroendocrine response, which increases capillary permeability and dilates arterioles. **Rationale:** Severe transfusion reactions can lead to shock and progress to cardiovascular collapse.

3. Impaired gas exchange related to ventilation–perfusion abnormality. **Rationale:** Catecholamine release as a response to the antigen–antibody reaction that produces vasoconstriction in the lungs.

4. Hyperthermia related to transfusion reaction. **Rationale:** The temperature is elevated as a result of alloimmunization.

Planning

1. Individualize the following goals for intervening in the event of a transfusion reaction:
   a. Limit the severity of the transfusion reaction. **Rationale:** The severity of a transfusion reaction is in part dependent on the amount of blood infused. If a reaction is suspected, *stop the transfusion immediately*.
   b. Adequate oxygenation. **Rationale:** Severe ven-

TABLE 27–4 ACUTE TRANSFUSION REACTIONS

Reaction Type	Onset	Signs and Symptoms	Clinical Action	Cause	Prevention
Mild allergic	Within 6 hours of transfusion	Localized urticaria (hives) Pruritus Rash	*Stop transfusion* Keep IV open with 0.9% NaCl Antihistamines may be administered (PO, IM, IV) If reaction subsides, transfusion may be completed Consult physician	Allergic reaction to plasma-soluble antigen contained in blood product	Treat prophylactically with antihistamines
Severe allergic (anaphylactic)	Immediately, with only a few milliliters of blood infused	Dyspnea, wheezing, tachypnea, cyanosis Hypotension Tachycardia Nausea, vomiting, cramping	*Stop transfusion* Keep IV open with 0.9% NaCl Epinephrine and/or steroids as prescribed *Caution:* May become medical emergency—support blood pressure and maintain open airway *Notify physician immediately*	Idiosyncratic reaction in patients with IgA deficiency; sensitization to IgA through previous transfusion or pregnancy	Transfuse thoroughly washed red blood cell products, from which all plasma has been removed. Consider using blood from IgA deficient donor.
Acute hemolytic	Usually during first 5 to 15 minutes, but may occur any time during transfusion	Rigors Fever Flank pain Hypotension Unexplained bleeding Oliguria Hemoglobinuria Hemoglobinemia	*Stop transfusion* Keep IV open with 0.9% NaCl Induce diuresis *Caution:* May become medical emergency; support blood pressure and maintain open airway *Notify physician immediately*	ABO group incompatibility	Thoroughly verify and document patient identification from type and crossmatch to component infusion.
Febrile	Within 6 hours of transfusion	Chills Unexpected fever [over 100.4°F (38°C) or > 1.8°F (1°C) rise]	*Stop transfusion* Keep IV open with 0.9% NaCl Febrile reactions usually respond to antipyretics. Avoid aspirin in thrombocytopenic patients	Allergic reaction to plasma-soluble antigen contained in blood product	Leukocyte-poor blood products may be considered.

tilation–perfusion abnormalities may result in respiratory distress requiring intubation and mechanical ventilation.

   c. Provide adequate intravenous hydration to prevent renal damage. **Rationale:** The antigen–antibody complex may cause acute tubular necrosis.

2. Prepare all necessary equipment and supplies. **Rationale:** Assembly of all the necessary equipment at the bedside ensures that the transfusion reaction will be treated efficiently.

   a. Intravenous solution (prescribed by physician).

   b. Intravenous administration set (macrodrip tubing).

   c. Flowmeter for oxygen.

   d. Nasal cannula or Venturi mask.

   e. Stethoscope.

   f. Blood pressure cuff or arterial line.

   g. Urine specimen container.

   h. Vacutainer holder and needle.

   i. Blood specimen tubes.

   j. Thermometer.

   k. Emergency drug box.

   l. Emergency cart.

   m. Exam gloves.

3. Prepare the patient.

   a. Explain that the patient may be having a reaction to the transfusion. **Rationale:** Promotes patient

understanding of the signs and symptoms being experienced.
b. Explain the procedure for treating transfusion

reaction. **Rationale:** Decreases anxiety and promotes cooperation.

Implementation

Steps	Rationale	Special Considerations
1. *Stop the transfusion.*	Prevents the patient from receiving additional blood/blood product.	Severity of the reaction is related to amount of product infused.
2. Wash hands.	Reduces transmission of microorganisms.	
3. Don gloves.	Universal precautions.	
4. Disconnect blood tubing from primary intravenous line.	Remaining blood/blood product should be sent back to the blood bank with tubing attached.	Institution policies and protocols regarding the disposition of the blood/blood product vary. Check with your blood bank.
5. Replace primary intravenous tubing with new tubing.	Prevents patient from receiving additional blood/blood product that may be in the primary tubing.	Macrodrip tubing is used should the patient become hypotensive and require rapid volume replacement.
6. Infuse primary intravenous solution at prescribed rate or as directed by the physician.	Ensures patency of intravenous catheter.	
7. Obtain urine specimen.	Determines presence of hemolysis.	Urine specimen is sent to blood bank with suspect unit of blood/blood products.
8. Obtain two blood specimens for type and crossmatch.	First sample is crossmatched with pretransfusion sample to determine if correct blood was administered. Second sample is examined for hemolysis.	Usually, blood specimens are sent to blood bank with the suspect unit of blood/blood products.
9. Complete specific forms for transfusion reaction.	Documents transfusion reaction and actions taken.	Most institutions have specific forms that are completed when a transfusion reaction is suspected.
10. Return blood/blood product to blood bank.	Allows blood bank to confirm presence or absence of a transfusion reaction.	Patient receiving multiple transfusions over time (AIDS, oncology) may demonstrate signs and symptoms of a transfusion reaction; however, laboratory analysis may not verify that a reaction has occurred. You may be instructed to rehang the unit of blood/blood product and monitor the patient closely.
11. Should the patient develop signs and symptoms of shock or cardiovascular collapse:		
a. Initiate another intravenous line.	Patient may require rapid administration of intravenous fluids.	
b. Prepare and administer intravenous solutions and emergency medications as directed.	Antihistamines and antibiotics are commonly administered in a transfusion reaction.	Emergency medications may be given IV push.
c. Monitor vital signs continuously.	Detects further respiratory/cardiovascular compromise.	Monitor blood pressure, heart rate/rhythm, respiratory rate/rhythm, breath sounds, and urine output.

Table continues on following page

Steps	Rationale	Special Considerations
d. Administer oxygen therapy as directed.	Corrects hypoxemia.	
e. Initiate CPR in the event of respiratory/cardiac arrest.	Life-threatening intervention.	
12. Remove and discard gloves.	Universal precautions.	
13. Wash hands.	Reduces transmission of microorganisms.	

Evaluation

Continue to assess the patient for fever with or without chills, rigor, dyspnea, hypotension, oliguria, shock, abnormal bleeding, chest pain, back/flank pain, and headache, and evaluate laboratory data for hemoglobinemia and hemoglobinuria. **Rationale:** These signs and symptoms indicate an acute hemolytic reaction. Lysis of red blood cells occurs and the body's intrinsic clotting cascade is activated, thus initiating DIC (disseminated intravascular coagulation). These reactions impair and may destroy renal function.

Expected Outcome

Vital signs remain within patient's baseline, and laboratory values are within normal limits. **Rationale:** Prompt recognition and treatment of a transfusion reaction will prevent damage to the cardiac, respiratory, and renal systems.

Unexpected Outcomes

1. Impaired renal function. **Rationale:** Hemolytic reactions may result in permanent damage to the renal tubules.
2. Respiratory/cardiac arrest. **Rationale:** Patient has an overwhelming response to the antigen–antibody reaction; early signs and symptoms of transfusion reaction were not detected with progression to complete cardiovascular collapse.

Documentation

Documentation in the patient record should include the date and exact time signs and symptoms of a transfusion reaction were observed, the assessment findings, the name of the physician notified, the interventions taken, and the patient's response. **Rationale:** Documents nursing interventions and patient responses.

Patient/Family Education

1. Explain transfusion reaction and that the patient and family should include this information when asked for medical/nursing histories. **Rationale:** Promotes patient and family understanding of transfusion reaction and will provide information of risk of transfusion reaction to future caregivers.
2. Evaluate the patient's need for long-term blood/blood product administration. **Rationale:** Patient may need to carry a record of transfusions, history/severity of transfusion reactions, and requirement for irradiated blood/blood products to prevent a reaction.

Performance Checklist
Skill 27–2: Transfusion Reaction

Critical Behaviors	Complies yes	no
1. Stop the transfusion.		
2. Wash hands.		
3. Don gloves.		
4. Disconnect blood tubing from primary intravenous line.		
5. Replace primary intravenous tubing with new tubing.		
6. Infuse primary intravenous solution at prescribed rate.		
7. Obtain urine specimen.		
8. Obtain two blood specimens for type and crossmatch.		
9. Complete specific forms for transfusion reaction.		

Table continues on following page

Critical Behaviors	Complies	
	yes	no
10. Return blood/blood product to blood bank.		
11. If shock or cardiovascular collapse ensues,		
a. Initiate another intravenous line.		
b. Prepare and administer intravenous solutions and emergency medications as directed.		
c. Monitor vital signs continuously.		
d. Administer oxygen therapy as directed.		
e. Initiate CPR as needed.		
12. Remove and discard gloves.		
13. Wash hands.		
14. Document in the patient record.		

SKILL 27–3

Use of a Blood Pump

A blood pump is used to infuse large amounts of blood/blood products rapidly in a patient with massive hemorrhage. The blood/blood product bag is placed in a device that can be pressurized to deliver a rapid flow rate. Blood pumps should be utilized with central line catheters. Caution must be exercised if a blood pump is used with a large-bore peripheral intravenous catheter to prevent damaging the vein.

Purpose

The nurse uses a blood pump for transfusion of blood/blood products to

1. Rapidly replace blood volume.
2. Infuse viscous whole blood or packed red blood cells within a prescribed time period.

Prerequisite Knowledge and Skills

Prior to using a blood pump, the nurse should understand

1. Principles of fluid and electrolyte balance.
2. Anatomy and physiology of the cardiovascular system.
3. Principles of hemodynamics.
4. Aseptic technique.
5. Principles of blood and blood product administration.
6. Universal precautions.

The nurse should be able to perform

1. Proper handwashing technique (see Skill 35–5).
2. Administration of blood and blood products (see Skill 27–1).
3. Vital signs assessment.

4. Cardiovascular system assessment.
5. Respiratory system assessment.
6. Assessment of fluid and electrolyte balance.
7. Universal precautions.

Assessment

1. Observe the patient for signs and symptoms of shock in the presence of massive hemorrhage (internal or external), including hypotension, decreased filling pressures (if applicable, CVP, PAP, and PCWP), tachycardia, cold and clammy extremities, pale skin color, tachypnea, dyspnea, and decreased urine output. **Rationale:** Massive hemorrhaging will result in signs and symptoms of a decreased circulating volume.
2. Assess the patient's complete blood count for hemoglobin and hematocrit values. **Rationale:** Prior to fluid resuscitation, the hemoglobin and hematocrit levels will provide an estimate of blood loss.

Nursing Diagnoses

1. Decreased tissue perfusion of major organs related to massive hemorrhage. **Rationale:** Major blood loss results in hypovolemic shock.
2. Decreased cardiac output related to hypovolemia. **Rationale:** Decreased circulating volume will impair stroke volume and thus the cardiac output.
3. Impaired gas exchange related to inadequate amounts of circulating hemoglobin. **Rationale:** Loss of hemoglobin decreases the oxygen-carrying capacity with resultant hypoxemia.

Planning

1. Individualize the following goals for use of a blood pump:

a. Maintain adequate circulating volume. **Rationale:** Major blood loss results in hypovolemic shock.
b. Maintain adequate tissue perfusion. **Rationale:** Shock state diminishes perfusion to vital organs and peripheral tissues.
c. Maintain adequate oxygenation. **Rationale:** Major blood loss decreases oxygen-carrying capacity.

2. Prepare all the necessary equipment and supplies. **Rationale:** Assembly of all necessary equipment and supplies allows for rapid infusion of blood/blood products with the blood pump.
a. Blood administration set.
b. Blood pump.
c. Blood/blood product for transfusion.

d. 0.9% normal saline for infusion (with whole blood or packed red blood cell transfusions).
e. Blood pressure cuff.
f. Stethoscope.
g. Thermometer.
h. Cardiac monitor.
i. Exam gloves.

3. Prepare the patient.
a. Explain the procedure to the patient. **Rationale:** Reduces anxiety and promotes cooperation.
b. Assess the intravenous site for redness, swelling, or pain. **Rationale:** Signs and symptoms of infiltration, which may be the cause of sluggish flow. The intravenous catheter must be restarted if infiltrated.

Implementation

Steps	Rationale	Special Considerations
1. Wash hands.	Reduces transmission of microorganisms.	
2. For peripheral administration, ascertain that the venous catheter is 18-gauge or larger.	Large-bore catheter allows for rapid administration and prevents hemolysis.	Blood pumps *cannot* be used on peripheral venous catheters smaller than 18 gauge.
3. Don gloves.	Universal precautions.	
4. Obtain and prepare blood/blood product for administration, insert into Y-port proximal to the insertion site, and open roller clamp on blood administration set (see Skill 27–1).	Administration rate will be adjusted with pressure of pump not roller clamp.	Blood/blood product should be assembled before inserting into pump.
5. Deflate the external blood pump cover.	Allows for easy placement of blood/blood product bag.	
6. Guide blood bag through mesh or plastic covering of the blood pump so that the *entire* blood bag remains behind the mesh/plastic panel.	Allows pressure to be evenly applied to blood/blood product bag.	Do *not* allow the top of the unit to appear above the mesh or plastic covering since it will interfere with flow.
7. Secure unit in place with fabric strap or Velcro closure, and hang from IV pole.	Prevents unit from slipping out of blood pump when hung from IV pole.	
8. Inflate blood pump to achieve the desired rate of flow.	Pressure of blood pump is used to adjust flow rate.	*Pressure should not exceed 300 mmHg to avoid damaging the red blood cells, rupturing the blood bag, dislodging the intravenous catheter, or injuring the vein.* Patient may complain of discomfort in his or her extremity if a peripheral catheter is used (as with administration of viscous blood). If appropriate, decrease pressure to maintain patient comfort.
9. Assess the IV site for redness, swelling, or pain.	Pressurized infusion can cause catheter dislodgment.	If signs or symptoms of infiltration occur, *stop the infusion*, remove the catheter, and initiate another intravenous catheter infusion site.

Table continues on following page

10. Monitor vital signs and urine output.	Rapid transfusion of cold blood can cause cardiac dysrhythmias.	Note any signs and symptoms of a transfusion reaction (see Skill 27–2).
11. When transfusion is complete, deflate the blood pump infusion device, close the roller clamp to the blood bag, and open the roller clamp to the 0.9% normal saline.	Pressure is not needed to infuse normal saline.	Normal saline is the only intravenous solution compatible with blood and blood components.
12. Flush primary infusion tubing with normal saline.	Allows patient to receive all the blood.	
13. For transfusion of additional units of blood/blood products, repeat steps 5 through 10.	Multiple transfusions will be required to treat hemorrhagic shock.	Blood administration set/filter can be used to infuse a *maximum* of 2 units.
14. When all transfusions are completed, remove the unit of blood/blood product from the blood pump, and discard the remainder and the administration set in appropriate receptacle or as per your institution's policy.	Universal precautions.	
15. Regulate primary intravenous infusion at prescribed rate.	Provides fluid resuscitation.	Administration of crystalloids and colloids is used in conjunction with blood replacement.
16. Remove and discard gloves.	Universal precautions.	
17. Wash hands.	Reduces transmission of microorganisms.	

Evaluation

1. Continuously monitor the patient's blood pressure, filling pressures (CVP, PAP, and PCWP, if applicable), heart rate/rhythm, urine output, and respiratory rate/rhythm. **Rationale:** Transfusion therapy should adequately restore circulating volume.
2. Assess the patient's hemoglobin and hematocrit. **Rationale:** Verifies effectiveness of transfusion or need for additional replacement.
3. Assess the patient for signs and symptoms of a transfusion reaction (see Skill 27–2). **Rationale:** Blood/blood product transfusions are foreign to the patient's immune system.

Expected Outcomes

1. Restoration of the circulating volume. **Rationale:** Whole blood or packed red blood cell transfusion increases intravascular volume.
2. Improved oxygenation status. **Rationale:** Blood replacement increases hemoglobin level and thus oxygen-carrying capacity.

Unexpected Outcomes

1. Signs and symptoms of a transfusion reaction. **Rationale:** Blood replacement constitutes an infusion of a foreign substance.
2. Cardiopulmonary arrest. **Rationale:** Rate of transfusion is not adequate to replace hemorrhage at rate of loss, resulting in a circulating volume incompatible with life.
3. Cardiac dysrhythmias. **Rationale:** Rapid replacement with cold blood can affect the cardiac conduction system.

Documentation

Documentation in the patient record should include date and time infusion is initiated and completed, the type and amount of blood/blood product infused, use of the blood pump, patient's response to the transfusion, and signs and symptoms of any unexpected outcomes and interventions taken. **Rationale:** Documents nursing interventions and patient responses.

Patient/Family Education

1. Explain the rationale for using a blood pump to both patient and family. **Rationale:** Reassures the patient and family that aggressive resuscitation measures are being instituted.
2. Explain that the patient may feel discomfort in his or her extremity if the blood pump is used with a peripheral intravenous catheter. **Rationale:** Pressure is applied to the vein, which may be uncomfortable for the patient.

Performance Checklist
Skill 27–3: Use of a Blood Pump

Critical Behaviors	Complies yes	no
1. Wash hands.		
2. Ascertain that the peripheral venous catheter is 18-gauge or larger.		
3. Don gloves.		
4. Obtain and prepare blood/blood product as per Skill 27–1.		
5. Deflate the blood pump.		
6. Guide blood bag through mesh or plastic covering of the blood pump so that the entire blood bag remains behind the mesh/plastic panel.		
7. Secure unit in place with fabric strap or Velcro closure, and hang from IV pole.		
8. Inflate blood pump bag to achieve the desired flow rate.		
9. Assess the IV site for infiltration.		
10. Monitor vital signs and urine output.		
11. When transfusion is complete, deflate the blood pump infusion device, close the roller clamp to the blood bag, and open the roller clamp to the 0.9% normal saline.		
12. Flush primary infusion tubing with normal saline.		
13. For infusion of additional units, repeat steps 5 through 10.		
14. When all transfusions are complete, remove unit and discard the remainder of the equipment in appropriate receptacle.		
15. Regulate the primary intravenous line at prescribed rate.		
16. Remove and discard gloves.		
17. Wash hands.		
18. Document procedure in the patient record.		

SKILL 27–4

Determination of Microhematocrit via Centrifuge

Hematocrit measures the percent of the total volume of red blood cells within a given blood sample. It is the ratio of the volume of red blood cells to that of whole blood expressed as a percentage. The hematocrit is determined by centrifuging an anticoagulated blood sample under standardized conditions. Hematocrit is useful in evaluating fluid and electrolyte status, in evaluating and classifying various types of anemia, and in evaluating fluid resuscitation in shock.

Microhematocrit via centrifuge uses a capillary tube of blood to obtain the hematocrit value. The procedure is usually done within the critical-care unit and takes approximately 5 minutes to complete. The quick result provides assessment data for immediate intervention.

Purpose

The nurse determines the microhematocrit by centrifuge to

1. Ascertain the hematocrit.
2. Provide data for assessing fluid and electrolyte balance.

Prerequisite Knowledge and Skills

Prior to determining the microhematocrit by centrifuge, the nurse should understand

1. Principles of fluid and electrolyte balance.
2. Principles of transfusion therapy.
3. Universal precautions.

The nurse should be able to perform

1. Proper handwashing technique (see Skill 35–5).
2. Universal precautions (see Skill 35–1).
3. Phlebotomy.

Assessment

1. Observe the patient for signs and symptoms of fluid and electrolyte imbalance. Signs of fluid volume deficit include dry mucous membranes, decreased skin turgor, lethargy, hyperventilation, decreased pulmonary artery pressures, increased urine specific gravity, and hypotension. Signs of fluid volume excess include edema, dyspnea, normal skin turgor, crackles, jugular vein distension, hypertension, decreased urine specific gravity, and elevated pulmonary artery pressures. **Rationale:** Hematocrit is below normal with fluid volume excess and above normal with dehydration or massive red blood cell hemolysis (major burn).

2. Observe the patient for signs and symptoms of anemia or hemorrhage, including restlessness, dizziness, syncope, severe headaches, disorientation, pallor, diaphoresis, rapid thready pulse, hypotension, and rapid and deep respirations that progress to shallow respirations. **Rationale:** Hematocrit provides a relative indication of the degree of anemia or hemorrhage. The hemoglobin level more accurately measures the red blood cell count.

Nursing Diagnoses

1. Fluid volume deficit related to decreased intravascular volume. **Rationale:** Decreased circulating volume can result from hemorrhage or loss of intravascular fluid to the extracellular compartment.

2. Decreased cardiac output related to hypovolemia. **Rationale:** Hypovolemia leads to inadequate preload and stroke volume.

3. Fluid volume excess related to an increased circulating volume. **Rationale:** Congestive heart failure, overinfusion of intravenous fluids, or return of "third-spaced" fluids to the intravascular compartment increases the circulating volume and may have a "dilutional effect" on the hematocrit.

Planning

1. Individualize the following goals for determining the patient's microhematocrit:
   a. Maintain fluid balance. **Rationale:** Hematocrit level contributes to the assessment of fluid and electrolyte status.
   b. Maintain an adequate intravascular volume. **Rationale:** Hematocrit provides assessment data for determining fluid volume deficit/excess and/or therapeutic effects of transfusion therapy.

2. Prepare all necessary equipment and supplies. **Rationale:** Assembly of all the necessary equipment ensures that the microhematocrit will be determined quickly and efficiently.
   a. Two heparinized capillary tubes (75 × 1.55 mm internal diameter).
   b. Standardized high-speed centrifuge.
   c. Sealing clay.
   d. Hematocrit linear scale for direct reading (Fig. 27–1 for Adams Micro-Hematocrit Reader).
   e. One 3-cc syringe.
   f. One 21-gauge needle.
   g. Tourniquet (if venipuncture is required).
   h. Exam gloves.

3. Prepare the patient and family by explaining the procedure and the potential for discomfort (if venipuncture is necessary). **Rationale:** Minimizes anxiety and promotes patient cooperation.

Implementation

Steps	Rationale	Special Considerations
1. Wash hands.	Reduces transmission of microorganisms.	
2. Don gloves.	Universal precautions.	
3. Obtain blood sample. If patient does not have an arterial line, perform venipuncture or fingerstick.	Provides blood for analysis.	
4. Keeping the index finger of the dominant hand over one end of the capillary tube, place the other end at hub of syringe to fill with blood, remove index finger, and reposition it again when the tube is filled within 5 to 10 mm of the end of the tube. Repeat with second capillary tube.	The small diameter of the capillary tube creates a pressure that causes the tube to fill. Proper amount is necessary for accuracy. Two tubes are necessary to balance the centrifuge.	

Table continues on following page

Steps	Rationale	Special Considerations
5. Place one end of each capillary tube into special sealing clay.	Capillary tubes must be sealed to centrifuge.	Make sure sealing clay forms a straight edge across interior of the tube.
6. Place one capillary tube in the centrifuge with the sealed end directed outward, and then place the second tube directly opposite the first tube on the centrifuge head.	Avoids spillage of blood and balances the machine.	
7. Place the cover on the centrifuge, turn the machine on, and set the automatic timer to 5 minutes at 10,000 to 15,000 × gravity.	Separates packed red blood cells from plasma so that hematocrit can be determined.	
8. After the indicated period of time, remove the capillary tubes from the centrifuge and obtain the graphic reader (see Fig. 27–1).	Graphic reader is used to read the hematocrit.	
9. Place a capillary tube in the holder on the graphic reader.	Correct placement of the tube is necessary.	
10. Align the bottom of the packed red cells with the line on the holder (Fig. 27–2).	The tube is now adjusted for the amount of blood in this specific tube.	
11. Take the plastic capillary tube holder and move it until the top of the plasma (not red blood cells) coincides with the 100 percent line that is the top of the white triangle.	Prepares the tube so that the hematocrit can be read.	
12. Now take the knob to the right of the reader and move it until the line coincides with the line where the plasma and packed red blood cells separate.	Identifies the microhematocrit.	
13. Read the microhematocrit (percentage of packed red blood cells) in the window.	The patient's hematocrit that is to be documented.	
14. For second capillary tube, repeat steps 11 through 13.	Duplicate results should agree to within ± 1 percent.	
15. Remove and discard gloves.	Universal precautions.	
16. Wash hands.	Reduces transmission of microorganisms.	
17. Document the determined value in the patient record.	Provides a record of the data for future evaluation.	Compare your results with that of the hematology laboratory.

Evaluation

1. Evaluate the patient's hematocrit level to determine the fluid and electrolyte balance in conjunction with other assessment findings. **Rationale:** To support or negate nursing diagnosis of fluid volume deficit or excess; provides direction for further interventions.

2. Assess the patient's hematocrit level in relation to blood volume loss. **Rationale:** Contributes to decision making with regard to blood/blood product transfusion requirements.

Expected Outcome

Accurate identification of hematocrit. **Rationale:** Performing procedure correctly will provide assessment data for patient's treatment plan.

Unexpected Outcome

Inability to identify hematocrit level or validate with the hematology laboratory result. **Rationale:** Centrifugal force must be strictly standardized for maximal packing of red blood cells to occur, which results in an accurate

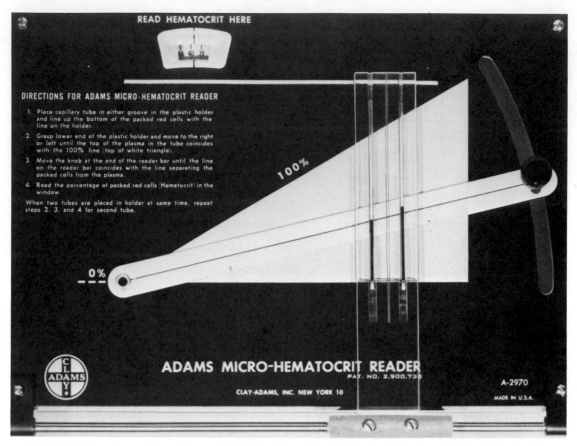

FIGURE 27–1. Adams Micro-Hematocrit Reader. (Reproduced with permission from Arthur Simmons, *Hematology: A Combined Theoretical and Technical Approach*. Philadelphia, Saunders, 1989. p. 205.)

hematocrit; if the red blood cells are pathologic in size and shape, the amount of trapped plasma increases the percentage of error.

Documentation

Documentation in the patient record should include the date and time of the procedure, the hematocrit obtained by centrifuge, pertinent assessment findings contributing to medical/nursing diagnosis, interventions taken based on microhematocrit obtained, and the assessment findings and the patient's response. **Rationale:** Documents nursing actions and interventions taken.

Patient/Family Education

Explain to both patient and family why microhematocrit is being performed. **Rationale:** Promotes patient and family understanding of the treatment plan and encourages patient and family questions.

Performance Checklist
Skill 27–4:   Determination of Microhematocrit via Centrifuge

	Complies	
Critical Behaviors	**yes**	**no**
1. Wash hands.		
2. Don gloves.		
3. Obtain blood sample.		
4. Fill two capillary blood tubes.		
5. Seal one end of each tube with special sealing clay.		
6. Appropriately place each capillary tube in the centrifuge.		

Table continues on following page

Critical Behaviors	Complies	
	yes	no
7. Place cover on centrifuge, and set timer to 5 minutes at 10,000 to 15,000 × gravity.		
8. Remove capillary tube from centrifuge and obtain a graphic reader.		
9. Place a capillary tube in the holder of the graphic reader.		
10. Align the bottom of the packed red cells with the line on the holder.		
11. Align the top of the plasma in tube with the 100 percent line on the graphic reader.		
12. Move the knob so that the line coincides with the line where the plasma and packed red blood cells separate.		
13. Read the microhematocrit.		
14. For second capillary tube, repeat steps 9 through 13.		
15. Remove and discard gloves.		
16. Wash hands.		
17. Document procedure in patient record.		

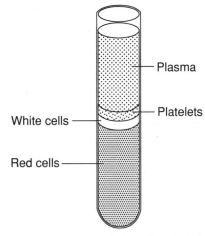

Plasma

Platelets

White cells

Red cells

FIGURE 27–2. Cell layers in centrifuged whole blood.

SKILL 27–5

Autotransfusion (with Disposable Device)

Autotransfusion is a process in which blood is collected from an active bleeding site and transfused back into the same patient. It is commonly used in trauma victims and patients undergoing cardiovascular and orthopedic procedures. Autotransfusion eliminates the need for a type and crossmatch, decreases dependence on the blood bank, and reduces the risk of transfusion reactions.

Purpose

The nurse performs autotransfusion to

1. Replace blood loss in trauma or surgical situations.
2. Reduce the possibility of a transfusion reaction.
3. Eliminate dependence on the blood bank.
4. Eliminate the incidence of transfusion-related disease (hepatitis, HIV).

Prerequisite Knowledge and Skills

Prior to performing autotransfusion with a disposable device, the nurse should understand

1. Anatomy and physiology of the cardiovascular system.
2. Principles of fluid and electrolyte balance.
3. Principles of hemodynamic monitoring.
4. Anatomy and physiology of the respiratory system.
5. Principles of aseptic technique.
6. Principles of intravenous therapy administration.
7. Principles of transfusion therapy.
8. Principles of chest drainage collection systems.
9. Universal precautions.

The nurse should be able to perform

1. Proper handwashing technique (see Skill 35–5).
2. Administration of intravenous therapy.
3. Administration of blood/blood products (see Skill 27–1).
4. Hemodynamic monitoring (see Skill 10–1).
5. Assessment of fluid and electrolyte status.
6. Assessment of the cardiovascular system.
7. Assessment of the respiratory system.
8. Collection of chest drainage (see Skill 5–1 and 5–2).
9. Assessment of vital signs.
10. Universal precautions (see Skill 35–1).

Assessment

1. Observe the patient for signs and symptoms of massive hemorrhage, including pale, clammy skin; hypotension (MAP < 60 mmHg); sinus tachycardia; tachypnea (RR > 30); dyspnea; overt blood loss (estimated in cc's; decreased filling pressures (PAD < 2 mmHg,

PCWP < 2, and CVP < 2 mmHg); decreased cardiac index (<2.5 L/min); and hourly urine output (<30 cc/h). **Rationale:** Significant loss of blood will require replacement with either whole blood or packed red blood cells.

2. Assess the patient's complete blood count for oxygen-carrying capacity, i.e., hemoglobin < 8 to 9 g/dl; hematocrit < 25 percent, in relation to the respiratory status and arterial blood gas analysis. **Rationale:** Significant improvement of hypoxemia may be seen by raising the hemoglobin level to more than 10 g/dl.

3. Assess the patient's platelet count and coagulation studies, i.e., prothrombin time (1 ½ to 2 times greater than control), partial prothrombin time (1 ½ to 2 times greater than control), and fibrin split product, when assessing for disseminated intravascular coagulopathy (elevated to greater than 1:8 dilution). **Rationale:** Specific clotting constituents may be required to stop bleeding. Transfusion of packed red blood cells alone will not provide appropriate clotting factors.

Nursing Diagnoses

1. Fluid volume deficit related to major blood loss. **Rationale:** Hemorrhage results in a decreased circulating volume.

2. Decreased tissue perfusion to major organs related to major blood loss. **Rationale:** Hemorrhage results in a decreased circulating volume.

3. Decreased cardiac output related to hypovolemia. **Rationale:** Decreased circulating volume diminishes stroke volume. Inadequate oxygen-carrying capacity may result in cardiac dysrhythmias.

Planning

1. Individualize the following goals for performing autotransfusion:
   a. Maintain adequate circulating volume. **Rationale:** Ensures adequate tissue perfusion.
   b. Enhance oxygen-carrying capacity. **Rationale:** Improves oxygenation status and cardiac output.
   c. Correct coagulation deficits. **Rationale:** Promotes hemostasis.

2. Prepare all necessary equipment and supplies. **Rationale:** Assembly of all necessary equipment and supplies facilitates prompt institution of autotransfusion.
   a. Autotransfusion set.
   b. Blood administration set.
   c. 0.9% normal saline for infusion.
   d. Hemodynamic monitoring equipment: blood pressure cuff/arterial line, central venous pressure manometer or pulmonary artery catheter, transducers, pressurized infusion system.
   e. Cardiac monitor.
   f. Stethoscope.
   g. Thermometer.
   h. One set of examination gloves.
   i. Source of suction.
   j. Connecting tubing, 6 ft.

3. Ensure the patency of an 18-gauge (or larger) peripheral intravenous catheter or central line for fluid administration. **Rationale:** Provides an infusion site for the blood/blood products to be transfused.

4. Prepare the patient, explaining the procedure and rationale for its use. **Rationale:** Reduces anxiety and provides an opportunity for the patient to ask questions.

Implementation

Steps	Rationale	Special Considerations
1. Wash hands.	Reduces transmission of microorganisms.	
2. Don exam gloves.	Universal precautions.	
3. Set up autotransfusion water-seal unit (Fig. 27–3).	Suction is required to drain blood into drainage unit.	
4. If prescribed, inject anticoagulant into the self-sealing port on the connector of the patient's drainage tubing prior to collecting blood from the patient.	CPDA-1 is the recommended agent; instill 1 ml for every 7 ml of blood.	Use of the anticoagulant remains controversial.
5. Prior to disconnecting the filled collection bag and infusing into the patient, a new collection system must be ready for attachment to the drainage system.	Allows for collection of additional blood as well as keeping the system closed and sterile.	Obtain new collection bag before removing the filled bag.

Table continues on following page

Steps	Rationale	Special Considerations
6. Clamp the tubes (attached to the tubing by the manufacturer) on the new bag. The new collection bag is now prepared for attachment.	Clamping eliminates the risk of air entering the system.	
7. Press the high negativity valve located on the top of the water-seal drainage system.	This is a relief valve that allows for disconnect.	
8. Close the clamp on the patient's drainage tube.	Stops further drainage of blood into bag.	
9. Close the clamps on the tubing that is attached to water-seal drainage unit.	Prepares for disconnect of system.	
10. Take the previously prepared new collection bag, and attach the connector to the water-seal unit and the second connector to the patient's chest tube (Fig. 27–4A).	Allows for continued collection of blood.	Check with individual manufacturers as to the color of tubing that is to be connected to the patient and to the water-seal unit.
11. Make sure that all connections are secure, and then open the clamps on the autotransfusion bag and the patient's drainage tubing (Fig. 27–4B).	Connections must be secured to create suction for drainage.	
12. Attach the patient's drainage tubing connector to the water-seal drainage unit tubing (Fig. 27–4C).	Closes the filled autotransfusion bag.	A sterile, closed system must be maintained.
13. Slide the collection bag out of the frame by pushing down on the frame and pulling up on the bag (Fig. 27–5A).	The bag will be put on the IV pole for reinfusion.	Reinfuse within 4 hours (check institution's policy).
14. Attach the new collection bag to the water-seal unit.	Secures bag to unit to ensure that it will remain upright.	
15. Assemble filled collection bag and blood administration set with microfilter, and prime the tubing for administration (Fig. 27–5B,C).	Filter is used to remove aggregates that form in stored blood.	
16. Initiate infusion as prescribed (see Skill 27–1).	Restores blood volume.	Patients receiving autotransfusions are at very low risk for transfusion reactions because the threat of blood incompatibility does not exist.
17. Repeat procedure until the patient has stabilized or as directed.		
18. To terminate, see Figure 27–6:		
a. Press the high negativity valve.	Relief valve for disconnect.	
b. Close the clamp on the patient's drainage tube.	Stops further drainage into bag.	
c. Close the clamps on the filled autotransfusion bag that is attached to water-seal unit.	Prepares for disconnect of the system.	
d. Remove the patient's drainage tube from the collection bag and attach it to the chest drainage unit.	Allows for drainage to enter water-seal unit. This drainage cannot be transfused.	

Table continues on following page

Steps	Rationale	Special Considerations
e. Process the filled autotransfusion bag as above.		
20. Remove and discard gloves.	Universal precautions.	
21. Wash hands.	Reduces transmission of microorganisms.	

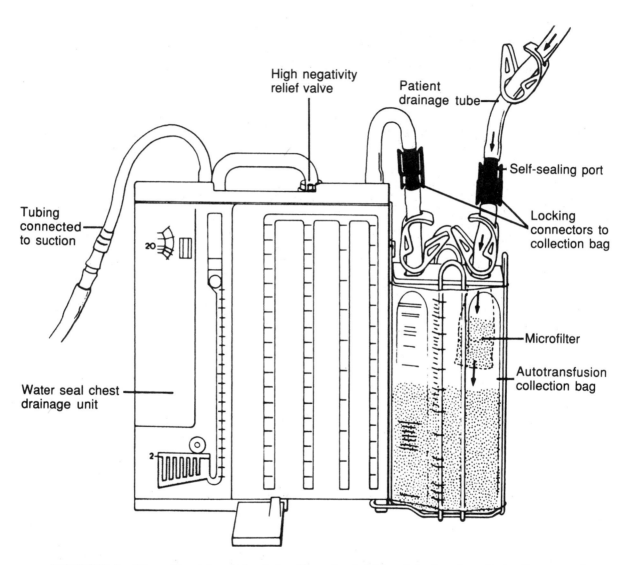

FIGURE 27–3. Disposable autotransfusion device. (Reproduced with permission from Susan Butler, Current trends in autologous transfusion. *RN* [Medical Economics Company, Inc.] 1989:59, 5–8.)

Evaluation

Evaluate the patient's hemoglobin and hematocrit levels, intravascular volume (i.e., blood pressure, filling pressures, cardiac index, heart rate, and urine output), and oxygenation/respiratory status. **Rationale:** Autotransfusion improves hematocrit, hemoglobin, and oxygen-carrying capacity.

Expected Outcomes

1. Stability of vital signs, hemoglobin, and hematocrit. **Rationale:** Autotransfusion has adequately replaced intravascular volume loss.
2. Increased PaO$_2$. **Rationale:** Infusion of packed red blood cells improves oxygen-carrying capacity.

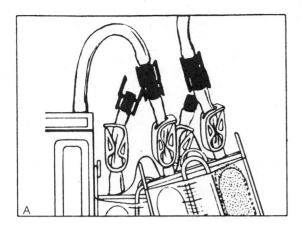

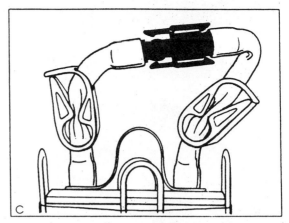

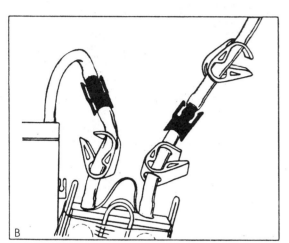

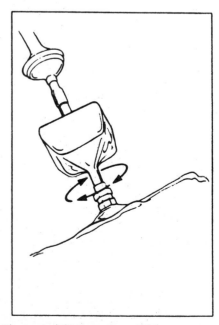

FIGURE 27–4. Preparing for reinfusion. (*A*) Attach the tubings from the water-seal unit and the patient to those on the new bag. (*B*) Make sure all connections are secure. Then open the clamps on the autotransfusion bag and the patient's drainage tube. (*C*) Close the filled autotransfusion bag by attaching the connectors to each other. (Reproduced with permission from Susan Butler, Current trends in autologous transfusion. *RN* [Medical Economics Company, Inc.] 1989:59, 5–8.)

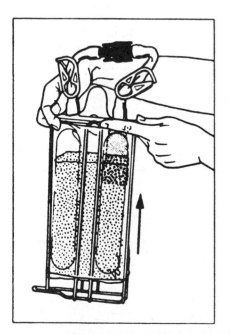

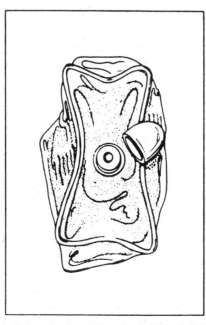

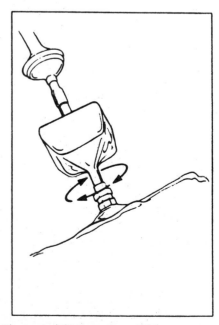

FIGURE 27–5. Setting up for transfusion of salvaged blood. (*A*) Slide the filled bag out of the frame by pushing down on the frame with your thumbs and pulling up on the bag with your fingers. (*B*) Assemble the microfilter and IV tubing for reinfusion. Then turn the bag upside down and remove the cap from the spike port. (*C*) Insert the top of the microfilter into the spike port, using a twisting motion. Gently squeeze the bag to fill the filter with blood. (Reproduced with permission from Susan Butler, Current trends in autologous transfusion. *RN* [Medical Economics Company, Inc.] 1989:59, 5–8.)

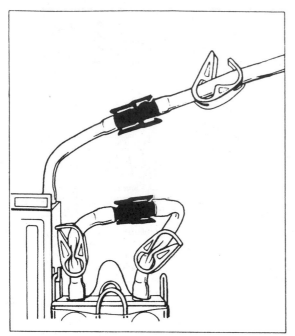

FIGURE 27–6. Terminating collection of blood for autotransfusion. When autotransfusion is no longer needed, remove the patient's
drainage tube from the collection bag and attach it to the chest drainage
unit. Before making the switch, press the relief valve and close all
clamps. Be sure to unclamp the patient's tube afterward. (Reproduced
with permission from Susan Butler, Current trends in autologous transfusion. *RN* [Medical Economics Company, Inc.] 1989:59, 5–8.)

tachypnea. **Rationale:** Left ventricular failure secondary
to overaggressive blood/fluid administration.

2. Infiltration of intravenous catheter. **Rationale:**
Catheter has become dislodged.

Documentation

Documentation in the patient record should include
the date and time the autotransfusion was initiated and
completed, the amount of anticoagulants instilled (if appropriate), the amount of blood collected and reinfused,
the patient's response to the procedure, and any unexpected outcomes encountered and interventions taken.
Rationale: Documents nursing care provided, unexpected outcomes, and interventions taken.

Patient/Family Education

1. Instruct the patient and family regarding the rationale for utilizing autotransfusion. **Rationale:** Promotes
patient and family participation in the treatment plan
and encourages the patient and family to ask questions.

2. If appropriate, suggest that the family consider
donating blood/blood products for the patient in the face
of continuing transfusion needs. Advise the family that
direct donation may take 7 to 14 days of processing before
the transfusion can be done. **Rationale:** Encourages family participation in care.

Unexpected Outcomes

1. Fluid volume excess manifested by increased filling pressures, crackles, dyspnea, frothy sputum, and

Performance Checklist
Skill 27–5: Autotransfusion (with Disposable Device)

Critical Behaviors	Complies	
	yes	no
1. Wash hands.		
2. Don exam gloves.		
3. Set up autotransfusion water-seal unit.		
4. Add anticoagulant to collection bag.		
5. Obtain a new collection bag prior to disconnecting filled collection bag.		
6. Clamp the tubes on the new collection bag.		
7. Press the high negativity valve on top of water-seal unit.		
8. Close the clamp on the patient's drainage tube.		
9. Close the clamps on the filled autotransfusion tube.		
10. Take the new drainage bag and attach the tubing to the water-seal unit and the patient chest tube.		
11. Secure all connections, and then open the clamps on the autotransfusion bag and the patient's drainage tube.		

Table continues on following page

	Complies	
Critical Behaviors	**yes**	**no**
12. Close the filled autotransfusion bag by attaching the patient's drainage tube connector to the water-seal drainage unit tubing.		
13. Slide the collection bag out of the frame.		
14. Attach the new collection bag to the water-seal unit.		
15. Assemble filled collection bag and administration set, and prime tubing of set.		
16. Administer autotransfusion.		
17. Repeat procedure as necessary until patient has stabilized.		
18. Terminate autotransfusion by pressing high negativity valve, closing clamps on the patient's drainage tube and autotransfusion bag, and reconnecting patient's chest tube to chest drainage unit.		
19. Remove and discard gloves.		
20. Wash hands.		
21. Document procedure in the patient record.		

BIBLIOGRAPHY

Brown, B. (1984). *Hematology: Principles and Procedures*. Philadelphia: Lea & Febiger.

Butler, S. (1989). Current trends in autologous transfusion. *RN* 59(11):44–55.

Callery, M.F., Culhane, M.B., Francis, C.K., et al. (1990). *Transfusion Therapy Guidelines for Nurses*. Washington, D.C.: NIH (publication No. 90-2668a).

DeLoor, R.M. and Schreiber, M.J. (1985). Blood and Blood Component Administration. In S. Millar, L. K. Sampson, and M. Soukup (Eds.), *AACN Procedure Manual for Critical Care* (pp. 409–430). Philadelphia: Saunders.

Huestis, D.W., Bore, J.R., and Case, J. (1988). *Practical Blood Transfusions*. Boston: Little, Brown.

Persons, C.P. (1987). *Critical Care Procedures*. Philadelphia: Lippincott.

Simmons, A. (1989). *Hematology: A Combined Theoretical and Technical Approach*. Philadelphia: Saunders.

Sorensen, K.C., and Luckmann, J. (1979). *Basic Nursing: A Psychophysiologic Approach*. Philadelphia: Saunders.

Widmann, F. (Ed.) (1985). *Technical Manual of the American Association of Blood Banks*. Arlington, Va.: American Association of Blood Banks.

UNIT VIII

THE INTEGUMENTARY SYSTEM

28

WOUND MANAGEMENT

BEHAVIORAL OBJECTIVES

After completing this chapter, the nurse will be able to

- Define the key terms.
- Describe the phases of wound healing.
- List the factors that affect the wound-healing process.
- Explain the purpose of wound dressings based on the type of wound.
- Discuss local wound care for various types of wounds.
- Perform the skills involved in wound management.

A wound, described as an interruption in tissue integrity, is managed through skills that affect the process and timeliness of healing. Wound healing occurs in a complex series of steps. The healing process can be summarized using the following model:

Phase I: Inflammatory phase. Vascular constriction occurs with formation of a platelet plug to stop the bleeding. Fibrin formation occurs to stabilize the plug. As the inflammatory response occurs, leukocytes and macrophages (monocytes) travel from the intravascular space to the wound to ingest and destroy wound debris. Epithelialization begins within 24 hours.

Phase II: Proliferative phase. Inflammation is followed by fibroblast migration within the wound. Collagen is formed during this phase, filling and giving tensile strength to the wound. Rapid capillary networking occurs.

Phase III: Remodeling or maturation phase. Remodeling occurs as the wound gains tensile strength. Collagen fibers mature, and contraction and scarring occur. (The wound never regains 100 percent of its original strength.)

Although the healing process is essentially the same for all wounds, variance in healing times is based on a number of internal and external factors. Internal host factors that can compromise healing include decreased circulation, anemia, poor nutrition, obesity, diabetes, advanced age, stress, smoking, and drugs, especially immunosuppressive drugs such as steroids. External factors that affect healing include the type of wound, the mechanism of healing (i.e., primary, secondary, or tertiary), any contamination or infection present, and local wound care.

Most clean or clean/contaminated surgical wounds heal by primary intention. The wound edges are approximated by suturing each layer of tissue. These wounds heal quickly and require minimal local wound care (Table 28–1).

Contaminated surgical or traumatic wounds are closed by secondary or tertiary intention. Wounds healed by secondary intention are left open to allow granulation tissue to fill in from the wound base. Wounds healed by tertiary intention are left open for several days to allow

TABLE 28–1 Phases in Primary Intention Healing

Phase	Activity
Initial phase (3–5 days)	Incision edges approximated Migration of epithelial cells Clot serves as meshwork for starting capillary growth
Granulation (fibroplasia) (5 days–4 weeks)	Migration of fibroblasts Secretion of collagen Capillary buds abundant Wound is fragile
Scar contracture (maturation) (7 days–several months)	Remodeling of collagen Scar gains in strength

Source: From S. M. Lewis and I. C. Collier, *Medical-Surgical Nursing: Assessment and Management of Clinical Problems*, 2d Ed. New York: McGraw-Hill, 1987, p. 135. Copyright C. V. Mosby, St. Louis, with permission.

for wound drainage, as in the case of a dirty wound; then the edges are sutured together. In secondary and tertiary healing, wounds are slow to heal and develop more granulation tissue (Fig. 28–1).

The presence of necrotic debris and/or infection in these slow granulating wounds will further impede healing, requiring aggressive local wound care and often systemic antibiotic therapy. A moist environment free of debris is necessary for granulation and epithelialization. The healing process will be halted if the tissue is allowed to dehydrate or if undue tension is caused by an accumulation of drainage or an infectious process.

Cleaning and dressing techniques support optimal healing. Cleaning removes debris and provides a moist environment. Dressings provide absorption, debridement, support and protection, hemostasis, and aesthetic security for the patient. Dressings also promote a moist environment for healing.

The focus of this chapter is the nursing skills vital for the promotion of an optimal wound-healing environment.

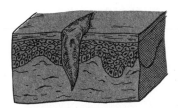 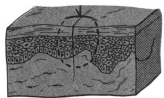 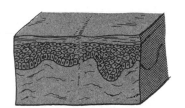

Incision with blood clot Edges approximated with suture Fine scar

A. PRIMARY INTENTION

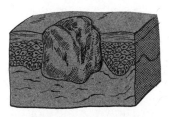 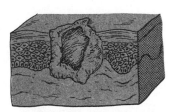 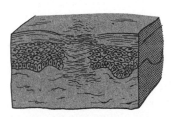

Irregular, large wound with blood clot Granulation tissue fills in wound Large scar

B. SECONDARY INTENTION

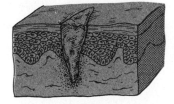 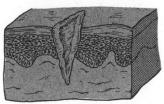 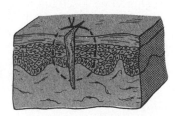

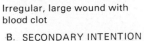
Contaminated wound Granulation tissue Delayed closure with suture

C. TERTIARY INTENTION

FIGURE 28–1. Types of wound healing. (Reproduced with permission from S. M. Lewis and I. C. Collier, *Medical-Surgical Nursing: Assessment and Management of Clinical Problems*, 2nd ed. New York: McGraw-Hill, 1987, p. 135. Copyright C.V. Mosby, St. Louis.)

KEY TERMS

anaerobic culture   *granulation*
antiseptic   *infected wound*
clean wound   *maceration*
clean/contaminated wound   *mechanical debridement*
contaminated wound   *necrotic debris*
epithelialization

SKILLS

28–1   Cleaning and Irrigating Wounds
28–2   Culturing Wounds
28–3   Dressing Wounds with Drains
28–4   Dressing Open Wounds

GUIDELINES

The following assessment guidelines assist the nurse in formulating a nursing diagnosis and an individualized plan of care to maintain optimal wound healing:

1.   Assess the host factors that could compromise wound healing.
2.   Know the type of wound-healing mechanism (primary, secondary, tertiary intention).
3.   Know if infection is present (wound culture reports, vital signs, WBC reports).
4.   Know what type of drainage is expected.

SKILL 28–1 _____

Cleaning and Irrigating Wounds

Cleaning a wound removes debris to facilitate general wound assessment, provides a clean wound bed for cell proliferation, and reduces the incidence of skin maceration by removing drainage and excess moisture. Cleaning techniques range from gentle mechanical washing with gauze on a surgically sutured wound to irrigation with a syringe or jet spray in a contaminated, necrotic wound.

Surgically sutured wounds are not usually disturbed for cleaning unless a large amount of drainage is present. Once the original surgical dressing is removed, the surrounding skin may be cleaned with mild soap and water. A grossly contaminated, necrotic wound may need aggressive mechanical cleaning using a combination of gauze with the syringe method of irrigation. Jet-spray irrigations (i.e., Water Pik) are sometimes used but have been found to be cumbersome and can be contaminated by bacteria. Rogness (1985) reports studies that show that irrigations using a 35-ml syringe and a 19-gauge needle will produce sufficient pressure for adequate cleaning and removal of debris. A bulb syringe should not be used because it does not produce sufficient pressure to remove debris.

The choice of cleaning solution is determined by the type of wound and goal of care. Cleaning, *not* disinfecting the wound, is the focus. Studies have shown that certain cleaning and antiseptic agents (i.e., hydrogen peroxide, povidone-iodine) are caustic to new granulating tissue. Normal saline is generally the cleaning solution of choice. Even in the presence of wound infection, systemic antibiotics are prescribed instead of treating the wound locally with antiseptics.

The use of antiseptic agents is limited to grossly contaminated wounds that need debridement of devitalized tissue. Once the wound is clean and free of debris, these agents are discontinued.

Purpose

The nurse cleans and irrigates a wound to

1.   Visualize and assess the wound.
2.   Prepare the wound for obtaining a culture.
3.   Remove debris.
4.   Protect surrounding skin from maceration.
5.   Promote a clean, moist wound bed for granulation and epithelialization.

Prerequisite Knowledge and Skills

Before performing wound cleaning and irrigation, the nurse should understand

1.   Principles of wound healing.
2.   Principles of aseptic technique.
3.   Universal precautions.

The nurse should be able to perform

1.   Proper handwashing technique (see Skill 35–5).
2.   Wound assessment.
3.   Dressing techniques (see Skills 28–3 and 28–4).
4.   Universal precautions (see Skill 35–1).

Assessment

1.   Observe the wound for type and amount of drainage. **Rationale:** Determines the amount of solution necessary for cleaning.
2.   Observe for necrotic debris within the wound. **Rationale:** Determines the amount of mechanical debridement necessary when cleaning.
3.   Assess surrounding skin for maceration and inflammation. **Rationale:** Excessive drainage and moisture will cause the breakdown of surrounding skin; determines the frequency of cleaning necessary.
4.   Assess for pain on palpation of surrounding area. **Rationale:** Patient may require an analgesic before procedure.

Nursing Diagnoses

1.   Impaired tissue integrity related to accumulation of drainage and/or necrotic debris. **Rationale:** Devitalized tissue and debris inhibit wound healing.
2.   Potential for infection related to retention of bac-

terial contamination in wound. **Rationale:** Impaired tissue integrity provides a medium for potential invasion of microorganisms.

Planning

1. Individualize the following goals for cleaning and irrigating the wound:
   a. Provide a clean, moist bed for granulation and epithelialization. **Rationale:** A moist wound surface that is free of debris provides an optimal environment for development of new granulation tissue and epithelium.
   b. Protect surrounding skin and tissue from maceration. **Rationale:** Drainage and necrotic debris can cause the breakdown of surrounding skin.
2. Determine the procedure that will be used for cleaning. **Rationale:** Allows the nurse to choose appropriate equipment. Nondraining or slightly draining sutured wounds can be cleaned with gauze. Highly draining wounds and contaminated/necrotic open wounds will need the syringe technique for irrigation.
3. Assemble all supplies and the cleaning solution. **Rationale:** Assembling necessary supplies provides organization and timely implementation of procedure.
   a. One pair exam gloves.
   b. One pair of sterile gloves.
   c. One plastic bag for soiled dressings.
   d. One waterproof pad.
   e. Sterile normal saline (or other solution as appropriate).
   f. One sterile basin.
   g. One sterile forceps (optional).
   h. All-gauze 4 × 4's (number is determined by the wound size and should be recorded in the nursing care plan).
   i. One sterile 35-ml syringe and a 19-gauge needle (for irrigation only).
   j. One collecting basin for irrigation returns.
   k. Sterile dressings/paper tape.
4. Prepare the patient.
   a. Administer pain medication as prescribed 30 minutes prior to treatment, if necessary. **Rationale:** Reduces discomfort and anxiety and encourages cooperation.
   b. Explain procedure to the patient. **Rationale:** Reduces anxiety and provides information should the patient be discharged with the wound.

Implementation

Steps	Rationale	Special Considerations
1. Wash hands.	Reduces transmission of microorganisms.	
2. Position patient to facilitate drainage of cleaning solution from least contaminated area of wound to most contaminated.	Gravity directs flow of solution.	
3. Place waterproof pad under patient, and position collecting basin to collect contaminated irrigation solution if necessary.	Waterproof pad and collecting basin keep patient comfortable and linen clean.	
4. Warm cleaning solution to body temperature.	Warm solution is more comfortable on wound and skin.	Solution may be warmed by placing unopened bottle under hot running tap or in basin of hot water. Check comfort of temperature by pouring small amount of solution over your own hand.
5. Place opened plastic bag within reach for soiled disposable items.	Prevents spread of microorganisms.	
6. Don clean gloves (and goggles, gown, and apron, if indicated).	Universal precautions.	Eye wear should be worn if there is a potential for splashing, as with syringe irrigation.
7. Remove soiled dressing and discard in plastic bag. Then remove and discard gloves.	Universal precautions.	
8. Assess wound bed for the need for culture.	Determines the need for culturette tube or syringe for obtaining culture.	See Skill 28–2.

Table continues on following page

Steps	Rationale	Special Considerations
9. Open sterile all-gauze 4 × 4 dressings onto a sterile field or into a sterile basin. If using syringe irrigation method for cleaning, open 35-ml syringe and 19-gauge needle onto a sterile field.	Maintains aseptic technique.	All-gauze 4 × 4's contain no cotton fibers, which could leave residue in the wound while cleaning.
10. Pour solution over 4 × 4's or in a sterile basin.	Prepares for cleaning.	
11. Don sterile gloves.	Maintains aseptic technique.	
Sutured Wound		
12. If using gauze method of cleaning, wash from top to bottom or center outward. Clean from least contaminated area to most contaminated area. Discard gauze with each wipe.	Prevents cleaned area from becoming recontaminated.	When cleaning around a drain, clean from drain site outward in a circular motion, discarding gauze with each circle (Fig. 28–2).
Open Wound		
13. If irrigation of wound is indicated, draw solution into syringe from sterile basin, attach needle, and direct solution onto wound surface approximately 1 in (2.5 cm) away. Direct flow from least contaminated area to most contaminated area. Continue with irrigation until returns are clear.	Irrigation removes drainage and wound debris.	Sufficient pressure must be used to release debris, but care must be taken to avoid splashing solution from wound by using excess pressure. Excess pressure also can cause trauma to wound tissue.
14. Dry surrounding skin with dry sterile gauze.	Prevents maceration of skin from excess moisture.	
15. Apply sterile dressing (see Skills 28–3 and 28–4).	Absorbs drainage and immobilizes and protects the wound.	
16. Dispose of all soiled equipment into appropriate receptacle.	Universal precautions.	
17. Remove and discard gloves.	Universal precautions.	
18. Wash hands.	Reduces transmission of microorganisms.	

Evaluation

1. Evaluate the wound for the condition of wound bed and epithelium. **Rationale:** Identifies the effect of cleaning and progress of wound healing.

2. Measure wound length, width, and depth (wound may appear larger after debris is removed) the first time the wound is seen and then at planned intervals. **Rationale:** Provides baseline wound size and monitors progress of wound healing.

3. Evaluate the surrounding skin for inflammation and maceration. **Rationale:** Drainage and necrotic tissue on surrounding skin will cause skin breakdown.

Expected Outcomes

1. Excess necrotic debris and drainage are removed from the wound bed. **Rationale:** Debris and drainage impede wound healing and foster infection.

2. Surrounding skin is clean and protected from maceration. **Rationale:** Clean dry skin is necessary for an optimal wound-healing environment.

3. Increased amounts of healthy granulation tissue and epithelium are visible. **Rationale:** Wound is healing.

Unexpected Outcomes

1. Wound hemorrhage. **Rationale:** Overaggressive irrigation pressure or mechanical debridement could cause excessive bleeding.

2. Wound dehiscence with or without evisceration. **Rationale:** Excessive mechanical trauma can dislodge sutures.

3. Wound infection. **Rationale:** Inadequate removal of contaminated debris or contamination from improper technique could foster infection.

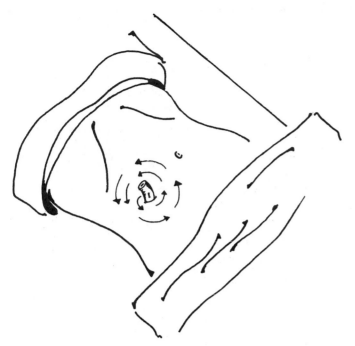

FIGURE 28–2. Cleaning around a drain. (Courtesy of Arturo Sanchez.)

Documentation

Documentation in the patient record should include the date and time of the procedure; the appearance of the wound bed and surrounding skin and the amount of drainage and necrotic debris prior to cleaning; the appearance of wound bed after cleaning; if sutures are intact; any remaining necrotic tissue; the condition of surrounding skin; the size of the wound, including length, width, and depth (on a periodic basis); the type and number of dressings applied; the patient's response to the procedure; and any unexpected outcomes and interventions taken. **Rationale:** Documents progress of wound healing and nursing care given.

Patient/Family Education

1. Explain and demonstrate the procedure to both the patient and family if the need for discharge wound cleaning/irrigation is likely. **Rationale:** Understanding of the procedure allays fears and encourages involvement in self-care activities.

2. Explain the technique of wound assessment. **Rationale:** Teaches skills that can be reinforced by practice. Teaches the patient and family the changes that must be reported to a professional.

3. Encourage the patient and family to assist in certain aspects of the procedure as warranted. **Rationale:** Reduces anxiety and builds skills.

4. Assess the need for long-term wound care. **Rationale:** Helps the nurse determine teaching needs and follow-up wound care.

5. Make appropriate referrals. **Rationale:** Early discharge planning facilitates continuity of care by addressing physical and educational needs of the patient and family.

Performance Checklist
Skill 28–1: Cleaning and Irrigating Wounds

Critical Behaviors	Complies	
	yes	no
1. Wash hands.		
2. Position patient.		
3. Place waterproof pad under patient, and position collecting basin under wound if necessary.		
4. Warm cleaning solution.		
5. Open plastic bag for soiled items.		
6. Don clean gloves, and don goggles, gown, and apron, if necessary.		
7. Remove soiled dressing and discard in plastic bag, and then remove and discard gloves.		

Table continues on following page

Critical Behaviors	Complies	
	yes	no
8. Assess wound bed for the need for culture.		
9. Open sterile dressings and sterile basin as necessary, and open 35-ml syringe and 19-gauge needle onto sterile field (if appropriate).		
10. Pour solution over dressings or into sterile basin.		
11. Don sterile gloves.		
Sutured Wound 12. Gauze method: Wash from top to bottom or center outward, discarding gauze with each wipe.		
Open Wound 13. Irrigation method: Draw solution into syringe from sterile basin, and direct solution onto wound surface from 1 in (2.5 cm) away, directing flow from least contaminated to most contaminated area. Continue with irrigation until returns are clear.		
14. Dry surrounding skin.		
15. Apply sterile dressing.		
16. Dispose of soiled equipment in appropriate receptacle.		
17. Remove and discard gloves.		
18. Wash hands.		
19. Document procedure in the patient record.		

SKILL 28–2

Culturing Wounds

All open wounds are considered contaminated but not necessarily infected. If the normal cell response in the wound can keep bacterial counts under control, infection will be prevented. When the body defenses cannot control the growth of microorganisms, local and systemic signs of infection occur.

Wound cultures are taken when a patient begins to show signs of clinical infection or if the potential for infection is highly suspect. Assessment of an infected wound will demonstrate signs that include purulent drainage, usually with a foul odor, increased pain and heat at the wound site, and increased inflammation and edema of the wound and surrounding skin. Infection is also suspected when the patient shows such systemic signs as fever and increased white blood cell (WBC) count.

Wound cultures may be taken initially in highly contaminated or necrotic wounds (i.e., traumatic wounds) or in contaminated or infected surgical cases (i.e., abscess drainage), particularly if the patient exhibits other clinical indicators, such as fever and/or a high white blood cell count.

Wound cultures validate evidence of wound infection and isolate the causative organism so that appropriate antibiotic therapy can be prescribed. Proper technique in obtaining the culture is extremely important to ensure a good specimen and to prevent contamination of the specimen. A culture can be taken by swab technique or aspiration technique. The wound should be assessed for the need to culture more than one location, especially if stab wounds and/or drains are present. Identification of the site is paramount for the laboratory to rule out normal flora.

Purpose

The nurse obtains a wound culture to

1. Determine the presence of infection in suspect wounds.
2. Determine the causative organism in an infected wound.

Prerequisite Knowledge and Skills

Prior to taking a wound culture, the nurse should understand

1. Principles of aseptic technique.
2. Universal precautions.
3. Pathological progression of inflammatory and infectious processes.

The nurse should be able to perform

1. Proper handwashing technique (see Skill 35–5).
2. Wound assessment.
3. Proper wound cleansing and irrigating technique (see Skill 28–1).
4. Proper wound dressing technique (see Skills 28–3 and 28–4).
5. Universal precautions (see Skill 35–1).

Assessment

1. Observe the wound for areas of drainage. **Rationale:** Determines if more than one culture site is necessary.

2. Assess the wound for swelling, which may contain pockets of drainage. Gentle palpation of the area may help express the drainage for culture. **Rationale:** Obtains accurate culture results.

3. Assess for pain on palpation of surrounding area. **Rationale:** Patient may need an analgesic before the procedure. Local pain may also be symptomatic of an infectious process.

Nursing Diagnosis

Potential for (actual) infection related to retention of microorganisms in the wound. **Rationale:** Impaired tissue integrity provides a medium for potential (actual) invasion of microorganisms.

Planning

1. Individualize the following goals for obtaining a wound culture:
    a. Validation of an infectious process within the wound. **Rationale:** Timely identification of an infectious process promotes early interventions to prevent complications.
    b. Identification of causative organism of wound infection. **Rationale:** Proper identification of organism ensures appropriate antibiotic therapy.

2. Prepare all appropriate supplies. **Rationale:** Assembling supplies ensures that a culture will be obtained quickly and efficiently.
    a. One sterile culturette tube or sterile 20-cc syringe with a 19-gauge needle and one cork for capping the needle after aspiration.
    b. Two pairs of exam gloves.
    c. Two pairs of sterile gloves.
    d. One plastic bag for soiled dressings.
    e. Sterile normal saline for cleaning.
    f. Sterile dressings.
    g. Label(s) for specimen container(s).
    h. Plastic bag for transporting specimen to laboratory.

3. Prepare the patient.
    a. Administer pain medication as prescribed 30 minutes prior to procedure, if necessary. **Rationale:** Reduces discomfort and anxiety and encourages cooperation.
    b. Explain the procedure. **Rationale:** Encourages patient cooperation.

Implementation

Steps	Rationale	Special Considerations
1. Wash hands.	Reduces transmission of microorganisms.	
2. Don clean gloves (and gown, if necessary).	Maintains universal precautions.	
3. Remove soiled dressings and discard in plastic bag. Then remove and discard gloves.	Prevents contamination and spread of microorganisms.	
4. Don sterile gloves, clean wound and surrounding skin with normal saline (see Skill 28–1), and remove and discard gloves.	Cleaning removes contaminated debris.	
Culturette Swab Method		
5. Don clean gloves, and remove swab from culturette tube, taking care not to touch swab or inside of tube.	Maintains universal precautions and aseptic technique.	
6. Swab inside of wound using a rolling motion.	Ensures collection of a good specimen.	
7. Use separate swabs if taking more than one specimen.	Ensures good culture specimen and prevents cross-contamination.	Care must be taken to swab inside of wound instead of wound edges to prevent contamination by skin flora and contaminated debris.
8. Carefully place swab into culturette tube without touching swab or inside of container.	Prevents contamination.	

Table continues on following page

Steps	Rationale	Special Considerations
9. Crush ampule of medium in culturette and close securely, making sure swab is surrounded by medium.	Keeps specimen from drying out and provides growth supporting medium.	

Anaerobic Culture Method

10. If collecting a specimen for anaerobic culture, care must be taken to keep anaerobic transport culture tube in an upright position to prevent carbon dioxide from escaping. Close container securely after swab is placed in tube (Fig. 28–3).	Maintains an anaerobic environment.	

Syringe Method

11. Insert sterile needle into drainage, and aspirate approximately 5 to 10 cc of drainage into sterile syringe.	Ensures good specimen and prevents contamination from skin flora.	Syringe method is used when large amounts of pus or drainage are present or for collecting anaerobic specimens from deep inside wounds.
12. Express excess air out of syringe.	Prevents contamination.	
13. Cork needle to send syringe/needle to laboratory as one unit containing specimen. Do not recap or attempt to disconnect needle from syringe.	Universal precautions. Prevents injury from needle stick and spread of microorganisms.	
14. Remove and discard gloves in plastic bag.	Prevents spread of microorganisms.	
15. Wash hands.	Reduces transmission of microorganisms.	
16. Don sterile gloves, and apply sterile dressing to wound.	Dressing absorbs drainage and immobilizes and protects the wound.	
17. Label specimen container(s) with patient name, room number, date, time, and exact source of specimen.	Ensures proper identification of specimen.	Proper source of specimen is important for laboratory to rule out normal flora from location.
18. Place container in clean plastic bag, and have specimen transported to laboratory as soon as possible.	Plastic bag prevents spread of microorganisms. Immediate transport prevents overgrowth of microorganisms that can occur if specimen is left at room temperature for an extended length of time.	
19. Dispose of all soiled equipment into appropriate receptacle.	Universal precautions.	
20. Wash hands.	Reduces transmission of microorganisms.	

Evaluation

1. Assess any drainage obtained for type, color, odor, and amount. **Rationale:** Gives baseline description/comparison of drainage.

2. Assess the condition of wound bed. **Rationale:** Identifies any trauma done to tissue during culturing procedure.

3. Assess the surrounding skin and tissue for inflammation, pain, heat, and edema. **Rationale:** Gives baseline data for progress of wound healing.

Expected Outcome

Specimen obtained will validate and identify causative organism of infection. **Rationale:** Appropriate antibiotic therapy can then be initiated.

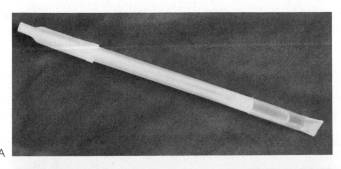

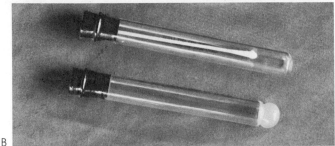

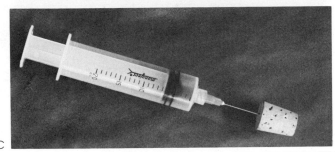

FIGURE 28–3. (*A*) Culturette. (*B*) Anaerobic culture tubes. (*C*) Needle and syringe with cork.

Unexpected Outcomes

1. Wound trauma. **Rationale:** Too aggressive swabbing/aspirating for culture could traumatize granulating wound bed or sutures.

2. Contamination of specimen. **Rationale:** Improper technique could contaminate specimen by introducing skin flora or contamination at wound edges.

Documentation

Documentation in the patient record should include that normal saline was used for cleaning to prepare wound for culture; condition of the wound before and after cleaning/culturing; type, amount, color, and odor of drainage; the area of wound from which specimen was collected; culture technique used; the date and time of specimen collection and time specimen was taken to laboratory; the type of dressing applied and the response of the patient to the procedure; and any unexpected outcomes and interventions taken. **Rationale:** Documents nursing care, the condition of the wound, and any expected or unexpected outcomes.

Patient/Family Education

1. Explain the need for wound culture to both patient and family. **Rationale:** Understanding of the procedure helps allay fears and encourages cooperation.

2. Teach wound-assessment skills to both patient and family. **Rationale:** Patient and family will be alert for any changes that should be reported to a professional.

Performance Checklist
Skill 28–2: Culturing Wounds

Critical Behaviors	Complies	
	yes	**no**
1. Wash hands.		
2. Don gloves (and gown, if necessary).		
3. Remove and discard dressing, and then remove and discard gloves.		
4. Don sterile gloves and clean wound.		
CULTURETTE METHOD 5. Don clean gloves, and remove swab from tube.		
6. Obtain specimen by rolling swab in wound.		
7. Use separate swabs for each specimen.		
8. Place swab into culturette tube.		
9. Crush ampule in culturette tube and close tube securely, making sure swab is surrounded by medium.		
ANAEROBIC CULTURE 10. Hold transport tube in an upright position, place swab into tube, and close tube securely.		
SYRINGE METHOD 11. Insert needle into drainage, and aspirate 5 to 10 cc.		

Table continues on following page

Critical Behaviors	Complies	
	yes	no
12. Express excess air from syringe.		
13. Cork needle.		
14. Remove and discard gloves.		
15. Wash hands.		
16. Don sterile gloves, and apply sterile dressing.		
17. Label all specimens with name, room number, date, time, and exact source.		
18. Place specimens in plastic bag.		
19. Dispose of soiled equipment in appropriate receptacle.		
20. Wash hands.		
21. Document procedure in the patient record.		

SKILL 28–3

Dressing Wounds with Drains

Drains facilitate the healing process by providing an exit for any drainage from a wound site. If pus, body fluids, blood, or necrotic debris does not drain freely from the site, wound healing will be compromised as pressure builds within the tissues. The collection of drainage also provides a source for proliferation of microorganisms. Even with a drain, the wound is still at risk for infection, since microorganisms can enter the deeper tissues of the body through the site and drain.

Surgeons insert drains in wounds that are expected to produce significant amounts of drainage. In most cases, surgeons prefer closed drainage systems (tubings that are attached to a suction apparatus or a collecting device for gravity drainage) over open drains (Penrose) (Figs. 28–4 through 28–10) that drain directly into a dressing (Table 28–2). Open drains tend to provide access for the migration of bacteria into the wound. Soule (1983) reports that studies have shown a slightly higher incidence of infections with open drains.

Drains are generally inserted in stab wounds distant from the primary wound site to reduce the risk of infec-

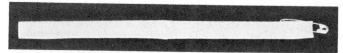

FIGURE 28–4. Penrose drain. (From Long, Barbara & Phipps, Wilma, *Medical Surgical Nursing: A Nursing Process Approach*, 2nd Ed. St. Louis: C. V. Mosby, 1989, with permission.)

FIGURE 28–5. Cigarette drain. (From Long, Barbara & Phipps, Wilma, *Medical Surgical Nursing: A Nursing Process Approach*, 2nd Ed. St. Louis: C. V. Mosby, 1989, with permission.)

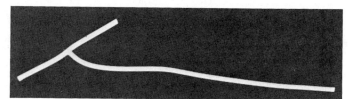

FIGURE 28–6. T-tube. (From Long, Barbara & Phipps, Wilma, *Medical Surgical Nursing: A Nursing Process Approach*, 2nd Ed. St. Louis: C. V. Mosby, 1989, with permission.)

FIGURE 28–7. Abramson. (From Long, Barbara & Phipps, Wilma, *Medical Surgical Nursing: A Nursing Process Approach*, 2nd Ed. St. Louis: C. V. Mosby, 1989, with permission.)

FIGURE 28–8. Saratoga sump. (From Long, Barbara & Phipps, Wilma, *Medical Surgical Nursing: A Nursing Process Approach*, 2nd Ed. St. Louis: C. V. Mosby, 1989, with permission.)

tion. For highly contaminated or infected wounds, the primary incision is left open to allow for drainage.

Dressing the wound with drains requires techniques that will facilitate drainage as well as protect the wound and deeper tissues from infection. Wound dressings also should protect the surrounding skin from maceration and the drains from tension that might cause them to dislodge from the wound.

Purpose

The nurse dresses a wound with drains to

1. Maintain aseptic conditions in the wound and drain site.

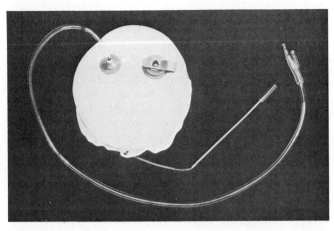

FIGURE 28–9. Hemo-drain. (From Long, Barbara & Phipps, Wilma, *Medical Surgical Nursing: A Nursing Process Approach*, 2nd Ed. St. Louis: C. V. Mosby, 1989, with permission.)

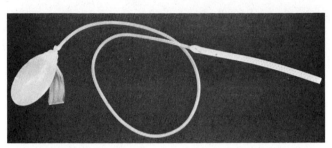

FIGURE 28–10. Jackson-Pratt drain. (From Long, Barbara & Phipps, Wilma, *Medical Surgical Nursing: A Nursing Process Approach*, 2nd Ed. St. Louis: C. V. Mosby, 1989, with permission.)

2. Prevent cross-contamination from drain site to wound.
3. Prevent obstruction of the drainage system.
4. Prevent maceration of the surrounding skin.
5. Prevent dislodging of drains.

Prerequisite Knowledge and Skills

Prior to dressing wounds with drains, the nurse should understand

1. Principles of aseptic technique.
2. Rationale for specific types of drains used (i.e., where the drain goes and how it is secured).
3. Principles of wound healing.
4. Universal precautions.

The nurse should be able to perform

1. Proper handwashing technique (see Skill 35–5).
2. Wound assessment.
3. Proper wound cleaning and irrigation techniques (see Skill 28–1).
4. Universal precautions (see Skill 35–1).

Assessment

1. Assess the wound for the locations of drains and the condition of sutures anchoring the drains. **Rationale:** Proper function of drains requires that they are intact, patent, and secure.
2. Note the positions of drains at the exit site from the wound. **Rationale:** Drains must be free of kinks, twists, debris, or clots for proper drainage; determines where to place dressings for optimal function of drains.
3. Assess the type and amount of drainage. **Rationale:** May determine frequency of dressing changes; changes in drainage may indicate alteration in patient condition.
4. Assess the condition of the wound bed. **Rationale:** Gives progress of wound healing; identifies need for wound culture.
5. Assess the surrounding skin for maceration and inflammation. **Rationale:** Excessive drainage and moisture will cause skin breakdown.
6. Assess for pain on palpation of area surrounding wound. **Rationale:** Patient may need an analgesic before

TABLE 28–2 Types of Drains

Type	Description
Penrose drain (Fig. 28–4) Cigarette drain (Fig. 28–5)	Open gravity drainage into a sterile dressing
T-tube (Fig. 28–6)	Closed gravity drainage of bile from common bile duct; attached to bag or bottle
Abramson (Fig. 28–7)	Triple-lumen drain for suction/irrigation/airway; used with low intermittent suction
Saratoga sump (Fig. 28–8)	Double-lumen tube within another tube; used with low intermittent suction
Hemo-drain (Fig. 28–9)	Self-contained low-pressure drainage; inner spring expands slowly, creating suction
Jackson-Pratt (Fig. 28–10)	Self-contained low-pressure drainage; compressed bulb expands slowly, creating suction

the procedure. Pain is also symptomatic of an infectious process.

Nursing Diagnoses

1. Potential for impaired tissue integrity related to accumulation of drainage and/or necrotic debris. **Rationale:** As debris and drainage accumulate within tissues, excess pressure compromises tissue integrity.
2. Potential for infection related to retention of bacterial contamination in wound. **Rationale:** Excess debris and drainage provide a medium for proliferation of microorganisms.
3. Potential for impaired skin integrity related to maceration of surrounding skin. **Rationale:** Excessive drainage and moisture will cause skin breakdown.

Planning

1. Individualize the following goals for dressing a wound with drains:
   a. Promote wound healing. **Rationale:** Proper wound healing requires a wound free of drainage accumulation. Inadequate drainage causes pressure within tissues and provides a growth medium for bacteria.
   b. Maintain the integrity of the surrounding skin. **Rationale:** Excessive drainage and moisture will cause skin breakdown.

Rationale: Excessive drainage and moisture will cause skin breakdown.

2. Assemble and prepare all necessary equipment and supplies. **Rationale:** Assembling supplies will provide for an organized approach to the procedure.
   a. All-gauze sterile 4 × 4's, ABD dressings (amount/number is determined by the wound size and should be recorded in the nursing care plan).
   b. Two pairs of exam gloves.
   c. One pair of sterile gloves.
   d. Sterile normal saline for cleaning.
   e. One sterile suture set or one pair of sterile scissors.
   f. One plastic bag for soiled dressings.
   g. One roll paper tape or one set of Montgomery straps.
   h. Liquid skin barrier (with application of Montgomery straps).
3. Prepare the patient.
   a. Administer pain medication as prescribed 30 minutes prior to treatment, if necessary. **Rationale:** Reduces discomfort and anxiety.
   b. Explain the procedure to patient. **Rationale:** Reduces anxiety and encourages cooperation.
   c. Position patient for optimal wound exposure. **Rationale:** Necessary for wound assessment and ease of access.

Implementation

Steps	Rationale	Special Considerations
1. Wash hands.	Reduces transmission of microorganisms.	
2. Prepare sterile field for cleaning/irrigating the wound.	Maintains aseptic technique.	
3. Don clean gloves (and goggles, gown, and apron, if indicated).	Universal precautions.	
4. Remove soiled dressing and discard in plastic bag. Then remove and discard gloves in plastic bag.	Prevents contamination and spread of microorganisms.	Take special care when removing dressing to prevent dislodging drain. Some drains (i.e., Penrose) may be hidden beneath the dressing.
5. Don clean gloves and clean/irrigate wound as indicated (see Skill 28–1).	Removes contaminated drainage and debris from wound.	
6. Remove gloves after cleaning and discard in plastic bag.	Prevents spread of microorganisms.	
7. Open sterile all-gauze 4 × 4's and ABD dressings onto sterile field.	Provides accessibility to dressings and maintains aseptic technique.	All-gauze 4 × 4's provide a wicking effect to absorb drainage and do not leave cotton fibers in the wound.
8. Don sterile gloves.	Maintains aseptic technique.	
9. Open 4 × 4's and fold lengthwise into narrow strips to place around drains (Fig. 28–11).	Absorbs drainage and protects surrounding skin.	

Table continues on following page

Steps	Rationale	Special Considerations
10. Apply 4× 4's to wound and around drains, dressing from least contaminated areas to most contaminated areas.	Prevents cross-contamination.	Apply enough 4 × 4's to absorb drainage but not so thick that drainage will be trapped under hidden dressings causing maceration to skin. Be careful to prevent kinking or twisting of drains by dressings.
11. Apply ABD dressing or other absorbent dressing over gauze.	Supports and immobilizes 4 × 4's and provides added absorption.	
12. Tape dressing with paper tape or Montgomery straps.	Secure dressing.	Montgomery straps are recommended to prevent skin stripping from tape if frequent dressing changes are necessary.

Tape

13. Using paper tape, tape across dressing, overlapping each layer of tape; extend tape approximately 2 in beyond dressing onto skin all around dressing, avoiding excess tension on skin or on drains; look for kinks or twists in tubing.	Paper tape is less traumatic to skin than adhesives. Limited use of tape reduces skin trauma. Freely draining tubes promote wound healing.	A liquid skin barrier may be applied under tape for skin protection.

Montgomery Straps

14. Apply liquid skin barrier to skin lateral to dressing at site of Montgomery strap placement; allow to dry thoroughly.	Protects skin from adhesive.	
15. Peel paper backing off of one Montgomery strap, and apply to skin, pressing gently; repeat with other strap.	Secures Montgomery strap to skin.	
16. Lace cotton tape (i.e., umbilical tape or trach ties) through holes in Montgomery strap and tie in a bow (Fig. 28–12).	Secures dressing in place.	
17. Dispose of soiled equipment in appropriate receptacle.	Universal precautions.	
18. Wash hands.	Reduces transmission of microorganisms.	

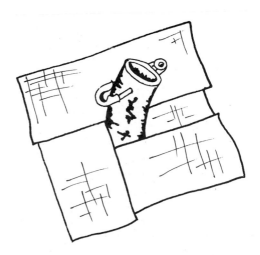

FIGURE 28–11. Dressing around a drain. (Courtesy of Arturo Sanchez.)

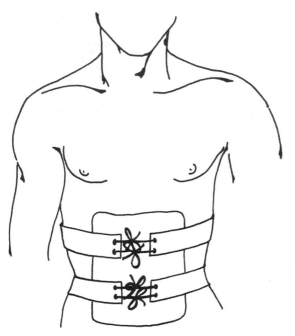

FIGURE 28–12. Montgomery straps. (Courtesy of Arturo Sanchez.)

Evaluation

1. Observe the incision and drain sites for the condition of the sutures. **Rationale:** Improper handling can dislodge drains.

2. Observe the patency of the drains to suction or gravity. **Rationale:** Kinking of drains may occur when new dressing is applied.

3. Check the suction apparatus for function. **Rationale:** Inadequate drainage will impede healing.

4. Monitor the type and amount of drainage. **Rationale:** Excessive amount of drainage may result in fluid and electrolyte imbalance and/or a change in the patient's condition.

5. Monitor the surrounding skin for inflammation or maceration. **Rationale:** Moisture on surrounding skin will cause skin breakdown.

Expected Outcomes

1. Evidence of wound healing. **Rationale:** Wound free of drainage is necessary for optimal wound healing.

2. Drains will remain intact. **Rationale:** Drains must remain in place to remove drainage from desired location.

3. Integrity of surrounding skin is maintained. **Rationale:** Drains and dressings contain drainage, protecting surrounding skin from breakdown/trauma.

Unexpected Outcomes

1. Dislodged drains from wound. **Rationale:** Loosened sutures around drains could result in removal of drain from site.

2. Excessive drainage from wound site with improperly functioning drain. **Rationale:** Clogged or kinked drains allow drainage to escape through wound onto surrounding skin.

3. Surrounding skin maceration. **Rationale:** Drainage from wound site of improperly functioning drain is trapped under dressing. Frequent dressing changes using paper tape will cause stripping of skin layers causing breakdown.

Documentation

Documentation in the patient record should include the date and time of the procedure, the location and position of the drain, the condition of the sutures securing drain, the amount and type of drainage through drain, any leakage around drain, the condition of the wound and surrounding skin, the function of suction apparatus, the type of dressing applied, how drains were secured to prevent dislocation, and any unexpected outcomes and interventions taken. **Rationale:** Documents nursing care given, progress of wound healing, status of drain/drainage, and expected and unexpected outcomes.

Patient/Family Education

1. Instruct the patient and family to notify the nurse of any discomfort or pulling sensations from wound site. **Rationale:** Improperly functioning drains could cause pain from collection of drainage in wound; tension on tubing could pull drain out of wound.

2. Assess the possibility for long-term drainage of wound. **Rationale:** Helps the nurse to determine teaching needs and wound-care needs should patient be discharged with drains.

Performance Checklist
Skill 28–3: Dressing Wounds with Drains

Critical Behaviors	Complies	
	yes	**no**
1. Wash hands.		
2. Prepare sterile field for cleaning/irrigating wound.		

Table continues on following page

Critical Behaviors	Complies	
	yes	no
3. Don clean gloves (and goggles, gown, and apron, if indicated).		
4. Remove soiled dressing and discard in plastic bag, and then remove and discard gloves.		
5. Don clean gloves and clean wound and around drains.		
6. Remove gloves used for cleaning and discard.		
7. Open appropriate dressings onto sterile field.		
8. Don sterile gloves.		
9. Open 4 × 4's and fold into narrow strips.		
10. Apply 4 × 4's to wound and around drains.		
11. Cover with ABD dressing.		
12. Secure dressing and drains with paper tape or Montgomery straps.		
Tape 13. Tape across dressing, overlapping each layer of tape; extend tape approximately 2 in onto skin; and secure drain to skin, avoiding tension on drain or skin.		
Montgomery Straps 14. Apply liquid skin barrier to skin lateral to dressing.		
15. Peel off paper backing from Montgomery straps, and apply straps to skin.		
16. Lace cotton tape through holes in Montgomery straps to secure dressing in place.		
17. Dispose of soiled equipment in appropriate receptacle.		
18. Remove and discard gloves.		
19. Wash hands.		
20. Document procedure in the patient record.		

SKILL 28–4

Dressing Open Wounds

Surgical incisions or traumatic wounds are left open in cases of contamination or in the presence of infection. Open wounds facilitate discharge of accumulated drainage and debris from deeper tissues. These wounds heal by secondary intention, granulating from the base upward. Special care must be taken to allow for uniform granulation to occur, preventing open pockets in the wound that will interfere with healing or allow space for collection of drainage. Cleaning and debridement are crucial to proper healing.

Granulating wounds are slow to heal. A moist wound environment is necessary to promote the migration of cells within the wound. If the wound is allowed to dry, granulation will be halted. Sufficient dressing material must be placed within the wound to avoid open spaces between the tissues without producing excessive pressure that could impede circulation.

Moderate to heavy draining wounds may require frequent dressing changes or the application of a pouch to collect excessive drainage (see Skill 20–2). Skin care must be impeccable to prevent maceration from excess moisture either from overzealous wet dressings or wound drainage.

Purpose

The nurse dresses an open wound to

1. Clean and debride necrotic tissue.
2. Absorb drainage.
3. Provide a moist environment for healing.
4. Protect the wound.
5. Protect the surrounding skin from maceration.

Prerequisite Knowledge and Skills

Before dressing an open wound, the nurse should understand

1. Principles of aseptic technique.
2. Principles of wound healing.
3. Universal precautions.

The nurse should be able to perform

1. Proper handwashing technique (see Skill 35–5).
2. Proper wound cleaning techniques (see Skill 28–1).
3. Wound assessment.
4. Universal precautions (see Skill 35–1).

Assessment

1. Observe the current dressings for the amount and type of drainage. **Rationale:** Determines adequacy of dressing and frequency of changes or the need for a drainage collecting pouch.
2. Observe the wound for drainage and necrotic debris. **Rationale:** Determines the type of cleaning and/or degree of mechanical debridement necessary.
3. Assess the size and condition of the wound bed. **Rationale:** Determines progress of wound healing.
4. Assess the surrounding skin for evidence of maceration. **Rationale:** Excessive drainage and moisture will cause breakdown of surrounding skin.
5. Assess for pain on palpation of area surrounding the wound. **Rationale:** Patient may require an analgesic before the procedure. Pain may also be a symptom of an infectious process.

Nursing Diagnoses

1. Impaired tissue integrity related to accumulation of drainage and/or necrotic debris. **Rationale:** Devitalized tissue and debris inhibit wound healing.
2. Potential for infection related to retention of bacterial contamination in the wound. **Rationale:** Impaired tissue integrity provides a medium for potential growth of microorganisms.
3. Potential for impaired skin integrity related to maceration of surrounding skin. **Rationale:** Excessive drainage and moisture will cause skin breakdown.

Planning

1. Individualize the following goals for dressing an open wound:
   a. Promote wound healing. **Rationale:** Proper wound healing requires a wound free of drainage accumulation. Inadequate drainage causes pressure within tissues and provides a growth medium for bacteria.
   b. Maintain the integrity of the surrounding skin. **Rationale:** Excessive drainage and moisture will cause skin breakdown.
2. Assemble and prepare all necessary equipment and supplies. **Rationale:** Assembling supplies will provide for an organized approach to the procedure.
   a. All-gauze sterile 4 × 4's, ABD dressings (amount/number is determined by wound size and should be recorded in the nursing care plan).
   b. Two pairs of exam gloves.
   c. One pair of sterile gloves.
   d. Sterile normal saline for cleaning wound and for moistening dressings (amount is determined by the size of the wound and the number of dressings needed and should be recorded in the nursing care plan).
   e. One sterile basin.
   f. One plastic bag for soiled dressings.
   g. One roll of paper tape or one set of Montgomery straps.
   h. Liquid skin barrier (for use with Montgomery straps).
3. Prepare patient.
   a. Administer pain medication as prescribed 30 minutes prior to treatment, as necessary. **Rationale:** Reduces discomfort and anxiety and encourages cooperation.
   b. Explain the procedure to the patient. **Rationale:** Reduces anxiety and provides information to patient.

Implementation

Steps	Rationale	Special Considerations
1. Wash hands.	Reduces transmission of microorganisms.	
2. Prepare sterile field for cleaning/ irrigating the wound.	Maintains aseptic technique.	
3. Don clean gloves (and goggles, gown, and apron, if indicated).	Universal precautions.	
4. Remove soiled dressing and discard in plastic bag. Then remove and discard gloves.	Prevents spread of microorganisms.	
5. Don clean gloves, and clean/ irrigate wound as indicated (see Skill 28–1).	Removes debris and drainage.	
6. Remove gloves and discard in plastic bag.	Prevents cross-contamination and spread of microorganisms.	

Table continues on following page

Steps	Rationale	Special Considerations
7. Open sterile all-gauze 4 × 4's for packing into wound into sterile basin, and open 4 × 4's and ABD dressings for top dressing onto sterile field.	Maintains aseptic technique.	All-gauze 4 × 4's provide a wicking effect to absorb drainage and prevent leaving cotton fibers in wound.
8. Pour normal saline over 4 × 4's in basin.	Moisture must be maintained to all granulating surfaces to promote cell proliferation.	
9. Don sterile gloves.	Maintains aseptic technique.	
10. Unfold each 4 × 4, and wring out excess moisture. Pack gauze one by one loosely but completely into all spaces of wound. Continue until wound is packed to the edges but not on surrounding skin.	Open gauze is easier to line the wound without creating pockets of open space. Excessively wet dressings will drip onto surrounding skin causing maceration.	Gauze should be moist, not wet. *Do not* overpack wound—excessive pressure of dressings will compromise tissue circulation.
11. Place dry 4 × 4 and ABD dressings over moist dressings.	Supports and immobilizes moist 4 × 4's and provides added absorption.	Dressings within wound must remain moist for wound healing.
12. Secure dressing with paper tape or Montgomery straps.	Secures dressing.	Montgomery straps are recommended to prevent skin stripping from tape if frequent dressing changes are necessary.
Tape		
13. Using paper tape, tape across dressing, overlapping each layer of tape; extend tape approximately 2 in beyond dressing onto skin all around dressing, avoiding excess tension on skin.	Paper tape is less traumatic to skin than adhesives. Limited use of tape reduces skin trauma.	Liquid skin barrier may be applied under tape for skin protection.
Montgomery Straps		
14. Apply liquid skin barrier to skin lateral to dressing at site of Montgomery strap placement, and allow to dry thoroughly.	Protects skin from adhesive.	
15. Peel paper backing off of one Montgomery strap, and apply to skin, pressing gently; repeat with other strap.	Secures Montgomery strap to skin.	
16. Lace cotton tape (i.e., umbilical tape or trach ties) through holes in Montgomery strap and tie in a bow (Fig. 28–12).	Secures dressing in place.	
17. Dispose of soiled equipment in appropriate receptacle.	Universal precautions.	
18. Wash hands.	Reduces transmission of microorganisms.	

Evaluation

1. Evaluate the wound bed. **Rationale:** Identifies effectiveness of cleaning/irrigation and amount of necrotic debris remaining.

2. Measure wound length, width, and depth at least once a week. **Rationale:** Monitors progress of wound healing.

3. Monitor the surrounding skin for inflammation or maceration. **Rationale:** Moisture on surrounding skin will cause breakdown.

Expected Outcomes

1. Debridement of necrotic tissue. **Rationale:** Necrotic debris impedes wound healing.

2. Granulation from the base upward within a beefy red, moist wound. **Rationale:** Optimal wound healing requires healing in a uniform manner from the bottom upward.

3. Integrity of surrounding skin is maintained. **Rationale:** Dressings contain drainage, protecting surrounding skin from breakdown or trauma.

Unexpected Outcomes

1. Desiccation of wound tissue. **Rationale:** Dry tissue halts cell proliferation.

2. Inadequate debridement of necrotic tissue. **Rationale:** Debris impedes healing; an increase in debris over time indicates that the wound tissue is not healthy and that there is a need to assess other factors influencing wound healing.

3. Wound edges close before the base of the wound fills in. **Rationale:** Open space within the wound allows for accumulation of drainage and debris, providing a reservoir for infection.

4. Surrounding skin maceration. **Rationale:** Drainage from the wound site of improperly functioning drain is trapped under dressing. Frequent dressing changes using paper tape will cause stripping of skin layers causing breakdown.

Documentation

Documentation in the patient record should include the date and time of the procedure, the amount of necrotic debris in wound before and after cleaning, the size of the wound (length, width, and depth), the condition of the wound bed and granulation tissue, the condition of the surrounding skin; the type of dressing applied and the number of 4 × 4's packed into the wound, and any unexpected outcomes and interventions taken. **Rationale:** Documents nursing care given and progress of wound healing.

Patient/Family Education

1. Demonstrate the procedure to both patient and family because open wounds heal slowly and the procedure will most likely need to be repeated following discharge. **Rationale:** Allays fears and encourages participation in self-care activities.

2. Explain wound-assessment techniques. **Rationale:** Teaches the patient and family to recognize changes that should be reported to a health care professional.

3. Encourage the patient and family to assist with certain aspects of the procedure as warranted. **Rationale:** Reduces anxiety and builds skills.

Performance Checklist
Skill 28–4: Dressing Open Wounds

Critical Behaviors	Complies	
	yes	no
1. Wash hands.		
2. Prepare sterile field for cleaning/irrigating the wound.		
3. Don clean gloves (and goggles, gown, and apron, if indicated).		
4. Remove soiled dressing and discard in plastic bag, and then remove and discard gloves.		
5. Don clean gloves, and clean/irrigate the wound.		
6. Remove and discard gloves.		
7. Open sterile all-gauze 4 × 4's for packing into wound into sterile basin, and open 4 × 4's and ABD dressings for top dressing onto sterile field.		
8. Pour normal saline over 4 × 4's in basin.		
9. Don sterile gloves.		
10. Completely unfold each moistened 4 × 4, wring out excess normal saline, and pack wound with 4 × 4's.		
11. Place dry 4 × 4's and ABD dressings over moist dressings.		
12. Secure dressing with paper tape or Montgomery straps.		
TAPE 13. Tape across dressing, overlapping each layer of tape, and extend tape approximately 2 in onto skin.		
MONTGOMERY STRAPS 14. Apply liquid skin barrier to skin, and dry thoroughly.		
15. Peel off paper backing on Montgomery strap, and apply strap to skin.		

Table continues on following page

Critical Behaviors	Complies	
	yes	no
16. Lace cotton tape through holes in Montgomery straps and tie in a bow.		
17. Dispose of soiled equipment in appropriate receptacle.		
18. Wash hands.		
19. Document procedure in the patient record.		

BIBLIOGRAPHY

Atwater, E. E. (1989). Care of the surgically created granulating wound. *Dermatol. Nurs.* 1(1):43–46.

Brown, C. V. (1986). Nursing tips and techniques, collecting viable culture specimens. *Curr. Concepts Wound Care* 9(4):15.

Harding, K. G. (1990). Wound care: Putting theory into practice. *Wounds* 2(1):21–31.

Long, B. C., and Phipps, W. J. (1989). Postoperative intervention. In *Medical-Surgical Nursing*, 2d Ed. (pp. 380–384). St. Louis: Mosby.

Martinez, J. A., and Burns, C. R. (1987). Wound management. *Curr. Concepts Wound Care* 10(2):9–16.

Marvin, J. A. (1989). The physiologic responses of the trauma patient. *J. Enterostomal Ther.* 16(2):65–71.

Neuberger, G. B., and Reckling, J. B. (1987). Preventing wound complications in an age of DRGs. *Ostomy/Wound Management* 17:20–30.

Neuberger, G. B. (1987). Wound care: What's clear, what's not. *Nursing 87* 17(2):34–37.

Simmons, B. P. (1982). Guideline for prevention of surgical wound infections. *Surg. Wound Infect.* March, 1–8.

Taylor, C., Lillis, C., and LeMone, P. (1989). Care of wounds. In *Fundamentals of Nursing* (pp. 1200–1226). Philadelphia: Lippincott.

Thomas, C. (1988). Nursing alert: Wound healing halted with the use of povidone-iodine. *Ostomy/Wound Management* 22:30–33.

Timberlake, G. A. (1986). Wound healing: The physiology of scar formation. *Curr. Concepts Wound Care* 1(1):4–14.

Wysocki, A. B. (1989). Surgical wound healing. *AORN J.* 49(2):502–518.

REFERENCES

Rogness, H. (1985). High-pressure wound irrigation. *J. Enterostomal Ther.* 12(1):27–28.

Soule, B. M. (Ed.) (1983). *The APIC Curriculum for Infection Control Practice.* Dubuque, Iowa: Kendall/Hunt.

29

MANAGEMENT OF PRESSURE SORES

BEHAVIORAL OBJECTIVES

After completing this chapter, the nurse will be able to

- Discuss the causative factors of pressure sore development.
- Discuss nursing interventions for pressure sore prevention.
- Describe treatment modalities for pressure sores.
- Demonstrate the skills involved in the management of pressure sores.

Pressure sores, also referred to as *decubitus ulcers* or *bedsores*, are areas of localized trauma to the skin that occur as a result of insufficient blood supply due to pressure. Determinants of pressure sore development include the intensity and duration of pressure and the tolerance of the tissue to pressure. Several aspects of critical illness, such as immobility, malnutrition, dehydration, diaphoresis, and incontinence, increase the risk of pressure sore formation.

Pressure sores can range from an epidermal irritation to full-thickness craters. The extent is usually classified by stages (Table 29–1).

This chapter includes procedures for prevention and treatment of pressure sores. Prevention is accomplished through assessment of risk factors; implementation of measures to reduce or relieve pressure, moisture, friction, and shear; and promotion of adequate nutrition and hydration. Treatment includes all the preceding, as well as cleansing, debriding, and covering the pressure sore.

KEY TERMS

capillary closing pressure	pressure reduction
debride	pressure relief
dermis	semipermeable occlusive
enzyme preparations	dressings
epidermis	shear
eschar	sinus tracts
hydrocolloid wafer	transparent adhesive
dressings	dressings
maceration	undermining

SKILLS

29–1 Pressure Sore Prevention
29–2 Management of Pressure Sores: Semipermeable Occlusive Dressings
29–3 Management of Pressure Sores: Enzyme Preparations

GUIDELINES

The following assessment guidelines assist the nurse in formulating a nursing diagnosis and an individualized plan of care for patients with actual or potential pressure sores:

1. Assess the patient's general health and underlying disease state(s).
2. Assess the patient's history for previous pressure sores and circulatory impairments.
3. Assess the patient's mobility status.
4. Assess the patient's ability to sense and communicate skin discomfort.
5. Assess the patient's nutritional status, including previous and current eating patterns, height and weight, and laboratory data, including serum albumin and serum transferrin.

SKILL 29–1

Pressure Sore Prevention

Pressure sore prevention is particularly important in the critical-care unit. Critically ill patients possess a combination of factors that significantly increases their risk for pressure sore development. Minor skin irritations that begin in the ICU can progress to major complications and delay the patient's discharge.

Purpose

The nurse performs pressure sore interventions to

1. Prevent pressure sore development by reducing or relieving pressure, friction, shear, and moisture to the skin.
2. Avert patient discomfort associated with impaired skin integrity.
3. Decrease the potential for infection related to impaired skin integrity.

Prerequisite Knowledge and Skills

Prior to instituting measures for pressure sore prevention, the nurse should understand

1. Anatomy and physiology of the skin.
2. Principles of circulation and tissue oxygenation.

TABLE 29–1 PRESSURE SORE STAGES

Stage	Definition	Presentation	Expected Outcome
I	Epidermal erythema; skin intact	Redness remains 15 minutes or more after pressure relief; may be painful	Reverse process; prevent further damage
II	Partial-thickness tissue loss involving epidermis and possibly dermis	Blisters or cracks with erythema and/or induration; painful	Epithelialization
III	Full-thickness tissue loss through epidermis, dermis, and into subcutaneous tissue	Shallow crater with distinct margins, exudate (usually); may include necrotic tissue; usually not painful	Granulation, contraction, epithelialization
IV	Full-thickness tissue loss through subcutaneous tissue; may involve muscle and bone	Deep crater; often includes necrotic tissue, exudate, and/or infection; usually not painful	Debridement of necrosis, granulation, contraction, epithelialization; prevent osteomyelitis

3. The negative impact of pressure sores on patient comfort, healing, and length/cost of hospitalization.

4. The negative impact of pressure sores on health care provider workload, liability, image, and expenditures.

The nurse should be able to perform

1. Risk-factor assessment for pressure sore development.
2. Skin assessment.
3. Nutritional assessment.
4. General health assessment.
5. Patient turning and positioning.
6. Proper handwashing technique (see Skill 35–5).

Assessment

1. Assess for the presence of the following risk factors: mobility limitations, activity limitations, sensory deficits, altered circulation and/or oxygenation, presence of excessive moisture (diaphoresis or incontinence), friction, shear, debilitated condition, old age, history of previous pressure ulcers, and malnutrition. Several pressure sore risk assessment tools have been developed and tested by nurses (Bergstrom et al., 1987; Goldstone and Goldstone, 1982; and Gosnell, 1987). An example of a pressure sore risk assessment tool is presented in Table 29–2. **Rationale:** All these factors have been found to increase the risk of pressure sore development.

2. Inspect the patient's entire body surface area, particularly bony prominences such as the sacrum, coccyx, heels, trochanters, and occiput for changes in color, actual pressure sores (stages I, II, III, or IV) (see Table 29–1), scar tissue from previous pressure sores, and other skin integrity impairments such as cracks, blisters, rashes, and abrasions. **Rationale:** Bony prominences are the most common sites for pressure sore development. Pressure can intensify existing skin integrity impairments.

3. Assess the patient's nutritional status, including weight and recent gains or losses; oral, enteral, and parenteral intake; serum albumin; serum transferrin; and total lymphocyte count. If nutritional depletion is suspected, consult dietician for more extensive assessment and recommendations. **Rationale:** Nutritional parameters associated with increased risk for pressure sore development include recent unintentional weight loss, NPO or clear liquid diet for more than 3 days, serum albumin less than 3.5 g/dl, serum transferrin less than 150 mg/dl, total lymphocyte count less than 1500 cells/mm^3. Malnutrition is often associated with total lymphocyte counts of less than 1500 cells/mm^3.

Nursing Diagnosis

Potential impaired skin integrity related to pressure-induced ischemia. **Rationale:** Prolonged pressure to the skin, particularly over bony prominences, causes capillary compression, ischemia, and tissue death.

Planning

1. The goal for pressure sore prevention is to maintain skin integrity. **Rationale:** Skin integrity impairments are caused by pressure, friction, shear, and prolonged moisture to the skin. Interventions for pressure sore prevention are directed toward alleviating these variables.
2. The preparation of equipment and supplies will be dependent on the individual patient's risk potential. Table 29–3 lists the most common products and equipment used as interventions for pressure sores. **Rationale:** Patients who are at low risk may require no additional supplies. Patients who are at extreme risk may require therapeutic mattresses, beds, or other devices.

TABLE 29–2 PRESSURE SORE RISK-FACTOR ASSESSMENT

Select one category for each assessment parameter. Add the points assigned to the selected categories to yield the total risk assessment score.

	Points 1	2	3	
MENTAL STATUS	Alert, oriented, communicative	Disoriented and/or unable to communicate needs	Comatose, nonresponsive	_____
ACTIVITY	Ambulatory	Out of bed with assistance	Bedfast	_____
MOBILITY	Major, independent position changes	Some limitations to movement	Immobile without assistance	_____
MOISTURE	Fully continent, skin dry	Occasional incontinence	Totally incontinent and/or usually diaphoretic	_____
NUTRITION	Eats most of all meals, normal weight for height	Oral, enteral, and/or parenteral intake, inadequate	NPO, enteral/parenteral intake < 50 percent of needs	_____
AGE	< 55 years	55–69 years	70 or more years	_____
			TOTAL SCORE	_____

Risk for Pressure Sore Development

Total Score	Risk
6–9 points	Low risk
10–13 points	Moderate risk
14–18 points	High risk

3. Prepare the patient and family.
   a. Explain what pressure sores are, how they develop, and outcomes related to pressure sores. **Rationale:** Teaches patient and family the need for preventive measures.
   b. Explain expectations for patient and family participation in promoting mobility, nutrition, and continence. **Rationale:** Encourages cooperation.

Implementation

Steps	Rationale	Special Considerations
1. Wash hands.	Reduces transmission of microorganisms.	
2. Establish a plan for position changes and weight shifts. Major repositioning (30 degrees or more) should occur at least every 2 hours, with minor position changes (i.e., ROM of an extremity) between.	Pressure sores can develop as a result of high pressure over a short time or low pressure over a long time. Ischemia can develop within 30 minutes in the severely compromised patient.	Many critically ill patients cannot tolerate major position changes without hemodynamic instability. In these patients, frequent, minor position changes can still be effective.
3. Select pressure-reducing device (i.e., block foam) specific for risk-factor assessment (see Table 29–3)	Pressure-reducing devices augment positioning schedules.	
4. Utilize devices for pressure relief (see Chapter 23) if it cannot be accomplished with positioning.	Capillary closing pressure is 25 to 32 mmHg. Pressure-relieving devices must reduce pressure below this level.	These devices are expensive and therefore are recommended for patients who cannot be turned or who have breakdown involving more than one surface.

Table continues on following page

Steps	Rationale	Special Considerations
5. Keep the head of the bed at 30 degrees or lower unless contraindicated.	Reduces potential for shear and friction from patient sliding down in bed.	
6. Use assistive devices for positioning (i.e., drawsheets, trapeze, lifts, and transfer boards).	Facilitates mobility and reduces friction in bedridden patient.	
7. Contain urinary and/or fecal incontinence by anticipating and providing for elimination needs, padding the bed with natural-fiber sheets or blankets, and providing perineal care as needed.	Protects skin from maceration and bacterial contamination.	Waterproof sheets with plastic or vinyl coatings, such as "blue pads" or "chux," increase the maceration potential by containing moisture close to the skin and blocking the action of low and high air loss beds. Adult diapers (i.e., Attends) have the same effect and can negatively affect patient esteem.
8. Contain diaphoresis with bathing as needed and bed padding.	Diaphoretic patients can develop maceration over bony prominences and in skin folds.	
9. Protect bony prominences of high-risk patients by covering (i.e., heel and elbow protectors, transparent or hydrocolloid dressings).	Protects areas from friction.	
10. Support nutrition and hydration status by monitoring daily intake and output and weight gains/ losses, encouraging oral intake, consulting with the dietician and physician to obtain orders for enteral or parenteral nutrition to meet caloric and protein requirements.	NPO or clear liquid diet for more than 3 days, unintentional weight loss, serum albumin < 3.5 g/dl, and serum transferrin < 150 mg/dl are associated with increased risk for pressure sore development.	
11. Wash hands.	Reduces transmission of microorganisms.	

Evaluation

1. Continually monitor patient's skin for areas of redness that do not resolve within 15 minutes of pressure reduction/relief. Investigate any patient complaints of skin discomfort. **Rationale:** Redness is the first visible sign of ischemia, but tissue destruction can develop at the bone–tissue interface before symptoms are visible on the skin surface.

2. Evaluate the patient's nutritional status with daily monitoring of intake and output, weight, and serum albumin and transferrin levels when available. **Rationale:** Risk of pressure sore development increases with nutritional depletion.

3. Evaluate the adequacy of the patient's turning and positioning schedule by changes in skin color, patient comfort/discomfort, hours of sleep/rest, and hemodynamic stability. **Rationale:** Repositioning should occur frequently enough to prevent pressure-induced ischemia without compromising other patient needs.

Expected Outcomes

1. Patient maintains skin integrity. **Rationale:** Alter-ations in skin integrity increase discomfort and the potential for infection.

2. Patient accomplishes or maintains adequate nutritional intake. **Rationale:** Pressure sore development is correlated with malnutrition.

Unexpected Outcomes

1. Impaired skin integrity. **Rationale:** Some critically ill patients develop skin integrity impairments even with extensive precautions.

2. Sleep deficit. **Rationale:** Frequent turning or positioning may disrupt sleep cycles.

Documentation

Documentation in the patient record should include date and time of skin assessment findings and specific preventive intervention(s) instituted, and patient's tolerance of interventions and ability to participate in self-care activities for pressure relief/reduction. **Rationale:** Accurate documentation will help promote continuity of care, prevent liability, and maximize reimbursement.

TABLE 29–3 PRESSURE SORE PRODUCTS AND EQUIPMENT

	Prevention			Treatment			
	Risk Potential			Stage			
	Low	Moderate	High	I	II	III	IV
Pressure reduction/relief:							
Mattresses/overlays:							
Foam*	X	X		X			
Air		X	X	X	X		
Water		X	X	X	X		
Gel		X	X	X	X		
Flotation		X	X	X	X	X	X
Air fluidized			X			X	X
Friction/shear control:							
Turning sheets	X	X	X	X	X	X	X
Trapeze		X	X	X	X	X	X
Moisture control:							
Cornstarch powder	X	X	X	X			
Aeration devices		X	X	X		X	X
Moisture barrier Creams		X	X	X	X		
Topical therapy†:							
Saline				X	X	X	X
Wound gels					X	X	X
Nonirritating cleansers (i.e., Cara-Klenz)				X	X	X	X
Sharp debridement						X	X
Enzymatic agents						X	X
Wound coverings‡:							
Plasticized coatings			X	X			
Transparent dressings			X	X	X	X	
Hydrocolloid dressings			X	X	X	X	
Absorptive dressings					X	X	X
Gauze					X	X	X

*Foam overlays should be at least 4 in thick to provide pressure reduction.

†Hydrogen peroxide, povidone-iodine, Dakin's solution, and acetic acid all destroy fibroblasts in granulating wounds.

‡Wet-to-dry dressings provide nonselective debriding, which can remove healthy granulating tissue along with necrotic tissue.

Note: This chart lists the most common indications and usages. Additional approaches may be used based on individualized patient needs and physician preferences.

Patient/Family Education

1. Explain the basic pathology related to pressure sore development to both patient and family. **Rationale:** Helps the patient and family understand the need for repositioning and other interventions.

2. Explain the rationale for devices related to pressure sore prevention, such as pressure-relief mattresses or specialty beds. **Rationale:** Overwhelming, unfamiliar technology can increase the stress of the ICU environment.

3. Reinforce the patient's and family's participation in promoting mobility, nutrition, hygiene, and continence. **Rationale:** Stresses that the patient's and family's participation in care may be simple but very important in preventing serious complications.

4. Evaluate the need for continued interventions to prevent pressure sores during convalescence and following discharge. **Rationale:** In some patients, such as those with spinal cord injuries, the need for long-term care can be identified during the ICU stay. Planning should be initiated as soon as possible to provide for round-the-clock assistance with pressure relief and moisture control, etc.

5. Make appropriate referrals as soon as long-term need is identified (i.e., social service, discharge planning nurse). **Rationale:** Acquisition of assistive personnel and/or devices, such as a trapeze or specialty mattresses, may require considerable time to investigate available fiscal resources.

Performance Checklist
Skill 29–1: Pressure Sore Prevention

Critical Behaviors	Complies	
	yes	no
1. Wash hands.		
2. Institute frequent position changes or weight shifts.		
3. Select and institute pressure-reduction or pressure-relief interventions.		
4. Lower head of bed to patient tolerance.		
5. Utilize assistive devices for turning and positioning.		
6. Contain urinary and/or fecal incontinence.		
7. Contain diaphoresis.		
8. Cover bony prominences.		
9. Maintain adequate nutrition and hydration.		
10. Wash hands.		
11. Document all interventions in the patient record.		

SKILL 29–2

Management of Pressure Sores: Semipermeable Occlusive Dressings

In recent years, two types of semipermeable occlusive dressings have shown great promise in the management of pressure sores: hydrocolloid wafer dressings and transparent adhesive dressings. These products provide several advantages over traditional gauze and tape dressings. Because the dressings have only one component, they can be applied quickly and easily. Once applied, they can be left in place for 5 to 7 days, thereby reducing nursing time and patient discomfort associated with frequent dressing changes. Both dressings promote a moist wound surface that protects the wound bed and promotes cellular migration. They both also support clean wound beds because they are impermeable to external environmental contaminants and bacteria. They also protect the area from external friction.

Both types of dressings are used to protect and promote healing of existing stage I or II pressure sores (stage III and IV sores usually require more extensive therapy). Transparent adhesive dressings have the added advantage of allowing for continuous visibility of the wound and maintaining oxygen permeability. Most hydrocolloid wafers are impermeable to oxygen and should not be used if the potential for anaerobic infection exists. Deep wounds and wounds with undermining or sinus tracts pose a greater risk for development of anaerobic infections and therefore should not be covered with occlusive dressings. Both types of occlusive dressings are contraindicated for use on infected wounds.

These dressings are frequently used to protect and promote healing of existing stage I or II pressure sores. They also can be used as a preventive intervention by applying them as protective coverings over the bony prominences of high-risk patients.

Purpose

The nurse uses semipermeable occlusive dressings to
1. Maintain intact skin over bony prominences.
2. Promote healing of Stage I or II pressure sores.

Prerequisite Knowledge and Skills

Prior to applying semipermeable occlusive dressings, the nurse should understand
1. Anatomy and physiology of the skin.
2. Principles of aseptic technique.
3. Universal precautions.
4. Principles of wound healing.
5. Principles of circulation and tissue oxygenation.

The nurse should be able to perform
1. Proper handwashing technique (see Skill 35–5).
2. Universal precautions (see Skill 35–1).
3. Risk-factor assessment for pressure sore development.
4. Nutritional assessment.
5. Skin assessment.
6. Pressure sore assessment and classification (see Skill 29–1).

Assessment

1. Assess the patient for the presence of the following risk factors: mobility limitations, activity limitations, sen-

sory deficits, altered circulation and/or oxygenation, presence of excessive moisture (diaphoresis or incontinence), friction, shear, old age, history of previous pressure ulcers, and malnutrition (see Table 29–2). **Rationale:** All these factors have been found to increase the risk of pressure sore development and deter pressure sore healing.

2. For each area of impaired skin integrity, identify location, size (length, width, and depth in centimeters), stage of pressure sore development (see Table 29–1), presence of exudate or necrotic tissue, presence of undermining or sinus tracts, pain/discomfort or absence thereof, and symptoms of infection. **Rationale:** Occlusive dressings are recommended for stage I and II pressure sores; they are contraindicated for infected wounds.

3. Assess the patient for a history of allergic reactions or hypersensitivity to tapes. **Rationale:** Patients with a history of tape allergies may develop a reaction to this type dressing.

4. Assess the patient's nutritional status, including weight and recent gains or losses; oral, enteral, and parenteral intake; serum albumin; serum transferrin; and total lymphocyte count. If nutritional depletion is suspected, consult dietitian for more extensive assessment and recommendations. **Rationale:** Nutritional parameters associated with increased risk of pressure sore development include recent unintentional weight loss, NPO or clear liquid diet for more than 3 days, serum albumin less than 3.5 g/dl, serum transferrin less than 150 mg/dl, and total lymphocyte count less than 1500 cells/mm^3.

Nursing Diagnoses

1. Actual impaired skin integrity related to pressure-induced ischemia. **Rationale:** Prolonged pressure over bony prominences compresses capillaries, leading to ischemia and cellular death.

2. Potential for infection related to epidermal destruction. **Rationale:** Intact skin is the body's first line of defense against infection; therefore, alteration provides a portal of entry for microorganisms.

Planning

1. Individualize the following goals based on the patient's identified risk potential and skin assessment:
   a. Prevent tissue destruction. **Rationale:** Cellular death will progress downward through skin layers.
   b. Promote wound healing. **Rationale:** Reverse the process of pressure-induced ischemia.

2. Prepare all necessary equipment and supplies. **Rationale:** Saves time and interruptions.
   a. Select a dressing that exceeds the size of the wound by 1 in on all sides.
   b. Soap, water, and washcloth (for stage I pressure sores) or saline and gauze (for stage II) or prescribed cleansing solution.
   c. One roll of 1-in paper tape.
   d. Mineral oil.
   e. Two pairs of exam gloves and gown (if potential exists for body fluid exposure).

3. Prepare the patient.
   a. Explain the procedure to patient. **Rationale:** Decreases anxiety and promotes cooperation.
   b. Assist the patient in achieving a position that is comfortable and sufficiently exposes the site. **Rationale:** Avoids turning/repositioning during procedure.

Implementation

Steps	Rationale	Special Considerations
1. Wash hands.	Reduces transmission of microorganisms.	
2. Don gloves (and gown if potential for body fluid exposure exists).	Universal precautions.	
3. If a dressing is in place, anchor the skin with nondominant hand, and peel the dressing in the direction of hair growth with the dominant hand.	Minimizes discomfort.	If necessary, mineral oil will soften the adhesive, easing removal.
4. Discard soiled dressing and gloves in appropriate receptacle.	Universal precautions.	
5. Don clean gloves.	Universal precautions.	
6. Cleanse the site with water, saline, or prescribed cleaning agent.	Removes debris and reduces microorganisms. Water or saline is preferable to topical antiseptics, which can impair wound healing.	Creams, oils, or ointments can impede dressing adhesion.

Table continues on following page

Steps	Rationale	Special Considerations
7. If excessive hair is present, clip with scissors.	Hair contributes to infection and sticks to dressing, causing pain when dressing is removed.	Shaving can cause small lacerations, increasing potential for infection.
8. Peel liner or backing from the dressing slightly.	Exposes adhesive.	Packaging of various brands differ.
9. Hold dressing by the outer edges, and avoid touching the portion that will contact the wound.	Avoids contamination and maintains adhesive.	
10. Gently lay the dressing on the skin/pressure sore, and smooth from center to edges.	Stretching the dressing can cause the skin to shear.	If applying to the sacrum, spread the gluteal fold first.
11. Frame edges with tape, if desired.	Prevents rolling and may extend wear time.	May be left in place for up to 7 days if clean and intact and showing no signs of infection.
12. Document date and time on dressing with a felt-tipped pen.	Helps communicate when change is due and avoids premature removal.	
13. Discard soiled equipment and gloves in appropriate receptacles.	Universal precautions.	
14. Wash hands.	Reduces transmission of microorganisms.	

Evaluation

1. Assess the dressed area every 4 hours for adherence, contamination or soiling, and evidence of infection. **Rationale:** Determines the need for a dressing change. It is important to note that a collection of exudate beneath a transparent adhesive dressing is not necessarily indicative of an infection. The use of transparent dressings over nonviable tissue can promote a healthy autolytic process that results in a collection of exudate from the breakdown of debris. An infection should be suspected if the exudate is accompanied by odor, induration, or increased temperature.
2. Monitor the surrounding skin for inflammation. **Rationale:** May indicate tape sensitivity.
3. Evaluate wound healing, including size, color, moisture, and type of tissue (i.e., granulation, slough, eschar). **Rationale:** Supports appropriateness of intervention and indicates the need for other interventions.

Expected Outcomes

1. Evidence of wound healing. **Rationale:** Provision of a moist wound bed and protection from external contamination and friction promotes healing of existing pressure sores.

Unexpected Outcomes

1. Anaerobic infection. **Rationale:** Hydrocolloid wafers are impermeable to oxygen and are contraindicated in the presence of anaerobic infections.
2. Dressing nonadherence. **Rationale:** Occlusive dressings may not adhere sufficiently if the patient is diaphoretic or has excessive wound drainage or incontinence.

Documentation

Documentation in the patient record should include the date and time of skin assessment findings and when the dressing was applied, for an existing pressure sore (and location if more than one site is involved); size, stage, and presence or absence of exudate and/or necrotic tissue; evidence of wound healing; complaints of or absence of discomfort; type and size of dressing selected; and patient's tolerance of procedure. **Rationale:** Accurate documentation promotes continuity of care, aids in following wound progress, and maximizes reimbursement.

Patient/Family Education

1. Explain the purpose and demonstrate the procedure with implications and contraindications to both patient and family. **Rationale:** Understanding of procedure reduces anxiety and encourages involvement.
2. Encourage the patient and family to report discomfort, burning, itching, or redness at the site. **Rationale:** May be caused by allergic reaction to dressing or infection.
3. Explain that dressing will be left in place for up to 7 days and that a moderate accumulation of drainage under the dressing will promote healing. **Rationale:** Prevents patient fears of neglect.
4. Evaluate the patient's need for dressings after discharge. **Rationale:** Helps determine teaching and referral needs. Hydrocolloid wafers and transparent adhesive dressings are frequently used in long-term and home care because of their ease of application and infrequent need for changing.

Performance Checklist
Skill 29–2: Management of Pressure Sores: Semipermeable Occlusive Dressings

Critical Behaviors	Complies	
	yes	no
1. Wash hands.		
2. Don gloves (and gown, if necessary).		
3. Peel off existing dressing (if present) in the direction of hair growth.		
4. Discard soiled dressing and gloves.		
5. Don clean gloves.		
6. Cleanse the site with appropriate solution.		
7. Clip excess hair.		
8. Peel liner or backing from dressing.		
9. Handle dressing by outer edges.		
10. Apply dressing, smoothing outward from center.		
11. Frame dressing with tape, if desired.		
12. Document date and time on dressing.		
13. Discard soiled supplies and gloves.		
14. Wash hands.		
15. Document the procedure in the patient record.		

SKILL 29–3

Management of Pressure Sores: Enzyme Preparations

The presence of necrotic debris in pressure sores impedes wound healing. Eschar (thick, dark-colored necrotic tissue) and slough (stringy, light-colored necrotic tissue) are types of debris commonly found in pressure sores. An important step in pressure sore management is the removal of this nonviable tissue.

Several mechanisms can be used for removal of debris. Options include promotion of autolysis, vigorous irrigation, sharp debridement, and enzyme preparations. Proteolytic enzymes digest and/or liquefy necrotic tissue and purulent exudate without affecting healthy granulation tissue. If a thick black eschar covers the wound, it should be surgically debrided or cross-hatched with a sharp instrument prior to initiating enzyme therapy.

Purpose

The nurse uses enzyme preparations to loosen and digest necrotic tissue and exudate.

Prerequisite Knowledge and Skills

Prior to applying enzyme preparations, the nurse should understand

1. Anatomy and physiology of the skin.
2. Principles of aseptic technique.
3. Universal precautions.
4. Principles of circulation and tissue oxygenation.
5. Principles of wound healing.
6. Principles of proteolytic enzyme debridement.

The nurse should be able to perform

1. Proper handwashing technique (see Skill 35–5).
2. Universal precautions (see Skill 35–1).
3. Risk-factor assessment for pressure sore development.
4. Nutritional assessment.
5. Skin assessment.
6. Wound/pressure sore assessment and classification (see Skills 29–1 and 29–2).
7. Clean and sterile dressing change (see Skills 28–1 and 28–4).

Assessment

1. Assess the patient for the presence of the following risk factors: mobility limitations, activity limitations, sensory deficits, altered circulation and/or oxygenation, presence of excessive moisture (diaphoresis or incontinence), friction, shear, old age, history of previous pressure ulcers, and malnutrition. **Rationale:** All these factors have been found to increase the risk of pressure sore development and deter pressure sore healing.

2. Assess the wound for type and amount of moisture/exudate. **Rationale:** Enzymes are inhibited by a dry wound bed.

3. Assess the type, amount, and density of necrotic debris within the wound. **Rationale:** Determines the amount of debridement necessary.

4. Assess the surrounding skin for inflammation or discomfort. **Rationale:** Excess moisture/drainage may cause maceration of surrounding skin.

Nursing Diagnoses

1. Impaired skin integrity related to pressure-induced ischemia. **Rationale:** Prolonged pressure over bony prominences compresses capillaries, leading to ischemia and cellular death.

2. Potential for infection related to epidermal destruction. **Rationale:** Intact skin is the body's first line of defense against infection.

Planning

1. Individualize the following goals for enzyme therapy:
   a. Remove necrotic tissue. **Rationale:** Impedes wound healing.

   b. Promote the development of a pink, granulating wound bed. **Rationale:** Denotes healthy wound progression.

2. Prepare all necessary equipment and supplies. **Rationale:** Saves time and interruptions.
   a. Enzyme preparation (specific formula is usually prescribed by physician).
   b. Cleansing solution (see Table 29–3).
   c. Irrigation solution (see Table 29–3).
   d. Sterile 30-ml syringe.
   e. Sterile 19-gauge needle.
   f. Two pairs of exam gloves.
   g. One gown and eyegear.
   h. Two to four sterile tongue blades (quantity depends on wound size).
   i. Dressings (nonadherent for Elase ointment, moist fine-mesh gauze for Elase solution or Travase).
   j. Waterproof sheets.

3. Prepare the patient.
   a. Explain the procedure to the patient. **Rationale:** Decreases anxiety and promotes cooperation.
   b. Assist the patient in achieving a position that is comfortable and sufficiently exposes the site. **Rationale:** Avoids turning/repositioning during procedure.

Implementation

Steps	Rationale	Special Considerations
1. Wash hands.	Reduces transmission of microorganisms.	
2. Position waterproof sheets under pressure sore to be treated.	Contain liquid runoff from cleansing and irrigation.	
3. Don exam gloves, gown, and eyegear.	Universal precautions.	Irrigation of large wounds will create high risk for body fluid exposure.
4. Remove old dressing.	Exposes the wound.	
5. Discard old dressing in appropriate receptacle.	Universal precautions.	
6. Discard soiled gloves, and don clean gloves.	Maintains aseptic technique.	Depending on location and characteristics of the wound, clean or sterile technique may be used.
7. Cleanse wound area using prescribed solution and technique.	Removes surface drainage and debris.	
8. Aspirate irrigation fluid into 30-ml syringe with a 19-gauge needle attached.	Large-capacity syringe connected to the 19-gauge needle will produce a high-pressure stream of irrigation fluid to facilitate removal of debris.	
9. Forcefully irrigate areas of slough and necrotic tissue.	Dislodges loose debris. Wound must be moist for enzyme to work.	If antimicrobial solutions are used for cleansing or irrigation, rinse with saline. Antimicrobials will denature the enzyme.

Table continues on following page

Steps	Rationale	Special Considerations
10. Use tongue blade(s) to apply a thin layer of enzyme preparation covering wound surface and extending ¼ in beyond wound edge.	Must be in contact with all eschar or slough.	Will not harm surrounding intact skin.
11. Apply appropriate moist dressing (nonadherent for Elase ointment, moist fine-mesh gauze for Elase solution or Travase).	Protects wound and contains debris. Enzymes are inhibited by a dry wound bed.	
12. Document date and time on dressing with felt-tipped pen.	Helps communicate when change is due.	
13. Remove and discard gloves.	Universal precautions.	
14. Wash hands.	Reduces transmission of microorganisms.	
15. Repeat procedure three to four times per day.	Changing and peeling of the moist dressing aids debridement.	
16. Discontinue enzyme therapy when the wound bed is pink with granulation tissue.	Debridement complete.	

Evaluation

1. Monitor the color, consistency, and amount of necrotic tissue with each application. **Rationale:** Evaluates effectiveness of therapy.
2. Evaluate wound length, width, and depth and the presence of granulation tissue with each application. **Rationale:** Wound size and shape may change with removal of debris.
3. Monitor the surrounding skin for evidence of maceration. **Rationale:** Skin may be damaged by continuous exposure to irrigation fluids and moist dressings.

Expected Outcome

Viable granulating wound bed. **Rationale:** Debris impedes wound healing.

Unexpected Outcomes

1. Wound infection. **Rationale:** Necrotic tissue often harbors bacteria. Poor debridement technique may result in infection.
2. Necrotic tissue remains or increases. **Rationale:** Effectiveness of enzyme preparations is highly dependent on appropriate application.

Documentation

Documentation in the patient record should include pressure sore size, stage, and color; character and amount of exudate and necrotic tissue; condition of wound bed and surrounding tissue; type of cleansing solution and process used; date, time, location, and type of dressing applied; and patient's response to procedure. **Rationale:** Accurate documentation promotes continuity of care and maximizes reimbursement.

Patient/Family Education

1. Explain the purpose of the procedure, demonstrate, and encourage participation if patient and family express interest. **Rationale:** Understanding of procedures reduces anxiety.
2. Instruct the patient and family to report discomfort, burning, itching or redness at the site to the nurse. **Rationale:** May be caused by allergic reaction to dressing or infection.
3. Explain the purpose for dressing changes three to four times per day. **Rationale:** Patient and family may perceive this as excessive.

Performance Checklist
Skill 29–3: Management of Pressure Sores: Enzyme Preparations

Critical Behaviors	Complies yes	no
1. Wash hands.		
2. Place waterproof sheets under the patient.		
3. Don clean gloves, gown, and eyegear.		

Table continues on following page

Performance Checklist
Skill

Critical Behaviors	Complies yes	no
4. Remove old dressing.		
5. Discard old dressing.		
6. Discard soiled gloves, and don clean gloves.		
7. Cleanse wound using appropriate solution and technique.		
8. Assemble irrigation fluid and equipment.		
9. Forcefully irrigate areas of debris.		
10. Apply enzyme using tongue blade to cover wound surface and extend $\frac{1}{4}$ in beyond edge.		
11. Apply a moist dressing.		
12. Document date and time on dressing.		
13. Remove and discard gloves.		
14. Wash hands.		
15. Repeat procedure three to four times per day.		
16. Discontinue enzyme therapy when wound is pink with granulation tissue.		
17. Document in the patient record.		

REFERENCES

Bergstrom, N., Braden, B., Laguzza, A., and Holman, V. (1987). The Braden scale for predicting pressure sore risk. *Nurs. Res.* 36(4):205–210.

Goldstone, L., and Goldstone, J. (1982). The Norton score: An early warning of pressure sores? *J. Adv. Nurs.* 7:419–426.

Gosnell, D. (1987). Assessment and evaluation of pressure sores. *Nurs. Clin. North Am.* 22(2):399–416.

BIBLIOGRAPHY

Alterescu, V., and Alterescu, K. (1988). Etiology and treatment of pressure ulcers. *Decubitus* 1(1):28–35.

Andrews, J., and Balai, R. (1988). The prevention and treatment of pressure sores by use of pressure distributing mattresses. *Decubitus* 1(4):14–21.

Barnes, S. (1987). Patient/family education for the patient with a pressure necrosis. *Nurs. Clin. North Am.* 22(2):463–474.

Bristow, J., Goldfarb, E., and Green, M. (1987). Clinitron therapy: Is it effective? *Geriatr. Nurs.* 8(3):120–124.

Conforti, C. (1989). Pressure sores: Dressed for successful healing. *Nursing 89* March, 58–61.

Cuzzell, J., and Stotts, N. (1990). Trial and error yields to knowledge. *Am. J. Nurs.* 10:53–63.

Fowler, E. (1987). Equipment and products used in management and treatment of pressure ulcers. *Nurs. Clin. North Am.* 22(2):449–461.

International Association of Enterostomal Therapists (1987). *Standards of Care: Dermal Wounds: Pressure Ulcers.* Irvine, Calif.: IAET.

30

BURN WOUND MANAGEMENT

BEHAVIORAL OBJECTIVES

After completing this chapter, the nurse will be able to

- Define the key terms.
- Identify factors affecting burn wound healing.
- Assess and describe the extent, depth, and condition of the burn wound.
- Demonstrate the skills involved in burn wound management.
- Identify measures to promote motor function.
- Identify measures to promote comfort.

Skin, the largest organ of the body, is the first-line barrier between the internal homeostatic environment and external environmental forces. Alterations in this system affect the body's ability to fight infection, maintain fluid and electrolyte balance, control temperature and pain, and maintain structural integrity.

Anatomically, the skin is comprised of two layers: the epidermis and dermis (Fig. 30–1). The epidermis is comprised of densely packed cells that create a physical barrier. Melanocytes, responsible for protection from the sun, and Langerhans' cells, a defense against foreign organisms, are found in this layer. Destruction at this level is a first-degree burn. Epidermal elements are damaged or destroyed, but regeneration is rapid (Table 30–1).

The dermis consists mainly of fibroblasts necessary for healing and extracellular materials, including collagen and elastin that provide the structure to this layer. The dermis also contains hair follicles, blood vessels, nerve endings, and sebaceous and sweat glands. A second-degree or partial-thickness burn, which involves epidermal and varying degrees of dermal destruction, relies on regeneration of the epidermal elements lining the hair follicles and other structures. Healing time depends on the depth of the injury and the number of proliferative cells available.

Below the dermis lies subcutaneous tissue rich in blood vessels. Destruction through the dermis into the subcutaneous tissue results in a third-degree or full-thickness burn. Because of the lack of supportive dermis and all epidermal elements in such burns, permanent closure of the wound is accomplished with skin grafting.

The healing and care of a burn wound depend on the extent and depth of the injury and the condition of the patient. The depth of the burn wound is directly related to the temperature intensity and duration of contact with the burning agent. Characterization of burns is related to the burning agent and includes thermal, chemical, and electrical. Thermal burns result from contact with a heat source, i.e., flame, steam or scalding water, or radiators. Thermal burns usually result in partial- and full-thickness burns. Immediate care should be directed to airway and circulatory stabilization, since inhalation injuries and hypovolemic shock are life-threatening.

Chemical injuries resulting from contact with alkali or acidic substances or fumes range from skin irritation to full-thickness burns. Immediate dangers include continued destruction of tissue and systemic absorption. Assess damage related to ingestion, inhalation, and contact with eyes.

Injuries resulting from electricity are usually extensive within the body. Entry and exit sites of the electricity can be seen. Thermal injuries resulting from clothing igniting also may be visible. Emergency care should include assessment of the cardiac and circulatory status of the patient, with special attention to renal failure resulting from extensive myoglobinuria.

Assessment of burn wounds is most accurately determined by using the Lund and Browder burn chart (Fig. 30–2), which incorporates age versus area in calculating the extent and depth of a burn. Criteria determining transfer to a specialized burn-care facility include inhalation injury; burns over greater than 20 percent of the total body surface area (TBSA); burns of the face, hands, or genitalia; burns to pediatric or geriatric patients; chemical burns; and electrical burns.

Complicating factors that affect healing include (1) the amount of edema from initial capillary permeability, (2) decreased circulation resulting from the initial decrease in intravascular volume and destruction of blood vessels, (3) increased caloric needs resulting from increased metabolism, (4) pain resulting from exposed nerve endings, (5) alterations in gas exchange with an inhalation injury, (6) multisystem failure associated with sepsis, and (7) continued trauma to the wound from poor wound care and/or wound sepsis. Successful wound healing with optimal function incorporates all these factors in the care of the patient.

This chapter addresses the care of the first-degree burn, superficial partial-thickness burn, deep partial-thickness and full-thickness burn, and care of the skin graft and donor site.

KEY TERMS

debridement	*eschar*
donor site	*escharotomy*
epithelialization	*full-thickness burn*

granulation tissue   *partial-thickness burn*
heterograft   *split-thickness skin graft*
homograft   *total body surface area*
interstices   *(TBSA)*

SKILLS

30–1   Care of the First-Degree Burn
30–2   Care of the Second-Degree or Third-Degree Burn
30–3   Care of the Donor Site
30–4   Care of the Skin Graft

GUIDELINES

The following assessment guidelines assist the nurse in formulating nursing diagnoses and an individualized plan of care for a patient with a burn wound:

1.   Identify the patient's past medical history with attention to specific factors that may affect wound healing, including diabetes and cardiovascular or peripheral vascular disease.

2.   Determine the degree of burn severity (see Table 30–1).

3.   Identify the patient's baseline weight, since all calculations are based on this weight.

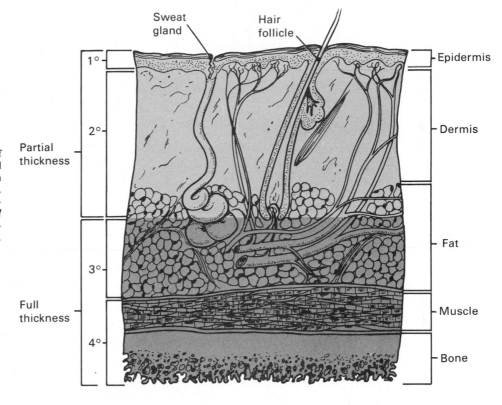

FIGURE 30–1. Cross section of skin with areas affected by partial- and full-thickness burns. (Reproduced with permission from S. M. Lewis and I. C. Cox, *Medical-Surgical Nursing: Assessment and Management of Clinical Problems*, 2nd ed. New York: McGraw-Hill, 1987, p. 408. Copyright C.V. Mosby, St. Louis.)

TABLE 30–1   Description of First-, Second-, and Third-Degree Burn Wounds

Type	Depth	Appearance	Mode of Healing
First degree	Epidermis	Red, sunburn-like; no blisters; painful	Rapid regeneration of epidermis in 3 to 7 days
Second-degree, superficial partial-thickness burn	Epidermis and upper dermis	Pink/red; blisters; wet; painful	Regeneration depends on number of epidermal elements present; heals in 7 to 14 days
Deep partial-thickness burn	Epidermis through to lower dermis	Red, wet, painful; may present with white or black eschar, depending on depth	Slow regeneration of epidermal elements; split-thickness skin graft preferred to reduce infection and scarring
Third-degree, full-thickness burn	Epidermis, dermis, and may involve underlying structures	Dry, black, leathery eschar; may have dry, cherry-red appearance with thrombosed vessels	Split-thickness skin graft

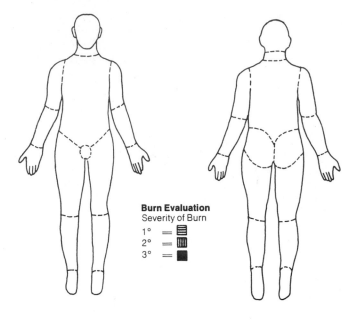

Burn Evaluation
Severity of Burn

1° = ▤
2° = ▥
3° = ■

Lund and Browder chart

AREA	AGE—YEARS					% 2°	% 3°	% TOTAL
	0–1	1–4	5–9	10–15	ADULT			
Head	19	17	13	10	7			
Neck	2	2	2	2	2			
Ant. Trunk	13	17	13	13	13			
Post. Trunk	13	13	13	13	13			
R. Buttock	2 1/2	2 1/2	2 1/2	2 1/2	2 1/2			
L. Buttock	2 1/2	2 1/2	2 1/2	2 1/2	2 1/2			
Genitalia	1	1	1	1	1			
R.U. Arm	4	4	4	4	4			
L. U. Arm	4	4	4	4	4			
R.L. Arm	3	3	3	3	3			
L.L. Arm	3	3	3	3	3			
R. Hand	2 1/2	2 1/2	2 1/2	2 1/2	2 1/2			
L. Hand	2 1/2	2 1/2	2 1/2	2 1/2	2 1/2			
R. Thigh	5 1/2	6 1/2	8 1/2	8 1/2	9 1/2			
L. Thigh	5 1/2	6 1/2	8 1/2	8 1/2	9 1/2			
R. Leg	5	5	5 1/2	6	7			
L. Leg	5	5	5 1/2	6	7			
R. Foot	3 1/2	3 1/2	3 1/2	3 1/2	3 1/2			
L. Foot	3 1/2	3 1/2	3 1/2	3 1/2	3 1/2			
					Total			

FIGURE 30–2. Graphically document areas of burned skin (i.e., degree, redness, preexisting wounds or pressure ulcers, intravenous sites, tracheostomy, ostomies, etc.).

4. Determine the patient's caloric requirements for age, weight, and size of burn.

5. Determine the patient's level of function prior to injury.

6. Identify the indications for and side effects of all topical agents used (Table 30–2).

SKILL 30–1

Care of the First-Degree Burn

The damaged epidermal cell layer resulting in a first-degree burn appears swollen, red, is painful to touch, and is usually likened to a sunburn. When the affected area (i.e., extremity, head, or genitalia) is in a dependent position, the patient may describe a throbbing pain. The patient may complain of chills and thirst. Any blister formation noted indicates a conversion to a superficial partial-thickness. First-degree burns heal spontaneously and rapidly. Moderate to severe pruritus often accompanies healing.

Purpose

The nurse performs wound care on the first-degree burn to

1. Reduce edema formation.
2. Decrease pain.
3. Prevent progression to a partial-thickness injury.

Prerequisite Knowledge and Skills

Prior to caring for the first-degree burn wound, the nurse should understand

1. Anatomy and physiology of the skin.
2. Principles of wound healing.
3. Principles of infection control and universal precautions.
4. Principles of pain relief.

The nurse should be able to perform

1. Proper handwashing technique (see Skill 35–5).
2. Universal precautions (see Skill 35–1).
3. Correct application of dressings and/or creams.

Assessment

1. Determine the postburn day to evaluate healing time. Observe for signs of healing, including reepithelialization, decreased pain, and decreased edema. Observe for complications, including blister formation, cellulitis, fever, and purulent drainage. **Rationale:** Healing should occur within 3 to 7 days. Complications prolong healing.

2. Graphically document areas of burned skin (see Fig. 30–2), including degree, redness, preexisting wounds or pressure ulcers. **Rationale:** Provides objective baseline for determining progression of healing or complications.

3. Know the etiology of pain and the patient's previous response to pain medications and therapies. **Rationale:** Pain is individualized, and medications should be administered in response to the patient's need. Peak action should correlate with the procedure for effective pain reduction.

TABLE 30-2 Burn Wound Topicals and Dressings

Type	Indications	Special Considerations
Silver sulfadiazine	Routine care of second- and third-degree burns	Easily applied; painless; poor eschar penetration; ineffective against most gram-negative bacteria; may cause neutropenia
Mafenide acetate	Infected second- and third-degree burns	Penetrates eschar well; effective against gram-negative and gram-positive bacteria; painful; may cause metabolic acidosis
Silver nitrate	Infected burns with eschar removed and granulation tissue	Effective against gram-negative and gram-positive bacteria; does not penetrate eschar well; cold, wet dressings; must wet q2h to avoid increase in concentration from evaporation; electrolyte disorders; stains everything black
Dakin's solution	Infected burns with eschar removed and granulation tissue	Poor eschar penetration; wet, cold dressings; effective against most gram-negative and gram-positive bacteria; can macerate surrounding unburned skin
Biologic dressings	Exposed granulation tissue; excised wounds	Protects granulation tissue; prepares for graft; difficult to apply and anchor; may not be easily available
Synthetic dressings (Biobrane, Duoderm)	Aseptic partial-thickness wounds	Occlusive dressing; reduces pain; good on donor sites

Nursing Diagnoses

1. Impaired skin integrity related to damaged epidermis. **Rationale:** Burning agent interrupts the integrity of the skin.
2. Pain related to exposed nerve endings and edema. **Rationale:** Destruction of protective epidermis exposes nerve endings to increased stimulation.

Planning

1. Individualize the following goals for care of the first-degree burn wound:
   a. Verbalization of an acceptable level of comfort on a scale of 0 to 10. **Rationale:** This reflects individualized pain relief and fosters cooperation with further care.
   b. Healing will occur within 3 to 7 days. **Rationale:** Reepithelialization within this time frame indicates absence of complications.
2. Medicate the patient for pain, as prescribed, 20 to 30 minutes prior to wound care. **Rationale:** Allows peak action of medication to coincide with wound care for optimal pain relief.
3. Prepare all necessary equipment and supplies. **Rationale:** Assembly of all equipment and supplies at the bedside ensures that wound care will be completed quickly and efficiently.
   a. Tepid tap water to wash entire body.
   b. Mild liquid soap to wash entire body.
   c. Soft wash cloth (nonsterile).
   d. Two pairs of exam gloves.
   e. Towels to dry entire body.
   f. Towels/pads moistened with cool water (for two applications).
   g. Six to ten 15 × 30 in waterproof sheets.
   h. Pillows or elastic net sling for elevation of affected extremities or dependent areas.
   i. Nonsterile wash basin.
4. Prepare the patient by explaining the procedure. **Rationale:** Diminishes fears related to the unknown. Patient learns the steps in wound care.

Implementation

Steps	Rationale	Special Considerations
1. Wash hands.	Reduces transmission of microorganisms.	
2. Don exam gloves.	Universal precautions.	

Table continues on following page

Steps	Rationale	Special Considerations
3. Remove burning agent, and apply towels moistened with cool water for 5 to 10 minutes (usually at the scene or in the emergency department). Continued use may cause vasoconstriction and/or hypothermia. Apply clean, dry wrap if transporting patient.	Prevents further destruction of tissue.	The burning agent is usually on the patient's clothing. As long as the skin is in contact with the burning agent, it will continue to destroy cell layers. An exception to this is tar, which should be softened with a Neosporin or Bacitracin ointment. This step should be implemented upon initial presentation of the burn victim in the prehospital or emergency department.
4. Remove and discard gloves, and wash hands.	Reduces transmission of microorganisms.	
5. Don exam gloves.	Universal precautions.	
6. Gently wash the affected area with tepid water and soap, and pat dry with towel.	Cleanses wound of debris and reduces surface microorganisms.	Make sure area surrounding burn is clean as well. The patient may wish to cleanse his or her own wounds. Since he or she knows his or her own pain threshold, it is often higher when the patient is in control. Areas of increased sensitivity include the hands, feet, and face.
7. Elevate burned extremities using pillows or loose elastic net slings. Keep the head of the bed elevated if the face or head is burned.	Elevation decreases edema formation.	If possible, keep patient from lying on burned area. If burns are circumferential, turn patient q2h. Rotate pillows to prevent prolonged pressure to an area. Patient may experience tingling in the extremities with elevation.
8. Arrange waterproof barriers on clean bed under burned areas.	Keeps bed dry for comfort.	
9. Apply towels moistened with tepid water for patient comfort.	Tepid water reduces throbbing and pain.	Patient may experience chills from wet towels. Monitor for hypothermia.
10. During the first 3 days postburn, do not apply any ointments.	Clogs pores and holds in the heat, potentially increasing pain and the depth of the burn.	After the wound is healed, a water-soluble, alcohol-free lotion should be used on healed, dry areas.
11. Remove and discard gloves.	Universal precautions.	
12. Wash hands.	Reduces transmission of microorganisms.	

Evaluation

1. Evaluate the progression of wound healing daily: reepithelialization within 3 to 7 days. **Rationale:** Usual progression of wound healing without complications.

2. Evaluate the type and effectiveness of pain-relief medications and therapies used. **Rationale:** Ensures patient's comfort.

3. Evaluate peripheral pulses in burned extremities every 2 hours. **Rationale:** Ensures adequate circulation.

Expected Outcomes

1. Wound heals without infectious complications. **Rationale:** Indicative of proper wound care.

2. Patient verbalizes comfort. **Rationale:** Indicative of effective pain relief.

Unexpected Outcome

Wound converts into a superficial partial-thickness injury with blistering or thin yellow eschar. **Rationale:** Impaired wound healing secondary to poor wound care, poor nutrition, or wound sepsis.

Documentation

Documentation in the patient record should include the date and time of wound care, postburn day, appearance of the wound (color, size, odor, depth, and drainage), if there is evidence of cellulitis around the wound (red, warm, and tender area surrounding wound), progression toward healing, results of circulation checks, level of pain before and after the procedure, the type of comfort measures used, patient's tolerance of the procedure, and any unexpected outcomes encountered and interventions taken. **Rationale:** Provides evidence of nursing care given, status of wound healing, and expected and unexpected outcomes.

Patient/Family Education

1. Assess the family's cognitive and motor abilities to provide care and comfort at home. **Rationale:** Depending on the extent or location of the burn, most patients are not hospitalized for more than a day with a first-degree burn. During the healing process, the patient will experience moderate to severe pruritus.

2. Stress the importance of reporting the signs and symptoms of infection to a health care professional (i.e., fever, edema, purulent drainage, and unusual redness and warmth in skin). Provide a phone number to call for questions or problems. **Rationale:** Patient and family need to recognize the necessity for an immediate assessment by a health care professional.

3. Discuss the importance of mobility and self-care in the activities of daily living during the healing phase. With a first-degree burn, the patient should be functioning close to or at the preinjury level of activity. **Rationale:** Self-care and exercise prevent the tightening associated with healing skin.

4. Inform the patient and family that with this type of burn, healing is rapid and there will probably be no scars. However, there will be discoloration for up to 1 year in some patients. **Rationale:** Alleviates anxieties about appearance.

5. Evaluate the patient's need for pain and pruritus medications. **Rationale:** Ensures the patient's comfort at home.

6. Provide the patient and family with the name of a water-based lotion to apply to the healed area. **Rationale:** Alleviates dryness and pruritus.

7. Provide any specific wound care instructions in writing, such as, "Cleanse daily with a nondrying soap and tepid water. Rinse and dry thoroughly. Apply lotion as needed, and monitor for areas of skin breakdown." If possible, have patient and family demonstrate wound care prior to discharge. **Rationale:** Patient may be treated in the emergency department and released. Patients less than 2 years of age may be hospitalized with a first-degree burn if it involves the hands, face, feet, or perineal area.

Performance Checklist
Skill 30–1: Care of the First-Degree Burn

Critical Behaviors	Complies yes	no
1. Wash hands.		
2. Don exam gloves.		
3. Remove burning agent, and apply towels moistened with cool water for 5 to 10 minutes.		
4. Remove and discard gloves, and wash hands.		
5. Don exam gloves.		
6. Gently wash burned area with tepid water and soap, and pat dry with a towel.		
7. Elevate burned extremity.		
8. Arrange waterproof barrier as appropriate.		
9. Apply tepid water–moistened towel for comfort, and monitor for hypothermia.		
10. Apply only water-based, nondrying lotion to healed areas.		
11. Remove and discard gloves.		
12. Wash hands.		
13. Document procedure in the patient record.		

SKILL 30–2

Care of the Second-Degree or Third-Degree Burn

Partial-thickness (second-degree) burns range from superficial to deep. Superficial partial-thickness burns appear as wet, pink tissue. Blisters may be present. Small blisters may be kept intact as the body's natural dressing. In order to decrease the risk of infection of the protein-rich fluid and consequently the dermis and to better evaluate the wound and its progression, blisters larger than 1 in (2 cm) should be opened and debrided. A superficial partial-thickness burn, having many epidermal elements, heals spontaneously in 7 to 14 days (Fig. 30–3).

Deep partial-thickness burns involve destruction of most of the dermis. The wound may appear deep red and present with a tight yellow-white eschar covering. These wounds will heal through the same principles as more superficial wounds, but the potential for complications with healing is greater. Since there are fewer epidermal elements, healing takes longer and the risk of infection is greater. In this time, fibroblasts begin generating collagen, forming granulation tissue. This appears as pink, nodular tissue that is the tensile strength of the wound. Therefore, the longer it takes to reepithelialize, the more the wound will contract and form scar tissue. A skin graft may be preferable to decrease the risk of infection and to minimize scarring in a deep partial-thickness wound that has not healed in approximately 2 weeks (Fig. 30–4).

Partial-thickness wounds are very painful. In the first few days, the wound will be "weeping" as a result of capillary leak. This leak causes edema, which can affect the circulation. Cell survival depends on the vascular supply being adequate. Therefore, reducing edema by elevation of the extremities and/or longitudinal incisions through constricting eschar to relieve pressure (escharotomies) is required. In addition, aggressive fluid replacement ensures an adequate circulating intravascular volume. Diminished circulation in a burned area may cause it to convert to a full-thickness wound.

In a full-thickness (third-degree) burn, complete destruction of the dermis renders the wound incapable of regeneration. Therefore, a skin graft is the only permanent means for wound closure. Third-degree burns appear as black, leathery eschar. In some cases, a dry, deep red, leathery eschar can be seen, often with thrombosed vessels. These wounds are not painful until the eschar begins to separate (Fig. 30–5).

Separation of the eschar occurs with the release of enzymes by migrating leukocytes to the point of demarcation between living and necrotic tissue. This process is slow, and the wound often becomes colonized with bac-

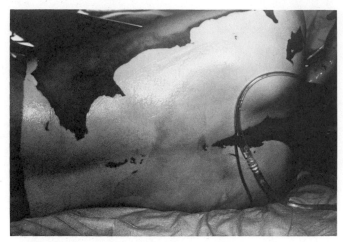

FIGURE 30–4. Deep partial-thickness burn with a thin layer of white eschar covering wound.

teria. Although the bacteria speed up the separation of the eschar, the moist, dark environment of necrotic tissue promotes bacterial proliferation and invasion. Before the eschar begins to separate, early excision and grafting of the wound are an option. This option is usually chosen if there is available unburned skin to use as donor sites or if there is a threat of wound sepsis. This type of graft is an autograft. It is often meshed to allow for expansion and greater wound coverage. Homografts or donated skin (usually from a cadaver) may be used to graft over the autograft if the expansion is large (1:6 meshing) (Herndon and Parks, 1986). As the autograft fills in, the homograft separates until it is completely removed.

If early excision is not indicated, debridement, in the form of wet-to-dry dressings or with sharp instruments, is necessary. As the granulation tissue exposed by the separation of eschar becomes red and healthy, a biologic dressing, such as a homograft, may be applied to protect and promote further vascularization of the wound. As this is accomplished, the next step, an autograft, provides permanent closure of the wound.

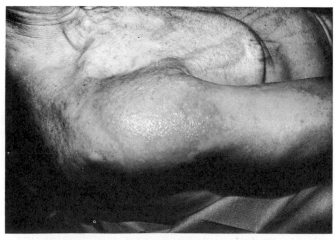

FIGURE 30–3. Superficial partial-thickness burn with epithelial buds indicating healing.

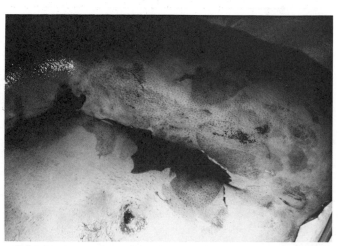

FIGURE 30–5. Full-thickness burn with dry, leathery eschar covering wound.

In many cases, electrical and chemical burns result in deep partial- and/or full-thickness burns. Electricity enters the body through a point of contact. At the entry site, one visualizes a thermal burn. Electricity is conducted through the body, primarily via the nerves, blood vessels, and bone, causing destruction along its course. It exits with tremendous force. This type of burn exhibits an "iceberg effect," whereby most of the destruction lies within the body. Serial assessments of peripheral pulses are imperative. Unfortunately, amputation is indicated in many cases (Fig. 30–6).

Cardiac dysrhythmias are a primary concern since an electrical burn can affect the heart's conduction system and initial stabilization may have included CPR. Renal function must be closely monitored because of the tremendous amount of circulating myoglobin from extensive muscle damage. This appears as port wine–colored urine. Fluid resuscitation must take into consideration the unseen internal damage. Urine output should be maintained from 100 to 150 cc in an adult until it becomes clear of myoglobin (Madden et al., 1990).

A chemical burn may vary in depth depending on the burning agent and the length of contact. Therefore, the primary concern upon presentation of a patient with a chemical burn is to remove the agent and clothing. Neutralization of the chemical is not recommended because such a chemical reaction causes heat production, thereby increasing the depth of the burn. Immediate care should

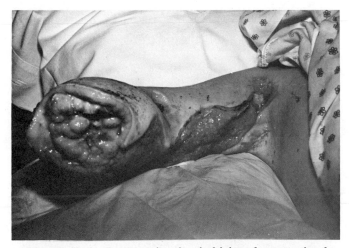

FIGURE 30–6. Postoperative electrical injury demonstrating devasting "iceberg effect." Escharotomy to remainder of limb.

include irrigation with copious amounts of running water for at least 1 to 2 hours. Treatment of specific chemicals is required to prevent further damage (Saydjazri et al., 1986) (Table 30–3). Chemical burns to the eyes should be continuously flushed, since blindness may result. Ophthalmic antibiotics are often used to prevent infection.

After initial treatment, care is standardized for the specific depth of burn. In addition, it should be noted that some of the chemicals may be absorbed into the body system, causing further systemic damage, including destruction to blood vessels, muscle, and nerves.

Purpose

The nurse performs wound care to the second or third-degree burn to

1. Promote healing.
2. Prevent infection.
3. Decrease pain.
4. Promote function.
5. Assess progression of wound healing.
6. Prevent wound sepsis.

Prerequisite Knowledge and Skills

Prior to caring for the second- or third-degree burn, the nurse should understand

1. Anatomy and physiology of the skin.
2. Principles of wound healing.
3. Principles of infection control and universal precautions.
4. Principles of pain relief.

The nurse should be able to perform

1. Proper handwashing technique (see Skill 35–5).
2. Universal precautions (see Skill 35–1).
3. Correct application of dressings and/or creams.
4. Clean and aseptic technique.

Assessment

1. Determine the postburn day to evaluate healing. Observe for signs of healing, including reepithelialization, decreased pain, and decreased edema. Observe for complications, including eschar formation, cellulitis, pu-

TABLE 30–3 Care with Specific Chemicals

Agent	Special Considerations
Alkali powders: Anhydrous ammonia Lime	Brush from skin before irrigation; potential increased tissue damage when wet
Phenol	Remove with glycerol or polyethelyne glycol; poor solubility in water
White phosphorous	Use copper sulfate to remove or keep wet until removed mechanically; dry powder ignites spontaneously

Note: Use gloves and instruments when providing care in order to decrease the risk of self-contact with the chemical.

rulent drainage, and fever. **Rationale:** Healing should occur within 7 to 14 days. Complications prolong healing.

2. Graphically document areas of burned skin, redness, preexisting wounds or pressure ulcers, intravenous sites, tracheostomy, ostomies, etc. **Rationale:** Provides objective baseline for determining progression of healing or complications.

3. Identify the edematous areas, and assess the peripheral pulses. **Rationale:** Edema formation impedes circulation, thus increasing cell death and conversion of the burn.

4. Know the etiology of the patient's pain and the patient's previous response to pain medications and therapies. **Rationale:** Pain is individualized, and medications should be administered in response to the patient's needs. Peak action should correlate with the procedure for effective pain reduction.

5. Observe for contracture formation, and note the level of function (i.e., hand movement, ability to walk, and ability to perform the activities of daily living). **Rationale:** Burns contract during the healing phase if not correctly splinted and exercised.

Nursing Diagnoses

1. Impaired skin integrity related to damaged epidermis and superficial dermis. **Rationale:** Burning agent interrupts the integrity and function of the skin.

2. Pain related to exposed nerve endings and edema. **Rationale:** Destruction of protective epidermis and superficial dermis exposes nerve endings to increased stimulation.

3. Potential for infection related to damaged epidermal elements and superficial dermal layers. **Rationale:** Risk of invasion by microorganisms is proportional to the depth and extent of the body surface area burned.

4. Impaired tissue perfusion related to edema formation. **Rationale:** Fluid shifts into interstitial tissue as a response to the burn injury compromise the peripheral circulation. Mobilization of fluid back into the vascular system usually begins after the first 72 hours.

5. Alteration in body temperature related to damaged epidermal and superficial dermal layers. **Rationale:** Burning agent destroys the thermoregulation function of intact skin.

6. Impaired physical mobility related to pain and edema. **Rationale:** Exposed nerve endings and edema formation from the burn injury make moving painful and difficult.

Planning

1. Individualize the following goals for care of the patient with a superficial partial-thickness burn wound:
   a. Verbalization of an acceptable level of comfort on a scale of 0 to 10. **Rationale:** Reflects individualized pain relief and fosters cooperation with further care.
   b. Healing occurs within 7 to 14 days in a superficial partial-thickness burn wound. **Rationale:** Reepithelialization within this time frame indicates an absence of complications.
   c. Promote eschar separation within 5 to 14 days in deep partial-thickness or full-thickness injury. **Rationale:** Formation of granulation tissue and/or some epithelialization indicates viable tissue capable of accepting a skin graft.
   d. Maintain range of motion at a level of function. **Rationale:** Contracture formation results from lack of exercise, improper positioning, and splinting and/or poor wound care.

2. Medicate the patient for pain, as prescribed, allowing for peak action of the medication to coincide with wound care. Because of poor absorption related to edema, subcutaneous or intramuscular injections should not be the route of medication administration. Intravenous administration is the method of choice. Oral medications should be given only in noncritical patients with a functioning gastrointestinal system. **Rationale:** Allows for optimal absorption of medication and optimal pain relief.

3. Prepare all necessary equipment and supplies. **Rationale:** Assembly of all equipment and supplies at the bedside ensures that wound care will be completed quickly and efficiently.
   a. Warm sterile normal saline.
   b. Sterile wash basin.
   c. Mild liquid soap to wash entire body.
   d. Sterile debridement instruments (four curved scissors, four forceps).
   e. Ten 4 × 4 sterile gauze pads for every 10 percent TBSA.
   f. Washcloth (nonsterile) to wash unburned areas.
   g. Two pairs sterile gloves.
   h. One sterile glove.
   i. Antimicrobial cream.
   j. Splints as prescribed.
   k. Nonsterile combine pads to pad splints.
   l. Gauze roll to wrap on splints.
   m. Sterile, nonadherent dressing (Adaptic) to cover wound if using splints.
   n. Pillows for elevation of burned extremities.
   o. Twenty-ply gauze sheets to cover wound with two layers.
   p. Gauze rolls to wrap dressings.

4. Prepare the patient by explaining the procedure. **Rationale:** Diminishes fears related to the unknown. Patient will learn the steps in wound care.

5. Coordinate all other appropriate care activities and health care professionals related to the wound being exposed (i.e., quantitative wound biopsies, assessment of wound by physician, and evaluation of level of function by physical or occupational therapists). **Rationale:** Organization of care prevents wound trauma and pain associated with multiple manipulations.

Implementation

Steps	Rationale	Special Considerations
1. Wash hands.	Reduces transmission of microorganisms.	
2. Don sterile gloves.	Prevents transmission of microorganisms.	
3. Gently wash the affected area with warm sterile normal saline. Patient may take a shower with tap water and soap.	Cleanses wound of debris and reduces microorganisms.	Make sure area surrounding burn is clean as well. The patient may wish to cleanse his or her own wounds. Since he or she knows his or her own pain threshold, it is often higher when the patient is in control. Areas of increased sensitivity include the hands, feet, and face.
4. With curved scissors and forceps, remove loose necrotic tissue and/or unroof separating eschar.	Aids in preventing infection.	In units not specializing in burns, this may be the responsibility of the physician.
5. Assess the wound for complications and stages of healing.	Validates healing process and identifies complications.	At this time, allow for evaluation by other disciplines.
6. Gently wrap patient in warm towels.	Supports maintenance of body temperature.	
7. Remove and discard gloves.	Universal precautions.	
8. Don single sterile glove on dominant hand.	Reduces transmission of microorganisms.	
9. Prepare adequate amount of antimicrobial cream to cover wound.	Prevents contamination of entire jar of cream.	
10. With sterile-gloved hand, reapply a ⅛-in layer of antimicrobial cream to completely cover wound.	Reduces proliferation of microorganisms and pain.	Gentle application is recommended to reduce pain and trauma.
11. *For open method, do not* apply gauze dressing.		For the open method, reapplication of cream is necessary as the wound becomes exposed.
12. Remove and discard single sterile glove, and don sterile gloves.	Universal precautions.	
13. *For closed method*, apply a single layer of sterile nonadherent gauze and combine padding over antimicrobial cream.	Provides comfort and prevents padding from sticking to wound.	Combine padding is used if splints are to be applied.
14. Loosely wrap wound with bulky gauze dressing if splints are not to be applied.	Keeps antimicrobial cream intact on wound.	
15. If wound requires wet dressings, pour sterile saline or prescribed solution into sterile basin and drop in sterile twenty-ply gauze pads.	Maintains aseptic technique.	Wet dressings must be moistened every 4 hours. Wet-to-dry dressings over eschar are removed dry, every 8 to 12 hours. Before removing, wet if it is adherent to epithelial buds or granulation tissue.
16. Don sterile gloves.	Maintains sterile technique.	
17. Squeeze excess solution from gauze and place on wound.	Protects wound and decreases pain.	
18. Wrap wound with gauze roll.	Maintains gauze pads in place.	

Table continues on following page

Steps	Rationale	Special Considerations
19. Apply splints in position of function, and secure with gauze roll or Velcro straps (see Fig. 30–9).	Prevents contracture formation and promotes function.	
20. Elevate burned extremities with loose elastic net and/or pillows, and elevate the head of the bed as indicated.	Reduces edema formation and decreases pain.	If possible, keep the patient from lying on burned area. If burns are circumferential, turn patient q2h. Patient may experience tingling in the extremities with elevation.
21. Remove and discard gloves in appropriate receptacle.	Universal precautions.	
22. Wash hands.	Reduces transmission of microorganisms.	

Evaluation

1. Evaluate the progression of wound healing daily (i.e., reepithelialization within 7 to 14 days) and range of motion. **Rationale:** Determines progression of wound healing and identifies onset of contracture formation.

2. Evaluate the type and effectiveness of pain-relief medications and therapies used. **Rationale:** Ensures the patient's comfort.

3. Evaluate peripheral pulses in burned extremities every 2 hours. **Rationale:** Determines adequacy of circulation.

4. Monitor for signs and symptoms of wound sepsis, including rapid separation of eschar (within 3 to 5 days), purulent pockets of exudate, foul odor, focal blackening, green or yellow discoloration, increasing necrosis, and positive quantitative wound biopsies or cultures (Table 30–4). **Rationale:** Identifies complicating factors necessitating intervention.

Expected Outcomes

1. Wound heals without infectious complications. **Rationale:** Indicative of proper wound care.

2. Patient verbalizes comfort. **Rationale:** Indicative of effective pain relief.

3. Position of optimal function is maintained. **Rationale:** Reduces mobility complications.

Unexpected Outcomes

1. Wound converts to a deeper injury. **Rationale:** Impaired wound healing secondary to poor wound care, poor nutrition, or wound sepsis.

2. Wound sepsis. **Rationale:** Poor wound care resulting from insufficient debridement, incorrect use of dressings, cross-contamination, immunocompromised host, or poor nutritional status.

Documentation

Documentation in the patient record should include the date and time of wound care, the postburn day, the appearance of the wound (color, size, odor, depth, and drainage), if there is evidence of cellulitis around the wound (red, warm, and tender area surrounding wound), progression toward healing, serial assessments of peripheral pulses, level of pain before and after procedure, the type of comfort measures used, the patient's tolerance of the procedure, and any unexpected outcomes encountered and interventions taken. **Rationale:** Provides evidence of nursing care given, status of wound healing, and expected and unexpected outcomes.

Patient/Family Education

1. Assess the family's cognitive and motor abilities to provide care and comfort at home. **Rationale:** Continued wound and skin care is usually necessary following discharge. During the healing process, the patient may experience moderate to severe pruritus.

2. Stress the importance of reporting the signs and symptoms of infection to a health care professional (i.e.,

TABLE 30–4 Signs of Wound Infection

Level	Manifestations
Superficial colonization	Presence of infectious agent on wound; no local or systemic effects
Local tissue cellulitis	Local toxic effects include edema, pain, redness, warmth in tissue surrounding wound; can progress to invasion
Wound invasion	Rapid separation of eschar; purulent subeschar pockets; eschar discoloration; foul odor; conversion to a deeper wound; may see systemic septic effects

fever, edema, purulent drainage, and unusual redness and warmth in skin). Provide a phone number to call for questions or problems. **Rationale:** Patient and family need to recognize the necessity for an immediate assessment by a health care professional if this occurs.

3. Discuss the importance of mobility and self-care in the activities of daily living during the healing phase. With a superficial second-degree burn, the patient should be functioning close to a preinjury level at discharge. **Rationale:** Self-care and exercise prevent contractures associated with healing skin.

4. Inform the patient and family that with a superficial partial-thickness burn, healing is rapid and there may be minimal scarring. However, there may be discoloration for up to 1 year in some patients, especially in patients with darker skin. **Rationale:** Alleviates anxieties about appearance.

5. Stress the importance of compliance with wearing pressure garments and splints. The patient should not be exposed to the sun for up to 1 year after the burn. **Rationale:** Reduces scar formation. Reconstructive surgery may be considered after 1 year; however, this may not restore the patient to the preburn state.

6. Inform the family that nightmares, alterations in body image, and psychological problems may occur. Provide the family and the patient with a name and phone number for follow-up counseling. **Rationale:** Common problems in patients experiencing burns.

7. Provide pain and pruritus medications if needed. **Rationale:** Supports patient's comfort at home.

8. Provide the patient and family with the name of a water-based lotion to apply to the healed area. **Rationale:** Alleviates dryness and pruritus.

9. Provide specific wound care instructions, in writing, such as, "Cleanse daily with a nondrying soap and tepid water. Rinse and dry thoroughly. Apply prescribed cream or ointment to open areas with clean hand. Apply lotion to healed areas as needed, and monitor for areas of skin breakdown." Have the patient and family demonstrate wound care prior to discharge. **Rationale:** Validates patient and family understanding of and ability to perform wound care and encourages questions and provides an opportunity to reinforce important points.

10. Provide the patient and family with follow-up appointments. **Rationale:** Continued professional evaluation of wound/skin healing is necessary.

Performance Checklist
Skill 30–2: Care of the Second-Degree or Third-Degree Burn

Critical Behaviors	Complies	
	yes	no
1. Wash hands.		
2. Don sterile gloves.		
3. Gently wash wound.		
4. Debride loose necrotic tissue.		
5. Assess the wound.		
6. Gently wrap patient in warm towels.		
7. Remove and discard gloves.		
8. Don single sterile glove.		
9. Remove adequate amount of antimicrobial cream from jar.		
10. Apply antimicrobial cream to wound.		
11. For open method, do not apply gauze dressing to wound but reapply cream as wound becomes exposed.		
12. Remove and discard single glove, and don sterile gloves.		
13. For closed method, apply nonadherent gauze.		
14. Wrap wound loosely with bulky gauze.		
15. If wound requires wet dressing, aseptically prepare sterile saline and twenty-ply gauze.		
16. Don sterile gloves.		
17. Squeeze excess solution from gauze, and apply gauze to wound.		
18. Wrap wound with gauze roll.		

Table continues on following page

Critical Behaviors	Complies	
	yes	no
FOR APPLICATION OF SPLINTS 19. Apply splints in position of function, and secure by wrapping with gauze roll or Velcro straps.		
20. Elevate burned extremities with elastic net and/or pillow, and elevate the head of the bed.		
21. Remove and discard gloves.		
22. Wash hands.		
23. Document procedure in the patient record.		

SKILL 30–3

Care of the Donor Site

Closure of a burn wound with a split-thickness skin graft (STSG) is the surgical treatment of choice for a deep second- or third-degree burn. Skin removed from intact areas of the same person are called *autografts*. *Homografts* (human skin from donors) or *heterografts* (nonhuman skin) may be used as biologic dressings, but permanent closure is only accomplished with autografts. An STSG is comprised of the epidermis and part of the dermis, simulating a second-degree burn. Donor sites heal spontaneously in 7 to 10 days.

Donor sites are surgically created wounds that can be considered sterile. The dressing of choice is a hydrocolloid sheet or Duoderm (Madden et al., 1989). This occlusive dressing is applied in the operating room at the time of removal of donor skin and may be replaced at the bedside as needed. Excessive leakage of exudate indicates a need for a dressing change. Other types of dressings used on a donor site include fine-meshed gauze, Xeroform gauze, Biobrane, Op-Site, or biologic dressings. Signs and symptoms of infection, such as purulent drainage, cellulitis, fever, or any disruption in the dressing, indicate a need for a dressing change. These dressings should be kept dry (Fig. 30–7).

If a donor site becomes infected, the dressing must be removed, and an antimicrobial cream, solution, or ointment should be applied.

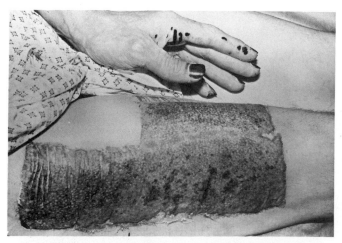

FIGURE 30–7. Dry, intact fine-meshed gauze covering donor site.

Purpose

The nurse performs wound care to the donor site(s) to

1. Promote healing.
2. Prevent infection.
3. Decrease pain.
4. Promote function.
5. Assess progression of wound healing.
6. Prevent progression to a deep partial- or full-thickness injury.

Prerequisite Knowledge and Skills

Prior to caring for a donor site, the nurse should understand

1. Anatomy and physiology of the skin.
2. Principles of wound healing.
3. Principles of infection control and universal precautions.
4. Principles of pain relief.

The nurse should be able to perform

1. Proper handwashing technique (see Skill 35–5).
2. Universal precautions (see Skill 35–1).
3. Correct selection of dressings and/or creams.
4. Clean and aseptic technique.

Assessment

1. Determine the postgraft day to evaluate healing. Observe for signs of healing, including reepithelialization and decreased pain. Observe for complications, including eschar formation, cellulitis, purulent drainage, and fever. **Rationale:** Healing should occur within 7 to 10 days. Complications prolong healing.
2. Graphically document donor-site changes. **Rationale:** Provides objective baseline for determining progression of healing or complications.
3. Know the patient's previous response to pain medications and therapies. **Rationale:** Pain is individualized, and medications should be administered in response to the patient's needs. Peak action should correlate with the procedure for effective pain reduction.
4. Observe and note the patient's level of function and ability to perform the activities of daily living. **Ra-

tionale: Healing donor sites are painful because of exposed nerve endings and tightening of healing skin.

Nursing Diagnoses

1. Impaired skin integrity related to donor site. **Rationale:** The surgical removal of the epidermis and superficial dermis interrupts the integrity and function of the skin.
2. Pain related to exposed nerve endings. **Rationale:** Removal of protective epidermis and superficial dermis exposes nerve endings to stimulation.
3. Potential for infection related to removed epidermis and superficial dermis. **Rationale:** Risk of invasion by microorganisms is increased with a break in skin integrity.
4. Impaired physical mobility related to pain. **Rationale:** Exposed nerve endings make moving painful and difficult.

Planning

1. Individualize the following goals for care of the donor site:
   a. Verbalization of an acceptable level of comfort. **Rationale:** Reflects individualized pain relief and fosters cooperation with further care.
   b. Healing occurs within 7 to 14 days. **Rationale:** Reepithelialization within this time frame indicates an absence of complications.
   c. Level of function is maintained at pregraft state. **Rationale:** Contracture formation results from lack of mobility and poor wound care.
2. Medicate the patient for pain, as prescribed, allowing for peak action of medication to coincide with wound care. **Rationale:** Allows for optimal absorption of medication and optimal pain relief.

3. Prepare all necessary equipment and supplies. **Rationale:** Assembly of all equipment and supplies at the bedside ensures that wound care will be completed quickly and efficiently.
   a. Waterproof pads.
   b. One roll of 2-in cloth or paper tape.

DRESSING CHANGES

   a. Dressing to cover donor site.
   b. Sterile saline (1 L for each $\frac{1}{4}$ ft^2 of donor site).
   c. Two sterile scissors.
   d. Two sterile forceps.
   e. One sterile field.
   f. Sterile gloves, two pairs.
   g. Exam gloves, three pairs.
   h. Ten to twenty sterile 4 × 4 gauze pads.
   i. Sterile wash basin.

FOR INFECTED DONOR SITES

   a. Warm sterile normal saline (1 L for each $\frac{1}{4}$ ft^2 donor site).
   b. Sterile wash basin.
   c. Mild liquid soap.
   d. Sterile debridement instruments (four curved scissors, four forceps).
   e. Ten 4 × 4 sterile gauze pads for every 10 percent TBSA.
   f. Washcloth for unburned areas.
   g. Two pairs of exam gloves.
   h. Two pairs of sterile gloves.
   i. One sterile glove for dominant hand.
   j. Antimicrobial cream.
   k. Elastic net and/or pillows for elevation of affected extremities.
4. Prepare the patient by explaining the procedure. **Rationale:** Diminishes fears related to the unknown. Patient learns the steps in wound care.

Implementation

Steps	Rationale	Special Considerations
General Donor-Site Care		
1. Wash hands.	Reduces transmission of microorganisms.	
2. Don exam gloves.	Universal precautions.	
3. Wrap donor site and intact dressing in waterproof pad, and seal edges with tape.	Protects integrity of dressing while care of the graft and other burned areas is accomplished.	
4. Remove and discard gloves.	Universal precautions.	
5. Wash hands.	Reduces transmission of microorganisms.	
Dressing Changes		
1. Wash hands.	Reduces transmission of microorganisms.	
2. Prepare sterile field, and place instruments on field.	Maintains aseptic technique.	

Table continues on following page

Steps	Rationale	Special Considerations
3. Don exam gloves.	Universal precautions.	
4. Remove old dressing and dispose in appropriate receptacle.	Exposes wound and maintains universal precautions.	
5. Remove and discard gloves.	Universal precautions.	
6. Don sterile gloves.	Maintains aseptic technique.	
7. Gently cleanse donor site of any crusty or loose exudate with wet gauze. Use forceps and scissors if necessary.	Removes debris and decreases microbial growth.	
8. Pat edges of wound and skin surrounding it dry with 4 × 4 gauze pads.	Enhances adherence of dressing.	
9. Cut dressing to the size of donor site.	Ensures correct fit.	
10. Apply dressing to wound, and secure edges of border.	Promotes adherence.	
11. Remove and discard gloves.	Universal precautions.	
12. Wash hands.	Reduces transmission of microorganisms.	
Care of the Infected Donor Site		
1. Wash hands.	Reduces transmission of microorganisms.	
2. Don exam gloves.	Universal precautions.	
3. Remove old dressing, and dispose in appropriate receptacle.	Exposes wound and maintains universal precautions.	
4. Remove and discard gloves.	Universal precautions.	
5. Don sterile gloves.	Maintains aseptic technique.	
6. Gently wash the affected area with warm sterile normal saline and soap.	Cleanses wound of debris and reduces microorganisms.	Make sure area surrounding wound is clean as well. The patient may wish to cleanse his or her own wounds. Since he or she knows his or her own pain threshold, it is often higher when the patient is in control.
7. With curved scissors and forceps, remove any loose necrotic tissue.	Reduces medium for bacterial infection.	In units not specializing in burns, this may be the responsibility of the physician.
8. Remove and discard gloves.	Universal precautions.	
9. Don single sterile glove on dominant hand.	Reduces transmission of microorganisms.	
10. Prepare an adequate amount of antimicrobial cream to cover wound.	Prevents contamination of entire jar of cream.	
11. With sterile-gloved hand, apply a ⅛-in layer of antimicrobial cream to completely cover donor site.	Reduces proliferation of microorganisms and pain.	Gentle application is recommended to reduce pain and trauma.
12. Elevate the affected area with loose elastic net and/or pillows. Elevate the head of the bed.	Promotes comfort.	If possible, keep patient from lying on affected area. If donor sites are circumferential, turn patient every 2 hours. Patient may experience tingling due to elevation.

Table continues on following page

Steps	Rationale	Special Considerations
13. Remove and discard glove.	Universal precautions.	
14. Wash hands.	Reduces transmission of microorganisms.	

Evaluation

1. Evaluate the progression of donor-site healing. **Rationale:** Reepithelialization occurs within 7 to 14 days.
2. Evaluate the type and effectiveness of pain-relief medications and therapies used. **Rationale:** Ensures patient comfort.

Expected Outcomes

1. Donor site heals within 7 to 14 days. **Rationale:** Indicative of proper wound care.
2. Verbalization of comfort. **Rationale:** Indicative of effective pain relief.

Unexpected Outcomes

1. Donor site converts to a deep second-degree injury. **Rationale:** Impaired wound healing secondary to poor wound care, poor nutrition, or wound sepsis.
2. Infected donor site. **Rationale:** Poor wound care.

Documentation

Documentation in the patient record should include the date and time of donor-site care, the postgraft day, the appearance of the site (color, size, odor, depth, and the presence of any drainage or cellulitis), and the progression toward healing, type of dressing applied, comfort measures used, patient's tolerance of the procedure, and any unexpected outcomes encountered and interventions taken. **Rationale:** Provides evidence of nursing care given, status of donor-site healing, and expected and unexpected outcomes.

Patient/Family Education

1. Assess the family's cognitive and motor abilities to provide care and comfort at home. **Rationale:** Continued wound and skin care is usually necessary following discharge. During the healing process, the patient will experience moderate to severe pruritus.
2. Stress the importance of reporting signs and symptoms of infection to a health care professional (i.e., fever, edema, purulent drainage, and unusual redness and warmth in skin). Provide a phone number to call for questions or problems. **Rationale:** Patient and family need to recognize the necessity for an immediate assessment by a health care professional if this occurs.
3. Discuss the importance of mobility and self-care in the activities of daily living during the healing phase. With a deep second- and/or third-degree burn, the patient should maintain a level of function based on the severity of the injury. **Rationale:** Self-care and exercise prevent contractures associated with healing skin.
4. Provide pain and pruritus medications, if needed. **Rationale:** Supports patient's comfort.
5. Provide the patient and family with the name of a water-based lotion to apply to the healed area. **Rationale:** Alleviates dryness and pruritus.
6. Provide specific wound care instructions in writing, such as, "Cleanse daily with a nondrying soap and tepid water. Rinse and dry thoroughly. Apply prescribed cream or ointment to open areas with clean hands. Apply lotion to healed areas as needed, and monitor for areas of skin breakdown." Have the patient and family demonstrate wound care prior to discharge. **Rationale:** Validates patient and family understanding of and ability to perform wound care. Encourages questions and provides opportunity to reinforce important points.
7. Provide the patient and family with follow-up appointments. **Rationale:** Continued professional evaluation of wound/skin care is necessary.

Performance Checklist
Skill 30–3: Care of the Donor Site

Critical Behaviors	Complies	
	yes	no
General Donor-Site Care 1. Wash hands.		
2. Don exam gloves.		
3. Wrap donor site and intact dressing in waterproof pads, and seal edges.		
4. Remove and discard gloves.		
5. Wash hands.		

Table continues on following page

Critical Behaviors	Complies	
	yes	no
DRESSING		
1. Wash hands.		
2. Prepare sterile field.		
3. Don exam gloves.		
4. Remove and discard old dressing.		
5. Remove and discard gloves.		
6. Don sterile gloves.		
7. Cleanse wound.		
8. Pat edges of wound and skin surrounding it dry.		
9. Cut dressing to appropriate size.		
10. Apply dressing, and secure edges.		
11. Remove and discard gloves.		
12. Wash hands.		
13. Document in the patient record.		
CARE OF THE INFECTED DONOR SITE		
1. Wash hands.		
2. Don exam gloves.		
3. Remove and discard old dressing.		
4. Remove and discard gloves.		
5. Don sterile gloves.		
6. Cleanse wound.		
7. Debride loose necrotic tissue.		
8. Remove and discard gloves.		
9. Don single sterile glove on dominant hand.		
10. Remove an adequate amount of antimicrobial cream from jar.		
11. Apply antimicrobial cream to wound.		
12. Elevate affected area with net and/or pillow, and elevate the head of the bed.		
13. Remove and discard glove.		
14. Wash hands.		
15. Document in the patient record.		

SKILL 30–4

Care of the Skin Graft

The most common type of split-thickness skin graft (STSG) for closure of a burn is a meshed graft. Meshing allows the graft to be stretched over an area larger than the actual donor site. The graft is usually held in place with staples. The spaces created by meshing, or the interstices, heal in from the edges of the graft. Therefore, these grafts are usually covered with a nonadherent dressing until the interstices heal, usually within 7 to 10 days (Fig. 30–8). Research is aimed at closure of the burn wound with cultured composite grafts (Cuono et al., 1987; Heck et al., 1985; Madden et al., 1986). The use of cultured allogeneic or autologous grafts over allogenic or artificial dermis is currently under study.

Sheet grafts are used for cosmetic or functional reasons. These grafts are usually secured in place and are

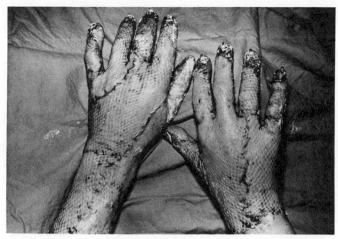

FIGURE 30–8. Meshed, split-thickness skin graft to hands with healed interstices.

kept open to air. With these grafts, pockets of serous fluid may accumulate under the graft. This must be reported to the physician for aspiration to prevent graft loss.

Purpose

The nurse performs skin-graft care to

1. Promote graft take.
2. Prevent infection.
3. Decrease pain.
4. Promote function.
5. Prevent graft loss.

Prerequisite Knowledge and Skills

Prior to caring for a skin graft, the nurse should understand

1. Anatomy and physiology of the skin.
2. Principles of grafting.
3. Principles of infection control and universal precautions.
4. Principles of pain relief.

The nurse should be able to perform

1. Proper handwashing technique (see Skill 35–5).
2. Universal precautions (see Skill 35–1).
3. Correct application of dressings and/or creams (see Skill 30–2).
4. Clean and aseptic technique.

Assessment

1. Assess graft take, as evidenced by vascularization of the graft, reepithelialization of the interstices, decreased pain, and adherence of graft. Observe for complications, including graft necrosis, sloughing, cellulitis, purulent drainage, and fever. **Rationale:** Healing should occur within 7 to 10 days. Complications will prolong healing.

2. Graphically document grafted areas. **Rationale:** Provides objective baseline for determining graft take or complications.

3. Know the patient's previous response to pain medications and therapies. Pain decreases as interstices close and nerve endings are covered. **Rationale:** Pain is individualized, and medications should be administered in response to the patient's needs. Peak action should correlate with the procedure for effective pain reduction.

4. Assess the position/immobilization method of the grafted body part. **Rationale:** Areas of the graft should be immobilized until there is evidence of graft take.

Nursing Diagnoses

1. Impaired skin integrity related to graft and open interstices. **Rationale:** The surgical removal of the epidermis and superficial dermis and meshing to form interstices interrupt skin integrity.

2. Pain related to exposed nerve endings. **Rationale:** Surgical debridement of the grafted burn and open areas of the graft expose nerve endings to increased stimulation.

3. Potential for infection related to interstices and unhealed burn. **Rationale:** Risk of invasion by microorganisms is increased with disrupted skin integrity.

4. Impaired physical mobility related to immobilization for graft take. **Rationale:** Grafted areas are often immobilized for 5 to 7 days after surgery.

Planning

1. Individualize the following goals for care of the skin graft:
   a. Verbalization of an acceptable level of comfort. **Rationale:** Reflects pain relief and fosters cooperation with further care.
   b. Maintain immobilization of grafted area for 5 to 7 days. **Rationale:** Fosters graft take and reduces risk of shearing.
   c. Promote vascularization of graft. **Rationale:** Encourages adequate circulation and graft take.

2. Medicate the patient for pain, as prescribed, allowing for peak action of medication to coincide with wound care. **Rationale:** Allows for optimal absorption of medication and optimal pain relief.

3. Prepare all necessary equipment and supplies. **Rationale:** Assembly of all equipment and supplies at the beside ensures that graft care will be completed quickly and efficiently.
   a. Warm sterile normal saline (1 L for each $\frac{1}{4}$ ft^2 graft).
   b. Sterile wash basin.
   c. Mild liquid soap.
   d. Sterile debridement instruments (four curved scissors, four forceps).

e. Ten 4 × 4 sterile gauze pads per 10 percent TBSA.
f. Washcloth for unburned areas.
g. Two pairs of examination gloves.
h. Two pairs of sterile gloves.
i. Pillows for elevation of affected extremities.
j. Staple remover.
k. Nonadherent gauze (Adaptic or Xerofoam).
l. Ten-ply sterile gauze sheets.
m. Bulky gauze roll to wrap dressings.
n. Combine pads for one layer of padding.
o. Gauze roll to wrap splints.

4. Prepare the patient by explaining the procedure. **Rationale:** Diminishes fear related to the unknown.
5. Organize all other appropriate care related to the graft being exposed (i.e., assessment by physician, therapists). **Rationale:** Organization of care prevents trauma to the graft.

Implementation

Steps	Rationale	Special Considerations
1. Wash hands.	Reduces transmission of microorganisms.	
2. Don exam gloves.	Universal precautions.	
3. Remove old bulky dressing using a continuous irrigation.	Exposes graft and prevents traumatic elevation.	
4. Remove and discard gloves.	Universal precautions.	
5. Don sterile gloves.	Maintains aseptic technique.	
6. Gently remove nonadherent gauze covering from grafted site. As dressing is being removed, hold down graft to prevent traumatic removal.	Exposes and protects graft.	
7. Gently rinse graft with saline and gauze pads.	Cleanses wound of debris and reduces microorganisms.	Make sure area surrounding wound is clean as well. Use washcloth and soap.
8. With curved scissors and forceps, carefully remove loose necrotic tissue.	Aids in preventing infection.	In units not specializing in burns, this may be the responsibility of the physician.
9. Remove scabs and staples as indicated.	Prevents complications of embedding and infection.	The first dressing change is usually on the third to fifth postoperative day. Staples are gradually removed starting on day 4 or 5.
10. Assess graft for complications and take.	Allows for further comparisons.	At this time, allow for evaluation by other disciplines.
11. Gently wrap patient in warm towels, keeping away from grafted areas.	Reduces loss of body temperature.	
12. Apply nonadherent dressing (if interstices are open) and ten-ply gauze, and wrap with bulky gauze roll.	Protects graft for healing.	
13. Apply splints and combine pads, and wrap with gauze roll (Fig. 30–9).	Decreases the risk of contractures and promotes function.	
14. Elevate grafted area with pillows.	Reduces edema and decreases pain.	If possible, keep patient from lying on grafted area. If grafts are circumferential, turn patient q2h. Patient may experience tingling due to elevation.
15. Remove and discard gloves.	Universal precautions.	
16. Wash hands.	Reduces transmission of microorganisms.	

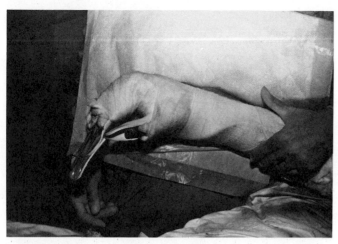

FIGURE 30–9. Example of closed method of wound dressing with hand splinted in position of function.

Evaluation

1. Evaluate the progression of wound healing (i.e., reepithelialization and graft take within 7 to 10 days). **Rationale:** Determines progression toward healing without complications.

2. Evaluate the type and effectiveness of pain-relief medications and therapies used. **Rationale:** Ensures patient comfort.

3. Maintain optimal level of range of motion/function. **Rationale:** Indicates proper splinting and positioning.

Expected Outcomes

1. Graft take within 7 to 10 days. **Rationale:** Indicative of proper wound care.

2. Patient verbalizes comfort. **Rationale:** Indicative of effective pain relief.

Unexpected Outcome

Graft loss. **Rationale:** Complicating factors of graft shearing, poor wound care, inadequate nutrition, inadequate circulation, and wound sepsis.

Documentation

Documentation in the patient record should include the date and time of care, the postgraft day, the appearance of the graft (vascularization, drainage, take, and number of staples) and size of interstices, type of dressing removed and replaced, amount and type of comfort measures used, patient's tolerance of the procedure, and any unexpected outcomes encountered and interventions taken. **Rationale:** Provides evidence of nursing care given, status of graft and expected and unexpected outcomes.

Patient/Family Education

1. Assess the family's cognitive and motor abilities to provide care and comfort at home. **Rationale:** Continued wound and skin care is usually necessary following discharge. During the healing process, the patient will experience moderate to severe pruritus.

2. Stress the importance of reporting signs and symptoms of infection to a health care professional (i.e., fever, edema, purulent drainage, and unusual redness and warmth in skin). Provide a phone number to call for questions or problems. **Rationale:** Patient and family need to recognize the necessity for an immediate assessment by a health care professional if this occurs.

3. Discuss the importance of mobility and self-care in the activities of daily living during the healing phase. With a skin graft, the patient should maintain a level of function based on the severity of the injury. **Rationale:** Self-care and exercise prevent contractures associated with healing grafts.

4. Inform the patient and family that with grafts, there may be some scarring. There will be discoloration for up to 1 year, and it may be permanent in some patients. **Rationale:** Anxieties about body image need to be addressed.

5. Inform the patient and family of the importance of compliance with wearing pressure garments and splints. The patient should not be exposed to the sun for up to 1 year after the burn. **Rationale:** Reduces scar formation. Reconstructive surgery may be considered after 1 year, but this will not restore the patient to the preburn state.

6. Inform the family that nightmares, alterations in body image, and psychological problems may occur. Provide the family and the patient with a name and phone number for follow-up counseling. **Rationale:** Common problems in patients experiencing burns.

7. Provide pain and pruritus medications, if needed. **Rationale:** Supports patient's comfort at home.

8. Provide the patient and family with the name of a water-based lotion to apply to the healed area. **Rationale:** Alleviates dryness and pruritus.

9. Provide specific wound care instructions in writing, such as, "Cleanse daily with a nondrying soap and tepid water. Rinse and dry thoroughly. Apply prescribed cream or ointment to open areas with clean hands. Apply lotion to healed areas as needed, and monitor for areas of skin breakdown." Have the patient and family demonstrate wound care prior to discharge. **Rationale:** Validates patient and family understanding of and ability to perform wound care. Encourages questions and provides an opportunity to reinforce important points.

10. Provide the patient and family with follow-up appointments. **Rationale:** Continued professional evaluation of wound/skin care is necessary.

Performance Checklist
Skill 30–5: Care of the Skin Graft

Critical Behaviors	Complies	
	yes	no
1. Wash hands.		
2. Don exam gloves.		
3. Remove and discard old dressing.		
4. Remove and discard gloves.		
5. Don sterile gloves.		
6. Remove nonadherent gauze.		
7. Rinse graft with saline.		
8. Remove loose necrotic tissue.		
9. Trim scabs and remove staples.		
10. Assess site for graft take or complications.		
11. Wrap patient in warm towels, leaving graft exposed.		
12. Apply nonadherent dressing and ten-ply gauze, and wrap with bulky gauze roll.		
13. Apply combine pads and splints, and wrap with gauze roll.		
14. Elevate grafted extremity.		
15. Remove and discard gloves.		
16. Wash hands.		
17. Document in the patient record.		

REFERENCES

Cuono, C. B., Langdon, R., Birchall, N., et al. (1987). Composite autologous-allogeneic skin replacement: Development and clinical application. *Plast. Reconstr. Surg.* 80(4):626–637.

Heck, E. L., Bergstresser, P. R., and Baxter, C. R. (1985). Composite skin graft: Frozen dermal allografts support the engraftment and expansion of autologous epidermis. *J. Trauma* 25(2):106–112.

Herndon, D. N., and Parks, D. H. (1986). Comparison of serial debridement and autografting and early massive excision with cadaver skin overlay in the treatment of large burns in children. *J. Trauma* 26:149.

Madden, M. R., Finkelstein, J., Marano, M. A., and Goodwin, C. W. (1990). The acute management and surgical treatment of the burned patient, part 1. *Surg. Rounds* 13(6):41–45.

Madden, M. R., Finkelstein, J., Hefton, J. M., et al. (1986). Grafting of cultured allogenic epidermis on second- and third-degree burn wounds on 26 patients. *J. Trauma* 26(11):955–961.

Madden, M. R., Nolan, E., Finkelstein, J., (1989). Comparison of an occlusive and a semiocclusive dressing and the effect of the wound exudate upon keratinocyte proliferation. *J. Trauma* 55(7):924–931.

Saydjazri, R., Abston, S., et al. (1986). Chemical burns. *J. Burn Care Rehabil.* 17(5):405–407.

UNIT IX

NUTRITIONAL SUPPORT

BEHAVIORAL OBJECTIVES

After completing this chapter, the nurse will be able to

- Define the key terms.
- Describe methods for infusing total parenteral nutrition.
- Discuss the nurses's role during insertion or guidewire exchange of a central venous catheter.
- Describe techniques for venous access maintenance.
- Demonstrate the skills involved in the administration of total parenteral nutrition.

Strict adherence to aseptic technique and close patient monitoring are required when administering total parenteral nutrition (TPN). Critically ill patients may need TPN to meet nutritional needs because of hypermetabolism or inadequate function of the gastrointestinal (GI) tract. Safe administration of TPN is dependent on adequate assessment of the patient, consistency in the infusion rate, and careful monitoring for potential complications.

The focus of this chapter is the procedures for the administration of TPN and the related patient care.

KEY TERMS

amino acids	guidewire exchange
anthropometric	hyperosmolar
measurement	in-line IV filter
catheter colonization	lipid emulsions
catheter infection	nitrogen balance
catheter-related septicemia	occlusive thrombosis
central venous access	parenteral nutrition
central venous catheter	parietal thrombosis
dextrose	peripheral parenteral
guidewire	nutrition (PPN)

stylet	TPN cycle
superior vena cava	Valsalva maneuver
total parenteral	venous thrombosis
nutrition (TPN)	

SKILLS

31–1 Assisting with Insertion of a Percutaneous Central Venous Catheter
31–2 Insertion of a Peripheral Central Venous Catheter
31–3 Assisting with Exchange of a Percutaneously Placed Central Venous Catheter
31–4 Central Venous Catheter Site Care
31–5 Infusion, Care, and Monitoring of a Total Parenteral Nutrition System
31–6 Removal of a Percutaneously Placed Central Venous Catheter

GUIDELINES

The following guidelines assist the nurse in formulating a nursing diagnosis and an individualized plan of care to provide TPN:

1. Assess the patient's respiratory, cardiovascular, and gastrointestinal function.
2. Determine the patient's baseline nutritional status.
3. Review the patient's medical and diet history.
4. Review the patient's current medical treatment plan and medication profile.
5. Determine appropriate interventions based on assessment findings.
6. Become adept with the equipment used for delivery of TPN.

SKILL 31–1 _____

Assisting with Insertion of a Percutaneous Central Venous Catheter

Central venous access is required for the infusion of total parenteral nutrition. The superior vena cava and the inferior vena cava afford high flow rates and volumes for rapid dilution of hypertonic solutions. Access to the superior vena cava or the inferior vena cava may be accomplished through any tributary sufficient in size to accommodate a catheter. Common access sites are the subclavian, jugular, basilic, cephalic, and antecubital veins. Because of the extreme risk of catheter-related septicemia, the femoral approach is rarely used for infusion of parenteral nutrition. The risk of catheter septicemia also may be increased with TPN infusion through multilumen catheters. A single-lumen catheter dedicated solely to TPN administration is optimal.

Access of the subclavian or jugular vein is a blind procedure utilizing anatomic landmarks as guidance. Therefore, the risk of injury to structures adjacent to the great veins is increased. Resulting complications are associated with high morbidity and mortality. Analysis of data from the Food and Drug Administration's Medical Device Reporting System (1988) determined that the cause of complications contributing to death or serious injury is not device related but most often related to the health care practitioner.

Although this is a medical procedure, the nurse significantly affects the outcome. Nursing interventions focus on patient education, maintenance of sterility, safety, and patient comfort.

Purpose

The nurse assists with insertion of a central venous catheter to

1. Provide preprocedural patient education.
2. Ensure sterility of the procedure.
3. Ensure patient safety and comfort.
4. Provide nursing intervention and medical support in the event of a complication.
5. Provide technical assistance.

Prerequisite Knowledge and Skills

Prior to assisting with insertion of a central venous catheter, the nurse should understand

1. Anatomy and physiology of the vascular system.
2. Principles of infection control.
3. Universal precautions.
4. Principles of aseptic technique.
5. Proper patient positioning for the procedure.
6. Design, use, and indications for the selected catheter.
7. The methods and techniques of insertion.
8. Potential complications of the procedure and the medical and nursing interventions for each.

The nurse should be able to perform

1. Proper handwashing technique (see Skill 35–5).
2. Aseptic technique.
3. Universal precautions (see Skill 35–1).
4. Proper patient positioning.
5. Respiratory system assessment.
6. Cardiovascular system assessment.
7. Dysrhythmia identification.
8. Application of a sterile occlusive dressing (see Skill 31–4).
9. Cardiopulmonary resuscitation.

Assessment

1. Review the nutritional assessment (Table 31–1), which should be completed prior to catheter placement. Identify the appropriateness of parenteral nutrition as the modality for therapy. **Rationale:** Central venous catheterization is not without serious risk (Table 31–2) and should not be done without clear indications.
2. Determine the appropriate site and vein for cannulation and the appropriate catheter for TPN administration. **Rationale:** Decreases the risk of insertion and postinsertion complications.
3. Assess the patient's fluid status, heart rate, blood pressure, intake and output, breath sounds, hematocrit, and serum electrolytes. **Rationale:** Low venous pressure and hypovolemia prevent adequate venous distension, increasing the risk of complications.
4. Check the patient's platelet count. A platelet count of less than 100,000/mm³ may require infusion of blood products prior to CVC insertion. **Rationale:** Platelet counts less than 100,000/mm³ increase the risk of bleeding complications, i.e., hematoma or hemothorax, with inadvertent venous or arterial injury.
5. Assess the patient's baseline vital signs, i.e., blood pressure, heart rate and rhythm, and respiratory rate, rhythm, and depth. **Rationale:** Baseline data provide information for assessment of the patient's tolerance of the procedure, evaluation of a suspected complication, and are a guide for intervention.
6. Assess the patient's history for sensitivity to lidocaine or antiseptic solutions. **Rationale:** Decreases the risk of allergic reactions.

TABLE 31-1 NUTRITIONAL ASSESSMENT PARAMETERS

History	Medical history
	Surgical history
	Social history
	Dietary history
Physical Examination	Clinical assessment
	Anthropometric measurements:
	Height and weight
	Skinfold thickness
	Arm circumference
Laboratory Data	Electrolyte balance
	Renal, hepatic, hematopoietic and
	pulmonary functions
	Cell-mediated immunity: total
	lymphocyte count
	Visceral protein compartment: albumin,
	prealbumin, total iron-binding
	capacity, transferrin
	Somatic protein compartment: nitrogen
	balance
	Nutrient requirements:
	Protein requirements:
	Nitrogen balance
	Energy requirements:
	Predicted: basal energy expenditure
	(BEE) and resting energy expenditure
	(REE)
	Measured: indirect calorimetry
	Fluid requirements: intake and output

TABLE 31-2 COMPLICATIONS OF CENTRAL VENOUS CATHETER INSERTION

Complication	Clinical Manifestation	Treatment	Prevention

Pneumothorax	Sudden respiratory distress
	Chest pain
	Hypoxia/cyanosis
	Decreased breath sounds
	Resonance to percussion
		Confirmation by chest x-ray
		Symptomatic treatment
		Small pneumothorax:
		  Bed rest
		  O_2
		Pneumothorax > 25%:
		  Chest tube
		  Cardiopulmonary support
			Proper patient preparation
			Sedation as necessary
			Proper patient positioning
			Adequate hydration status
			Low acuity of the angle of the
			  needle on venipuncture
			Avoid multiple passes with the
			  needle
			Clinician skilled and experienced in insertion technique
			Use of peripherally inserted
			  central venous catheter

Tension pneumothorax	Most likely to occur in patients on ventilatory support
	Respiratory distress
	Rapid clinical deterioration:
	  Cyanosis
	  Venous distension
	  Hypotension
	  Decreased cardiac output
		Treatment must be rapid and
		  aggressive
		Immediate air respiration followed by chest tube
		Cardiopulmonary support
			Proper patient preparation
			Sedation as necessary
			Proper patient positioning
			Adequate hydration status
			Reduction of PEEP $\leq$ 5
			  cmH_2O at time of venipuncture
			Low acuity of the angle of the
			  needle on venipuncture
			Avoid multiple passes with the
			  needle
			Clinician skilled and experienced in insertion technique
			Use of peripherally inserted
			  central venous catheter

Table continues on following page

Complication	Clinical Manifestation	Treatment	Prevention
Delayed pneumothorax	Slow onset of respiratory symptoms Subcutaneous emphysema Persistent pleuritic chest or back pain	Confirmation by chest x-ray Chest tube Cardiopulmonary support	Proper patient preparation Sedation as necessary Proper patient positioning Adequate hydration status Low acuity of the angle of the needle on venipuncture Avoid multiple passes with the needle Clinician skilled and experienced in insertion technique Use of peripherally inserted central venous catheter
Hydrothorax hydromediastinum	Dyspnea Chest pain Muffled breath sounds High glucose level of chest drainage Low-grade fever	Stop infusion Confirmation by chest x-ray; contrast injection may be helpful Cardiopulmonary support	Proper patient preparation Sedation as necessary Proper patient positioning Adequate hydration status Low acuity of the angle of the needle on venipuncture Avoid multiple passes with the needle Clinician skilled and experienced in insertion technique Use of peripherally inserted central venous catheter Placement of catheter tip in lower superior vena cava
Hemothorax	Respiratory distress Hypovolemic shock Hematoma in the neck with jugular insertions	Confirmation by chest x-ray Chest tube Thoracotomy for arterial repair if indicated	Correct coagulopathies before insertion Adequate hydration status Avoid multiple passes with the needle Evaluation by venogram of suspected thrombosis from prior cannulation before insertion

Arterial puncture/laceration	Return of bright red blood in the syringe under high pressure
	Pulsatile blood flow on disconnection of the syringe
	Deterioration of clinical status:
	  Hemorrhagic shock
	  Respiratory distress
	Bleeding from catheter site may or may not be observed
	Deviation of trachea with large hematoma in the neck
	Hemothorax may be detected on chest x-ray
		Application of pressure for 3 to 5 minutes following removal of the needle
		Elevate head of bed
		Chest tube as indicated
		Thoracotomy for arterial repair if indicated
			Correct coagulopathies before insertion
			Adequate hydration status
			Avoid multiple passes with the needle
			Evaluation by venogram of suspected thrombosis from prior cannulation before insertion
			Use of small-gauge needle to first locate the vein

Bleeding/hematoma, venous or arterial bleeding	Bleeding from insertion site Hematoma formation; not likely to be seen with subclavian approach Bleeding may occur internally without visible evidence Tracheal compression Respiratory distress Carotid compression	Application of pressure to the insertion site Thoracotomy for arterial repair Tracheostomy for tracheal deviation from hematoma	Correct coagulopathies before insertion Adequate hydration status Avoid multiple passes with the needle at venipuncture Use of small-gauge needle to first locate the vein
Cardiac dysrythmias	Cardiac dysrythmias: Premature ventricular contractions	Withdraw the guidewire or catheter from the heart Pharmacologic treatment of	Avoid entry into the heart with guidewire or catheter Observe cardiac monitor; tall

Table continues on following page

Complication	Clinical Manifestation	Treatment	Prevention
Cardiac dysrythmias cont'd.	Supraventricular trachycardia Ventricular trachycardia Premature arterial contractions Refractory arterial flutter Sudden cardiovascular collapse	persistent arrythmias	peaked P waves can be identified as the catheter tip enters the right atrium Palpation of peripheral pulse (if not on ECG monitor)
Air embolism	Symptoms dependent on amount of air drawn in Sudden cardiovascular collapse Tachypnea, apnea, tachycardia Hypotension, cyanosis, anxiety Diffuse pulmonary wheezes "Mill wheel" churning heart murmur Neurologic deficits, paresis, stroke, coma Cardiac arrest	Stop airflow Position patient on left side with head down (Durant position) Oxygen administration Air aspiration; transthoracic needle or intracardiac catheter Cardiopulmonary support	Adequate hydration status Head-down tilt or Trendelenburg position during catheter insertion Use of small-bore needle for insertion Application of thumb over needle or catheter hub during disconnection; needle or hub should not be exposed longer than 1 second Advancement of catheter during positive-pressure cycle in patients on ventilatory support Avoid nicking of catheter with careful suturing technique Avoid catheter exchange from large-bore catheter (Swan-Ganz) to smaller catheter Use of Luer-lok connections Minimal risk with peripherally inserted central venous catheter
Catheter malposition	Pain in ear or neck Swishing sound in ear with infusion Sharp anterior chest pain Pain in ipsilateral shoulder blade Cardiac dysrythmia Observation on chest x-ray Signs or symptoms may be absent No blood return on aspiration	Position the patient in a high Fowler's position to allow gravity to correct jugular tip malposition Repositioning of catheter with guidewire under fluoroscopy or new venipuncture Catheter removal	Proper patient positioning Anthropometric measurement for accurate intravascular catheter length Avoid use of force when advancing the catheter Use of a guidewire or blunt-tipped stylet
Catheter embolism	Cardiac dysrythmias Chest pain Dyspnea Hypotension Tachycardia May be clinically silent	Location of fragment on x-ray Transvenous retrieval of catheter fragment Thoracotomy	Use of "over a guidewire" (Seldinger) insertion technique Extreme caution with use of through-the-needle catheter designs; *never* withdraw a catheter through the needle Use of guidewire or stylet within a catheter that is inserted through a needle
Pericardial tamponade	Retrosternal or epigastric pain Dyspnea Venous engorgement of face and neck Restlessness, confusion Hypotension, paradoxical pulse Muffled heart sounds Mediastinal widening Pleural effusion Cardiac arrest	Treatment must be rapid and aggressive Discontinuation of infusions Aspiration through the catheter Emergency pericardiocentesis Emergency thoracotomy Slow withdrawal of catheter with contrast injection to detect residual myocardial leak	Catheter tip position: Parallel to the walls of the superior vena cava 1 to 2 cm above the junction of the superior vena cava and right atrium Use of soft, flexible catheters Minimal risk with peripherally inserted central venous catheter

Table continues on following page

Complication	Clinical Manifestation	Treatment	Prevention
Tracheal injury	Subcutaneous emphysema Pneumomediastinum Air trapping between the chest wall and the pleura Respiratory distress with puncture of endotracheal tube cuff	Emergency reintubation (for punctured endotracheal tube cuff) Aspiration of air in mediastinum	Clinician skilled and experienced in insertion techniques Use of peripherally inserted central venous catheter
Nerve injury	Patient complaints of tingling/numbness in arm or fingers Shooting pain down the arm Paralysis Diaphragmatic paralysis (phrenic nerve injury)	Remove catheter if suspected brachial plexus injury	Clinician skilled and experienced in insertion technique Minimal risk with peripherally inserted central venous catheter
Sterile thrombophlebitis	Potential complication of the peripherally inserted central venous catheter Redness, tenderness, swelling along the course of the vein Pain in the upper extremity or shoulder	Application of heat for 48 to 72 hours Removal of catheter	Thorough washing of gloves prior to handling Silastic catheters Strict aseptic technique during catheter insertion Adequate skin preparation Atraumatic insertion
Pulmonary embolism	Potential complication of catheter exchange Often clinically silent Chest pain Dyspnea Coughing Tachycardia Anxiety Fever	Chest x-ray Lung perfusion scan Cardiopulmonary support	Avoid catheter exchange in veins with thrombosis

Nursing Diagnoses

1. Potential for injury related to catheter insertion. **Rationale:** Venipuncture of the great veins is a blind procedure. Structures in proximity to the central vasculature may be injured by aberrant passage of the needle, guidewire, or catheter.

2. Potential for infection related to contamination during the insertion procedure. **Rationale:** Catheter insertion is an invasive procedure requiring surgical asepsis. Inadequate skin preparation or inadvertent contamination of the sterile field may result in catheter-related septicemia.

Planning

1. Individualize the following goals for assisting with insertion of a central venous catheter:
   a. Maintain sterility of the procedure. **Rationale:** The patient is at risk for infection if aseptic technique is not utilized.
   b. Ensure patient comfort and safety. **Rationale:** An anxious, uncomfortable, uncooperative patient increases the risk of complications.
2. Prepare necessary equipment and supplies. **Rationale:** Collection and organization of the equipment at the bedside ensure that the procedure will be completed quickly and efficiently.

Prep Items

a. Face masks (for each person in attendance).
b. One moisture-proof underpad.
c. One antiseptic scrub sponge.
d. One pair nonsterile gloves.
e. One sterile towel.
f. One pair of goggles.
g. One cap or head covering.
h. One towel roll (for subclavian approach only).
i. Isotonic solution, 250 to 1000 cc, with Luer-lok administration set for IV infusion.

Sterile Items

a. One sterile gown.
b. One pair of sterile gloves.
c. Three povidone-iodine swabsticks.
d. Catheter of choice, usually supplied with insertion needle, syringe, and guidewire.
e. 1% lidocaine, 30 cc.
f. One 25-gauge ⅝-in needle.
g. 0.9% sodium chloride, 10 to 30 cc.
h. One 10- to 12-cc non-Luer-lok syringe.
i. Two 3- to 5-cc syringes.
j. Two 22-gauge 1½-in needles.
k. Six 4 × 4 gauze sponges.
l. Heparin 100 U/cc (for multilumen catheters), 1 to 2 cc.
m. One hemostat.

n. One pair of scissors.
o. One needle holder.
p. One pack of 3-0 or 4-0 nylon suture with curved needle.
q. One Luer-lok extension tubing.

DRESSING MATERIALS

a. Three alcohol swabsticks.
b. Three povidone-iodine swabsticks.
c. One single-dose packet of povidone-iodine ointment.
d. Two 2 × 2 gauze sponges.
e. One skin protectant swabstick.
f. One roll of 2-in tape or transparent dressing.

3. Prepare the patient.
a. Explain the procedure to the patient and reinforce information given during informed consent. **Rationale:** Minimizes risk and reduces anxiety.
b. Explain the patient's expected participation and importance of maintaining sterility. **Rationale:** Minimizes risk of contamination and encourages cooperation.
c. Explain the required positioning for the procedure. **Rationale:** Encourages cooperation and reduces anxiety.
d. Instruct the patient to report symptoms of pain. **Rationale:** Reduces anxiety and facilitates cooperation. Quick, unexpected movements by the patient increase the risk of injury while the needle is advanced (see Table 31–2).
e. Acquire orders for sedation for highly anxious or combative patients. **Rationale:** Quick, unexpected movements by the patient increase the risk of injury while the needle is advanced (see Table 31–2).
f. Perform endotracheal or tracheostomy suctioning on ventilated patients (see Skill 1–9). **Rationale:** Minimizes risk of complications and contamination of the sterile field from coughing or interruption of the procedure (see Table 31–2).
g. Position the patient flat, arms straight at the side, pillows removed, and head turned away from the insertion side. **Rationale:** Proper body alignment for catheter insertion.
h. For subclavian insertions, place a towel roll longitudinally between the scapulae along the upper thoracic spine. The towel roll should be large enough to allow the shoulders to drop back toward the bed. **Rationale:** This position lowers the clavicle to allow a parallel approach on advancement of the needle under the clavicle, reducing the risk of pneumothorax.

4. Prepare a clean, dry work surface for a sterile field. **Rationale:** Reduces the transmission of microorganisms.

Implementation

Steps	Rationale	Special Considerations
1. Wash hands with antiseptic hand wash.	Reduces transmission of microorganisms.	
2. Prepare the IV solution, and prime the new IV tubing.	Enables immediate connection when vascular access is obtained.	
3. Don face mask and nonsterile gloves.	Prevents transmission of microorganisms; universal precautions.	
4. Place moisture-proof pad under the shoulder of the selected side of insertion.	Avoids soiling of the bed.	
5. Clip or shave heavy hair growth at and surrounding the insertion site.	Heavy hair growth may inhibit an occlusive seal of the dressing and may be painful with tape removal.	Skin nicks and abrasions are potential sites for infection; perform with care.
6. Scrub the operative area with antiseptic scrub. a. *For subclavian insertion*, scrub shoulder to contralateral nipple line and from neck to nipple line. b. *For jugular insertion*, scrub midclavicle to opposite border of the sternum and ear to a few inches above the nipple line (Fig. 31–1).	Mechanical friction physically removes microbes. Antiseptics chemically destroy microbes.	The patient's skin should be physically clean before the application of an antiseptic solution. Organic material may inactivate antiseptic agents. Antiseptic scrub solutions may include povidone-iodine scrub 7.5%, chlorhexidine gluconate 4%, and isopropyl alcohol, 70%.

Table continues on following page

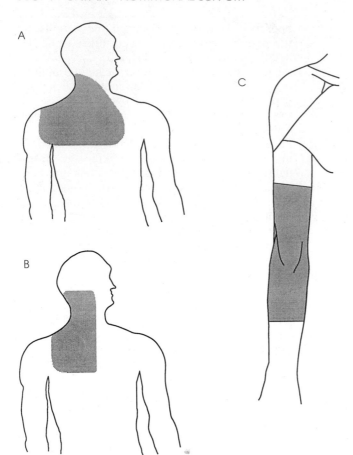

FIGURE 31–1. Area of preoperative skin prep for central venous catheter insertions. (*A*) *Subclavian insertions*: Scrub from shoulder to contralateral nipple line and from neck to nipple line. (*B*) *Jugular insertions*: Scrub midclavicle to opposite border of the sternum and from the ear to a few inches above the nipple line. (*C*) *Peripherally inserted central venous catheters (PICC)*: Scrub the entire arm circumference from midforearm to mid-upper arm. (Courtesy of Suredesign.)

Steps	Rationale	Special Considerations
7. Pat dry, and cover with a sterile towel.	Removes soap, dirt, and moisture. Protects from contamination until the insertion procedure begins.	
8. Mask any person in the immediate area of the bedside.	Prevents transmission of microorganisms.	
9. Assist the physician with donning sterile garb.	Maintains aseptic technique.	
10. Turn or instruct the patient to turn his or her head away from the insertion site.	Prevents transmission of microorganisms.	
11. Remove the towel from the insertion site.	Exposes the area for the sterile prep.	
12. While the physician completes the skin prep, ensure patient comfort by a. Explaining that application of the antiseptic solution will be wet and may be cold. b. Explaining that the injection of local anesthetic may burn or sting as the tissue is infiltrated.	Reduces anxiety and encourages cooperation.	Holding the patient's hand usually provides a great deal of comfort and security. Continue providing support and comfort throughout the procedure.
13. After the physician injects the local anesthetic, place the bed in a 10 to 45 degree head-down tilt.	Provides venous dilatation and increases central venous pressure to reduce the risk of air embolism.	May be contraindicated in certain patients, i.e., increased intracranial pressure, elevated venous pressure, respiratory or cardiac compromise.

Table continues on following page

Steps	Rationale	Special Considerations
14. Reduce the positive end expiratory pressure (PEEP) to a maximum of 5 cm H₂O at the time of venipuncture, as prescribed.	PEEP greater than 5 cm H₂O greatly increases the risk of pneumothorax.	Assess patient tolerance by observing pulse oximetry.
15. Ensure that adequate time has been given to allow the local anesthetic to take effect before the physician performs the venipuncture.	Minimizes risk, comforts the patient, and reduces anxiety.	
16. Explain that there may be a feeling of pressure as the physician now inserts and advances the needle.	Minimizes risk of injury and reduces anxiety.	This should not be painful if patient is adequately anesthetized.
17. Monitor the heart rate, respiratory rate and rhythm, and the patient's comments or complaints.	Assessment may indicate occurrence of complication (see Table 31–2) or inadequate pain control.	
18. *For subclavian insertions*, instruct the patient to turn his or her head toward the ipsilateral side while the guidewire and the catheter are advanced.	Avoids malpositioning of the catheter into the jugular vein.	
19. Observe the cardiac monitor or palpate a peripheral pulse while the physician advances the guidewire and catheter, and then	Advancement of the guidewire or catheter into the heart may induce cardiac dysrhythmias.	Tall, peaked P waves can be identified as the catheter tip enters the right atrium.
a. Inform the physician immediately if a dysrhythmia occurs.		Arrythmias typically resolve with withdrawal of the guidewire or catheter.
b. Prepare to administer antidysrhythmics.		
20. Assist with connection of IV administration set and sterile extension tubing to the catheter.	Maintains aseptic technique. Immediate connection of the IV administration set to the catheter prevents air embolism.	Ensure a tight connection to prevent accidental disconnection. Luer-lok devices prevent an accidental disconnection.
21. Begin infusion at a "keep vein open" rate.	Avoids infusion of large amounts of solution into the thoracic cavity if the catheter has perforated the vein.	
22. Lower the IV solution below the level of the heart, and observe for backflow of venous blood.	Aids in verification of venous catheter placement.	Does not confirm tip position, since the blood may originate from a branch vessel or hematoma.
23. Encourage placement of only a single suture at the immediate insertion site.	Prevents inward or outward migration of the catheter and allows for cleaning the skin under the catheter.	
24. Reposition the patient in a supine or low semi-Fowler's position, and remove the towel roll.	Head-tilt position is no longer necessary. Provides patient comfort.	
25. Readjust PEEP settings as prescribed.	Returns PEEP to therapeutic levels.	
26. Don sterile gloves.	Maintains sterile technique.	
27. Gently tug on the catheter to evaluate the integrity of the suture.	Avoids dislodgment of the catheter.	A loose suture should be corrected before application of dressing.
28. Apply sterile dressing (Skill 31–4).	Prevents catheter-related infection.	

Figure continues on following page

Steps	Rationale	Special Considerations
29. Irrigate the additional lumens of a multilumen catheter with heparin as prescribed.	Prevents clotting of lumens.	Common dosage is 2 to 3 cc of heparin 100 U/cc.
30. Prepare the patient for chest x-ray.	Chest x-ray confirms accurate tip position and detects complications.	Infusions (especially TPN) should not be initiated until tip placement is confirmed.
31. Remove and discard gloves.	Universal precautions.	
32. Wash hands.	Reduces transmission of microorganisms.	

Evaluation

1. Monitor the patient's vital signs, i.e., temperature, heart rate and rhythm, blood pressure, and respiratory rate and rhythm. **Rationale:** Identifies signs and symptoms of complications and allows for immediate intervention.
2. Confirm catheter tip location in the distal superior vena cava (SVC) on chest x-ray before initiating infusions. **Rationale:** Ensures accurate catheter tip placement for the infusion of hypertonic solutions.
3. Assess the catheter for venous blood return and patency before initiating infusions. **Rationale:** Indicates position of the catheter tip in the vascular space and detects signs and symptoms of catheter occlusion before attempting infusion.
4. Observe the dressing and catheter site for bleeding or hematoma every 30 minutes for the first 4 hours after insertion. **Rationale:** Postinsertion bleeding may occur in patients with coagulopathies, arterial punctures, multiple attempts at vein access, or with the use of through-the-needle introducer designs for insertion.

Expected Outcomes

1. The catheter is inserted without complication. **Rationale:** Utilization of proper technique minimizes the risk of complications.
2. Parenteral nutrition solutions infuse without interruption. **Rationale:** The catheter remains patent for continuous infusion.
3. Insertion site, catheter, and systemic circulation remain free of infection. **Rationale:** Maintenance of asepsis with catheter insertion, accessing, and dressing management diminishes the risk of infection.
4. The catheter remains in place without dislodgment. **Rationale:** Movement of the catheter in and out of the skin increases the risk of infection; retraction of the catheter out of the skin results in repositioning of the tip. Infusion of hypertonic solutions in the proximal SVC, innominate, or subclavian vein increases the risk of venous thrombosis.

Unexpected Outcomes

1. Pain or severe discomfort during the procedure. **Rationale:** Pain on insertion may be related to improper administration of local anesthetic, patient positioning, or lack of patient preparation, comfort, and support.
2. Complications of catheter insertion, i.e., arterial puncture, pneumothorax, tension pneumothorax, hydrothorax, hemothorax, catheter malposition, cardiac tamponade, cardiac dysrhythmia, air embolism, venous or arterial injury, arteriovenous fistula, lymphatic fistula, tracheal injury, hydromediastinum, nerve injury, catheter embolism, or death (see Table 31–2). **Rationale:** Lack of compliance with recommended procedures significantly increases the risk of insertion complications.
3. Local or systematic infection. **Rationale:** Infection related to catheter insertion may be the result of improper skin preparation or contamination of equipment.

Documentation

Documentation in the patient record should include vital signs, vein and catheter selection criteria, patient and family education, known allergies, medications administered, date and time of procedure, catheter type, lumen size, length inserted, and length remaining outside the insertion site, nursing interventions, fluids administered, patient tolerance of the procedure, type of dressing applied, confirmation of catheter tip position, any unexpected outcomes encountered and interventions taken. **Rationale:** Provides evidence of nursing care and baseline data for future evaluation.

Patient/Family Education

1. Explain to the patient and family the necessity for central venous access for administration of parenteral nutrition solutions. **Rationale:** Decreases anxiety, improves acceptance and cooperation, and encourages questions.
2. If indicated, discuss the potential use of a long-term venous access device for the delivery of parenteral nutrition solutions in the home. **Rationale:** Prepares the family for the potential need for home parenteral nutrition support and potential expectations of care.
3. Evaluate the need for long-term parenteral nutri-

tion. **Rationale:** Allows the nurse to begin teaching related to the treatment modality, device management, and potential complications related to parenteral nutrition and central venous access.

4. If the patient is a likely candidate for home therapy, begin discharge planning with discharge planning coordinators and home infusion therapists. **Rationale:** Discharge coordinators and home infusion therapists make assessments of the appropriateness of the home environment and support groups, financial considerations, and learning needs.

Performance Checklist
Skill 31–1: Assisting with Insertion of a Percutaneous Central Venous Catheter

Critical Behaviors	Complies yes	no
1. Wash hands.		
2. Prepare the IV solution, and prime tubing.		
3. Don face mask and nonsterile gloves.		
4. Place moisture-proof pad.		
5. Clip or shave heavy hair growth as indicated.		
6. Scrub the operative area.		
7. Pat dry, and cover with sterile towel.		
8. Ensure that all persons in the area are masked.		
9. Assist the physician with donning sterile garb.		
10. Instruct the patient on head position.		
11. Remove the sterile towel from the insertion site.		
12. Ensure patient comfort during the procedure.		
13. Position the patient in a head-down tilt position.		
14. Reduce PEEP as prescribed.		
15. Assess effectiveness of local anesthetic.		
16. Instruct and assist with head positioning on catheter advancement during subclavian insertion.		
17. Observe for cardiac dysrhythmias on passage of guidewire and catheter.		
18. Assist with connection of the IV tubing, begin the IV infusion at KVO, and evaluate blood return.		
19. Reposition the patient and remove the towel roll.		
20. Readjust PEEP setting as prescribed.		
21. Don sterile gloves.		
22. Assess the integrity of the suture.		
23. Apply sterile dressing.		
24. Irrigate the additional lumens of the multilumen catheter.		
25. Prepare the patient for a chest x-ray.		
26. Confirm catheter tip position before initiating intravenous solutions.		
27. Remove and discard gloves.		
28. Wash hands.		
29. Document procedure in the patient record.		

SKILL 31–2

Insertion of a Peripheral Central Venous Catheter

The peripherally inserted central venous catheter (PIC catheter) is a small-gauge Silastic or polyurethane catheter that is inserted by venipuncture of the basilic, medial cubital, or cephalic vein at or above the antecubital space. The catheter is advanced until the tip is positioned in the lower one-third of the superior vena cava.

The peripheral approach for central venous access has significant benefits in the critically ill patient, including (1) elimination of high morbidity and mortality complications of neck and chest insertions, especially in patients with cardiac and pulmonary compromise, (2) reduced risk of catheter sepsis, since the catheter site is distant to endotracheal tubes, tracheostomies, and contaminating secretions, (3) reduced risk of air embolism, (4) suspected catheter sepsis is easily evaluated by catheter exchange or removal with reduced risk of reinsertion, (5) preservation of the peripheral vasculature, since the necessity for repeated venipuncture is eliminated, and (6) decreased pain and suffering from frequent venipuncture. An additional advantage for the patient requiring parenteral nutrition is the use of a single dedicated line for TPN administration.

Advancements in technology have provided catheter materials and introducing devices that have significantly reduced the potential for insertion and postinsertion complications. Nurses desiring to insert these catheters should confirm with their state board of registered nursing that the performance of this procedure is within the scope of nursing practice, have strong technical IV skills, have a good working knowledge of vascular access devices, participate in an educational program designed for instruction in catheter insertion, complications, management, and care of the catheter, and demonstrate competency in the clinical setting.

Purpose

The nurse inserts a PIC catheter to

1. Provide central venous access for the administration of intravenous solutions, drug therapy, parenteral nutrition, antibiotics, chemotherapy, and blood sampling.
2. Avoid complications of neck and chest insertions (see Table 31–2).
3. Reduce the risk of catheter-related septicemia.
4. Reduce the risk of air embolism.
5. Preserve the peripheral vasculature.
6. Decrease pain and suffering from frequent venipuncture.

Prerequisite Knowledge and Skills

Prior to the insertion of a PIC catheter, the nurse should understand

1. Anatomy and physiology of the vasculature and adjacent structures in the upper extremity, neck, and chest.
2. The design, material, and insertion technique of the selected catheter.
3. Principles of aseptic technique.
4. Prevention and management of potential complications.
5. Principles of intravenous therapy.
6. Principles of infection control.
7. Principles of administration of local anesthesia.
8. Principles of suturing.
9. Methods of measurement for accurate catheter tip placement.
10. Rationale for proper patient positioning.
11. Vein selection criteria.
12. Patient selection criteria.
13. Legal implications and regulations of the board of registered nursing in the state in which the nurse practices.
14. Policies of the institution.

The nurse should be able to perform

1. Accurate anthropometric measurement of the anatomic pathway of the selected vein.
2. Proper patient positioning.
3. Assessment of the vasculature for vein selection.
4. Measurement of mid-upper arm circumference.
5. Application of surgical garb.
6. Aseptic technique.
7. Surgical skin preparation.
8. Surgical handwashing technique.
9. Vital signs assessment.
10. Hemodynamic and cardiac rhythm assessment.
11. A venipuncture (see Skill 9–1).
12. Administration of local anesthetic.
13. Placement of a skin suture for catheter fixation (optional).
14. Application of a sterile dressing (see Skill 31–4).
15. Assessment of and intervention for complications.

Assessment

1. Review the patient's nutritional assessment (see Table 31–1), which should be completed prior to catheter exchange for the TPN. Identify the appropriateness of parenteral nutrition as the modality for therapy. **Rationale:** Central venous catheterization is not without serious risk (see Table 31–2) and should not be done without clear indications.
2. Obtain the patient's baseline vital signs, i.e., blood pressure, respiratory rate, and heart rate and rhythm. **Rationale:** Cardiac dysrhythmias may occur if the catheter is advanced into the heart. Although very rare, pneumothorax may occur. Baseline data facilitate identification of suspected problems and provide a guide for intervention.
3. Assess the vasculature of the antecubital space of both arms. Priority of vein selection is the basilic vein, the medial cubital vein, and the cephalic vein. Criteria

for vein selection include length of catheter required for accurate tip placement compared with the length of the available catheter, size and status of the vein, dominant versus nondominant arm, activity level of the patient, ability to visualize or palpate the vein, and condition of the skin to be covered by the dressing. **Rationale:** Proper vein selection increases the success of insertion and decreases the incidence of postinsertion complications.

4. Evaluate the patient's past medical history, previous IV therapy history, and current diagnosis for evidence of coagulopathies, vascular surgery or injury, IV-related complications, and contraindications for use of the extremity, i.e., mastectomy, severe thrombophlebitis, thrombosis, A-V fistula, or skin problems. **Rationale:** Provides additional information for appropriate vein selection and prevention of complications.

5. Assess the patient's level of understanding of the need for central venous access for administration of parenteral nutrition solutions. **Rationale:** The procedure requires informed consent.

6. Assess the patient's history for sensitivity to lidocaine or antiseptic solutions. **Rationale:** Decreases the risk of allergic reactions.

Nursing Diagnoses

1. Knowledge deficit related to the necessity of central venous access for infusion of parenteral nutrition solutions and potential complications of device insertion and management. **Rationale:** This is an invasive procedure that requires patient education for informed consent.

2. Potential for injury related to insertion of the PIC catheter. **Rationale:** Complications may occur as a result of the insertion procedure.

3. Potential for infection related to contamination during the insertion procedure. **Rationale:** The placement of a catheter through the skin and into the central vasculature provides a mode of transmission and direct access to the systemic circulation. Inadequate skin preparation or inadvertent contamination of the sterile field may result in catheter-related septicemia.

Planning

1. Individualize the following goals for PIC catheter insertion:
   a. Provide access to the central venous system. **Rationale:** Hypertonic parenteral nutrition solutions require central venous access for administration.
   b. Insert the catheter without complication. **Rationale:** Utilization of proper technique and equipment minimizes the risk of complications.

2. Identify a second nurse or physician who will assist with the procedure as needed. **Rationale:** Sterile procedures can be performed with greater ease, efficiency, safety, and comfort for the patient when additional assistance is utilized.

3. Prepare a clean, dry work surface for a sterile field. **Rationale:** Reduces the transmission of microorganisms.

4. Prepare all necessary equipment and supplies. **Rationale:** Collection and organization of the equipment at the bedside ensure that the procedure will be completed quickly and efficiently.

PREP ITEMS

a. One measuring tape.
b. One waterproof underpad.
c. One blood pressure cuff or tourniquet.
d. Face masks (for each person in attendance).
e. One pair of exam gloves.
f. Two antiseptic scrub sponges.
g. One sterile towel.
h. One heat pack (optional).
i. One cap or head covering.
j. One pair of goggles.

STERILE ITEMS

a. One sterile gown.
b. One pair of sterile gloves.
c. One bottle of normal saline or sterile water (at least 100 cc).
d. One sterile towel.
e. Two nonabsorbent barriers.
f. Three povidone-iodine swabsticks.
g. One fenestrated drape.
h. 1% lidocaine, 1 to 2 cc.
i. One 1-cc 25-gauge, ⅝-in needle syringe.
j. One measuring tape.
k. Catheter of choice with guidewire or stylet (should be blunt tipped) and introducing device (angiocatheter introducer, peel-away angiocatheter, or break-away needle).
l. Three to four 4 × 4 noncotton gauze sponges.
m. 0.9% sodium chloride, 30 cc.
n. One 10-cc syringe with 20-gauge 1-in needle.
o. One Luer-lok injection cap.
p. One Luer-lok extension tubing (optional).
q. One 3-cc syringe with 20-gauge 1-in needle or 5-cc syringe if inserting a double-lumen catheter.
r. Heparin 100 U/cc, 2 cc.
s. One needle holder (optional).
t. One 3-0 or 4-0 nylon suture on a small curved cutting needle (optional).

DRESSING MATERIALS

a. One pair of scissors.
b. Three alcohol swabsticks.
c. Three povidone-iodine swabsticks.
d. One single-dose packet of povidone-iodine ointment.
e. One 2 × 2 gauze sponge.
f. One skin protectant swabstick.
g. One roll of 2-in tape or transparent dressing.
h. One packet of Steri-Strips (if not suturing).

5. Prepare the patient
   a. Obtain consent from the patient. Discussion for the informed consent should include an expla-

nation of the necessity for therapy and vascular access, the procedure, risks and benefits, and alternative vascular access devices and an adequate opportunity for questions. **Rationale:** Central venous catheterization is an invasive procedure that requires consent of the patient.

b. Explain the patient's participation during the procedure and the importance of maintaining sterility. **Rationale:** Encourages cooperation and prevents accidental contamination of the sterile field or equipment.

c. Perform endotracheal or tracheostomy suctioning on ventilated patients. **Rationale:** Minimizes the risk of contamination of the sterile field from coughing and avoids disruption of procedure.

d. Assist the patient in achieving a position that facilitates the procedure:

(1) Position in a Fowler, semi-Fowler, or flat position depending on the patient's condition and comfort. **Rationale:** The upright position allows gravity to assist in directing the catheter downward when advancing the catheter into the innominate vein and superior vena cava. It may also avoid mis-

direction of the catheter into the jugular vein.

(2) Position the selected arm at 45 degrees of extension from the body for anthropometric measurement. **Rationale:** Allows for displacement of the catheter with arm motion.

(3) Maintain the desired position of the arm with a towel or pillow. **Rationale:** Patient comfort and ease of vein access.

(4) Instruct the patient on head positioning. The head is positioned facing the contralateral side throughout the procedure, except when advancing the catheter from the axillary vein to the superior vena cava, when the head is positioned toward the ipsilateral side with the chin dropped to the shoulder. **Rationale:** Avoids misdirection of the catheter into the jugular vein.

(5) Select the vein and site of venipuncture. **Rationale:** The site of venipuncture is the distal point to begin measurement for the desired length of catheter to be inserted.

Implementation*

Steps	Rationale	Special Considerations
1. Wash hands.	Reduces the transmission of microorganisms.	
2. Measure from the site of venipuncture directly over the course of the selected vein to the lower one-third of the superior vena cava (Fig. 31–2).	Accurate measurement ensures proper tip position for administration of hypertonic solutions and determines the length of catheter to be inserted.	Catheter tip position 2 to 3 cm above the right atrium avoids tip migration, dysrythmias, and perforation of the vein or myocardium.
3. Measure mid-upper arm circumference.	Provides baseline for evaluation of suspected thrombosis.	Increases greater than 2 cm over baseline are suggestive of venous occlusion.
4. Place moisture-proof pad under the arm.	Avoids soiling the bed.	
Steps 5 through 9 may be performed by the assistant while the nurse performing the insertion begins at step 10.		
5. Position the blood pressure cuff as high as possible on the upper extremity, or position the tourniquet under the upper arm near the axilla.	Placement high on the extremity avoids contamination of the sterile field.	
6. Don face mask, head covering, goggles, and nonsterile gloves.	Universal precautions.	Blood splashing may occur with use of guidewires, stylets, and break-away or peel-away introducers.

*The procedure described is performed with the use of an assistant.

Table continues on following page

Steps	Rationale	Special Considerations
7. Scrub the entire arm circumference from midforearm to mid-upper arm with antiseptic scrub sponge (see Fig. 31–1).	Mechanical friction physically removes microbes. Antiseptics chemically destroy microbes.	The patient's skin should be physically clean before the application of an antiseptic solution. Organic material may inactivate antiseptic agents. Antiseptic scrub solutions may include chlorhexidine gluconate 4%, povidone-iodine scrub 7.5%, and isopropyl alcohol 70%.
8. Pat dry and cover with sterile towel.	Removes soap, dirt, and moisture. Protects from contamination until prepared to begin the sterile skin prep.	
9. Apply heat pack over towel (optional).	Increases and maintains vasodilation.	
10. Scrub hands and forearms with antimicrobial soap × 5 minutes.	Primary action of antimicrobial soap includes mechanical removal and chemical killing or inhibition of contaminating and colonizing flora.	Surgical hand scrub antiseptics include chlorhexidine gluconate 4%, povidone-iodine scrub 7.5%, and isopropyl alcohol 70%.
11. Don sterile gown and sterile gloves.	Maintains aseptic technique and compliance with universal precautions.	Blood splashing may occur with use of guidewires, stylets, and break-away or peel-away introducers.
12. Wash gloves with sterile water or saline, and dry with a sterile noncotton towel.	Silastic material attracts various particles such as talc, dust, and cotton fibers, which may adhere to the catheter and induce sterile phlebitis.	
13. Prepare all items on a sterile field.	Maintains aseptic technique.	Sterile barrier and gauze pads should be of noncotton material.

Table continues on following page

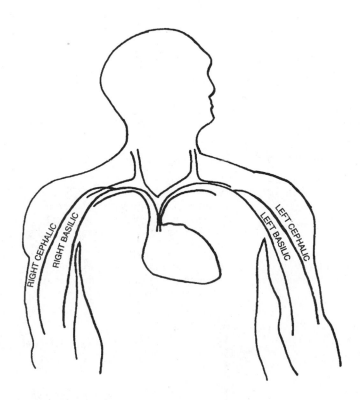

FIGURE 31–2. Anthropometric measurement of the basilic and cephalic venous pathway for accurate tip placement of peripherally inserted central venous catheter. Measurement begins at the point of venipuncture and ends in the distal third of the superior vena cava. (Courtesy of Suredesign.)

Steps	Rationale	Special Considerations
14. Measure the catheter using a sterile measuring tape:	Catheters are made in variable lengths.	
a. Subtract the predetermined length for insertion plus an additional 1 to 3 cm to be left outside the skin.		
b. If the remaining length is excessive, remove the guidewire and cut the catheter straight across with sterile scissors.	Cutting the catheter tip with a bevel may increase the incidence of clotting at the tip.	Closed-tipped catheters would be cut at the opposite end.
c. Flush the catheter with normal saline.	Facilitates guidewire removal.	
d. Reinsert the guidewire so that the guidewire/stylet tip is covered by approximately 0.5 to 1 cm of the catheter.	Provides softness and flexibility at the tip, thus preventing perforation of the vein.	A guidewire or blunt-tipped stylet should be used to reduce the risk of catheter shearing and fragmentation (with a through-the-needle design), to reduce the incidence of coiling or knotting in the vein, and for ease of insertion.
e. Irrigate the additional lumens of a multilumen catheter with heparin as prescribed.	Prevents clotting of lumens.	Common dosage is 2 to 3 cc of heparin 100 U/cc.
15. Request assistant to remove the heatpack and towel.	For access to the arm.	Maintains aseptic technique.
16. Instruct the patient to lift the arm, place a sterile drape underneath, and position the arm at 45 to 90 degrees of extension from the body.	Prevents contamination in the event of dropping items through the fenestration. Arm extension increases the ability to advance the catheter at the shoulder.	
17. Beginning at the venipuncture site, apply povidone-iodine in concentric circles extending outward from midforearm to midupper arm and from side to side of the arm to drape.	Povidone-iodine solution is an antibacterial, antifungal antiseptic.	The solution should not be removed. Drying is not necessary. Application time is for chemical kill.
18. Place the fenestrated drape over the prepared area leaving the venipuncture site exposed, and tuck the drape under the arm to hold the drape in place.	Maintains aseptic technique.	
19. Palpate and establish the location of the brachial artery.	Prevents inadvertent puncture of the artery.	
20. Instruct the assistant to tie the tourniquet or inflate the blood pressure cuff.	Provides vasodilation of the vein for venipuncture.	Constriction should effectively cause venous distension without arterial occlusion. The blood pressure cuff is most effective, especially on obese patients.
21. Inject a skin weal of approximately 0.5 cc of 1% lidocaine at or adjacent to the venipuncture site (optional).	Provides local anesthesia for venipuncture with large-gauge needles and introducers.	Lidocaine may produce stinging, burning, obliteration of the vein, or venospasm. Use sparingly.
22. Perform the venipuncture according to catheter design and manufacturer's instructions.	Catheters are available in multiple designs and introducing techniques.	
23. Insert the catheter approximately 6 to 8 in (15 to 20 cm).	Establishes venous access.	

Table continues on following page

Steps	Rationale	Special Considerations
24. Instruct the assistant to release the tourniquet or blood pressure cuff.	Vasodilation is not required for catheter advancing.	
25. Turn or instruct the patient to turn his or her head toward the cannulated arm and drop his or her chin to the shoulder.	Avoids malpositioning of the catheter in the jugular vein.	
26. Gently advance the remainder of the catheter and guidewire to the predetermined length, and observe or palpate the heart rate and rhythm.	Cardiac dysrythmias may occur if the catheter is advanced into the heart.	Never advance catheter against resistance. Excessive pushing or torque force could lead to perforation of the vein or myocardium. If cardiac dysrythmias occur, pull the catheter back and reassess the heart rate. Contact a physician immediately if dysrhythmias persist.
27. Turn or instruct the patient to turn his or her head facing the contralateral side.	Prevents contamination of the field by organisms of the respiratory tract.	
28. Measure the length of the catheter remaining outside the skin, and reposition if necessary to the predetermined length.	Ensures proper catheter tip position.	
29. Slowly and gently remove the guidewire.	Prevents recoiling of the catheter.	
30. Attach the 10-cc syringe with saline, aspirate blood, flush with 5 to 10 cc of saline, remove the syringe, and attach a Luer-lok injection cap or Luer-lok extension tubing with cap.	Affirms patency of the catheter. Luer-Lok devices prevent inadvertent disconnection.	
31. Inject 2 to 3 cc of heparin 100 U/cc into the catheter, and withdraw the needle while injecting the last 0.5 cc.	Maintains patency and prevents backflow of blood in the catheter.	Flush both lumens if the catheter is a double lumen.
32. Secure the catheter at the insertion site with one suture (optional): a. Inject a skin weal of 0.5 cc of 1% lidocaine to one side of the insertion site. b. Tie one loose loop through the skin. c. Then tie the suture around the catheter so that the catheter does not slip but not so tight that the catheter is occluded, or secure the catheter with Steri-Strips directly at the insertion site.	Prevents inward or outward migration of the catheter.	Nylon suture is recommended. Silk suture may support bacterial growth. Do not suture catheters that are 2.8 French or smaller. Do not tie suture tight to the skin.
33. Apply sterile dressing (see Skill 31–4).	Decreases catheter-related infections.	
34. Prepare the patient for a chest x-ray.	Chest x-ray confirms accurate tip position and detects complications.	Infusions (especially TPN) should not be initiated until tip placement is confirmed.
35. Remove and discard gloves.	Universal precautions.	
36. Wash hands.	Reduces transmission of microorganisms.	

Evaluation

1. Confirm catheter tip position in the distal SVC by chest x-ray before initiating intravenous drugs or solutions. **Rationale:** Ensures accurate catheter tip placement for the infusion of hypertonic solutions.
2. Observe the dressing and insertion site every 30 minutes for the first 4 hours after insertion for bleeding or hematoma formation. **Rationale:** Postinsertion bleeding may occur in patients with coagulopathies, arterial punctures, multiple attempts at vein access, or with the use of through-the-needle/introducer designs for insertion.
3. Assess the insertion site and upper arm every 8 hours for signs and symptoms of thrombophlebitis, i.e., pain, redness (streaking), and swelling. **Rationale:** Sterile thrombophlebitis may occur within 0 to 10 days of catheter insertion.
4. Assess the catheter for venous blood return and patency before infusing solutions. **Rationale:** Indicates position of catheter tip in the vascular space and ensures patency before attempting infusion.

Expected Outcomes

1. Catheter tip is positioned in the lower one-third of the superior vena cava. **Rationale:** Malpositioned catheters increase the risk for thrombophlebitis and thrombosis.
2. Insertion site and upper arm remain free of thrombophlebitis. **Rationale:** Aseptic technique and proper handling of the catheter reduce the incidence of mechanical phlebitis.
3. Insertion site, catheter, and systemic circulation remain free of infection. **Rationale:** Maintenance of asepsis with catheter insertion, accessing, and dressing management minimizes the risks of infection.

Unexpected Outcomes

1. Pain and severe discomfort during the procedure. **Rationale:** Pain on insertion may be alleviated by the use of local anesthesia, good technical skills, arm positioning in proper alignment, and retraction of the catheter on meeting resistance.
2. Complications of catheter insertion, such as arterial puncture, catheter embolism, pneumothorax, tension pneumothorax, hydrothorax, cardiac dysrhythmia, nerve or tendon damage, air embolism, venous or arterial laceration, or postinsertion mechanical phlebitis. **Rationale:** Lack of compliance with recommended procedures significantly increases the risk of insertion complications (Table 31–2).
3. Malposition of the catheter. **Rationale:** Malposition of the catheter may be alleviated by proper positioning of the patient and accurate anthropometric measurement.
4. Local or systematic infection. **Rationale:** Incidence of infection related to catheter insertion may be the result of improper preparation or contamination of equipment.

Documentation

Documentation in the patient record should include the completed informed consent, any known allergies, abnormal coagulation laboratory values (PT, PTT, platelet count), date and time of procedure, catheter make, lumen size, length inserted, length of catheter remaining outside the insertion site, length of catheter trimmed, mid-upper arm circumference, use of aseptic technique, amount and type of local anesthetic used, vein accessed and location of insertion site, method of securing catheter (i.e., Steri-Strips or suturing), problems or complications encountered during insertion and nursing or medical interventions, and location of catheter tip confirmed by x-ray. **Rationale:** Documents nursing assessment, performance of the procedure, and any unexpected outcomes and the interventions taken.

Patient/Family Education

1. Explain the risks, benefits, and alternatives of vascular devices for parenteral nutrition solution administration. **Rationale:** Decreases anxiety, improves acceptance and confidence, and encourages questions.
2. Evaluate the patient's need for long-term parenteral nutrition. **Rationale:** Allows the nurse to begin teaching related to the treatment modality, device management, and potential complications related to parenteral nutrition and the peripherally inserted central venous catheter.
3. If indicated, discuss the potential use of a long-term arm venous access device for the delivery of parenteral nutrition solutions in the home. **Rationale:** Prepares the family for the potential need for home parenteral nutrition support and potential expectations of care.
4. If the patient is a likely candidate for home therapy, begin discharge planning with discharge planning coordinators and home infusion therapists. **Rationale:** Discharge coordinators and home infusion therapists can make assessments for appropriateness of home environment and support groups, financial considerations, and learning needs. Teaching plans should be coordinated with the home infusion therapist.

Performance Checklist
Skill 31–2: Insertion of a Peripheral Central Venous Catheter

Critical Behaviors	Complies	
	yes	no
1. Wash hands.		

Table continues on following page

Critical Behaviors	Complies	
	yes	**no**
2. Measure to determine length of catheter to be inserted.		
3. Measure mid-upper arm circumference.		
4. Place moisture-proof pad under the arm.		
5. Place tourniquet or blood pressure cuff near the axilla.		
6. Don head covering, face mask, goggles, and nonsterile gloves.		
7. Scrub the operative area.		
8. Pat the arm dry and cover with sterile towel.		
9. Apply heat as necessary.		
10. Perform surgical hand scrub.		
11. Don sterile gown and sterile gloves.		
12. Wash gloves with sterile water or saline.		
13. Prepare all items on the sterile field.		
14. Measure, irrigate, and trim the catheter as necessary, and adjust the guidewire/stylet within the catheter.		
15. Remove headpack and towel.		
16. Place sterile drape under the arm.		
17. Apply povidone-iodine.		
18. Place fenestrated drape over the arm.		
19. Establish location of brachial artery.		
20. Instruct the assistant to tie the tourniquet or inflate the blood pressure cuff.		
21. Administer local anesthetic (optional).		
22. Perform the venipuncture according to catheter design and manufacturer's instructions.		
23. Advance the catheter 6 to 8 in (15 to 20 cm).		
24. Instruct the assistant to release the tourniquet or blood pressure cuff.		
25. Instruct the patient in head positioning.		
26. Advance the catheter to premeasured length.		
27. Instruct the patient in head positioning.		
28. Measure the length remaining outside the skin, and adjust accordingly.		
29. Remove the guidewire/stylet.		
30. Aspirate blood with syringe, flush the catheter with 5 to 10 cc of saline, and attach a Luer-lok injection cap or extension tubing.		
31. Irrigate with heparin.		
32. Secure the catheter at the insertion site.		
33. Apply sterile dressing.		
34. Prepare the patient for a chest x-ray.		
35. Confirm catheter tip position before initiating intravenous solution.		
36. Remove and discard gloves.		

Table continues on following page

Critical Behaviors	Complies	
	yes	**no**
37. Wash hands.		
38. Document procedure in the patient record.		

SKILL 31–3

Assisting with Exchange of a Percutaneously Placed Central Venous Catheter

Catheter exchange is accomplished by the advancement of a spring-tipped guidewire through a preexisting catheter, followed by removal of the catheter with the guidewire left in place. The new catheter is then threaded over the wire through the insertion site, followed by removal of the guidewire. This procedure can be accomplished with single-lumen or multilumen catheters. Although this is a medical procedure, specially trained nurses can perform a guidewire exchange of a peripherally inserted central venous catheter.

The ability to exchange a catheter over a wire has a distinct advantage over removing the catheter and reinserting by venipuncture in a new site. In many instances, a complication of central venous catheter placement could contribute to a detrimental outcome in a critically ill patient. The ability to evaluate a catheter as a potential source of sepsis is of critical importance, especially in cases of sepsis with clinical deterioration when vascular access is crucial for treatment. Of value in the TPN patient is the ability to continue administration of solutions without lengthy disruption. Discontinuation and restarting TPN result in loss of caloric intake in high-expenditure states as well as potential glucose intolerance in unstable metabolic states.

Decisions in the management of vascular access devices are at times very difficult, and the nurse can give valuable input when nursing interventions are focused on collection of appropriate cultures, thorough assessment, and maintenance of sterility.

Purpose

The nurse assists with a guidewire exchange of a central venous catheter to

1. Provide preprocedure patient education.
2. Provide technical assistance.
3. Ensure sterility of the procedure.
4. Ensure patient safety and comfort.
5. Obtain cultures of the catheter for evaluation of catheter-related infection.
6. Provide nursing interventions and medical support in the event of a complication.

Prerequisite Knowledge and Skills

Prior to performing or assisting with the exchange of a central venous catheter, the nurse should understand

1. Principles of aseptic technique.
2. Anatomy and physiology of the vascular system.
3. Principles of infection control.
4. Design, use, and indications for the selected catheter.
5. The method and technique of the exchange procedure.
6. Potential complications of the procedure and the medical and nursing interventions for each.

The nurse should be able to perform

1. Proper handwashing technique.
2. Aseptic technique.
3. Proper patient positioning.
4. Aspiration of blood from the catheter for culture.
5. Respiratory system assessment.
6. Cardiovascular system assessment.
7. Dysrhythmia identification.
8. Cardiopulmonary resuscitation.
9. Semiquantitative culturing of the catheter.
10. Application of a sterile occlusive dressing (see Skill 31–4).

Assessment

1. Review the patient's nutritional assessment (see Table 31–1), which should be completed prior to catheter exchange for the initiation of TPN. Identify the appropriateness of parenteral nutrition as the modality for therapy. **Rationale:** Central venous catheterization is not without serious risk (see Table 31–2) and should not be done without clear indications.

2. Assess the patient's baseline vital signs, i.e., heart rate and rhythm, blood pressure, and respiratory rate, rhythm, and depth. **Rationale:** Baseline data provide information for assessment of the patient's tolerance of the procedure, the evaluation of suspected complications, and a guide for intervention.

3. Assess the need for catheter exchange. **Rationale:** Common clinical situations indicating a need for catheter exchange include initiation of TPN, redirection of a malpositioned catheter, correction of a mechanical problem, or for suspected catheter-related septicemia.

4. Inspect the existing catheter site. **Rationale:** A new site should be chosen if redness, tenderness, or purulent drainage is observed.

5. Evaluate the patient's temperature. **Rationale:** If fever exists, the existing catheter should be considered a potential source of sepsis; however, the absence of fever does not eliminate the possibility of catheter infection.

6. Evaluate the location of the catheter site. **Rationale:** A new site may be indicated if the existing site is at risk for cross-contamination from wounds, tracheostomy, etc.

7. Use caution in exchanging a large diameter catheter for a smaller catheter, i.e., Swan-Ganz to multi- or single-lumen catheter. **Rationale:** The large remaining subcutaneous tract increases the risk of infection and air embolism.

8. Determine the need for cultures. **Rationale:** Evaluation of suspected sepsis may be indicated at the time of exchange.

9. Assess the patient's history for sensitivity to lidocaine or antiseptic solutions. **Rationale:** Decreases the risk of allergic reactions.

Nursing Diagnoses

1. Potential for injury related to the catheter exchange. **Rationale:** Cardiac dysrythmias or myocardial or venous perforation may result from aggressive passage of a guidewire. Pulmonary emobolism may result from the release of a thrombus or fibrin sheath on catheter removal or on advancement of the guidewire or the new catheter.

2. Potential for infection related to contamination during the catheter exchange procedure or with advancement of a catheter through an infected site or subcutaneous tract. **Rationale:** Catheter exchange is an invasive procedure requiring surgical asepsis. Inadequate skin and device preparation or inadvertent contamination of the sterile field may result in septicemia. Passage of a catheter through an infected site or dermal tract carries microorganisms into the bloodstream.

Planning

1. Individualize the following goals for assisting with the exchange of the central venous catheter:
   a. Maintain sterility of the procedure. **Rationale:** The patient is at risk for infection if aseptic technique is not utilized.
   b. Ensure patient comfort and safety. **Rationale:** An anxious, uncomfortable, uncooperative patient increases the risk of complication.
   c. Maintain serum glucose levels during the procedure until parenteral nutrition can be restarted. **Rationale:** Rebound hypoglycemia can occur with rapid or abrupt discontinuation of TPN.
2. Decrease the TPN infusion rate to one half for at least 1 hour prior to beginning the procedure (a longer time may be indicated in patients with glucose intolerance) or begin $D_{10}W$ infusion at current rate through another IV access. **Rationale:** Tapering the glucose infusion prevents rebound hypoglycemia during the procedure while the TPN is disconnected.
3. Prepare all necessary equipment and supplies. **Rationale:** Collection and organization of the equipment at the bedside support aseptic technique and ensures that the procedure will be completed quickly and efficiently.

Prep Items

a. Face masks (for each person in attendance).
b. One moisture-proof underpad.
c. One antiseptic scrub sponge.
d. One pair of examination gloves.
e. One sterile towel.
f. One pair of goggles.
g. One cap or head covering.
h. Isotonic saline solution with Luer-lok administration set for IV infusion, 250 to 1000 cc.
i. Two blood culture bottles.
j. Two sheep blood agar plates.
k. One povidone-iodine prep pad.

Sterile Items

a. One sterile gown.
b. Two pairs of sterile gloves.
c. Three povidone-iodine swabsticks or 30 cc povidone-iodine solution.
d. Catheter of choice, usually supplied with insertion needle, syringe, and guidewire.
e. Spring-tipped guidewire of appropriate size, at least 10 cm longer than the selected catheter.
f. 0.9% sodium chloride, 10 to 30 cc.
g. Two (one or both non-Luer-lok) 10- to 12-cc syringes.
h. Two 3- to 5-cc syringes.
i. Two 22-gauge 1 ½-in needles.
j. Six 4 × 4 gauze sponges.
k. Heparin 100 U/cc (for multilumen catheters), 1 to 2 cc.
l. One hemostat.
m. Two pairs of scissors.
n. One needle holder.
o. One pair of 3-0 or 4-0 nylon suture on a curved needle.
p. One Luer-lok extension tubing.

Dressing Materials

a. Three alcohol swabsticks.
b. Three povidone-iodine swabsticks.
c. One single-dose packet of povidone-iodine ointment.
d. Two 2 × 2 gauze sponges.
e. One skin protectant swabstick.
f. One roll of tape or transparent dressing.

3. Prepare the patient.
   a. Explain the procedure to the patient and reinforce information given during informed consent. **Rationale:** Minimizes risk and reduces anxiety.
   b. Explain the patient's expected participation and importance of maintaining sterility. **Rationale:** Minimizes risk of contamination and encourages cooperation.

c. Explain required positioning for the procedure. **Rationale:** Encourages cooperation and reduces anxiety.
d. Instruct the patient to report symptoms of pain. **Rationale:** Reduces anxiety and facilitates cooperation. Quick, unexpected movements by the patient increase the risk of injury (see Table 31–2).
e. Acquire orders for sedation for highly anxious or combative patients. **Rationale:** Quick, un-

expected movements by the patient increase the risk of injury (see Table 31–2).
f. Perform endotracheal or tracheostomy suctioning on ventilated patients. **Rationale:** Minimizes risk of complications and contamination of the sterile field from coughing or interruption of the procedure (see Table 31–2).
4. Prepare a clean, dry work surface for a sterile field. **Rationale:** Reduces the transmission of microorganisms.

Implementation

Steps	Rationale	Special Considerations
1. Wash hands with antiseptic hand wash.	Reduces transmission of microorganisms.	
2. Prepare the IV solution, and prime the new IV tubing.	Provides immediate connection after the new catheter is advanced.	
3. Don face mask and nonsterile gloves.	Prevents transmission of microorganisms; universal precautions.	
4. Scrub the catheter hub and tubing connection for 30 to 60 seconds with povidone-iodine.	Povidone-iodine is a bactericidal and fungicidal agent. Prevents entry of organisms into the catheter on disconnection.	Parenteral nutrition solutions support fungal growth.
5. Disconnect the tubing from the catheter hub, and quickly attach a 10-cc syringe.	During inspiration, negative intrathoracic pressure is transmitted to the catheter in the central veins; any opening of the system may result in aspiration of air through the catheter into the central venous system.	Disconnection should be done while the patient is performing the Valsalva maneuver or at the beginning of the expiratory phase of the respiratory cycle (both ventilated and nonventilated patients). The catheter hub should not be open longer than 1 second.
6. Aspirate 10 cc of blood for culture.	Blood culture results aid in diagnosis of catheter sepsis and subsequent management.	Send the initial 10-cc blood sample for culture and sensitivity. Do not draw a discard sample. Blood should be drawn from the most frequently used port if exchanging for the initiation of TPN or from the TPN port if previously used.
7. Flush the catheter with 3 to 5 cc of normal saline, leave the syringe attached, or place a new injection cap on the hub.	Prevents clotting of the catheter, maintains sterility of the catheter hub, and prevents air embolism.	
8. Cleanse, disconnect, and cap all ports of a multilumen catheter.	Prepares catheter for antiseptic prep.	Consider need for alternate IV access for drugs (i.e., antidysrythmics, vasopressors, etc.) that cannot be intermittently disconnected during this procedure.
9. Place moisture-proof pad under the patient's shoulder.	Avoids soiling the bed.	
10. Reclip or reshave hair growth as indicated.	Heavy hair growth may prevent formation of an occlusive seal around dressing and may be painful with tape removal.	Shaving should be avoided or performed with care because skin nicks and abrasions are potential sites for infection. Caution should be used to avoid nicking or cutting the catheter with the razor.

Table continues on following page

Steps	Rationale	Special Considerations
11. Scrub the operative area and entire catheter with antiseptic scrub (see Fig. 31–1).	Mechanical friction physically removes microbes. Antiseptics chemically destroy microbes.	The patient's skin should be physically clean before the application of an antiseptic solution. Organic material may inactivate antiseptic agents. Antiseptic scrub solutions may include povidone-iodine scrub 7.5%, chlorhexidine gluconate 4%, and isopropyl alcohol 70%.
12. Pat dry and cover with a sterile towel.	Removes soap, dirt, and moisture. Protects from contamination until the insertion procedure begins.	
13. Mask any persons in the immediate area of the bedside.	Prevents transmission of microorganisms.	
14. Assist the physician with donning sterile garb.	Maintains aseptic technique.	
15. Turn or instruct the patient to turn his or her head away from the insertion site.	Prevents transmission of microorganisms.	
16. Remove the towel from the insertion site.	Exposes the area for the sterile prep.	
17. Ensure patient comfort by a. Explaining that application of the antiseptic solution will be wet and may be cold. b. Explaining that only minor discomfort should be experienced and to report any symptoms of pain.	Reduces anxiety and encourages cooperation.	Holding the patient's hand usually provides a great deal of comfort and security. Continue providing support and comfort throughout the procedure.
18. Monitor the heart rate, respiratory rate and rhythm, and the patient's comments or complaints during the exchange.	Assessment may indicate occurrence of complication (see Table 31–2).	
19. Observe the cardiac monitor or palpate a peripheral pulse during passage of the guidewire and catheter: a. Inform the physician immediately if a dysrhythmia occurs. b. Prepare to administer antidysrythmics if the dysrhythmia does not subside.	Advancement of the guidewire or catheter into the heart may induce cardiac dysrythmias.	Tall, peaked P waves can be identified as the catheter tip enters the right atrium. Dysrythmias typically subside with withdrawal of the guidewire or catheter out of the heart.
20. Ensure that the original catheter is placed on the sterile field.	Preserves for semiquantitative culturing.	
21. Assist with connection of the IV administration set and sterile extension tubing to the catheter.	Maintains aseptic technique. Immediate connection of the IV administration set to the catheter prevents air embolus.	Ensure a tight connection to prevent accidental disconnection. Luer-lok devices prevent inadvertent disconnection.
22. Begin infusion at a "keep vein open" rate.	Avoids infusion of large amounts of solution into the thoracic cavity if the catheter has perforated the vein.	
23. Lower the IV solution below the level of the heart, and observe for backflow of venous blood.	Aids in verification of venous catheter placement.	Does not confirm tip position, since the blood may originate from a branch vessel or hematoma.

Table continues on following page

Steps	Rationale	Special Considerations
24. Encourage placement of a single suture at the immediate insertion site.	Prevents inward and outward migration of the catheter. Allows for cleaning the skin under the catheter.	
25. Don sterile gloves.	Maintains sterile technique.	
26. Gently tug on the catheter to evaluate the integrity of the suture.	Avoids dislodgment of the catheter.	A loose suture should be corrected before application of the dressing.
27. Apply sterile dressing (see Skill 31–4).	Discourages catheter-related infection.	
28. Irrigate the additional lumens of a multilumen catheter with heparin.	Prevents clotting of lumens.	Common dosage is 2 to 3 cc heparin 100 U/cc.
29. Complete the semiquantitative culturing of the catheter.	Provides diagnostic information.	
30. Prepare the patient for chest x-ray.	Chest x-ray confirms tip position and detects complications.	Infusions should not be initiated until tip placement is confirmed.
31. Remove and discard gloves.	Universal precautions.	
32. Wash hands.	Reduces the transmission of microorganisms.	

Evaluation

1. Monitor the patient's vital signs, i.e., temperature, heart rate and rhythm, blood pressure, and respiratory rate and rhythm. **Rationale:** Identifies signs and symptoms of complications and allows for immediate intervention.

2. Confirm catheter tip location in the distal SVC by chest x-ray before initiating infusions. **Rationale:** Ensures accurate catheter tip placement for the infusion of hypertonic solutions.

3. Assess the catheter for venous blood return and patency before initiating infusions. **Rationale:** Indicates position of the catheter tip in the vascular space and detects signs and symptoms of catheter occlusion before attempting infusion.

Expected Outcomes

1. The catheter exchange is completed without complication. **Rationale:** Utilization of proper technique minimizes the risk of complications.

2. Insertion site, catheter, and systemic circulation remain free of infection. **Rationale:** Maintenance of asepsis with catheter exchange, accessing, and dressing management diminishes the risk of infection.

3. The catheter remains in place without dislodgment. **Rationale:** Movement of the catheter in and out of the skin increases the risk of infection; retraction of the catheter out of the skin results in repositioning the tip. Infusion of hypertonic solutions in the proximal SVC, innominate, or subclavian vein increases the risk of venous thrombosis.

4. Serum glucose level is maintained. **Rationale:** Proper tapering of TPN solutions or infusion of D_{10} prevents hypoglycemic episodes.

Unexpected Outcomes

1. Pain or severe discomfort during the procedure. **Rationale:** Pain during catheter exchange may indicate the occurrence of a complication such as venous or cardiac perforation, pneumothorax, cardiac tamponade, malposition, or pulmonary embolism.

2. Complications of catheter exchange, i.e., catheter malposition, perforation, cardiac dysrhythmia, or air embolism (see Table 31–2). **Rationale:** Lack of compliance with recommended procedure significantly increases the risk of insertion complications.

3. Local or systemic infection. **Rationale:** Infection related to catheter exchange may be a result of improper skin and catheter preparation, contamination of equipment, or exchange of a large-diameter catheter with a smaller one.

4. Air embolism. **Rationale:** Large-diameter catheters (such as a Swan-Ganz) create a large skin tract. When exchanging with a smaller-diameter catheter, the unoccupied portion of the skin tract may allow the introduction of air into the venous system.

5. Pulmonary embolism. **Rationale:** Introduction of a guidewire, removal of the catheter, and reintroduction of a catheter may dislodge or strip fibrin sheath or thrombus into the circulation resulting in embolism to the lung.

Documentation

Documentation in the patient record should include completed informed consent, vital signs, catheter selection criteria, patient and family education, any known allergies, medications administered, date and time of the procedure, catheter type, lumen size, length inserted, and length remaining outside the insertion site, nursing interventions, fluids administered, patient tolerance of the procedure, type of dressing applied, and confirmation of catheter tip position. **Rationale:** Provides evidence of nursing care and baseline data for future evaluation.

Patient/Family Education

1. Explain the rationale for catheter exchange to both patient and family. **Rationale:** Enhances patient and family's understanding of care and encourages questions.

2. Explain to the patient and family the necessity for central venous access for administration of parenteral nutrition solutions. **Rationale:** Decreases anxiety, improves acceptance and cooperation, and encourages questions.

Performance Checklist
Skill 31–3: Assisting with Exchange of a Percutaneously Placed Central Venous Catheter

Critical Behaviors	Complies	
	yes	no
1. Wash hands.		
2. Prepare the IV solution, and prime tubing.		
3. Don face mask and nonsterile gloves.		
4. Scrub the catheter hub and tubing junction.		
5. Disconnect the IV tubing, and attach a 10-cc syringe.		
6. Aspirate 10 cc of blood for culture.		
7. Flush the catheter with 3 to 5 cc of normal saline, leave the syringe attached, or place a new injection cap on the hub.		
8. Cleanse, disconnect, and cap additional hubs of a multilumen catheter.		
9. Place a moisture-proof pad under the patient's shoulder.		
10. Clip or shave heavy hair growth as indicated.		
11. Scrub operative area and catheter.		
12. Pat dry and cover with a sterile towel.		
13. Ensure that all persons in attendance are masked.		
14. Assist the physician with donning sterile garb.		
15. Instruct the patient on head positioning.		
16. Remove the sterile towel from the insertion site.		
17. Ensure patient comfort during the procedure.		
18. Perform continuous assessment of patient's cardiac status, respiratory status, and tolerance.		
19. Observe for cardiac dysrythmias on passage of guidewire and catheter.		
20. Secure the original catheter for culturing.		
21. Assist with the connection of the IV tubing.		
22. Begin the IV infusion at KVO rate and evaluate blood return.		
23. Encourage placement of a single suture at insertion site.		
24. Don sterile gloves.		
25. Assess integrity of the suture.		
26. Apply sterile dressing.		
27. Irrigate the additional lumens of a multilumen catheter.		

Table continues on following page

Critical Behaviors	Complies	
	yes	no
28. Complete the culturing of the catheter.		
29. Prepare the patient for chest x-ray.		
30. Confirm catheter tip position before initiating intravenous solutions.		
31. Remove and discard gloves.		
32. Wash hands.		
33. Document procedure in the patient record.		

SKILL 31–4

Central Venous Catheter Site Care

Percutaneous catheters are inserted through the skin and subcutaneous tissue directly into the vein. Migration of bacteria from the skin surface along the subcutaneous tract to the bloodstream has been designated as the primary mechanism in the pathogenesis of catheter-related septicemia. Prior to insertion, the skin is disinfected with antiseptics. After insertion, recolonization of the skin occurs to a normal or even greater level. Repeated disinfection of the skin is necessary to prevent recolonization of the skin and catheter infection. An occlusive dressing is applied to prevent environmental contamination of the skin and insertion site.

Transparent dressings have been associated with an increased rate of colonization of the catheter and an increased rate of infection when used with central lines. Moisture tends to collect under the dressing, promoting microbial growth. The presence of moisture is increased in the critical-care patient with frequent suctioning and use of high humidification in ventilatory support and oxygen therapy. The thorax has a greater density of cutaneous flora and a higher skin temperature than the arm. These factors play a major role in the risk of infection with central venous catheters placed in the chest or neck versus peripherally inserted central venous catheters.

The frequency of dressing change is dependent on the condition of the catheter site; the presence of contaminating drainage, secretions, or excessive perspiration; the type of dressing material; the activity level of the patient; and the integrity of the dressing on inspection. Some patients may require daily dressing changes, while others need dressing changes only two to three times per week. High-risk intensive care unit patients should have dressing changes every 48 hours, at which time the site is recleansed with antiseptics. The key factor is a dry, sterile, and intact dressing. Ongoing observation of the dressing and daily assessment for potential catheter sepsis are essential.

Purpose

The nurse changes the central venous catheter dressing to

1. Prevent catheter-related infections.
2. Assess the catheter insertion site for signs of infection or catheter dislodgment.
3. Observe and maintain skin integrity under the dressing.
4. Assess the integrity of the suture.

Prerequisite Knowledge and Skills

Prior to changing the dressing, the nurse should understand

1. Principles of infection control.
2. Principles of clean and aseptic technique.
3. Signs and symptoms of catheter infection and septicemia.
4. Design, purpose, and function of the catheter in place.

The nurse should be able to perform

1. Proper handwashing technique (see Skill 35–5).
2. Clean and aseptic technique.
3. Assessment of the catheter, skin, and insertion site.

Assessment

1. Evaluate the patient's clinical status for signs and symptoms of infection or sepsis, i.e., fever, chills, change in mental status, hypotension, leukocytosis with left shift, respiratory alkalosis, metabolic acidosis, or glucose intolerance. **Rationale:** Careful assessment of clinical status and the catheter site is performed to evaluate for catheter sepsis.
2. Assess the patient's arm, shoulder, neck, and chest on the ipsilateral side of the catheter insertion site for signs of pain, swelling, or collateral circulation. **Rationale:** Assessment is made to evaluate for thrombophlebitis or venous thrombosis.
3. Assess the patient's history for sensitivity to antiseptic solutions. **Rationale:** Decreases risk of allergic reactions.

Nursing Diagnoses

1. Potential for infection related to the presence of a catheter inserted through the skin and into the bloodstream. **Rationale:** The placement of a catheter through the skin and into the central vasculature provides a mode of transmission for microorganisms and direct access to the systemic circulation, which significantly increases the risk of septicemia. The risk is reduced with the peripherally inserted central venous catheter because there is a greater density of skin flora on the thorax than on the arm and the peripheral site has little or no subcutaneous tract as a potential space for infection.

2. Potential for impaired skin integrity related to frequent replacement of the dressing. **Rationale:** Irritated or excoriated skin from frequent adhesive or tape removal increases the risk of infection.

Planning

1. Individualize the following goals for care of the catheter insertion site:
   a. Evaluate and prevent catheter-related infections. **Rationale:** Preventing contamination at the catheter site reduces the risk of infection. Early recognition and treatment of site infections may prevent septicemia.
   b. Maintain skin integrity under the dressing. **Rationale:** Reduces the risk of infection and maximizes catheter indwelling time.
2. Prepare all supplies and equipment. **Rationale:** Assembly of all the necessary equipment and supplies at the bedside facilitates quick and efficient completion of the procedure.

   a. One face mask (optional for peripheral sites).
   b. One pair of exam gloves.
   c. One pair of sterile gloves (optional for peripheral sites).
   d. Three alcohol swabsticks.
   e. Three povidone-iodine swabsticks.
   f. One-unit dose packet of povidone-iodine ointment.
   g. One transparent dressing or 2 × 2 gauze sponge.
   h. One skin protectant swabstick.
   i. One roll of 2-in tape.
3. Prepare the patient.
   a. Explain the patient's participation during the procedure and the importance of maintaining sterility. **Rationale:** Encourages cooperation and prevents accidental contamination of the sterile field or equipment.
   b. Suction the patient on ventilatory support (Skill 1–9). **Rationale:** Prevents contamination of the catheter site and avoids disruption of the procedure.
   c. Assist the patient in achieving a comfortable position that facilitates the procedure:
      (1) Position the patient in a flat or head-down tilt position if the tubing is changed as part of this procedure (not required for peripheral sites). **Rationale:** Prevents air embolism on disconnection of the catheter hub and tubing.
      (2) Instruct or turn the patient's head toward the contralateral side of insertion (not required for peripheral sites). **Rationale:** Prevents contamination of the site with microorganisms of the patient's respiratory tract.

Implementation

Steps	Rationale	Special Considerations
1. Wash hands with antiseptic handwash.	Reduces transmission of microorganisms; universal precautions.	
2. Don face mask and exam gloves.	Prevents transmission of microorganisms.	
3. Remove the dressing and discard in appropriate receptacle.	Exposes the catheter site for inspection and cleansing. Universal precautions.	
4. Inspect the catheter, insertion site, suture, and surrounding skin.	Detects signs of infection, catheter dislodgment, leakage, or loose sutures.	Observations should include evaluation of signs of infection (erythema, tenderness, swelling, exudate), leakage around the catheter, condition of the skin, and length of catheter external to the skin. The physician should be notified of signs of infection, leakage, skin breakdown, or catheter dislodgment.
5. Remove and discard gloves, and don sterile gloves.	Maintains aseptic technique.	Dressing changes on peripheral sites can be done with clean technique.

Table continues on following page

Steps	Rationale	Special Considerations
6. Gently tug on the catheter to evaluate the integrity of the suture.	Avoids dislodgment of the catheter.	A loose suture should be replaced.
7. Starting at the insertion site, using concentric circles, cleanse the catheter and skin around the insertion site with the alcohol swabsticks.	Removes soap, dirt, and moisture. Protects from contamination until prepared to begin sterile technique.	
8. Cleanse the catheter and skin with the povidone-iodine swabsticks as described in the previous step, and allow to dry.	Reduces the rate of recolonization of skin microflora.	
9. Apply a small amount of povidone-iodine ointment to the insertion site.	Ointment provides continued microbial action.	
10. Apply skin protectant to the skin.	Protects the skin from injury upon tape removal.	Do not apply within 1 in (2.5 cm) around the insertion site.
11. Apply transparent dressing or cover site with 2 × 2 gauze sponge.		
12. Cover gauze with at least a ½-in (1.25 cm) border of tape, leaving the catheter hub and tubing connection exposed (Fig. 31–3A).	Provides occlusive seal to prevent site contamination.	
13. Split a piece of tape in a Y configuration (Fig. 31–3B).	Prepares for application to the dressing.	
14. Slip the tape under the catheter hub and tubing connection until the end of the split is tight against the tape covering the gauze or the transparent dressing (Fig. 31–3C).	Prevents catheter dislodgment.	
15. Chevron cross the wings of the tape over the dressing (see Fig. 31–3C).	Secures the tape to prevent dislodgment.	
16. Place a second piece of tape covering the tape wings and catheter hub and tubing connection (Fig. 31–3D to F).	Secures connections and prevents inadvertent dislodgment.	
17. Tape the tubing to the arm or loop the tubing and tape to the chest or neck dressing.	Discourages inadvertent disconnection.	
18. Remove and discard gloves.	Universal precautions.	
19. Wash hands.	Reduces the transmission of microorganisms.	

Evaluation

1. Monitor the dressing for maintenance of the occlusive seal and the presence of moisture. **Rationale:** Loss of occlusive seal or moist dressings increase the risk of infection. Leakage of fluid from the catheter site is suggestive of venous thrombosis or lymphatic fistula.

2. Monitor the dressing and catheter site for evidence of catheter dislodgment. **Rationale:** Dislodgment of the catheter out of the skin displaces the catheter tip. Administration of hypertonic solutions proximal to the distal superior vena cava increases the risk of thrombosis.

Expected Outcomes

1. The dressing will remain dry, sterile, and intact. **Rationale:** Dry sterile, intact dressings reduce the risk of catheter infection and catheter dislodgment.

2. The catheter site remains free from infection. **Ra-

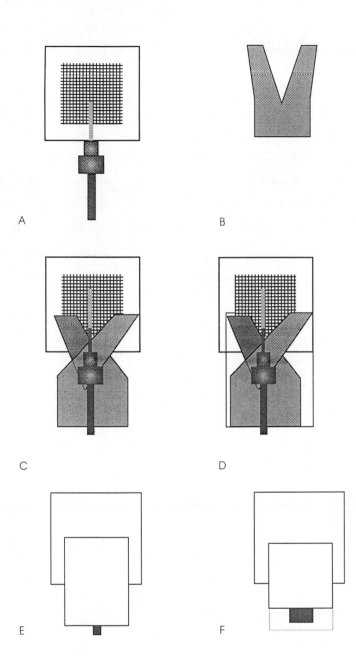

FIGURE 31–3. Taping technique for central venous catheter dressings. (*A*) Cover site with transparent dressing or 2 × 2 gauze sponge. Cover gauze with ½-in border, leaving catheter hub and tubing connection/injection cap exposed. (*B*) Split a piece of 2-in tape in a Y configuration. (*C*) Slip the tape under the catheter hub tubing/cap connection until the end of the split is tight against the transparent dressing or tape covering the gauze. Chevron cross the wings of the tape over the dressing. (*D*) Place a second piece of tape covering the tape wings and catheter hub connection. (*E*) Appearance of completed dressing with extension tubing or IV administration tubing. (*F*) Appearance of completed dressing with Luer-lok injection cap. Allows for easy cleansing of the cap and stability for accessing with a needle. (Courtesy of Suredesign.)

tionale: Colonization of the skin at the insertion site is the most important source of organisms causing central venous catheter-related bacteremias.

3. The catheter remains in place without dislodgment. **Rationale:** Repositioning of the catheter tip increases the risk of venous thrombosis. Accidental removal of the catheter places the patient at risk for complication with insertion of a new catheter.

Unexpected Outcomes

1. Catheter-related septicemia. **Rationale:** There are multiple mechanisms of catheter-related septicemia, but violations in meticulous care of the catheter are the leading cause of catheter-related infections.

2. Accidental removal of the catheter or malpositioning of the tip. **Rationale:** Loss of the catheter or tip malposition requires catheter exchange or reinsertion of a new catheter.

3. Impaired integrity of the skin under the dressing.

Rationale: Impaired skin integrity increases the risk of infection.

Documentation

Documentation in the patient record should include date and time of the procedure, date of catheter insertion, condition of the catheter site, condition of the surrounding skin, length of catheter external to the skin, and type of dressing applied. **Rationale:** Provides evidence of nursing care and observations for comparison on future evaluation.

Patient/Family Education

Explain the indications for repeated catheter site care to both patient and family. **Rationale:** Increases the understanding of the care provided.

Performance Checklist
Skill 31–4: Central Venous Catheter Site Care

Critical Behaviors	Complies yes	no
1. Wash hands.		
2. Don exam gloves and face mask.		
3. Remove the dressing.		
4. Inspect the catheter, insertion site, suture, and surrounding skin.		
5. Remove and discard gloves, and don sterile gloves.		
6. Evaluate suture integrity.		
7. Cleanse the catheter, insertion site, and skin with alcohol swabsticks.		
8. Cleanse the catheter, insertion site, and skin with povidone-iodine swabsticks.		
9. Apply povidone-iodine ointment.		
10. Apply skin protectant.		
11. Apply transparent dressing, or cover site with a 2 × 2 gauze sponge.		
12. Apply tape with an occlusive seal.		
13. Secure the tubing to the arm or chest.		
14. Remove and discard gloves.		
15. Wash hands.		
16. Document the procedure in the patient record.		

SKILL 31–5

Infusion, Care, and Monitoring of a Total Parenteral Nutrition System

Total parenteral nutrition (TPN) consists of an intravenous infusion of a hyperosmolar solution of dextrose, amino acids, and lipid emulsions via a large-bore catheter. The administration of these components, along with vitamins, minerals, electrolytes, and water, provides nutrients essential to the repair and maintenance of the body's tissues. The critically ill patient may be unable to ingest sufficient nutrition by mouth or may have a dysfunctional GI tract thus requiring TPN to meet nutritional needs. Peripheral parenteral nutrition (PPN) consists of the same components as TPN, except for a lower concentration of dextrose to provide a formula that is less hyperosmolar. The PPN solution must be lower than 900 mOsmol/L to prevent thrombosis of the peripheral vein (Hoheim et al., 1990). Because of the lower concentration of dextrose used in PPN, the solution does not provide as many calories as TPN and is frequently used as supplemental nutrition.

The initiation of TPN is performed with a continuous infusion of the solution, with a constant flow rate regulated with an electronic infusion device. This allows for regulation of the patient's fluid status and serum glucose level. The TPN may be cycled over a shorter period of time to allow the patient to be free from the infusion device, to encourage oral intake by stimulation of appetite, or to prepare the patient for long-term TPN (Gil et al., 1991). A TPN cycle is generally the infusion of the same volume of solution over a shorter period of time (e.g., 2 L over 12 hours). Assessment of the patient's fluid balance, respiratory and cardiovascular status, and serum glucose levels is essential to prevent complications prior to initiation of a TPN cycle.

Patients with burns, trauma, or sepsis may require large amounts of protein and calories to repair tissues and meet the needs of their hypermetabolic state (Vermeij et al., 1989). Patients with an ileus, enteric fistulas, or decreased small bowel length with loss of an absorptive surface are candidates for TPN. These patients may require prolonged therapy with TPN to provide bowel rest and adaptation. Acute inflammatory processes (e.g., pancreatitis, Crohn's disease) also may require bowel rest and have the potential for prolonged TPN. TPN is also indicated in patients who are unable to tolerate enteral tube feedings because of loss of GI tract function or when their metabolic needs exceed their oral intake (Edes, 1991).

Principles of TPN administration include hydration, provision of nutrients, sterile technique, heparinization of the catheter, and site care. TPN not only provides essential nutrients (e.g., fats, carbohydrates, and protein), but also water to maintain the patient's fluid balance. Sterile technique is essential to prevent infection while delivering TPN because of the use of hypertonic dextrose and access to the patient's vasculature with central venous catheters. Heparinization of the catheter will prevent clotting between TPN infusions when the patient may be cycled. Site care to the venous access reduces microorganisms on the skin and assists in preventing ascending infection via the catheter tract (Ryder, 1988a and 1988b).

TPN prevents or reverses malnutrition and related morbidity and mortality by providing nutrients to tissues to promote wound healing, improve immunocompetence, and support the patient's rehabilitation (Young, 1988). It is an important adjunct therapy during the acute phase of a critical illness and may become a chronic therapy for patients with permanent impairments of the GI tract.

Purpose

The nurse infuses TPN to

1. Provide essential nutrients with an intravenous solution of carbohydrates, fats, amino acids, electrolytes, minerals, vitamins, and water.
2. Maintain a positive fluid and nitrogen balance.
3. Maintain muscle mass and provide calories for metabolic demands.

Prerequisite Knowledge and Skills

Prior to infusing TPN, the nurse should understand

1. Anatomy and physiology of the gastrointestinal and cardiovascular systems.
2. Principles of digestion and absorption.
3. Principles of aseptic technique.
4. Principles of universal precautions.
5. Principles of intravenous therapy.
6. Principles of fluid and electrolyte balance.
7. Principles of carbohydrate, protein, and fat metabolism.

The nurse should be able to perform

1. Proper handwashing technique (see Skill 35–5).
2. Universal precautions (see Skill 35–1).
3. Vital signs assessment.
4. Gastrointestinal and cardiovascular assessment.
5. Assessment of fluid balance status.
6. Operation of an electronic infusion device (see Chapter 33).

Assessment

1. Obtain the patient's baseline weight, and note the presence or absence of edema (pedal, sacral, or generalized). Note the patient's admission weight and current weight. **Rationale:** Admission weight and initial fluid balance assessment will provide a baseline for evaluating the effectiveness of nutritional support.
2. Assess the patient for indications of protein-calo-rie malnutrition, including weight loss, muscle atrophy, temporal wasting, edema, weakness, lethargy, and possible failure to wean from ventilatory support. **Rationale:** Physical signs and symptoms provide indicators of severity of malnutrition and baseline for subsequent evaluation.
3. Assess the patient's medical history for the presence of chronic cardiac, hepatic, renal, or pulmonary disease. **Rationale:** Chronic illness may dictate restrictions in volume of fluid or amounts and types of amino acids, dextrose, and lipid emulsions added to TPN.
4. Assess the patient's serum proteins indicative of nutritional deficits (albumin < 3.5 g/dl, total protein < 6.0 g/dl, serum transferrin < 150 mg/dl, prealbumin < 200 μg/dl). Assess for nitrogen balance calculated from 24-hour urine collection. **Rationale:** Decreases in circulating proteins are indicative of the degree of malnutrition. Negative nitrogen balance will indicate the use of somatic and visceral proteins for energy.
5. Assess the patient for food allergies and intolerances, especially allergies to eggs. **Rationale:** Lipids are emulsified fats derived from soybean or safflower oils. Use in patients with egg allergies is contraindicated.
6. Assess the patient's serum triglyceride levels and history of hyperlipidemia. **Rationale:** Serum triglyceride levels will be elevated after infusion of lipid emulsions if lipid clearance is inadequate.
7. Assess the patient's endocrine function, history of diabetes, and baseline serum glucose. **Rationale:** Infusion of large amounts of carbohydrates may cause or exacerbate hyperglycemia.

Nursing Diagnoses

1. Potential for infection related to indwelling catheter. **Rationale:** Catheter placed in central vasculature provides direct access to bloodstream for microorganisms. High concentrations of dextrose and lipid emulsions in TPN support bacterial growth if system is contaminated.
2. Alteration in nutrition less than body requirements related to physiologic deficits. **Rationale:** Inadequate ingestion of protein and calories will result in malnutrition.

Planning

1. Individualize the following goals for TPN therapy:
   a. Maintain body weight at baseline or to achieve 1- to 2-pound weight gain per week in the patient with weight loss. **Rationale:** TPN provides sufficient calories for metabolic demands and weight maintenance or gain.
   b. Maintain serum proteins within normal range (total protein 6.0 to 8.0 mg/dl, albumin 3.5 to 5.0 g/dl). **Rationale:** Adequate protein intake will spare visceral proteins and assist in wound healing.
2. Prepare all necessary equipment and supplies. **Ra-

tionale: Assembly of equipment and supplies at bedside ensures that TPN will be initiated quickly and efficiently.
   a. TPN solution.
   b. Prescribed lipid emulsion bottle (for separate infusion).
   c. IV administration set for lipid emulsion.
   d. 20-gauge 1-in needle.
   e. IV administration set appropriate for electronic infusion device.
   f. IV filter (optional, depending on institution's policy), 1.2-μm filter for TPN containing lipid emulsions, 0.22-μm filter for TPN without lipid emulsions.
   g. One roll of 1-in paper or silk tape.
   h. Four povidone-iodine prep pads or swabsticks.
   i. Two 5-ml syringes with 22-gauge 1-in needles.
   j. 10-ml vial of 0.9% sodium chloride.
   k. 10-ml vial of heparin (10 to 100 U/ml) or prefilled syringes.
3. Prepare the patient by explaining the procedure. Rationale: Minimizes anxiety and fear.
4. Remove TPN bag from refrigeration 1 hour prior to initiation of infusion. Rationale: Warms TPN to room temperature, which increases patient comfort.

Implementation

Steps	Rationale	Special Considerations
1. Verify physician's orders with pharmacy label on TPN bag.	Reduces risk of error.	Order should include volume to be infused, rate of delivery, and time period for infusion if TPN is to be cycled. If rate is to be gradually increased and/or tapered, length of time at each setting should be indicated. Note the date and time solution will expire.
2. Wash hands.	Reduces transmission of microorganisms.	
3. Compare patient's ID band with label on TPN bag.	Prevents inadvertent administration of TPN to wrong patient.	
4. Aseptically spike TPN bag with IV administration set.	Prepares tubing for priming.	Volume-controlled infusion devices are more accurate than gravity-controlled infusion devices in the delivery of TPN solutions. Gravity-controlled infusion devices may not deliver highly viscous solutions accurately.
5. If indicated by hospital policy, add appropriate filter to IV administration set, prime, and then close clamp on set.	Traps particulate matter, bacteria, endotoxins, and vents air from IV tubing.	If using three-in-one TPN (lipid emulsions added to TPN bag) and filtering the solution, use a 1.2-μm filter to prevent clogging.
6. Clamp central venous or peripheral catheter.	Prevents air embolism and blood backup.	Final concentration of dextrose should be 10 percent or less if solution is to be administered via a peripheral catheter.
7. Don exam gloves.	Reduces exposure to blood and body fluids.	
8. Cleanse connection of catheter hub and injection cap or IV administration set with povidone-iodine prep pad.	Reduces microorganisms at catheter hub connection to reduce risk of infection.	The catheter lumen should not have been used previously for other IV fluids. If it has been used, it should be changed over a guidewire prior to TPN initiation. Use of a catheter lumen for other IV fluids increases the risk of contamination of the lumen. Subsequent infusion of TPN via the lumen may promote bacterial growth because of the presence of hypertonic dextrose.

Table continues on following page

Steps	Rationale	Special Considerations
9. Remove injection cap or "keep open" IV tubing from catheter hub, and attach IV administration set from TPN bag to catheter hub using Luer-lok connector.	Luer-lok connector prevents inadvertent disconnection of IV tubing from catheter.	Use of a needle into an injection cap for continuous infusion of TPN is not recommended because of an increased risk of accidental disconnection of TPN with resulting hypoglycemia. A needle should be used only if secured with a locking device.
10. Tape the IV tubing/catheter hub connection.	Secondary safety measure to prevent accidental disconnection.	
11. Open catheter clamp.	Allows TPN to flow into catheter.	
12. Place IV administration set into infusion device according to manufacturer's directions.	Use of an infusion device ensures accurate, consistent delivery of TPN.	
13. Label IV administration set with date.	Identifies timeframe for changing IV administration set.	Change set every 24 to 72 hours according to hospital policy to reduce risk of infection.
14. Set prescribed rate of infusion on pump, and start pump.	Consistent delivery of TPN prevents metabolic complications (see Table 31–3).	If TPN needs to be suddenly interrupted, notify physician. $D_{10}W$ should be infused at the same rate as TPN prescribed to prevent hypoglycemia.
For Cycled TPN		
15. Infuse TPN at prescribed rate; physician may order rate to be increased over 1 to 2 hours, or to begin at full rate.	Gradual increase in TPN rate may improve patient tolerance to glucose load.	Cycled TPN is infused over 10 to 14 hours. This may be performed to decrease incidence of hepatic complications and to help stimulate the patient's appetite.
16. One to 2 hours prior to end of TPN cycle, decrease rate of TPN infusion by half.	Decreases glucose load, thus decreasing pancreatic secretion of insulin to prevent rebound hypoglycemia.	
17. At end of TPN infusion, turn off infusion device, clamp IV tubing, and proceed with heparinization of catheter.	Discontinues TPN infusion at end of cycle.	
Separate Lipid Emulsion Infusion		
18. Compare label on lipid emulsion bottle with the physician's order.	Prevents infusion of incorrect concentration or amount of lipid emulsion.	Lipid emulsions may be infused separately as a piggyback infusion. Lipid emulsions are available as 10% or 20% solutions in 250- and 500-ml bottles.
19. Remove metal tab from top of lipid emulsion bottle, and cleanse rubber stopper with povidone-iodine prep pad.	Reduces microorganisms on stopper prior to insertion of IV set.	
20. Clamp tubing on emulsion administration set, and attach 20-gauge 1-in needle to end connector.	Provides method to piggyback lipid emulsion into TPN administration set.	
21. Spike lipid emulsion bottle, and prime tubing.	Prevents infusion of air into patient.	
22. Cleanse the Y-site on TPN administration set closest to patient with povidone-iodine prep pad.	Reduces microorganisms on Y-site.	If a filter smaller than 1.2 μm is on the TPN set, lipids must be infused below filter to prevent clogging the filter.

Table continues on following page

Steps	Rationale	Special Considerations
23. Insert needle of lipid emulsion set into Y-site, and tape in place or use locking device.	Secures needle to prevent inadvertent disconnection.	
24. Open roller clamp on lipid emulsion administration set, and adjust to prescribed rate of infusion.	Provides for controlled delivery of lipid emulsions.	An electronic infusion device may be used to control delivery rate. Lipids may flow retrograde into the TPN tubing if they are infused via gravity because of positive pressure of TPN on volumetric pump.
25. When infusion of lipids is complete, remove needle from Y-site.	Prevents air infusion from lipid bottle when infusion is complete.	Lipid emulsions may be infused over 4 to 6 hours.

Heparinization

Steps	Rationale	Special Considerations
26. Clamp catheter with slide clamp attached to catheter or nonserrated clamp.	Prevents blood backup or air embolism when catheter is disconnected from IV administration kit.	
27. Remove tape from IV administration set/catheter hub connection, and clean connection with povidone-iodine prep pad.	Reduces the number of microorganisms at connection.	
28. Remove IV administration set, and place injection cap on end of catheter.	Closes catheter system to prevent blood backup or air embolism.	
29. Cleanse rubber on injection cap with povidone-iodine prep pad.	Reduces number of microorganisms on injection cap.	
30. Fill syringe with 3 to 5 cc 0.9% sodium chloride, and fill a second syringe with 1 to 5 cc heparin (10 to 100 U/ml).	Sodium chloride flushes catheter lumen of TPN solution and prevents drug-nutrient interactions with heparin and TPN.	Prefilled syringes of sodium chloride and heparin may be used.
31. Flush catheter with sodium chloride.	Irrigates TPN solution from catheter to prevent drug interaction with heparin.	Filling volume of short-term multilumen catheters is less than 1 ml. Filling volume of long-term Silastic catheters is less than 2 ml. Between 3 and 5 ml is an adequate volume to flush any size lumen.
32. Flush catheter with heparin (100 U/ml).	Prevents blood from clotting in catheter between infusions.	Heparin concentrations may range from 10 to 100 U/ml depending on hospital policy. Flush volumes vary with hospital policy. Percutaneously placed central venous catheter lumen fill volumes are less than 1 ml.
33. Tape injection cap to catheter hub.	Secures injection cap to catheter and prevents inadvertent disconnection.	
34. Heparinize other lumens of multilumen catheters if not being used for infusions every 24 hours.	Prevents blood from clotting in lumens.	In patients with sensitivity to heparin or in cases where heparin is contraindicated, saline flushing is adequate if performed every 8 to 12 hours.
35. For catheter site care, see Skill 31–4.		
36. Remove and discard gloves.	Universal precautions.	
37. Wash hands.	Reduces the transmission of microorganisms.	

TABLE 31-3 METABOLIC COMPLICATIONS OF TPN

Complication	Etiology	Symptoms	Treatment
Carbohydrate Metabolism			
Hypoglycemia	Abrupt decrease or cessation of glucose infusion Too much insulin	Blood glucose less than 80 mg/dl Lethargy Diaphoresis Headache Pallor	Give glucose bolus by vein or orally depending on patient condition
Hyperglycemia	Too rapid initiation of TPN Diabetes mellitus Infection Steroids	Elevated blood glucose Glycosuria Diuresis Thirst	Decrease rate or stop infusion Addition of regular insulin to TPN
Hyperglycemic hyperosmolar nonketotic dehydration	Uncontrolled hyperglycemia	Blood glucose level > 500 mg/dl Increased BUN Lethargy Coma	Stop TPN Hydrate with free water Accurate I&O Administer insulin and potassium
Fat			
Essential fatty acid deficiency	Lack of fat intake or supplement	Dry, flaky skin Hair loss Coarse hair Impaired wound healing	Administer 10% to 20% lipid emulsion IV
Essential fatty acid overload	Overinfusion of lipid emulsions	Increased serum cholesterol, triglycerides, phospholipids Exacerbation of atherosclerotic heart disease	Decrease amount or concentration of lipid emulsions or discontinue and monitor serum lipid levels
Protein			
Prerenal azotemia	Impaired renal or liver disease	Increased serum BUN	Decrease protein intake in TPN
Water			
Hypovolemia	Inadequate free water or large glucose infusion	Increased serum BUN, decreased output, dehydration, thirst	Increase free water in TPN, decrease glucose calories
Hypervolemia	Fluid volume overload in renal, cardiovascular, pulmonary, or hepatic disease	Jugular vein distension, dyspnea, pedal and sacral edema, increased CVP	Concentrate fluids in TPN, decrease free water in TPN or other IV fluids
Electrolytes			
Hypokalemia	Inadequate administration or increased losses	Cardiac dysrhythmias Muscle weakness	Increase potassium in TPN
Hyperkalemia	Excess administration or failure to excrete K^+ as in renal failure	Cardiac dysrhythmias	Stop current TPN and reduce K^+ in subsequent order
Hypocalcemia	Inadequate calcium administration or excess phosphorus administration	Paresthesia Positive Chvostek's sign	Increase calcium in TPN
Hypomagnesemia	Inadequate administration of Mg^+	Tingling around mouth, dizziness, paresthesias	Add or supplement Mg^+ in TPN solution
Hypophosphatemia	Inadequate phosphate administration Excessive use of antacids (phosphate binders)	Lethargy, paresthesias, respiratory distress, coma	Add phosphate as K^+ or Na^+ salts in TPN
Anemia, iron deficiency	Excessive blood loss, inadequate iron, copper, B_{12}, folate replacement	Pallor, fatigue, exertional dyspnea	Addition of iron to TPN Blood transfusion as needed
Trace element deficiencies (copper, zinc, chromium)	Inadequate administration of trace elements, excessive losses	Dependent on specific element deficiency, impaired wound healing, glucose intolerance, hair loss	Appropriate replacement of trace elements

Evaluation

1. Monitor the patient's urine output and/or serum glucose and insulin requirements every 6 hours. Use of a bedside glucose monitor will facilitate assessment of the patient's serum glucose level. **Rationale:** High carbohydrate intake in TPN solution may lead to glucose

intolerance. Glucosuria may occur as later symptom of hyperglycemia. Sudden increase in insulin requirements in TPN and glucose intolerance are early indicators of sepsis.

2. Weigh the patient daily, compare with baseline weight, and note trends in weight changes (Ireton-Jones and Turner, 1991). Assess skin turgor every 8 hours. Auscultate breath sounds every 8 hours. **Rationale:** Weight changes are indicative of dehydration or fluid overload. Dehydration may occur as a result of fluid losses and/or inadequate fluid intake. Overhydration may occur in patient with cardiac, hepatic, or renal failure.

3. Monitor the patient's intake and output. Quantitate all output, including drains, ostomies, and stool. Observe for increased or decreased urine output. **Rationale:** Intake and output amounts reflect fluid balance. Trends demonstrated over a 2- to 3-day period may reveal a negative or positive fluid balance, indicating need for change in volume of TPN and other fluids.

4. Assess the appearance of the catheter exit site daily. Assess for pain, tenderness, erythema, and drainage from site. **Rationale:** Purulent drainage, erythema, warmth, or pain may be an indication of catheter site infection, which could lead to systemic infection.

5. Monitor the patient's serum electrolytes frequently (usually daily at initiation of therapy and three times a week thereafter). Assess for signs of electrolyte imbalance (e.g., muscle cramps, dysrhythmias, weakness, or lethargy). **Rationale:** Infusion of TPN may alter patient's serum electrolytes if amounts of electrolytes are not adjusted according to patient's serum levels. Protein metabolism may elevate serum BUN and should be monitored for sharp increases after initiation of TPN, particularly in the patient with renal or liver disease (see Table 31–3).

6. Monitor the patient's liver function studies at initiation of therapy and weekly thereafter. Assess the patient for signs of tenderness over right upper quadrant, jaundice of skin or sclera, or increasing lethargy. **Rationale:** Infusion of TPN may elevate liver function studies as a result of metabolism of amino acids, dextrose, and/or lipids.

7. Monitor the patient's hematology studies and iron, ferritin, vitamin B_{12}, and folate levels two to three times per week. Assess for weakness, fatigue, exertional dyspnea, and pallor. **Rationale:** Excessive blood loss and inadequate administration of iron, copper, and vitamins may result in anemia and iron and vitamin deficiencies (see Table 31–3).

8. Assess the patient for impaired wound healing, glucose intolerance without signs of sepsis, hair loss, acneiform lesions on skin, anemia, and abnormalities in blood coagulation. **Rationale:** Deficiencies in trace minerals (e.g., copper, zinc, and chromium) may cause abnormalities in metabolism and impairments in skin integrity. Trace minerals should be added to TPN daily to prevent deficiencies.

9. Monitor the patient's temperature and vital signs every 4 hours. Monitor white cell count three times a week for any elevation. **Rationale:** Elevated temperature and white cell count may indicate development of systemic infection. Central venous catheter and/or TPN solution should be considered as potential source of infection until ruled out.

Expected Outcomes

1. Maintenance of baseline body weight or weight gain of 1 to 2 pounds per week in the patient with weight loss. **Rationale:** Indicates adequate caloric intake.

2. Maintenance or repletion of serum proteins (albumin, transferrin, and prealbumin), normal or improved wound healing, maintenance of muscle mass, and positive nitrogen balance. **Rationale:** Indicates adequate protein intake to meet metabolic needs.

3. Fluid balance slightly positive (approximately 500 ml), serum sodium within normal limits, breath sounds clear, and absence of jugular vein distension and dyspnea. **Rationale:** Fluid needs being met with TPN without cardiac or respiratory compromise.

4. Catheter exit site clean, dry, and without pain or tenderness on palpation of site. **Rationale:** Catheter site without signs of infection.

Unexpected Outcomes

1. Weight gain of more than 3 pounds in 1 week. Presence of dyspnea, jugular vein distension, and sacral or pedal edema. **Rationale:** Cardiac, hepatic, or renal failure may result in fluid overload.

2. Dehydration, as evidenced by negative fluid balance, poor skin turgor, furrowed tongue, dry oral mucosa, and elevated serum sodium and blood urea nitrogen. **Rationale:** Use of hyperosmolar TPN solutions, inadequate infusion of additional water, and fluid losses will result in a negative fluid balance.

3. Hyperosmolar hyperglycemic nonketotic (HHNK) dehydration, as evidenced by elevated serum glucose (>600 mg/dl), osmotic diuresis, lethargy, and/or coma. **Rationale:** Use of hyperosmolar solutions and large concentrations of dextrose with an inadequate insulin supply and fluid intake will cause osmotic diuresis leading to severe dehydration.

4. Catheter site infection, as evidenced by erythema pain, warmth, tenderness, and purulent drainage at the site. **Rationale:** Catheter entry into skin may become infected by skin's microorganisms.

5. Systemic infection, as evidenced by leukocytosis, fever, chills, positive blood cultures, septic shock, and glucose intolerance. **Rationale:** Central venous catheter breaks integrity of skin and serves as a portal of entry for pathogens to the vasculature.

Documentation

Documentation in the patient's record should include date and time each TPN bag is initiated; infusion rate; volume infused; lipid emulsion infusion volume and date and time if infused separately; patient tolerance to therapy; gastrointestinal, cardiovascular, and pulmonary assessments; presence or absence of edema; intake and output; results of urine and bedside serum glucose tests;

vital signs, including temperature; daily weight, and mouth and skin care; catheter site appearance, including presence or absence of erythema, drainage, and tenderness; dressing change date and time; heparinization of lumens of catheter; date and time of IV administration set and filter change (Maki et al., 1987); injection cap change; and any unexpected outcomes and interventions taken. **Rationale:** Documents nursing care provided, expected outcomes, and any unexpected outcomes and interventions taken.

Patient/Family Education

1. Explain the purpose of venous access and TPN to both patient and family. **Rationale:** Promotes patient and family understanding of treatment plan and encourages questions.

2. Explain potential length of time TPN will be used and goals to be met indicating weaning from TPN. **Rationale:** Promotes understanding of treatment regimen and goals.

Performance Checklist
Skill 31–5: Infusion, Care, and Monitoring of a Total Parenteral Nutrition System

Critical Behaviors	Complies yes	no
1. Verify physician order with pharmacy label on TPN bag.		
2. Wash hands.		
3. Accurately identify patient with TPN bag.		
4. Spike and prime IV administration set aseptically.		
5. Add appropriate IV filter to administration set.		
6. Clamp catheter before opening hub.		
7. Don exam gloves.		
8. Cleanse catheter hub and injection cap or IV set with povidone-iodine.		
9. Aseptically connect IV set to catheter before opening hub.		
10. Tape connection of IV administration set to catheter hub.		
11. Open catheter clamp.		
12. Correctly load IV set into electronic infusion device.		
13. Label IV administration set with date.		
14. Accurately set delivery rate on infusion device.		
15. Taper/discontinue TPN appropriately.		
16. Change IV administration set and filter every 24 hours.		
17. Assemble lipid emulsions correctly.		
18. Piggyback lipid emulsions below IV filter.		
19. Regulate lipid emulsions with roller clamp or infusion pump.		
20. Discontinue lipid emulsions prior to bottle emptying.		
21. Flush catheter with normal saline after discontinuing TPN/lipids.		
22. Flush lumens of catheter with heparin when not in use.		
23. Apply catheter dressing using aseptic technique.		
24. Remove and discard gloves.		
25. Wash hands.		
26. Document in the patient record.		

SKILL 31–6

Removal of a Percutaneously Placed Central Venous Catheter

Removal of a percutaneously placed central venous catheter by the nurse may be prohibited, restricted to certified nurses, or permissible for all unit registered nurses, as dictated by hospital policy. Restrictions on performance of this procedure are the result of potential but rare serious complications associated with catheter removal.

Air embolism can occur during insertion, during the course of therapy, or with or after removal of the catheter. Catheters remaining in place for extended periods of time form fibrous tracts around the catheter from the skin entry site to the vein. Patients with long-duration therapies, muscle wasting, and decreased subcutaneous fat have a diminished distance from the skin to the vein and thus may be at greater risk for this complication.

Air embolism following removal of the catheter is a result of air drawn in along the subcutaneous tract and into the vein. During inspiration, negative intrathoracic pressure is transmitted to the central veins; therefore, any opening external to the body to one of these veins may result in aspiration of air into the central venous system. This is more likely to occur on deep inspiration when the patient is in an upright position, dehydrated, or hypovolemic. Coughing may initiate entry of air into the venous system by associated pressure changes that dislodge the sealing thrombus and separate soft tissues along the tract. The pathologic effects depend on the volume and rate of air aspirated. Death may occur quickly as a result of air obstruction of the pulmonary outflow tract. If not immediately fatal, local hypoxia with pulmonary hypertension may predispose the patient to a fluid leak and subsequent pulmonary edema or adult respiratory distress syndrome. The risk of air embolism on removal is reduced with peripherally inserted central venous catheters, since a skin tract is not usually formed and the pressure gradients do not exist at peripheral sites.

Fibrin deposition in the form of a fibrin tail on the catheter tip, a fibrin sleeve partially or totally encasing the catheter, mural thrombi, or complete venous thrombosis occurs to some degree on most venous catheters. Although rare, the stripping or dislodgment of this material on catheter removal may result in pulmonary emboli.

Purpose

The nurse removes the central venous catheter as a result of

1. Completion of therapy.
2. The occurrence of mechanical malfunction, catheter occlusion, or malposition.
3. Catheter-related infection or septicemia.
4. The development of a lymphatic fistula.

Prerequisite Knowledge and Skills

Prior to removing a catheter, the nurse should understand

1. Anatomy and physiology of the central venous system.
2. Type, design, and material of the catheter.
3. Principles of aseptic technique.
4. Universal precautions.
5. Potential associated complications.
6. Nursing interventions for potential complications.

The nurse should be able to perform

1. Proper handwashing technique (see Skill 35–5).
2. Aseptic technique.
3. Universal precautions (see Skill 35–1).
4. Vital signs assessment.
5. Proper patient positioning in the event of air embolism.
6. Cardiopulmonary resuscitation.

Assessment

1. Review laboratory data for platelet counts. **Rationale:** Pressure on the catheter site may be required for a longer period of time.
2. Determine if the patient is receiving anticoagulant therapy. **Rationale:** Pressure on the catheter site may be required for a longer period of time.
3. Observe the catheter site for signs and symptoms of infection, i.e., redness, warmth at site, tenderness, or presence of drainage. **Rationale:** Culturing of the catheter site, hub, skin segment, catheter tip, intravenous solutions, blood, and other potential sites of infection may be indicated for diagnosis and treatment of catheter-related septicemia.

Nursing Diagnoses

1. Potential for injury related to bleeding. **Rationale:** Direct pressure cannot be applied to the subclavian vein.
2. Potential for injury related to air embolism. **Rationale:** Air can be aspirated into the venous system along a subcutaneous tract.
3. Potential for injury related to pulmonary embolism. **Rationale:** Catheter removal may strip or dislodge fibrinous thrombi resulting in a pulmonary embolus.
4. Decreased cardiac output related to the occurrence of air or pulmonary embolism. **Rationale:** Air embolism causes obstruction of the right pulmonary outflow tract or the pulmonary vasculature. Pulmonary embolism may result in pulmonary hypertension, right ventricular strain, and decreased gas exchange. A massive air or pulmonary embolism may result in cardiopulmonary arrest.

Planning

1. Individualize the following goals for removing a central venous catheter:
   a. Maintain integrity of the catheter on removal. **Rationale:** Breaking the catheter with excessive tension or accidental cutting of the catheter may result in catheter embolism.
   b. Prevent infection of the site after removal of the catheter. **Rationale:** Antiseptic cleansing and application of a dressing allow for healing and protection against environmental contamination.
   c. Prevent air embolism through the remaining skin tract. **Rationale:** The wound must be occluded to prevent the entry of air.
2. Prepare all necessary equipment and supplies. **Rationale:** Assembly of all appropriate supplies ensures that procedure will be completed quickly and efficiently.
   a. Three each of alcohol and povidone-iodine swabsticks.
   b. One suture removal kit or sterile scissors.
   c. One pair of exam gloves.
   d. One petroleum gauze dressing.
   e. Two 2 × 2 sterile gauze pads.
   f. One roll of 2-in tape or transparent dressing.
3. Prepare the patient.
   a. Explain the procedure to the patient. **Rationale:** Minimizes risk of complications, reduces anxiety, and elicits cooperation from the patient.
   b. Position patient in horizontal or 10°–15° head-down tilt position unless contraindicated (i.e., patients with risk of spontaneous bleeding from elevated venous pressure or elevated intracranial pressure). **Rationale:** A normal pressure gradient exists between atmospheric air and the central venous compartment that promotes air entry if the compartment is open. The lower the site of entry below the heart, the lower is the pressure gradient and the less is the likelihood of venous air embolism.

Implementation

Steps	Rationale	Special Considerations
1. Wash hands.	Reduces transmission of microorganisms.	
2. Prepare clean work surface.	Reduces transmission of microorganisms.	
3. Open sterile packages: suture removal kit, petroleum gauze, and sterile gauze pads.	Prepares supplies for use.	
4. Turn IV infusion off.	Prevents saturating the bed with intravenous solution upon catheter removal.	Tapering of TPN should be completed *prior* to removal of catheter.
5. Remove the catheter dressing and discard in the appropriate receptacle.	Exposes the catheter site. Universal precautions.	
6. Don exam gloves.	Reduces the transmission of microorganisms; universal precautions.	
7. Starting with the insertion site, using concentric circles, cleanse the skin with alcohol and/or povidone-iodine.	Prevents contamination of the wound by skin microorganisms.	Cleanse an area approximately 2 in (5 cm) in diameter.
8. Carefully cut the suture, pull the suture through the skin, and discard in the appropriate receptacle.	Allows for removal of the catheter.	Be sure that all the suture is removed. Retained sutures can form epithelialized tracts that can lead to infection.

Table continues on following page

Steps	Rationale	Special Considerations
9. Remove the catheter:		
a. Instruct the patient to perform the Valsalva maneuver or hold his or her breath as the catheter is withdrawn. If the patient is on a ventilator, withdraw the catheter during the expiratory cycle.	Decreases the pressure gradient between the atmosphere and the central vascular compartment.	The Valsalva maneuver may be contraindicated in patients with compromised cardiac status or increased intracranial pressure.
b. Grasp the catheter with the dominant hand and slowly withdraw the catheter in one continuous motion. The distal end of a multilumen catheter should be removed quickly, since the exposed proximal and medial openings could permit air entry.	Prevents breakage of the catheter and injury to the vein wall.	Do not force removal. Catheter may be knotted or lodged. If unable to remove, *do not* apply force. Secure the catheter, apply sterile dressing, and notify physician.
c. With the nondominant hand, quickly apply pressure over the puncture site with a sterile gauze pad.	Controls bleeding and prevents air embolism.	If indicated, send catheter tip to laboratory for culture and sensitivity.
10. Maintain pressure for 2 to 3 minutes until hemostasis is achieved.	Prevents bleeding and hematoma formation.	
11. Immediately apply petroleum gauze over the catheter site, and cover with sterile gauze.	Prevents air embolism through catheter tract. Prevents entry of microorganisms from the environment.	Any air occlusive dressing may be used. *Note*: Air embolism through the subcutaneous tract has been reported with use of ointment on the site.
12. Tape over the gauze providing a minimum ½-in (1.25 cm) border around the edges of the gauze.	Maintains dressing in place. Prevents contamination of the site.	
13. Inspect and measure catheter.	Ensures that entire catheter has been removed.	
14. Remove and discard gloves.	Universal precautions.	
15. Wash hands.	Reduces transmission of microorganisms.	

Evaluation

1. Inspect and measure the catheter to ensure that catheter breakage has not occurred. Catheter length and tip configuration are variable. Notify physician immediately if breakage has occurred. **Rationale:** Catheters can rupture or break while in the body or on removal. Silastic catheters may have been cut to length before insertion.

2. Observe the dressing every 2 to 3 minutes for the first 15 minutes and every 15 minutes for the next hour for excessive bleeding. **Rationale:** Hemostasis may not have been achieved.

3. Remove dressing and assess for closure of the catheter site in 48 to 72 hours. An air occlusive dressing should be reapplied if the wound is not closed. **Rationale:** Verifies healing and closure of insertion site.

4. Observe the catheter site for signs of infection, i.e., redness, tenderness, or drainage. **Rationale:** Infection of the skin tract or site may occur after removal.

Expected Outcome

Closure of catheter site without infection. **Rationale:** The wound will close and heal quickly with proper care.

Unexpected Outcomes

1. Air embolism, i.e., sucking sound, tachypnea, air hunger, wheezing, hypotension, loud "churning" or "mill wheel" murmur over the pericardium, chest pain, nonspecific neurologic changes, loss of consciousness, or cardiac arrest. May result in pulmonary edema or adult respiratory distress syndrome. **Rationale:** Obstruction of venous flow reduces cardiac output.

2. Pulmonary embolism, i.e., hypoxia, hypotension, tachypnea, dyspnea, or chest pain. **Rationale:** Obstruc-

tion of the pulmonary vasculature prohibits perfusion of the alveoli and gaseous exchange.

3. Local catheter infection (i.e., redness, tenderness, or drainage) after removal. **Rationale:** Improper site care can result in migration of skin organisms into wound and establishment of infection.

Documentation

Documentation in the patient record should include date and time of the procedure, site assessment, ease of catheter removal, evaluation of the catheter, length of time pressure was applied, application of air occlusive dressing, patient tolerance to the procedure, and any unexpected outcomes and interventions taken. **Rationale:** Provides evidence of nursing care.

Patient/Family Education

1. Explain the rationale for catheter removal to both patient and family. **Rationale:** Enhances patient and family understanding of care and encourages questions.

2. Instruct the patient and family to report signs of pulmonary or air embolism, i.e., shortness of breath or chest pain. **Rationale:** Patient or family may recognize signs and symptoms before they are clinically evident.

Performance Checklist
Skill 31–6: Removal of a Percutaneously Placed Central Venous Catheter

Critical Behaviors	Complies	
	yes	no
1. Wash hands.		
2. Prepare clean work surface.		
3. Prepare required supplies.		
4. Turn IV infusion off.		
5. Remove the catheter dressing.		
6. Don gloves.		
7. Prep the catheter insertion site with selected antiseptic.		
8. Cut and remove the suture.		
9. Remove the catheter: a. Instruct the patient to perform Valsalva maneuver or hold his or her breath as the catheter is withdrawn. Withdraw during expiration if patient is on ventilator. b. Withdraw the catheter slowly in one continuous motion. c. Apply pressure over the puncture site with a sterile gauze pad.		
10. Maintain pressure until hemostasis is achieved.		
11. Apply petroleum gauze over the catheter site, and then cover with sterile gauze.		
12. Tape over the gauze with at least ½-in border over all the edges of the gauze.		
13. Inspect and measure the catheter to assure that the catheter has been removed intact.		
14. Remove and discard gloves.		
15. Wash hands.		
16. Document procedure in the patient record.		

REFERENCES

Edes, T. E. (1991). Nutrition support of critically ill patient. *Postgrad. Med.* 89(5):193–200.

FDA Medical Device Reporting System (1988).

Gil, K. M., Skeie, B., Kvetan, V., Askanazi, J., and Freidman, M. I. (1991). Parenteral nutrition and oral intake: Effect of glucose and fat infusions. *J. Parenter. Enter. Nutr.* 15(4):426–432.

Hoheim, D. F., O'Callaghan, R. A., Joswick, B. J., Boysen, D. A., and Bommarito, A. A. (1990). Clinical experience with three-in-one admixtures administered peripherally. *Nutr. Clin. Pract.* 5(3):118–122.

Ireton-Jones, C. S., and Turner, W. W., Jr. (1991). Actual or ideal body weight: Which should be used to predict energy expenditure? *J. Am. Diet. Assoc.* 91(2):193–195.

Maki, D. G., Botticelli, J. T., LeRoy, M. L., and Thielke, T. S. (1987). Prospective study of replacing administration sets for IV therapy at 48 vs. 72 hour intervals. *J.A.M.A.* 258(13):1777–1781.

Ryder, M. (1988a). Parenteral Nutrition. In C. Kennedy-Caldwell and J. A. Grant (Eds.), *Nutrition Support Nursing*. Philadelphia: Grune and Stratton.

Ryder, M. (1988b). Parenteral Nutrition Delivery Systems. In C. Kennedy-Caldwell and J. A. Grant (Eds.), *Nutrition Support Nursing*. (pp. 133–189). Philadelphia: Grune and Stratton.

Vermeij, C. G., Feenstra, B. W. A., van Lanschot, J. J. B., and Bruining, H. A. (1989). Day-to-day variability of energy expenditure in critically ill surgical patients. *Crit. Care Med.* 17(7):623–626.

Young, M. E. (1988). Malnutrition and wound healing. *Heart Lung* 17(1):60–67.

BIBLIOGRAPHY

Callahan, J. L., and Wesorick, B. (1987). Bacterial growth under a transparent dressing. *Am. J. Infect. Control* 15(6):231–237.

Kashuk, J. L., and Penn, I. (1984). Air embolism after central venous catheterization. *Surg. Gynecol. Obstet.* 159:249–252.

Norwood, S., Ruby, A., Civetta, J., and Cortes, V. (1991). Catheter-related infections and associated septicemia. *Chest* 99:968–975.

Santoro, I. H., and Lang, R. M. (1989). Iatrogenic air embolism causing the adult respiratory distress syndrome. *Catheter. Cardiovasc. Diagn.* 17:84–86.

Scott, W. L. (1988). Complications associated with central venous catheters: A survey. *Chest* 94:1221–1224.

Preventing central venous catheter-related complications: A roundtable discussion. (1990). *Infect. Med.* 7(10):9–23.

ENTERAL NUTRITION

BEHAVIORAL OBJECTIVES

After completing this chapter, the nurse will be able to

- Define the key terms.
- Describe the insertion of a feeding tube.
- Describe methods for confirming placement of a feeding tube.
- State the differences in design and placement of gastrostomy, jejunostomy, and percutaneous endoscopic gastrostomy (PEG) tubes.
- Describe methods for administering enteral nutrition via a variety of feeding tubes.
- Demonstrate the skills involved in enteral nutrition support.

Enteral nutrition support is indicated in the patient who is unable to meet his or her own nutritional needs with an oral diet. It is also a means of transitioning a patient from total parenteral nutrition to an oral diet. The gastrointestinal tract must be functioning (i.e., bowel sounds audible and peristalsis occurring) for enteral nutrition to be digested and absorbed. Provision of nutrition via the gastrointestinal (GI) tract has theoretical benefits in maintaining gut barrier structure and function and possibly preventing bacterial translocation and its morbidity and mortality.

Currently, there are over 130 enteral products available. They provide carbohydrates, protein, fat, vitamins, and minerals to meet a patient's needs, provided they are administered in adequate volumes. Formulas vary according to their protein source, although the primary consideration in selecting an enteral formula is the calorie and protein needs of the patient. A common method of delivery is continuous feeding using an enteral feeding pump to control delivery. Intermittent feeding (usually 100 to 400 cc over 30 to 60 minutes via gravity drip) is often used for gastrostomy feeding. Overall, intermittent gravity feeding is a simpler delivery system. The bolus method (i.e., feeding a volume of formula via syringe over a few minutes) has been found to cause more adverse effects (e.g., cramping, nausea, and abdominal distension) than continuous feeding.

This chapter focuses on the feeding accesses and the delivery of enteral nutrition.

KEY TERMS

aspiration
bolus feeding
continuous feeding
duodenum
gastric residual
intermittent feeding
jejunum
nasoenteric feeding
nasogastric feeding
percutaneous endoscopic gastrostomy (PEG) tube
peristalsis
pylorus
Silastic tube
stylet

SKILLS

32–1   Feeding Tube Insertion and Confirmation of Placement
32–2   Enteral Nutrition via Feeding Tube
32–3   Jejunostomy, Gastrostomy, and Percutaneous Endoscopic Gastrostomy Tubes

GUIDELINES

The following assessment guidelines will assist the nurse in caring for a patient receiving enteral nutrition:

1. Know the patient's gastrointestinal function.
2. Determine the patient's baseline nutritional status.
3. Know the patient's medical and diet history.
4. Know the patient's current medical treatment plan and medication profile.
5. Perform periodic assessments to determine the effectiveness of therapy.
6. Become adept in the use of equipment for the provision of enteral feedings.

SKILL 32–1

Feeding Tube Insertion and Confirmation of Placement

Enteral feeding tubes have developed over recent years with advanced technology to a more safe, efficient, and comfortable means of providing nutrition support. In the past, it was common practice to bolus the feeding formulas into no. 14, 16, or 18 French polyvinyl chloride tubes. These tubes can cause nasal necrosis and sinusitis, increase the risk of aspiration, and are generally uncomfortable for the patient. The bolus method of enteral feeding can cause abdominal distension, cramping, nausea, and diarrhea as a result of the rapid administration. An alternative to the bolus method is the intermittent method, in which 100 to 400 cc of formula is gravity infused for 30 to 60 minutes. It is useful in gastric feeding and when the accuracy of a pump is not mandatory.

The development of small-bore Silastic or polyurethane feeding tubes reduced the incidence of rhinitis and nasal necrosis. The tube sizes range from no. 5 to no. 12 French. Most adults require a no. 8 or 10 French. The tube has a weighted tip, usually tungsten segments, that curve the tip of the tube through the nasopharynx on insertion. The tube has a flexible stylet to stiffen it for insertion, and then the stylet is removed after confirmation of placement. Clogging of these tubes is common, primarily when crushed medications are administered through them. The tubes come in various lengths for placement in the stomach or duodenum. Nasally placed feeding tubes are generally meant for short-term use (less than 4 weeks), after which time an alternative tube placement (e.g., gastrostomy, PEG, or jejunostomy) should be performed.

Purpose

The nurse inserts an enteral feeding tube to

1. Provide an access to the gastrointestinal tract.
2. Administer nutrients, medications, and fluid into the gastrointestinal tract.

Prerequisite Knowledge and Skills

Prior to inserting an enteral feeding tube, the nurse should understand

1. Anatomy and physiology of the upper and lower gastrointestinal tract.
2. Principles of clean technique.

The nurse should be able to perform

1. Proper handwashing technique (see Skill 35–5).
2. Gastrointestinal system assessment.
3. Respiratory assessment.
4. Universal precautions (see Skill 35–1).

Assessment

Review the patient's medical history for risk factors for insertion of an enteral feeding tube, including head and neck cancer, nasal surgery, tracheostomy, esophageal cancer, decreased level of consciousness, and decreased pharyngeal reflexes. An absolute contraindication for insertion of a nasoenteric feeding tube is basal skull fracture. Assess the patency of the nares for potential obstructions to feeding tube passage (i.e., deviated septum, masses, bleeding, or copious secretions). **Rationale:** Physical deformities or obstructions of the nasopharynx or esophagus may make passage of the tube difficult or impossible. Respiratory disease may hamper placement because of the patient's lack of tolerance.

Nursing Diagnosis

1. Alteration in nutrition: less than body require-

ments. **Rationale:** The patient is unable to meet caloric and protein requirements orally secondary to physiologic deficits, such as dysphagia, decreased level of consciousness, tumors of the oropharynx, or anorexia.

2. Potential for injury related to aspiration. **Rationale:** Risk of vomiting and aspiration with gastric feedings secondary to decreased level of consciousness and poor gag reflex.

Planning

1. Individualize the following goals for inserting a feeding tube:
   a. Provide access to the gastrointestinal tract for enteral nutrition and oral medications. **Rationale:** A feeding tube provides a means to deliver nutrition and medications to patients who are unable to do so orally.
   b. Analyze gastric contents. **Rationale:** Feeding tube provides access to stomach for aspiration of contents to monitor gastric pH.
2. Prepare all necessary equipment and supplies. **Rationale:** Assembly of all the necessary equipment at the bedside will allow the procedure to be completed quickly and efficiently.
   a. One small-bore weighted enteral feeding tube of appropriate size for patient. **Rationale:** Size of feeding tube is based on patient's weight/size for comfort. Infants and children up to approximately 30 kg body weight will need a no. 5 or 6 French feeding tube. Feeding tubes for adults range in size from no. 8 to no. 12 French. The smaller lumen size of the feeding tube will promote patient comfort. Tube length ranges from 36 to 54 in (91 to 137 cm). The 36-in (91 cm) tube is indicated for gastric placement. Duodenal placement in an adult requires a tube at least 43 in (109 cm) in length.
   b. One package (½ oz) of water-soluble lubricant if the tube is not prelubricated.
   c. One pair of exam gloves.
   d. One 60-cc syringe with Luer-slip tip.
   e. Glass of water and drinking straw.
   f. One roll of 1-in hypoallergenic tape.
   g. Tincture of benzoin, 5 cc.
   h. One 4 × 4 gauze pad.
3. Prepare the patient.
   a. Explain the procedure to the patient. **Rationale:** Reduces patient's anxiety.
   b. Explain the need for the patient's participation and the importance of swallowing water during tube insertion. **Rationale:** Enhances patient's cooperation and facilitates feeding tube progression into the GI tract.
   c. Assist the patient into a comfortable position, usually semi-Fowler's or high Fowler's position. **Rationale:** Promotes patient comfort and facilitates tube insertion.

Implementation

Steps	Rationale	Special Considerations
Gastric Placement		
1. Wash hands.	Reduces transmission of microorganisms.	
2. Don exam gloves.	Universal precautions.	
3. Assist the patient to semi-Fowler's or high Fowler's position with the neck slightly flexed.	Facilitates tube passage into esophagus.	
4. Measure the approximate length to be inserted by measuring from the ear to the nose to the xiphoid process, and mark the length to be inserted with a piece of tape on the tube (Fig. 32–1).	Ensures probability of placing feeding port of the tube into the stomach and not the esophagus.	Measure from the feeding port of the tube and not from the weighted portion of the tube.
5. Assess patency of the patient's nares.	Will facilitate passage of the tube through the patient nares.	
6. Attach a 60-cc syringe filled with water to the end connector of the feeding tube, flush with 10 cc water, and remove.	Activates lubricant in tube to promote removal of the stylet.	Most tubes can be flushed with the stylet in the tube.
7. Lubricate the outer portion of the tube by placing the weighted end in water or by squeezing lubricant onto the distal 6 in (15 cm) of the tube.	External lubrication facilitates passage of the tube through the nasopharynx.	Tubes have a lubricant on their outer surface that is activated by placing the tube in water.
8. Insert the tube into the nares, and pass it into the posterior pharynx while patient sips water through a straw. For the intubated, mechanically ventilated, or trached patient, ask the patient to swallow, if able, as you advance the feeding tube.	Swallowing facilitates tube passage and obviates the gag reflex. For such patients and/or the obtunded patient, the stylet may be removed once the tube is advanced into the posterior pharynx.	Flexing the patient's neck slightly aids in tube passage into the esophagus.

Table continues on following page

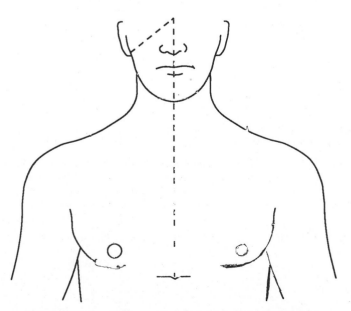

FIGURE 32–1. Measuring for placement of nasogastric tube.

Steps	Rationale	Special Considerations
9. Continue passing the tube while the patient swallows water until predetermined mark reaches the nares.	Achieves correct tube placement.	
10. Attach an empty 60-cc syringe to the end connector of the tube, and aspirate 10 to 30 cc of gastric contents.	Assists in confirming placement of the tube in the stomach.	Auscultation or insufflation of air is not an accurate method of feeding tube placement confirmation. Tubes collapse easily, and gastric returns may not be obtained. If unable to aspirate gastric returns, obtain radiologic confirmation of tube placement.
11. Observe the characteristics of the gastric returns (i.e., color, consistency, and odor).		Frank bleeding or fecal returns require further evaluation.
12. Apply tincture of benzoin to the bridge of the nose, and allow to dry.	Benzoin will assist in maintaining tape secured to nose to prevent tube dislodgment and also will "toughen" the skin to prevent breakdown from shearing forces of tape removal.	Ascertain that the patient is not allergic to benzoin or adhesives. *Do not* use benzoin on infants or children.
13. Secure the tube to the nose using hypoallergenic tape or "nose bandaids." *Do not* allow the tube to press or pull tightly against nasal mucosa.	Pressure against nasal mucosa can cause irritation, breakdown, and necrosis.	
a. Tape: tear a piece of 1 in tape 3-4 in in length. Tear half of the tape to bridge of nose. Wrap halved tapes around tube below nares.	Secures tube to prevent inadvertent dislodgment.	
b. Nose band-aid: Place broad section of nose bandaid on bridge of nose. Wrap narrower section of bandaid around tube below nares.		
14. Apply tincture of benzoin to cheek, and tape the tube to the cheek, taking care not to pull the tube at a sharp angle to the nares, which could cause pressure on the nares.	Removes tension from the tube and prevents inadvertent dislodgment.	
15. Remove and discard gloves.	Universal precautions.	
16. Wash hands.	Reduces transmission of microorganisms.	
17. Obtain an abdominal x-ray.	Feeding tubes are radiopaque, and x-ray will demonstrate tube placement.	
18. Remove stylet by gently pulling on hub of stylet connector.	Stylet is needed during insertion to stiffen tube for passage only.	Do not reinsert the stylet into the tube after the tube is inserted into patient. The stylet may puncture the pleura with a misguided reinsertion.
Duodenal/Postpyloric Placement		
1. Proceed with steps 1 through 13 under Gastric Placement, except add an additional 10 to 15 cm to the distance measured for placement. Promote passage into the duodenum by one of the following methods.	Allows the tube to be passed beyond the pylorus.	Tube needs to be at least 43 in (109 cm) in length.

Table continues on following page

Steps	Rationale	Special Considerations
Method I		
1. Assist the patient to a right-side semi-Fowler's position.	Aids in passage of the tube through the pylorus.	
2. Secure tube as under Gastric Placement with extra loops free for tube advancement, and remove stylet.	Prevents dislodgment of tube. Removal of the stylet allows the tube to be flexible for passage past the pylorus.	
3. Obtain an abdominal x-ray 12 to 24 hours after placement to confirm tube placement.	Peristalsis should carry the tube beyond the pylorus after 12 to 24 hours.	
Method II		
1. If the tip of the tube remains in the stomach after positioning, an order for 10 mg metoclopramide IV may be given and a repeat abdominal x-ray should be done in 4 hours.	Metoclopramide increases gastrointestinal motility, which may assist in tube advancement.	Ascertain patient's allergies prior to administering metoclopramide.
Method III		
1. Proceed as in steps 1 and 2 under Method I, and then send patient to radiology for fluoroscopic placement of the tube past the pylorus.	Ensures accurate placement and prevents delay in initiating feeding.	
2. Remove and discard gloves.	Universal precautions.	
3. Wash hands.	Reduces transmission of microorganisms.	

Evaluation

1. Compare the patient's respiratory status before and after insertion, and verify the radiology report for confirmation of feeding tube placement. **Rationale:** Identifies inadvertent intubation of trachea with feeding tube.
2. Monitor the feeding tube placement every 2 hours, noting the length of tube extending from the nares and the integrity of the tape securing the tube. **Rationale:** Evaluates for inadvertent dislodgment of tube.

Expected Outcomes

1. Distal tip of feeding tube is placed in stomach or duodenum as prescribed. **Rationale:** Enteral feeding is tolerated in the stomach or duodenum.
2. Maintenance of feeding tube placement. **Rationale:** Provides monitoring of tube placement for dislodgment and/or skin breakdown.

Unexpected Outcomes

1. Intubation of tracheobronchial tree. Patient becomes cyanotic, has difficulty speaking, and evidences sudden coughing or choking. **Rationale:** Feeding tube inserted into trachea interferes with respiratory status.
2. Tube coils in oropharynx, as evidenced by gagging and choking. **Rationale:** Feeding tube has not advanced past the epiglottis into the esophagus but has advanced into the mouth.

3. Failure of the tube to pass into the duodenum. Feeding tube will need to be placed via fluoroscopy. **Rationale:** Gastric motility in some individuals is inadequate for passage of the tube into the small intestine. Such individuals will need physical intervention to facilitate passage.

Documentation

Documentation in the patient record should include the date and time of the procedure, the size and length of tube inserted, the nares the tube was inserted in, the ease of insertion or difficulties encountered during insertion, gastric returns obtained, characteristics of the gastric returns, verification that x-ray confirmation was ordered/obtained, patient position for duodenal placement, patient tolerance of the procedure, respiratory status after insertion, and any unexpected outcomes and interventions taken. **Rationale:** Documents nursing care given and expected and unexpected outcomes.

Patient/Family Education

1. Explain the purpose of the enteral feeding tube to both patient and family. **Rationale:** Promotes patient and

family understanding of treatment plan and encourages questions.

2. Explain the potential length of time the tube will remain in place and the goals to be met indicating removal of tube. **Rationale:** Promotes understanding of treatment regimen and goals.

3. Evaluate the patient's need for long-term nutritional support. **Rationale:** Allows the nurse to anticipate and plan for the patient's needs after discharge. If long-term nutritional support is indicated (>1 month), a more stable, permanent access should be anticipated.

Performance Checklist
Skill 32–1: Feeding Tube Insertion and Confirmation of Placement

Critical Behaviors	Complies yes	Complies no
GASTRIC PLACEMENT 1. Wash hands.		
2. Don exam gloves.		
3. Position patient.		
4. Measure length of tube to be inserted.		
5. Assess patency of the nares.		
6. Attach a 60-cc syringe-filled with water to end connector and flush tube.		
7. Lubricate the tube.		
8. For the conscious/unintubated patient, insert the tube while the patient sips water. For the unconscious or intubated patient, flex the patient's neck during insertion and remove the stylet after passage into posterior pharynx.		
9. Continue passing the tube until predetermined mark reaches nares.		
10. Aspirate gastric contents to confirm placement.		
11. Observe the characteristics of the gastric returns.		
12. Apply tincture of benzoin to nose, and allow to dry.		
13. Secure the tube to the nose.		
14. Apply tincture of benzoin to the cheek, and tape the tube to the cheek.		
15. Remove and discard gloves.		
16. Wash hands.		
17. Obtain an abdominal x-ray for confirmation of placement.		
18. Remove stylet (if left in).		
19. Document procedure in patient record.		
DUODENAL/POSTPYLORIC PLACEMENT 1. Proceed with steps 1 to 13 under Gastric Placement. *Method I*		
1. Position patient in right-side semi-Fowler's position.		
2. Secure tube with extra loops free for advancement.		
3. Obtain an abdominal x-ray 12 to 14 hours later. *Method II*		
1. If tip remains in stomach, obtain an order for metoclopramide, and repeat x-ray in 4 hours. *Method III*		
1. Proceed as in steps 1 and 2 under Method I, and then send patient to radiology for fluoroscopic placement of tube.		
2. Remove and discard gloves.		

Table continues on following page

Critical Behaviors	Complies yes	no
3. Wash hands.		
4. Document procedure in patient record.		

SKILL 32–2

Enteral Nutrition via Feeding Tube

A nasoenteric feeding tube is inserted via the patient's nasopharynx and esophagus, with the distal tip placed in either the stomach or the duodenum. Enteral nutrition via a feeding tube is indicated in the individual who is unable to ingest adequate nutrients orally. An individual who is unable to eat because of a decreased level of consciousness or who is unable to eat adequate amounts of food to meet caloric and protein needs is a candidate for enteral feedings. The gastrointestinal tract must be functioning when nutrition is delivered enterally to ensure absorption of the nutrients. Enteral feeding is preferred over parenteral nutrition whenever possible because of decreased cost and a lower risk for complications (e.g., sepsis, thrombophlebitis, technical complications of catheter insertion).

Provision of adequate amounts of calories, protein, carbohydrates, fats, and vitamins enterally will prevent the development of or worsening of malnutrition. Malnutrition results in lower serum proteins and is accompanied by weight loss, fat loss, skeletal muscle atrophy, poor wound healing, increased susceptibility to infection, and increased morbidity and mortality.

There are three types of malnutrition: kwashiorkor, marasmus, and mixed. Kwashiorkor is characterized by a decreased intake of protein with a resultant drop in serum proteins. There may be minimal weight loss, which may be masked by edema due to lowered oncotic vascular pressure from decreased serum proteins. The individual may have an adequate intake of calories from carbohydrates and fats that contributes to weight maintenance. Typically, the patient identified with kwashiorkor is hospitalized and undergoing acute metabolic stress. The patient's acute protein deficiency is aggravated by catabolism from stress and the use of dextrose solutions infused intravenously without the addition of protein.

Marasmus is a reduction in caloric intake with gradual wasting of fat and muscle. Marasmus is seen in prolonged starvation, chronic illness, and anorexia. Serum proteins may remain at normal levels, but the patient may still have extreme wasting.

A mixed protein-calorie malnutrition state occurs with decreased protein and calorie intake. There is a wasting of muscle and visceral protein, loss of fat stores, and mineral and vitamin deficiencies. This type of malnutrition is associated with the highest risk of morbidity and mortality.

Commercially available enteral formulas are prepared to meet a variety of patient needs. Formulas may be categorized as blenderized, lactose free, fiber containing, milk based, modular, elemental, and disease specialized.

Blenderized formulas are essentially beef, vegetables, corn oil, and additives that are prepared to be delivered via tube. Because of lactose intolerance, many patients better tolerate a lactose-free formula. The carbohydrate source is usually maltodextrin, corn syrup, or sucrose. The caloric concentration of these formulas ranges from 0.5 to 2.0 cal/ml, increasing in 0.5-cal/ml increments. These formulas are supplied premixed in liquid form, and many come in prefilled, ready-to-use bottles that become part of the enteral delivery system.

Fiber-containing formulas range from 1.0 to 1.2 cal/ml. The use of fiber-containing formulas has been promoted to provide bulk in the stool, and some studies have associated improved glucose tolerance in patients receiving fiber-enriched enteral feedings.

Milk-based formulas are primarily used as oral supplements and should only be provided to those individuals who can tolerate milk products. Modular enteral components are currently used to supplement other enteral formulas with individual nutrients. A patient requiring additional protein intake because of increased needs may have a protein powder component added to their enteral formula. Most of the modular components are in powder form, although a few of the fat and carbohydrate supplements are liquid.

Elemental formulas are hydrolyzed nutrients for ease in digestion and absorption. Protein is provided in the form of free amino acids or peptides. Carbohydrates are generally supplied as oligosaccharides, and fat is minimally supplied as long-chain or medium-chain triglycerides. Elemental diets are generally unpalatable and are usually administered via feeding tube. They are low in residue but high in osmolarity, which may contribute to diarrhea and dehydration.

Specialized formulas are available for specific disease states. Differences in the specialized formulas vary on the basis of the metabolic aberration associated with a specific disease. For the trauma patient, there are several enteral formulas available with a high percentage of branched-chain amino acids (BCAA) as the protein source. The development of these "trauma" formulas was based on research demonstrating the need for provision of BCAAs in the stressed patient.

Increased intake of calories from carbohydrates has been shown to increase the respiratory quotient of patients with chronic obstructive pulmonary disease (COPD) and resultant deterioration of their respiratory status. Increasing the calorie intake from fat sources and reducing carbohydrates reduce the respiratory quotient below 1.0, with improvement in respiratory status. A specific enteral formula is available for patients with COPD, and it contains a greater percentage of calories from fat.

Other formulas have been developed for specific patient populations, including formulas for immunosuppressed, glucose-intolerant, renal failure, and hepatic failure patients. All these developments are based on a need to either restrict or supplement a specific nutrient because of an alteration in a patient's metabolism as a result of a disease.

Most patients require additional free water to be delivered via the feeding tube to prevent dehydration and a hyperosmolar state. Placement of the feeding tube must be confirmed by x-ray prior to administration of a tube feeding, and measures to prevent aspiration during feeding need to be anticipated and provided.

Purpose

The nurse initiates enteral tube feedings to

1. Administer nutrients to achieve calculated nutritional requirements.
2. Administer nutrients to achieve the recommended daily allowance (RDA) of vitamins and minerals.
3. Administer free water for fluid balance.

Prerequisite Knowledge and Skills

Prior to administering enteral tube feedings, the nurse should understand

1. Principles of clean technique.
2. Anatomy and physiology of the upper and lower gastrointestinal tract.
3. Principles of digestion and absorption.

The nurse should be able to perform

1. Proper handwashing technique (see Skill 35–5).
2. Gastrointestinal assessment.
3. Insertion of an enteral feeding tube (see Skill 32–1).
4. Flushing of an enteral feeding tube.
5. Respiratory assessment.

Assessment

1. Obtain the patient's baseline weight, and note the presence or absence of edema (pedal, sacral, generalized). Note the patient's weight on admission. **Rationale:** Admission weight and fluid balance assessment will provide evidence of effectiveness of nutrition support after intervention.
2. Assess the patient for indications of protein-calorie malnutrition, including weight loss, muscle atrophy, temporal wasting, edema, weakness, lethargy, or failure to wean from ventilatory support. **Rationale:** Physical signs and symptoms provide an indication of the severity of malnutrition and baseline for later evaluation.
3. Assess the patient's medical history for the presence of chronic cardiac, hepatic, renal, or pulmonary disease. **Rationale:** Chronic illness may dictate restrictions in volume of fluid or type of enteral formula administered.

4. Assess the patient's serum proteins indicative of nutritional deficits (i.e., albumin less than 3.5 g/dl, protein less than 6.0 mg/dl, serum transferrin less than 150 mg/dl, prealbumin less than 200 μg/dl, and assess nitrogen balance calculated from 24-hour urine collection for urine urea nitrogen and total urine creatinine. **Rationale:** Depressed levels indicate patient at risk.
5. Assess the patient's past and current medication profile for use of catabolic steroids (e.g., prednisone, dexamethasone). **Rationale:** Catabolic steroids increase protein requirements.
6. Observe the patient for signs of infection or sepsis, which increases metabolic demands and subsequently protein and caloric needs. **Rationale:** Enteral formula delivery is based on protein and calorie requirements of patient.
7. Assess the patient's GI tract function, including the presence of bowel sounds on auscultation, abdomen soft and nondistended, and patient passing flatus/stool. **Rationale:** Enteral tube feeding tolerance is improved when administered via a functioning gastrointestinal tract.
8. Calculate the patient's resting energy expenditure and prescribed formula's caloric content. **Rationale:** Awareness of resting energy expenditure promotes delivery of optimal nutrition.

Nursing Diagnoses

1. Alteration in nutrition: less than body requirements related to decreased oral intake of nutrients. **Rationale:** Patients who are NPO or have decreased their oral intake are not able to maintain nutritional status.
2. Potential for aspiration related to decreased or absent gag reflex. **Rationale:** Patients receiving enteral nutrition are at risk for aspiration with decreased/absent gag reflex, supine position, or high residuals.
3. Potential fluid volume deficit related to use of hyperosmolar enteral formulas. **Rationale:** Use of hyperosmolar formulas and inadequate fluid intake may lead to hyperosmolar hyperglycemic non-ketotic dehydration.

Planning

1. Individualize the following goals for administering enteral tube feeding.
   a. Maintain or increase body weight, except in the obese patient. **Rationale:** Indicates adequate caloric intake to meet energy/metabolic needs.
   b. Maintain serum proteins within normal range (i.e., protein 6.0 to 8.0 mg/dl, albumin 3.5 to 5.0 g/dl). **Rationale:** Adequate protein intake will protect visceral proteins and assist in wound healing.
   c. Protect patient's airway. **Rationale:** Enteral feedings into the stomach may predispose a patient to aspiration.
2. Prepare all necessary equipment and supplies. **Rationale:** Assembly of all equipment and supplies at

the bedside ensures that enteral tube feedings will be initiated quickly and efficiently.

a. One enteral feeding bag and administration set. (Some administration sets are preattached to the bag, while others have twist-on caps or spike into feeding container. Enteral bag may be a flexible or semirigid container.)

b. One 60-cc Luer-slip tip syringe.

c. One clean graduated measuring cup.

d. Stethoscope.

e. Blue food coloring or methylene blue, 5 cc (optional).

f. Prescribed enteral formula.

g. One enteral feeding pump.

h. One roll of 1-in paper tape.

3. Prepare the patient.

a. Explain the procedure. **Rationale:** Minimizes anxiety and enhances tolerance to feeding.

b. Assist the patient into a semi-Fowler's or high Fowler's position. Head of the bed should be elevated 30 degrees during infusion of enteral feeding. Patients who must remain supine (e.g., unstable neck fracture) must be monitored closely for aspiration during enteral tube feedings. **Rationale:** Prevents aspiration of gastric contents if the patient vomits.

Implementation

Steps	Rationale	Special Considerations
1. Verify physician's order for enteral tube feedings.	Reduces risk of error.	Physician order should include type of formula, volume to be delivered, and rate or length of time of infusion.
2. Wash hands.	Reduces transmission of microorganisms.	
3. Elevate the head of the bed 30 degrees.	Discourages aspiration of gastric contents during feeding.	If patient must be supine (e.g., unstable neck fracture), extreme caution must be exercised to monitor for aspiration.
4. For continuous feeding, close clamp on enteral feeding bag, and pour 4 hours' worth of formula into bag or hang prepackaged closed system container of prescribed formula. For intermittent feeding, hang 100 to 480 ml of formula in bag (Fig. 32–2).	Hanging only 4 hours' worth of formula prevents bacterial overgrowth in formula.	Because of the high carbohydrate concentration and frequent exposure of formula to multiple personnel, bacterial growth can occur rapidly, leading to gastritis, nausea, vomiting, and diarrhea. Limiting hang time or using a closed delivery system will reduce risk of contamination.
5. Add 5 cc of blue food coloring or methylene blue to each 250 cc of formula.	Serves as a marker of formula aspiration.	Food coloring and methylene blue also will tint patient's stool and urine a blue-green color.
6. Hang bag on IV pole, and prime tubing. For continuous enteral feeding, load administration set into enteral feeding pump.	Priming of tubing will purge system of air.	
7. Attach a 60-cc syringe to the feeding tube, and aspirate gastric contents. If greater than 60 cc, place returns in clean cup at bedside.	To confirm tube placement and to determine stomach's readiness for feeding. If gastric residue is more than 125 cc, feeding should be delayed 1 hour.	Gastric residual may be elevated due to formula intolerance, delayed gastric emptying, sepsis, or gastrointestinal disease. Residual is also dependent on infusion rate and gastric emptying time. Notify physician if residual is greater than 125 cc after 2 hours.
8. Heme test and pH gastric aspirate.	To assess for gastric bleeding.	Gastric bleeding indicates the need for further assessment and intervention. Enteral feeding usually is not tolerated if the patient is bleeding.
9. After determining volume of gastric residual, return up to 125 cc of gastric aspirate to stomach using same syringe.	Gastric aspirate contains enzymes and secretions essential for digestion of nutrients to be administered. Returning more than 125 cc of gastric aspirate may overfill stomach when enteral feeding is started.	If gastric residual heme test is positive, do not reinstill.

Table continues on following page

Steps	Rationale	Special Considerations
10. Flush feeding tube with 30 to 50 cc water.	Prevents clogging of tube and provides additional free water to patient.	Patients on fluid restrictions (e.g., renal failure, congestive heart failure) should have 10- to 20-cc flush to clean tube.
11. Elevate head of bed 30 degrees.	Discourages aspiration.	
12. Connect end connector of feeding bag administration set to distal end of feeding tube with safety-tape connection.	Prevents inadvertent disconnection.	
13. Set prescribed infusion flow rate for continuous feeding, and begin infusion via pump. Adjust roller clamp to infuse formula via gravity over 30 to 60 minutes for intermittent feeding.	Initiates administration of feeding.	For intermittent feeding, infuse 100 to 480 ml of formula every 4 to 6 hours depending on total volume prescribed for gastric feedings.
14. Label enteral feeding bag and administration set with date and time bag is hung. Change bag and set every 24 hours.	Indicates to nursing staff when bag needs to be changed.	Changing enteral administration set every 24 hours prevents bacterial overgrowth in set.
15. Administer mouth care every 2 hours.	Prevents drying and cracking of oral mucosa.	Moisten mouth with water-soaked sponge/gauze. Apply petroleum-based ointment to lips.
16. Administer water boluses as prescribed by physician.	Enteral formulas do not contain sufficient water to meet some patient's needs. High-osmolality formulas could lead to dehydration.	Adults require 25 to 35 ml/kg water each day (e.g., for a 70-kg patient receiving 2000 ml of an isotonic formula, 600 cc of additional water will need to be administered). Water boluses can be given with a syringe into the feeding tube in 100-cc increments every 4 hours. The formula could be diluted with necessary water and infusion rate increased. The greater the formula's osmolality, the less free water in the formula. This may necessitate increased water boluses in addition to the formula (Table 32–1).
17. Wash hands.	Reduces transmission of microorganisms.	
18. Prior to administration of medications via feeding tube, determine drug–nutrient incompatibilities.	Medications and enteral formulas may interact reducing effectiveness of medication or causing enteral side effects.	See Table 32–2.

Evaluation

1. Monitor the patient's urine glucose level every 6 hours. May need to monitor serum glucose using bedside glucose monitor for patients with consistently abnormal serum glucose levels. **Rationale:** High carbohydrate concentration of formula may exceed endogenous insulin supply. In hyperosmolar hyperglycemic nonketotic dehydration, patient will have glucosuria with an osmotic diuresis.

2. Weigh the patient daily, and compare with base-line weight. Note trends of weight gain/loss. Check skin turgor every shift. **Rationale:** Dehydration can occur as a result of hyperosmolar formulas, patient fluid losses, and inadequate water intake. Overhydration can occur in the patient with cardiac, hepatic, or renal failure. Fluid needs are increased in the patient with an elevated temperature.

3. Monitor the patient's intake and output carefully. Quantitate diarrheal stool output. Observe for decreased or increased urine output. Stool culture should be obtained with persistent diarrhea to rule out pseudomem-

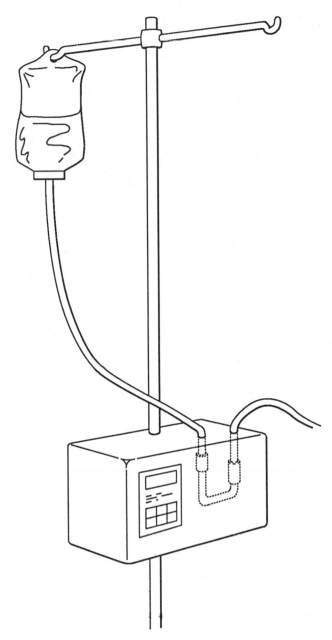

FIGURE 32–2. Closed enteral delivery system.

branous colitis due to *Clostridium difficile* toxin. **Rationale:** Diarrhea can occur as a result of the use of hyperosmolar formulas, lactose intolerance, prolonged use of antibiotics, bacterial contamination of formulas, severe hypoalbuminemia (less than 2.5 g/dl), or medications, resulting in dehydration.

4. Assess the patient's medication profile for potential cause of or relationship to persistent diarrhea. **Rationale:** Osmolality of medications may cause diarrhea. Antibiotics cause bacterial overgrowth in gastrointestinal tract, resulting in diarrhea. Medications in elixir form (e.g., theophylline, acetaminophen) contain large amounts of sorbitol, which has a strong cathartic action.

5. Monitor the frequency of diarrhea, and administer antidiarrheals as indicated, using nonnarcotic antidiarrheal or bulk-forming agent. **Rationale:** Control of diarrhea will prevent dehydration and improve absorption of nutrients.

6. Auscultate the patient's bowel sounds every 8 hours for motility. **Rationale:** Gastrointestinal function will affect patient's tolerance to enteral feedings.

7. Aspirate the patient's gastric residuals every 4 hours. If residual is more than 125 to 150 cc, hold feeding for 1 hour and recheck residual. If residual remains elevated (more than 125 cc), notify physician. Patient may be placed on metoclopramide 10 mg q.i.d. to increase gastrointestinal motility. **Rationale:** Residuals greater than 150 cc indicate decreased gastric motility and/or emptying. Continued feeding with high residuals increases the risk of vomiting and aspiration. Residuals may be increased because of formula intolerance, indicating a need for reevaluation of formula.

8. Hold feeding for 30 to 60 minutes prior to patient having procedure requiring supine position. **Rationale:** Decreases risk of aspiration.

Expected Outcomes

1. Maintenance of baseline weight or weight gain of ½ to 1 pound per week. **Rationale:** Indicates adequate caloric intake.

2. Maintenance or elevation of serum and visceral proteins, improved wound healing, maintenance of muscle mass, and positive nitrogen balance. **Rationale:** Indicates adequate protein intake to meet protein needs.

3. Fluid balance stable, as evidenced by serum sodium within normal limits, absence of diarrhea, and balanced or slightly positive fluid intake. **Rationale:** Fluid needs being met without excessive losses.

Unexpected Outcomes (See Table 32–3)

1. Intolerance of tube feeding, as evidenced by nausea, vomiting, diarrhea, abdominal distension, and high gastric residues. **Rationale:** Patient's tolerance is related to disease, osmolality of formula, rate of infusion, type of formula, and decreased gastric emptying.

2. Aspiration, as evidenced by suctioning of blue secretions from trachea. **Rationale:** Decreased gag reflex and supine position and high gastric residuals increase

TABLE 32–1   FREE WATER IN ENTERAL FORMULAS

Formula	Cal/ml	Percent Free Water
Ensure, Entrition, Isocal, Nutren	1.0	80 to 85
Ensure Plus, Nutren 1.5, Sustacal HC	1.5	77 to 79
Isocal HCN, Magnacal, Nutren 2.0	2.0	69 to 71

TABLE 32—2   DRUG-NUTRIENT INTERACTIONS

Type of Incompatibility	Characteristics	Medications Known to be Incompatible	Actions to Prevent Incompatibilities
Physical	Visible changes when drug and formula are mixed together: Formula curdled, gritty Viscosity increased/decreased Suspension may layer out	Acidic syrups (pH 4.0 or less): Sudafed, Neocalglucon, liquid pectin Water in oil preparations: MCT oil, mandelamine suspension, cyclosporine Calcium over 130 mEq/L	Do not mix medication with enteral formula. Use an alternate dosage form. Use an alternate route of administration. Use a therapeutic equivalent.
Pharmaceutical	Alteration of a dosage form for administration is contrary to design of dosage form (e.g., crushing coated tablets)	Enteric-coated tablets Sublingual tablets Sustained-release preparations: Spansules Extentabs, SR, SA, LA	Use an alternate dosage form. Use an alternate route of administration. Use a therapeutic equivalent.
Pharmacologic	Mechanism of action of medication alters GI tolerance of enteral feeding. May be manifested by altered GI motility, vomiting, altered GI flora, altered metabolism, antagonistic activity	Increased GI motility: metoclopramide, cholinergics Decreased GI motility: narcotics, anticholinergics Vomiting: opiates, antineoplastic agents (cisplatin, adriamycin, nitrogen mustard) Altered GI flora: antibiotics, histamine-2 blockers Altered metabolism: glucocorticoids Antagonistic activity: warfarin-vitamin K	Use a therapeutic equivalent. Use adjunct medication to treat adverse effect.
Physiologic	Tolerance to enteral feeding is related to nonpharmacologic actions of medication. May be related to osmolality of medication or excipients of medications (additives to drugs). May be manifested by diarrhea or GI tract irritation.	Osmolality of medications: KCl elixir (10%), cimetidine liquid, theophylline elixir Diarrhea: antibiotics, quinidine, methyldopa, antacids GI tract irritation: KCl, erythromycin, iron preparations, NSAIDs and aspirin Excipients: lactose, gluten, sorbitol (in theophylline and acetaminophen elixirs)	Use an alternate enteral formula. Use an alternate dosage form. Use an alternate route of administration. Use a therapeutic equivalent. Use adjunct medication to treat adverse effect. Dilute medication.
Pharmacokinetic	Bioavailability, distribution, metabolism, or elimination of the medication is altered by enteral formula.	Phenytoin, digoxin, morphine sulfate, carbamazepine	Do not mix medication with enteral formula. Use an alternate enteral formula. Use an alternate dosage form. Use an alternate route of administration. Use a therapeutic equivalent.

the risk of aspiration. Secretions are tinted blue from food coloring/methylene blue in enteral formula.

3. Dehydration, as evidenced by negative fluid balance, poor skin turgor, furrowed tongue, dry oral mucosa, elevated serum sodium, decreased urine output, and increased blood urea nitrogen. **Rationale:** Use of

TABLE 32–3 COMMON PROBLEMS RELATED TO ENTERAL TUBE FEEDINGS

Problem	Cause	Intervention
Intolerance of feeding (i.e., nausea, cramps, abdominal distension, high gastric residues)	Decreased gastric emptying	Measure residuals q4h on continuous feedings. If less than 125 cc, continue feeding. If more than 125 cc, hold feeding for 1 hour. If more than 125 cc for more than 2 hours, notify physician. Obtain order for metoclopramide if not contraindicated (10 mg IV or PO q6h).
	Rapid infusion of enteral formula	Reduce rate of infusion and/or concentration of formula. Auscultate bowel sounds q8h. Palpate abdomen q8h for distension.
	Obstruction	Discontinue enteral feeding. Obtain abdominal x-ray to verify obstruction. Assess for impaction, and assess stool frequency.
	Gastrostomy tube or jejunostomy tube migration causing outlet obstruction	Reposition gastrostomy tube.
Hyperglycemia	Carbohydrate content/infusion exceeds endogenous insulin supply or exogenous insulin therapy	Increase insulin dose. Decrease carbohydrate content of diet. Increase fat content of diet.
	Sepsis	Sepsis workup (panculture to determine source of sepsis).
	Medications (i.e., steroids)	
Hyperosmolar hyperglycemic nonketotic dehydration	Carbohydrate content of formula exceeds endogenous insulin supply or exogenous insulin therapy. Glucosuria occurs with osmotic diuresis leading to dehydration	Discontinue enteral feeding. Hydrate patient. Administer insulin.
Diarrhea	Hyperosmolar formula; rapid infusion rate	Build to desired infusion rate over 2 to 3 days. Increase in increments of 25 cc/h every 12 to 24 hours until reaching goal volume (e.g., day 1 = 25 cc/h full strength osmolite; day 2 = 50 cc/h full strength osmolite; day 3 = goal: 90 cc/h). Avoid rapid intermittent or bolus feedings.
	Prolonged use of antibiotics causing bacterial overgrowth in gastrointestinal tract and/or pseudomembranous colitis	Review patient's medication profile for causative agents. Culture stool for *Clostridium Difficile* and other enteric pathogens. Administer nonnarcotic antidiarrheal agents.
	Addition of medications to formula that increase osmolality	Hang only 4 hours' worth of formula at time.

Table continues on following page

Problem	Cause	Intervention
Aspiration	Use of medications in elixir form with high sorbitol content; bacterial contamination of formula; intolerance to formula ingredients (i.e., lactose, fat)	Change enteral delivery system q24h. Change formula to lactose-free and/or low-fat formula.
	Patient in supine position	Place patient in semi-Fowler's or high Fowler's position with HOB elevated at least 30 degrees during infusion. Discontinue feeding 30 minutes prior to any procedure requiring patient to be placed in supine position. Add 5 ml of blue food coloring or methylene blue to each 250 ml of formula to serve as marker of aspiration of stomach contents.
	Improper placement of tube	Aspirate stomach contents of nasally placed feeding tubes prior to and after every 4 hours of enteral infusion. Obtain abdominal x-ray to verify placement prior to initial use.
	Migration of tube after initial placement	
Clogged feeding tube	Inadequately crushed medications delivered via tube	Administer medications in liquid form when available. Finely crush medications and dissolve in 20 ml of warm water. Flush tube with 30 to 50 ml of warm water before and after medication administration via tube, whenever enteral infusion is discontinued, and every 8 hours for continuous feedings. With 30- to 60-ml syringe filled with water, use piston-like motion to dislodge clogged material. If unsuccessful, flush tube with carbonated beverage (e.g., cola) or instill with cola, clamp for 1 hour, then flush with warm water. May also use ½ tsp. of meat tenderizer in 10 ml of water. Clamp tube for 1 hour; then flush with water. Frequent use of meat tenderizer or inadequate flushing after its use could cause tissue injury in the esophagus or gastric mucosa.
	Inadequate flushing of tube before and after medication administration	
	Enteral formula congeals within feeding tube	
	Kinking of feeding tube	
	Highly viscous fiber-containing formulas in tubes smaller than no. 10 French	
Dehydration	Inadequate free water administration	Assess fluid intake and output q8h. Adults require 25 to 35 ml/kg per day of water. Infants and chil-
	Use of hyperosmolar formulas	

Table continues on following page

Problem	Cause	Intervention
		dren under 3 years of age require 120 to 160 ml/kg per day of water. Enteral formulas contain 70 to 85 percent water (see Table 32–1). Calculate water based on patient's weight and cardiac, renal, and hepatic function. Administer water boluses via syringe incrementally distributed throughout the day. Monitor electrolytes three times per week.
Overhydration	Hepatic, cardiac, and/or renal failure	Monitor intake and output q8h. Weigh patient daily. Change formula to more concentrated solution (1.5 or 2 cal/ml). Restrict free water intake. Administer diuretics as ordered.
	Excessive infusion of fluid	
Rhinitis, otitis media, nasal necrosis	Use of stiff polyvinyl chloride tubes	Change tube to small-bore polyurethane or silicone tube.
	Excessive pressure on nares	Secure tube to nose without pulling on nares. Apply petrolatum-based ointment to nares q8h.
	Prolonged use of naso-esophageal route for enteral infusions	Consider alternative placement of tube: gastrostomy, jejunostomy, PEG tube.

hyperosmolar formulas, inadequate administration of additional water, and patient fluid losses will cause dehydration.

4. Hyperosmolar hyperglycemic nonketotic dehydration, as evidenced by elevated serum glucose (>600 mg/dl), osmotic diuresis, and lethargy or coma. **Rationale:** Use of hyperosmolar formulas and inadequate fluid intake causing osmotic diuresis leading to severe dehydration.

5. Clogged feeding tube, as evidenced by occlusion alarm on enteral pump, inability to flush tube with water-filled syringe, and inability to aspirate from tube. **Rationale:** Enteral formula or medications administered via feeding tube occlude internal lumen or opening orifice of tube, prohibiting infusion or aspiration via tube (see Table 32–2).

6. Feeding tube rupture, as evidenced by sudden release of pressure on irrigating syringe, eruptation, and aspiration of formula from infusion of formula through ruptured tube in esophagus. **Rationale:** Feeding tube may rupture as a result of excessive pressure on irrigating syringe if tube is clogged.

7. Persistent elevated glucose level, as evidenced by serum glucose level greater than 200 mg/dl. **Rationale:** High carbohydrate content of formula may not be tolerated because of low levels of endogenous insulin.

8. Diarrhea, as evidenced by four or more loose or liquid stools per day. **Rationale:** Prolonged use of antibiotics, medications with high sorbitol content, and high-osmolality enteral formula and the presence of *Clostridium difficile* toxin may result in diarrhea.

Documentation

Documentation in the patient record should include the gastrointestinal assessment prior to initiation of feeding, skin turgor, date and times feeding was initiated, volumes of gastric residuals, strength and type of formula, infusion rate, tolerance to feeding, total volume delivered, condition of oral cavity and times mouth care is provided, amount of free water instilled, glucose level, daily weight, intake and output, number of stools/amount of diarrhea, bowel sound(s) assessment, and any unexpected outcomes and interventions taken. **Rationale:** Documents nursing care given, tolerance to feedings, expected and unexpected outcomes, and interventions taken.

Patient/Family Education

1. Explain the rationale for the feeding to both patient and family. **Rationale:** Alleviates anxiety and pro-

motes understanding of treatment regimen and possible length of therapy.

2. Tell the patient to report signs and symptoms of nausea, abdominal cramping, and abdominal fullness. **Rationale:** Indicates potential intolerance to rate of in-

fusion or type of formula and decreased patient comfort.

3. Evaluate the patient's need for long-term enteral nutrition support. **Rationale:** Allows for planning of long-term access if indicated. Consult nutritional support nurse if long-term enteral feedings are anticipated.

Performance Checklist
Skill 32–2:   Enteral Nutrition via Feeding Tube

Critical Behaviors	Complies	
	yes	no
1. Verify physician order for feedings.		
2. Wash hands.		
3. Elevate HOB to 30 degrees.		
4. Fill enteral feeding bag with formula.		
5. Add 5 cc of food coloring or methylene blue per 250 cc of formula.		
6. Prime tubing on enteral administration set, and correctly load administration set in feeding pump.		
7. Aspirate gastric contents prior to feeding and every 4 hours during feeding (except for jejunostomy tubes).		
8. Heme test and pH gastric contents.		
9. Return gastric contents if not heme test–positive.		
10. Flush feeding tube with 30 to 50 cc water prior to feeding.		
11. Elevate HOB 30 degrees.		
12. Connect and secure administration set to feeding tube.		
13. Set infusion rate accurately, and start pump.		
14. Label enteral feeding bag with date and time hung.		
15. Administer mouth care q2h.		
16. Administer water boluses, as prescribed.		
17. Wash hands.		
18. Determine drug–nutrient incompatibilities prior to administration of medications via feeding tube.		
19. Document procedure in the patient record.		

SKILL 32–3

Jejunostomy, Gastrostomy, and Percutaneous Endoscopic Gastrostomy Tubes

Patients requiring enteral nutrition support for greater than 4 weeks should be considered as candidates for a long-term enteral access. Some patients are not able to have enteral feeding tubes nasally placed because of head and neck surgery or trauma. Tumors of the esophagus also prevent passage of an enteral feeding tube. Such patients would benefit from placement of a gastrostomy, jejunostomy, or percutaneous endoscopic gastrostomy (PEG) tube. The gastrostomy, jejunostomy, and PEG

tubes are placed directly into the stomach, jejunum, or duodenum (Table 32–4).

The gastrostomy tube is inserted during a surgical procedure through the abdominal wall, with the tip placed in the stomach (Fig. 32–3). Many gastrostomy tubes are Foley or mushroom catheters, although there are commercially designed tubes made of Silastic that have features not found in the Foley or mushroom catheter. Most gastrostomy tubes are secured by inflating a balloon (5 to 30 cc) on the end of the tube once it is placed in the stomach. A few tubes have disks that rest on the skin to secure the tube's position. If removed, reinsertion of the gastrostomy tube is a routine procedure once the gastric tunnel/stoma is healed, which usually requires 2 weeks.

TABLE 32–4 COMPARISON OF LONG-TERM FEEDING TUBES

	Advantages	**Disadvantages**
Gastrostomy tube	Promotes patient comfort by preventing nasal necrosis, otitis media, rhinitis, and other complications of a nasally-inserted feeding tube. Can be easily replaced by patient/family/nursing staff once tract is well established. Large bore of tube allows easy aspiration and delivery of medication.	Need intact gag reflex to prevent aspiration. May migrate and obstruct pylorus, causing gastric outlet obstruction. May migrate into duodenum causing dumping syndrome with bolus feeding. Stoma around tube may leak.
Percutaneous Endoscopic Gastrostomy (PEG)	Placed endoscopically under local anesthesia. Acceptable alternative when laparotomy and general anesthesia are not optional. Secures with bolster or flange in stomach, making dislodgment difficult. Most tubes made of Silastic material that is biocompatible. Can be modified to gastrojejunal tube for gastric decompression and concurrent jejunal feeding.	Prior gastric surgery may preclude placement of PEG. Possible increased risk of infection from oral flora introduced during insertion. Disk or bumper on skin surface may be too tight against skin, causing skin irritation and pressure on underlying gastric mucosa.
Jejunostomy tube	Reduced risk of aspiration in patient with absent gag reflex. Tube may be easily replaced by nursing staff/patient/family after tract well established. May feed immediately postoperatively.	Usually requires continuous or cycled feeding via pump to prevent dumping syndrome. Requires laparotomy and general anesthesia for insertion. Must be secured appropriately to prevent migration, which may cause small bowel obstruction. Obstruction of catheter common with highly viscous or fiber-enriched formulas, or medications due to small lumen size of catheter.

The PEG tube is placed endoscopically in the stomach without general anesthesia. A guidewire is threaded through the oropharynx, esophagus, and stomach and brought out through the abdominal wall. The PEG tube is then threaded over the guidewire and passed into the stomach. The tapered end of the tube is brought through the abdominal wall until the distal end is snug against the gastric mucosa. A retention disk or bumper is placed on the skin surface to secure the tube and prevent excess motion of the tube in the tract (Fig. 32–4). An adapter

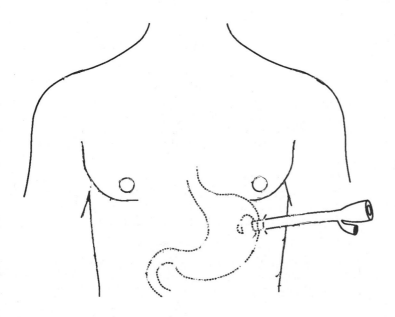

FIGURE 32–3. Gastrostomy tube.

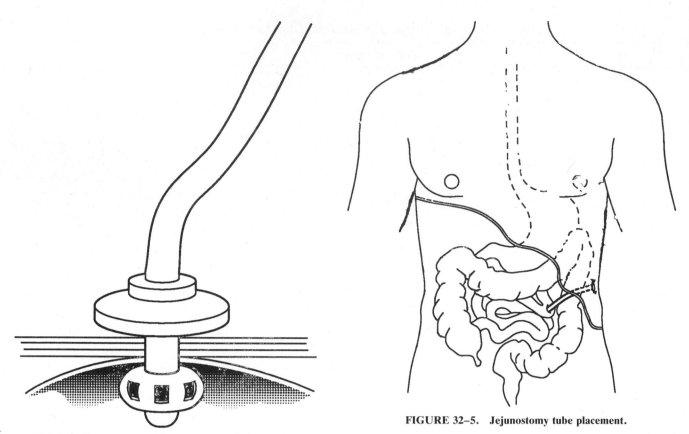

FIGURE 32–4. Percutaneous endoscopic gastrostomy.

FIGURE 32–5. Jejunostomy tube placement.

is placed on the end of the tube for attaching a feeding administration set. Previous gastric resections, tumors blocking passage of the endoscope, ascites, morbid obesity, and esophageal or gastric varices are contraindications for placement of a PEG tube.

The jejunostomy tube is indicated in those patients who are at increased risk of aspiration or who are unable to tolerate enteral feedings into the stomach. Unconscious patients or those patients without a gag reflex are at the greatest risk of aspiration. Early enteral feedings after surgery are promoted with the use of this tube. The jejunostomy tube bypasses the stomach, with the tip placed in the jejunum (Fig. 32–5). These tubes come in a variety of designs. The needle catheter jejunostomy is meant as a temporary access and is more prone to clogging because of the small lumen size of the catheter. A no. 10 to no. 16 French Foley catheter is frequently used for jejunostomy tubes, but the balloon should not be inflated because peristalsis may carry the tube further into the small bowel and cause an obstruction.

Silastic jejunostomy tubes are also available with Luer-Loc end connectors. All these tubes must be placed surgically, approaching through the abdominal wall and locating the tip of the catheter about 8 in (20 cm) distal to the ligament of Treitz in the jejunum. Because of tube placement in the small intestine, high-osmolality formulas may not be tolerated well if they are given in a bolus form. Tolerance is greatly enhanced by administering the formula via a pump. Close monitoring of the patient is necessary when enteral feedings are initiated

via a jejunostomy tube to determine the patient's tolerance.

Purpose

The nurse administers enteral nutrition via a gastrostomy, jejunostomy, or PEG tube to

1. Maintain a patient's nutritional status and body weight.
2. Provide long-term nutrition support while reducing a patient's risk of aspiration and nasal tissue necrosis.

Prerequisite Knowledge and Skills

Prior to administering enteral nutrition via a gastrostomy, jejunostomy, or PEG tube, the nurse should understand

1. Principles of clean technique.
2. Anatomy and physiology of the upper and lower gastrointestinal system.
3. Principles of digestion and absorption.

The nurse should be able to perform

1. Proper handwashing technique (see Skill 35–5).
2. Gastrointestinal assessment.
3. Respiratory assessment.

Assessment

1.   Assess the need for long-term enteral access as a result of the patient's inability to meet nutritional needs orally for at least 4 weeks. **Rationale:** To maintain patient's nutritional status and body weight.

2.   Observe the skin around jejunostomy, gastrostomy, or PEG tube for erythema, tenderness, or drainage. **Rationale:** Infection could develop at the tube insertion site or tract from the skin to the gastrointestinal tract.

3.   Assess the patency of the feeding tube for clogging from formula or medications administered via the tube. **Rationale:** Ensures that feeding will be delivered to the gastrointestinal tract and decreases risk of aspiration.

Nursing Diagnoses

1.   Alteration in nutrition: less than body requirements related to physiologic deficits. **Rationale:** Patient is unable to meet metabolic needs with oral diet for extended length of time.

2.   Potential for fluid volume deficit related to administration of hyperosmolar formulas. **Rationale:** Hyperosmolar formulas may cause osmotic diuresis leading to dehydration.

3.   Potential for aspiration related to decreased or absent gag reflex. **Rationale:** Gastric feedings may be vomited and aspirated by patient.

Planning

1.   Individualize the following goals for administering enteral nutrition via a gastrostomy, jejunostomy, or PEG tube:
   a.   Maintain fluid balance. **Rationale:** Administration of hyperosmolar formulas could lead to dehydration.
   b.   Provide nutritional requirements to meet metabolic needs. **Rationale:** Sepsis, burns, and trauma increase the metabolic rate, requiring additional calories and protein.

   c.   Maintain serum proteins within normal range (i.e., albumin 3.5 to 5.0 mg/dl, protein 6.0 to 8.0 mg/dl). **Rationale:** Adequate protein intake will protect visceral proteins, prevent muscle wasting, and assist in wound healing.
   d.   Protect the patient's airway. **Rationale:** Enteral feedings into the stomach may predispose a patient to aspiration.

2.   Prepare all necessary equipment and supplies. **Rationale:** Assembly of all equipment and supplies at the bedside ensures that enteral tube feeding will be initiated quickly and efficiently.
   a.   One enteral feeding bag and administration set (Some administration sets are preattached to the bag, while others have twist-on caps or spike into the feeding container. Enteral bag may be a flexible or semirigid container.)
   b.   One 60-ml Luer-slip tip syringe for Luer-end connector jejunostomy or PEG tube or one 60-ml catheter-tip syringe for gastrostomy or PEG tube.
   c.   One clean graduated measuring cup.
   d.   Blue food coloring or methylene blue, 5 cc (optional).
   e.   4 hours' volume of prescribed enteral formula.
   f.   One enteral feeding pump.
   g.   One roll of 1-in paper tape.
   h.   Dressing supplies:
      (1)   30 ml half-strength hydrogen peroxide
      (2)   60 ml tap water
      (3)   Two small clean basins
      (4)   Three cotton-tip applicators
      (5)   Two 4 × 4 gauze sponges
      (6)   One roll of 1-in hypoallergenic tape
      (7)   One 4 × 4 split gauze sponge
      (8)   One 60-ml catheter-tip syringe (optional).

3.   Prepare the patient.
   a.   Explain the procedure to patient. **Rationale:** Reduces anxiety and enhances the tolerance to enteral feeding.
   b.   Assist the patient into a comfortable position, usually a semi-Fowler's or high Fowler's position. **Rationale:** Improves tolerance of feeding and reduces risk of aspiration.

Implementation

Steps	Rationale	Special Considerations
1. Wash hands.	Reduces transmission of microorganisms.	
2. For administration of formula, see Skill 32–2.		
3. Perform dressing site care everyday and as needed:		
a. Pour 1 ounce of hydrogen peroxide into basin, and add an equal amount of water.	Reduces microorganisms on skin that may cause breakdown of skin or inflammation.	

Table continues on following page

Steps	Rationale	Special Considerations
b. Saturate distal end of a cotton tip applicator in hydrogen peroxide, and cleanse around feeding tube with applicator starting from tube insertion site outward in a circular pattern.	Half-strength hydrogen peroxide removes crusts that could harbor bacteria and break down skin.	For gastrostomy tubes with disks, cleanse under the disk with cotton applicator. Dry with 4 × 4 gauze. For PEG tubes, cleanse carefully under T-bar or bumper. Excessive pulling on flange in stomach causes pain and irritation to gastric mucosa.
c. Continue cleansing in the same manner as needed with remaining applicators saturated with hydrogen peroxide until crusts and drainage are removed.	Prevents infection and breakdown of skin.	May use povidone-iodine solution to cleanse skin if erythema or drainage is present.
d. Rinse insertion site with water by either pouring water from clean basin or irrigating with 60-ml catheter-tip syringe.	Removes hydrogen peroxide from skin, which may cause excessive drying or irritation if left in contact with skin.	
e. Dry site with sterile gauze.	Drying site reduces moisture, which could promote bacterial growth.	
4. Place split gauze dressing around tube over skin, and secure loosely with tape.	Loose dressing promotes air circulation to skin, reducing moisture at site. Dressing protects site from irritation from clothing.	*Do not* place gauze under bumper or disk of PEG tube, which would cause tension on flange in gastric mucosa.
5. Secure tube to patient's skin with a piece of tape at another site on abdomen.	Reduces tension on tube.	If no drainage is present around feeding tube, you may leave dressing off. *Do not* use occlusive dressing, since this prevents air circulation to skin.
6. Wash hands.	Reduces transmission of microorganisms.	

Evaluation

1. Monitor the patient's urine glucose level every 6 hours. Monitor the serum glucose level using a bedside glucose monitor for patients with consistently abnormal serum glucose levels. **Rationale:** High carbohydrate concentration of formula may exceed endogenous insulin supply. In hyperosmolar hyperglycemic nonketotic dehydration, patient will have glucosuria with an osmotic diuresis.

2. Weigh the patient daily, and compare with baseline weight. Note trends of weight gain/loss. Assess skin turgor every shift. **Rationale:** Dehydration can occur as a result of the use of hyperosmolar formulas, patient's fluid losses, and inadequate water intake. Overhydration can occur in the patient with cardiac, hepatic, or renal failure. Fluid needs are increased in the patient with an elevated temperature.

3. Monitor the patient's intake and output carefully. Quantitate diarrheal stool output. Observe for decreased or increased urine output. A stool culture should be obtained with persistent diarrhea to rule out pseudomembranous colitis due to *Clostridium difficile* toxin. **Rationale:** Diarrhea can occur as a result of the use of hyperosmolar formulas, lactose intolerance, prolonged use of antibiotics, bacterial contamination of formulas, severe hypoalbuminemia (<2.5 mg/dl), or medications resulting in dehydration.

4. Assess the medication profile of the patient for a potential cause or relationship to persistent diarrhea. **Rationale:** Osmolality of medications may cause diarrhea. Antibiotics cause bacterial overgrowth in gastrointestinal tract, resulting in diarrhea. Medications in elixir form (e.g., theophylline, acetaminophen) contain large amounts of sorbitol, which has a strong cathartic action.

5. Monitor the frequency and amount of diarrhea, and administer antidiarrheals as indicated, using a non-narcotic antidiarrheal or a bulk-forming agent. **Rationale:** Control of diarrhea will prevent dehydration and improve absorption of nutrients.

6. Auscultate the patient's bowel sounds every 8 hours for motility. **Rationale:** Gastrointestinal function will affect the patient's tolerance to enteral feedings.

7. Aspirate the gastric residuals every 4 hours on a tube placed in the stomach. If the residual is more than 125 to 150 cc, hold feeding for 1 hour and recheck residual. If residual remains elevated, notify physician. Patient may be placed on metoclopramide 10 mg q.i.d. to increase gastrointestinal motility. **Rationale:** Residuals greater than 150 cc indicate decreased gastric motility and/or emptying. Continued feeding with high residuals increases the risk of vomiting and aspiration. Residuals

may be increased because of formula intolerance, indicating the need for evaluation of the formula and perhaps a change to an isotonic or elemental formula.

8. Hold the feeding for 30 to 60 minutes prior to the patient having a procedure requiring the supine position. **Rationale:** Decreases risk of aspiration.

Expected Outcomes

1. Maintenance of baseline weight or weight gain of ½ to 1 lb per week in the nonobese patient. **Rationale:** Indicates adequate caloric intake.

2. Maintenance or elevation of visceral proteins (prealbumin), improved wound healing, maintenance of muscle mass, and positive nitrogen balance. **Rationale:** Indicates adequate protein intake to meet protein needs.

3. Fluid balance stable, as evidenced by serum sodium within normal limits, absence of diarrhea, and balanced or slightly positive fluid intake. **Rationale:** Fluid needs being met without excessive losses.

Unexpected Outcomes (See Table 32–3)

1. Intolerance of tube feeding, as evidenced by nausea, vomiting, diarrhea, abdominal distension, and high gastric residuals. **Rationale:** Patient's tolerance is related to disease, osmolality of formula, rate of infusion, type of formula, decreased gastric emptying, and tube position.

2. Aspiration, as evidenced by suctioning of blue secretions from trachea. **Rationale:** Decreased gag reflex and supine position and high gastric residuals increase the risk of aspiration.

3. Dehydration, as evidenced by negative fluid balance, poor skin turgor, furrowed tongue, dry oral mucosa, and elevated serum sodium and blood urea nitrogen. **Rationale:** Use of hyperosmolar formulas, inadequate administration of additional water, and patient fluid losses will cause dehydration.

4. Hyperosmolar hyperglycemic nonketotic dehydration, as evidenced by elevated serum glucose (>600 mg/dl), osmotic diuresis, and lethargy or coma. **Rationale:** Use of hyperosmolar formulas and inadequate fluid intake cause osmotic diuresis leading to severe dehydration.

5. Clogged feeding tube, as evidenced by occlusion alarm on enteral pump, inability to flush tube with water-filled syringe, and inability to aspirate from tube. **Rationale:** Enteral formula or medications administered via feeding tube occlude internal lumen or opening orifice of tube, prohibiting infusion or aspiration via tube.

6. Tube dislodgment and/or malposition, as evidenced by tube removed from stoma, tube length from stoma shorter, distended abdomen, and high-pitched bowel sounds indicating obstruction. **Rationale:** Feeding tubes with balloons inflated can float into gastric outlet, or with jejunal tubes, block the lumen of the small bowel, causing a gastric outlet or small bowel obstruction. Three to four weeks after placement, gastrostomy or jejunostomy tubes can be replaced at bedside.

7. Persistent elevated glucose level, as evidenced by a serum glucose greater than 200 mg/dl. **Rationale:** High

carbohydrate content of formula may not be tolerated because of low levels of endogenous insulin.

8. Diarrhea, as evidenced by four or more loose or liquid stools per day. **Rationale:** Prolonged use of antibiotics, medications with high sorbitol content, high osmolality of enteral formula, and presence of *Clostridium difficile* toxin may result in diarrhea.

9. Drainage, pus, erythema, and tenderness at catheter insertion site. **Rationale:** Invasive catheter is site for bacterial growth.

Documentation

Documentation in the patient record should include the date and time the feeding was initiated; gastrointestinal assessment; volume of gastric residuals, strength of formula; volume of formula infused; presence or absence of cramping, nausea, vomiting, diarrhea, and/or abdominal distension; condition of catheter insertion site, including presence or absence of tenderness, drainage, and erythema; results of urine glucose tests; intake and output; daily weight; blood glucose level; number of stools/amount of diarrhea; bowel sounds assessment; amount of gastric residuals, condition of oral cavity and times mouth care is provided; amount of free water instilled; and any unexpected outcomes and interventions taken. **Rationale:** Documents nursing care given, tolerance to feedings, expected and unexpected outcomes, and interventions taken.

Patient/Family Education

1. Assess the patient and family for readiness to learn enteral feeding procedures. **Rationale:** Psychomotor and cognitive impairment may delay teaching.

2. Describe the steps for initiating/discontinuing enteral feedings, and encourage patient and family questions. **Rationale:** Reduces anxiety and promotes understanding of treatment regimen.

3. Instruct the patient and family to report signs and symptoms of intolerance to enteral feedings (i.e., abdominal cramping, abdominal fullness, and nausea). **Rationale:** Indicates intolerance to rate of infusion or type of formula and decreased patient comfort.

4. Evaluate the need for home enteral nutritional support. **Rationale:** Provides time for patient and family to learn procedures and/or explore discharge options.

5. Initiate a consultation with a nutritional support nurse (if available). **Rationale:** Further assessment and discharge planning related to enteral feedings are needed to determine formula, schedule, equipment, and learning needs.

6. If the patient is to be discharged with enteral feedings, initiate teaching plan for home enteral nutrition. **Rationale:** Meeting the patient's and family's learning needs allays anxiety and facilitates transition from hospital to home care.

Performance Checklist
Skill 32–3:   Jejunostomy, Gastrostomy, and Percutaneous Endoscopic Gastrostomy Tubes

Critical Behaviors	Complies yes	no
1. Wash hands.		
2. For administration of formula, see Skill 32–2.		
3. Perform dressing site care: a. Prepare half-strength hydrogen peroxide. b. Using saturated cotton tip applicator, cleanse around feeding tube. c. Continue cleansing as needed until crusts and drainage are removed. d. Rinse hydrogen peroxide from skin. e. Dry skin thoroughly.		
4. Apply dry, sterile nonocclusive dressing.		
5. Secure tube to skin.		
6. Wash hands.		
7. Document procedure in the patient record.		

BIBLIOGRAPHY

Altman, E., and Cutie, A. J. (1984). Compatibility of enteral products with commonly employed drug additives. *Nutrition Support Services* 4:8–17.

Bowman, M., Eisenberg, P., Katz, B., and Metheny, N. (1988). Effect of tube-feeding osmolality on serum sodium levels. *Crit. Care Nurs.* 9(1):22–28.

Caswell, C. S. (1988). Confirmation of feeding-tube placement complications. *Nutritional Support Services* 8(7):7–8.

Cerra, F. B., Shronts, E. P., Raup, S., and Konstantinides, N. (1989). Enteral nutrition in hypermetabolic surgical patients. *Crit. Care Med.* 17(7):619–662.

Curtas, S. (1988). In C. Kennedy-Caldwell and P. Guenter (Eds.), *Nutrition Support Nursing: Core Curriculum* (pp. 29–42). Silver Spring, Md.: American Society for Parenteral and Enteral Nutrition.

Edes, T. E., Walk, B. E., and Austin, J. L. (1990). Diarrhea in tube-fed patients: Feeding formula not necessarily the cause. *Am. J. Med.* 88(2):91–93.

Flynn, K. T., Norton, L. C., and Fisher, R. L. (1987). Enteral tube feeding: Indications, practices and outcomes. *Image* 19(1):16–19.

Forlaw, L. Enteral Nutrition. In C. Kennedy-Caldwell and P. Guenter (Eds.), (1988). *Nutrition Support for Parenteral and Enteral Nutrition: Core Curriculum* (pp. 457–484). Silver Spring, Md.: American Society for Parenteral and Enteral Nutrition.

Fox, A. D., Kripke, S. A., DePaula, J. et al. (1988). Effect of a glutamine-supplemented enteral diet on methotrexate-induced enterocolitis. *J. Parenter. Enter. Nutr.* 12(4):325–331.

Gottschlich, M. M., Warden, G. D., Michel, M., et al. (1988). Diarrhea in tube-fed burn patients: Incidence, etiology, nutritional impact, and prevention. *J. Parenter. Enter. Nutr.* 12(4):338–345.

Hansen, B. C. (1984). Feeding Methods and Gastrointestinal Function. In J.L. Rombeau and M.D. Caldwell (Eds.), *Enteral and Tube Feeding* (pp. 253–260). Philadelphia: Saunders.

Heymsfield, S. B., Hoff, R. D., Gray, T. F., et al. (1988). In J.M. Kinney, K.N. Jeejeebhoy, G. L. Hill, and O. E. Owen (Eds.), *Nutrition and Metabolism in Patient Care* (pp. 477–509). Philadelphia: Saunders.

Irwin, M. M., and Openbrier, D. R. A delicate balance: Strategies for feeding ventilated COPD patients. *Am. J. Nurs.* 85(3):275–280.

Jones, T. N., Moore, F. A., Moore, E. E., and McCroskey, B. L. (1989). Gastrointestinal symptoms attributed to jejunostomy feeding after major abdominal trauma: A critical analysis. *Crit. Care Med.* 17(11):1146–1150.

Kalfarentzos, F., Alivizatos, V., Kostas, P., and Androulakis, J. (1987). Nasoduodenal intubation with the use of metoclopramide. *Nutritional Support Services* 7(9):33–34.

Marcuard, S. P., and Perkins, A. M. Clogging of feeding tubes. *J. Parenter. Enter. Nutr.* 12(4):403–405.

Metheny, N., Eisenberg, P., and McSweeney, M. (1988). Effect of feeding tube properties and three irrigants on clogging rates. *Nurs. Res.* 37(3):165–169.

Petrosino, B. M., Meraviglia, M., and Becker, H. (1988). Mechanical problems with small-diameter enteral feeding tubes. *J. Neurosci. Nurs.* 19(5):15–22.

Rombeau, J. L. (1989). Manual Placement of Nasoenteric Tube. In J. L. Rombeau, M. D. Caldwell, L. Forlaw, and P. A. Guenter (Eds.), *Atlas of Nutritional Support Techniques* (pp. 81–84). Boston: Little, Brown.

Smith, C. E., Marian, L., Brogdon, C., et al. (1990). Diarrhea associated with tube feeding in mechanically ventilated critically ill patients. *Nurs. Res.* 39(3):149–152.

Souba, W. W. (1988). The gut as a nitrogen-processing organ in the metabolic response to critical illness. *Nutritional Support Services* 8(5):15–22.

Wilson, M. F., and Haynes-Johnson, V. Cranberry or water? A comparison of feeding-tube irrigants. *Nutritional Support Services* 7(7):23–24.

UNIT X

![gray bars]

PHARMACO-THERAPEUTICS

33

BEHAVIORAL OBJECTIVES

After completing this chapter, the nurse will be able to

- Define the key terms.
- Describe infusion devices and techniques for administration of intravenous pharmacotherapy.
- Discuss indications for using an intravenous infusion device or a specific technique for medication administration.
- Demonstrate the skills involved in using infusion devices.
- Formulate a teaching plan for the patient receiving patient-controlled analgesia.

INFUSION DEVICES AND TECHNIQUES FOR ADMINISTRATION

Patients in the critical care unit commonly require infusions of vasoactive agents, antiarrhythmic drugs, and other potent medications as part of their plan of care. A continuous infusion at the prescribed rate of flow must be ensured to achieve the desired therapeutic effect and to prevent serious sequelae from an inconsistent or incorrect administration rate. Gravity infusions with a roller clamp often provide an uncertain and inconsistent rate of flow. Thus a number of infusion devices and techniques have been developed to safely administer pharmacotherapy, and this chapter addresses such administration techniques.

KEY TERMS

bolus	IVBP (intravenous
Buretrol	piggyback)
delay	PCA dose
IV push (intravenous	primary tubing
push)	

SKILLS

33–1 Buretrol Administration
33–2 Bolus Administration
33–3 Gravity-Controlled Infusion Device
33–4 Volume-Controlled Infusion Device
33–5 Patient-Controlled Analgesia Device

GUIDELINES

The following assessment guidelines assist the nurse in formulating a nursing diagnosis and an individualized plan of care to administer pharmacotherapy:

1. Know the patient's baseline respiratory assessment.
2. Know the patient's baseline cardiovascular profile.
3. Know the patient's medical history.
4. Identify the patient's drug allergies and sensitivities.
5. Know the patient's baseline vital signs.
6. Become adept with equipment and techniques used to administer intravenous therapy and medications.

SKILL 33–1

Buretrol Administration

Administration of intravenous fluid and medications with a Buretrol administration set provides an accurate accounting of the volume infused and prevents inadvertent administration of large volumes of intravenous fluid. Buretrol administration of medications and intravenous fluid is frequently utilized for antibiotics, loading doses of bronchodilator and vasoactive agents, antifibrinolytic agents, and electrolyte boluses. Generally, patients requiring fluid restriction and all pediatric patients will receive intravenous therapy and medications via a Buretrol administration set.

Purpose

The nurse utilizes a Buretrol administration set to

1. Accurately measure intravenous fluid for administration.
2. Infuse medications.
3. Infuse small volumes of intravenous fluid.

Prerequisite Knowledge and Skills

Prior to assembling a Buretrol administration set, the nurse should understand

1. Principles of aseptic technique.
2. Principles of intravenous therapy.
3. Principles of medication administration.
4. Principles of fluid balance.

The nurse should be able to perform

1. Proper handwashing technique (see Skill 35–5).
2. Respiratory system assessment.
3. Cardiovascular system assessment.
4. Assessment of fluid balance status.

Assessment

1. Assess the patient's fluid status, including heart rate, blood pressure, urine output, filling pressures (central venous pressure, pulmonary artery pressure, pulmonary capillary wedge pressure), breath sounds, serum electrolytes, hematocrit, daily weights, and intake and output. **Rationale:** Infusion of intravenous fluids and medications will affect the patient's fluid balance and hemodynamic status.

2. Monitor the patient's pulmonary artery pressure and pulmonary capillary wedge pressure during fluid administration. **Rationale:** Increases in the pulmonary artery pressure and pulmonary capillary wedge pressure may be the first indicators of fluid overload.

Nursing Diagnoses

1. Potential for fluid volume excess related to labile cardiovascular status and/or rapid administration of intravenous fluids. **Rationale:** Patients receiving intravenous therapy and medications via a Buretrol administration set may tolerate minimal amounts of fluid.
2. Potential for injury related to inappropriate administration of intravenous fluids. **Rationale:** Medications administered too rapidly may cause the patient to develop undesirable side effects.

Planning

1. Individualize the following goals for administering intravenous therapy and medications via a Buretrol administration set:
   a. Maintain fluid balance. **Rationale:** Buretrol administration set allows for accurate administration of fluid volumes.
   b. Provide route for medication administration. **Rationale:** Medications may be administered via the Buretrol administration set when the maintenance intravenous infusion should not be interrupted.
2. Prepare all necessary equipment and supplies. **Rationale:** Assembly of all the necessary equipment and supplies ensures that the Buretrol administration of intravenous fluids and medications will be accomplished quickly and efficiently.
   a. Intravenous fluid (prescribed by physician).
   b. Buretrol administration set.
   c. One sterile 19-gauge needle.
   d. One alcohol prep.
   e. One roll of 2-in paper tape.
   f. Syringe with medication for infusion (if applicable).
3. Prepare the patient by explaining the procedure. **Rationale:** Enhances patient cooperation and reduces anxiety.

Implementation

Steps	Rationale	Special Considerations
1. Wash hands.	Reduces transmission of microorganisms.	

Table continues on following page

Steps	Rationale	Special Considerations
2. Verify physician prescription for intravenous fluid and/or medication for administration.	Prevents errors in intravenous fluid and/or medication administration.	Intravenous fluids: Note type, amount, and duration of infusion. Medications: Note drug, dose, amount of fluid in which drug should be administered, and duration of infusion.
3. Insert tubing spike into intravenous fluid bag/bottle.	Accesses Buretrol administration set to fluid or medication source.	Maintain aseptic technique.
4. Open vent and main clamp between Buretrol administration set and tubing spike, and allow fluid to fill chamber of Buretrol administration set with the desired amount of fluid. Then close the clamp.	Fills Buretrol set with intravenous fluid.	
5. Gently squeeze the drip chamber.	Opens diaphragm.	Aggressive squeezing of Buretrol administration set may cause the diaphragm to rupture. The diaphragm will close when the chamber is emptied.
6. Prime tubing. *Do not* remove cap from end of tubing.	Eliminates air from tubing while maintaining aseptic technique. Prevents patient from receiving an air bolus.	
7. Remove cap from tubing, and attach sterile needle. If the primary intravenous solution is to be administered with a Buretrol administration set, remove the cap and connect directly to the catheter hub.	Allows for connection to primary intravenous line.	Pediatric patients and adult patients with rigid fluid restrictions commonly receive their primary intravenous infusion via the Buretrol administration set.
8. For medication administration:		
a. Cleanse injection site with alcohol prep.	Reduces transmission of microorganisms.	
b. Inject medication through injection site into prescribed amount of fluid within the Buretrol administration set.	Dilutes medication for administration.	
c. Label Buretrol administration set with name and dose of medication.	Safety precaution.	
d. Cleanse Y-port injection site on primary intravenous tubing, and insert needle attached to Buretrol administration set.	Allows medication to be administered without interruption of primary intravenous infusion.	
9. Secure needle insertion site with paper tape.	Prevents accidental disconnection.	
10. Adjust roller clamp to prescribed rate.	Fluid will be administered within prescribed time period.	When determining flow rate, consider the drop factor of the administration set. Buretrol administration sets usually deliver microdrops: 60 gtts/cc.
11. Wash hands.	Reduces transmission of microorganisms.	

Evaluation

1. Monitor the patient's vital signs as patient's condition dictates, including blood pressure, heart rate, respiratory rate, urine output, and hemodynamic pressure (if a Swan-Ganz or central venous catheter is placed). **Rationale:** Intravenous fluids or medications may need to be titrated based on patient's response.

2. Monitor the patient's intake and output as patient's condition dictates. **Rationale:** Intravenous fluids/medications may need to be increased/decreased based on hourly intake and output balance.

3. Assess the patient for desired response to pharmacologic agents. **Rationale:** Intravenous administration of medications effects a rapid response.

4. Monitor the patient's electrolyte values as prescribed or as needed based on the patient's condition. **Rationale:** Intravenous fluid and medication administration will affect electrolyte balance.

Expected Outcomes

1. Patient will achieve/maintain fluid and electrolyte balance. **Rationale:** Achieves homeostasis.

2. Patient will achieve desired effects of medication being administered. **Rationale:** Intravenous medication administration usually achieves an immediate response when compared with other routes of administration.

Unexpected Outcomes

1. Fluid and/or medication will not infuse. **Rationale:** Aggressive squeezing of the drip chamber has ruptured the diaphragm. The Buretrol administration set will need to be replaced.

2. Patient receives too rapid infusion of intravenous solution and/or medication resulting in signs and symptoms of fluid overload and/or untoward side effects of drug. **Rationale:** Incorrect calculation of the drip rate will allow rapid infusion of fluid and/or medication.

Documentation

Documentation in the patient record should include the type and amount of intravenous solution infused; the duration of the infusion; the name, dose, and time of medication administered; the patient's response to fluid/medication administration; actions taken in the event of signs/symptoms of fluid overload or undesirable side effects of the drug; and changes in electrolyte values secondary to fluid/medication administration. Check your institution's policies/procedures for documenting intravenous therapy and medication administration. **Rationale:** Documents nursing care given, expected and unexpected outcomes, and interventions taken.

Patient/Family Education

1. Explain the rationale for fluid administration via the Buretrol administration set. **Rationale:** Decreases patient/family anxiety.

2. Explain the medication(s) to be administered, focusing on the expected action and potential side effects. **Rationale:** Encourages the patient and family to ask questions and participate in the treatment plan.

Performance Checklist
Skill 33–1:   Buretrol Administration

Critical Behaviors	Complies	
	yes	no
1. Wash hands.		
2. Verify physician order for intravenous fluids/medications.		
3. Insert tubing spike into IV fluid bag or bottle.		
4. Accurately fill Buretrol chamber.		
5. Gently squeeze the drip chamber.		
6. Prime the IV tubing.		
7. For primary IV solution administration, remove cap from set and connect directly to catheter.		
8. For medication administration		
a. Cleanse injection site with alcohol prep.		
b. Inject medication through site into prescribed amount of fluid in set.		
c. Label set with name and dose of medication.		
d. Cleanse Y-port injection site on tubing, and insert needle attached to set.		
9. Secure connection site with tape.		

Table continues on following page

Critical Behaviors	Complies	
	yes	no
10. Accurately adjust the flow with roller clamp.		
11. Wash hands.		
12. Document procedure in the patient record.		

SKILL 33–2

Bolus Administration

Bolus administration refers to the infusion of intravenous fluids and/or medications usually over a short period of time. In an effort to expand intravascular volume, it is common to administer a *bolus* of 250 to 500 cc of crystalloid or colloid solutions over a 20- to 30-minute period. Should the patient fail to respond to the fluid challenge, either a second bolus is administered to correct the fluid-depleted state or other causes of the hypovolemia are determined.

Loading doses of medications are given as a *bolus*, meaning IV push, to push the medication contained in a syringe directly into the primary infusion over a recommended period of time. This is commonly done in the treatment of cardiac dysrhythmias and in cardiopulmonary resuscitation.

Supplemental doses of electrolytes are also administered as a *bolus* to correct electrolyte imbalances. The electrolyte is diluted in a prescribed amount of fluid and administered over a specified time interval. The more common electrolytes to be administered as a bolus are potassium chloride, potassium phosphate, magnesium sulfate, calcium gluconate, and calcium chloride.

Most critical care units have policies and protocols for bolus administration. Be aware that *bolus* has different interpretations with regard to fluids, antidysrhythmic agents, electrolytes, and other medications to be administered.

Purpose

The nurse utilizes bolus administration to

1. Provide fluid resuscitation to the volume-depleted patient.
2. Provide a loading dose of a medication.
3. Deliver a supplemental dose of an electrolyte.

Prerequisite Knowledge and Skills

Prior to utilizing bolus administration, the nurse should understand

1. Principles of intravenous therapy.
2. Principles of fluid and electrolyte balance.
3. Principles of medication administration.
4. Principles of aseptic technique.

The nurse should be able to perform

1. Vital signs assessment.
2. Assessment of fluid balance and electrolyte status.
3. Proper handwashing technique (see Skill 35–5).
4. Cardiovascular system assessment.
5. Respiratory system assessment.

Assessment

1. Observe the patient for signs of fluid volume deficit, including decreased blood pressure, tachycardia, decreased filling pressures (central venous pressure, pulmonary artery pressures, and pulmonary capillary wedge pressure), decreased cardiac output, and decreased urine output. **Rationale:** Fluid volume deficit results in signs and symptoms of a decreased circulating volume.
2. Monitor the patient's cardiac rhythm and rate for disturbances. **Rationale:** The first dose of an antidysrhythmic drug is commonly given as a bolus followed by a continuous infusion.
3. Assess the patient's electrolyte status. **Rationale:** Electrolyte imbalances are treated with bolus administration of supplementation.
4. Verify the patency of the venous catheter. **Rationale:** Bolus administration is usually "piggybacked" into an existing intravenous line.

Nursing Diagnoses

1. Fluid volume deficit related to a decreased circulating volume. **Rationale:** Decreased circulating volume may occur secondary to hemorrhage, "third spacing," sepsis, or cardiogenic shock.
2. Decreased cardiac output related to inadequate fluid resuscitation/administration. **Rationale:** Inadequate circulating volume, pump failure, congestive heart failure, dysrhythmias, etc. contribute to a decreased cardiac output.
3. Potential for injury related to electrolyte imbalance. **Rationale:** Electrolyte imbalances may cause dysrhythmias/cardiac standstill.

Planning

1. Individualize the following goals for performing

bolus administration of intravenous fluids and/or medications:
   a. Expand intravascular volume. **Rationale:** Volume-depleted patients require fluid replacement for resuscitation.
   b. Replenish electrolyte losses. **Rationale:** Electrolyte balance is required for proper functioning of all body systems.
   c. **Provide a loading dose of a medication. Rationale:** Required to establish a therapeutic blood level, followed by a continuous infusion.
2. Prepare all necessary equipment and supplies. **Rationale:** Assembly of all necessary equipment and supplies at the bedside ensures that the bolus of fluid and/or medication will be accomplished quickly and efficiently.

   a. Intravenous fluid (if applicable).
   b. Medication (if applicable).
   c. Buretrol administration set (for electrolyte replacement).
   d. Two alcohol preps.
   e. One 19-gauge, $1\frac{1}{2}$-in needle.
   f. One syringe (appropriate size for medication bolus).
   g. One roll of 1-in paper tape.
3. Prepare the patient by explaining the procedure and the rationale for administering the prescribed fluid/medication/electrolyte. **Rationale:** Decreases patient and family anxiety.

Implementation

Steps	Rationale	Special Considerations
For Fluid Bolus		
1. Wash hands.	Reduces transmission of microorganisms.	
2. Verify physician order for fluid bolus.	Reduces the possibility of error in fluid administration.	Physician order should include the patient's name, type and amount of intravenous solution, and duration of infusion.
3. Assemble intravenous solution and tubing, and prime the tubing.	Eliminates possibility of patient receiving an air emboli.	Maintain aseptic technique.
4. Connect needle to distal end of intravenous tubing.	Large-bore needle facilitates rapid infusion of intravenous fluid.	Maintain aseptic technique.
5. Cleanse Y-port on the primary infusion tubing with an alcohol prep.	Reduces transmission of microorganisms.	Y-port should be the one most proximal to the venous catheter insertion site.
6. Insert needle into Y-port, and tape connection.	Allows for infusion of fluid bolus. Prevents accidental disconnection.	Maintain aseptic technique.
7. Adjust roller clamp to infuse fluid bolus within prescribed period of time.	Corrects fluid deficit.	
8. Monitor vital signs as patient condition dictates.	Validates efficacy of fluid administration.	Monitor heart rate, blood pressure, urine output, filling pressures (CVP, PAP, PCWP), and breath sounds.
For Bolus Medication Administration		
1. Wash hands.	Reduces transmission of microorganisms.	
2. Verify physician order for medication to be administered as a bolus.	Reduces possibility of medication error.	Physician order should be *written* and include name of the patient, name of drug, dose, and duration of infusion. In emergency situations, verify the drug and dose upon receipt of the verbal order and a second time before administering the medication.
3. Draw up medication in appropriate size syringe, and label syringe with name and dose of drug.	Prepares medication for instillation. Reduces possibility of medication error.	Be aware of which medications *may not* be given as a bolus (IV push).

Table continues on following page

Steps	Rationale	Special Considerations
4. Verify physician order again before IV push administration.	Reduces possibility of medication error.	
5. Cleanse Y-port on primary intravenous tubing most proximal to venous catheter insertion site with an alcohol prep.	Reduces transmission of microorganisms.	The most proximal Y-port is selected to allow medication to enter the bloodstream quickly and also reduces the possibility of drug incompatibilities within the tubing.
6. Insert needle into Y-port, inject medication over the recommended period of time.	Corrects underlying physiologic instabilities.	Know the recommended period of time for administration of all emergency medications. Be familiar with your unit's policies and protocols regarding IV push or bolus administration of medications.
7. Monitor vital signs as the patient's condition dictates.	Most medications given as a bolus have serious side effects that require continuous monitoring.	Monitor heart rate/rhythm, blood pressure, filling pressures (CVP, PAP, PCWP), and other indicators of physiologic imbalance being treated.
8. Wash hands.	Reduces transmission of microorganisms.	

For Electrolyte Replacement

Steps	Rationale	Special Considerations
1. Wash hands.	Reduces transmission of microorganisms.	
2. Verify physician order for electrolyte replacement.	Reduces possibility of medication error.	Physician order should include patient's name, name and dose of electrolyte to be administered, the amount and type of intravenous fluid for dilution, and the duration of the infusion.
3. Assemble Buretrol administration set, and prime the tubing (see Skill 33–1).	Electrolyte supplementation is *never* administered by IV push but is infused over a specified period of time.	Maintain aseptic technique. Make certain the Buretrol administration set is equipped with a microdrop infusion and contains the amount of fluid prescribed for dilution.
4. Attach needle to the administration set.	Provides for infusion of electrolyte.	Maintain aseptic technique.
5. Cleanse Y-port on the primary tubing proximal to venous catheter insertion site with an alcohol prep.	Reduces transmission of microorganisms.	Electrolyte boluses can be very irritating to the vein.
6. Insert needle into Y-port, tape the connection, and keep the roller clamp in the closed position.	Administration set is now ready for infusion.	Infusion should not be initiated until electrolyte replacement is instilled into the Buretrol chamber.
7. Cleanse the injection port of Buretrol administration set with an alcohol prep.	Reduces transmission of microorganisms.	
8. Inject the prescribed amount of electrolyte replacement into the Buretrol.	Dilutes electrolyte replacement for infusion.	Electrolyte replacements *must always* be diluted prior to administration.
9. Adjust the roller clamp to allow infusion over the prescribed period of time.	Rapid administration of electrolytes can lead to cardiac dysrhythmias and/or cardiac standstill.	Know your unit's policies and protocols for electrolyte replacement as a bolus.
10. Monitor vital signs as patient's condition dictates.	Detects side effects of replacement therapy.	Be familiar with the side effects of the electrolyte being administered. Monitor cardiac rate and rhythm (see Skill 7–1).

Table continues on following page

Steps	Rationale	Special Considerations
11. Wash hands.	Reduces transmission of microorganisms.	

Evaluation

1. Monitor the patient's vital signs every hour or as needed, including blood pressure, heart rate, respiratory rate, urine output, and hemodynamic pressures (if a Swan-Ganz or central venous catheter is placed). **Rationale:** Intravenous fluids or medications may need to be titrated based on patient's response.

2. Monitor the patient's intake and output every hour or as needed. **Rationale:** Intravenous fluids/medications may need to be increased/decreased based on intake and output balance.

3. Assess the patient for desired response to intravenous fluid administration/pharmacologic agents. **Rationale:** Intravenous administration of medications effects a rapid response.

4. Monitor the patient's electrolyte values as prescribed or as needed based on the patient's condition. **Rationale:** Intravenous fluid and medication administration will affect electrolyte balance.

Expected Outcomes

1. Hemodynamic parameters will return to patient's baseline. **Rationale:** With adequate fluid resuscitation, patient's vital signs and urine output should be life-sustaining.

2. Electrolyte values will be within normal limits. **Rationale:** Patients with intra- and extracellular electrolyte depletion may require several boluses before serum electrolyte concentrations are replenished.

3. Medication bolus resolves physiologic instability. **Rationale:** Most medications given by IV push are administered in life-threatening situations. Common exceptions are narcotics, paralyzing agents, and sedatives.

Unexpected Outcomes

1. Vital signs do not return to baseline or life-sustaining parameters. **Rationale:** Hemodynamic instability is caused by something other than or in addition to a fluid volume deficit.

2. Serum electrolyte values do not return to normal. **Rationale:** Ascertain that laboratory report is not spurious. Additional bolusing may be required in the presence of total body depletion.

3. Patient experiences serious side effects of IV push medication administration. **Rationale:** Administration may have been infused too rapidly; the patient may be sensitive to the drug. Prepare to administer appropriate antidote.

Documentation

Documentation in the patient record should include the type, dose, and the amount of solution for dilution (for electrolyte replacement) of fluid/drug/electrolyte bolus, the duration of the infusion, the patient's response to the bolus, and any untoward side effects manifested and actions taken. If the physician order has been given verbally, make *certain* the order is *written and signed* by the prescribing physician. **Rationale:** Documents nursing care given, expected and unexpected outcomes, and interventions taken.

Patient/Family Education

1. Explain the rationale for bolus administration of fluid, medication, or electrolyte to both patient and family. **Rationale:** Decreases patient and family anxiety.

2. Provide an opportunity for patient and family to ask questions about medications and physiologic status. **Rationale:** Responds to patient and family fears and possible misperceptions of patient's status.

Performance Checklist
Skill 33–2: Bolus Administration

Critical Behaviors	Complies	
	yes	no
FOR FLUID BOLUS 1. Wash hands.		
2. Verify physician order.		
3. Assemble and prime IV administration set.		
4. Connect needle to distal end of IV tubing.		
5. Cleanse Y-port on primary infusion line.		
6. Connect fluid bolus line into primary infusion line, and tape connection.		

Table continues on following page

Critical Behaviors	Complies	
	yes	**no**
7. Adjust roller clamp to desired rate.		
8. Monitor vital signs.		
9. Wash hands.		
10. Document in the patient record.		
FOR BOLUS MEDICATION ADMINISTRATION 1. Wash hands.		
2. Verify physician order.		
3. Draw up medication in syringe, and label syringe with name and dose of drug.		
4. Verify physician order again before IV push.		
5. Cleanse Y-port on primary IV tubing proximal to venous catheter insertion site.		
6. Insert needle into Y-port, inject medication over recommended/prescribed period of time.		
7. Monitor vital signs.		
8. Wash hands.		
9. Document in the patient record.		
FOR ELECTROLYTE REPLACEMENT 1. Wash hands.		
2. Verify physician order.		
3. Assemble and prime Buretrol administration set.		
4. Attach needle to administration set.		
5. Cleanse Y-port on primary tubing proximal to venous catheter insertion site.		
6. Insert needle into Y-port, tape the connection, and keep roller clamp closed.		
7. Cleanse the injection port of the Buretrol set.		
8. Inject the prescribed amount of electrolyte into set.		
9. Adjust the roller clamp to desired rate.		
10. Monitor vital signs.		
11. Wash hands.		
12. Document in the patient record.		

SKILL 33–3

Gravity-Controlled Infusion Device

A gravity-controlled infusion device ensures the rate of flow by the counting of drops by a drop sensor. Flow of fluid will cease and an alarm will sound when an infusion is complete or when the selected rate of infusion cannot be maintained. Table 33–1 lists some commonly used gravity-controlled infusion devices.

TABLE 33–1   BRAND NAMES OF GRAVITY-CONTROLLED INFUSION DEVICES

Critikon Rateminder IV
Gemini PC-1
Gemini PC-2 (dual chamber)
IVAC 230 Drop Counting Controller
IVAC Volumetric Controller Model 260i
IVAC Site Saver Volumetric Controller Model 280/280+

Purpose

The nurse uses a gravity-controlled infusion device to
1. Ensure an accurate flow of fluid.
2. Accurately administer fluids when an infusion control device using positive pressure is contraindicated.

Prerequisite Knowledge and Skills

Prior to using a gravity-controlled infusion device, the nurse should understand
1. Principles of gravity infusion.
2. Principles of intravenous therapy.
3. Principles of aseptic technique.
4. Principles of fluid balance.

The nurse should be able to perform
1. Proper handwashing technique (see Skill 35–5).
2. Universal precautions (see Skill 35–1).
3. Vital signs assessment.
4. Hemodynamic assessment.
5. Assessment of the vascular access site.

Assessment

1. Identify indications for using a gravity-controlled infusion device. **Rationale:** Certain medications and/or intravenous therapies must have their rate of flow delivered in a consistent, accurate manner to avoid life-threatening consequences.
2. Assess the patient's fluid status, including heart rate, blood pressure, urine output, breath sounds, serum electrolytes, hematocrit, daily weights, and intake and output records. **Rationale:** Infusion of intravenous fluids and medications will affect the patient's fluid balance and hemodynamic status.
3. Assess the patient's artery pressures and pulmonary capillary wedge pressure during fluid administration. **Rationale:** Increases in the pulmonary artery pressures and pulmonary capillary wedge pressure may be the first indicators of fluid status changes.
4. Assess the venous catheter for patency and signs and symptoms of infiltration and/or phlebitis. **Rationale:** Ensures administration of fluid intravenously.

Nursing Diagnoses

1. Potential fluid volume excess related to overzealous fluid administration. **Rationale:** Patients receiving intravenous therapy and medications may tolerate only minimal amounts of fluid in light of a labile cardiovascular status.
2. Potential for injury related to equipment failure. **Rationale:** Medications administered too rapidly may cause the patient to develop undesirable side effects or if delivered too slowly not achieve the desired effect.

Planning

1. Individualize the following goals for administering intravenous therapy and medications via a gravity-controlled infusion device:
   a. Maintain fluid balance. **Rationale:** Gravity-controlled infusion device allows for accurate administration of fluid volumes.
   b. Maintain a consistent, accurate rate of flow. **Rationale:** Gravity-controlled infusion device facilitates an accurate, consistent delivery.
2. Assemble and prepare all equipment. **Rationale:** Ensures that intravenous fluids/medications administered via a gravity-controlled infusion device will be initiated quickly and efficiently.
   a. IV pole.
   b. Gravity-controlled infusion device.
   c. Intravenous administration set (specific for gravity-controlled infusion device selected).
   d. Intravenous fluid/medications (prescribed by physician).
   e. One sterile 19-gauge needle.
   f. One alcohol prep pad.
   g. One roll of 2-in paper tape.
3. Determine the infusion rate (drops per minute) based on the administration set selected and drop factor of tubing. **Rationale:** Infusion rate errors are commonly attributed to the incorrect selection of macro- versus microdrip tubing.
4. Prepare the patient.
   a. Explain the procedure to the patient. **Rationale:** Reduces patient anxiety and enhances cooperation.
   b. Explain the medication(s) to be administered, including action and side effects, if appropriate. **Rationale:** Patient should be instructed in the pharmacotherapeutic aspects of the treatment plan.

Implementation

Steps	Rationale	Special Considerations
1. Verify physician order for IV fluid to be administered and the rate of infusion.	Prevents errors in intravenous and medication administration.	Physician order should include type, amount, rate, and duration of infusion. For medication administration: drug, dose, amount of fluid in which drug should be diluted, and rate of infusion or titration parameters.

Table continues on following page

Steps	Rationale	Special Considerations
2. Wash hands.	Reduces transmission of microorganisms.	
3. Insert tubing spike into intravenous bag/bottle.	Accesses fluid source.	
4. Squeeze drip chamber and allow fluid to fill half of chamber.	Prevents air from entering the tubing.	Do not fill more than half of drip chamber because the sensor will not be able to detect the drop.
5. Prime the tubing. *Do not* remove the cap from the end of the tubing.	Eliminates air from system while maintaining aseptic technique. Prevents patient from receiving an air bolus.	
6. Thread the tubing through the gravity-controlled infusion device as described by the manufacturer.	Required for the device to operate properly.	Information is often listed on the device. Refer to operating manual.
7. Remove the cap from the tubing, and attach the sterile needle. If primary intravenous solution is to be administered with the device, remove the cap and connect directly to the catheter hub.	Allows for connection to primary intravenous line.	Pediatric and adult patients with rigid fluid restrictions commonly receive their primary intravenous infusion via a gravity-controlled infusion device.
8. Using an alcohol prep, cleanse the Y-port injection site on the primary intravenous tubing, and insert needle.	Allows fluid to be administered.	
9. Secure needle insertion site with paper tape.	Prevents accidental disconnection.	
10. Open roller clamp completely.	Prevents obstruction to flow.	Device will control rate of fluid to be administered.
11. Apply drop sensor above the fluid level in the drip chamber.	Allows for counting or "sensing" of drops.	If drop sensor is placed too low on the drip chamber, the machine will alarm because the sensor will not be able to detect the drops. If the drops splash (drip chamber is less than half filled), the drops may be counted twice, leading to an inaccurate rate and volume of fluid administered.
12. Set infusion rate as prescribed by the physician.	Ensures correct rate of flow.	Be sure the drop factor has been correctly determined; the gravity-controlled infusion device counts *drops* per minute.
13. Plug gravity-controlled infusion device into an electrical outlet.	Required for device to operate.	Most devices can run by battery for a limited time *only*; battery operation should be utilized when transporting the patient.
14. Turn on gravity-controlled infusion device.	Permits fluid to be administered at set rate.	
15. Monitor device for accurate functioning. If alarm sounds, check for the following causes: a. Infusion is complete. b. Flow is occluded by bending of the extremity, clot formation at catheter tip, clogging/kinking of the IV tubing, roller clamp in the closed position, or local infiltration.	Ensures accurate delivery of fluid/medication at the prescribed rate.	If unable to isolate or correct the problem, obtain another gravity-controlled infusion device. Tag the malfunctioning device with a statement of the problem, the date, time, and your initials.

Table continues on following page

Steps	Rationale	Special Considerations
c. Battery not functional.		
16. Wash hands.	Reduces transmission of microorganisms.	

Evaluation

1. Monitor the patient's vital signs every hour or as needed, including blood pressure, heart rate, respiratory rate, urine output, and hemodynamic pressures (if Swan-Ganz or central venous catheter is placed). **Rationale:** Intravenous fluids or medications may need to be titrated based on patient's response.

2. Monitor the patient's intake and output every hour or as needed. **Rationale:** Intravenous fluids/medications may need to be increased/decreased based on hourly intake and output balance.

3. Assess the patient for desired response to pharmacologic agents. **Rationale:** Intravenous administration of medications effects a rapid response.

4. Monitor the patient's electrolyte values as prescribed or as needed based on the patient's condition. **Rationale:** Intravenous fluid and medication administration will affect electrolyte balance.

Expected Outcomes

1. Fluid and electrolyte balance is maintained. **Rationale:** Intravenous therapy/medication administration achieves immediate response compared with other routes of administration.

2. Hemodynamic pressures are maintained/titrated as prescribed by the physician. **Rationale:** Potent pharmacotherapy for a labile/unstable hemodynamic/cardiovascular status is administered via an infusion device.

Unexpected Outcomes

1. Fluid overload or fluid deficit. **Rationale:** Equipment malfunction or inaccurate calculation of flow rate or use of incorrect tubing will result in too much or too little fluid being infused.

2. Inability to maintain hemodynamic parameters secondary to IV fluid/medication administration. **Rationale:** Difficulty in troubleshooting device malfunction or equipment failure can adversely affect patient status.

Documentation

Documentation in the patient record should include the type and amount of intravenous solution infused; the duration of the infusion; the name, dose, date, and time of medication administered; the patient's response to fluid/medication administration; and actions taken in the event of signs and symptoms of fluid overload or undesirable side effects of the drug. Check your institution's policies and procedures for documenting intravenous therapy and medication administration. **Rationale:** Documents nursing care given, expected and unexpected outcomes, and interventions taken.

Patient/Family Education

1. Discuss the rationale for using a gravity-controlled infusion device with both patient and family. **Rationale:** Decreases anxiety and facilitates understanding of procedures implemented to manage patient care.

2. Explain the causes for device alarm. **Rationale:** Decreases anxiety.

3. Instruct the patient in activity restrictions (i.e., bending of arm). **Rationale:** Promotes patient cooperation.

Performance Checklist
Skill 33–3:   Gravity-Controlled Infusion Device

Critical Behaviors	Complies	
	yes	no
1. Verify physician order for IV fluid/medication to be administered.		
2. Wash hands.		
3. Insert tubing spike into IV bag/bottle.		
4. Half fill drip chamber.		
5. Prime tubing.		
6. Thread tubing through device.		
7. Attach needle to distal end of tubing or attach tubing to catheter hub.		

Table continues on following page

Critical Behaviors	Complies	
	yes	**no**
8. Cleanse Y-port on peripheral intravenous tubing, and insert needle.		
9. Secure needle to tubing.		
10. Open roller clamp completely.		
11. Apply drop sensor to drip chamber.		
12. Set infusion rate.		
13. Plug device into an electrical outlet.		
14. Turn device on.		
15. Monitor device for accurate functioning.		
16. Wash hands.		
17. Document procedure in the patient record.		

SKILL 33–4

Volume-Controlled Infusion Device

A volume-controlled infusion device is indicated when accurate administration of intravenous fluid and/or medications is required. Volume infusion devices use positive pressure to deliver intravenous fluids as opposed to a gravity-controlled infusion device, which uses gravity. The volume of fluid to be delivered is preset. The device then regulates the flow rate to achieve the preset volume. The device also detects resistance to flow, which triggers an alarm. These devices commonly require tubing manufactured specifically for each type of device that is not interchangeable. Table 33–2 lists some commonly used volume-controlled infusion devices.

Purpose

The nurse uses a volume-controlled infusion device to

1. Ensure a consistent rate of flow.
2. Titrate pharmacotherapy based on prescribed parameters.
3. Deliver accurate volumes of intravenous fluid.

TABLE 33–2 BRAND NAMES OF VOLUME-CONTROLLED INFUSION DEVICES

Abbott Lifecare 5000 Infusion System
Abbott LifeCare Model 4P
Omni-Flow 4000 (multichannel)
AVI 200A (Micro 210A) Infusion Pump
AVI 400A Infusion Pump
Baxa Corp. Exacta-Med Pharmacy Pump No. 10
Baxter Flo-Gard 6200 Volumetric Infusion Pump
Baxter Flo-Gard 6300 Dual Channel Volume Infusion Pump
Baxter Flo-Gard 8000 Volume Infusion Pump
Baxter Flo-Gard 8100 Volume Infusion Pump
Baxter Flo-Gard 8500 Volume Infusion Pump
Critikon Rateminder V Volume Infusion Pump
Gemini PC-1
Gemini PC-2 (dual chamber)
IMED 965A Micor-Volumetric Infusion Pump
IMED 980 Volume Infusion Pump
IVAC 262 + , 570, 599
IVAC Variable Pressure Volume Infusion Pump Model 560/560 +
IVAC Neo-Mate Variable Pressure Microinfusion Pump Model 565
IVAC Star-Flow Volumetric Pump Model 590
Ivy Medical Commander 500
Kendall 520 Intelligent Pump
Kendall 522 Intelligent Pump
Schoch Electronics VoluMed uVP2001
Siemens Life Support Systems Mini-Med II
Smith & Nephew Sigma 6000 +
Valleylab 7000/7200 Volumetric Pump

Prerequisite Knowledge and Skills

Prior to using a volume-controlled infusion device, the nurse should understand

1. Principles of positive-pressure infusion.
2. Principles of intravenous therapy.
3. Principles of aseptic technique.
4. Principles of fluid balance.

The nurse should be able to perform

1. Proper handwashing technique (see Skill 35–5).
2. Universal precautions (see Skill 35–1).
3. Vital signs assessment.
4. Hemodynamic assessment.
5. Assessment of vascular access site.

Assessment

1. Assess the need for a volume-controlled infusion device, such as medications requiring titration or a consistent rate of flow (commonly, vasoactive agents, continuous narcotic infusions, neuromuscular blockades, anticoagulant or bronchodilator therapy), labile cardiovascular status, severe fluid restrictions, or labile fluid balance status. **Rationale:** Volume-controlled infusion devices are used when accurate administration of fluids and/or titration of medications is essential.

2. Assess the patient's fluid status, including heart rate, blood pressure, urine output, breath sounds, serum electrolytes, hematocrit, daily weights, and intake and output records. **Rationale:** Infusion of intravenous fluids and medications will affect patient's fluid balance and hemodynamic status.

3. Monitor the patient's pulmonary artery pressures and pulmonary capillary wedge pressure during fluid administration. **Rationale:** Increases in the pulmonary artery pressures and pulmonary capillary wedge pressure may be the first indicators of fluid overload.

4. Assess the venous catheter for patency and signs and symptoms of infiltration and/or phlebitis. **Rationale:** Ensures administration of fluid intravenously.

Nursing Diagnoses

1. Potential for volume deficit/excess related to intravenous fluid administration. **Rationale:** Preset volume/amount may have been set incorrectly, equipment malfunction, and/or change in the hemodynamic status will affect the state of fluid balance.

2. Potential for injury related to pharmacotherapy. **Rationale:** Potent medications titrated incorrectly or which extravasate in the peripheral tissues may result in life/limb-threatening complications. These medications are preferentially administered through central venous access.

Planning

1. Individualize the following goals for titration of fluids and/or medications:
   a. Maintain mean arterial pressure as prescribed. **Rationale:** Necessary to maintain adequate organ perfusion.
   b. Maintain other hemodynamic parameters as prescribed by the physician. **Rationale:** Volume-controlled infusion devices are commonly employed for titration of intravenous fluids and pharmacotherapy.

2. Assemble and prepare all necessary equipment. **Rationale:** Assembly of all necessary equipment ensures that intravenous/medication infusion will be initiated quickly and efficiently.
   a. IV pole.
   b. Volume-controlled infusion device.
   c. IV administration set (specific for volume-controlled infusion device selected).
   d. IV fluid/medications (prescribed by physician).
   e. One sterile 19-gauge needle.
   f. One alcohol prep pad.
   g. One roll of 2-in paper tape.

3. Prepare the patient.
   a. Explain the procedure to the patient. **Rationale:** Reduces patient anxiety and enhances cooperation.
   b. Explain the medication(s) to be administered, including action and side effects, if appropriate. **Rationale:** Patient should be instructed in the pharmacotherapeutic aspects of the treatment plan.

Implementation

Steps	Rationale	Special Considerations
1. Verify physician order for IV fluid to be administered and the rate of infusion.	Prevents errors in intravenous and medication administration.	Physician order should include type, amount, rate, and duration of infusion. For medication administration: drug, dose, amount of fluid in which drug should be diluted, and rate of infusion or titration parameters.
2. Wash hands.	Reduces transmission of microorganisms.	

Table continues on following page

Steps	Rationale	Special Considerations
3. Insert tubing spike into the intravenous bag/bottle.	Accesses fluid source.	
4. Squeeze drip chamber and allow fluid to fill half of chamber.	Prevents air from entering the tubing.	Do not fill more than half of drip chamber because sensor will not be able to detect the drop.
5. Prime the tubing as per manufacturer's instructions. *Do not* remove the cap from the end of the tubing.	Eliminates air from system while maintaining aseptic technique. Prevents patient from receiving an air bolus.	Priming instructions are device specific.
6. Thread the tubing through the device as described by the manufacturer.	Required for the device to operate properly.	Refer to operator's manual.
7. Remove the cap from the tubing, and attach the sterile needle. If primary intravenous solution is to be administered with the device, remove the cap and connect directly to the catheter hub.	Allows for connection to primary intravenous line.	Pediatric and adult patients with rigid fluid restrictions may receive their primary intravenous infusion via a volume-controlled infusion device.
8. Using an alcohol prep, cleanse the Y-port injection site on the primary intravenous tubing, and insert the needle.	Allows fluid to be administered.	
9. Secure needle insertion site with paper tape.	Prevents accidental disconnection.	
10. Open roller clamp completely.	Device will control rate of fluid to be administered.	
11. Apply flow sensor above the fluid level in the drip chamber.	Ensures correct rate of flow.	Measured in cc's per hour.
12. Set infusion rate as prescribed or titrate for maintenance of hemodynamic parameters.	Ensures correct rate of flow.	
13. Plug infusion device into an electrical outlet.	Required for device to operate.	Most devices can run by battery for a *limited time only*.
14. Turn infusion device on.	Permits fluid to be administered at set rate.	
15. Monitor device for accurate functioning. If alarm sounds, check for the following causes: a. Infusion is complete. b. Flow is occluded by bending of the extremity, clot formation at catheter tip, clogging/kinking of the IV tubing, roller clamp in the closed position, or local infiltration. c. Battery not functional.	Ensures accurate delivery of fluid/ medication at the prescribed rate.	If unable to isolate or correct the problem, obtain another volume-controlled infusion device. Tag the malfunctioning device with a statement of the problem, the date, time, and your initials.
16. Monitor the patient for signs of fluid overload and/or untoward side effects of the medication(s).	Assesses response to therapy.	Monitor the cardiovascular, hemodynamic, and respiratory status. Note specific therapeutic or undesirable side effects of the drug.
17. Wash hands.	Reduces transmission of microorganisms.	

Evaluation

1. Monitor the patient's vital signs every hour or as needed, including blood pressure, heart rate, respiratory rate, urine output, and hemodynamic pressures (if Swan-Ganz or central venous catheter is placed). **Rationale:** Intravenous fluids or medications may need to be titrated based on patient's response.

2. Monitor the patient's intake and output every hour or as needed. **Rationale:** Intravenous fluids/medications may need to be increased/decreased based on hourly intake and output balance.

3. Assess the patient for desired response to pharmacologic agents. **Rationale:** Intravenous administration of medications effects a rapid response.

4. Monitor the patient's electrolyte values as prescribed or as needed based on the patient's condition. **Rationale:** Intravenous fluid and medication administration will affect electrolyte balance.

Expected Outcomes

1. Fluid and electrolyte balance is achieved. **Rationale:** Intravenous therapy/medication administration achieves immediate response compared with other routes of administration.

2. Hemodynamic pressures are maintained/titrated as prescribed by the physician. **Rationale:** Potent pharmacotherapy for a labile/unstable hemodynamic/cardiovascular status is administered via an infusion device.

Unexpected Outcomes

1. Fluid overload or fluid deficit. **Rationale:** Equipment malfunction or inaccurate calculation of flow rate or use of incorrect tubing will result in too much or too little fluid being infused.

2. Inability to maintain hemodynamic parameters secondary to IV fluid/medication administration. **Rationale:** Difficulty in troubleshooting device, malfunction, or equipment failure can adversely affect patient status.

3. Extravasation of vasoactive/chemotherapeutic medication(s) into peripheral tissues resulting in tissue necrosis. **Rationale:** Venous catheter has infiltrated, with delivery of medications under positive pressure significant extravasation with limb-threatening complications may ensue.

Documentation

Documentation in the patient record should include the type and amount of intravenous solution infused; the duration of the infusion; the name, dose, date, and time the medication was initiated; assessment of the insertion site; the patient's response to fluid/medication administration; and actions taken in the event of signs and symptoms of fluid overload or undesirable side effects of the drug. Check your institution's policies and procedures for documenting intravenous therapy and medication administration. **Rationale:** Documents nursing care given, expected and unexpected outcomes, and interventions taken.

Patient/Family Education

1. Discuss the rationale for using a volume-controlled infusion device with both patient and family. **Rationale:** Decreases anxiety and facilitates understanding of procedures implemented to manage patient care.

2. Explain the causes for device alarm. **Rationale:** Decreases anxiety.

3. Instruct the patient in activity restrictions (i.e., bending of arm). **Rationale:** Promotes patient cooperation.

Performance Checklist
Skill 33–4: Volume-Controlled Infusion Device

Critical Behaviors	Complies	
	yes	no
1. Verify physician order for IV fluid/medication to be administered.		
2. Wash hands.		
3. Insert tubing spike into IV bag/bottle.		
4. Half fill drip chamber.		
5. Prime tubing.		
6. Thread tubing through device.		
7. Attach needle to distal end of tubing or attach tubing to catheter hub.		
8. Cleanse Y-port on peripheral intravenous tubing, and insert needle.		
9. Secure needle to tubing.		
10. Open roller clamp completely.		
11. Apply sensor to drip chamber.		

Table continues on following page

Critical Behaviors	Complies	
	yes	no
12. Set infusion rate.		
13. Plug device into an electrical outlet.		
14. Turn device on.		
15. Monitor device for accurate functioning.		
16. Monitor patient for therapeutic/untoward effects of IV fluid/medication administration.		
17. Wash hands.		
18. Document procedure in the patient record.		

SKILL 33–5

Patient-Controlled Analgesia Device

Patient-controlled analgesia (PCA) is an alternate method for administering pain medication. It is designed to maintain therapeutic blood levels of analgesia by having the patient depress a control button when pain relief is required, thereby activating a physician-prescribed dose of narcotic. The system prevents overdosing by using a preset time delay when no narcotic infusion is possible and a 1-hour dosage limit.

Patient-controlled analgesia decreases the peaks and valleys of serum narcotic concentration associated with conventional intravenous and intramuscular methods. It can be used for moderate to severe pain. Advantages of patient-controlled analgesia include patient titration for effective analgesia without excessive sedation, relief of pain with lower dosages of medication, immediate delivery of medication, patient's sense of self-control (which lowers anxiety), and less nursing time spent preparing medications.

Disadvantages of PCA include the high cost of the pump necessary to deliver the drug, the necessity of the patient's having a clear mental status, and health care professionals' resistance to a patient's activation of the device.

Purpose

The nurse uses a patient-controlled analgesia device to

1. Provide pain relief/control.
2. Promote patient participation and control in securing pain relief.
3. Decrease patient waiting time for pain medication.

Prerequisite Knowledge and Skills

Prior to utilizing a patient-controlled analgesia device, the nurse should understand

1. Principles of pain and pain control/relief.
2. Principles of aseptic technique.
3. Principles of intravenous therapy.
4. Principles of positive-pressure infusion.
5. Principles of patient-controlled analgesia.
6. Patient selection criteria for patient-controlled analgesia.

The nurse should be able to perform

1. Proper handwashing technique (see Skill 35–5).
2. Universal precautions (see Skill 35–1).
3. Assessment of pain.
4. Assessment of vascular access site.
5. Respiratory assessment.
6. Neurologic assessment.

Assessment

1. Assess the patient's baseline vital signs, including heart rate, blood pressure, and respiratory rate, rhythm, and depth. **Rationale:** Narcotic administration may depress respirations and cause vasodilation with decreased preload. Provides a baseline to evaluate effectiveness of therapy.
2. Assess the patient's level of consciousness and cognitive ability. **Rationale:** Patient must be mentally competent and alert to operate the PCA device.
3. Assess the patient for nonverbal indicators of pain, including facial expression (masklike, grimace, tension), guarding or protective behaviors, restlessness or increase in motor activity, withdrawal or decrease in motor activity, skeletal muscle tension, short attention span, irritability, anxiety, and sleep disturbance. **Rationale:** Patient may not verbalize or be able to verbalize pain.
4. Assess the patient for autonomic indicators of pain, including diaphoresis, vasoconstriction, increased systolic and diastolic blood pressure, increased heart rate, pupillary dilatation, change in the respiratory rate, and muscle tension or spasm. **Rationale:** Objective indicators that validate the patient's report of pain. Useful in assessing pain in the aphasic patient. Note that patients with chronic pain (>6 months' duration) may not exhibit an autonomic response.
5. Assess the patient's history for alcohol and/or drug (prescription and over-the-counter) use. **Rationale:** History of drug and/or alcohol use affects effective dosages of analgesic (patient may require more or less).

6. Assess the vascular access for patency, infiltration, and phlebitis. **Rationale:** Ensures administration of narcotic medication into the vascular system.

Nursing Diagnoses

1. Pain related to surgical procedure or pathophysiologic condition. **Rationale:** Patients undergoing surgical procedures are the most common candidates for PCA.
2. Pain related to hesitancy to medicate self. **Rationale:** Occasionally, a patient may fear overdosing himself or herself or fears communicating inadequate pain relief and thus becomes noncompliant with the device.
3. Potential ineffective breathing pattern related to overdose of narcotics. **Rationale:** Respiratory depression can result with PCA.
4. Potential decreased cardiac output related to overdose of narcotics. **Rationale:** Decreased preload secondary to venous vasodilation may result with narcotic administration.

Planning

1. Individualize the following goals for utilizing a PCA device:
   a. Achieve and maintain pain control/relief. **Rationale:** Patient receives a prescribed dosage of medication when *the patient* determines the need for pain relief.
   b. Provide the patient with a sense of control. **Rationale:** Patient depresses a control button to receive a prescribed dosage of medication when *the patient* determines the need for pain relief.
2. Assemble and prepare all necessary equipment. **Rationale:** Assembly of all necessary equipment ensures that intravenous/medication infusion will be initiated quickly and efficiently.
   a. IV pole.
   b. Patient-controlled analgesia device.
   c. Tubing/administration set (specific for patient-controlled analgesia device selected).
   d. Syringe or a cassette with prescribed narcotic (prescribed by physician).
   e. IV maintenance solution (as prescribed by the physician).
   f. One sterile 19-gauge needle.
   g. One alcohol prep pad.
   h. One roll of 2-in paper tape.
3. Assist the patient to assume a comfortable position that facilitates optimal lung expansion. **Rationale:** Respiratory depression is a side effect of narcotic administration.
4. Prepare the patient by explaining the rationale for using a PCA device. **Rationale:** PCA may be a new concept and unfamiliar to the patient. Facilitates understanding and acceptance of this modality.

Implementation

Steps	Rationale	Special Considerations
1. Verify physician order for PCA.	Reduces possibility for error.	Physician order should include medication, concentration, reservoir size, route, delay interval, patient-controlled dose, and dosage limit per hour.
2. Wash hands.	Reduces transmission of microorganisms.	
3. Install syringe or reservoir into device.	Allows compartment door to close.	
4. Secure and lock device.	Prevents tampering with infusion.	
5. Secure filled narcotic reservoir to PCA tubing.	For priming the tubing.	
6. Turn PCA device on.	Required to set codes within the device.	The setup and operation are specific for each type/brand of PCA device. Manufacturer's directions *must* be consulted to ensure correct operation of the device.
7. Prime PCA tubing according to manufacturer's directions.	Eliminates bolus of air into vascular system.	
8. Enter security code.	Infusion is a controlled substance.	
9. Set infusion mode.	Required for operation.	

Table continues on following page

Steps	Rationale	Special Considerations
10. Set dosage as prescribed by physician.	For pain relief.	
11. Set time delay as prescribed by physician.	Prevents overdosing.	This is also referred to as the "lockout time."
12. Set the 1-hour dosage limit.	Additional security to prevent overdosing.	
13. Remove cap from tubing, and attach sterile needle.	Allows for connection to primary intravenous line.	
14. Using an alcohol prep, cleanse Y-port injection site on primary intravenous tubing, and insert the needle.	Maintains aseptic technique. Allows for narcotic administration.	
15. Secure needle insertion site with paper tape.	Prevents accidental disconnection.	
16. Press "start."	Initiates infusion.	
17. Provide patient with control button.	Allows patient to receive a prescribed dosage of medication.	
18. Wash hands.	Reduces transmission of microorganisms.	

Evaluation

1. Monitor the patient for verbalization or evidence of pain or discomfort. Use a pain scale, rating discomfort on a scale of 0 (no discomfort) to 10. **Rationale:** Adjustments to device settings can be made to secure adequate pain relief.

2. Monitor the patient for nonverbal and autonomic responses to pain. **Rationale:** Patient may not feel comfortable expressing pain/discomfort or may be aphasic.

3. Monitor the patient's vital signs every hour or in accordance with hospital policy, including respiratory rate, rhythm, and depth, heart rate and blood pressure, and level of consciousness. **Rationale:** Provides physical evidence of effectiveness and/or adverse side effects of PCA.

4. Monitor the vascular access site for signs and symptoms of infiltration. **Rationale:** Infusion of narcotic into subcutaneous tissue will diminish pain relief.

5. Monitor the patient's comfort level and ability to use the device. **Rationale:** Occasionally a patient will not be comfortable with the device and will desire traditional pain-relief methods.

Expected Outcomes

1. Verbalization of comfort. **Rationale:** Demonstrates effectiveness of modality.

2. Absence of nonverbal and autonomic indicators of pain. **Rationale:** Demonstrates effectiveness of modality.

Unexpected Outcomes

1. Lethargy, confusion, hypotension, tachycardia, and decrease in respiratory rate and depth. **Rationale:** Indicates overdosing of narcotic. Narcan may be administered to reverse sedation.

2. Verbalization of inadequate pain relief, as evidenced by pain scale. **Rationale:** Patient may not be using the device correctly; inadequate dosing, prolonged lockout time, or equipment malfunction may contribute to inadequate pain relief.

Documentation

Documentation in the patient record should include date and time of baseline and serial vital signs and level of consciousness, degree of pain relief according to the pain scale, patient's response to PCA, total narcotic dose per shift, cumulative narcotic dose received, expected and unexpected outcomes, and the interventions taken. Check your institution's policies and procedures for documenting PCA therapy and narcotic administration. **Rationale:** Documents nursing care given, expected and unexpected outcomes, and interventions taken.

Patient/Family Education

1. Explain the operation of the PCA device to both patient and family. Have the patient do a return demonstration. **Rationale:** Decreases anxiety, encourages questions, and improves patient acceptance and confidence.

2. Explain the rationale for the lockout mechanism. Emphasize that narcotics are *not* delivered unless the patient depresses the control button. **Rationale:** Reduces

anxiety patient may have about overdosing himself or herself or becoming narcotic dependent.

3. Instruct the patient that other methods of pain relief are available should he or she feel uncomfortable or overanxious with PCA. **Rationale:** Reduces anxiety when patient attempts a new skill.

4. Instruct the patient to report inadequate pain relief. **Rationale:** Dosage or frequency may need to be changed, or device may not be functioning properly.

5. Instruct the patient and family that a dose of analgesia is recommended prior to an activity (i.e., cough and deep breathing, ambulating, or transferring out of bed). **Rationale:** Physical exertion frequently exacerbates pain. Adequate analgesia encourages greater compliance with pulmonary toileting procedures and mobility interventions.

Performance Checklist
Skill 33–5:   Patient-Controlled Analgesia Device

Critical Behaviors	Complies	
	yes	no
1. Verify physician order.		
2. Wash hands.		
3. Install reservoir into device.		
4. Secure and lock device.		
5. Secure narcotic reservoir to PCA tubing.		
6. Turn PCA device on.		
7. Prime PCA tubing.		
8. Enter security code.		
9. Set infusion mode.		
10. Set dosage as prescribed.		
11. Set time delay as prescribed.		
12. Set the 1-hour dosage limit.		
13. Attach sterile needle to tubing.		
14. Cleanse Y-port injection site on primary tubing, and insert needle.		
15. Secure needle insertion site with tape.		
16. Press "start" to initiate infusion.		
17. Provide patient with control button.		
18. Wash hands.		
19. Document procedure in the patient record.		

BIBLIOGRAPHY

Drain, C. B., and Christoph, S. S. (1987). *The Recovery Room: A Critical Approach to Post Anesthesia Nursing*, 2d Ed. Philadelphia: Saunders.

Lange, M. P., Dahn, M. S., and Jacobs, L. A. (1988). Patient-controlled analgesia versus intermittent analgesia dosing. *Heart Lung* 17:495–498.

Layon, A. J., and Kirby, R. R. (1988). Fluids and Electrolytes in the Critically Ill. In J. M. Civetta, R. W. Taylor, and R. R. Kirby (Eds.), *Critical Care*. Philadelphia: Lippincott.

White, P. F. (1987). Mishaps with patient-controlled analgesia. *Anesthesiolgy* 68:81–83.

White, P. F. (1988). Use of patient-controlled analgesia for management of acute pain. *J.A.M.A.* 259:243–247.

BEHAVIORAL OBJECTIVES

After completing this chapter, the nurse will be able to

- Define the key terms.
- Discuss the indications for placement of a long-term venous access device.
- Differentiate between the various types of long-term venous access devices and the appropriate clinical indications for each.
- Demonstrate the skills involved in the use of long-term venous access devices.

Long-term venous access to the central venous system allows for systemic treatment as well as sampling of blood to monitor the efficacy of therapeutic interventions. These devices increase the efficiency of treatment while minimizing the psychological and physical trauma of repeated venipuncture.

There are two basic types of long-term venous access devices: the external right atrial Silastic catheter (Fig. 34–1) and the totally implanted venous access port (Fig. 34–2). Although they serve the same purpose, the patient's underlying condition, the indications for using a venous access device, and the capabilities of the patient and family to perform self-care activities necessary for home maintenance will determine which device is appropriate for insertion.

The external right atrial Silastic catheter is used more commonly in acute-care settings, such as for administration of antibiotics (i.e., osteomyelitis, endocarditis), or for patients who would not be able to tolerate repeated punctures through the skin (i.e., therapies that result in severely lowered platelet counts). The implanted venous access port is more suitable for patients requiring prolonged (at least 6 months) intermittent care or for patients receiving therapy that is not likely to lead to prolonged periods of severe immunosuppression.

Right atrial Silastic catheters are multipurpose devices that can be used simultaneously for several different purposes. These devices have become widely accepted by patients and health care personnel. With the current knowledge of therapeutic interventions for venous access device complications, the benefits outweigh the risks. These devices provide patient comfort and optimal quality of life. With a venous access device, the patient may receive a continuous infusion of chemotherapy, hyperalimentation, pain medication, etc. at home using an ambulatory infusion pump. This decreases time spent in the hospital and the overall cost of treatment and allows the patient to maintain his or her independence.

Right atrial catheters are inserted surgically, usually under local anesthesia for adults and general anesthesia for pediatric patients. The catheter is trimmed to the desired length before placement. The surgeon isolates a large central vein. Forceps are then passed through the subcutaneous tissue from the entrance site of the vessel to an exit site on the midchest area, thereby forming the subcutaneous tunnel.

The implanted venous access port is surgically placed under the skin in a subcutaneous pocket (usually in the chest) that holds the port reservoir (Figs. 34–3 and 34–4). It is usually inserted under local anesthesia for adults and general anesthesia for pediatric patients and frequently in an outpatient surgical setting. The Silastic catheter is then tunneled from the port pocket to a large central vein. When it is not being used for treatment and there is no needle in place, the port is fairly inconspicuous, visible only as a bump under the skin. This leaves the patient's body image intact and allows complete freedom of activity. Because the system is completely closed and there is no manipulation of the device by the patient, the risk of infection is decreased in relation to the external Silastic catheter.

KEY TERMS

external right atrial Silastic catheter
extravasation
Huber point needle
port
implanted venous access

intralumenal catheter occlusion
one-way valve effect
urokinase
venous thrombosis

SKILLS

34–1 Access to and Administration through a Totally Implanted Venous Access Port

34–2 Obtaining Blood Specimens through a Totally Implanted Venous Access Port

34–3 Removing the Huber Point Needle Administration Set from a Totally Implanted Venous Access Port

34–4 Luer-lok Cap Change and Irrigation of a Right Atrial Silastic Catheter

34–5 Site Care and Dressing Change for a Right Atrial Silastic Catheter

GUIDELINES

The following assessment guidelines assist the nurse in

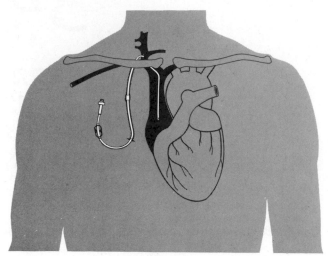

FIGURE 34–1. External right atrial Silastic catheter. (Courtesy of Davol, Inc.)

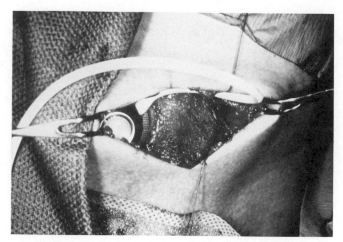

FIGURE 34–3. Surgical placement of the totally implanted venous access port. (Courtesy of Strato Medical Corporation.)

formulating a nursing diagnosis and an individualized plan of care to maintain maximal function of a long-term venous access device:

1. Know the type of implanted device, the location of the port reservoir, and/or the location of the Silastic catheter tip.

2. Know the indications for placement of the long-term venous access device in this patient.

3. Know the patient's medical history and current therapy involving the long-term venous access device.

4. Perform a skin assessment of the area overlying the implanted venous access port or the exit site of the right atrial Silastic catheter.

5. Know the baseline level of function and associated problems of the patient's long-term venous access device.

6. Determine the appropriate intervention(s) for the assessed findings.

7. Become adept with the equipment used to access

and withdraw blood from the long-term venous access device.

SKILL 34–1

Access to and Administration through a Totally Implanted Venous Access Port

Access to an implanted venous access port is performed to administer blood/blood products and/or intravenous therapy. Only a Huber point noncoring needle should be used, since any other needle will cause damage to the silicone septum (Fig. 34–5). Huber point needles come in various gauges and lengths, right-angled and

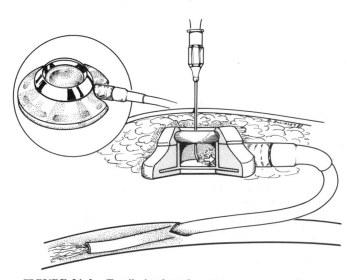

FIGURE 34–2. Totally implanted venous access port. (Courtesy of Davol, Inc.)

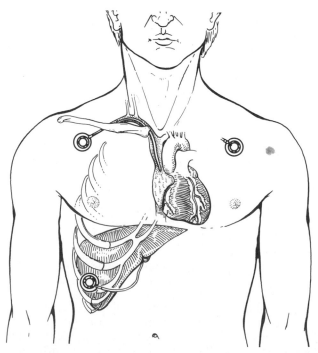

FIGURE 34–4. Typical locations for totally implanted venous access port. (Courtesy of Davol, Inc.)

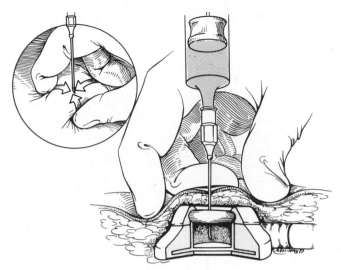

FIGURE 34–5. Huber point needle access into the totally implanted venous access port. (Courtesy of Davol, Inc.)

straight, either with or without an attached administration set. The most commonly used needle is ¾ in in length, although patients with an excess of subcutaneous tissue or a deeply implanted port may require a 1- or 1½-in needle. In the adult population, a 20-gauge needle is used for most purposes; in pediatric patients, a 22-gauge needle is used. For blood and blood product administration, a 19-gauge needle is preferred. Difficulty may occur transfusing blood/blood products through a right-angled needle because of red blood cell occlusion at the bend of the needle. Should this occur, a straight needle is used.

Purpose

The nurse accesses a totally implanted venous port to

1. Administer intravenous therapy.
2. Administer intravenous medications.
3. Provide total parenteral nutrition.
4. Deliver chemotherapy.
5. Infuse blood/blood products.
6. Withdraw blood specimens for laboratory analysis.

Prerequisite Knowledge and Skills

Prior to accessing an implanted venous access port, the nurse should understand

1. Anatomy and physiology of the vascular system.
2. Design, purpose, and function of the implanted venous access port.
3. Principles of aseptic technique.
4. Principles of infection control.
5. Principles of intravenous therapy.
6. Principles of blood/blood product administration.
7. Universal precautions.

The nurse should be able to perform

1. Proper handwashing technique (see Skill 35–5).

2. Setup of a sterile field.
3. Palpation of the port septum.
4. Skin assessment of the trunk and neck.
5. Universal precautions (see Skill 35–1).

Assessment

1. Assess the skin overlying the implanted venous access port and the tissues surrounding the port, noting erythema, inflammation, exudate, supraclavicular swelling, venous distension, and development of collateral circulation. **Rationale:** Access to the venous access port will not be performed through compromised skin; detects signs and symptoms of local infection or venous thrombosis.
2. Assess the patient's vital signs, including temperature, heart rate, blood pressure, and respiratory rate. **Rationale:** Supports diagnosis of local and/or systemic infection.

Nursing Diagnoses

1. Potential impaired skin integrity related to presence of foreign body within the subcutaneous tissue. **Rationale:** Repeated venipuncture through the skin overlying the implanted venous port, risk of infusate extravasation into the subcutaneous tissue surrounding the implanted venous port, and irritation caused by cleansing of the site with povidone-iodine solution increase the risk for impaired skin integrity.
2. Potential for infection related to presence of a foreign body within the subcutaneous tissue. **Rationale:** Direct access into the central venous vasculature and the presence of a needle within the implanted port septum provide a portal of entry for microorganisms.

Planning

1. Individualize the following goals for utilizing a totally implanted venous access port:
   a. Maintain central venous access. **Rationale:** Allows for administration of intravenous therapy, medications, TPN, chemotherapy, and blood/blood products as well as withdrawal of blood specimens for laboratory analysis.
   b. Maintain optimal function of the implanted venous access port. **Rationale:** Skin integrity and patency of the totally implanted venous port are maintained by adhering to established procedures.
2. Prepare all necessary equipment and supplies. **Rationale:** Assembly of all the necessary equipment at the bedside ensures that the procedure will be completed quickly and efficiently.
   a. Central venous catheter dressing kit. If kit is unavailable, obtain
      (1) One sterile barrier
      (2) Two pairs sterile gloves

    (3) Three povidone-iodine swab sticks
    (4) One sterile 2 × 2 in gauze pad.
  b. Appropriately sized Huber point needle with attached administration set.
  c. Two 5-cc syringes.
  d. Two 20-gauge 1-in needles.
  e. Normal saline solution for injection, 10 cc.
  f. One 3 × 5 in transparent dressing.
  g. One roll of 1-in paper tape.
  h. Two alcohol preps.
  i. Intravenous solution (prescribed by physician) with primed intravenous administration set.

If converting to a heparin lock:
  j. One 3-cc syringe.
  k. One 20-gauge 1-in needle.
  l. Heparin saline solution (100 units/cc), 3 cc.

  m. One male Luer-lok adapter.
3. Prepare the patient.
  a. Explain the procedure to the patient. **Rationale:** Minimizes risks and reduces anxiety.
  b. Describe the sensations (palpation, wetness of povidone-iodine, pressure and needle stick during access) that the patient is likely to experience during the procedure. **Rationale:** Encourages cooperation and reduces the risk of unexpected activity by the patient during the procedure, which could contaminate the sterile field.
  c. Assist the patient in achieving a position (usually supine) that is comfortable for the patient and the nurse. **Rationale:** Promotes patient comfort and supports good body mechanics for the nurse.

Implementation

Steps	Rationale	Special Considerations
1. Wash hands with antiseptic solution.	Reduces transmission of microorganisms.	
2. Identify the implanted venous port by palpation, and confirm the silicone septum location within the perimeter of the port.	Verifies that the port is in proper position for use and ensures that it has not "flipped" within its pocket.	If swelling, tenderness, and/or inflammation exist or you are unable to palpate the septum of the port, notify the physician (see Table 34–1).
3. Prep the port using povidone-iodine swab sticks (start at the septum of the port and move outward in concentric circles 2 in beyond the perimeter of the port), repeat twice, and allow the povidone-iodine to air dry.	Reduces transmission of microorganisms.	Use friction to enhance the antifungal and antibacterial effects of the povidone-iodine. To avoid contamination once an area has been cleaned, do not cleanse that area with the same povidone-iodine swab.
4. Wash hands again with antiseptic solution.	Reduces transmission of microorganisms.	Handwashing is repeated because hands become contaminated during port palpation.
5. Create a sterile field using the sterile barrier.	Access to the implanted venous access port is a sterile procedure.	
6. Place the following items onto the sterile field: a. Appropriately sized Huber point needle administration set. b. Two 5-cc syringes. c. Two 20-gauge 1-in needles. d. A 2 × 2 in sterile gauze pad. If converting to heparin lock, also obtain e. One 3-cc syringe. f. One additional 20-gauge 1-in needle. g. One male Luer-lok adapter.	Maintains sterility of all items.	A newly developed alternative to the Huber needle for accessing implanted ports, the Surecath system, uses an introducer spike to pass a flexible Teflon catheter through the septum into the port reservoir. When the introducer unit is removed, the catheter is left in place. The principles of the access procedure are unchanged.
7. Cleanse the top of the normal saline vial with an alcohol prep.	Infection control.	
8. Don sterile gloves.	Maintains sterile technique.	

Table continues on following page

Steps	Rationale	Special Considerations
9. Attach needles to syringes, and return to sterile field.	Prepares syringes for use.	Some institutions carry prefilled syringes with needles attached. Check what your institution supplies.
10. Withdraw 5 cc of normal saline into each 5-cc syringe. If converting to a heparin lock, withdraw 3 cc of heparin saline solution into the 3-cc syringe. Then return syringes to the sterile field.	Prepares syringes.	The normal saline vial and the heparin saline vials are not sterile. *Do not* contaminate syringes or the sterile field with the hand used to hold the vials.
11. Don a new pair of sterile gloves.	Maintains sterile technique.	
12. Remove 20-gauge needles from filled syringes, attach one of the syringes to the Huber point needle administration set, and flush with 1 cc of normal saline. Leave syringe attached.	Clears the needle administration set of air and primes it for insertion into the port.	The Huber point needle administration set is changed routinely every 7 days whether it is being used for continuous or intermittent infusion. If erythema or inflammation occurs at the site, it should be changed as needed.
13. Stabilize the port with the thumb and index finger of the nondominant hand.	Port must be stabilized because firm pressure is required to penetrate the silicone septum.	
14. With the dominant hand, use the forefinger to support the needle bend, insert the Huber point needle directly perpendicular to the port septum, and apply steady pressure until you feel the needle "hit" the base of the port reservoir (Fig. 34–6).	Prevents deflection of needle upon entry into the port septum.	Do not rock or rotate the needle once in place because this will damage the silicone septum.
15. Pull back on syringe plunger until the blood enters the syringe.	Confirms needle placement in the port reservoir.	If blood return is brown with fibrin clots (as may occur when the port has not been used recently), continue to aspirate until bright red blood appears in the syringe. Detach the syringe and flush with the other 5-cc saline-filled syringe. If no blood return is obtained, notify the physician (see Table 34–1).
16. Slowly inject the 5 cc of normal saline into the port, clamp the administration set, and remove the syringe.	Flushes blood from port reservoir and Silastic catheter and prevents occlusion.	If resistance is met, verify needle placement by applying pressure on the needle until the base of the reservoir is felt. If resistance is still met, remove Huber point needle administration set and reaccess port with a sterile Huber point needle (as per procedure steps 10 to 14). If resistance is met a second time, notify the physician.
17. Observe for signs of extravasation, such as swelling in the port pocket or complaints of pain over the port site.	Extravasation requires removal of Huber point needle and reaccess.	In a newly inserted port there may be tenderness and accumulation of fluid subcutaneously for up to 1 week postoperatively.
18. If the port is to be used for a *continuous* intravenous infusion, connect the Huber point needle administration set directly to the intravenous solution administration set, and seal the connection with paper tape.	Prevents accidental disconnection.	

Table continues on following page

Steps	Rationale	Special Considerations
19. If the port is to be used *intermittently*, attach a male Luer-lok adapter to the Huber point needle administration set, and seal the connection with paper tape. To heparin lock the port, inject 3 cc of heparin saline solution through Luer-lok adapter.	Prevents accidental separation. Maintains patency of port reservoir and Silastic catheter.	Incompatible solutions *cannot* be administered simultaneously through a single-lumen port (the most common port in use). *Consecutive* administration is permitted when the port is flushed with 20 cc of normal saline between incompatible solutions. This prevents "mixing" in the port reservoir. Incompatible solutions *may* be administered through a dual-lumen port because there are two distinct port reservoirs and mixing will not occur. However, two products that the patient may react to (e.g., blood products and amphotericin) should not be given simultaneously.
20. If there is a ¼-in or greater gap between the skin and the Huber point needle, place a folded 2 × 2 in gauze under the hub of the Huber point needle.	Supports the Huber point needle and prevents motion at the insertion site.	
21. Apply a sterile transparent dressing over the port, the Huber point needle, and the upper portion of attached administration set, and pinch dressing around the administration set.	Maintains sterility and allows for observation of needle position and the site.	Pinching the dressing makes an occlusive seal and maintains the position of the needle at a 90-degree angle. The transparent dressing is necessary only when the port is accessed. It is changed every 7 days along with the needle administration set and as needed if it becomes wet or nonocclusive. The patient may shower while the port is accessed if the transparent dressing is covered with another waterproof dressing.
22. Remove sterile gloves.	Sterile technique is no longer necessary.	
23. For *continuous* infusion, adjust the roller clamp to infuse intravenous solution at prescribed rate.	Administers intravenous therapy.	
24. Form a safety loop with the Huber point administration set tubing, and secure to the chest with paper tape.	Prevents accidental needle dislodgment.	The majority of extravasation incidents are caused by inadvertent needle dislodgment from strain on the catheter tubing. This is prevented by providing the appropriate length of intravenous tubing and securing it well.
25. Discard used equipment in appropriate manner.	Universal precautions.	
26. Wash hands.	Reduces transmission of microorganisms.	

TABLE 34-1 MANAGEMENT OF COMPLICATIONS OF VENOUS ACCESS DEVICES

Problem	Rationale	Action to be Taken
Extravasation of fluid into subcutaneous tissue surrounding the venous access device	Displaced Huber point needle	Verify needle placement by applying direct pressure on the needle until contact is made with the base of the port reservoir, and check for blood return.

Table continues on following page

Problem	Rationale	Action to be Taken
		If needle placement is not verifiable, remove existing needle, and gently express fluid from the pocket if able. If unable to express fluid, apply warm compresses to aid in fluid reabsorption. When fluid has been expressed or reabsorbed, palpate and stabilize the perimeter of the port, and reaccess according to the procedure.
	Damaged venous access device	Gently flush with 10 cc of normal saline solution, and observe for increased swelling or leakage at the site. If present, stop procedure and notify physician. Damage of the port septum or Silastic catheter can be confirmed by radiographic dye study through the device.
	Thrombus at the tip of the catheter causing retrograde flow of infusate along the outer wall of the catheter until the fluid is deposited into the subcutaneous tissue	If presence of a thrombus is confirmed by radiographic dye study, a heparin infusion or lytic therapy (urokinase) may be instituted to attempt to lyse the thrombus as prescribed or as according to institutional policy.
Inability to withdraw blood from the venous access device when the device is irrigated without resistance	Incorrectly placed Huber point needle with needle bevel within the septum of the implanted port rather than in the port reservoir	Verify needle placement by applying pressure on the needle until contact is made with the base of the reservoir. Remove needle and reinsert sterile Huber point needle according to the procedure if it is placed too close to the sides of the septum rather than in the center.
	Catheter tip lying against the wall of the blood vessel	Instruct patient to: Raise arms above head and inhale and exhale deeply or cough. Change position (e.g., lying to sitting). Bear down in a Valsalva maneuver with mouth open.
	Formation of fibrin sheath at tip of catheter causing a one-way valve effect during blood withdrawal attempt	Attach a 10-cc syringe with 5 cc of heparin saline solution, and attempt to alternately flush and aspirate *gently* using a push–pull technique. Aspirate fibrin and clotted blood into syringe and discard. Attach a sterile syringe of normal saline solution and flush. If inability to withdraw blood persists, confer with physician about Radiographic dye study to verify correct catheter placement, to rule out catheter kinking, or to document presence of fibrin sheath. Administration of a lytic agent (e.g., urokinase) to attempt to lyse the fibrin sheath as per physician order on unit protocol.
Catheter occlusion: Inability to irrigate the implanted port or the right atrial catheter.	Intralumenal clotting. Intralumenal clotting is almost always caused by an interruption in the intravenous	Attach a 10-cc syringe with 5 cc of heparin saline solution, and attempt to alternately flush and aspirate

Table continues on following page

Problem	Rationale	Action to be Taken
First assume that inability to irrigate the port is caused by a malpositioned or occluded Huber point needle. If after the needle is changed, irrigation is still not possible, the probability of occlusion is high.	flow to the catheter either by pump malfunction, by a problem with the intravenous tubing, or by unrecognized completion of the infusion.	gently using a push–pull technique. (Selection of a 10-cc syringe is essential because this will ensure that a high pressure is not exerted on the occluded catheter, which may cause it to rupture or separate from the port.) If preceding attempts are not successful, confer with physician about administration of a lytic agent (e.g., urokinase) to attempt to lyse the clot.
	Intralumenal drug precipitation	In the case of drug precipitation, prevention is often the only course of action. Once drug crystals have lodged within the catheter lumen, they are extremely difficult to dissolve.

	Venous thrombosis.
	Note: The most frequent signs and symptoms of venous thrombosis include
	Discomfort or pain in the area of the shoulder, neck, or arm.
	Supraclavicular swelling.
	Pattern of venous distension in the neck, shoulder, or chest wall.
	Development of collateral circulation on the chest wall or arm.
	Less frequent signs and symptoms of venous thrombosis include
	  Dysphagia.
	  Superior vena cava syndrome.
	  Pain in the ear.
	  Headache.
	These symptoms usually occur on the same side as the catheter but occasionally may occur contralaterally.
		Attach a 10-cc syringe with 5 cc of heparin saline solution. Attempt to flush gently. If the patient complains of pain or if complete resistance is met, stop procedure and confer with physician about a radiographic dye study and/or systemic thrombolytic therapy.

Local infection	Alteration in skin integrity overlying the venous access port or surrounding the exit site of right atrial Silastic catheter	Evaluate the patient's temperature; if elevated, notify physician. Assess skin overlying the port or surrounding the catheter for signs and symptoms of infection:
		  erythema
		  inflammation
		  tenderness
		  exudate.
		If local infection is suspected in an implanted port and a Huber point needle is already in place:
		  Draw blood culture through the port using existing needle.
		  Draw peripheral blood culture.
		  Culture needle site.
		  Apply povidone-iodine ointment to the site.
		  Administer systemic antibiotics as prescribed.
		Note: Blood cultures should be done through the port only if a Huber point needle is already in place at the time the infectious process is noted. Otherwise, a potentially infected port pocket should never be accessed with a needle to decrease

Table continues on following page

Problem	Rationale	Action to be Taken
		the risk of tracking organisms into the port reservoir, into the catheter, and subsequently into the systemic circulation.
		If local infection is suspected in a right atrial catheter: Culture the exit site. Cleanse the exit site with hydrogen peroxide and saline, and swab with povidone-iodine. Apply povidone-iodine ointment to the exit site. Obtain peripheral and/or device cultures as prescribed.
		If the subcutaneous tunnel of the venous access device is inflamed, notify the physician and apply warm saline soaks continuously to the area.
Systemic infection	Signs and symptoms of systemic infection when a long-term venous access device is implanted lead to suspicion that the venous access device may be the source of infection.	Evaluate the patient's temperature; if elevated, notify physician. Assess skin around the device for signs and symptoms of infection: erythema inflammation tenderness exudate.
		If local infection is suspected, follow preceding guidelines for action to be taken with a local infection.
		If the patient is febrile and the area around the port does not appear to be infected, the port may be accessed according to procedure: Obtain blood culture via the port or the right atrial catheter. Obtain peripheral blood cultures. Administer systemic antibiotics as prescribed.
Port extrusion through the skin	Therapy through the venous port may cause damage to the skin integrity, as in the case of fluid extravasation, or the results of therapy may cause loss of body tissue, as in the case of cachexia related to chemotherapy, which causes the metal or plastic port reservoir to extrude through the skin.	Notify physician to determine if the venous access port requires removal.
Catheter slippage out of the skin	Excessive tension on intravenous tubing or the catheter itself or unintentional pulling on the catheter may cause it to slip out of the exit site, especially if the Dacron cuff has not fully engrafted. This may be recognized by the presence of the Dacron cuff at the exit site or by the appearance of the catheter itself. The portion of the catheter that was originally under the surface of the skin will be a slightly different color than the external portion of the catheter.	Notify physician to determine if the external catheter requires removal. The catheter may be stitched in place if a chest x-ray verifies that the catheter tip remains in the proper location for use.

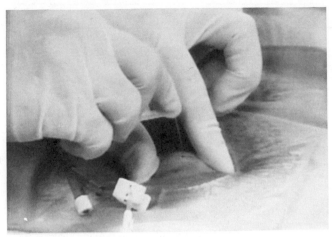

FIGURE 34–6. Insertion of right-angle Huber point needle into the totally implanted venous access port. (Courtesy of Strato Medical Corporation.)

Evaluation

1. Compare the patient's skin assessments before and after accessing the totally implanted venous access port. **Rationale:** Identifies the effects of the access procedure on the patient's skin integrity.

2. Monitor the patient's vital signs, including temperature, heart rate, blood pressure, and respiratory rate every 4 hours. **Rationale:** Identifies signs and symptoms of infection related to access of the totally implanted venous access port.

3. Monitor the site for signs and symptoms of extravasation. When the implanted port is used for continuous infusions, the site is assessed every 2 to 4 hours. **Rationale:** Enables early detection of extravasation and minimizes trauma to the tissue surrounding the port.

Expected Outcomes

1. Intact skin overlying and surrounding the implanted venous access port. **Rationale:** The presence of the totally implanted venous access port and repeated access increase the risk for impaired skin integrity.

2. Intravenous pharmacotherapy and/or transfusions continue as prescribed without interruption. **Rationale:** Totally implanted venous access port remains patent for therapeutic intervention.

3. Patient is free of signs and symptoms of infection. **Rationale:** Maintenance of sterile technique when accessing and utilizing the port and minimizing strain on the catheter tubing (thereby decreasing the risk for needle dislodgment/extravasation) diminishes the risks for infection.

Unexpected Outcomes

1. Extravasation of fluid into subcutaneous tissue surrounding the implanted venous access port. **Rationale:** Displaced Huber point needle, damaged venous access port, or thrombus at the tip of the catheter.

2. Inability to withdraw blood from the implanted venous access port. **Rationale:** Incorrectly placed Huber point needle with needle bevel within the septum of the implanted port rather than in the port reservoir, catheter tip lying against the wall of the blood vessel, or formation of a fibrin sheath at the tip of the catheter causing a one-way valve effect during blood withdrawal attempt.

3. Inability to irrigate the implanted venous access port. **Rationale:** Catheter occlusion: intralumenal clot, intralumenal drug precipitate, or venous thrombosis.

4. Impaired skin integrity overlying the implanted venous access port. **Rationale:** Fluid extravasation, irritation related to skin care procedures, presence of the needle in the implanted port septum, local infection, or port extrusion.

5. Systemic infection. **Rationale:** An implanted venous access port is a potential source of infection.

6. Port extrusion through the skin. **Rationale:** Therapy through the implanted venous access port may cause damage to the skin integrity (e.g., extravasation) or the results of therapy may cause loss of body tissue (e.g., cachexia related to chemotherapy), which causes the titanium or plastic port reservoir to extrude through the skin.

Documentation

Documentation in the patient record should include the date and time of the procedure, position of the port upon palpation, condition of the overlying skin and surrounding tissue, ease of insertion of the Huber point needle, needle gauge and length, degree of patency of the port, presence or absence of blood return, any signs of extravasation, the patient's tolerance of the procedure, any unexpected outcomes encountered and interventions taken. **Rationale:** Documents nursing care given, functional status of the implanted venous port, and expected and unexpected outcomes.

Patient/Family Education

1. Assess patient and family understanding of the indications for placement of the totally implanted venous access port and its function. **Rationale:** The patient and family require knowledge of the indications for use and function of the totally implanted venous access port to ensure that the port is used appropriately and to notify health care professionals that the port is in situ, since its presence may not be apparent with visual inspection only.

2. Educate the patient and family about the necessity for routine heparinization of the implanted venous access port by a health care professional when it is not in use (e.g., every 4 to 6 weeks), and stress the importance of keeping scheduled appointments. **Rationale:** The patient and family must comply with the maintenance requirements of the implanted venous access port to facilitate its optimal function.

3. Have the patient and family state the signs and symptoms of local infection versus systemic infection (e.g., fever, chills, flulike symptoms, erythema, tenderness, exudate at the needle insertion site) and how to contact the physician when these symptoms are present.

Rationale: Facilitates immediate assessment/intervention when signs and symptoms of an infection are present.

4. Provide the patient and family with a patient education booklet and a completed medical alert identification card (to be carried with the patient *at all times*) indicating the type of implanted venous access port and

its location. **Rationale:** Provides the patient and family with written materials for reference should problems or questions arise. Also provides a source of information about the implanted venous access port to health care personnel.

Performance Checklist
Skill 34–1 Access to and Administration through a Totally Implanted Venous Access Port

Critical Behaviors	Complies	
	yes	no
1. Wash hands.		
2. Identify port system and silicone septum by palpation.		
3. Prep the port, and allow the povidone-iodine to air dry.		
4. Rewash hands.		
5. Create a sterile field.		
6. Place appropriate equipment onto the sterile field.		
7. Cleanse the top of the normal saline vial.		
8. Don sterile gloves.		
9. Attach needles to syringes.		
10. Fill syringes with normal saline or heparin saline solution as appropriate.		
11. Don second set of sterile gloves.		
12. Prime Huber point needle administration set and leave syringe attached.		
13. Stabilize port with nondominant hand.		
14. Insert Huber point needle into the port septum.		
15. Aspirate blood into the syringe.		
16. Inject normal saline into the port, clamp the administration set, and remove the syringe.		
17. Observe for signs of extravasation.		
18. For *continuous infusion*, connect primed intravenous tubing directly to the Huber point needle administration set, and seal the connection with paper tape.		
19. For *intermittent use*, attach a male Luer-Loc adapter to the Huber point administration set, seal the connection with paper tape, and heparin lock the port.		
20. Place a folded 2 × 2 in gauze pad under the hub of the Huber point needle (if needed).		
21. Apply a sterile transparent dressing.		
22. Remove sterile gloves.		
23. Adjust intravenous solution to prescribed rate (for continuous infusion).		
24. Form a safety loop with the Huber point needle administration set tubing, and secure to the chest.		
25. Discard used equipment appropriately.		
26. Wash hands.		
27. Document procedure in the patient record.		

SKILL 34–2

Obtaining Blood Specimens through a Totally Implanted Venous Access Port

A Huber port needle must be placed in the septum of the totally implanted venous access port to obtain blood specimens (see Skill 34–1). Blood specimens may be obtained from an implanted venous access port when a continuous intravenous infusion is in progress or when the port is accessed and heparin locked. Coagulation studies *may not* be drawn through a "locked" implanted venous access port because it is heparinized or through a continuous infusion line containing heparin because the results would not reflect the true coagulation status of the patient.

When the venous port has been implanted for a period of time (usually more than 6 months), there is a tendency for fibrin sheath formation at the tip of the Silastic catheter. Infusion through the port is usually not compromised. However, the fibrin sheath can occlude the opening of the catheter tip when blood withdrawal is attempted, causing what is known as a one-way valve effect. Administration of a thrombolytic agent (e.g., urokinase) is often useful in dissolving this sheath, and blood withdrawal can again be achieved. In the event that blood withdrawal is still not possible, administration through the port is permissible when radiographic studies confirm the integrity and correct placement of the implanted venous access port and the attached Silastic catheter.

Purpose

The nurse obtains blood specimens from an implanted venous access port to

1. Provide assessment data related to the medical/nursing diagnosis.
2. Evaluate the efficacy of the medical/nursing interventions and treatment plan.

Prerequisite Knowledge and Skills

Prior to obtaining blood specimens from an implanted venous access port, the nurse should understand

1. Anatomy and physiology of the vascular system.
2. Design, purpose, and function of the implanted venous access port.
3. Principles of aseptic technique.
4. Principles of infection control.
5. Universal precautions.

The nurse should be able to perform

1. Proper handwashing technique (see Skill 35–5).
2. Universal precautions (see Skill 35–1).
3. Verification of proper placement of the Huber point needle within the reservoir of the implanted venous access port (see Skill 34–1).
4. Peripheral blood specimen collection.

Assessment

Assess the port site for signs and symptoms of fluid extravasation (swelling in the port pocket, complaints of pain over the port site), venous thrombosis (discomfort/pain in the area of the shoulder, neck, or arm; supraclavicular swelling; venous distension; or development of collateral circulation), and impaired skin integrity (erythema, inflammation, or exudate). **Rationale:** Determines that the implanted venous access port meets criteria enabling blood specimens to be obtained.

Nursing Diagnoses

1. Potential impaired skin integrity related to the presence of a foreign body within the subcutaneous tissue. **Rationale:** Repeated venipuncture through the skin overlying the implanted venous port, infusate extravasation into the subcutaneous tissue surrounding the implanted venous port, and irritation caused by cleansing the skin with povidone-iodine solution increase the risk for impaired skin integrity.
2. Potential for infection related to interruption of closed system to obtain blood specimens. **Rationale:** There is a direct relationship between the number of interruptions of the system and the increased risk of infection.

Planning

1. Individualize the following goals for obtaining blood specimens:
   a. Monitor treatment. **Rationale:** Laboratory analysis of blood specimens allows evaluation of effects of treatment.
   b. Prevent additional venipuncture procedures. **Rationale:** Decreases patient trauma.
   c. Maintain infection-free state. **Rationale:** Decreases patient morbidity.
2. Prepare all necessary equipment and supplies. **Rationale:** Assembly of all the necessary equipment at the bedside ensures that the procedure will be completed quickly and efficiently.
   a. Plastic vacutainer holder.
   b. One 21-gauge 1½-in two-way vacutainer needle.
   c. Three alcohol preps.
   d. Appropriate tubes for specimen collection and an extra tube marked with an X (identifies discard tube).
   e. Appropriate requisitions and patient identification labels.
   f. One 5-cc syringe.
   g. One 3-cc syringe.
   h. Two 20-gauge 1-in needles.
   i. Sterile normal saline solution for injection, 10 cc.
   j. One hemostat (if continuous intravenous infusion is in progress).
   k. Heparin saline solution 100 units/cc (for heparin-locked port), 3 cc.
   l. One pair of nonsterile gloves.

3. Prepare the patient.
   a. Explain the procedure to the patient. **Rationale:** Minimizes risks and reduces anxiety.
   b. Assist the patient in achieving a position, usually supine or sitting, that is comfortable for the patient and the nurse. **Rationale:** Promotes patient comfort and supports good body mechanics for the nurse.
4. Verify the physician request for laboratory specimens. **Rationale:** Eliminates unnecessary laboratory tests.

Implementation

Steps	Rationale	Special Considerations
1. Wash hands with antiseptic solution.	Reduces transmission of microorganisms.	A Huber point needle administration set must be in place prior to performing this procedure (see Skill 34–1).
2. Cleanse the top of the normal saline vial with an alcohol prep.	Infection control.	
3. Using the 5-cc syringe, draw up 5 cc of normal saline.	The 5-cc syringe identifies the normal saline.	It is *essential* to standardize the size of the syringes used (e.g., 5 cc for normal saline and 3 cc for heparin saline solution) to readily differentiate them from each other.
4. For heparin-locked ports, cleanse the top of the heparin saline vial with an alcohol prep.	Infection control.	
5. Using the 3-cc syringe, draw up 3 cc of heparin saline solution.	The 3-cc syringe identifies the heparin saline solution.	
6. Assemble vacutainer holder and needle.	For obtaining blood specimen.	
7. Don nonsterile gloves.	Universal precautions.	
8. Using a hemostat, clamp the intravenous tubing proximal to the Y-port nearest to the Huber point needle, and cleanse the diaphragm with an alcohol prep.	Minimizes the amount of intravenous fluid to be discarded before obtaining the blood specimens.	
9. Insert 1 to 2 cm of the vacutainer needle into the rubber diaphragm of the Huber point administration set.	Inserting only 1 to 2 cm of the needle prevents puncturing the administration set.	
10. Insert specimen tube marked with the X (discard tube) into the end of the vacutainer holder, puncturing the rubber stopper. Maintain the tube in an upright position.	Approximately 10 cc of blood is discarded to ensure accurate laboratory results.	A discard tube is not necessary if the first specimen is sent for culture and sensitivity or type and crossmatch.
11. If unable to obtain blood, remove the specimen tube, irrigate the port with 5 cc of normal saline, and reattempt obtaining specimen.	A vigorous flush with normal saline may eliminate intralumenal fibrin sludge, which may be causing a one-way valve effect.	If still unable to obtain blood, notify physician.
12. Set aside discard tube.	Reduces risk of confusion of discard tube with laboratory specimens.	
13. Insert second specimen tube into vacutainer holder, and puncture rubber stopper. Continue in this manner until all specimens are obtained.	Allows for specimen collection.	PT/PTT samples *cannot* be obtained from a heparinized port with a capped Huber point needle administration set. PT/PTT samples *can* be obtained from a port connected to a continuous intravenous infusion provided the infusion does *not* contain heparin.

Table continues on following page

Steps	Rationale	Special Considerations
14. Remove the vacutainer needle from the rubber diaphragm, insert the 5-cc syringe containing normal saline into the same rubber diaphragm used for blood drawing, and flush the port with 5 cc of normal saline.	It is *essential* to flush the port with normal saline after the last blood specimen is obtained even if the patient has a continuous intravenous infusion to prevent intralumenal clotting or blood clot formation within the port reservoir.	
15. If the patient has a continuous intravenous infusion, remove the hemostat, and resume intravenous fluid administration at the prescribed rate.	The port is not heparinized after blood specimen collection if the patient has a continuous intravenous infusion.	
16. If the patient does not have a continuous infusion, heparinize the port by injecting the 3 cc of heparin saline solution.	Prevents intralumenal clotting or blood clot formation within the port reservoir.	
17. Label the tubes of blood in accordance with institutional policy.	Promotes proper identification of blood specimens.	
18. Discard used equipment in appropriate manner.	Universal precautions.	
19. Remove and discard gloves.	Universal precautions.	
20. Wash hands with antiseptic solution.	Reduces transmission of microorganisms.	

Evaluation

Compare the patency assessments before and after obtaining blood specimens. **Rationale:** Identifies the development of any signs and symptoms of device occlusion related to obtaining blood specimens.

Expected Outcomes

1. Blood specimens are obtained. **Rationale:** The implanted venous access port is patent and does not demonstrate evidence of one-way valve effect.
2. The implanted venous access port remains patent. **Rationale:** Failure to flush and/or heparinize the implanted venous access port may lead to catheter and/or port reservoir occlusion.

Unexpected Outcomes

1. Inability to withdraw blood specimens. **Rationale:** Incorrectly placed Huber point needle with bevel within the septum of the implanted port rather than in the port reservoir, catheter tip lying against the wall of the blood vessel, or formation of a fibrin sheath at the tip of the catheter causing a one-way valve effect during withdrawal attempt.
2. Inability to irrigate the implanted venous access port. **Rationale:** Catheter occlusion: intralumenal clot, intralumenal drug precipitate, or venous thrombosis.

3. Extravasation of fluid into the subcutaneous tissue surrounding the implanted venous access port. **Rationale:** Displaced Huber point needle, damaged venous access port, or thrombus at the tip of the catheter.

Documentation

Documentation in the patient record should include the degree of patency of the port; the presence or absence of blood return; date, time, and type of specimen(s) obtained; the patient's tolerance of the procedure; and any unexpected outcomes encountered and interventions taken. **Rationale:** Documents nursing care given, functional status of the implanted venous port, and expected and unexpected outcomes.

Patient/Family Education

Explain to the patient and family what tests will be performed with the specimen(s) and the relationship to the treatment plan. **Rationale:** Encourages patient and family questions and understanding of treatment plan.

Performance Checklist
Skill 34–2: Obtaining Blood Specimens through a Totally Implanted Venous Access Port

Critical Behaviors	Complies yes	no
1. Wash hands.		
2. Cleanse top of normal saline vial.		
3. Draw up 5 cc of normal saline.		
4. If port is heparin locked, cleanse top of heparin saline solution vial.		
5. Draw up 3 cc of heparin saline solution.		
6. Assemble vacutainer holder and needle.		
7. Don nonsterile gloves.		
8. Clamp the intravenous tubing using a hemostat, and cleanse the rubber diaphragm.		
9. Insert the vacutainer needle into the rubber diaphragm.		
10. Obtain discard specimen.		
11. If unable to obtain blood, irrigate port with normal saline, and reattempt obtaining the blood specimen.		
12. Set discard tube aside.		
13. Obtain blood specimens for laboratory analysis.		
14. Flush the port with normal saline.		
15. If the patient has a continuous intravenous infusion, remove hemostat to resume intravenous fluid administration.		
16. If the patient does not have a continuous intravenous infusion, heparinize the port.		
17. Label the tubes of blood appropriately.		
18. Discard used equipment in appropriate manner.		
19. Remove and discard gloves.		
20. Wash hands.		
21. Document procedure in the patient record.		

SKILL 34–3

Removing the Huber Point Needle Administration Set from a Totally Implanted Venous Access Port

Patients receiving treatment through a totally implanted venous access port usually have the Huber point needle removed prior to discharge. If the patient will be receiving a continuous infusion at home via an ambulatory infusion pump, as is occurring more and more frequently, he or she will return to an ambulatory care facility to have the infusion discontinued and the implanted venous access port heparinized, or a home health agency may provide this service in the patient's home.

Purpose

The nurse removes the Huber point needle adminis-

tration set from a totally implanted venous access port to

1. Terminate intravenous treatments/interventions.
2. Eliminate access to the central venous system.

Prerequisite Knowledge and Skills

Prior to removing the Huber point needle administration set from a totally implanted venous access port, the nurse should understand

1. Anatomy and physiology of the vascular system.
2. Design, purpose, and function of the totally implanted venous access port.
3. Rationale for heparinization of the totally implanted venous access port.
4. Principles of aseptic technique.
5. Principles of infection control.
6. Universal precautions.

The nurse should be able to perform

1. Proper handwashing technique (see Skill 35–5).
2. Skin assessment of the trunk and neck.
3. Irrigation of the implanted venous access port (see Skill 34–1).
4. Universal precautions (see Skill 35–1).

Assessment

Assess the port site for signs and symptoms of fluid extravasation (swelling in the port pocket, complaints of pain over the port site), venous thrombosis (discomfort/pain in the area of the shoulder, neck, or arm; supraclavicular swelling; venous distension; or development of collateral circulation), and impaired skin integrity (erythema, inflammation, or exudate). **Rationale:** Identifies complications that require intervention prior to removing the Huber point needle administration set.

Nursing Diagnoses

1. Potential for impaired skin integrity related to the presence of a foreign body in the subcutaneous tissue. **Rationale:** Presence of a Huber point needle within the implanted port septum, infusate extravasation into the subcutaneous tissue surrounding the implanted venous port, and irritation caused by removing excess povidone-iodine or adhesive from the skin place the patient at increased risk for impaired skin integrity.

2. Potential for infection related to the presence of a foreign body in the subcutaneous tissue. **Rationale:** Presence of direct access into the central venous vasculature places the patient at increased risk for infection.

Planning

1. Individualize the following goals for implanted venous access port deaccession procedure:
   a. Terminate direct access into the central venous system. **Rationale:** Treatment is complete, and continued access is no longer necessary.
   b. Maintain optimal function of the implanted venous access port. **Rationale:** Skin integrity and patency of the totally implanted venous access port are maintained by adhering to established procedures.

2. Prepare all necessary equipment and supplies. **Rationale:** Assembly of all the necessary equipment at the bedside ensures that the procedure will be completed quickly and efficiently.
   a. One 5-cc syringe.
   b. One 3-cc syringe.
   c. Two 20-gauge 1-in needles.
   d. Normal saline solution for injection, 5 cc.
   e. Heparin saline solution (100 units/cc), 3 cc.
   f. Three alcohol preps.
   g. One sterile 2 × 2 in gauze pad.
   h. One pair of nonsterile gloves.
   i. Adhesive remover.
   j. One Band-Aid.

3. Prepare the patient.
   a. Explain the procedure to the patient. **Rationale:** Minimizes risks and reduces anxiety.
   b. Assist the patient in achieving a position (usually supine) that is comfortable for the patient and the nurse. **Rationale:** Promotes patient comfort and supports good body mechanics for the nurse.

Implementation

Steps	Rationale	Special Considerations
1. Wash hands with antiseptic solution.	Reduces transmission of microorganisms.	
2. Cleanse the top of the normal saline vial with an alcohol prep.	Infection control.	
3. Using the 5-cc syringe, draw up 5 cc of normal saline, recap needle, and set aside.	The 5-cc syringe identifies the normal saline.	It is *essential* to standardize the sizes of the syringes used (e.g., 5-cc for normal saline and 3 cc for heparin saline solution) in order to readily differentiate them from each other.
4. Cleanse the top of the heparin saline solution vial with an alcohol prep.	Infection control.	
5. Using the 3-cc syringe, draw up 3 cc of heparin saline solution, recap needle, and set aside.	The 3-cc syringe identifies the heparin saline solution.	
6. Don nonsterile gloves.	Universal precautions.	This procedure utilizes clean technique. Sterile gloves are not necessary.
7. Clamp the extension tubing.	Prevents backflow of blood.	

Table continues on following page

Steps	Rationale	Special Considerations
8. Cleanse the rubber diaphragm of the Y-port of the Huber point needle administration set with an alcohol prep.	Infection control.	
9. Insert the needle of the 5-cc syringe into the rubber diaphragm, and irrigate the port with normal saline.	The normal saline clears the port reservoir and catheter lumen of residual blood and/or intravenous fluid.	Observe for signs of extravasation.
10. Insert the needle of the 3-cc syringe into the rubber diaphragm of the Y-port, and irrigate the port with the heparin saline solution. Keep the extension tubing clamped to avoid blood backflow.	Prevents blood clot formation within the port reservoir and Silastic catheter.	The implanted port is irrigated after each use or every 4 to 6 weeks when not in use.
11. Gently remove the transparent dressing.	Abrupt movement of the Huber point needle will damage the port septum.	Be careful not to dislodge the Huber point needle while removing the dressing.
12. If present, remove the rolled gauze from under the needle and discard.	Facilitates visualization of needle insertion site.	
13. Stabilize the port with the thumb and forefinger of the nondominant hand, and with the dominant hand, firmly hold the hub of the Huber point needle and withdraw at a perpendicular angle to the skin.	Deaccesses port.	To prevent skin and septum damage, avoid angling or rotating the needle in the port septum.
14. Apply pressure to the puncture site with a sterile 2 × 2-in gauze for 5 minutes.	Prevents hematoma formation.	
15. Remove remaining povidone-iodine solution from the skin with an alcohol prep.	Prevents irritation caused by the povidone-iodine and promotes skin integrity.	
16. Remove adhesive left on the skin by the transparent dressing with adhesive remover.	Prevents irritation caused by the adhesive and promotes skin integrity.	
17. Observe the port site for tenderness or erythema.	Signs of local inflammation/infection.	Report to the physician any signs of infection/inflammation (see Table 34–1).
18. Apply Band-Aid over needle puncture site.	Prevents contamination of recent puncture site.	
19. Discard used equipment in the appropriate manner.	Universal precautions.	
20. Remove and discard gloves.	Universal precautions.	
21. Wash hands with antiseptic solution.	Reduces transmission of microorganisms.	

Evaluation

Compare the patient's skin assessment before accession of the implanted venous access port with the skin assessment at the time of the removal of the Huber point needle administration set. **Rationale:** Identifies the effects of the access and maintenance procedures on patient's skin integrity.

Expected Outcomes

1. Intact skin overlying and surrounding the implanted venous access port. **Rationale:** Utilizing proper

procedures to access and maintain the implanted venous access port promotes optimal skin integrity.

2. The implanted venous access port remains patent. **Rationale:** Failure to flush and/or reheparinize the implanted venous access port may lead to catheter and/or port reservoir occlusion.

Unexpected Outcomes

1. Extravasation of fluid into the subcutaneous tissue surrounding the implanted venous access port. **Rationale:** Displaced Huber point needle, damaged venous access port, or thrombus at the tip of the catheter.

2. Inability to irrigate the implanted venous access port. **Rationale:** Catheter occlusion: intralumenal clot, intralumenal drug precipitate, or venous thrombosis.

3. Impaired skin integrity overlying the implanted venous access port. **Rationale:** Fluid extravasation, irritation related to skin care procedures, local infection, or port extrusion.

Documentation

Documentation in the patient record should include the date and time of procedure, assessment of skin integrity, ease of removal of the Huber point needle, degree of patency of the implanted venous access port, signs of extravasation, the patient's tolerance of the procedure, and any unexpected outcomes encountered and interventions taken. **Rationale:** Documents nursing care given, functional status of the implanted venous access port, and expected and unexpected outcomes.

Patient/Family Education

1. Educate the patient and family about the necessity for routine heparinization of the implanted venous access port by a health care professional when it is not in use (e.g., every 4 to 6 weeks), and stress the importance of keeping scheduled appointments. **Rationale:** The patient and family must comply with the maintenance requirements of the implanted venous access port to facilitate its optimal function.

2. Have the patient and family state the signs and symptoms of local infection versus systemic infection (e.g., fever, chills, flulike symptoms, erythema, tenderness, or exudate at the needle insertion site) and how to contact the physician when these symptoms are present. **Rationale:** Facilitates immediate assessment/intervention when signs and symptoms of an infection are present.

3. Provide the patient and family with a patient education booklet and a completed medical alert identification card (to be carried with the patient *at all times*) indicating the type of implanted venous access port and its location. **Rationale:** Provides the patient and family with written materials for reference should problems or questions arise. Also provides a source of information about the implanted venous access port to health care personnel.

Performance Checklist
Skill 34–3: Removing the Huber Point Needle Administration Set from a Totally Implanted Venous Access Port

Critical Behaviors	Complies yes	no
1. Wash hands.		
2. Cleanse top of normal saline vial.		
3. Draw up 5 cc of normal saline, recap needle, and set aside.		
4. Cleanse top of heparin saline vial.		
5. Draws up 3 cc of heparin saline solution, recap needle, and set aside.		
6. Don nonsterile gloves.		
7. Clamp extension tubing.		
8. Cleanse the rubber diaphragm of the Y-port of the Huber point needle administration set.		
9. Irrigate the port with normal saline.		
10. Irrigate the port with heparin saline solution.		
11. Remove the transparent dressing.		
12. If present, remove the rolled gauze.		
13. Withdraw the Huber point needle.		
14. Apply pressure to the puncture site.		
15. Remove remaining povidone-iodine solution.		

Table continues on following page

Performance Checklist
Skill

Critical Behaviors	Complies	
	yes	no
16. Remove remaining adhesive.		
17. Observe port site for tenderness or erythema.		
18. Apply Band-Aid.		
19. Discard used equipment in appropriate manner.		
20. Remove and discard gloves.		
21. Wash hands.		
22. Document procedure in the patient record.		

SKILL 34–4

Luer-lok Cap Change and Irrigation of a Right Atrial Silastic Catheter

Right atrial Silastic catheters require routine maintenance to promote optimal function. At this point in time there are no standardized catheter care protocols based on controlled studies indicating which solution the catheter should be irrigated with (normal saline solution versus heparin saline solution), the concentration of heparin if heparin saline solution is used (10 units/cc versus 100 units/cc), the amount of solution for irrigation (3, 5, 10, or 20 cc), and the frequency of irrigation (daily, twice weekly, or weekly). The exception to this statement is the Groshong right atrial catheter. This catheter has a unique slit valve at the tip that remains closed when the catheter is not in use and thus prevents blood backup. Normal saline is used to routinely irrigate this catheter on a weekly basis. Most hospital maintenance protocols are based on recommendations from the manufacturers of the Silastic catheters. Regardless of protocol used, the procedure remains the same.

Purpose

The nurse performs the right atrial Silastic catheter Luer-lok cap change and irrigation to maintain catheter patency.

Prerequisite Knowledge and Skills

Prior to performing the right atrial Silastic catheter Luer-lok cap change and irrigation, the nurse should understand

1. Anatomy and physiology of the vascular system.
2. Design, purpose, and function of the right atrial Silastic catheter.
3. Principles of aseptic technique.
4. Principles of infection control.
5. Universal precautions.

The nurse should be able to perform

1. Proper handwashing technique (see Skill 35–5).
2. Assessment of catheter integrity.
3. Assessment of the skin surrounding the right atrial catheter.
4. Universal precautions (see Skill 35–1).

Assessment

1. Assess the skin surrounding the catheter for pain, swelling, venous distension, and development of collateral circulation. **Rationale:** Detects signs and symptoms of venous thrombosis.
2. Assess the patient's vital signs, including temperature, heart rate, blood pressure, and respiratory rate. **Rationale:** Supports diagnosis of local and/or systemic infection.

Nursing Diagnoses

1. Potential for infection related to the presence of a foreign body in the subcutaneous tissue. **Rationale:** Direct access into the central venous vasculature, the venous access device exiting from the skin, and the necessity for specific home maintenance procedures increase the risk for infection.
2. Body image disturbance related to the presence of a skin-exiting venous access device. **Rationale:** Patients will have varying degrees of comfort/coping skills with this adjustment to a changed body image.

Planning

1. Individualize the following goals for maintaining optimal function of the right atrial Silastic catheter:
   a. Maintain venous access. **Rationale:** Allows for administration of intravenous therapy, medications, TPN, chemotherapy, and blood/blood products and withdrawal of blood specimens for laboratory analysis.

b. Maintain optimal function of the right atrial Silastic catheter. **Rationale:** Skin integrity and patency of the right atrial Silastic catheter are maintained by adhering to established procedures.

2. Prepare all necessary equipment and supplies. **Rationale:** Assembly of all the necessary equipment at the bedside ensures that procedure will be completed quickly and efficiently.
   a. Atraumatic catheter clamp.
   b. Luer-lok catheter cap.
   c. One roll of 1-in paper tape.
   d. One syringe prefilled with prescribed amount/concentration of irrigation solution.
   e. One 25-gauge ⅝-in needle.
   f. Two alcohol preps.
   g. One pair of nonsterile gloves.
   If a prefilled syringe is not available:
   h. One 10-cc syringe.
   i. One 20-gauge 1-in needle.
   j. One vial of prescribed amount/concentration of irrigation solution.

3. Prepare the patient.
   a. Explain the procedure to the patient. **Rationale:** Minimizes risk and reduces anxiety.
   b. Assist the patient in achieving a position (usually supine or sitting) that is comfortable for the patient and nurse. **Rationale:** Promotes patient comfort and supports good body mechanics for the nurse.

Implementation

Steps	Rationale	Special Considerations
1. Wash hands with antiseptic solution.	Reduces transmission of microorganisms.	
2. Prepare a clean area upon which to work (a sterile field is not necessary).	Infection control.	Catheter care should *never* be performed in the bathroom.
3. Don nonsterile gloves.	Universal precautions.	
4. Apply atraumatic catheter clamp to reinforced area of the external catheter.	Prevents damage to the friable Silastic material.	If the catheter does not have a reinforced area upon which to clamp, apply a piece of paper tape and wrap it around the catheter so that the opposite edges adhere. Clamp over the paper tape. Change the location of the paper tape every time you clamp the catheter to avoid repeated clamping on the same area.
5. Remove tape from catheter tubing/Luer-lok cap connection.	Allows for Luer-lok cap removal.	
6. Open Luer-lok cap package, and remove cover on new cap.	Prepares for cap replacement.	Do not contaminate the exposed end of the catheter cap.
7. Twist off old cap counterclockwise, and twist on new cap clockwise.	Maintains closed system to prevent infection.	The Luer-lok cap should be changed once or twice per week depending on usage; if it is punctured frequently, change the cap more often. The catheter should only be capped when it is not being used or only being used for intermittent infusions. Continuous intravenous infusions should be *connected directly* to the Silastic catheter tubing.
8. Fold down the edges of a piece of paper tape, and wrap the tape around the connection so that the opposite edges adhere.	Prevents accidental separation of the cap from the catheter tubing.	Folding down the edges of the paper tape facilitates removal of the tape at the next Luer-lok cap change.
9. Remove atraumatic catheter clamp.	Allows for infusion of irrigation solution.	
10. For *prefilled syringes*, attach the 25-gauge ⅝-in needle to the syringe.	Use of a 25-gauge needle will make the smallest possible core in the rubber tip Luer-lok cap upon insertion.	If syringe comes prepackaged with a larger-bore needle, replace it with the 25-gauge needle.

Table continues on following page

Steps	Rationale	Special Considerations
11. If not already in place, insert the plunger into the syringe.	Prepares syringe for use.	Maintain sterility of needle and syringe.
12. *If prefilled syringes are unavailable*, attach the 20-gauge 1-in needle to the 10-cc syringe, cleanse top of irrigation solution vial with an alcohol prep, draw up the prescribed amount of irrigation solution, and replace the 20-gauge needle with the 25-gauge ⅝-in needle.		
13. Cleanse the rubber diaphragm of the Luer-lok cap with an alcohol prep.	Reduces transmission of microorganisms.	
14. Insert the needle into the rubber diaphragm of the Luer-lok cap, and inject the prescribed amount/concentration of irrigation solution.	It is only necessary to irrigate the catheter when it is not in use in order to maintain patency.	Be absolutely sure that the atraumatic catheter clamp has been removed from the catheter before injecting the irrigation solution to avoid catheter rupture.
15. Discard used equipment in appropriate manner.	Universal precautions.	
16. Remove and discard gloves.	Universal precautions.	
17. Wash hands with antiseptic solution.	Reduces transmission of microorganisms.	

Evaluation

1. Monitor the patient's vital signs, including temperature, heart rate, blood pressure, and respiratory rate, every 4 hours. **Rationale:** Identifies signs and symptoms of infection related to irrigation of the right atrial Silastic catheter.
2. Compare patency assessments before and after performing the Luer-lok cap change and irrigation. **Rationale:** Detects signs and symptoms of catheter occlusion.
3. Monitor the skin surrounding the catheter for evidence of infection, extravasation, venous distension, and the development of collateral circulation. **Rationale:** Allows for immediate intervention.

Expected Outcomes

1. Right atrial Silastic catheter is patent. **Rationale:** Promotes maximum catheter indwelling time.
2. Right atrial Silastic catheter remains infection free. **Rationale:** Performing Luer-lok cap change and irrigation according to established procedures diminishes risk of infection.

Unexpected Outcomes

1. Extravasation of fluid into subcutaneous tissue surrounding the right atrial Silastic catheter. **Rationale:** Damaged Silastic catheter or thrombus at the tip of the catheter.
2. Inability to irrigate the right atrial Silastic catheter.

Rationale: Catheter occlusion: intralumenal clot, intralumenal drug precipitate, or venous thrombosis.
3. Systemic infection. **Rationale:** A right atrial Silastic catheter is a potential source of infection.

Documentation

Documentation in the patient record should include the date and time of the procedure, the condition of the catheter and the skin overlying the catheter, the degree of patency of the catheter, signs of extravasation, the patient's tolerance of the procedure, and any unexpected outcomes encountered and interventions taken. **Rationale:** Documents nursing care given, functional status of the right atrial Silastic catheter, and expected and unexpected outcomes.

Patient/Family Education

1. Assess patient and family understanding of the indications for placement of the right atrial Silastic catheter and its function. **Rationale:** The patient and family require knowledge of the indications for use and function of the right atrial Silastic catheter to ensure that the catheter is used appropriately.
2. Have the patient and family state the signs and symptoms of local infection versus systemic infection (e.g., fever, chills, flulike symptoms, erythema, tenderness, or exudate at the catheter exit site) and how to contact the physician when these symptoms are present.

Rationale: Facilitates immediate assessment/intervention when signs and symptoms of an infection are present.

3. Have the patient and family state the signs and symptoms of catheter occlusion and venous thrombosis (e.g., inability to irrigate catheter, pain, swelling, venous distension, and development of collateral circulation in the area surrounding the catheter) and how to contact the physician when these symptoms are present. **Rationale:** Facilitates immediate assessment/intervention when signs and symptoms of an occlusion/venous thrombosis are present.

4. Provide the patient and family with a patient ed-

ucation booklet and a completed medical alert identification card (to be carried with the patient *at all times*) indicating the type of right atrial Silastic catheter in place. **Rationale:** Provides the patient and family with written materials for reference should problems or questions arise. Also provides a source of information about the right atrial Silastic catheter to health care personnel.

5. Evaluate the need for the patient and family to perform right atrial Silastic catheter home maintenance procedures. **Rationale:** Allows the nurse to anticipate the need for the patient's discharge home with a right atrial Silastic catheter.

Performance Checklist
Skill 34–4 Luer-lok Cap Change and Irrigation of a Right Atrial Silastic Catheter

Critical Behaviors	Complies	
	yes	no
1. Wash hands.		
2. Prepare a clean area on which to work.		
3. Don nonsterile gloves.		
4. Apply atraumatic catheter clamp.		
5. Remove tape from catheter tubing/Luer-lok cap connection.		
6. Open Luer-lok cap package, and remove cap cover.		
7. Remove old cap, and apply new cap.		
8. Apply paper tape to catheter tubing/Luer-lok cap connection.		
9. Remove atraumatic catheter clamp.		
10. For prefilled syringes, attach the 25-gauge ⅝-in needle to the syringe.		
11. If not already in place, insert the plunger into the syringe.		
12. If prefilled syringes are unavailable, attach the 20-gauge 1-in needle to the 10-cc syringe, cleanse the top of the irrigation solution vial, draw up irrigation solution, and replace 20-gauge needle with the 25-gauge ⅝-in needle.		
13. Cleanse the rubber diaphragm of the Luer-lok cap.		
14. Irrigate catheter with prescribed amount/concentration of irrigation solution.		
15. Discard used equipment in appropriate manner.		
16. Remove and discard gloves.		
17. Wash hands.		
18. Document procedure in the patient record.		

SKILL 34–5

Site Care and Dressing Change for a Right Atrial Silastic Catheter

A standard research-based protocol for right atrial Silastic catheter site care and dressing change does not exist. The results of small studies indicate no significant

difference in the use of transparent dressings versus gauze dressings versus no dressing related to local catheter site colonization and infection. The frequency of dressing changes and the skin-preparation procedure vary from institution to institution. Since the goal is to minimize irritation to the skin surrounding the catheter exit site and maintain skin integrity, individualized care protocols based on patient assessment are appropriate.

Purpose

The nurse performs right atrial Silastic catheter site care and dressing change to

1. Maintain skin integrity surrounding the right atrial Silastic catheter.
2. Reduce the incidence of catheter-related infections by preventing contamination at the exit site.
3. Promote maximum catheter indwelling time.

Prerequisite Knowledge and Skills

Prior to performing the right atrial Silastic catheter site care and dressing change, the nurse should understand

1. Design, purpose, and function of the right atrial Silastic catheter.
2. Principles of aseptic technique.
3. Principles of infection control.

The nurse should be able to perform

1. Proper handwashing technique (see Skill 35–5).
2. Skin assessment of the exit site of the right atrial catheter and the tissue overlying the catheter tunnel.

Assessment

1. Assess the skin surrounding the exit site of the right atrial Silastic catheter and the tissue overlying the catheter tunnel for pain, swelling, erythema, discharge, venous distension, or the development of collateral circulation. **Rationale:** Routine care will not be performed on compromised skin; detects signs and symptoms of local infection or venous thrombosis.
2. Assess the patient's vital signs, including temperature, heart rate, blood pressure, and respiratory rate. **Rationale:** Supports the diagnosis of local and/or systemic infection.

Nursing Diagnoses

1. Potential for impaired skin integrity related to the presence of a foreign body in the subcutaneous tissue.

Rationale: The presence of a skin-exiting venous access device, infusate extravasation into the subcutaneous tissue surrounding the right atrial Silastic catheter, and irritation caused by cleansing of the exit site with povidone-iodine solution increase the risk for impaired skin integrity.

2. Potential for infection related to the presence of a foreign body in the subcutaneous tissue. **Rationale:** Direct access into the central venous vasculature and presence of a skin-exiting venous access device increase the risk for infection.
3. Body-image disturbance related to the presence of a skin-exiting venous access device. **Rationale:** Patients will have varying degrees of comfort/coping skills with this adjustment to a changed body image.

Planning

1. Individualize the following goals for catheter site care and dressing change:
   a. Prevent catheter-related infections. **Rationale:** Preventing contamination at the exit site reduces the risk of catheter-related infection.
   b. Maintain skin integrity surrounding the catheter exit site. **Rationale:** Promotes maximum catheter indwelling time.
2. Prepare all equipment and supplies. **Rationale:** Assembly of all the necessary equipment at the bedside ensures that the procedure will be completed quickly and efficiently.
   a. Three povidone-iodine swab sticks.
   b. One sterile 4 × 4 air permeable, absorbent dressing.
   c. One roll of 1-in paper tape.
   d. Skin prep.
   e. One pair of nonsterile gloves.
3. Prepare the patient.
   a. Explain the procedure to the patient. **Rationale:** Minimizes risks and reduces anxiety.
   b. Assist the patient in achieving a position (usually supine or sitting) that is comfortable for the patient and the nurse. **Rationale:** Promotes patient comfort and supports good body mechanics for the nurse.

Implementation

Steps	Rationale	Special Considerations
1. Wash hands with antiseptic solution.	Reduces transmission of microorganisms.	
2. Prepare a clean area on which to work.	Infection control.	Catheter care should *never* be performed in the bathroom.
3. Don nonsterile gloves.	Universal precautions.	

Table continues on following page

Implementation

Steps	Rationale	Special Considerations
4. While stabilizing the catheter to avoid dislodging it, remove the old dressing by pulling the skin away from the tape rather than pulling the tape away from the skin, and discard the old dressing.	Less trauma occurs to the skin by pulling it away from the tape.	Scissors should *not* be used in removing the old dressing because the catheter may inadvertently be cut.
5. Inspect the catheter exit site and surrounding skin.	Detects early signs of impaired skin integrity.	Observations should include signs of infection (i.e., erythema, inflammation, tenderness, exudate), leakage around the catheter, and general condition of the skin. If appropriate, culture the site. The physician should be notified of any sign of skin breakdown or infection (see Table 34–1).
6. Remove gloves, and wash hands with antiseptic solution.	Gloves are contaminated from handling the old dressing.	
7. Cleanse the exit site and surrounding skin with a povidone-iodine swab stick. Start at the exit site and move outward in concentric circles 2 in beyond the exit site. Use friction to enhance the antifungal and antibacterial effects of the povidone-iodine. Repeat twice, and allow the povidone-iodine to air dry.	Reduces transmission of microorganisms.	To avoid contamination, once an area has been cleaned, do not cleanse that area with the same povidone-iodine swab stick.
8. Apply skin prep to the area that will be underneath the adhesive part of the dressing.	Enhances adhesion of dressing and may prevent skin irritation.	
9. Apply air-permeable dressing over the catheter exit site, taking care to touch only the outer edges.	Maintains sterility of the portion of the dressing that interfaces with the catheter exit site.	After the first month, if the skin is intact with good tissue granulation and without signs and symptoms of local site infection, the site is still cleansed with povidone-iodine daily, but the dressing becomes optional.
10. Pinch the adhesive portion of the dressing around the catheter.	Makes an occlusive seal around the catheter.	
11. Loop catheter, and secure to dressing using paper tape.	Prevents pulling or kinking of the catheter at the exit site.	Support of the catheter is mandatory at all times to prevent dislodgment.
12. Wash hands with antiseptic solution.	Reduces transmission of microorganisms.	

Evaluation

1. Monitor the patient's vital signs, including temperature, heart rate, blood pressure, and respiratory rate, every 4 hours. **Rationale:** Identifies signs and symptoms of infection related to the catheter presence and exit site care procedures.

2. Monitor the skin surrounding the catheter for evidence of infection, extravasation, venous distension, and the development of collateral circulation. **Rationale:** Allows for immediate intervention.

Expected Outcomes

1. The skin surrounding the right atrial Silastic catheter is intact. **Rationale:** The patient's skin integrity has not been disrupted by the presence of the catheter or by the procedures performed to maintain the catheter exit site.

2. Catheter tunnel and exit site remain free of signs and symptoms of infection. **Rationale:** Promotes maximum catheter indwelling time.

Unexpected Outcomes

1. Impaired skin integrity surrounding the exit site of the right atrial Silastic catheter and/or catheter tunnel. **Rationale:** Irritation related to skin care procedure or local infection.

2. Systemic infection. **Rationale:** A right atrial Silastic catheter is a potential source of infection.

Documentation

Documentation in the patient record should include the date and time of the procedure, the condition of the skin surrounding the catheter exit site and the tissue overlying the catheter tunnel, the patient's tolerance of the procedures, and any unexpected outcomes encountered and interventions taken. **Rationale:** Documents nursing care given, degree of skin integrity, and expected and unexpected outcomes.

Patient/Family Education

1. Have the patient and family state the signs and symptoms of local infection versus systemic infection (e.g., fever, chills, flulike symptoms, erythema, tenderness, and exudate at the catheter exit site) and how to contact the physician when these symptoms are present. **Rationale:** Facilitates immediate assessment/intervention when signs and symptoms of an infection are present.

2. Provide the patient and family with a patient education booklet and a completed medical alert identification card (to be carried with the patient *at all times*) indicating the type of right atrial Silastic catheter in place. **Rationale:** Provides the patient and family with written materials for reference should problems or questions arise. Also provides a source of information about the right atrial Silastic catheter to health care personnel.

Performance Checklist
Skill 34–5: Site Care and Dressing Change for a Right Atrial Silastic Catheter

Critical Behaviors	Complies	
	yes	no
1. Wash hands.		
2. Prepare a clean area on which to work.		
3. Don nonsterile gloves.		
4. Remove and discard old dressing.		
5. Inspect catheter exit site and surrounding skin.		
6. Remove gloves, and wash hands.		
7. Cleanse exit site and surrounding skin, and allow the povidone-iodine to air dry.		
8. Apply skin prep.		
9. Apply sterile dressing.		
10. Pinch the adhesive portion of dressing around catheter.		
11. Loop catheter, and secure it to the dressing.		
12. Wash hands.		
13. Document procedure in the patient record.		

BIBLIOGRAPHY

Brown, J. M. (1990). Evaluation of Surecath access device. *J. Intravenous Nurs.* 5(12):298–301.

Camp-Sorrell, D. (1990). Advanced central venous access: Selection, catheters, devices, and nursing management. *J. Intravenous Nurs.* 6(13):361–370.

Carter, P., Engelking, C. H., Fiscus, J. A., et al. (1989). *Access Device Guidelines: Module I: Catheters.* Pittsburgh: Oncology Nursing Society.

Carter, P., Engelking, C. H., Fiscus, J. A., et al. (1989). *Access Device Guidelines: Module II: Implanted Ports and Reservoirs.* Oncology Nursing Society.

Goodman, M. S., and Wickham, R. (1984). Venous access devices: An overview. *Oncol. Nurs. Forum* 11(5):16–23.

Groeger, J. S., and Lucas, A. (1990). Implanted Ports and Catheters: The Memorial Sloan-Kettering Cancer Center Experience (1630 Devices). In *Proceedings of Eurochirurgie 90, First European Surgical Congress.* Paris.

Groeger, J. S., Lucas, A., and Brown, A. (1988). Venous Access Device Infections in Adult Cancer Patients: Catheters vs. Ports. In *28th Interscience Conference on Antimicrobial Agents and Chemotherapy* (ICAAC) (p. 158). Los Angeles.

Groeger, J. S., Lucas, A., Brown, A., et al. (1990). Hickman Catheters and Totally Implanted Ports: A Prospective Evaluation of Infectious Morbidity in 1434 Patients. In *International Consensus on Supportive Care in Oncology.* Brussels.

Groeger, J. S., Lucas, A., Coit, D., et al. (1990). Totally Implanted Venous Access Ports in Cancer Patients: A Prospective Evaluation of Morbidity. In *Proceedings of the American Society of Clinical Oncology* (p. 320). Washington.

Hadaway, L. C. (1989). Evaluation and use of advanced IV technology: I. Central venous access devices. *J. Intravenous Nurs.* 12(2):73–82.

Handy, C. M. (1989). Vascular access devices: Hospital to home care. *J. Intravenous Nurs.* 12(1, Supplement):s10–s17.

Howser, D. M., and Meade, C. D. (1987). Hickman catheter care: Developing organized teaching strategies. *Cancer Nurs.* 10(2):70–76.

Jones, P. M. (1987). Indwelling central venous catheter-related infections and two different procedures of catheter care. *Cancer Nurs.* 10(3):123–130.

Lucas, A. B., and Groeger, J. S. (1990). A Prospective Evaluation of Hickman Catheter Morbidity with Twice Weekly Flushing Compared to Daily Flushing. In *International Consensus on Supportive Care in Oncology*. Brussels.

Moore, C. L. (1987). Nursing Management of Infusion Catheters. In J. Lokich (Ed.), *Cancer Chemotherapy by Infusion* (pp. 78–90). Chicago: Precept Press.

Moore, C. L., Erikson, K. A., Yanes, L. B., et al. (1986). Nursing care and management of venous access ports. *Oncol. Nurs. Forum* 13(3):35–39.

Petrosino, B., Becker, H., and Christian, B. (1988). Infection rates in central venous catheter dressings. *Oncol. Nurs. Forum* 15(6):709–717.

Wachs, T., Watkins, S., and Hickman, R. (1987). "No more pokes": A review of parenteral access devices. *Nutritional Support Services* 18:12–13.

Winters, V. (1984). Implantable vascular access devices. *Oncol. Nurs. Forum* 11(6):25–30.

UNIT XI

SAFETY

INFECTION PREVENTION AND CONTROL IN THE CRITICAL CARE UNIT

BEHAVIORAL OBJECTIVES

After completing this chapter, the nurse will be able to

- Define the key terms.
- Identify the need for protective barriers based on patient assessment and planned patient interaction.
- Describe the indications for handwashing and the preferred product to use.
- Determine the level of disinfection necessary for equipment, and identify appropriate agents.
- Discuss the role of the employee health program in reducing risks of acquisition and transmission of infectious agents.
- Discuss the role of the inanimate environment as a reservoir for potentially infectious agents.
- Demonstrate the skills involved in infection prevention and control.

Nosocomial infection is one of the most frequent complications for patients in critical care units. In adult units, nosocomial infection rates from 10 to 50 percent have been reported. This high risk for infection is due to the combination of severe underlying disease, compromised host defenses, the routine use of multiple medical devices, and frequent and prolonged contact with numerous health care personnel.

Infection prevention and control measures in the critical care unit can reduce some of the risks of nosocomial infection. These measures need to be evaluated regularly and revised as needed to reflect current scientific research. Employee compliance with risk-reduction measures should be monitored and the results incorporated into the employee's performance appraisal.

This chapter focuses on generic procedures to reduce the risks of nosocomial infection. It does not address the infection risks and prevention measures related to the management of invasive devices, clearly the major risks for infection in critical care patients.

KEY TERMS

antiseptic agents
aseptic technique
barrier precautions
colonization
disinfection
inapparent infection
infectious waste
nosocomial infection
personal protective
  equipment
sterilization
transient and resident flora

SKILLS

35–1 Infection Prevention and Control Measures: Barrier Precautions
35–2 Infection Prevention and Control Measures: Personnel
35–3 Infection Prevention and Control Measures: Environment
35–4 Infection Prevention and Control Measures: Equipment

35–5 Infection Prevention and Control Measures: Handwashing

GUIDELINES

The following assessment guidelines assist the nurse in identifying risks for infection and implementing measures to decrease that risk:

1. Know the patient's medical history.
2. Know the patient's current medical treatment.
3. Determine appropriate handwashing.
4. Determine the appropriate use of protective barriers.
5. Determine how medical equipment will be used and the level of disinfection required.

SKILL 35–1 _____

Infection Prevention and Control Measures: Barrier Precautions

Barrier precautions are necessary to reduce the risks for transmission of infectious agents among patients, from patients to personnel, and from personnel to patients. *Barrier precautions* are the use of personal protective equipment (gloves, masks, eye protection, and aprons/gowns) for contact with a patient's blood, any moist body substance, mucous membranes, or nonintact skin. Previously, barrier precautions were used only for patients with known or suspected infections (traditional diagnosis-driven isolation); now, however, they are recommended for all patients regardless of their diagnosis.

Consistent, appropriate use of barrier precautions *eliminates* the need for traditional isolation techniques, for which there is no scientific documentation of efficacy. Using this approach, universal precautions that are intended to reduce the risk of transmission of blood-borne pathogens will be followed. However, this approach goes beyond universal precautions because it is intended to reduce the risks of cross-transmission among patients as well as protect health care workers.

Purpose

The nurse uses barrier precautions to

1. Reduce the risk of transmission of infectious agents to patients and personnel.
2. Reduce the risk of transmission of infectious agents from a clinically inapparent case.

Prerequisite Knowledge and Skills

Before initiating barrier precautions, the nurse should understand

1. That hands are the most important vehicle for the transmission of microorganisms in hospitals.

2. That infectious agents frequently colonize the mucous membranes, secretions, and tissues of patients.
3. That clinically inapparent infections are a major reservoir for infectious agents.
4. That nurses, as well as patients, may be at risk for nosocomial infections.

The nurse should be able to perform

1. Appropriate handwashing technique.
2. Proper barrier use.

Assessment

1. Assess the likelihood of contact with blood, moist body substances, mucous membranes, or nonintact skin before beginning any patient care procedure. **Rationale:** The need for barriers is dependent on the procedure to be performed and the likelihood of contact with blood, moist body substances, mucous membranes, or nonintact skin while performing the procedure. The nurse is expected to exercise independent judgment in making decisions about when to use particular barriers.
2. Assess the amount of patient excretions and secretions. **Rationale:** Gloves are the only barriers that are *routinely* necessary. However, additional barriers, such as plastic aprons, may be necessary depending on the condition of the patient, the procedure to be performed, and the likelihood of contact with blood and/or moist body substances.

Nursing Diagnosis

Potential for infection related to compromised host defenses, invasive technology, antibiotic use, and critical care environment. **Rationale:** Patients in critical care units have multiple risk factors predisposing them to nosocomial infection.

Planning

1. Individualize the following goals for using barrier precautions:
   a. Decrease nosocomial transmission of infectious agents among patients. **Rationale:** Patients in critical care units are colonized or infected with nosocomial pathogens. Use of protective barriers, especially gloves, reduces the risk of transmission of microorganisms.
   b. Reduce the risk of transmission of infectious agents to nurses. **Rationale:** Protective barriers can block potential portals of entry for microorganism, thus, reducing the risk of infection to nurses.
2. Prepare all necessary equipment and supplies. Personal protective equipment (barriers) should be available at each bedside. **Rationale:** Easy access to

barriers facilitates use on a routine basis for all patients.
a. Gloves, clean latex or vinyl.
b. Masks.
c. Protective eyewear.
d. Plastic aprons or gowns.

e. Hair covers (usually only necessary for burn units).
3. Prepare the patient explaining the routine use of barriers for patient care procedures. **Rationale:** Reduces anxiety.

Implementation

Steps	Rationale	Special Considerations
1. Wash hands.	Handwashing is the single most important infection-control measure.	Antiseptic soap is recommended for critical care units. The availability of more than one product should be considered to reduce the possibility of intolerance to any specific agent.
2. Wear *gloves* for anticipated contact with blood, mucous membranes, nonintact skin, or any moist body substance.	Hands are the most efficient vehicle for the transmission of microorganisms. Gloves are an important barrier to reduce the risk of transmission of infectious agents among patients.	Glove use is determined by the patient–nurse interaction, *not* the patient's diagnosis.
3. Change gloves between patients.	Gloves can become contaminated with microorganisms.	Gloves should not be washed because washing may alter the composition and result in leaks.
4. Wash hands after removal of gloves.	Microorganisms on the hands can multiply rapidly in the warm, moist environment of the glove, even when no external contamination has occurred.	
5. Wear eye protection and masks during any patient care activity where splashing or aerosolization of blood or moist body substances is likely.	Mucous membranes of nurses can be a portal of entry for infectious agents.	Corrective eyeglasses are usually adequate eye protection, since they serve as a barrier to protect the eyes.
6. Wear plastic aprons or gowns for any patient care activity where clothing is likely to become soiled with blood or moist body substances.	Serves as a barrier to blood and moist body substances.	Clothing does not play a direct role in the transmission of infectious agents, but hands may become contaminated from blood or moist body substances on clothing.
7. Place patients with diseases, known to be transmitted by the airborne route in a private room, keep the door closed, and susceptible personnel should wear masks at all times.	Use of masks for airborne disease is not dependent on patient interaction.	Few diseases are truly airborne. Those most likely to be encountered in the hospital include tuberculosis, measles, and influenza.
8. Use hair covers during invasive procedures performed in the critical care unit.	Hair covers prevent the dissemination of microorganisms into an open wound.	Hair covers may be indicated for all patient care activities in burn units.
9. Remove and discard protective barriers in appropriate receptacles.	State and local laws will determine how medical waste is disposed.	
10. Wash hands.	Reduces the risk of transmission of microorganisms among patients, from patients to personnel, and from personnel to patients.	Hands are considered the most important vehicle for the transmission of microorganisms.

Evaluation

1. Monitor handwashing practices to determine if handwashing is occurring at appropriate times and to identify factors that may be preventing handwashing. **Rationale:** Monitoring compliance with patient care policy is an essential part of quality assessment. Feedback of information on compliance can influence individual performance.

2. Monitor the appropriate use of protective barriers. **Rationale:** Failure to use appropriate barriers can increase the risk of infection transmission. Overuse of barriers is costly.

Expected Outcome

Personnel will comply with infection precautions as described by the policy/procedures of the agency. **Rationale:** The risk of transmission of infectious agents is reduced by appropriate barrier use.

Unexpected Outcome

Personnel do not comply with infection precautions as described by the policy/procedure of the agency. **Rationale:** Appropriate barrier use may reduce the risk of nosocomial infection, but barriers will not prevent all nosocomial infections, since many result from the patient's condition and/or treatment and are independent of appropriate barrier use.

Documentation

Documentation of routine barrier use in the patient record is not necessary. Appropriate barrier use and handwashing should be reflected in the nurses' performance evaluation. **Rationale:** Provides feedback to nurse, which reinforces the routine use of barrier precautions.

Patient/Family Education

1. Reinforce the routine use of barriers to the patient and family. **Rationale:** Reduces anxiety and corrects myths regarding disease transmission. Maintains confidentiality of disease diagnosis.

2. Evaluate the need for barriers in the home setting (e.g., gloves may be needed for wound care or suctioning), instruct the patient and family about when and what barriers to use and about handwashing, and identify where barriers may be purchased. **Rationale:** Reduces the risk of infection transmission to family members.

Performance Checklist
Skill 35–1:   Infection Prevention and Control Measures: Barrier Precautions

Critical Behaviors	Complies	
	yes	no
1. Wash hands.		
2. Put on appropriate personal protective equipment.		
3. Identify the need for additional protective equipment or change of equipment during procedure.		
4. Remove and discard protective equipment in appropriate receptacle.		
5. Wash hands.		

SKILL 35–2 _____

Infection Prevention and Control Measures: Personnel

Health care workers have the potential for becoming infected both within the hospital setting and in the community. Some of these infections may then be transmitted to patients in the hospital or to other health care workers. This skill focuses on the employee health program and *its* role in reducing risks of acquisition and transmission of infectious agents.

Purpose

The nurse participates in an employee health program to decrease the risk of transmission of infectious agents to patients and to decrease the risk of transmission of infectious agents from the patients to the nurse.

Prerequisite Knowledge and Skills

Prior to participating in an employee health program, the nurse should understand

1. Diseases that have the potential for transmission to patients.
2. Methods that effectively decrease the employee's risk of acquiring/transmitting such diseases.

The nurse should be able to

1. Communicate preemployment and current personal health status.

2. State her/his immunization and communicable disease history.

3. Identify exposure(s) to communicable disease(s).

Assessment

Assess the essential components of an employee health program including preemployment/periodic health assessments, immunizations, exposure follow-up and work restrictions for personnel with communicable diseases. **Rationale:** Most health care facilities include at least these four components to promote employee and patient safety.

Planning

Become familiar with your institution's policies and procedures for preemployment/periodic health assessments, immunization history and requirements, exposure follow-up, and work restrictions. **Rationale:** Compliance with the institution's policies and procedures for employee health can decrease the risk of transmission of infection to others and provides protection and early detection of infections among employees.

Implementation

Steps	Rationale	Special Considerations
1. Adhere to institutional preemployment/periodic health assessment requirements:		
a. Preemployment physical examination and health assessment.	Preemploymet assessments and examinations may detect infectious diseases that require treatment prior to patient contact.	Preemployment examinations should be completed prior to the employee having patient contact.
b. Periodic health assessments.	Periodic assessments may detect infections not present on the employment examination.	Each facility will determine the frequency of periodic assessments. Consider state requirements.
c. Laboratory testing.	Some infectious diseases may be subclinical and detected only by laboratory testing.	Hepatitis B and rubella testing are sometimes done on employment, but it is acceptable for immunization to be provided without testing first.
d. Tuberculosis skin testing.	Tuberculosis skin tests can detect TB infection. A baseline test on employment is helpful in later determining infection resulting from occupational exposure.	Mantoux testing is preferable over Tine tests.
2. Maintain a record of immunizations and antibody titers: a. Hepatitis B. b. Measles, mumps, rubella. c. Influenza.	Immunization is available for hepatitis B, measles, mumps, rubella, and influenza.	
3. Adhere to institutional policies and procedures for exposure follow-up:		
a. Communicable diseases.	Exposures must be assessed to provide appropriate prophylactic treatment and/or implement work restrictions.	See Figure 35–1.
b. Needlestick injuries.	Needlestick injuries must be assessed to determine if employee testing or source testing for hepatitis B or HIV is recommended.	
c. Blood or moist body substance exposures.	Exposures must be assessed to determine if a significant exposure occurred and if follow-up action must be taken.	Significant exposures include parenteral or mucous membrane exposure.
4. Institute work restrictions as recommended by the employee health program.	Certain communicable diseases and exposures may dictate the need for work restrictions.	See Table 35–1.

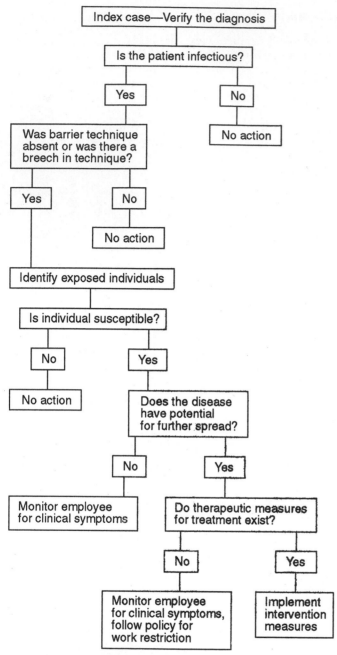

FIGURE 35–1 Algorithm for management of an employee exposure. (From Soule, B. Ed.: APIC Curriculum, Iowa, Kendall-Hunt Publishers, 1983.)

Evaluation

Evaluate compliance with employee health policies and incorporate into the employee's annual performance appraisal. **Rationale:** This will ensure annual review of compliance and correction of noncompliance at least yearly.

Expected Outcome

Compliance with employee health policies. **Rationale:** To prevent transmission of infectious agents from employee to patient and to prevent employee acquisition of infectious agents.

Unexpected Outcomes

1. Infection in patients or health care workers transmitted by an employee. **Rationale:** Compliance with employee health policies decreases the risk of transmission of infectious agents from employees.
2. Noncompliance with employee health policies. **Rationale:** Understanding of the rationale behind specific employee health policies should encourage compliance.
3. Infection in employee secondary to an occupational exposure. **Rationale:** Compliance with employee health policies should lead to early detection and treatment of exposures and therefore reduce the risk of employee infection.

Documentation

Employee health information is considered confidential and should be maintained in the individual's employee health record. **Rationale:** Documentation provides evidence of employee follow-up and evaluation by the employee's health service; of particular importance in workman compensation cases.

Employee Education

1. Reinforce the need for compliance with periodic health assessments. **Rationale:** May detect infections that present a risk to patients and/or other health care workers.
2. Stress the importance of complying with laboratory and TB testing. **Rationale:** May detect subclinical infectious disease states.
3. Reinforce the necessity of identifying and reporting exposures (communicable diseases, needlestick injuries, and blood/moist body substances). **Rationale:** Identifies the potential for infection transmission to/from patients and other health care workers.

TABLE 35–1 SUMMARY OF IMPORTANT RECOMMENDATIONS AND WORK RESTRICTIONS FOR PERSONNEL WITH INFECTIOUS DISEASES

Disease/Problem	Relieve from Direct Patient Contact	Work Restriction	Duration	Category
Conjunctivitis, infectious	Yes		Until discharge ceases	II
Cytomegalovirus infection	No			II
Diarrhea:	Yes		Until symptoms resolve and/or infection with *Salmonella* is ruled out	II
Acute stage (diarrhea with other symptoms)				
Convalescent stage: *Salmonella* (nontyphoidal)	No	Personnel should not take care of high-risk patients.	Until stool is free of the infecting organism on two consecutive cultures not less than 24 hours apart	II
Other enteric pathogens	No			II
Enteroviral infections	No	Personnel should not take care of infants and newborns.	Until symptoms resolve	II
Group A streptococcal disease	Yes		Until 24 hours after adequate treatment is started	I
Hepatitis, viral:				
Hepatitis A	Yes		Until 7 days after onset of jaundice	III
Hepatitis B				
Acute	No	Personnel should wear gloves for procedures that involve trauma to tissues or contact with mucous membranes or nonintact skin.	Until antigenemia resolves	II
Chronic antigenemia	No	Same as acute illness.	Until antigenemia resolves	II
Hepatitis NANB	No	Same as acute hepatitis B.	Period of infectivity has not been determined	II
Herpes simplex:				
Genital	No			
Hands (herpetic whitlow)	Yes	(*Note*: It is not known whether gloves prevent transmission.)	Until lesions heal	I
Orofacial	No	Personnel should not take care of high-risk patients.	Until lesions heal	II
Measles:				
Active	Yes		Until 7 days after the rash appears	I
Postexposure (susceptible personnel)	Yes		From the fifth through the twenty-first day after exposure and/or 7 days after the rash appears	II
Mumps:				
Active	Yes		Until 9 days after onset of parotitis	I
Postexposure	Yes*		From the twelfth through the twenty-sixth day after exposure or until 9 days after onset of parotitis	III
Pertussis:				
Active	Yes		From the beginning of the catarrhal stage through the third week after onset of paroxysms or until 7 days after start of effective therapy	I
Postexposure (asymptomatic personnel)	No			II
Postexposure (symptomatic personnel)	Yes		Same as active pertussis	I

Disease/Problem	Relieve from Direct Patient Contact	Work Restriction	Duration	Category
Rubella:				
Active	Yes		Until 5 days after the rash appears	I
Postexposure (susceptible personnel)	Yes		From the seventh through the twenty-first day after exposure and/or 5 days after rash appears	II
Scabies	Yes		Until treated	I
Staphylococcus aureus (skin lesions)	Yes		Until lesions have resolved	II
Upper respiratory infections (high-risk patients)	Yes	Personnel with upper respiratory infections should not take care of high-risk patients.	Until acute symptoms resolve	II
Zoster (shingles), active	No	Appropriate barrier desirable; personnel should not take care of high-risk patients.	Until lesions dry and crust	II
Varicella (chickenpox):				
Active	Yes		Until all lesions dry and crust	I
Postexposure	Yes		From the tenth through the twenty-first day after exposure or if varicella occurs until all lesions dry and crust	I

*Mumps vaccine may be offered to susceptible personnel. When given after exposure, mumps vaccine may not provide protection. However, if exposure did not result in infection, immunizing exposed personnel should protect against subsequent infection. Neither mumps immune globulin nor immune serum globulin (ISG) is of established value in postexposure prophylaxis. Transmission of mumps among personnel and patients has not been a major problem in hospitals in the United States, probably due to multiple factors, including high levels of natural and vaccine-induced immunity.
Source: Adapted from W. Williams, *Guidelines for Infection Control in Hospital Personnel*. Washington: U.S. Public Health Service, 1983, pp. 21–22.

Performance Checklist
Skill 35–2:   Infection Prevention and Control Measures: Personnel

Critical Behaviors	Complies yes	Complies no
1. Adhere to institutional requirements for preemployment/periodic health assessments, laboratory testing, and TB skin testing.		
2. Maintain a record of immunizations and antibody titers for hepatitis B, measles, mumps, rubella, and influenza.		
3. Adhere to institutional policies and procedures for exposure follow-up of communicable diseases, needlestick injuries, and blood/moist body substances.		
4. Institute work restrictions as recommended by the employee health program.		

SKILL 35–3 _____

Infection Prevention and Control Measures: Environment

The environment, although frequently contaminated with microorganisms, rarely contributes to human infection. Elaborate cleaning procedures are not necessary in a critical care unit. This skill addresses ventilation, housekeeping, and waste disposal in the critical care unit.

Purpose

The nurse institutes environmental measures to

1. Reduce the risk of transmission of microorganisms from the inanimate environment to patients and hospital staff.
2. Reduce the number of microorganisms from surfaces that may come in contact with patients or patient care equipment.
3. Ensure adequate ventilation.

Prerequisite Knowledge and Skills

Before implementing environmental measures, the nurse should understand

1. The limited role of the environment in transmitting infectious agents.
2. Principles of segregation of "clean" and "dirty" areas.
3. Principles of barrier precautions (see Skill 35–1).

The nurse should be able to

1. Collaborate with the Engineering Department to ensure adequate ventilation.
2. Assess the cleanliness of the physical environment.
3. Dispose of medical waste consistent with local, state, or federal regulations.
4. Institute barrier precautions as needed.

Assessment

1. Assess the cleanliness of horizontal surfaces (e.g., bedside tables and noncarpeted floors). **Rationale:** Soiled areas can serve as a reservoir for microorganisms that could contaminate patient care equipment.
2. Assess the procedure for cleaning the environment immediately after contamination with blood. **Rationale:** All blood should be considered infectious. Blood spills should be cleaned up immediately using a hospital-grade detergent/disinfectant registered with the Environmental Protection Agency (EPA).
3. Assess air exchanges and frequency of ventilation filter changes. **Rationale:** Prevents the cumulative buildup of airborne organisms.
4. Assess the flow direction in rooms with regulated airflow. **Rationale:** Contaminated room air is not allowed to exit to the hall or other rooms (negative pressure).
5. Assess the segregation and disposal of infectious and noninfectious waste. **Rationale:** Medical waste disposal is regulated by local, state, and federal laws. Improper disposal results in environmental contamination and possible fines against a hospital.
6. Assess the functional appropriateness of "clean" and "dirty" work/utility areas. **Rationale:** Segregation reduces the likelihood of contamination of sterile or clean items.

Planning

1. Collaborate with the Housekeeping Department to develop cleaning procedures that will not interfere with patient care. **Rationale:** Ensures a clean environment.
2. Develop a schedule to change air filters and monitor air exchanges. **Rationale:** Clean filters enhance efficiency.
3. Define infectious waste and develop procedures for segregation and disposal. **Rationale:** Compliance with local, state, and/or federal laws.
4. Designate "clean" and "dirty" work/utility areas. **Rationale:** Reduce risks for cross-contamination.
5. Develop tools for monitoring compliance with procedures. **Rationale:** An essential part of quality assessment and risk management.

Implementation

Steps	Rationale	Special Considerations
1. Clean horizontal surfaces and noncarpeted floors daily using any EPA-registered detergent/disinfectant.	Decreases microbial contamination of surfaces.	"Elbow grease" is the most important factor in environmental cleaning. Cleaning should not interfere with patient care, however.
2. Refrain from the use of carpeting in the immediate patient care areas of the critical care units.	Frequent wetting, spillage, and heavy soiling make cleaning difficult and contribute to odors.	Carpets impregnated with antimicrobial substances have *not* been demonstrated to reduce infection risk.
3. Use high-efficiency air filtration systems and change filters on a regular basis.	Prevents cumulative buildup and loss of efficiency.	Compared with other reservoirs, air is an infrequent source of nosocomial organisms in critical care units.
4. Keep the doors of regulated-airflow rooms closed.	Maintains a negative pressure and keeps most air inside the room.	
5. Keep windows closed.	Insects and/or fumes may enter.	
6. Immediately clean up any spill of blood and/or moist body substances using an EPA-registered germicide.	Decreases microbial contamination of surfaces.	Protective barriers should be available in all patient care areas and used for cleaning up spills.
7. Segregate infectious from noninfectious waste, and place in appropriate containers.	Local, state, and federal regulations.	Inappropriately disposed waste can result in environmental contamination and monetary fines for the institution.
8. Keep linen and clean supplies separate from dirty areas and used supplies.	Reduces the risk of cross-contamination.	

Evaluation

Monitor compliance with policies and procedures that address the critical care environment. **Rationale:** Identify and correct factors that may influence compliance. Noncompliance may result in fines against the institution.

Expected Outcomes

1. A clean, adequately ventilated critical care unit. **Rationale:** The environment may be a reservoir for pathogenic microorganisms.
2. Designation and use of disposal containers for infectious and noninfectious waste. **Rationale:** Medical waste disposal is regulated by law.
3. Designation and use of "clean" and "dirty" utility areas. **Rationale:** Prevents contamination of sterile and clean items.

Unexpected Outcomes

1. A visibly dirty environment. **Rationale:** A dirty environment is a reservoir for pathogenic microorga-

nisms. A dirty environment may be "perceived" as substandard care.
2. Environmental contamination. **Rationale:** Improper disposal of biohazardous waste will taint the environment.
3. A fine from a regulatory agent for improper disposal of medical waste. **Rationale:** Cost and potentially adverse publicity.
4. Clean and dirty supplies and equipment stored and/or used in the same area. **Rationale:** Clean/sterile supplies may be contaminated before use.

Documentation

Documentation is done with a compliance monitoring tool and by the individual departments (e.g., records of filter changes, health department inspections, etc.). **Rationale:** Documentation is part of an overall quality-assessment and risk-management program.

Performance Checklist
Skill 35–3: Infection Prevention and Control Measures: Environment

Critical Behaviors	Complies yes	Complies no
1. Keep horizontal surfaces and noncarpeted floors clean.		
2. Refrain from the use of carpeting in critical care units.		
3. Ensure that air filters are changed on a regular basis.		
4. Keep the doors of regulated-airflow rooms closed.		
5. Keep windows closed.		
6. Clean up any spill of blood or moist body substance immediately with an appropriate germicide and use protective barriers in the process.		
7. Segregate infectious wastes and dispose in designated container.		
8. Separate clean/sterile supplies from dirty areas and used supplies.		

SKILL 35–4 _____

Infection Prevention and Control Measures: Equipment

Patient care in the critical care unit requires the use of many types of equipment and devices, both invasive and noninvasive. Much of the equipment used must be sterile and is generally prepackaged for one-time use. Nursing actions focus on the appropriate use of the device and aseptic technique. Some of the equipment is maintained by other departments, e.g., Respiratory Therapy or Central Services. Still the critical care nurse makes decisions about certain equipment maintained in the unit as well as the preparation of equipment, instruments, and supplies processed in Central Services. The information included in this skill addresses cleaning, disinfection, and sterilization of equipment in the critical care environment.

Purpose

The nurse institutes measures for equipment to

1. Reduce risks for transmission of infectious agents secondary to use of contaminated equipment.
2. Provide for cleaning, disinfection, or sterilization of equipment appropriate for its intended use.

Prerequisite Knowledge and Skills

Prior to instituting cleaning, disinfection, and sterilization procedures, the nurse should understand

1. Principles of aseptic technique in handling sterile or disinfected equipment.
2. The intended use of the equipment.
3. Principles of barrier precautions.

The nurse should be able to perform

1. Appropriate cleaning/processing of contaminated objects/equipment.
2. Barrier precautions (see Skill 35–1).

Assessment

1. Determine the equipment used in critical care for which sterility is critical, less critical, and not critical. **Rationale:** Equipment must receive the appropriate level of decontamination and processing for its intended use to reduce the risks of transmission of infectious agents (Table 35–2).

2. Identify interchangeable patient items (e.g., monitors, infusion control devices, IV poles, etc.) and requirements for cleaning between patients. **Rationale:** Equipment that is used between patients must be adequately cleaned before reuse.

3. Identify equipment within the critical care unit maintained by other departments and their cleaning/distribution or sterilization standards. **Rationale:** The critical care nurse using the equipment needs to know that appropriate procedures have been used for cleaning, disinfecting, and sterilizing the equipment.

TABLE 35–2 METHODS OF ENSURING ADEQUATE PROCESSING OF INANIMATE OBJECTS IN THE HOSPITAL ENVIRONMENT

Object and Classification	Example	Method	Comment
Patient-Care Objects			
Sterility is critical: Sterilized in the hospital; reusable and single-use items.	Surgical instruments and devices, angiography catheters	Use before maximum safe storage time. Inspect package for integrity and for exposure of sterility indicator before use. Follow manufacturer's instructions for each sterilizer or use recommended protocol. Test sterilizers to find out whether they can kill resistant commercial spores.	Sterilization processes are designed to have a wide margin of safety. If spores are not killed, the sterilizer should be checked for proper use and function; if spore tests remain positive, discontinue use of the sterilizer and have it serviced.
Purchased as sterile	Intravenous fluids, needles, syringes	Use before expiration date if one is given. Inspect package for integrity before use. Culture only if clinical circumstances suggest infection related to use of the item.	Notify the U.S. Food and Drug Administration if factory-related (intrinsic) contamination is suspected.
Sterility is less critical, but should be free of most vegetative bacteria Usually disinfected rather than sterilized in the hospital	Respiratory therapy equipment and instruments for gastrointestinal endoscopy that will touch mucous membranes	Sterilize if possible; if not, follow a protocol for high-level liquid chemical disinfection or pasteurization. Culture equipment after any important changes in the disinfection process.	These devices come in contact with mucous membranes. Resistant spores can remain after liquid chemical disinfection, but these are not usually pathogenic. Culturing can verify that a disinfection process (or disinfectant) has not resulted in marked increases in recovery of bacteria from equipment.
Purchased	Water, including water for hemodialysis	Use an adequately treated source of hospital water. Store fluids with proper chlorination to avoid microbial proliferation. Perform routine culturing of hemodialysis water.	The risk of disease appears to be related to the number of organisms present (unless virulent organisms are present). Water for hemodialysis may require further processing, e.g., deionization.

Table continues on following page

Object and Classification	Example	Method	Comment
Sterility is not critical and can be expected to be contaminated with some bacteria.	Bedpans, crutches, bed rails, water glasses, linens, food utensils, ECG leads, bedside tables, radiology suites, hemodialysis centers	Follow a protocol for cleaning (use a disinfectant or disinfecting process).	
Non-Patient-Care Objects*			
Likely to be contaminated with virulent microorganisms	Laboratories handling patient specimens†	Follow a protocol for cleaning (use a disinfectant or disinfecting process).	Areas handling blood or microbiologic specimens are most important.
Unlikely to be contaminated with virulent microorganisms	Areas not involved in patient care: offices, storage areas	Perform routine cleaning.	Cleaning is aimed mainly at improving the appearance of and providing a proper atmosphere in which to work

*Adequate processing of non-patient-care objects is primarily aimed at protecting personnel and others who come in contact with these objects; sterility is not critical.

†For disposal of specimens from patients, see *Guidelines for Hospital Environmental Control: Housekeeping Services and Waste Disposal or Isolation Techniques for Use in Hospitals* when applicable.

Source: From B. P. Simmons, *Guidelines for Hospital Environmental Control: Cleaning, Sterilization, and Disinfection of Hospital Equipment.* Washington: U.S. Public Health Service, 1982, p. 3.

Planning

1. Develop procedures for care and cleaning/disinfection of specific items used and maintained by the critical care nursing staff (Table 35–3). **Rationale:** Serves as a reference for all nurses in the unit.

2. Develop tools for monitoring compliance with procedures. **Rationale:** Ensures compliance and therefore patient safety.

TABLE 35–3   METHODS OF STERILIZATION AND DISINFECTION

	Sterilization		Disinfection		
	Critical Items (Will Enter Tissue or Vascular System or Blood Will Flow Through Them)		**High Level (Semicritical Items; Will Come in Contact with Mucous Membrane or Nonintact Skin)**	**Intermediate Level (Some Semicritical Items and Noncritical Items)**	**Low Level (Noncritical Items; Will Come in Contact with Intact Skin)**
Object	**Procedure**	**Exposure Time (h)**	**Procedure (Exposure Time ≥ 20 min)[b,c]**	**Procedure (Exposure Time ≤ 10 min)**	**Procedure (Exposure Time ≤ 10 min)**
Smooth, hard surface[a]	A	MR	C	H	H
	B	MR	D	J	I
	C	MR	E	K	J
	D	6	F[d]		K
	E	6	G		L
Rubber tubing and catheters[c]	A	MR	C		
	B	MR	D		
	C	MR	E		
	D	6	F[d]		
	E	6			
Polyethylene tubing and catheters[c,e]	A	MR	C		
	B	MR	D		
	C	MR	E		
	D	6	F[d]		
	E	6			
Lensed instruments	B	MR	C		
	C	MR	D		
	D	6	E		
	E	6			

Table continues on following page

	Sterilization		Disinfection		
	Critical Items (Will Enter Tissue or Vascular System or Blood Will Flow Through Them)		**High Level (Semicritical Items; Will Come in Contact with Mucous Membrane or Nonintact Skin)**	**Intermediate Level (Some Semicritical Items and Noncritical Items)**	**Low Level (Noncritical Items; Will Come in Contact with Intact Skin)**
Object	**Procedure**	**Exposure Time (h)**	**Procedure (Exposure Time ≥ 20 min)**[b,c]	**Procedure (Exposure Time ≤ 10 min)**	**Procedure (Exposure Time ≤ 10 min)**
Thermometers (oral and rectal)[f]				H[i]	
Hinged instruments	A	MR	C		
	B	MR	D		
	C	MR	E		
	D	6			
	E	6			

Key: A, heat sterilization, including steam or hot air (see manufacturer's recommendations); B, ethylene oxide gas (see manufacturer's recommendations); C, glutaraldehyde-based formulations (2%) (a glutaraldehyde-phenate formulation at full strength also has been shown to sterilize items that are soaked for 6¾ hours. Caution should be exercised with all glutaraldehyde formulations when further in-use dilution is anticipated); D, demand-release chlorine dioxide (will corrode aluminum, copper, brass, series 400 stainless steel, and chrome, with prolonged exposure); E, stabilized hydrogen peroxide 6% (will corrode copper, zinc, and brass); F, wet pasteurization at 75°C for 30 minutes after detergent cleaning; G, sodium hypochlorite (1000 ppm available chlorine; will corrode metal instruments); H, ethyl or isopropyl alcohol (70% to 90%); I, sodium hypochlorite (100 ppm available chlorine); J, phenolic germicidal detergent solution (follow product label for use-dilution); K, iodophor germicidal detergent solution (follow product label for use-dilution); L, quaternary ammonium germicidal detergent solution (follow product label for use-dilution); MR, manufacturer's recommendations.
"See text for discussion of hydrotherapy.
ᵇThe longer the exposure to a disinfectant, the more likely it is that all microorganisms will be eliminated. Ten minutes' exposure is not adequate to disinfect many objects, especially those which are difficult to clean because they have narrow channels or other areas that can harbor organic material and bacteria. Twenty minutes' exposure may be the minimum time needed to reliably kill *M. tuberculosis* with glutaraldehyde.
ᶜTubing must be completely filled for disinfection; care must be taken to avoid entrapment of air bubbles during immersion.
ᵈPasteurization (washer disinfector) of respiratory therapy and anesthesia equipment is a recognized alternative to high-level disinfection. Some data challenge the efficacy of some pasteurization units.
ᵉThermostability should be investigated when indicated.
ᶠLimited data suggest that at least 20 minutes' exposure time is necessary. Do not mix rectal and oral thermometers at any stage of handling or processing.
Source: Modified from W. A. Rutala. In R. P. Wenzel, (Ed.), *Prevention and Control of Nosocomial Infections*. Baltimore: Williams & Wilkins, 1987, pp. 257–282; and from B. P. Simmons, *Am. J. Infect. Control* 11:96–115, 1983.

Implementation

Steps	Rationale	Special Considerations
1. Identify location within the hospital where processing will occur.	Various departments have equipment maintenance and processing responsibilities.	
2. Identify staff/department responsible for processing.	Assignment of responsibility provides consistency in processing.	
3. Educate nursing staff on individual responsibility regarding equipment cleaning, disinfection, and sterilization.	Training is necessary to ensure that policies and procedures are understood by responsible staff.	Disposable one-time-use patient care item should not be reused or reprocessed unless the procedure for doing so is available in writing from the manufacturer. If not available from the manufacturer, the facility must have clear, written policies.

Evaluation

Monitor compliance with established procedures using the tool(s) developed. Identify areas of noncompliance and reason(s) for noncompliance. Implement corrective action as appropriate. **Rationale:** Monitoring compliance is an essential aspect of a quality-assessment program.

Expected Outcome

Personnel compliance with procedures for care and

cleaning/disinfection of equipment. **Rationale:** Appropriate care of equipment is necessary to decrease the risk of infection to patients.

Unexpected Outcome

Lack of compliance with procedures for care of equipment. **Rationale:** Lack of compliance may indicate lack of knowledge of procedures, choice not to comply with procedures, or obstacles that prevent compliance with procedures. Unexpected outcomes may be corrected by determining the cause for lack of compliance and educating the nurse on the procedures, counseling the nurse regarding her or his choice, and identifying and removing the obstacle to appropriate practice.

Documentation

Documentation is done via the compliance monitoring tools and by individual departments. **Rationale:** Documentation becomes part of quality assessment program.

Performance Checklist
Skill 35–4: Infection Prevention and Control Measures: Equipment

Critical Behaviors	Complies	
	yes	no
1. Identify types of equipment used in critical care.		
2. Delineate type of processing needed for each piece of equipment.		
3. Identify location within the hospital where processing will occur.		
4. Identify staff responsible for processing.		
5. Educate staff on individual responsibilities.		
6. Monitor compliance with established procedures.		
7. Identify areas of noncompliance.		
8. Assess reasons for noncompliance.		
9. Implement corrective action.		
10. Reevaluate compliance.		

SKILL 35–5

Infection Prevention and Control Measures: Handwashing

Handwashing is the single most important procedure in reducing the risk of nosocomial infections because many infections are caused by organisms transmitted on the hands of health care workers. This skill focuses on handwashing as a means of reducing the risk of transmission of potentially infectious organisms among patients (usually via the hands of personnel), from patients to health care workers, and from health care workers to patients.

Purpose

The nurse performs appropriate handwashing to decrease the risk of transmission of potentially infectious agents.

Prerequisite Knowledge and Skills

Prior to performing handwashing, the nurse should understand

1. Principles of transient and resident microbial contamination of hands.
2. Appropriate selection and use of antiseptic products for handwashing.

Assessment

Prior to performing handwashing, the nurse should consider the following:

1. Is handwashing indicated? **Rationale:** If direct patient contact with secretions or nonintact skin or contact with contaminated objects occurs, handwashing is indicated.
2. Are facilities available for handwashing? **Rationale:** If facilities are not available, alternative means of handwashing should be considered.
3. Is a medicated or nonmedicated soap preferred for this patient care situation (Table 35–4)? **Rationale:** Certain patient care situations require the use of an antiseptic soap.
4. Is the handwashing product available? **Rationale:** Soap or antiseptic agents must be available to facilitate removal of soil and microorganisms from the hands.
5. Are there acceptable alternatives to routine hand-

TABLE 35–4   INDICATIONS FOR USE OF PLAIN OR ANTISEPTIC SOAP

Examples	Mechanical Cleaning*	Rapid Reduction of Contaminating and Colonizing Flora†	Residual Activity†
Routine patient bathing	X		
Routine handwashing in low-risk patient areas	X		
Routine handwashing in high-risk patient areas (e.g., newborn nursery, intensive care unit, severely immunocompromised, transplant unit)	X	X	X
Preparation of hands before invasive procedures (e.g., venipuncture)	X	X	
Preoperative preparation of patient skin	X	X	
Surgical hand scrub	X	X	X

*If only this column is checked, plain soap is recommended.
†If this column is checked, antiseptics may be desirable.
Source: From E. Larson, Guideline for use of antimicrobial agents. *Am. J. Infect. Control* 16:254, 1988.

washing if obstacles are present? **Rationale:** Various waterless products for handwashing may serve as a temporary substitute for handwashing when handwashing with soap and running water cannot be done.

Nursing Diagnosis

Potential for infection. **Rationale:** Patients are at an increased risk for infection when health care workers do not practice proper handwashing.

Planning

Prepare all necessary equipment and supplies:

1. Locate sink.
2. Handwashing product (Table 35–5).
3. Paper towels.

TABLE 35–5   CHARACTERISTICS OF SIX TOPICAL ANTIMICROBIAL INGREDIENTS

Agent	Mode of Action	Gram-Positive Bacteria	Gram-Negative Bacteria	Mycobacterium Tuberculosis	Fungi	Viruses	Rapidity of Action	Residual Activity	Usual Concentrations (%)	Affected by Organic Matter?	Safety/Toxicity
Alcohols	Denaturation of protein	Excellent	Excellent	Good	Good	Good	Most rapid	None	70–92	No data	Drying, volatile
Chlorhexidine	Cell wall disruption	Excellent	Good	Poor	Fair	Good	Intermediate	Excellent	4, 2 detergent base; 0.5 in alcohol	Minimal	Ototoxicity, keratitis
Hexachlorophene	Cell wall disruption	Excellent	Poor	Poor	Poor	Poor	Slow–intermediate	Excellent	3 by prescription only	Minimal	Neurotoxicity
Iodine/iodophors	Oxidation/substitution by free iodine	Excellent	Good	Good	Good	Good	Intermediate	Minimal	10, 7.5, 2, 0.5	Yes	Absorption from skin with possible toxicity; skin irritation more common
PCMX (chloroxylenol)	Cell wall disruption	Good	Fair*	Fair	Fair	Fair	Intermediate	Good	0.5–3.75	Minimal	More data needed
Triclosan (Irgasan, DP-300)	Cell wall disruption	Good	Good (except for *Pseudomonas*)	Fair	Poor	Unknown	Intermediate	Excellent	0.3–1.0	Minimal	More data needed

*Activity improved by addition of chelating agent such as EDTA.
Source: From E. Larson. Guideline for use of topical antimicrobial agents. *Am. J. Infect. Control* 16:253–266, 1988.

Implementation

Steps	Rationale	Special Considerations
1. Adjust water temperature.	Provides comfort in washing hands.	
2. Wet hands thoroughly.	Prepares skin for soap (decreases chapping).	Applying soap before water increases dryness of skin.
3. Select/dispense appropriate soap.	Facilitates removal of soil and microorganisms.	

Table continues on following page

Steps	Rationale	Special Considerations
4. Lather soap by using friction to wash all surfaces of the hands, fingers, and forearms.	Cleanses all surfaces.	A 10-second wash is generally acceptable between patient contacts.
5. Rinse hands and forearms thoroughly.	Removes soap and prevents dryness.	
6. Dry hands and forearms thoroughly.	Prevents chapping of skin.	
7. Use paper towel to turn faucet off.	Prevents recontamination of hands.	Wall-mounted blow dryers for hands are not acceptable in patient care areas unless paper towels are also provided to use to turn off the faucet.
8. Discard paper towel in trash receptacle.	Removes from access by others.	

Evaluation

1. Monitor compliance with handwashing before and after each patient contact. **Rationale:** Monitoring compliance is an essential part of a quality-assessment program.

2. Evaluate handwashing technique and selection of appropriate soap. **Rationale:** Appropriate technique and selection of soap have been shown to decrease contact transmission of microorganisms.

• Expected Outcome

Handwashing is performed consistently before and after each patient contact. **Rationale:** Consistent handwashing practices decrease the risk of transmission of infectious agents.

Unexpected Outcomes

1. Infection in a patient due to lack of ineffective handwashing. **Rationale:** Lack of handwashing has been implicated in the transmission of infectious agents.

2. Obstacle(s) prevent effective handwashing, e.g., lack of handwashing supplies. **Rationale:** Handwashing supplies should always be available. Assignment of responsibility for restocking supplies is necessary.

Documentation

Documentation of handwashing is not required be-cause it is a routine practice for the care of all patients. Documentation of handwashing will occasionally be done when monitoring of handwashing is a part of the department's quality-assessment compliance monitoring program.

Patient/Family Education

1. Assess whether the patient and family are participating in patient care that necessitates handwashing (e.g., dressing changes, colostomy care). **Rationale:** Activities that require contact with infected or heavily colonized sites will require handwashing.

2. Demonstrate handwashing technique to the patient and family, and request a return demonstration. **Rationale:** Enables patient and family to practice handwashing and ask questions.

3. Assess the patient's and family's ongoing need to provide patient care at home, and instruct about handwashing. Assess the home environment for sinks and running water. **Rationale:** Emphasizes the importance of handwashing during patient care in the home setting. Identify supplies needed and where they may be purchased.

Performance Checklist
Skill 35–5: Infection Prevention and Control Measures: Handwashing

Critical Behaviors	Complies	
	yes	no
1. Adjust water temperature.		
2. Wet hands thoroughly.		
3. Select an appropriate soap product.		
4. Lather soap by using friction to wash hands, fingers, and forearms.		

Table continues on following page

Critical Behaviors	Complies	
	yes	no
5. Wash at least 10 seconds.		
6. Rinse hands and forearms.		
7. Dry hands and forearms.		
8. Turn faucet off with paper towel.		
9. Discard paper towel in appropriate receptacle.		

BIBLIOGRAPHY

Bennett, G. (1983). Employee Health. In B. Soule (Ed.), *APIC Curriculum for Infection Control Practice*, Vol. 2 (pp. 990–1014). Iowa: Kendall/Hunt.

Berg, R. (Ed.) (1988). *APIC Curriculum for Infection Control Practice*, Vol. 3. Iowa: Kendall/Hunt.

Centers for Disease Control (1987). Recommendations for prevention of HIV transmission in health-care settings. *MMWR* 36:3S–18S.

Centers for Disease Control (1988). Update: Universal precautions for prevention of transmission of human immunodeficiency virus, hepatitis B virus and other bloodborne pathogens in healthcare settings. *MMWR* 37:377–388.

Department of Labor Occupational Safety and Health Administration (1989). Occupational exposure to bloodborne pathogens. *Fed. Reg.* 54:23042–23139.

Garner, J. S., and Favero, M. S. (1986). Guidelines for handwashing and hospital environmental control, 1985. *Am. J. Infect. Control* 14:110–126.

Jackson, M. M., and Lynch, P. (1990). In search of a rational approach. *Am. J. Nurs.* 90:73–76.

Jackson, M. M., and Lynch, P. (1985). Isolation practices: A historical perspective. *Am. J. Infect. Control* 13:21–31.

Jackson, M. M., and Lynch, P. (1984). Isolation control: Too much or too little? *Am. J. Nurs.* 84:208–210.

Larson, E. (1988). APIC guidelines for use of topical antimicrobial agents. *Am. J. Infect. Control* 16:253–266.

Larson, E. (1989). Handwashing: It's essential—Even when you use gloves. *Am. J. Nurs.* 89:934–941.

Lynch, P., Jackson, M. M., Cummings, J., and Stamm, W. E. (1987). Rethinking the role of isolation practices in the prevention of nosocomial infections. *Ann. Intern. Med.* 107:243–246.

Lynch, P., Cummings, M. J., Roberts, P. L., et al. (1990). Implementing and evaluating a system of generic infection precautions: Body substance isolation. *Am. J. Infect. Control* 18:1–12.

Maki, D. G., Alvarado, C., and Hassemer, C. (1986). Double-bagging of items from isolation rooms is unnecessary as an infection control measure: A comparative study of surface contamination with single- and double-bagging. *Infect. Control* 7:535–537.

Massanari, M. R., and Hierholzer, W. J. (1986). The Intensive Care Unit. In J. V. Bennett and P. S. Brachman (Eds.), *Hospital Infections*, 2d Ed. (pp. 285–297). Boston: Little, Brown.

Rhame, F. S. (1986). The Inanimate Environment. In J. V. Bennett and P. S. Brachman (Eds.), *Hospital Infections*, 2d Ed. (pp. 223–248). Boston: Little, Brown.

Rutala, W. A. (1990). APIC guidelines for selection and use of disinfectants. *Am. J. Infect. Control* 18:99–114.

Soule, B. M. (Ed.) (1983). *APIC Curriculum for Infection Control Practice*, Vols. 1 and 2. Iowa: Kendall/Hunt.

Williams, W. (1984). Guideline for infection control in hospital personnel. *Am. J. Infect. Control* 12:34–57.

36

ELECTRICAL SAFETY

BEHAVIORAL OBJECTIVES

After completing this chapter, the nurse will be able to

- Describe the basic principles of electricity and the associated precautions particular to the critical care patient and unit.
- Identify the need for electrical safety precautions based on patient assessment and environmental evaluation.
- Discuss the role of the Biomedical/Clinical Engineering Department in maintaining electrically safe equipment and environment.
- Define the key terms.

The responsibility for ensuring electrical safety within the critical care unit lies with the nurse, biomedical technician, and hospital administration. Local, state, and national ordinances set the standards for the design and maintenance of electrical components within the hospital. The National Fire Protection Association (NFPA) provides the most commonly used electrical code. Section 76B of the NFPA code categorizes areas of the hospital by patient risk.

Hospitals consistently employ the use of three-pronged plugs and three-wire cables and grounds to promote an electrically safe environment. Other safety installations include power-isolation transformers, line-isolation monitors, and ground-fault circuit interrupters. Power-isolation transformers and line-isolation monitors limit the strength of an electric shock. The ground-fault circuit interrupter limits the duration of an electric shock.

The power-isolation transformer transfers electrical energy electromagnetically without a direct mechanical or electrical connection between the wires leading in and out of it. This feature protects the patient when leakage current occurs secondary to defective insulation within a piece of equipment.

The line-isolation monitor detects leakage current in excess of 1 mA. Should this situation occur, the device enters an alarm state indicating that the critical care unit is no longer isolated from ground.

The electrical resistance of the human body drops precipitously when the skin is wet or the integrity is disrupted, thus increasing the electrical hazard. A ground-fault circuit interrupter (GFCI) is required in dialysis units and hydrotherapy rooms. Similar in function to a circuit breaker, the GFCI automatically disconnects power in these areas when the leakage current exceeds 5 mA.

All hospitals have guidelines for maintaining and monitoring the safety of electrical equipment. Generally, these inspections are conducted by a biomedical engineer or technician qualified to evaluate the equipment's function and safety.

The nurse should be advised of considerations and risks inherent in operating electrical equipment. Product or equipment instruction manuals provided by the manufacturer should be available and referred to when using a piece of equipment for the first time. Even the least indication of equipment malfunction should be reported to Biomedical Engineering or the appropriate hospital department.

KEY TERMS

circuit	leakage current
ground	microshock
ground fault	short circuit
insulator	

SKILL

36–1 Electrical Safety for Patients and Medical Device Operators

GUIDELINES

The following assessment guidelines will assist the nurse in implementing electrical safety precautions and maintaining an electrically safe environment:

1. Know the patient's medical history.
2. Know the patient's current medical treatment plan.
3. Determine which biomedical device(s) will be used, the rationale for use, and clinical function.
4. Identify the basic operating principles and mechanics of the biomedical device(s).
5. Identify the specific hazards and respective precautions to avoid adverse effects for each biomedical device(s) used.

SKILL 36–1 _____

Electrical Safety for Patients and Medical Device Operators

The amount of current needed to induce ventricular fibrillation is dependent on where the electric current is applied and the pathway it takes through the body. *Macroshock* is defined as the level of current that an individual *perceives* when an electrical stimulus is applied usually externally to the body. The minimum level of perception is generally considered to be 1 mA or 1000 μA. *Microshock* is defined as a current that passes *unperceived* along the surface of or through the body.

Externally applied currents may take different pathways through the body (Figs. 36–1 and 36–2). Thus even a large external current may not travel through the myocardium. The most vulnerable period in the ECG cycle is during the T wave. An electrical stimulus applied during the T wave may cause ventricular fibrillation, while the same stimulus applied during the other portions of the ECG cycle will have no effect.

Patients with external transvenous pacemakers and indwelling arterial lines are classified as *electrically sensitive* because the protective skin barrier has been bypassed. All electrically sensitive patients are vulnerable to microshock.

The saline solution infused through an arterial line or Swan-Ganz catheter conducts an electric current just as well as the wire of a pacemaker electrode. Even a small leakage current of 100 μA secondary to a grounding problem can cause ventricular fibrillation if the current bypasses the protective insulation of the skin and is transmitted directly to the heart. Sixty-cycle interference dis-played on an oscilloscope indicates a leakage-current problem that could result in microshock.

When using an external pacemaker, a minimum 10-mA electrical impulse is required to cause the myocardial muscle to contract. The external pacemaker emits *controlled synchronous* electric impulses one at a time. However, a leakage current of only 100 μA (or 0.1 mA) can cause ventricular fibrillation. This is possible because common household current (ac current) is emitted in 60 cycles per second (Hz). A grounding defect allows the rapid, *uncontrolled* impulses of ac current to be transmitted to the myocardium, potentially causing ventricular fibrillation. Specific measures are instituted to prevent an electrical accident in this vulnerable patient population.

All hospital electrical equipment employs the basic safety features of a three-wire power cord and three-pronged plug (Fig. 36–3). Additional features also have been developed to allow the critical care patient to be isolated from the electrical equipment. In telemetry monitoring, a battery-operated transmitter connected to the patient electrodes sends radio signals to the monitor. There is no direct electrical connection between the transmitter and the monitor. In cardiac monitoring, the signals from the patient electrodes and pressure transducers are coupled within the monitor via a magnetic or optical isolation circuit. The signals are then transferred as *magnetic* energy within a second circuit. No electric current passes between the patient and the monitor's 60-Hz power source. Within hemodynamic monitors, the signals are converted to light beams that are processed for display on the oscilloscope.

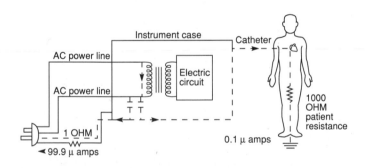

NORMAL PATH OF LEAKAGE CURRENT

FIGURE 36–1. **When ac powered equipment is properly grounded, leakage currents take the pathway of least resistance to ground.** (From S. Miodownik, Ensuring electrical safety in the critical care environment. *Crit. Care Monit.* **3**(3):8, 1983, with permission.)

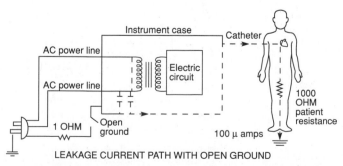

LEAKAGE CURRENT PATH WITH OPEN GROUND

FIGURE 36–2. **If the ground wire is opened or missing, the available chassis leakage will "seek" ground wherever it is available.** (From S. Miodownik, Ensuring electrical safety in the critical care environment. *Crit. Care Monit.* **3**(3):8, 1983, with permission.)

Purpose

The nurse implements the principles of electrical safety to

1.   Provide an electrically safe environment.
2.   Utilize biomedical devices in a safe manner.
3.   Prevent microshock and the resultant tachyarrhythmias.

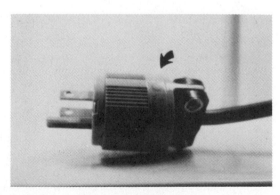

FIGURE 36–3. **Hospital-grade plug.**

Prerequisite Knowledge and Skills

Prior to implementing electrical safety precautions, the nurse should understand

1. Principles of electricity.
2. Electrical hazards particular to the critical care patient and environment.
3. The hospital department responsible for maintaining the electrical safety of biomedical equipment and the patient environment.

The nurse should be able to

1. Operate and troubleshoot biomedical equipment.
2. Perform cardiopulmonary resuscitation.
3. Report equipment/device malfunctions.

Assessment

1. Examine equipment in the patient care area, noting loose connections; cracked, frayed, or broken cords or cables; damaged or absent three-pronged plugs; broken or defective knobs and switches; and inadequate strain relief. **Rationale:** These conditions may result in a small amount of stray electric current or in a short-circuited electrical device.
2. Identify the safety inspection expiration date for each piece of biomedical equipment. **Rationale:** Most commonly, each hospital maintains a tag on each piece of biomedical equipment that indicates the date of the last inspection or when the device should be inspected again (generally every 6 months). The purpose of the safety inspection is to avoid the use of hazardous or deteriorating equipment that can still be operated with unobserved defective ground connections.
3. Determine if the patient is in a nonelectric bed. **Rationale:** A nonelectric bed is ideal. If this is not possible, have the electric bed checked for proper grounding and integrity of the electrical components before use. If a malfunction is suspected or detected, unplug the bed immediately and notify the biomedical engineer or your hospital's appropriate department, and place the patient in another bed.

4. Identify the electrically sensitive patient, including patients with wet skin or impaired skin integrity (disrupted by punctures or abrasions), external transvenous pacemakers, or intraarterial lines. **Rationale:** Electrically sensitive patients are at an increased risk for microshock.
5. Assess the patient's linen and environment for the presence of urine, blood, water, or other fluids. **Rationale:** Moist or wet linen, floor, surfaces, etc. are excellent conductors of electricity.

Nursing Diagnosis

Potential for injury related to microshock. **Rationale:** Stray electric current, static electricity, or current from a short-circuited electrical device may enter the myocardium resulting in tachyarrhythmias.

Planning

1. Individualize the following goals for implementing electrical safety precautions:
   a. Prevent microshock. **Rationale:** Lethal tachyarrhythmias can occur with as little as 100 μA (0.1 mA) of current directly through the heart. The accepted maximum level of leakage current set by most medical device manufacturers is 10 μA.
   b. Maintain an electrically safe environment and equipment. **Rationale:** Ischemia or drug toxicity can reduce the threshold to fibrillation allowing minute amounts of stray electric current that have entered the myocardium to cause tachyarrhythmias.
2. Prepare the patient by discussing the rationale for electrical safety precautions. **Rationale:** Encourages compliance and reduces anxiety.

Implementation

Steps	Rationale	Special Considerations
General Precautions:		
1. Use only three-pronged plugs in properly grounded wall outlets.	Protects from hazards associated with leakage current.	Avoid using a two-pronged plug or extension cord because these bypass the ground wire in the wall outlet.
2. Use a three-pronged extension cord only if absolutely necessary.	Extension cords increase the risk of leakage current.	If an extension cord is used, tape the cord to the floor to prevent falls and damage to the plug. Request that the equipment's cord be lengthened to avoid this necessity in the future.
3. Avoid plugging multiple devices that use high current into the same wall outlet.	Diminishes the possibility of overloading a circuit.	High-current devices include ventilators, radiant warmers, and televisions.
4. Turn equipment off before unplugging.	Prevents sparks that may cause a fire.	

Table continues on following page

Steps	Rationale	Special Considerations
5. Remove the plug from the outlet by grasping the plug itself rather than the cord.	Pulling on the cord may damage connections within the plug.	Pulling on the cord may result in the breaking of the ground connection.
6. Return any device that has been dropped to the Biomedical Engineering Department for inspection, and attach a note to the device indicating the incident date and that the device was dropped.	Ensures safety.	Even though the device may appear intact, the internal components may be damaged, posing a safety hazard.
7. Remove all discontinued or unused equipment from the patient environment.	Prevents accidental damage to the equipment resulting in an electrical hazard.	
8. Maintain the relative humidity at 50 to 60 percent in the clinical environment.	Minimizes the generation of electrostatic charges, reducing the possibility of injury to patient and staff or damage to the equipment.	
9. Ground all metal beds.	Metal is a good conductor.	
10. Make certain that all electric beds are either double-insulated or equipped with an isolation transformer.	Isolates the patient from any pathway to the power wiring provided by the bed.	

Precautions for Cardiac and Hemodynamic Monitors

1. Check for a clear, crisp tracing on the oscilloscope.	Indicates proper electrical functioning.	If 60-Hz interference is noted, check electrode pads for adequate conductive gel and good skin contact; check that the cable is intact, the plug is three-pronged, and the device is properly grounded. Determine if another device has leakage current. If unable to correct, use another monitor.
2. *Do not place* wet towels/linen, beverages, or solutions on top of monitors or other electrical equipment.	Decreases electrical hazard.	Intravenous solutions are good conductors of electricity.

Precautions for Indwelling Cardiac, Pulmonary, or Arterial Lines

1. Ensure that all cords and plugs are properly grounded.	Decreases potential for electrical hazard.	For indwelling hemodynamic monitoring lines, the electrical hazard occurs at the transducer site, where leakage current is most likely to enter. The plastic tubing and catheters do act as insulators, but the fluid column (especially normal saline) is an excellent conductor.

Precautions for External Pacemakers

1. Place all exposed parts of the lead's external electrode at the terminals in a rubber glove.	Provides insulation, which inhibits the conduction of electric current.	Newer external pacemakers conceal the leads and terminals inside the case. Additional protection is not necessary unless it is likely that the pacemaker may become wet.

Table continues on following page

Steps	Rationale	Special Considerations
2. If pacing leads are not in use or not attached to the external pacemaker, place them in a rubber glove or dry, glass phlebotomy tube, secure with tape, and tape the glove/tube and lead to the patient.	Provides insulation, which inhibits the conduction of electric current. Prevents inadvertent dislodging of the lead(s).	Insulate and label atrial and ventricular leads separately to facilitate correct identification if an emergency necessitating prompt cardiac pacing occurs.
3. Use only battery-powered external pacemakers.	Decreases the likelihood of transmitting leakage current.	
4. Wear rubber gloves when handling the leads or terminals of the external pacemaker.	Prevents electrical contact with other powered equipment.	Pacing leads provide low-resistance current pathways to the myocardium.
5. Ensure that all equipment and electrical devices in the patient environment are connected directly to a common ground.	Prevents an electrical potential from developing between pieces of equipment/devices. It decreases the likelihood of stray electric current or current flow between two pieces of electrical equipment.	Grounding systems connect all ground wires from all electric outlets to a common ground.
6. Avoid contact with the external pacemaker and its terminals when touching electrical equipment/ device/metal bed frame.	Minute amounts of alternating current can result in ventricular fibrillation.	
7. Ensure that a defibrillator and resuscitation equipment are immediately available.	Stimulation of the myocardium during the cell's vulnerable period may result in ventricular fibrillation.	

Evaluation

1. In the patient with an external pacemaker, monitor for strong electric fields: an erratic deflection of the sense/pace indicator needle to the left. **Rationale:** May interfere with the demand function of the external pacemaker.

2. Monitor equipment for any signs of malfunction, including tingling, smoke, or sparks. Should these signs be present, remove the device and notify the Biomedical Engineering Department immediately. **Rationale:** This device represents an electrical hazard to patient and staff.

3. Ensure that electrical safety inspection and preventive maintenance programs are performed. **Rationale:** Reduces electrical hazard risks to patients and staff. Meets JCAHO and state regulatory/licensing requirements.

4. Evaluate nursing procedures and techniques for electrical safety. **Rationale:** To identify any action/procedure that may increase the risk of electrical hazard to patients and staff.

5. Secure manufacturer's instruction manuals in a centralized, accessible location. **Rationale:** Equipment users need to refer to manuals for proper utilization and troubleshooting of equipment and for developing institution-specific policies and procedures for use.

6. Provide in-service education programs addressing electrical safety. **Rationale:** Meets JCAHO and state regulatory/licensing requirements.

Expected Outcomes

1. Electrically safe environment and equipment. **Rationale:** Electrically hazardous situations are minimized with the implementation of electrical safety precautions and an inspection program.

2. Absence of microshock. **Rationale:** Electrical safety inspections/precautions facilitate the detection of leakage-current levels of greater than 10 μA.

Unexpected Outcomes

1. Patient/staff injury. **Rationale:** Leakage current, inadequate grounds, frayed wires, loose connections, wet surfaces/linen, and damaged equipment contribute to an increased electrical hazard.

2. Microshock. **Rationale:** Stray electrical current, static electricity, or current from a short-circuited electrical device entering the myocardium may result in lethal tachyarrhythmias.

Documentation

1. Documentation of general electrical safety precautions in the patient record is not customary. Docu-

mentation providing evidence of an ongoing inspection program for biomedical equipment should be maintained. Attendance at an annual in-service program addressing electrical safety should be reflected in the nurse's performance evaluation. **Rationale:** Provides evidence of meeting common regulatory agency standards for patient/staff safety.

2. Documentation in the patient record should indicate that specific electrical safety precautions for the patient with a direct conduction pathway to the myocardium were instituted. Document any unexpected outcomes and interventions taken. **Rationale:** Documents nursing care provided, expected and unexpected outcomes, and interventions taken.

may be brought in from home or outside the hospital. **Rationale:** These devices may be improperly grounded, are potential sources of leakage current, and generally use a two-pronged plug.

2. Instruct the patient and family that smoking is absolutely *not allowed* in the critical care unit. **Rationale:** A lighted match and cigarette pose an electrical/fire hazard in the presence of oxygen.

3. If the patient is in an electrical bed, instruct him or her not to use the bed control. **Rationale:** May increase the risk of microshock.

4. Instruct the patient and family to avoid using or touching line-powered devices (i.e., cardiac monitor, radio, electrical razors) while the temporary pacing leads are in place. **Rationale:** Potential sources of leakage current, which increases the risk of microshock.

Patient/Family Education

1. Instruct the patient and family that no equipment

Performance Checklist
Skill 36–1: Electrical Safety for Patients and Medical Device Operators

Critical Behaviors	Complies	
	yes	no
1. Use only three-pronged plugs in grounded outlets.		
2. Use three-pronged extension cords only if absolutely necessary.		
3. Avoid plugging devices that use high current into the same outlet.		
4. Turn equipment off before unplugging.		
5. Grasp plug rather than cord to remove plug from outlet.		
6. Return defective equipment and equipment that has been dropped to the Biomedical Engineering Department. Attach a note stating the date and reason for the reevaluation.		
7. Remove all discontinued or unused equipment from patient environment.		
8. Maintain clinical environment humidity at 50 to 60 percent.		
9. Ground all metal beds.		
10. Validate electrical safety of all electric beds.		
11. Check for a clear, crisp tracing on oscilloscope of hemodynamic monitors.		
12. Do not place liquid or wet articles on top of monitors or other electrical equipment.		
PRECAUTIONS FOR ELECTRICAL PACEMAKERS: 1. Contain exposed parts of the lead's external electrode at the terminals in a rubber glove.		
2. If pacing leads are not in use, place them in a rubber glove, secure, and tape to the patient.		
3. Use only battery-powered external pacemakers.		
4. Wear rubber gloves when handling leads or terminals of the external pacemaker.		
5. Validate that all electrical devices and equipment are connected to a common ground.		
6. Avoid contact with external pacemaker and terminals when touching electrical equipment/device/ metal bed frame.		
7. Ensure that the defibrillator and emergency resuscitation equipment are readily available.		

BIBLIOGRAPHY

Buchsbaum, W. H., and Goldsmith, B. (1975). *Electrical Safety in the Hospital*. Oradell, N.J.: Medical Economic Company.

Guzzetta, C. E., and Dossey, B. M. (1984). *Cardiovascular Nursing: Bodymind Tapestry*. St. Louis: Mosby.

Meth, I. M. (1980). Electrical safety in the hospital. *Am. J. Nurs.* 80:1344–1345.

Miodownik, S. (1983). Ensuring electrical safety in the critical care environment. *Crit. Care Monit.* 3(3):1, 8–9.

Norris, B. W. (1985). Electrical Safety Precautions for the Patient with Direct Conduction Pathways to the Myocardium. In S. Millar, L. K. Sampson, and M. Soukup (Eds.), *AACN Procedure Manual for Critical Care*, 2d Ed. Philadelphia: Saunders.

Persons, C. B. (1987). *Critical Care Procedures and Protocols*. Philadelphia: Lippincott.

Stahler-Miller, K. (1985). Electrical Safety for Patients and Medical Device Operators. In S. Millar, L. K. Sampson, and M. Soukup (Eds.), *AACN Procedure Manual for Critical Care*, 2d Ed. Philadelphia: Saunders.

37

Radiation Safety

BEHAVIORAL OBJECTIVES

After completing this chapter, the nurse will be able to

- Define the key terms.
- Describe methods for limiting radiation exposure for staff and patients.
- Discuss nursing management related to care of the patient undergoing a radiopharmaceutical procedure or a diagnostic x-ray.

Historically, exposure to radiation has been associated with health risks. First, there seems to be a direct relationship between the amount of radiation exposure and health risks (Mancino, 1983). Chromosomal damage is known to result from radiation exposure. Other health risks include cancer, leukemia, congenital defects, and central nervous system defects. Since there is a lag period between the time of exposure and the development of symptoms, it is difficult to establish a direct cause–effect relationship. Secondarily, different age groups of people react differently to radiation exposure; a fetus is more sensitive to radiation than a child and a child is more sensitive than an adult as a result of the high growth index of babies and children. However, all ages remain at risk.

Efforts have been made in the past several years to protect health care workers from undue exposure to radiation. Measures such as the passage of the Health and Safety Act have been legislated to protect health care workers from the potential adverse effects of long-term radiation exposure. Standards have been set by the Joint Commission for Accreditation of Healthcare Organizations that address radiation safety, and the Nuclear Regulatory Commission has formulated strict guidelines for limiting exposure to radiation. In addition, local governments have established health codes to protect people from undue exposure (Mancino, 1983).

The basis for diagnostic roentgenology is the differential absorption of x-rays by various body tissues. Three elements will increase or decrease this absorption. First, as the atomic number of the material being radiated increases, absorption increases. Lead, which has a high atomic number, absorbs x-rays well. Bone, which has a higher atomic number than other body tissues, will absorb x-rays better than other tissues of the body. The second element affecting absorption is density. A lower-density substance such as air does not absorb x-rays as well as fluid. Third, absorption increases as thickness increases. X-rays that are not absorbed by tissues will pass through the body, forming an image on a photographic film (Lenihan, 1985).

Since critical care patients are frequently too acutely ill to be transported to the radiology department, health care workers in critical care environments are possibly exposed to ionizing radiation from portable x-ray equipment. Fluoroscopy, another common source of radiation, is routinely used in some units to assist in the insertion of pulmonary artery catheters and temporary pacing wires. In addition, nurses often accompany patients for radiologic procedures such as CT scans and cardiac catheterizations and remain with them during the procedure (Miracle and Wigginton, 1990).

Another potential source of exposure to radiation is caring for the patient who has received a radiopharmaceutical agent for a nuclear medicine procedure such as a multigated blood-pool analysis (MUGA), thallium scan, or a lung scan. A radiopharmaceutical agent is injected through a vein and localizes in an organ or system. The radioactive substance emits gamma rays that can be detected externally by cameras, scanners, or probes. The source of radiation in nuclear medicine is the patient, whereas the source of radiation in an ionizing-radiation procedure is the x-ray machine (Lenihan, 1985).

Radioactive implants, such an intrauterine devices, are yet another source of potential radiation exposure for health care workers. Implants emit higher levels of radiation than the aforementioned sources. The *patient* with a radioactive implant is *not* radioactive; the *source* is *radioactive*. Thus the worker is no longer at risk once the source is removed (Godwin et al., 1985).

The most frequently used method to measure the amount of radiation a health care worker has been exposed to is the film badge. This badge measures exposure to beta and gamma rays and x-radiation. The film badge is a device that holds a small section of radiation-sensitive film inside a plastic holder that can be attached to the health care worker's clothing. When the radiation-sensitive film is developed, the measurements of radiation exposure will be compared with standard film. Each health care worker should have his or her own film badge, which should only be worn at work. The badge should be worn between the waist and shoulders and under a lead apron if one is worn (Lenihan, 1985).

Four factors contribute to the degree of radiation exposure in health care personnel. The first factor is the time spent in contact with the radioactive source. The longer the amount of time, the greater is the amount of radiation to which one is exposed. The second factor is the degree of radioactivity present, which varies according to the strength of the specific radioactive material used. Distance is the third factor. The closer one remains to the source of radiation, the greater is the exposure (Jankowski, 1986). The last factor is shielding. Using an absorbing lead shield will decrease the amount of radioactive exposure to the health care worker (Lenihan, 1985).

This chapter presents an overview of the precautions one must take when caring for a patient who is receiving or who has undergone a radiologic procedure.

KEY TERMS

gamma rays
ionizing radiation
millirem (mrem)
radiation absorbed
 dosage (rad)

radioisotope
roentgen-equivalent-man
 period (rem)

SKILLS

37–1 Radiopharmaceutical Radiation Safety Precautions
37–2 Portable X-Ray Radiation Safety Precautions

GUIDELINES

The following assessment guidelines are useful for the nurse when caring for a patient undergoing a radiologic procedure:

1. Know which procedure the patient is undergoing.
2. Know the type of radiation used.
3. Know the factors necessary to limit exposure to radiation.
4. Identify the specific precautions necessary to limit radiation exposure to patients and health care workers.

SKILL 37–1

Radiopharmaceutical Radiation Safety Precautions

Radiopharmaceutical procedures are diagnostic or therapeutic nuclear studies. Examples of these procedures include radioactive iodine uptake tests, lung perfusion scans, and thallium imaging. A drug containing a radioactive tracer is administered to the patient. This radioactive substance localizes in an organ or system. As

the radioisotope decays, radiation is emitted that is detected externally by scanners, cameras, or probes. There do not need to be any changes in nursing care or assignments when caring for patients who have undergone a nuclear medicine study. There is very little radiation emitted from these patients (Jankowski, 1986). See Table 37–1 for a description of the most commonly used tracer radioisotopes (Taveras and Ferruisi, 1990).

Purpose

Health care workers must understand the principles of radiation safety precautions when caring for a patient who has undergone a nuclear medicine study.

Prerequisite Knowledge and Skills

The nurse should understand

1. Principles of radiopharmaceutical studies.
2. Principles of radiation safety.
3. Principles for limiting exposure.

The nurse should be able to

1. Identify the specific radioactive tracer administered.
2. Identify specific precautions for the radioactive tracer administered.

Assessment

1. Assess the patient's potential risk for exposure to radiation (i.e., history of previous exposure, type of radiation, pregnancy, and length of exposure). **Rationale:** Risk increases with repeated exposure, pregnancy, and length of exposure.
2. Assess the nurse's potential risk for radiation exposure (i.e., history of previous exposure, type of radiation, pregnancy, distance from source, and length of exposure). **Rationale:** Risk increases with repeated exposure, pregnancy, length of exposure, and proximity to source of radiation.

Nursing Diagnoses

1. Potential for injury related to exposure to radioisotopes. **Rationale:** Even though the amount of radia-

TABLE 37–1 COMMONLY USED TRACER RADIOISOTOPES

Radioisotope	Half-Life	Common Uses
Iodine-131	8 days	Thyroid, kidney
Iodine-123	13 hours	Kidney, thyroid
Technetium-99m	6 hours	Liver, bone, lung, heart, kidney, thyroid
Thallium-201	37 hours	Heart, parathyroid
Indium-111 DTPA	68 hours	Cysternograms

Source: Data from Taveras, J. M. and Ferrucci, J. T., *Radiology: Diagnosis-Imaging-Intervention*, Vol 1. Philadelphia: Lippincott, 1990, Chap. 1, p. 5 and Chap. 25, p. 5.

tion in radiopharmaceutical agents is minimal, a potential risk does exist.

2. Potential for anxiety related to fear of having a radioactive substance administered. **Rationale:** Information and education help allay anxiety by decreasing misconceptions and myths regarding nuclear diagnostic studies.

Planning

1. Explain the procedure to the patient. **Rationale:** Minimizes risk and reduces anxiety.

2. When wearing a lead apron, the film badge must be worn on the inside of the apron (Fig. 37–1). **Rationale:** To accurately record the amount of radiation to which one is exposed. The film badge merely monitors the amount of radiation exposure the body receives with the protective apron. A false body reading will be obtained if the badge is worn outside the apron.

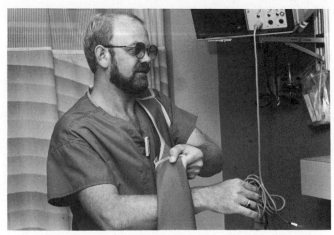

FIGURE 37–1. Critical care nurse showing proper placement of film badge under the lead apron.

Implementation

Steps	Rationale	Special Considerations
1. Wear your badge inside the apron.	Accurately records the amount of radiation exposure.	
2. Don exam gloves when disposing of urine according to hospital protocol.	Universal precautions.	Radioactive substances are excreted primarily through the kidneys.
3. Wash hands after removing gloves.	Decreases risk of contamination or possible ingestion.	
4. Have the patient wash his or her hands with soap and water after voiding.	Decreases risk of contamination.	

Evaluation

Level of radiation exposure will be exhibited on film badge if worn, but usually exposure is negligible. **Rationale:** The amount of radiation emitted from a patient who has undergone a radiopharmaceutical procedure is minimal.

Expected Outcome

Negligible exposure will be monitored if film badge is worn. **Rationale:** The amount of radiation emitted from a patient who has undergone a radiopharmaceutical procedure is minimal.

Unexpected Outcome

Radiation exposure greater than 100 mrem per week. **Rationale:** A possible breakdown in procedure has occurred. All aspects of the procedure need to be examined.

Documentation

1. Documentation in the patient record should include the date, time, and name of procedure; the patient's tolerance of the procedure; specific safety precautions utilized; and patient education. **Rationale:** Documents nursing care given.

2. Film badges, if worn, should be monitored according to hospital protocol. **Rationale:** Documents level of exposure.

Patient/Family Education

1. Discuss the procedure, any special preparation before the procedure, or special care afterward with both patient and family. **Rationale:** Patient and family education minimizes anxiety and increases cooperation.

2. Explain the precautions necessary with urine to

both patient and family (i.e., wash hands with soap and water after voiding). **Rationale:** Patient and family education minimizes anxiety and increases cooperation and also decreases possible exposure.

3. Tell the patient to continue washing hands with soap and water after voiding for 3 days after the procedure. Patient may wear gloves, if desired. Provide gloves, if necessary. **Rationale:** Half-life of some of the radioisotopes can last up to 78 hours.

Performance Checklist
Skill 37–1: Radiopharmaceutical Radiation Safety Precautions

Critical Behaviors	Complies	
	yes	no
1. Implement universal precautions.		
2. Wash hands after removing gloves.		
3. Tell patient to wash hands after voiding.		
4. Document procedure in patient record.		

SKILL 37–2

Portable X-Ray Radiation Safety Precautions

Potential sources of ionizing radiation within critical care nursing include portable x-rays, fluoroscopy, CT scans, and cardiac catheterizations. Radiation exposure from portable x-rays is unpredictable because of undetected leaks from faulty equipment and from radiation scatter. *Scatter* is the deflection of x-rays that are not absorbed by the patient (Godwin et al., 1985). Even though portable fluoroscopy emits less radiation than standard x-rays, it can be hazardous to nurses because of extended testing periods, potentially resulting in a higher absorbed dose.

Purpose

Nurses should institute safety precautions with procedures utilizing ionizing radiation to limit the degree of radiation exposure to self, other patients, and other health care workers.

Prerequisite Knowledge and Skills

The nurse should understand
1. Principles of ionizing radiation.
2. Principles of radiation safety.
3. Principles of limiting radiation exposure.

The nurse should be able to
1. Identify the specific radiologic procedure.
2. Identify specific precautions for the radiologic procedure.

Assessment

1. Assess the patient's potential risk for exposure to radiation (i.e., history of previous exposure, type of radiation, pregnancy, and length of exposure). **Rationale:** Risk increases with repeated exposure, pregnancy, and length of exposure.

2. Assess the health care worker's potential risk for exposure to radiation (i.e., history of previous exposure, type of radiation, pregnancy, distance from source, and length of exposure). **Rationale:** Risk increases with repeated exposure, pregnancy, length of exposure, and proximity to source of radiation.

Nursing Diagnoses

1. Potential for injury related to exposure to ionizing radiation. **Rationale:** Even though the amount of ionizing radiation is minimal, a potential risk does exist.

2. Potential for anxiety related to fear of the unknown or radiation exposure. **Rationale:** Information and education help allay anxiety by decreasing one's misconceptions and myths.

Planning

1. Explain the procedure to patient. **Rationale:** Minimizes risk and decreases anxiety.

2. If the nurse is pregnant or may be pregnant, she should try to find a substitute to stay with the patient. **Rationale:** Even though the amount of radiation is minimal, the effects of even low-dose radiation on the fetus are as yet unknown.

3. All personnel should wear lead aprons. A female patient of child-bearing age should have a lead apron covering the abdomen. **Rationale:** Even though the amount of radiation is minimal, the effects of even low-dose radiation are as yet unknown.

Implementation

Steps	Rationale	Special Considerations
1. Increase your distance from the source of radiation.	Radiation exposure is inversely proportional to the square of the distance ($D = 1/R^2$, where D = dose, R = distance).	Attempt to stay 2 to 4 ft away from the source of radiation, if possible. Stay behind the x-ray machine, if possible. Ask the technician to give ample warning before taking the x-ray.
2. If you must remain with the patient, wear protective shielding, such as a lead apron, that wraps around the entire body.	The wearing of protective clothing decreases absorption. Lead will absorb the x-rays because of its density.	Stand to the side away from the direct x-ray beam. Use mechanical restraints or chemical sedation, if needed, for the patient. Remain behind a lead-lined barrier if lead apron is not available. If wearing a film badge, wear it on the inside of the apron.
3. Decrease the length of time of exposure.	Exposure has a cumulative effect.	

Evaluation

Level of radiation exposure will be exhibited on film badge. **Rationale:** The amount of ionizing radiation to which one is routinely exposed is minimal.

Expected Outcome

Radiation exposure is minimal, less than 100 mrem per week (Miracle and Wigginton, 1990). **Rationale:** The amount of ionizing radiation to which one is routinely exposed is within an acceptable range as defined by the Nuclear Regulatory Commission.

Unexpected Outcome

Significant radiation exposure (>100 mrem per week). **Rationale:** A possible breakdown in procedure has occurred. All aspects of the procedure need to be examined. The film badge may have been worn in sunlight, thus giving a false-positive reading for significant radiation exposure.

Documentation

Documentation in the patient record should include the date, time, and type of procedure; the patient's tolerance of the procedure; specific safety precautions utilized; and patient education. **Rationale:** Documents nursing care given.

Patient/Family Education

Discuss the procedure and any special preparation or care before and after the procedure with the patient and family. **Rationale:** Patient and family education minimizes anxiety, increases cooperation and compliance, and minimizes risk.

Performance Checklist
Skill 37–2: Portable X-Ray Radiation Safety Precautions

Critical Behaviors	Complies yes	no
1. Increase distance from source of radiation.		
2. Wear lead apron for shielding.		
3. Limit length of exposure to smallest time possible.		
4. Document procedure in the patient record.		

REFERENCES

Godwin, C. L., Bucholtz, J. D., and Wall, S. L. (1985). Guide to hazards in the job: III. Radiation. *Nurs. Life* 5(6):43–47.
Jankowski, C. B. (1986). Preventing radiation exposure in critical care. *Dimens. Crit. Care Nurs.* 5:170–176.
Lenihan, E. (1985). Radiation safety. In S. Millar, L. K. Sampson, and M. Soukup (Eds.), *AACN Procedure Manual for Critical Care*, 2d Ed. Philadelphia: Saunders.
Mancino, D. (1983). Radiation in the nurses' workplace. *Imprint* 30:35–39.
Miracle, V. A., and Wigginton, M. A. (1990). Nurses and ionizing radiation: A study of two institutions. *Crit. Care Nurs.* 20(5):58–64.

Traveras, J. M., and Ferruisi, J. T. (1990). *Radiology: Diagnosis–Imaging–Intervention*. Philadelphia: Lippincott.

BIBLIOGRAPHY

Berger, M. E., and Hubner, K. F. (1983). Hospital hazards: Diagnostic radiation. *Am. J. Nurs.* 83:1155–1159.

Pilapil, F., and Studva, K. V. (1979). *Programmed Instruction: Radiation Safety*. New York: Masson.

Ritenour, E. R. (1984). Overview of the Hazards of Low Level Exposure to Radiation. In W. R. Hendre (Ed.), *Health Effects of Low Level Radiation*. Norwalk, Conn.: Appleton-Century-Crofts.

Shell, T. A., and Carter, J. (1987). The gynecological implant patients. *Semin. Oncol. Nurs.* 3(1):54–66.

Stringer, B. (1984). Nurse heal thyself: Your work could be killing you. *Can. Nurse* 8(9):18–22.

UNIT XII

ORGAN PROCUREMENT

38

ORGAN DONATION

BEHAVIORAL OBJECTIVES

After completing this chapter, the nurse will be able to

- Define the key terms.
- Describe the clinical criteria and methods for identifying potential organ donors.
- Discuss the process of obtaining consent.
- Develop a care plan for the multiple-organ donor.
- Describe the methods of organ preservation and the system in place for the sharing and distribution of the organs.

The significant growth and development in the field of transplantation may be attributed to the progress in the science of immunosuppression, the development of organ preservation, enabling long-distance procurement, and the refinement of surgical techniques. This progress has been coupled with increased public awareness and increased knowledge among health care professionals relating to organ donation, procurement, and transplantation. However, the limiting factor in the continued application of this therapeutic intervention is the shortage of donor organs. To maximize the availability of donor organs and tissues, the nurse must be skilled in identification of the potential donor, the mechanisms and methodologies for obtaining consent for donation, the referral process to organ procurement organizations, and the clinical care of the donor. This knowledge and these skills must be integrated with an understanding and trust of the national system and a commitment to the professional responsibility of the donation process as a means to save the lives of patients who are either severely limited or will otherwise die from end-stage organ failure.

The nurse should be aware of the legislative factors involved in the organ donation process. The Uniform Anatomical Gift Act was enacted in 1970 by all 50 states.

This act legally provides anyone above the age of 18 with the right to indicate willingness to become a donor at the time of death. The act also authorizes the next of kin to donate and protects the health care professional from liability related to participating in the donation process. Section 9318 of the Omnibus Budget Reconciliation Act of 1986 (PL 99-509) added a new section to the National Organ Transplant Act of 1984 (PL 98-507). This section allows hospitals that meet the conditions of participation in Medicare and Medicaid programs to participate only if

1. The hospital established written protocols to identify potential organ and tissue donors that

    a. Ensure that families of potential donors are made aware that they have an option to donate organs or tissue and an option to decline to donate.

    b. Encourage discretion and sensitivity with respect to the circumstances, views, and belief of the families of potential donors.

    c. Require that an organ procurement agency designated by the secretary of Health and Human Services be notified of potential donors.

2. In the case of a hospital that performs organ transplants, the hospital is a member of and abides by the rules of the Organ Procurement and Transplantation Network (OPTN), established in accordance with section 372 of the Public Health Service Act.

These laws constitute the framework for "required request" in addition to approximately 44 state laws that require that families be given the option to donate or to decline to donate. Ninety-five percent of all donor situations occur in critical care units.

The Joint Commission on Accreditation of Healthcare Organizations (JCAHO) established standards for accreditation related to organ donation in 1988. The sections addressing management and medical records within the JCAHO guidelines contain these standards.

This chapter focuses on the major groups into which donors are categorized, the specific evaluation of the potential donor, the consent process, the needs of the donor family, the clinical management of the organ donor, and the preservation of the organs.

KEY TERMS

brain death
metabolic homeostasis
neuroendocrine regulation
organ donor
organ perfusion

organ preservation
organ procurement
organization
organ oxygenation
required request

SKILLS

38–1 Identifying Potential Organ Donors
38–2 Facilitating Organ Donation
38–3 Organ Preparation for Retrieval

GUIDELINES

The following assessment guidelines assist the nurse in formulating a nursing diagnosis and an individualized plan of care to recognize and care for the organ donor and family:

1. Know the clinical criteria for multiple-organ donation.
2. Know the patient's medical history.
3. Know the patient's current injuries, hospitalization, and medical treatment.
4. Perform neurologic assessments in a systematic and timely fashion.
5. Perform organ perfusion and oxygenation assessments in a systematic and timely fashion.
6. Determine appropriate interventions for assessed findings.
7. Assess the potential donor family in terms of their knowledge of the situation.

SKILL 38–1

Identifying Potential Organ Donors

All donors of vascular organs are patients who have been declared brain dead utilizing criteria that have been established within a particular locale or institution (Simmons et al., 1984). The nurse must be familiar with the policy and procedure specific to his or her institution. There have been many criteria used to diagnose brain death, including those offered in 1968 by the Ad Hoc Committee of the Harvard Medical School for the Definition of Death and a Presidential Commission for the Study of Ethical Problems in Medicine and Biomedical Research in 1981. Flye (1989) has reviewed many of the criteria used and has found three principles common to all:

1. Coma of established cause: no toxins, physiologic abnormalities corrected.
2. Cerebral unresponsivity.
3. Absent brainstem reflexes: pupils, oculovestibular responses, respiration.

Identification of the potential organ donor is based on the recognition of a patient unlikely to survive because of the nature of his or her injuries or medical problem who meets the criteria for donation. The criteria for donation may be specific to the locale or to the receiving transplant team. Since criteria have become more liberal because of the donor shortage, many areas have routine referral policies by which all deaths are reported to the organ procurement organization (OPO) for consideration. Table 38–1 indicates one example of basic criteria that may be used. Each critical care nurse should be familiar with local practices.

The causes of brain death include head trauma, intracerebral hemorrhage, primary brain tumors, or cerebral anoxia after cardiac or respiratory arrest. After consultation with the responsible physician(s), the potential donor should be referred to the appropriate (OPO) to determine specific suitability as a donor. To avoid conflict of interest, the procurement team cannot participate in the care of the potential donor prior to the pronouncement of death and cannot itself make the determination of death. However, the team should be able to provide guidelines for declaring a person brain dead. The referral of the potential donor to the OPO does not change the current plan of clinical care or represent a commitment on the part of the health care team, but rather helps to prevent a needless approach to the family if there are no viable organs or tissues available. The OPO staff will indicate its opinion regarding the donation possibility based on a history of the injuries, hospitalization, and certain pertinent data such as age, blood group, vital signs, laboratory data, etc.

Purpose

The nurse participates in recognition and referral of the potential organ donor to

1. Provide the full continuum of care for the patient who is brain dead.

TABLE 38–1 LIFESOURCE, ORGAN DONOR REVIEW CHART

	Kidney	Heart	Liver	Pancreas	Heart for Valves	Bone	Skin	Eye	Ear
Age (years)	0–65	2–50	1 mo.–65	1–65	0–55	16–55	14–75	0–100+	8–100+
Cardiac arrest resuscitated	Prob. OK	No	Prob. OK	Prob. OK	OK	Heart-beating cadaver not mandatory	Heart-beating cadaver not mandatory	Heart-beating cadaver not mandatory	Heart-beating cadaver not mandatory
Chest/abdominal trauma	Important	Extremely important	Extremely important	Important	Little importance	Little importance	Little importance	Not important	Not important
No active systemic infections	Mandatory	Mandatory	Mandatory	Mandatory	Mandatory	Mandatory	Mandatory	N/A	Mandatory
No presence or history of communicable disease	Mandatory	Mandatory	Mandatory	Mandatory	Mandatory	Mandatory	Mandatory	Mandatory	Mandatory
Hypotension	Sensitive	Very sensitive	Very sensitive	Sensitive	N/A	N/A	N/A	N/A	N/A
Vasopressor, i.e., dopamine sensitive	Yes	Very	Very	Yes	N/A	N/A	N/A	N/A	N/A
Weight important	No	Yes	Yes	No	No	No	>100 lbs	N/A	N/A
Body build important	No	Yes	Yes	No	No	No	No	No	No
Blood type	Mandatory	Mandatory	Mandatory	Mandatory	N/A	N/A	N/A	N/A	N/A
Additional physician consults required	Usually not	Yes	Possibly	Usually not	No	No	No	No	No
Additional laboratory data needed	Yes, kidney specific	Yes, heart specific	Yes, liver specific	Yes, pancreas specific	No	No	No	No	No
Time needed to set up additional teams	No	Yes	Yes	Yes	No	No	Possible	No	No
Tissue may be retrieved after cardiac death	No	No	No	No	Yes, up to 12 hours after death. The whole heart is retrieved in the OR.	Yes, up to 24 hours in the OR under sterile conditions	Yes, up to 36 hours if refrigerated	Yes, up to 6 hours. Place ice packs on the eyes after closing them.	Yes, up to 48 hours. May be procured following embalming.

2. Meet the ethical responsibility to those patients awaiting transplants.

3. Meet the state, federal, and JCAHO requirements pertaining to organ donation.

Prerequisite Knowledge and Skills

Prior to participating in recognition and referral of the potential organ donor, the nurse should understand:

1. The technological, immunologic, and surgical advances that have made organ and tissue transplantation a viable therapeutic modality for patients with end-stage organ disease.

2. That thousands of Americans could potentially benefit from organ and tissue transplantation.

3. The organ procurement system in his or her locale.

4. The clinical criteria for brain death.

5. His or her personal feelings about life, death, and ethical issues surrounding transplantation (Heitman, 1987).

The nurse should be able to perform:

1. Neurologic, respiratory, and cardiovascular assessment.

2. Laboratory data analysis, including arterial blood gases, renal function, liver function, and electrolyte balance.

3. An interview with the family regarding medical history.

Assessment

1. Conduct a thorough history that includes current age, current injuries, diseases, treatments, familial health, and social habits via the patient chart, the attending physician, and the family. Of particular interest is a history of renal disease, hypertension, diabetes mellitus, malignant disease, hepatitis, recent blood transfusions, or recent pregnancy. **Rationale:** Provides information related to organ function or the possibility of transmissible diseases.

2. Document the level at which blood pressure has been maintained and the 24-hour fluid intake and urinary output since the occurrence of trauma or acute signs and symptoms of neurologic damage. **Rationale:** Indicators of adequate tissue perfusion.

3. Perform a physical assessment, observing for old surgical scars, needle track marks, congenital anomalies, injuries, and the placement and adequacy of venous access. **Rationale:** Indicators of physical or social aspects that may influence organ function or suitability for transplantation.

4. Monitor pertinent laboratory data, including blood, urine, and/or sputum cultures; VDRL, HIV antibody, hepatitis screening, and CMV serology should be performed. **Rationale:** Rules out transmissible diseases or active infection. Liver function and cardiac enzyme tests, serum creatinine, blood urea nitrogen level, and urinalysis are assessed to monitor organ function. Blood

type determination is mandatory for all vascular organ matching because ABO incompatibility compromises the viability of the transplanted organ.

5. Document an accurate measurement of height and weight. **Rationale:** Provides information for matching extrarenal organs to a recipient of corresponding body size.

6. The neurologic assessment must demonstrate that the patient has total unawareness to externally applied stimuli and that even the most noxious stimuli must evoke no vocal or other purposeful response (Flye, 1989). This assessment should be made in the presence of normothermia with no evidence of remediable exogenous or endogenous intoxication. There should be no brainstem function, with the following reflexes absent: pupillary light, corneal, oculocephalic (doll's eyes response), oculovestibular (caloric stimulation), and oral pharyngeal (gag reflex). There should not be motor response to central pain stimulation. There may be spinal reflex activity. The patient should have no spontaneous respirations. Total apnea is the final criteria for brain death that must be met. In a proper test for apnea, the patient should be removed from the ventilator and CO_2 should be allowed to accumulate while the thorax is observed and palpated carefully for spontaneous respiration. At the end of a period of time (usually 10 minutes) estimated to bring the $PaCO_2$ to above 50 mmHg, (a $PaCO_2$ rise of approximately 2.5 mmHg per minute can be expected in most patients), a blood gas sample is drawn and the patient is reconnected to the ventilator. If the $PaCO_2$ at the end of the test exceeds 50 mmHg and pH is below 7.35, apnea has been adequately demonstrated (Black and Todres, 1989). **Rationale:** Confirms brain death.

Nursing Diagnosis

Altered cerebral perfusion related to trauma, edema, hemorrhage, CVA, or masses. **Rationale:** The interruption of blood flow to the brain creates a loss of consciousness.

Planning

Develop a plan for performing potential donor recognition, assessment, and referral:

1. Recognize neurologic findings indicating brain death. **Rationale:** Most organ donors are in the intensive care unit demonstrating a clinical course that will lead to the diagnosis of brain death.

2. Document clinical criteria that will be pertinent to determining the ability to donate organs for transplantation. **Rationale:** Whereas all potential donors may be referred to OPOs, organs may not be viable for transplantation because of clinical history or findings.

3. Communicate information about the potential donor to the OPO per hospital policy. **Rationale:** The OPO provides the access to the national computer system necessary for matching donors with recipients and assists with the actual recovery and placement of the organs.

Implementation

Steps	Rationale	Special Considerations
1. Update personal information on the status of transplantation as a clinical entity.	Provides incentive for participating in donation process.	
2. Update personal information on the current need for donor organs.	Provides motivation for participating in donation process.	
3. Examine personal feelings related to organ donation.	Negative attitudes may interfere with effectiveness in dealing with the donor family and in caring for the donor.	
4. Be knowledgeable of donor criteria.	Age, disease, and trauma may rule out organ donation. Age may not rule out tissue donation.	If routine referral is the policy, all deaths would be referred to the OPO.
5. Obtain assessment data: medical and social history, physical examination, laboratory and neurologic status.	Provides accurate data to OPO.	
6. Collaborate with the physician to confirm neurologic status, and facilitate pronouncement of death according to standard medical practice.	When a patient is pronounced dead on the basis of neurologic evidence, organ removal can take place with proper consent.	Tissue and bone donation does not require a heart-beating cadaver. Special consideration must be given to the diagnosis of brain death in children.
7. Communicate all information relevant to organ donation to the OPO.	The OPO can assist in the assessment of the donor. The referral meets the requirement of PL 99-509.	

Evaluation

Expected Outcomes

1. In the presence of brain death, proper documentation of the declaration of death and consideration of organ donation should take place. **Rationale:** Federal law requires that all families be given the opportunity to donate or decline to donate the organs of their next of kin.

2. The OPO servicing the hospital should be notified of the potential donor. **Rationale:** Notification of the OPO is required by law. Additionally, the OPO can offer assistance relating to the recovery of organs and/or tissues.

3. Vital signs, organ perfusion, and oxygenation are monitored and maintained. **Rationale:** To maintain the viability of the organs for possible transplantation.

Unexpected Outcomes

1. The recognition and documentation of brain death does not take place. **Rationale:** The option for donation is not possible.

2. The recognition of a potential donor does not take place. **Rationale:** The option for donation is not possible.

3. The notification of the OPO or a potential donor does not take place. **Rationale:** Violates federal law.

Documentation

Documentation in the patient record should include pertinent patient history; physical and neurologic assessment findings; current clinical status, including vital signs and fluid intake and output; communication with other health care team members relating to the neurologic status of the patient and the potential for organ or tissue donation; and communication with the OPO. **Rationale:** This reflects the nursing care given, meets legal and JCAHO requirements, and sets the stage for progressing to the consent process with the patient's family.

Performance Checklist
Skill 38–1: Identifying Potential Organ Donors

Critical Behaviors	Complies	
	yes	no
1. Know the criteria for brain death and organ/tissue donation.		
2. Know the success rates for transplantation.		

Table continues on following page

Critical Behaviors	Complies	
	yes	no
3. Recognize the donor shortage.		
4. Have clarified personal feelings regarding organ donation and transplantation.		
5. Know the hospital's policies and procedures regarding brain death, notifying the organ procurement organization, and required request or routine referral.		
6. Obtain the patient's medical, social, and current clinical history.		
7. Perform and document physical and neurologic assessments.		
8. Confirm findings with medical colleagues.		
9. Make referral to OPO.		

SKILL 38–2

Facilitating Organ Donation

The organ procurement system is greatly a result of the positive attitudes of the American people. Many studies have demonstrated the high level of public support for organ donation and transplantation. A Gallup survey in 1985 indicated that 93 percent of Americans report they have heard or read about organ transplants and 73 percent of those aware of transplants say that they are very likely to give permission to have the organs of a loved one donated after that person's death (Ettner et al., 1988). It was also because of public input that donation and transplant-related legislation was enacted. Even though the public is positively inclined, the consent process, managed by health care professionals, is a major factor. Many medical personnel are reluctant to offer this opportunity to the family of a potential donor based on their own fears and perceptions and the common difficulty of dealing with the issue of their own mortality. In reality, organ donation may be the only positive event experienced by the family during the immediate period of grieving and loss related to the death of a loved one. Donation may provide them with tangible assistance in grieving and provide altruistic feelings about the opportunity to help another human being. Studies have shown that organ donation is viewed by the next of kin as the highest form of charity and a meaningful and helpful part of the normal grief process (Bartucci, 1987). Some families will seek out the health care practitioner and initiate the discussion in order to ensure that this opportunity is not overlooked. However, the family cannot be expected to initiate the idea of organ donation during this stressful time.

Each family must be assessed carefully with regard to offering the option of organ donation. If a religious or moral conflict is present, the health care professional must use judgment and discretion in making the request. Some state laws mandate that if prior knowledge of this objection is known, a request should not be made.

The subject of organ donation should never be raised in the same sentence as brain death; the family "just can't handle it then" (Crane, 1983). The reaction of family members depends not only on how they feel about organ donation, but also on their readiness to accept the finality of death. After brain death is explained, the family may need time to contemplate. Previously formed attitudes of the patient and the family also may be important. The nurse should help determine if the patient carried a signed donor card or had signed the organ donor proviso of a driver's license. If so, that information should be conveyed to the family of the patient. Family members might initially be opposed to donation if they are unaware that the patient wanted it, and they may desire to change their position after being presented with such information (Heitman, 1987).

The nurse, as well as all others involved in the consent process, should understand that the decision to donate an organ is a highly personal and emotional one. It is made under stressful conditions, and thus the discussion should take place in a nonthreatening, private environment. The topic should not be discussed at the patient's bedside, in the waiting area, or in open public places. The conversation may begin with an inquiry into the family's interest in donation. A family with reservations about donation will frequently verbalize them at this time. Reluctance may stem from a lack of knowledge or understanding of the processes utilized to care for their relative, the tests and procedures utilized to determine death, and/or the donation process itself. Written information may be a helpful reference for the family during the decision-making process. Many OPOs have prepared materials specifically for this purpose. The family should have a basic understanding of brain death and the implication that it is necessary to continue the mechanical support process through the surgical recovery procedure. The term *life support* should not be used because it may cause confusion for the family that has been told that their loved one is dead. The family should understand that this continuation of support does not represent a hope for recovery of their loved one or an attempt to create an opportunity for the premature donation of organs before death has occurred. Despite continuing organ support, the donor is neurologically, legally, and biologically dead.

The actual request for organ donation may be made by a physician, nurse, chaplain, social worker, or coordinator from the OPO. It is imperative that whoever makes the request be specifically trained in this area and have the ability to address questions that the family may have regarding timing, cost, distribution of the organs, the surgical procedure, and the effects on funeral plans.

The consent form utilized should specify the organs and tissues that the family wishes to be recovered and transplanted. The family should understand that all possible efforts will be made to successfully recover and transplant the organs and tissues for which they have consented and that no other organs or tissues will be recovered. They should understand that they are allowed to limit the recovery to specific purposes, such as transplantation and/or medical therapy and/or research if they so desire. The concept of informed consent is applicable in this situation.

There is no cost to the family of the organ donor for donor management after brain death has been declared and the consent for organ donation has been signed. It is necessary for the nurse to document the time these occur. All charges from that point on should be submitted to the OPO. There should be no delays in funeral plans and an open casket is still possible following donation. The local and national distribution networks ensure that the patient with the greatest need or the greatest possibility of success will receive the organs. The timing of the organ recovery process depends on where the transplant teams are coming from and which organs will be removed. The family should understand that their confidentiality as well as that of the recipients will be protected. The donor family will be informed that their gift has been utilized and may receive certain generic information regarding the transplant recipient(s). Donation is, for the most part, an act of anonymity.

The nurse will often play an important role in assisting physicians in make the diagnosis of brain death and may be involved in the request for donation. However, the nurse's most important role is in the clinical management of the organ donor. If the donor is not properly cared for, the organ(s) will not remain viable and the desired outcome of transplantation cannot take place. Once brain death has occurred, the viability of the patient is no longer the focus of care—the donor family and the viability of the organs become the objectives.

Purpose

The nurse participates in facilitating organ donation by

1. Providing supportive and factual information to the family of the brain dead patient.
2. Participating in the request process as appropriate.
3. Providing clinical maintenance of the donor in order to ensure the viability of the donated organs. The objectives of this clinical care are to maintain adequate organ perfusion to prevent ischemic injury, to maintain adequate tissue oxygenation to prevent hypoxic injury, and to prevent or treat complications that may occur secondary to the initial injury or during the course of donor maintenance which may compromise the organs.

Prerequisite Knowledge and Skills

Prior to participating in the request process or donor maintenance, the nurse should understand

1. Principles of communication with an acutely bereaved family.
2. Factual information regarding the recovery process.
3. The necessity of separating the discussion of brain death from the discussion of organ donation with a grieving family.
4. The policies and procedures for obtaining consent for donation.
5. The clinical care required to maintain viable organs for transplantation.

The nurse should be able to perform

1. Psychologically supportive interaction with potential donor family members.
2. Sterile technique.
3. Vital signs assessment.
4. Multisystem assessment.
5. Clinical care to maintain hemodynamic stability.

Assessment

1. Assess the family members for appropriate coping related to the loss of their loved one. **Rationale:** Inability to understand and acknowledge that their family member is dead will hinder the family's ability to grieve or deal with the possibility of donation.
2. Assess the donor for signs and symptoms of inadequate organ perfusion. **Rationale:** Poor perfusion may lead to ischemic injury.
3. Assess the donor for signs and symptoms of poor tissue oxygenation. **Rationale:** Decreased oxygenation may lead to hypoxic injury.
4. Assess the donor for signs and symptoms of infection. **Rationale:** Development of an infectious process could eliminate the possibility of organ donation.
5. Assess the donor vital signs and intake and output carefully. **Rationale:** The organs, particularly kidneys, can be damaged by inadequate perfusion secondary to hypotension or by tubular necrosis secondary to inadequate urinary output or dehydration.

Nursing Diagnoses

1. Decreased tissue perfusion related to failure of the autonomic nervous system in brain death. **Rationale:** The functional regulatory mechanisms no longer operate, and the sympathetic nervous system often becomes inactive. There may be an initial increase in blood pressure from the increased intracranial pressure and sympathetic discharge, but the subsequent failure of the sympathetic nervous system results in arterial vasodilation with a loss of vasomotor tone and usually will result in a dramatically decreased blood pressure. Hypotension also may be related to preexisting fluid deficits in patients who have

received diuretic agents in an attempt to reduce cerebral edema (Goldsmith, 1985) (Table 38–2). A situation exists where preload is inadequate, systemic vascular resistance is decreased, venous pooling occurs, and therefore, cardiac output is insufficient to adequately perfuse vital organs.

2. Decreased cardiac output related to chest trauma, hypovolemia, pulmonary edema, electrolyte imbalance, hypothermia, or cardiac rhythm disturbances. **Rationale:** Circulatory dynamics are affected by thoracic mechanics, circulating volume, electrolyte balance, body metabolism, and/or vasoactive drugs. Dysrhythmias may be a potential problem in the brain dead patient. Continuous ECG monitoring is necessary, and serial 12-lead ECGs may be requested. When cardiac problems are encountered, cardiac catheterization or an echocardiogram may be indicated prior to consideration of heart donation. Tachycardia is usually a result of increased sympathetic discharge during early management and later is most often associated with hypovolemia. The etiology must be determined and appropriate interventions applied because heart rates greater than 150 beats per minute are usually poorly tolerated and result in decreased stroke volume and thus cardiac output. Bradycardia may be seen in the later stages of increased intracranial pressure and may be an ominous sign both with regard to decreased cardiac output and to overall cardiovascular instability.

3. Ineffective breathing pattern or ineffective airway clearance related to lack of spontaneous respiration. **Rationale:** Intubation and mechanical ventilation are necessary to maintain a patent airway and promote respiratory gas exchange. Neurogenic pulmonary edema may develop with rapid onset after injury to the central nervous system (Goldsmith, 1985). Chest x-rays may reveal alveolar infiltrates, which cause severe disturbances in gas exchange.

4. Potential altered body temperature related to loss of temperature regulation that occurs with brain death. **Rationale:** Temperature regulation is a function of the central nervous system, which involves the hypothalamus, brainstem, and spinal cord. Normothermia is required to make the diagnosis of brain death and to preserve the viability of the donor organs.

5. Potential for infection related to the use of invasive procedures and devices for monitoring or therapeutic purposes. **Rationale:** Host defense mechanisms are altered and provide access for microorganisms into the body. Respiratory infections in the donor may be attributed to intubation or tracheostomy that bypasses the natural upper airway defense mechanisms.

6. Potential fluid volume deficit related to damage to the hypothalamus and inadequate ADH production resulting in the excretion of copious amounts of urine. **Rationale:** Regulation of body water depends on the formation and release of antidiuretic hormone (ADH) from the pituitary gland.

Planning

1. Develop a plan for discussing the diagnosis of brain death with the patient's family. **Rationale:** It may be difficult for the family to comprehend the concept of

---

TABLE 38–2   PATHOPHYSIOLOGY OF BRAIN DEATH

Hypovolemic Shock

↓ Intravascular volume
↓
↓ Venous return
↓
↓ Filling pressures
↓
↓ Stroke volume
↓
↓ Cardiac output/index
↓
↓ Tissue perfusion

Neurogenic Shock

Loss of vascular sympathetic tone
↓
↑ Vasodilation
↓
↓ Venous return
↓
↓ Cardiac output/index
↓
↓ Tissue perfusion

brain death in the presence of other signs of life (chest movement, heartbeat, and body warmth).

2.   Develop a plan for the actual request process. **Rationale:** Specifically trained professionals should be involved in the process. The process requires a commit-ment of time and knowledge as well as to the required legal policies and procedures.

3.   Develop a plan for clinical care of the donor. **Rationale:** The condition of brain death requires specific nursing care to maintain hemodynamic stability until the organs and tissues are recovered.

Implementation

Steps	Rationale	Special Considerations
1. Update personal information on facts regarding the organ recovery process.	The family should make an informed decision.	
2. Review the diagnosis of brain death with the family, and assess their understanding.	The diagnosis and concept of brain death must be separate from the request for donation.	
3. Institute the policies and procedures for obtaining the signed consent for donation if the family agrees, as per your institution.	This documentation is part of the legal patient record and allows the donation process to proceed.	Families have the ability to designate which organs and/or tissues they wish to donate for transplantation or research.
4. Coordinate organ recovery activities with the OPO.	The OPO staff will provide guidance as to which organs and tissues can be utilized and will coordinate placement.	The OPO may provide an onsite coordinator to assist with clinical care of the donor.

Evaluation

1.   Monitor the donor's hemodynamic status continuously, maintaining SBP > 80 mmHg and a CVP of 5 to 12 cmH$_2$O. **Rationale:** The donor may be unstable, compromising the viability of the organs. Organ perfusion is adequate with an SBP of 80 mmHg.

2.   Monitor the donor's intake and output hourly, maintaining adequate urinary output of 1 cc/kg/h. **Rationale:** Documents renal function and possible diabetes insipidus. Adequate urinary output is a sign of organ perfusion.

3.   Administer medications as necessary to maintain adequate urinary output and hemodynamic stability. Administer dopamine (2 to 10 mcg/kg/min) to maintain SBP. Nitroglycerine may be administered to prevent coronary artery spasm. Aqueous Pitressin (50 units/500 ml IV infusion at 50 ml/h) as necessary to control diabetes insipidus (titrate infusion to maintain urinary output of 100 to 200 ml/h). For sustained low urinary output in the presence of satisfactory rehydration, administer intravenous IV infusion of furosemide 100 mg or mannitol 12.5 g. **Rationale:** Low-dosage administration of dopamine increases heart stroke volume and perfusion pressure without causing vasoconstriction of the renal arteries. Administration of an antidiuretic hormone (Pitressin) will control urinary output and prevent electrolyte imbalances and dehydration. Diuretics stimulate diuresis through excretion of water, sodium, potassium, and chloride.

4.   Monitor cardiac rhythm continually. **Rationale:** Dysrhythmias may occur, compromising viable organs.

5.   Monitor ABGs and electrolytes every 2 hours and p.r.n. Maintain SaO$_2$ > 90 percent, pH of 7.35 to 7.45, and administer KCl for K$^+$ < 4.0 mEq/L. **Rationale:** This identifies electrolyte and acid–base imbalances, which may cause electrophysiologic instability and poor tissue oxygenation.

6.   Suction p.r.n. and turn every 2 hours. **Rationale:** Immobility and decreased respiratory effort may cause atelectasis and pooled secretions, which may lead to hypoxemia and bacterial infection.

7.   Auscultate the lungs every 2 hours. Administer diuretics as ordered. **Rationale:** Pulmonary edema may occur related to sympathetic discharge.

8.   Monitor rectal temperature every hour. Apply warming or cooling blanket to maintain temperature of 97 to 100°F (36.1 to 37.8°C). **Rationale:** Hypo- or hyperthermia may occur related to hypothalamic dysfunction.

9.   Monitor for infection. Obtain urine, sputum, blood cultures. Observe IV sites. Administer antibiotics as ordered. **Rationale:** Infection can compromise the ability to transplant donated organs. Prophylactic administration of antibiotics may guard against infection.

10.   Maintain sterile technique with insertion of monitoring lines, IVs, urinary catheters, and with suctioning. **Rationale:** Decreases the potential for infection.

11.   Monitor serum glucose level every 2 hours. Administer 50% glucose or insulin as ordered. **Rationale:** Hyperglycemia may occur secondary to sepsis or stress.

12.   Communicate with the family as to progress with the organ recovery process. The OPO coordinator may

assist with this. **Rationale:** Provides comfort and support for the family.

Expected Outcomes

1. Following consent for organ/tissue donation, the donor will receive clinical care to maintain the viability of the organs for transplantation. **Rationale:** Satisfactory cardiopulmonary status and organ perfusion are imperative to ensure organ viability.

2. The recovery process will be facilitated as quickly as possible, with the assistance of the OPO. **Rationale:** Expediency is helpful to the grieving family and decreases the opportunity for clinical complications that may exclude transplantation.

3. The donor family will receive the optimal amount of information and support. **Rationale:** Assists them with the grieving process.

Unexpected Outcomes

1. The donor becomes hemodynamically unstable and the organs are no longer acceptable for transplantation. **Rationale:** Satisfactory organ perfusion is necessary to ensure organ viability.

2. The donor family, OPO staff, and ICU staff are put under increased stress because of an extended time period for organ recovery. **Rationale:** The emotional aspects and clinical care demands for a patient who is dead may be difficult for the staff involved, as well as for the family.

3. The donor family is not kept informed as to the care of their loved one. **Rationale:** Adequate communication is necessary for all families.

Documentation

1. Documentation in the patient record should include the time the patient was pronounced dead and the time donor care was initiated. **Rationale:** Facilitates the avoidance of billing the donor family for care following the declaration of death.

2. The chronologic process of obtaining consent from the family should be documented in the patient record or where recommended by hospital policy. This includes who approached the family, at what time, the location

of the consent discussion, and the response of the family. **Rationale:** Facilitates monitoring of the consent process for evaluation purposes.

3. The proper forms and signatures should be obtained relating to the permission to recover organs/tissue for transplantation and/or research. **Rationale:** Meets legal requirements.

Family Education

1. Assess the family's understanding of the diagnosis of brain death. **Rationale:** This diagnosis may be difficult to understand because the patient does not "look" dead. Additionally, it is not possible to proceed with the request for organ donation until the family accepts that their loved one is dead.

2. Provide the emotional support the family needs to cope with the death of their loved one. **Rationale:** The suddenly bereaved family has special needs that may require the time and attention of a specially trained professional. This may be the critical care nurse or other member of the health care team.

3. Provide the information needed by the family related to the donation process and the placement of the donated organs and/or tissues. **Rationale:** Assists the family in progressing with the grieving process.

4. Maintain confidentiality with regard to the donor family and the recipient(s) of the organs/tissues. **Rationale:** Maintains professional practice and anonymity of donation act.

5. Allow the family adequate time to say goodbye to their loved one prior to going to the operating room for recovery of the organs. **Rationale:** Helps the family progress with grieving.

6. Give the family permission to leave the hospital when the donor goes to the operating room. **Rationale:** The family may be unsure of the procedure and whether it is all right to leave.

7. Provide information to the family regarding the recovery process and placement of organs. This can be done by phone following the surgery. **Rationale:** The family should have complete information regarding the care of their loved one.

Performance Checklist
Skill 38–2: Facilitating Organ Donation

Critical Behaviors	Complies	
	yes	no
1. Know the factual information regarding the donation process.		
2. Assess each potential donor family's understanding of brain death.		
3. Offer the option of organ donation to appropriate families or contact the appropriate colleague to do so.		
4. Know the institutional policies and procedures for documenting the consent process and the consent for donation.		

Table continues on following page

		Complies	
Critical Behaviors		**yes**	**no**
5. Perform and document clinical care for the organ donor.			
6. Collaborate with the OPO appropriately.			

SKILL 38–3

Organ Preparation for Retrieval

In previous years, before the era of multiple organ donation or transplantation, the majority of cadaveric kidneys were surgically removed by nonphysicians, usually procurement coordinators. Today, the complexity of the recovery procedures requires the entire professional surgical team, headed by the transplant surgeons. Two or three organ recovery teams may be involved with a single donor. In most cases, at least one of these teams will travel from their distant transplant hospital to participate in the recovery procedure. Thus the OPO and their staff must coordinate the timing and logistics of the process carefully and communicate clearly with the ICU staff that is caring for the donor.

Prior to admission of the donor to the operating room, the patient record must document the date and time of the declaration of death and contain a permit for the recovery of organs that is in compliance with the hospital's policy and procedure or, where defined, in compliance with state law. Many hospitals will require a signed death certificate also.

The protocol for management of the donor is similar for any patient in the operating room. The responsibilities of the anesthesiologist include safe transport of the donor to the operating room, monitoring and managing the donor's airway and gas exchange, and maintaining ventilation, circulation, and fluid and electrolyte balance, as well as providing whatever anesthesia, such as neuromuscular relaxants, the donor may require. Brain dead patients often require a variety of pharmacologic interventions to maintain hemodynamic stability and adequate organ perfusion. Occasionally, it may be necessary to treat reflex hemodynamic and muscle responses to surgical stimulation (Simmons et al., 1984).

Most recovery programs prefer to work with the donor hospital operating room staff and do not include nursing personnel on their team. The recovery teams will provide any specialized instruments, solutions, and apparatuses necessary. The hospital's responsibilities include normal instrumentation, supplies, and support. Operating times for the recovery procedure vary depending on donor anatomy, organs recovered, and the skill and experience of the recovery teams. The typical multiorgan recovery should require no more than 4 hours of operating time and will likely average 2 to 2 ½ hours.

The heart and liver are the organs most sensitive to in situ ischemia, and additionally, the life of the recipient depends on their immediate normal function. For these reasons, the heart and liver must be mobilized first, and the heart should be removed as soon as a cold perfusion system can be set up to cool the liver and kidneys in situ.

The concurrent donation of a liver and the whole pancreas cannot be done, but that of a segmental pancreas and liver is possible. Regardless of the organs to be removed, an incision extending from the suprasternal notch to the pubis provides the widest possible exposure for organs within the peritoneal cavity as well as the chest (Simmons et al., 1984).

When the heart, liver, distal pancreas, and kidneys are all to be transplanted, the order of removal is as follows: The great vessels in the chest are mobilized and a cardioplegia catheter is threaded through the innominate artery into the ascending aorta. The liver and pancreas are then mobilized, and the distal pancreas and spleen are removed; the pancreas is flushed ex vivo prior to preservation. Mobilization of the liver is then completed, and cannulas are placed in the splenic vein (or superior mesenteric vein), distal aorta, and distal vena cava. The kidneys are mobilized along with retroperitoneal fat and adrenal glands (Simmons et al., 1984).

The goal of organ preservation is to maintain the viability of an organ ex vivo for an amount of time that will accomplish the following objectives:

1. Allow transportation of the cadaveric organ to the transplant center.
2. Provide time for donor–recipient tissue matching, if necessary.
3. Yield good initial function following transplantation.

There are three methods used to preserve organs and tissues, and preservation research continues to hold widespread interest. The primary methods include continuous hypothermic perfusion, simple cold storage after vascular flushout, and cryopreservation below 0°C (Flye, 1989).

The potential benefit of lowering the temperature of an excised organ was grasped instinctively by early workers in the field of transplantation. Intestinal and cardiac grafts were preserved almost 30 years ago by simple immersion in ice-cold saline at the University of Minnesota. In the late 1960s, the first widely applicable technique for long-term (24-hour) renal preservation was utilized. This technique involved recirculating a cold (7°C), oxygenated plasma perfusate in a special circuit containing the kidney(s) (Belzer et al., 1967). During the 1970s, the static preservation methodology became available and gained wide acceptance. This technique involved an initial washout of the organ with a high-potassium, hyperosmolar solution at 4°C followed by subsequent storage of the organ by immersion in this same solution (Collins solution) at the same temperature (Matas et al., 1982). This technique provided for only 8 to 12 hours of preservation. Modification of this solution (Euro-Collins' solution) has improved preservation capability to approximately 72 hours and is used for both kidneys and livers. However, livers have been successfully perfused for 12 hours, but optimal cold ischemic time is up to 8 hours. Belzer and associates have recently devised a new solution that may preserve livers for up to 24 hours (Wisconsin solution).

Preservation of the excised heart utilizes a similar system. Most cardiac teams prefer to recover the heart after pharmacologically induced arrest is accomplished utilizing a highly concentrated potassium solution called cardioplegia. Effective preservation is now considered 4 to 6 hours utilizing this method.

Methods for the preservation for heart/lung blocs, lungs, and pancreati are variable. Common to all presently utilized methods for preservation is hypothermia to reduce metabolic activity and oxygen requirements.

Purpose

The nurse participates in the preparation of organs for transplantation to

1. Continue oxygenation and perfusion of the organ(s).
2. Anticipate and administer medications that may be necessary in organ preparation for subsequent donation.

Prerequisite Knowledge and Skills

Prior to the removal and transport of donated organs, the nurse should understand

1. Brain death criteria.
2. The necessity to continue ventilatory and hemodynamic support until the actual moment of organ removal.
3. Pharmacotherapy that may have a subsequent beneficial effect on the transplanted organs.
4. The necessity to perform cardiopulmonary resuscitation and prepare for emergency surgery if the donor suffers cardiac arrest while waiting for the retrieval operation.

Assessment

1. Assess the donor's organ oxygenation and perfu-

sion until surgical removal of the organs occurs. **Rationale:** Ensures organ viability.
2. Determine that all proper documentation is in place in the donor's chart prior to going to the operating room. **Rationale:** Meets legal requirements.

Nursing Diagnoses

1. Decreased tissue perfusion related to brain death. **Rationale:** The destruction of the sympathetic nervous system occurs in brain death.
2. Decreased cardiac output related to the loss of vascular sympathetic tone, vasodilation, and decrease in venous return. **Rationale:** The destruction of the sympathetic nervous system occurs in brain death.
3. Ineffective breathing pattern related to loss of the regulatory center's regulatory mechanism. **Rationale:** There is a loss of regulatory mechanisms in the brain with brain death.
4. Potential altered body temperature related to destruction of the hypothalamic thermostat. **Rationale:** There is a loss of regulatory mechanisms in the brain with brain death.

Planning

1. Communicate with the OPO coordinator to determine the timing and logistics of the retrieval surgery. **Rationale:** The OPO coordinator has the responsibility of organ placement and the coordination of the arriving surgical recovery teams.
2. Communicate with the operating room staff and anesthesiologist regarding transfer of the donor to the operating room. **Rationale:** All involved staff must coordinate the care of the donor to maximize stability.
3. Prepare medications for anticipated use (particularly with kidney donors): methylprednisolone (Solu-Medrol) 1 g, heparin 10,000 units, phenoxybenzamine hydrochloride (Dibenzylene) 100 mg. **Rationale:** Pretreatment of donors with select medications may have a subsequent beneficial effect on the transplanted organs.
4. Be prepared to institute cardiopulmonary resuscitation if necessary. **Rationale:** Every effort must be made to prevent tissue/organ ischemia.

Implementation

Steps	Rationale	Special Considerations
1. Ascertain that the donor has been pronounced dead according to neurologic criteria.	Prerequisite to admission to the operating room.	
2. Coordinate donor transfer to operating room with OPO coordinator, OR staff, and anesthesia.	Cooperation is necessary to progress efficiently.	Additional time may be necessary to allow for travel time of recovery teams.

Table continues on following page

Steps	Rationale	Special Considerations
3. Monitor the donor's hemodynamic status continuously.	The donor may be unstable, compromising the viability of the organs.	
4. Monitor the donor's respiratory status continuously.	Validates organ oxygenation.	
5. Maintain the donor's body temperature throughout transfer to maintain homeostatic environment for the organs.	Hypo- or hyperthermia may occur related to hypothalamic dysfunction.	
6. Communicate with the donor's family as to progress with the recovery process.	Provides comfort and support for the family.	The OPO coordinator may assist with this. The family may be at home during this time.

Evaluation

Expected Outcomes

1. The donor remains hemodynamically stable. **Rationale:** Maintains organ viability.
2. Coordination of the transfer of the donor to the operating room, arrival of the recovery team(s), retrieval of the organs, and completion of the process take place in an efficient, timely manner. **Rationale:** Provides for optimal system for organ retrieval.
3. The organs remain oxygenated, perfused, and preserved. **Rationale:** Maximizes organ function following transplant.
4. The donor family will receive the optimal amount of information and support. **Rationale:** Assists with the grieving process.

Unexpected Outcomes

1. The donor becomes hemodynamically unstable or suffers a cardiac arrest. **Rationale:** Compromises or ends the possibility of retrieval of organs for transplantation.
2. The period of time from the consent for organ donation and recovery of the organs is prolonged. **Rationale:** The viability of the organs is compromised and the family undergoes undue stress.
3. The donor family is not kept informed as to the care of their loved one. **Rationale:** Communication assists in the grieving process.

Documentation

1. Documentation in the patient record should include a completed preoperative checklist for all patients going to the operating room. **Rationale:** Ensures that standard procedures are being followed.
2. The proper consent forms must be in the patient record. This usually includes a signed death certificate. **Rationale:** Meets legal requirements for organ procurement.
3. The continuous monitoring and treatment of the clinical status of the donor should be documented. **Rationale:** This reflects the nursing care given.

Family Education

1. Assess the family's understanding of the retrieval process and timing. **Rationale:** The family will have a need to continue their knowledge of what is happening to their loved one.
2. Reinforce to the family that surgical removal of the organs takes place with respect and careful technique similar to any operation. **Rationale:** Provides comfort to the family as they envision the process.
3. Give the family permission to wait at home or outside the hospital for the information that the retrieval surgery is complete. **Rationale:** The family should have had the opportunity to say "goodbye" to their loved one prior to transferring him or her to the operating room. This also confirms that the donor is indeed dead and that funeral plans can proceed.

Performance Checklist
Skill 38–3: Organ Preparation for Retrieval

Critical Behaviors	Complies yes	no
1. Recognize the timing and logistics requirements for retrieval.		

Table continues on following page

Critical Behaviors	Complies	
	yes	no
2. Ensure that all appropriate documentation related to the declaration of brain death and preparation for the surgical procedure is in the patient record.		
3. Collaborate with OPO staff and visiting procurement teams appropriately.		
4. Facilitate or implement timely, therapeutic communication with family regarding the procurement process.		

REFERENCES

Bartucci, M. R. (1987). Organ donation: A study of the donor family perspective. *J. Neurosci. Nurs.* 19:305–309.

Belzer, F. O., Ashby, B. S., Dunphy, J. E. (1967). 24-hour and 72-hour preservation of canine kidneys. *Lancet* 2:536.

Black, P. Mc., and Todres, D. I. (1989). Brain Death in Children, Guidelines and Experience at the Massachusetts General Hospital. In H. Kaufman (Ed.), *Pediatric Brain Death and Organ/Tissue Retrieval.* New York: Plenum.

Chernow, B., and Anderson, D. M. (1985). Endocrine responses to critical illness. *Semin. Respir. Med.* 7(1):1–10.

Crane, M. (1983). Ready or not, you're on the transplant team. *Med. Econ. Surg.* 12:46.

Ettner, B. J., et al. (1988). Professional attitudes toward organ donation and transplantation. *Dialysis Transplant.* 17(2):72–76.

Flye, M. W. (1989). *Principles of Organ Transplantation.* Philadelphia: Saunders.

Goldsmith, J. (1985). Nursing care of the potential organ donor. *Crit. Care Nurs.* 5(6):22–29.

Heitman, L. K. (1987). Organ donation in community hospitals: A nursing perspective. *Curr. Concepts Nurs.* 1(3):2–5.

Matas, A. J., Sutherland, D. E., Payne, W. D., Van Hook, E. J., Simmons, R. L., Najarian, J. S. (1982). Retrieval of kidneys for transplantation from cadaver donors in Minnesota. *Minn. Med.* 65:163.

Simmons, R. L., Fulton, J., and Fulton, R. (1984). *Manual of Vascular Access: Organ Donation and Transplantation* (pp. 105–114). New York: Springer-Verlag.

BIBLIOGRAPHY

Plum, F., and Posner, J. B. (1972). *Diagnosis of Stupor and Coma,* 2d Ed. Philadelphia: F.A. Davis.

Posner, J. B. (1978). Coma and other states of consciousness: The differential diagnosis of brain death. *Ann. N.Y. Acad. Sci.* 315:215–223.

Sammons, B., and Pietroski, R. (1989). *Organ Donor Management: Pathophysiologic Principles.* East Hanover, N.J.: Sandoz Pharmaceuticals.

GLOSSARY

a-$_{AD}$CO$_2$—The arterial to alveolar difference for CO$_2$ (normally 2–5 mmHg; derived from subtracting PaCO$_2$ – PetCO$_2$).

Abdominal Girth—Measurement of the circumference of the body at the level of the abdomen, at or just below the umbilicus, to assess for the accumulation or reduction of fluid or air within the abdomen.

Action Potential—Rapid changes in the membrane potential which suddenly changes from the normal resting negative potential to a positive membrane potential and back again.

Afterload—Pressure in the aortic root against which the left ventricle must contract.

Air Breaks—In hyperbaric oxygen therapy, a period of time given off 100% oxygen. The two reasons for air breaks: (1) for patient comfort and (2) to decrease possibility of oxygen toxicity.

Air Fluidized Therapy—A dynamic pressure relieving treatment; a high air loss, bead, or sand bed.

Airway Adjunct—Special devices that help control the airway.

Airway Resistance (Raw)—Resistance to air flow; the pressure necessary to move a volume of gas per unit of time; ratio of the driving pressure to the flow; expressed in cmH$_2$O per liter per second; normal is 0.5–1.5 cmH$_2$O/L/s.

Albumin—Pooled from human plasma; used as an intravascular volume expander by increasing osmotic pressure.

Alignment—Arrangement in a straight line, as bones after a fracture.

Allen's Test—Test to assess occlusion of ulnar or radial arteries.

Alligator Clip—An insulated conducting wire which has clamps or connections at both ends, used to connect pacing lead to an ECG lead.

Alveolar-Arterial Oxygen Gradient Difference (A-aDO$_2$)—Difference in partial pressure between alveolar oxygen (PAO$_2$) and arterial oxygen (PaO$_2$); expressed in mmHg; normal is 50 mmHg.

Alveolar Plateau—The portion of the CO$_2$ waveform representing exhalation of alveolar gas.

Alveolar Ventilation—Ventilation of the alveolar sacs.

Amino Acids—Basic components of protein molecules.

Anaerobic Culture—Culture technique used to identify microorganisms that grow in the absence of oxygen.

Anthropometric Measurement—Comparative measurements of the human body.

Antiseptic—A product with antimicrobial activity that is designed for use on skin or other superficial tissues; removes resident as well as transient organisms.

Antitachycardiac Pacing—A method of interrupting a tachycardia by delivering critically timed paced stimuli.

Arcing—The disbursement of electrical current outside the intended directional flow through a critical mass of the myocardium.

Arterial Blood Gas (ABG)—The sampling of arterial blood to determine the oxygenation and the acid-base status of the patient.

Arterial Oxygen Tension to Fraction of Inspired Oxygen Ratio—(Respiratory index, PaO$_2$/FIO$_2$) expressed in mmHg; normal is 350 to 450 mmHg.

Arterial-Venous Oxygen Difference (a-$\bar{v}$DO$_2$)—Difference between arterial and mixed venous oxygen contents; expressed in ml of oxygen in 100 ml of blood (volume %); normal is 5 ml oxygen/100 ml blood or 5 vol %.

Arthrodesis—The fixation or stiffening of a joint by surgical means.

Artificial Airway—Any device that is inserted into patient to maintain the patency of air passages.

Ascites—Accumulation of fluid within the intraperitoneal space; transudate fluid which can occur secondary to cirrhosis or peritonitis.

Aseptic Technique—Practices designed to render and maintain objects and areas free from microorganisms; also referred to as "sterile technique."

Aspiration—Inhalation of foreign matter into lungs.

Assist-Control (A-C)—Ventilator mode that delivers preset tidal volume in response to patient's inspiratory effort; provides breaths automatically when patient fails to initiate inspiration.

Assisted Aortic End Diastolic Pressure—The lowest diastolic pressure produced after each augmented pressure. This pressure should be less than the patient's inherent diastolic pressure, thus demonstrating afterload reduction.

Assisted Systole—The patient's systolic pressure produced after IABP inflation and deflation. The assisted systolic pressure should be less than the unassisted systolic pressure due to afterload reduction.

Atelectasis—Collapse of lung tissue.

Atmospheres Absolute—Pressure at sea level of the atmosphere usually expressed as 14.7 PSI.

Atmospheric Pressure—The pressure exerted by the atmosphere at sea level, equivalent to that of a column of mercury 760 mmHg.

Augmentation—Increase in arterial diastolic pressure resulting from the displacement of the aortic blood volume as the balloon inflates.

Autologous—Related to the self.

Auto-Peep—Elevation of alveolar pressure from stacking of breaths, caused by inadequate time for complete expiration prior to the next inspiration.

Autonomic Dysreflexia—An abnormal sympathetic response in patients with spinal cord lesions at the sixth thoracic level and above; usually precipitated by distended bowel or bladder and results in an acute hypertensive crisis; resolved by removal of offending stimulus.

Autonomic Nervous System—That part of the nervous system that regulates and reacts without conscious control.

Autoregulation—The mechanism by which the brain maintains consistent pressure within specific limits. This is regulated by redistributing blood or CSF as needed.

Autotransfusion—The reinfusion of the patient's own blood which has been collected from a site.

AV Interval—The time between an intrinsic or paced atrial event and the subsequent ventricular paced event, comparable to the P-R interval of the normal heart rhythm.

AV Sequential—Pacing in which stimulation of the atria and ventricle occur in a synchronous fashion.

Barotrauma—Injury caused by increased barometric pressure manifested as pneumothorax, pneumomediastinum, pneumopericardium, and/or subcutaneous emphysema.

Barrier Precautions—Infection prevention practices used for all patients to reduce the risk of transmission of infectious agents among patients and to and from health care workers.

Baseline—The initial assessment parameter obtained.

Bedside Monitor—Monitor located at the patient's bedside.

Bevel—Slanting edge of the tip of a catheter.

Bipolar—A pacemaker circuit in which both the positive and negative poles of the circuit are in contact with the myocardium. May also refer to a lead which contains two points of conduction along a single lead.

Bivalve—To cut a cast into an anterior and posterior shell to relieve constriction, perform skin care or exercises.

Blister—A vesicle containing serum or blood.

Blood Pump—Used to rapidly infuse large amounts of blood/blood products during massive hemorrhaging; blood is placed into the device which can be pressurized to deliver a rapid flow rate.

Body Cast—A rigid structure that encloses the trunk from the neck to the groin.

Bolus—An amount of fluid/medication administered as an addition to the maintenance requirements; a dose of medication to either establish or increase serum level.

Bolus Feeding—Administration of enteral formula via syringe, using either gravity or syringe plunger, to instill formula into stomach via feeding tube over 5 to 15 minutes.

Bradycardia—Heart rate below 60 beats/minute.

Brain Death—The irreversible cessation of total brain function.

Bronchial Brushing—A diagnostic technique utilized in conjunction with fiberoptic bronchoscopy in which a brush tipped catheter is inserted through the channel of the fiberscope to the lower respiratory tract and swept over the mucosa to collect specimens.

Bronchoalveolar Lavage—A diagnostic and/or therapeutic technique utilized in conjunction with fiberoptic bronchoscopy in which a saline solution is instilled through the channel of the fiberscope to facilitate removal of secretions which are aspirated into a sterile container.

Bronchus—Large anatomical passegeway into the lower airways of the lungs, the right and left bronchi have their point of origin off the trachea.

Bruit—A humming or buzzing sound heard through a stethoscope when placed over a narrowed or bulging wall of an artery.

Buck's Traction—An apparatus for obtaining extension of and traction to a fractured hip or femur; consists of a system of weights, ropes, pulleys, and adhesive straps.

Buretrol—An intravenous tubing administration set with a pre-measured fluid chamber.

Burr Hole—Surgically drilled opening through the cranium to gain access to intracranial contents.

CaO$_2$—The volume of oxygen transported in arterial blood (both bound to hemoglobin and dissolved in plasma).

Calibrating—The process of adjusting the internal electronics of the monitoring system to insure accuracy of readings.

Callus—The osseous material formed between the ends of a fractured bone.

Cancellous Bone—Refers particularly to bony tissue that underlies or lies between layers of compact bone in epiphyses, sternum, ribs, vertebrae, and diploe of the skull; the interstices are filled with red bone marrow.

Cannulation—The accessing of the vascular system for the initiation of hemodialysis.

Capillary Closing Pressure—The pressure at which capillaries close; approximately 25 to 32 mmHg.

Capnography—The measurement and graphical display of carbon dioxide (CO_2) concentration in the airway over the course of each breath. Capnograph refers to the instrument while capnogram refers to the waveform.

Capture—The successful depolarization of the myocardium represented on the ECG by a pacemaker artifact followed by a P wave in atrial pacing or a wide QRS in ventricular pacing.

Carbon Dioxide Narcosis—Stuperous state induced by high levels of carbon dioxide.

Carbon Dioxide Toxicity—State of cellular toxicity due to elevated carbon dioxide levels.

Cardiac Dysrhythmia—Irregular heart action caused by disturbances in discharge transmission of cardiac impulses.

Cardiac Cycle—The combined periods of contraction and recovery dependent on the depolarization and repolarization of the myocardial cell membrane.

Cardiac Index—Expresses the cardiac output relative to body size; expressed in liters/minute/square meter of body surface area. Normal value is 2.5 to 4 L/min/M^2.

Cardiac Output—Amount of blood ejected by the ventricles each minute; expressed in liters/minute. Normal value is 4 to 8 L/min.

Cardiac Profile—Measurement and calculation of cardiac output, cardiac index, and systemic vascular resistance.

Cardiac Tamponade—Condition resulting from accumulation of excess fluid in the pericardium which compresses the heart and impairs normal heart function.

Carina—Site where trachea divides into right and left mainstem bronchi.

Cast—The rigid encasement of a part with plaster or plastic for the purpose of immobilization.

Cast Cutter—Saw used to bivalve a cast prior to removal.

Cast Syndrome—A cluster of patient signs and symptoms as a result of compression of the superior mesenteric artery in a body with a spica cast.

Catheter Colonization—Refers to organisms living within a host without producing either a local or systemic response. The subcutaneous skin tract of a venous catheter is considered colonized if there are fewer than 15 colonies present by semiquantitative catheter culture and there are no signs of local infection or systemic bacteremia.

Catheter Infection—Microbial growth from the catheter tip or from a blood culture drawn from the catheter with no growth of the same organisms in the peripheral blood culture.

Catheter-Related Septicemia—Diagnosis based on the isolation of the same organism from a catheter segment quantitative or semiquantitative culture and from a peripheral blood culture.

Cellular Metabolism—All energy and material transformations that occur within living cells.

Celsius—Temperature scale on which the freezing point of water is 0° and the boiling point is 100°.

Central Station—Monitoring station in a central location which receives input from multiple monitors.

Central Venous Catheter—A catheter introduced through a large peripheral vein, jugular or subclavian vein ending in the superior vena cava for the purpose of administering parenteral solutions, and obtaining blood samples.

Central Venous Pressure—The pressure measured from the tip of a catheter placed within the right atrium (RA) or superior vena cava which provides information about the volume status and right ventricular function.

Cerebral Edema—Net increase in intracellular or extracellular water content of brain.

Cerebral Metabolic Rate—The rate at which the brain utilizes glucose and oxygen.

Cerebral Perfusion—The ability of the cerebral circulation to deliver blood to cerebral structures.

Cerebral Perfusion Pressure—CPP = MAP − ICP, the force with which the brain is perfused. Considers mean arterial pressure (MAP), the pressure supplied by systemic circulatory structures, and the ICP, the resistance exerted by intracranial structures and contents.

Chemical Paralysis—Paralysis induced chemically, as with neuromuscular blocking agents (e.g., tubocurarine, pancuronium, etc.).

Chemical Pleurodesis—The instillation of therapeutic agents into the pleural space.

Chest Drainage System—A collection system that uses a water seal, gravity, and/or suction to restore negative pressure to the intrapleural space, and removes intrapleural accumulations of air, fluid, and/or blood so that a collapsed lung can reexpand.

Chest Tube—A thoracostomy tube or thoracic catheter inserted into the pleural space for the purpose of collecting drainage or allowing the escape of air.

Cholothorax—The collection in the intrapleural space of fluid which contains bile.

Chronic Obstructive Pulmonary Disease (COPD)—Disease process that causes decreased ability of the lungs to perform their function. Diseases that cause this are chronic bronchitis, pulmonary emphysema, and chronic asthma.

Chyle—The product of intestinal digestion which is absorbed into the lymphatic system, conveyed through the thoracic duct and emptied into the venous system at the base of the neck.

Chylothorax—The collection of chyle in the pleural space.

Circuit—A closed electrical pathway; current flows from the power source to the device and back to the power source or ground.

Circulatory Assist Device—Mechanical devices used to improve the function of a failing heart; includes the intraaortic balloon pump, left-, right-, and biventricular assist devices, and the total artificial heart.

Claustrophobia—Fear of being confined in a closed or confined space.

Clean/Contaminated Wound—Operative wound entering the respiratory, genitourinary, or alimentary tracts, performed under controlled conditions without break in aseptic technique or with any contamination.

Clean Wound—Operative wound made under aseptic conditions.

CO₂ Sensor/Optical Bench—The component of the capnograph which analyzes the respiratory gas for CO_2; placement varies according to measurement style (in-line vs. remote).

Colonization—The presence of microorganisms in or on a host with growth and multiplication but without tissue invasion or damage.

Coma—Clinical description of a state in which the person has severely impaired level of consciousness, is unresponsive or demonstrates abnormal responses to noxious stimuli.

Comminuted—Broken into pieces.

Compartment—The areas between muscle groups in the leg or forearm thighs.

Compartment Syndrome—A condition in which increased pressure within a compartment interferes with the circulation of blood to the contents of that space, often following musculoskeletal or vascular trauma and/or surgery.

Compression—Increasing the barometric pressure inside a pressure chamber by adding compressed air or oxygen.

Computerized Axial Tomography (CAT)—A painless diagnostic procedure for examining soft tissues; consists of x-ray pictures integrated through a computer.

Condyle—Bony outgrowths at ends of long bones which articulate with adjacent bones and provide anchorage for ligaments.

Congestive Heart Failure—Inability of the heart to meet metabolic demands due to decreased myocardial contractility with resulting fluid retention.

Conjugate—Referring to eye movements; ocular gaze is coordinated, symmetric, and directional.

Connecting Cable—An insulated extension wire which may be used to provide additional length between the pulse generator and the pacing lead.

Contaminated Wound—Operative or accidental wound with major breaks in aseptic technique or with gross contamination from spillage; bacteria is present but host defenses are not overwhelmed.

Content of Oxygen in the Arterial Blood (CaO₂)—Amount of oxygen actually carried in the arterial blood; includes oxygen attached to hemoglobin and dissolved oxygen; expressed as ml of oxygen in 100 ml of blood (volume %); normal is 20 ml/100 ml or 20 vol %.

Continuous Feeding—Administration of enteral formula via feeding tube into stomach, duodenum, or jejunum at a constant rate of infusion over 24 hours, via a pump.

Continuous Positive Airway Pressure (CPAP)—The application of positive pressure throughout inspiration and expiration during spontaneous breathing; expressed in cmH_2O.

Contraction—A reduction in size, especially applied to muscle fibers, a shortening or increase in tension.

Contracture—A permanent muscular contraction due to tonic spasm or fibrosis, or to loss of muscular equilibrium.

Controlled Mandatory Ventilation (CMV)—Ventilator mode that delivers preset tidal volume at a preset rate independent of patient's inspiratory effort.

Counterpulsation—Principle on which IABP therapy is based. The balloon deflates just prior to ventricular systole and inflates during diastole; this produces a "pulse" or movement of blood opposite to the cardiac cycle.

Countertraction—Force exerted in a direction opposite to the pull of traction.

Cranium—Bony enclosure surrounding the brain and brainstem structures.

Critical Closing Pressure—Arteriole pressure gradient at which microcirculation ceases.

Cryoprecipitate Antihemophilic Factor (AHF)—Primarily factor VIII with factor XIII removed from whole blood and 250 mg of fiberinogen; used primarily with classic hemophilia patients.

Crystalloid Fluid—Fluid which can diffuse through bodily membranes.

Cycler—An automated device used in intermittent peritoneal dialysis which times and controls the inflow and outflow of the dialysate.

Dampening—The steady diminution of the amplitude of vibration of a specific form of energy (mechanical, electrical, or sound).

Dead Space (Vd/Vt)—The ratio of dead space (wasted ventilation, or ventilation that does not participate in gas exchange) ventilation to tidal ventilation; expressed in ml, fraction, or percentage; normal is 150 ml, 0.30, or 30%.

Dead Space (Wasted) Ventilation—A physiologic condition in which ventilation exceeds perfusion within the lung; results in abnormally wide A-aDCO₂; extremely high V/Q relationship.

    A. Anatomic Dead Space—Volume of air in pulmonary conducting system that does not undergo molecular gas exchange with pulmonary blood (normal is approx. 150 ml).

    B. Alveolar Dead Space—Volume of air in alveoli that does not undergo molecular gas exchange with pulmonary blood.

Debride—Remove nonviable tissue.

Debridement—The surgical or enzymatic removal of necrotic tissue and debris from a wound.

Decompression—The opposite of compression, release of air or oxygen to a lower pressure.

Decubitus—A misnomer for a pressure sore, gradually being replaced by dermal ulcer, pressure sore, or pressure ulcer.

Defibrillation (External)—Electrical current passed across the chest wall to cause simultaneous depolarization of muscle fibers, the current is randomly delivered.

Defibrillation (Internal)—Electrical current delivered directly to the heart via open thoracotomy to cause simultaneous depolarization of muscle fibers, the current is randomly delivered.

Defibrillator (Automatic Implantable Device)—Device surgically implanted onto the myocardium which will respond to abnormal heart rhythms by delivering low level electrical energy directly to the myocardium to convert the dysrhythmia.

Delay—An inactivation time period when no analgesic will be infused.

Demand, Synchronous—Pacing in which the intrinsic electrical activity of the myocardium is sensed by the pacemaker and pacing only occurs when intrinsic rate falls below pacemaker set rate.

Denuded—Loss of epidermal layer of skin (usually peristomal area).

Deoxyhemoglobin—Hemoglobin not bound with oxygen (reduced hemoglobin).

Depolarization—An alteration in the cell membrane permeability allowing for rapid influx of ions into the cell so that the inside of the cell becomes positively charged with respect to the outside of the cell.

Dermal Wound—Loss of skin integrity, may be superficial or deep.

Dermis—The second layer of skin, immediately below the epidermis.

Dextrose—Carbohydrates provided in simplest form parenterally to be converted to energy as calories.

Dialysate—An electrolyte solution used for dialysis in which the composition can be altered based upon the patient's lab values.

Dialyzer—A semipermeable membrane through which solutes and water move from the blood to the dialysate or from the dialysate to the blood in accordance with the principles of diffusion, osmosis, and ultrafiltration.

Dicrotic Notch—Landmark of the arterial waveform that signifies closure of the aortic valve.

Diencephalon—Area that contains center structures of the brain, such as the thalamus and hypothalamus.

Diffusion—Movement of solutes from an area of greater concentration to an area of lesser concentration.

Diffusion Phase—The length of time that the dialysate remains in the peritoneal cavity during which osmosis and diffusion occur; same as dwell time.

2,3 Diphosphate Glycerate (2–3 DPG)—An organic phosphate that acts to decrease the affinity of hemoglobin for oxygen, thus increasing oxygen delivery to the tissues.

Disinfection—A process that eliminates many or all pathogenic organisms on inaminate objects, with the exception of bacterial spores.

Diuretics—Drugs used to decrease tubular reabsorption, thereby reducing total body sodium and water.

Doll's Eyes—Also called the oculocephalic response. This is a maneuver performed on the unconscious patient to evaluate reflex extraocular movement and brainstem function. The patient's head is turned briskly side to side, and the eyes are observed closely for movement. Doll's eyes are "present" if the eyes seem to "float" conjugately as the head is turned, which indicates functioning brainstem connections. Abnormal or absent response can be observed by dysconjugate or no eye movement during this procedure.

Donor Site—Area from which skin was removed to graft to another area.

Dry Weight—Patient's weight immediately following dialysis.

Duodenum—Section of small intestine distal to stomach.

Dura Mater—Outermost portion of the meninges; composed of inelastic fibrous tissue. Folds of dura form sinuses which assists in forming the venous drainage system of the brain.

Dwell Time—The amount of time the dialysate remains within the peritoneum, during which osmosis and diffusion occur; same as diffusion phase.

Dynamic Compliance (CMPdyn)—Representation of forces resisting expansion of the lung during flow; volume (tidal) divided by pressure (PIP); expressed in liters per cmH20; normal is 50 to 100 ml/cmH$_2$O.

Dynamic Device—Devices with moving parts which require energy or physical force in motion.

Dysconjugate—Referring to eye movements. The patient's gaze is not coordinated and symmetric. Each eye may seem to have a separate independent direction.

Dysfunctional Hemoglobin—Hemoglobin types that are unable to bind with O$_2$, i.e., carboxyhemoglobin, methemoglobin, sulfhemoglobin.

Edlich Tube—A single lumen nasogastric or oral tube of large diameter with an attached graduated syringe. The tube is passed into the stomach and used to evacuate large amounts of solid or liquid contents.

Effluent—The fluid drained from the peritoneal cavity in peritoneal dialysis.

Electrocardiogram (ECG or EKG)—The recording of the electrical activity of the myocardial cells.

Electrode—A lead wire transmitting an electrical impulse.

Electrode Gel—A water soluble colloidial substance used to increase conduction of electrical impulses.

Electrolyte—An element essential to bodily function which produces an electric current and is decomposed by the passage of an electric current. Examples are potassium and calcium.

Electromagnetic Interference (EMI)—Noncardiac electrical or electromagnetic signals that temporarily inhibit pacemaker function.

Embolism—Obstruction of a blood vessel by a foreign substance or blood clot. (Often referred to as thrombosis.)

Empyema—The presence of pus in a body cavity.

Encephalitis—Inflammation of the brain; is usually manifested by brain swelling and tissue dysfunction. Some causes of encephalitis are anoxia, toxic poisoning, uremia, and liver (metabolic) dysfunction.

Endoscope—A device used for visualization of the interior of a body cavity.

Endoscope Sclerotherapy—A nonoperative technique utilizing a sclerosing solution to cause obliteration of esophageal and gastric varices.

Endotracheal Tube—A tube inserted through the mouth or nose and terminating in the trachea.

Entrain—To draw room air into a mask and mix with oxygen.

Enzyme—Complex protein capable of causing chemical changes in another substance without changing itself. Essential for proper bodily functioning.

Enzyme Preparations—Proteolytic substances which break down and liquefy nonviable tissue.

Epicardial Pacemaker—Pacing leads attached to the outside of the heart during open heart surgical procedures.

Epidermis—The outermost layer of skin.

Epidural Catheter—Pressure sensing device placed between the dura and the cranium; is associated with less risk of infection because it does not penetrate the dura.

Epidural Space—The space between the cranium and the dura.

Epithelialization—Regeneration of the epidermal layer of skin across a wound surface.

Eschar—The necrotic tissue covering a burn wound.

Escharotomy—Longitudinal incisions, surgically created through eschar to relieve underlying pressure thereby restoring circulation.

Esophageal Obturator Airway (EOA)—An artificial airway used to provide an emergency method of ventilation and to prevent aspiration of stomach contents in an unconscious individual.

Ewald Tube—A single lumen tube of large diameter passed through the mouth into the stomach to evacuate large amounts of liquid or solid contents. This tube has a funnel device at the proximal end for installation of large amounts of fluid and a squeeze bulb at mid-tube.

Exchange—A cycle of peritoneal dialysis involving three phases: inflow, dwell, and drain.

External Right Atrial Silastic Catheter—A long-term indwelling catheter which is tunneled into a large blood vessel with the catheter tip location in superior vena cava or the right atrium of the heart; exits on the anterior chest; a dacron cuff anchors the catheter within the tunnel; may have one, two, or three lumens—the multilumen catheter allows incompatible solutions to be given simultaneously; provides venous access for continuous or intermittent systemic therapy for patients requiring prolonged drug and fluid administration.

Extracorporeal—Outside the body.

Extraocular Movements (EOMs)—Observed by asking the patient to move eyes upward, downward, laterally, and obliquely. This tests the function of cranial nerves III, IV, and VI.

Extravasation—Leakage of intravenous fluids into the subcutaneous tissues surrounding the implanted venous access port or tunneled right atrial silastic catheter.

Extubation—The act of removing a tube that has been placed into the trachea.

Fahrenheit—Temperature scale on which the freezing point of water is 32° and the boiling point is 212°.

Fat Embolism—Fat globules obstructing blood vessels.

Femur—The thigh bone; the longest and strongest bone in the body extending from the hip to the knee.

Fever—Elevation of temperature above a patient's normal body temperature.

Fiberglass—An open-weave tape saturated with polyurethane resin which when mixed with water forms a lightweight rigid cast.

Fiberoptic Bronchoscopy (FOB)—A procedure in which a flexible fiberscope containing high precision lenses is inserted via the oral or nasal cavity to the subsegmental level of the tracheobronchial tree for exploration, collection of specimens, drainage of secretions, removal of airway obstruction, or temporary control of bleeding.

Fistula—An abnormal opening between an internal cavity to the skin or another cavity.

Fixed-Rate, Asynchronous—Pacing in which intrinsic electrical activity of the myocardium is not sensed by the pacemaker.

Fluctuation—A wavelike motion or changing of position, usually of a liquid, which can be observed in the water seal chamber of a closed chest drainage system.

Foramen Magnum—Opening at the base of the skull; anatomically, the uppermost portion of the spinal cord is found here.

Foramen of Monro—Opening in the lateral ventricle which allows passage of CSF into the third ventricle.

Fraction of Inspired Oxygen (FIO$_2$)—Fractional concentration of oxygen in inspired gas; room air has a FIO$_2$ 0.21, or 21% oxygen.

Fracture—A break in the continuity of a bone, epiphyseal plate, or joint surface.

Fresh Frozen Plasma—Plasma rich in clotting factors removed from whole blood with the platelets removed; to replace clotting factors.

Frequency of Respiration (f)—Source of breaths should be designated, such as spontaneous, ventilation-delivered, and total (combined spontaneous and ventilator breaths), for example, 4 (spontaneous)/12 (IMV) (16) (Total); expressed in breaths per minute of frequency (f); normal is 12 to 20.

Frontal Plane Leads or Limb Leads—Leads which reveal variation in the electrical potential between the extremities. Consists of I, II, III, aVr, aVf, and aVl.

Full Thickness Burn—Burn wound whereby all epidermal and dermal elements are destroyed.

Functional Hemoglobin—Hemoglobin types that are able to reversibly bind with O_2.

Gastric Distention—Expansion or stretching of the stomach caused by the accumulation of fluids, solids, or gas.

Gastric Lavage—Instillation and retrieval of fluid from the stomach for the purpose of removing contents, usually blood or toxic substances.

Gastric Motility—Power of gastric system to spontaneously move foodstuffs.

Gastric Residual—Volume of stomach contents. Measured during enteral feeding to assess rate of gastric emptying.

Gauge—Dimension or caliber of an instrument.

Granulation—Formation and growth of connective tissue and capillaries within a healing wound.

Granulation Tissue—Pink, nodular collagen containing tissue formed in response to a deep second or third degree injury. This is the body's attempt to heal and contract the wound.

Granulocytes—Used to raise the leukocyte level and is prepared by centrifugation or filtration leukopheresis which removes granulocytes from whole blood.

Gravity-Infusion Device—A system that controls the infusion drop rate; rate is controlled by counting drops by a flow sensor.

Green Cast—A cast which has set but from which the excess water has not evaporated.

Ground—A low-resistance electrical pathway to the earth.

Ground Fault—A nonintact ground wire.

Guidewire—A flexible metallic wire over which a catheter is passed to advance it into proper position within the blood vessel.

Guidewire Exchange—Replacement of existing short-term central venous catheter by insertion of guidewire into catheter, removal of catheter, and placement of new catheter over guidewire.

Halo Ring—Circular support which surrounds the patient's head; guides four stabilizing pins (two anterior and two posterior) which are inserted to grip the outer table of the cranium.

Halo Struts—Sturdy rods attaching the halo ring to the halo vest.

Halo Vest (Halo External Fixator)—Plastic vest with form-fitting anterior and posterior pieces; anchors struts and opens at the sides for access.

Hardwire—Monitoring system which requires direct cable attachment from patient to monitor.

Heimlich Valve—A commercial one-way exit valve designed to allow air or fluid to escape without allowing atmospheric air to enter the pleural space.

Hematoma—A localized collection of blood, usually clotted, in an organ, space, or tissue, due to a break in the wall of a blood vessel.

Hemodialysis—Extracorporeal technique for removing waste products or toxic substances from the systemic circulation.

Hemolysis—Lysis or destruction of red cells by antibodies in the serum initiated by an antigen on the red cell.

Hemopneumothorax—The collection of blood (hemothorax) and air (pneumothorax) in the pleural space.

Hemothorax—The collection of blood in the pleural space.

Herniation—Forcing tissue through or against inelastic structures causing tissue ischemia and dysfunction.

Heterograft—Skin graft obtained from a species other than that being grafted onto.

High-Flow Oxygen Delivery Systems—An apparatus that supplies a total volume of inspired gas to the patient. All the gas the patient breathes is provided by the oxygen therapy device. Specific, consistent oxygen concentrations may be delivered.

High-Frequency Ventilation (HFV)—Mechanical ventilation provided at frequencies greatly in excess of normal respiratory rate; includes high-frequency positive pressure ventilation (HFPPV), high-frequency jet ventilation (HFJ), and high-frequency oscillation (HFO).

Homograft—Skin graft obtained from a member of the same species that it is being grafted into.

Horizontal Plane Leads or Precordial Chest Leads—Leads which reveal variation in the electrical potential from six different positions on the chest. Consists of V_1 through V_6.

Huber Point Needle—Made specifically for use with implanted venous access ports; is beveled with a deflected end point to prevent coring of the silicone port septum upon entry; makes a straight-line tear that seals itself when the needle is removed.

Humerus—The bone of the upper arm, between the elbow and shoulder joint.

Hydrocolloid Wafer Dressing—Occlusive dressing which interacts with wound exudate to form a moist substance which protects the wound bed.

Hydrothorax—The collection of noninflammatory, serous fluid within the pleural space.

Hyperbaric Oxygen Therapy—Breathing 100% oxygen under increased atmospheric pressure.

Hyperextension—Overextension of the cervical vertebrae.

Hyperflexion—Flexion of a body part beyond the normal limit.

Hyperinflated—Overinflation of the pulmonary system.

Hyperkeratosis—Overgrowth of the horny layer of the epidermis.

Hyperosmolar—High solute concentration in solution with osmolarity greater than 400 mOsm/L.

Hyperthermia—Unusually high fever above 106°F (41°C).

Hyperventilation—Increased rate and depth of ventilation, or both.

Hypothermia—Unusually low temperature—<95°F (35°C).

Hypoventilation—Decreased rate and/or irregular respiratory pattern with decrease in depth of ventilation and with $PaCO_2$ greater than 50 mmHg.

Hypothyroidism—Condition due to deficiency of thyroid secretion, resulting in lowered basal metabolism.

Hypovolemia—Diminished blood volume.

Hypoxemia—Arterial PO_2 less than 50 mmHg measured by arterial blood gas analysis.

Hypoxia—Diminished availability of oxygen for body tissues.

Ileal/Colon Conduit—A surgically created reservoir for urine after bladder removal.

Ileostomy—Fecal diversion with the opening into the small bowel making a connection between the small bowel and the abdominal wall. Drainage is thin to thick liquid, never solid.

Immobility—Inability to move separate parts of the body easily and without pain.

Immobilize—To render fixed or incapable of moving.

Immobilization—Preventing movement (extension, flexion, and rotation) of the spine.

Implanted Venous Access Port—A drug and fluid administration system consisting of a silicone septum (through which needle access is gained) which is encased in a metal or plastic port reservoir and attached to a silastic catheter; may have one or two lumens— the dual lumen port allows incompatible solutions to be given simultaneously; provides long-term venous access for continuous or intermittent systemic therapy.

Inapparent Infection—An infectious process running a course similar to that of clinical disease but below the threshold of clinical symptoms (asymptomatic, subclinical).

Inatropic Agents—Drugs which stimulate myocardial contractility and force of contraction.

Independent Lung Ventilation (ILV)—Differential, and often asynchronous, ventilation of the lungs with a double-lumen endotracheal tube.

Infarction—The formation of an area of coagulation necrosis in a tissue due to local ischemia resulting from obstruction of circulation to the area, most commonly by a thrombus or embolus.

Infected Wound—Wounds containing purulent material which overwhelm host defenses and cause a systemic response.

Infectious Waste—Biological waste which potentially contains infectious agents and requires special handling. (Infectious waste is usually defined by state or local law.)

Inflatable Splint—A plastic splint used as a first aid measure; it is inflated after application to conform and immobilize a fractured arm or leg.

Inflow Phase—The time required to infuse the prescribed volume of dialysate.

In-Line IV Filter—Porous fiber membrane placed in IV administration set to protect against particulate matter, bacterial contamination, and air embolism.

Insensate—Lack of sensation capabilities.

Inspiratory to Expiratory Ratio (I:E Ratio)—Ratio of inspiratory time and expiratory time during a breath expressed as a ratio of seconds; normal is 1:2.

Insulator—A material highly resistant to the flow of electricity.

Intercostal—Between two ribs.

Intercostal Space (ICS)—Space between two ribs.

Intermittent Feeding—Administration of 100 to 480 cc of enteral formula via feeding tube using gravity drip and infusing over 30 to 60 minutes.

Intermittent Mandatory Ventilation (IMV)—Ventilator mode that delivers breaths with a preset volume and rate, irrespective of patient's spontaneous breathing pattern; expressed as frequency per minute.

Intersticies—Holes created by meshing donor skin to allow for expansion of the graft over a larger wound.

Interstitial Tissue—That which lies between the pulmonary alveoli.

Intracranial Hypertension—Condition in which the pressure of the intracranial contents rises and is sustained at greater than normal pressures (ICP > 15 mmHg).

Intracranial Pressure—Refers to consistent pressure equilibrium between the contents within the cranium; blood, CSF, and brain. Normal is 0 to 15 mmHg.

Intracranial Pressure Monitoring—Assessment of generalized pressure forces within the cranium; can be measured in several locations: the epidural space, subarachnoid space, intraventricular, and intraparenchymal.

Intraluminal Catheter Occlusion—Inability to irrigate the venous access device.

Intrapleural—Within the pleural space.

Intrapulmonary Pressure—The pressure within the alveoli that equals the atmospheric pressure when the lungs are at rest; normally is slightly negative during inspiration and slightly positive during expiration.

Intrathecal—Within the subarachnoid space. Refers to route of administration for medications directly into the CNS.

Intraventricular—Within the lateral ventricles of the brain.

Intrinsic Rate—Underlying heart rate without pacemaker initiated depolarizations.

Intrinsic Rhythm—Underlying spontaneous myocardial electrical events; any cardiac depolarization not initiated by the pacemaker.

Introducer—A catheter used to gain access to the central circulation.

Intubation—The passage of a tube directly into the trachea.

Ionizing Radiation—Radiation capable of displacing electrons from atoms or molecules, thus producing electrically charged ions. This may, in turn, disrupt certain life processes.

Ischemia—A deficiency of blood flow due to functional constriction or obstruction of a blood vessel to a part.

Isoelectric Line—Flat line on oscilloscope or recorder showing no variation in electrical potential.

IV Piggyback (IVPB)—A method of infusing intravenous solution(s) in addition to the fluids infusing via the primary line.

Jejunum—Section of small intestine distal to duodenum.

Joule—Delivered energy contained in the electrical shock. One joule is equivalent to one watt/second.

Kirschner's Wire—A wire drilled into a bone to apply skeletal traction.

Koch Pouch (Continent Stoma)—A surgically created internal reservoir, or pouch, constructed from the patient's ileum with an internal valve mechanism. A plastic catheter is inserted through the valve (intubation) to release stool/urine.

Lead—A conductive wire which delivers electrical energy.

Lead Placement—Specific areas on the chest where electrodes are placed in order to determine the view of the electrical activity of the heart.

Lead Selector—Switch which determines the lead to be viewed on the monitor.

Lead Wire—Wire which attaches to the specific electrode and transfers the electrical activity to the monitor or recorder. These can be positive, negative, or neutral in polarity.

Leakage Current—Current that is coupled away from its usual pathway and is seeking ground.

LEDs—Light emitting diodes incorporated into the sensor that emits specific wavelengths of light in the red and infrared spectral range.

Left Atrial Pressure—The pressure exerted by the blood within the left atrium. LAP is measured using a catheter which is placed directly into the LA during heart surgery and connected to a pressure transducer system.

Leukocyte-Poor Packed Red Blood Cells—Red blood cells from which all leukocytes and plasma proteins are removed; often used with patients with a history of transfusion reactions.

Leveling—The process of raising or lowering the transducer in order to make it level with the approximate location of the right atrium or the tip of the catheter where ever it may be located. Leveling eliminates the effects of hydrostatic pressure on the transducer.

Levine Tube—A single lumen tube suitable for passage through the nose or mouth into the stomach or duodenum to instill or evacuate contents from the upper gastrointestinal tract.

Lipid Emulsions—Emulsified safflower or soybean oil to provide fat parenterally.

Logroll—To turn the head, thorax, and pelvis as one unit; requires the assistance of at least four (4) people.

Low Air Loss Therapy—A dynamic pressure relieving treatment.

Low Flow Oxygen Delivery Systems—A method of oxygen delivery which entrains room air to mix with oxygen when the patient inspires; FIO_2 is dependent upon changes in the tidal volume and ventilatory pattern.

Lower Airway—Passageway for gas consisting of the trachea, bronchi, bronchioles, and alveoli.

Lumen—The cavity or channel within a tube or tubular organ.

Maceration—Destructive softening of tissue caused by excessive exposure to moisture.

Magnetic Resonance Imaging (MRI)—A diagnostic technique which does not use ionizing radiation or contrast agents but uses a magnetic device to produce three-dimensional views of internal organs and tissues.

Malleoli—The rounded lateral projection at distal ends of bones of lower extremity at the ankle.

Malunion—Healing of a fracture in a faulty position.

Mandible—The lower jaw.

Maximum Voluntary Ventilation (MVV)—The volume of gas the patient can breathe in or out during one minute of maximum effort; usually measured for 15 seconds and multiplied by four; expressed in liter/minute; normal is 120 to 180 L/min.

Mechanical Debridement—Removal of devitalized tissue through physical means such as a surgical instrument, scrubbing, or irrigation.

Mechanical Sigh—Intermittent deep breaths which supplement the V_t to provide alveolar hyperinflation thus preventing microatelectasis; usually 1.5 to 2 times the V_t; may be delivered by a mechanical ventilator or self-inflating resuscitation bag.

Mediastinal Tube—A tube or catheter placed in the Mediastinum to drain fluid and/or blood.

Mediastinum—The space between the lungs, sternum, and vertebral column containing the heart, great vessels, and bronchi.

Meninges—Protective covering of the brain. Consists of three layers, the pia mater, arachnoid, and dura mater; surrounds both the brain and spinal cord structures.

Metabolic Homeostasis—Equilibrium in body chemistry which preserves the viability of organ(s) to be utilized for transplantation.

Microatelectasis—Pulmonary condition caused by elimination of nitrogen (nitrogen washout) and the negative effects of oxygen on pulmonary surfactant.

Microschock—An electrical injury from current leakage not sensed by a healthy individual; tachydythymias may be induced by current leakage entering the myocardium through a pacing lead.

Midaxillary—The imaginary vertical line that extends down the lateral thorax from the midpoint of the axilla.

Midclavicular—An imaginary vertical line that extends down the anterior thorax from the midpoint of the clavicle.

Milliamperes (mA)—A unit of measure of electrical energy delivered to the myocardium, regulated by the output dial of the pulse generator.

Millirem (MREM)—.001 rem.

Minute Ventilation (VE)—Volume of expired gas in one minute; equal to $V_t \times RR$ or F (tidal volume multiplied by the respiratory rate) expressed in L/min; normal is 5 to 6 L/min.

Mode—A programmed response of a medical device, such as a ventilator, pacemaker, etc.

Modified Allen's Test—Determines patency of ulnar artery and adequacy of blood flow to the hand; performed prior to the insertion of an arterial line.

Moleskin—A soft, usually adhesive-backed fabric applied to areas of the body to prevent irritation or abrasion.

Monoplace Chamber—A pressurized chamber utilized for hyperbaric oxygen therapy which only accommodates the patient.

Morbidity—State of being diseased.

Mortality—State of being subjected to death.

Mucocutaneous Junction—Incision where mucous membrane of colon and abdominal skin are sutured together to secure the stoma exteriorly.

Multichannel—An ECG machine which simultaneously records three consecutive leads automatically with correct lead placement.

Multiplace Chamber—A pressurized chamber utilized for hyperbaric oxygen therapy which can accommodate two or more patients and health care professionals.

Myocardium—Muscular portion of the heart.

Myelogram—Dye injected into the spinal canal is radiologically imaged to identify vertebral and soft tissue structures within the spinal canal.

Nasoenteric Feeding—Administration of enteral formula via a feeding tube inserted into the nose and positioned in small bowel, usually in the duodenum or jejunum.

Nasogastric Feeding—Administration of enteral formula via feeding tube inserted into the nose and positioned in stomach.

Nasogastric Tube—A generic term for a tube passed through the nose/mouth and esophagus into the stomach to instill or evacuate contents from the stomach.

Necrotic Debris—Avascular, devitalized tissue within a wound.

Negative Inspiratory Pressure/Force (NIP, NIF)—Amount of negative pressure the patient can generate with maximum inspiratory effort; expressed in cmH_2O; normal is 80 to 100 cmH_2O; parameter used to determine if a patient is ready for weaning from a ventilator.

Negative Pressure—A pressure having a value less than zero.

Neuroendocrine Regulation—The regulatory mechanisms (baroreceptors, osmoreceptors, and chemoreceptors) that are absent in the brain-dead patient due to the destruction of the hypothalamic, pituitary, and medullary regions of the brain.

Neurogenic Bladder—State of the urinary bladder when voluntary and reflex innervation is interrupted by injury/disease; results in expansion of bladder without reflexive emptying.

Neurogenic Bowel—State of the bowel when voluntary and reflex innervation is interrupted by injury/disease; results in indiscriminate bowel emptying.

Neurovascular Check—Series of assessments (pulse, pain, pallor, paresthesia, paralysis) required to measure neurological and circulatory status of peripheral tissues.

Neurovascular Status—Vascular and neurologic assessment of the limbs.

Nitrogen Balance—Calculation of amount of nitrogen intake (dietary, intravenous, enteral) and amount of nitrogen output (stools, urine, drainage) by a patient in a 24-hour period to determine protein metabolism.

Normothermia—Normal body temperature; usually 98.6 °F (37°C) orally; 0.5 to 1.0 degree higher rectally; 0.5 to 1.0 degree lower axillary.

Nosocomial Infection—An infection not present or incubating at the time of admission.

Nuchal Rigidity—Pain with neck flexion.

Nystagmus—An involuntary movement of the eyes that may be horizontal, vertical, rotary, or mixed in direction. The tempo of the movements may be regular, rhythmic, jerky, or pendular with a fast or slow component.

Occlusive Thrombosis—Thrombus totally occluding the lumen of a vessel with complete obstruction of flow.

One-Way Valve Effect—Inability to withdraw blood from a venous access device when the device is able to be irrigated without resistance; caused by fibrin sheath formation at the tip of the catheter which covers the entrance to the catheter upon blood withdrawal attempt.

Open Reduction—Reduction of a fracture after incision into the site of the fracture.

Optical Shunt—A phenomenon where some portion of emitted light reaches the photodetector without passing through an arteriolar bed; results in either erratic or stable but inaccurate measurements.

Organ Donor—A patient who has been pronounced dead by neurologic criteria, after having total, irreversible brain damage. Intact cardiopulmonary functioning exists which must be artificially maintained to minimize ischemia of donor organs.

Organ Oxygenation—The mechanical process of providing adequate exchange of respiratory gases, in the proper concentration, to preserve the viability of organs to be utilized for transplantation.

Organ Perfusion—The availability and movement of blood for exchange of gases, nutrients, and cellular metabolites to organs that will be utilized for transplantation.

Organ Preservation—The ability to maintain the viability of an organ ex vivo for an amount of time that will allow transportation of the cadaveric organ to the transplant center, provide time for donor-recipient matching, and yield good initial function following transplantation.

Organ Procurement Organization—A local or regional agency, certified by the Organ Procurement and Transplant Network (established by federal law), that coordinates the recovery and distribution of organs.

Oronasal Mask—A mask that covers both the mouth and nose.

Oropharynx—Middle third of the pharynx posterior to the soft palate and extends to the epiglottis; common pathway for food and solids.

Orthosis—General term for an external device applied to a patient for supportive, preventive, or corrective purpose.

Oscillating Support Therapy—A dynamic pressure relieving treatment; a rotating table or lateral rotation cushions.

Osmosis—Movement of fluid from an area of lesser to an area of greater concentration.

Osteomyelitis—Infection involving bone.

Osteostomy—Surgical opening of bone or cutting through a bone.

Ostomy—Surgically created opening into the gastrointestinal or genitourinary tract.

Outer Table (of the skull)—The portion of the cranium directly beneath the scalp and soft tissue.

Outflow Phase—The time required to drain the peritoneal cavity of infused dialysate plus excess extracellular fluid.

Output, Current—The amount of energy delivered to the myocardium, measured in milliamperes (MA).

Overdistraction—A stretching of the vertebrae and spinal cord usually resulting from application of excessive weights and manifested by a deterioration in motor/sensory function.

Overdrive Suppression—A method of inhibiting a tachycardia by pacing the myocardium at a rate faster than the rate of the tachycardia.

Oxygen Toxicity—A complication of oxygen therapy in which the lung parenchyma was damaged by microalveolar hemorrhage and hyperplasia of alveolar cells. The toxicity may be due to high oxygen concentrations or prolonged periods of oxygen therapy.

Oxyhemoglobin—Hemoglobin not bound with oxygen (reduced hemoglobin).

Pacing Artifact—Spike seen on the ECG, a perpendicular voltage deflection from the ECG baseline representing the delivery of energy from the pacemaker.

Packed Red Blood Cells—Centrifuged from whole blood; used to restore oxygen-carrying capacity and intravascular volume.

PaCO$_2$—The partial pressure of CO$_2$ in arterial blood.

Paracentesis—Insertion of a hollow needle or catheter into a body cavity to remove fluid; used as a diagnostic and therapeutic procedure.

Parenteral Nutrition—The administration of nutrients by the intravascular route.

Parietal Pleura—The serous membrane lining the walls of the thoracic cavity.

Parietal Thrombosis—Thrombus attached to the lumen wall partially obstructing flow.

Partial Pressure of Carbon Dioxide in the Arterial Blood (PaCO$_2$)—Expressed in mmHg; normal is 35 to 45 mmHg.

Partial Pressure of Oxygen in the Arterial Blood (PaO$_2$)—Expressed in mmHg; normal is 80 to 100 mmHg.

Partial Pressure of Oxygen in the Mixed Venous Blood (P$\overline{v}$O$_2$)—Expressed in mmHg; normal is 40 mmHg.

Partial Thickness Burn—Burn wound whereby epidermal and/or part of the dermal elements are destroyed.

Pathophysiological—Disease of bodily function.

Patient Cable—Electrical cable which attaches lead wires to the ECG machine, monitor, or recorder.

Patient-Controlled Infusion Device—A system in which the patient self-administers pharmacologic administration.

Patient-Ventilator Synchrony—Synchronous rise and fall of the chest with each breath.

PCA Dose—Amount of medication administered to the patient when the control button is pressed.

Peak Inspiratory Flow (PIF)—Peak speed of gas flow during ventilator delivery of the tidal volume; expressed in liters per minute.

Peak (Maximum) Inspiratory Pressure (PIP, MIP)—Highest pressure displayed on the ventilator gauge at the end of inspiration; expressed in cmH$_2$O.

PEG (Percutaneous Endoscopic Gastrostomy) Tube—A feeding tube inserted into the stomach using percutaneous endoscopic gastrostomy technique.

Pelvic Sling—A canvas support for suspension of the pelvis.

Percussion—The rhythmical striking of the skin over the lung to aid in mechanical movement of secretions using a cupped hand.

Pericardial Effusion—The abnormal accumulation of more than 50 cc fluid in the pericardial sac.

Pericardial Sac—Fibrous tissue that surrounds the heart and great vessels.

Pericardiocentesis—Surgical puncture of the pericardial cavity for aspiration of fluid.

Perifistula—Skin area surrounding the fistula.

Peristalsis—Waves of contraction in gastrointestinal tract that propel digested food from stomach to rectum.

Peripheral Parenteral Nutrition—The administration through a peripheral vein of energy substrates and other nutrients that partially or totally meet the patient's daily caloric and nitrogen requirements. Dextrose concentrations do not exceed 10% in adult solutions, and are generally considered temporary support.

Peripheral Vascular Resistance—Force applied by the capillaries to the blood passing through them.

Peristomal—Skin area surrounding the stoma.

Peritoneal Dialysis—The technique for the removal of metabolic waste products and fluid from the body via osmosis and diffusion through the peritoneal membrane.

Peritoneal Lavage—Instillation and removal of a physiologic solution into the peritoneal cavity to examine returns for the presence of blood, abnormal cells, or bacteria; may also be used to cleanse the peritoneal cavity of purulent material.

Personal Protective Equipment—Protective apparel (gloves, masks, eye protection, gowns/ aprons) used to reduce risks to health care workers of exposure to infectious agents.

Petalling—A particular method used to finish ragged edges of a plaster cast to prevent skin irritation or pressure.

PetCO$_2$—The measured CO$_2$ (in mmHg) at the end of exhalation. Also referred to as end-tidal partial pressure of CO$_2$.

pH—An expression of the alkalinity or acidity of a solution.

Phlebitis—Inflammation of a vein. The condition is marked by infiltration of the coats of the vein and the formation of a thrombus. The condition is also marked by edema, stiffness, and pain in the affected part.

Photodetector—The element in the sensor that functions as a collector of residual light which has passed through a pulsatile tissue bed.

Pierson Attachment—An additional attachment which converts Thomas splint to balanced suspension. In addition allows passive motion of knee without malalignment of the affected extremity.

Plasmanate—Pooled from human plasma; used as an intravascular volume expander by increasing osmotic pressure.

Plaster of Paris—Calcium sulfate impregnated bandage which when mixed with water forms a paste that dries to a rigid mass.

Plateau Waves—Noted when there is a dramatic and sustained rise in ICP. ICP associated with plateau waves is 50 to 100 mmHg; the patient may exhibit neurological deterioration with onset of these waves.

Platelet Concentrate—Platelets are removed from whole blood; used to increase the platelet count and improve hemostasis.

Pleural Space—The potential "space" between the parietal and visceral pleura; pressure within the pleural space under normal conditions is always negative.

Pleural Pressure—A pressure having a value greater than zero.

Pneumatic Counterpressure—Air is utilized to create pressure against something.

Pneumatic Splint—An inflatable splint which uses air to provide immobilization of an extremity.

Pneumothorax—The accumulation of air or gas in the pleural space resulting in the collapse of the lung.

Polarity—Identification of the electrical potential of a lead system. Either positive or negative in nature.

Positive End-Expiratory Pressure (PEEP)—Positive pressure at end-expiration which prevents intrathoracic pressure from returning to atmospheric pressure at the end of expiration; expressed in cmH$_2$O.

Positive Pressure—A pressure having a value greater than zero.

Positive Pressure Ventilation (PPV)—Volume or pressure assisted mechanical ventilation that produces positive intrathoracic pressure during inspiration.

Postural Drainage—The utilization of a series of positions to assist the gravitational movement of lung secretions.

Preload—Volume of blood in the ventricles prior to systole; also referred to as the amount of stretch on the heart muscle.

Pressure Reducing Devices—Devices that do not consistently keep interface pressure below 32 mmHg (foam overlay, air mattress).

Pressure Reduction—A decrease in skin surface pressure below the pressures normally created by the interface between skin and mattresses or other support surfaces, but not below the normal capillary closing pressure.

Pressure Relief—Consistent reduction of pressure to skin surfaces below 25 to 32 mmHg.

Pressure Relieving Devices—Devices that consistently reduce interface pressure below 25 to 32 mmHg (air-fluidized beds, low air loss beds, oscillating therapy tables and cushions).

Pressure Sore—An area of localized tissue damage caused by ischemia due to pressure.

Pressure Support (PS)—Pressure-limited mechanical ventilatory assistance which augments the patient's spontaneous breaths; expressed in cmH_2O.

Primary Tubing—IV tubing connected directly into the IV insertion site.

Pulley—A wheel with a grooved rim in which a piece of rope is placed; part of traction apparatus used to change point of application of the pulling face.

Pulmonary Artery—Blood vessel leading from the right ventricle past the pulmonic valve, on the venous side of the pulmonary circulation.

Pulmonary Artery Pressure—The pressure within the pulmonary artery measured by the pulmonary artery flow directed catheter. The PAP provides information about the pulmonary vasculature, the lung tissues, the intravascular volume status, and left ventricular function.

Pulmonary Artery Wedge Pressure—Indication of left ventricular pressure and at end of diastole; the average pressure in the left atrium measured in the capillary bed of the pulmonary artery reflects the pressure of the pulmonary vasculature downstream.

Pulmonary Edema—Effusion of fluid (either serous or blood) into interstitial tissue and alveoli of the lungs.

Pulmonary Wedge Pressure—Is a pressure obtained from the PA catheter when a balloon located on the tip of the catheter is inflated and allowed to carry the catheter into a capillary where the balloon wedges against the vessel wall. Provides an indirect measure of left ventricular end diastolic pressure, also known as left ventricular preload.

Pulse Generator—The source that initiates electrical activity and controls the rate and intensity of each energy discharge. It houses the energy source and controls.

Pulse Paradoxus—Greater than 10 mmHg decline in systolic arterial pressure with normal inspiration.

Pulse Pressure—The difference between the systolic and the diastolic pressure; expresses tone of the arterial walls.

Pulse Oximeter—A noninvasive method of measuring arterial hemoglobin oxygen saturation (SaO_2); normal SaO_2 is 95 to 100%.

Pulsus Alternans—Alternating strong and weak beats.

Pylorus—Distal portion of stomach where sphincter opens to gradually admit digested food into small bowel.

Pythorax—The presence of purulent exudate in the pleural cavity.

Quad-Assist Cough—A method of assisting the quadriplegic patient to cough. The nurse applies forceful pressure beneath the patient's diaphragm and supplements abdominal muscle function, thereby increasing cough effectiveness and productivity.

Radiation Absorbed Dose (RAD)—Measure of absorbed dose of ionizing radiation.

Radioisotope—An element which has radioactive properties; electromagnetic energy emitted by a radioactive substance which has strong penetrating capabilities.

Recorder—Equipment that prints out ECG data.

Reduce/Reduction—To restore something to its normal place or position, as in fracture or dislocation.

Refractory Period (Pacemaker)—A period of time when the pacemaker is unable to sense intrinsic electrical activity.

Repolarization—Return of cellular ions to their resting state.

Required Request—The legal requirement to ensure that families of potential donors are given the option to donate or to decline to donate, their deceased's organs and tissues for transplantation.

Resident Flora—Organisms that survive and multiply on the skin. These organisms can be cultured repeatedly and are not easily removed by handwashing.

Respiratory Failure—Arterial blood gas values of a PaO_2 less than 50 mmHg and/or $PaCO_2$ of greater than 50 mmHg when the patient is at rest and breathing room air.

Retrolental Fiberplasia—A bilateral disease of the retinal vessels present in premature infants who often received high oxygen concentrations. High oxygen concentration causes vasoconstriction of immature retinal vessels and eventually occlusion of the vessels which may lead to blindness.

Right Atrial Pressure (See also Central Venous Pressure)—The pressure exerted by the blood within the right atrium. Right atrial is often the same as central venous pressure.

Right Ventricular Pressure—The pressure within the right ventricle which can be measured during insertion of the PA catheter. RVP gives information about blood volume, right ventricular function, and pulmonary vascular or interstitial disease.

Roentgen-Equivalent-Man Period (REM)—Amount of potential damage of radiation exposure. It produces the same biologic effects as unit of ordinary x-rays. Occupational exposure is usually less than the recommended dosage limit of less than 5 REM a year or less than 100 MREM a week. This may vary from institution to institution.

Salem Sump—A two-lumen tube used to drain fluid from a space, usually the stomach; main lumen evacuates drainage; secondary lumen vents air down the tube through the drainage outlets along the main lumen to prevent occlusion of the drainage outlets.

Saturation of Hemoglobin with Oxygen in the Arterial Blood (SaO$_2$)—Amount of oxygen actually carried by the hemoglobin in proportion to the amount of oxygen that could be carried by the hemoglobin in arterial blood; expressed as a percentage; normal is >95%.

Saturation of Hemoglobin with Oxygen in the Mixed Venous Blood (S$\bar{v}$O$_2$)—Amount of oxygen actually carried by the hemoglobin in proportion to the amount of oxygen that could be carried by the hemoglobin in mixed venous blood; expressed as a percentage; normal is 75%.

Semipermeable Membrane—A membrane which allows for the movement of solutes and fluid according to the principles of osmosis and diffusion.

Semipermeable, Occlusive Dressing—Dressings which totally cover the wound surface and permit selective passage of gases and vapors.

Semirigid Collar—A collar made of hard plastic or foam which is utilized to maintain head and neck in neutral position. It has an anterior and posterior splint which adds stability at the chin and occiput. Does not provide total stability or immobilization (i.e., Philadelphia collar).

Sensing Threshold—The minimum electrical signal needed to activate the pacemaker's sensing circuit.

Setting Time—The interval required for the casting material to become a rigid dressing.

Sequester—Isolate blood in the extremities.

Shear—Tissue trauma below the skin surface, created by layers of tissue sliding against each other; commonly occurs when a patient slides down in bed.

Shivering—Tremoring of the skin and underlying muscles.

Short Circuit—An accidental electrical connection between a hot wire within the piece of equipment and the equipment housing; can occur through mechanical damage or insulation breakdown; excessive current generally causes arcing and sparks, which cause the circuit breaker or fuse to open, thus disrupting power to the equipment.

Shunt—A physiologic condition in which the lung unit is perfused but not ventilated.

Sigmoid Colon—Distal portion of the large intestine which begins at the termination of the descending colon and ends at the rectum; may be "S" or "V" shaped.

Silastic Tube—Catheter made of soft, flexible, durable rubber.

Single Channel—ECG machine which records in one single lead at a time as determined by the selector switch.

Sinus Tract—A narrow dead space extending distally under the skin from a wound bed.

Sling—A bandage that supports any part of the body, particularly the arm.

Sling and Swathe—Cradle type sling with body strap to prevent abduction of the shoulder.

Slit Catheter—A catheter used to measure compartment pressure; slits along tip of polyethylene tubing maintain continuity between tissue and saline within catheter.

Slough—Stringy, light colored, nonviable tissue, often seen in pressure sores.

SO$_2$—The percent of total hemoglobin bound with oxygen as measured by a laboratory co-oximeter or as calculated (estimated) using a standard blood gas analyzer; (SaO$_2$ = arterial O$_2$ saturation, S$\bar{v}$O$_2$ = mixed venous saturation).

Spasm—An involuntary muscle contraction.

Spica Cast—A rigid structure used to immobilize an extremity by incorporating part of the body along with the injured extremity.

Spinal Cord Injury—A manifestation of motor weakness or sensory disturbance due to injury or ischemia to the spinal cord.

Spinal Injury—Injury to the vertebrae usually resulting in spinal instability; may or may not be associated with spinal cord injury.

Spinal Stabilization—Providing support (externally or internally) to the spine in order to maintain spinal alignment.

Splint—An apparatus, usually rigid, used to support, protect, and immobilize an injured part temporarily.

Split Thickness Skin Graft—Skin graft comprised of epidermis and part of the dermis.

SpO$_2$—The percent of functional hemoglobin bound with oxygen as measured by a pulse oximeter.

Spreader Bar—Notched metal bar, used for pelvic traction; placement of traction ropes in specific notches allows for varying degrees of compression.

Stabilization—The seating of a fixed or movable body part so it will not tilt or be displaced under pressure.

Static (Effective) Compliance (CMPst)—Representation of forces resisting expansion of the lung measured at no flow; volume (tidal volume) divided by pressure (static); expressed in liters per cmH_2O; normal is 60 to 100 ml/cmH2O.

Static Device—Devices which are motionless and non-powered.

Steal Syndrome—Distal ischemia (to the A-V fistula) to the bypass of arterial blood.

Steinmann Pin—An alternative to the use of a Kirschner wire for applying skeletal traction to a limb, generally used in larger bones of lower extremity.

Sterilization—The complete elimination or destruction of all forms of microbial life.

Stimulation Threshold—The smallest amount of energy or millamperes required to consistently depolarize the myocardium.

Stockinette—Stretchable cotton material of various sizes and widths used immediately over the skin to protect the tissues from the irritation of casting materials.

Stoma—A surgically created opening in the intestine brought out to the abdomen and everted at skin level.

Stoma Necrosis—Dead, avascular stoma mucosa.

Stopcock—Device placed inline within a venous or arterial infusion system that allows access to selective points.

Stylet—A flexible metallic wire inserted in the lumen of a soft catheter to stiffen it and give it form during its passage.

Subarachnoid Space—Area between the arachnoid and pia mater in which CSF circulates.

Subcutaneous Emphysema—The abnormal presence of air or gas beneath the layers of the skin.

Superior Vena Cava—A large blood vessel communicating the subclavian and jugular veins and proximal to the right atrium.

Supplemental Oxygen—Delivery of oxygen to patients who require additional oxygen.

Swan-Ganz Catheter—Trade name for a type of flow-directed pulmonary artery catheter.

Sympathetic Nervous System—That portion of the nervous system which responds to stress by innervating the heart, smooth muscle, and glands.

Synchronized Cardioversion—Electrical current passed across chest wall to cause simultaneous depolarization of muscle fibers and synchronized to deliver the energy after the peak of the R wave, outside the vulnerable period.

Synchronized Intermittent Mandatory Ventilation (SIMV)—Ventilator mode that delivers breaths with a preset volume in synchrony with the patient's spontaneous breathing pattern to prevent stacking of spontaneous and mechanical breaths; expressed as frequency per minute.

Tachydysrhythmias—Rapid rhythms of the heart, including paroxysmal atrial tachycardia, atrial tachycardia, atrial fibrillation, atrial flutter, and ventricular tachycardia.

TBSA—Total body surface area.

Telemetry—Monitoring system which uses radio signals to transmit impulses to a monitoring station.

Tenodesis—A functional contracture of the wrist; allows for passive thumb opposition when wrist is extended.

Tension Pneumothorax—A life threatening form of pneumothorax that occurs due to a "one way valve" effect when air enters into the pleural space but cannot escape from it.

Tentorium Cerebri—A fold of dura which separates the cerebrum from the cerebellum. An opening in this fold, called the tentorial notch, allows for passage of the midbrain structures. Under increased pressure, parts of the cerebrum (specifically the temporal lobe margins) can be forced through this opening, resulting in herniation.

Thermal Burn—Tissue injury resulting from fire, hot objects, or fluids.

Thermodilution—A method of measuring ventricular blood volume and cardiac output in which a cold or cool indicator, such as a saline or dextrose solution is injected and sampled by a thermistor.

Thermoregulatory Balance—Balance of the body's temperature.

Thomas Splint—Used for fractures of the femoral shaft, hip, or lower-leg.

Thoracentesis—A surgical puncture and drainage of the thoracic cavity.

Thoracostomy—An incision of the chest wall with the maintenance of the opening for the purpose of drainage.

Thoracotomy—An incision of the chest wall.

Thorax—The part of the body between the neck and abdomen (i.e., the chest).

Thrill—A buzzing sensation palpated over the area of the anastomosis of the artery and vein in an arteriovenous fistula.

Thrombosis—The formation, development, or presence of a thrombus.

Thyrotoxicosis—Toxic condition due to hyperactivity of thyroid gland, causing elevated metabolism.

Tidal Volume (VT)—Volume of gas either inspired or expired with each breath; expressed in ml.; normal is 5 to 7 ml/kg (350 to 500 ml.).

Timing—Synchronization of counterpulsation with patient hemodynamics; utilizes ECG tracing and arterial pressure waveform.

Tomogram—Radiologic study allowing anterior, posterior, and oblique views of the spinal cord.

Tongs (Gardener-Wells, Crutchfield, Vinke)—A type of external fixation which incorporates a metal/graphite bow and 2 sharp pins to establish a firm grip on the outer table of the cranium to provide a means for cervical traction.

Torque—Torquing halo insertion pins comprises applying a rotary force to the pin (usually with a specialized wrench) until a specific force (measured in inch pounds) is achieved. Normal torque value for a halo pin is 4 to 8 inch pounds.

Total Parenteral Nutrition (TPN)—The administration of energy substrates and other nutrients that totally satisfy the requirements of the body. The amounts of energy and nutrients provided may be adjusted to cover only basal requirements or to satisfy an augmented need from increased losses, previous deficiencies, or increased energy needs.

Tourniquet—Band or cuff used to restrict blood flow in an extremity.

T-Piece (T-Bar, Blow-By)—Device that delivers supplemental oxygen and/or humidity to an artificial airway during spontaneous breathing.

TPN (Total Parenteral Nutrition) Cycle—Infusion of 24 hours of TPN in a reduced amount of time (e.g., 12 to 14 hours) to promote activity and stimulate appetite.

Traction—A steady drawing or pulling exerted manually or with a mechanical device to overcome muscle spasm, so that a fracture may be reduced, to keep the ends of fractured bones in position until healing can take place, to prevent deformities or contracture from fractures or other conditions, or to correct or lessen deformities such as scoliosis— many of these types of apparatus involve the use of pulleys and weights to produce a steady pulling on a part.

Trachea—Membranous tube, composed of cartilage, descending from the larynx and branching into the right and left bronchi.

Tracheal Tube—A tube inserted through an incision made in the trachea.

Transcutaneous External Pacemaker—A method of pacing in which energy is delivered through the chest wall via two patches applied to the chest.

Transcutaneous Ear Oximetry—Method used to determine the degree of oxygen saturation of blood flowing through the capillary bed of the ear by attaching an oximeter to the pinna of the ear.

Transducer—A device that translates one form of energy to another, e.g., the pressure, temperature, or pulse to an electrical signal.

Transfusion Reaction—An antigen-antibody reaction which causes an acute hemolytic transfusion reaction; mediated by neuroendocrine responses and activating the complement and coagulation cascades.

Transient Flora—Organisms not firmly attached to the skin that survive only a short time (<24 hours), do not multiply, and can be removed by handwashing.

Translaryngeal—Passing across the larynx.

Transmembrane (Negative) Pressure—The negative pressure set on the dialysis machine to remove desired ultrafiltrate.

Transmural Pressure—Pressure through the wall of a vessel, specifically the arteriole in compartment syndrome.

Transparent Adhesive Dressing—A semipermeable occlusive dressing which maintains wound visibility and a moist wound bed, and promotes autolysis when applied directly to a wound.

Transtracheal Biopsy—A diagnostic technique utilized in conjunction with fiber optic bronchoscopy in which a needle or forceps is inserted through the channel of the fiberscope to suspicious areas of the tracheobronchial tree and penetrated for collection of tissue-specimens.

Transvenous Endocardial Pacemaker—Pacing leads inserted via a central vein into the myocardial chambers.

Transverse Colostomy—Fecal diversion with the opening into the transverse colon. Drainage is thick liquid to pasty. The stoma may be double barrel, single end, or loop.

Trigger—Signal used by IAB console to synchronize inflation and deflation with the cardiac cycle; the patient ECG, arterial waveform, pacer spike, or an additional console generated signal can be used.

"Type and Crossmatch" (Compatibility Testing)—A test for incompatibilities between donor and recipient blood. It is carried out prior to transfusion to avoid potentially lethal hemolytic reactions between the donor's red blood cells and antibodies in the recipient's plasma.

Ultrafiltration—An alternative or adjunctive method of treating acute and chronic renal failure which allows for the removal of plasma water and non-protein solutes.

Ultrasound—Radiologic technique where deep structures are viewed by recording the reflection of sound waves directed at the tissues.

Unassisted Aortic End-Diastolic Pressure—The patient's inherent diastolic pressure without IAB effect.

Unassisted Systole—The patient's inherent systolic pressure without IAB effect.

Uncus—Portion of the temporal lobe which is forced against the tentorial notch when extreme pressures are applied. Uncus typically exerts pressure on the oculomotor nerve (cranial nerve III) and produces dilated pupil and extraocular movement impairment.

Undermining—Dead space under the skin at the margins of a wound.

Union—The process of healing or growing together, as occurs between the edges of a wound or the ends of fractured bones.

Unipolar—A pacemaker circuit in which only the negative pole of the circuit is in contract with the myocardium. May also refer to a lead which contains only a single point of conduction at the lead tip.

Upper Airway—Passageway for gas consisting of nasal cavity, pharynx, larynx, and structures above the larynx.

Urokinase—Is an enzyme (protein) produced by the kidney; acts on the endogenous fibrinolytic system by converting plasminogen to the enzyme plasmin, which degrades fibrin clots as well as fibrinogen and other plasma proteins; is indicated for the restoration of patency of venous access devices obstructed by clotted blood or fibrin.

Urostomy—A urinary diversion whereby the bladder is removed and the ureters are exteriorized.

VA Interval—The time between the last ventricular event, whether paced or intrinsic, and the next paced atrial event; also known as the atrial escape interval.

Vacuum—A space devoid of gas or air.

Vallecula—The space between the base of the tongue and the pharyngeal surface of the epiglottis.

Valsalva Maneuver—Forced expiratory effort with closed nose and mouth.

Varix/Varices—Enlarged and tortuous, submucosal blood vessel(s) caused by portal hypertension.

Vascular Access—The insertion of a cannula or shunt or the creation of a fistula which allows for entry into the circulation for hemodialysis.

Vasodilator—Agent which causes relaxation and dilatation of blood vessels.

Vasospasm—Spasm of the blood vessels, resulting in a decrease in their caliber.

Velpeau Sling—An upper extremity sling used to alleviate hand edema and prevent abduction of affected extremity.

Venous Admixture (% Shunt, $\dot{Q}s/\dot{Q}t$)—Fractional shunt per unit of time; blood shunted through the lungs without participating in alveolar gas exchange divided by the total blood flow through the lungs (cardiac output); expressed as percentage; normal is <5%.

Venous Return—Blood in the veins returning to the heart from the extremities.

Venous Thrombosis—Aggregation for blood factors, primarily platelets, fibrin, and other cellular elements within a blood vessel, that may lead to complete occlusion.

Ventricular Fibrillation—Random contraction of individual myocardial fibers produced by chaotic impulse conduction resulting in a loss of synchronicity and pumping action of the heart.

Vibration—The transmission of movements to a patient's chest from the shoulders and hands of the performer for the purpose of increasing mechanical movement of secretions in the lung.

Visceral Pleura—The serous membrane covering the surface of the lungs.

Vital Capacity (VC)—Maximal volume that can be expired after a maximal inspiration; expressed in ml; normal is 65 to 75 ml/kg (4,500 to 5,200 ml).

Volkmann's Contracture—A rapidly developing flexion deformity of the wrist and fingers caused by ischemia of the muscles.

Volume-Controlled Infusion Device—A system that uses positive pressure to deliver intravenous fluids accurately.

Vulnerable Period—The moment in the cardiac cycle when the heart is recovering from the previous biochemical changes and repolarization of the membrane is in progress.

$\dot{V}/\dot{Q}$ Relationship—The ratio of ventilation ($\dot{V}$) to perfusion ($\dot{Q}$) throughout the lung; ideal value is 1.0.

Water Seal—The use of water to create a one-way mechanism that allows air to escape from the pleural space while not allowing air from the atmosphere to enter.

Watt/Sec—Energy over time in seconds; one watt/sec is equivalent to one joule.

Weaning—Process of decreasing the assist frequency of the IABP or IAB volume as the patient's condition improves.

Webril—Stretchable cotton material applied over the skin to protect from plaster irritation when casting.

Weight—Metal object used to exert downward force on traction apparatus.

Weil Sling—A type of pelvic sling used to compress the bones of the pelvis following trauma.

Whole Blood—Red blood cells with platelets and/or white blood cells removed; used to restore oxygen-carrying capacity and intravascular volume.

Wick Catheter—A catheter used to measure compartment pressure; a cylindric wick allows a large fluid pick-up area without requiring infusion of saline.

Windowing—Cutting a small area of a cast to permit inspection of tissues below.

Work of Breathing [Inspiration] (WOB [WKIN])—Energy expended by the respiratory muscles to overcome the forces resisting expansion of the lung; expressed in kilogram-meters per liter (kg-m/L) or in joules per liter (j/L), with 1 kg-m equal to about 10 joules; normal is 0.073 kg-m/L or 0.73 j/L.

Xiphoid Process—Bony structure at distal end of sternum.

Zeroing—The process of opening the transducer stopcock to air in order to eliminate the effects of atmospheric pressure on a pressure transducer system.

INDEX

Dunlop's skeletal traction, 668t, *669*
Duodenum, feeding tube placement in, 816–817
  upper endoscopy and, 557
Duoderm, 753t
Dura, perforation of, 472
Dynamic compliance (CMP$_{dyn}$), 128–129
  implementation and, 130–131
Dynamic devices, 624
  air fluidized therapy beds as, 626–630
  alternating air mattresses as, 639–642
  low air loss therapy and, 630–633
Dysphagia, 472
Dysrhythmias, bolus administration and, 839
  brain death and, 919
  from tamponade tube, 539
  hypothermia/hyperthermia blankets and, 444
  in bronchoscopy, 221
  in central venous catheter insertion, 774–775t
    percutaneously placed, 791, 793
  in pericardiocentesis, 436
  in pulmonary artery catheterization, 335, 341
  intraaortic balloon pump and, 409
  monitoring for, 237
  postoperative, 377
  sustained, recurrent ventricular, 251
  transvenous temporary pacing and, 389

Echocardiography, 434
Edema, pulmonary, 429, 430
Edlich tube, 525, 530
Effective compliance, 129
Effusion, pericardial, 434
Eighth cranial nerve, function of, 511
Electrical activity, of myocardium, 368
Electrical burns, 757
Electrical plug, hospital-grade, *899*
Electrical resistance, 898
Electrical safety, 898–904, *899*
Electrocardiography, 232–250
  alternating current interference in, 243
  artifact in, 243
  at bedside, *233, 234*
  atrial electrogram with, 395–396, *396*
  false alarms in, 243
  hardware and telemetry in, *234–236, 234–244, 239–243*
  in asynchronous atrial pacing, *378*
  in external temporary pacing, 372, *373*
  in paroxysmal atrial tachycardia, *393*
  in right atrium, *384*
  in right ventricle, *384*
  monitoring of, central station for, *234*
  recording strips in, *242, 243*
  single-channel or multiple-channel recorder in, *236*
  60-cycle interference in, 243, *243*
  standard and augmented limb leads in, 244
  temporary pacing and, 369
  twelve-lead, 244, *244–246*
    electrodes for, *235*
    limb lead reversal on, 248, *248*
    recordings from, *248, 249*
    vena cava and, *383*
  wandering baseline in, 243
Electrodes, *233, 235*
  burns from, 261
  diameter of, 258t
  disposable defibrillator (DDE), 259
  in bedside monitoring, *234*
  in defibrillation, 257, 259–260

pacing, posterior, 371, *372*
  anterior, 372, *372*
  transvenous temporary, 375
  pregelled or adhesive-type of, 247, 259
Electrograms, atrial, 395–400, *396, 398, 399*
  unipolar or bipolar, 396, *396, 398,* 398–401, *399*
Electrolytes, administration of, infusion devices for. *See* Infusion devices.
  bolus administration of, 839, 841–842
  brain death and, 919
  hemodialysis and. *See* Hemodialysis.
  of cerebrospinal fluid, 502t
  total parenteral nutrition and, 805, 806t
Elemental diet (formula), 819
Embolism, air, in catheter insertion, 305, 308, 775t, 794
  in catheter removal, 808, 810
  in atrial pressure measurement, 305, 308
  fat, casts and, 652–653
    traction and, 664, 666, 672, 678
  in catheter insertion, 775t
  in catheter removal, 349, 351
  intraaortic balloon pump and, 422
  pulmonary, 776t, 791, 794, 808, 810–811
  rotating tourniquets and, 432
  transvenous temporary pacing and, 389
Emergency cuff inflation, for faulty inflating line, *49*
Empyema, 166
End-expiratory pressure waveform, 319
Endocarditis, 855
Endoscopy, gastrostomy tubes and, 828–834, *829,* 829t, *830*
  scleral therapy and, 541–545, *543*
  upper, at bedside, 557–560
Endotracheal tube, 23–39
  assessment of, 25
  bloody secretions from, 340–341, 344
  bronchoscopy and, 220
  care of, 26–27, 30–32
  parts of, 24, *25*
  securing of, *108*
  size of, 25t
  suctioning of, 39–44
  T-tube adaptor for, *146*
  unintentional extubation of, 37t
End-partial pressure of carbon dioxide, *206,* 206–212, *207, 208, 209, 210*
End-tidal carbon dioxide monitoring, continuous, *206–210,* 206–212
  decrease in, *208,* 208–209
  gradual increase and elevation in, 207, *208*
Enteral nutrition, 813–834
  closed delivery system for, 821, *823*
  drug-nutrient interactions in, 824t
  feeding tube in. *See* Feeding tube.
  formulas for, 813, 819
    free water in, 823t
  guidelines and indications for, 813
  jejunostomy, gastrostomy, and percutaneous endoscopic gastrostomy tubes in, 828–834, *829,* 829t, *830*
  problems in, 825–827t
  pump for, 813
  tubes for, 519
Environment, infection prevention and control in, 888–890
Enzymes, in pressure sore management, 746–749
Epicardial pacing, temporary, 376–378, *377,* 382
  atrial electrograms and, 395
Epidermal erythema, 739t
Epidural space, 480, *480,* 481t

Epinephrine, in arterial puncture, 278
  in tong or halo insertion, 459
Epithelialization, 739t
Equipment, in infection prevention and control, 890–894, 891–893t
  barrier precautions and, 882–884
Erythema, 739t
Eschar, 746, 756, *756, 757*
Escharotomy, *757*
Esophageal endoscopy, 557
Esophageal perforation, 544
Esophageal rupture, 539
Esophageal tamponade, balloon tube inflation in, 537, *538*
  complications of, 539, 544
Esophageal varices, 533
Esophagogastric tamponade, 533–541, *534, 537, 538*
Ethics, in organ donation, 912
Ethylene oxide, 892–893t
Evisceration, 722
Ewald tube, 525, *526,* 530
Exposure, employee, *886*
  radiation, 905–906
External access devices, temporary, 580–585
External counterpressure, with pneumatic antishock garments, 424–429, *425*
External fixation traction, 673–679, *674–677. See also* Traction.
  infection in, 670
  insertion of, 454–462, *455–458,* 456t, 458t, 459t, *462*
  maintenance of, 462–466
  wrenches for, *675*
External fixator, for lower extremity fracture, *676*
  for pelvic fracture, *674*
External pacemaker. *See* Cardiac pacemaker, temporary.
Extracorporeal circuit, for hemodialysis, 591–599, *592*
Extraocular movement, 511
Extravasation. *See also* Infiltration, venous.
  in volume-controlled infusion devices, 850
  venous access device and, 860t–861t, 864, 868, 869, 872
  right atrial Silastic catheter in, 881
Extremities, compartments in, 680, 681t
  external fixation devices for, *674*
  lower. *See* Leg.
  upper, venous system anatomy in, *270*
  volar compartment of, 681t
Extubation, 51–54
  unintentional, 32, 37t
Eye, infection of, prevention and control in, 882–884
  injury to, cervical pins or tongs in, 468

Family, organ donation and, 916–917
Fat, in total parenteral nutrition, 805, 806t
Fat emboli, casts and, 652–653
  traction and, 664, 666, 672, 678
Febrile reaction, from transfusion, 700, 701t
Feeding tube, 819–828, *821,* 823t, 824t, 825–827t. *See also* Nasogastric tube.
  assessment and, 820
  clogged, 826t, 827, 832
  coiled, in oropharynx, 817
  common problems with, 825–827t
  dislodged or malpositioned, 827, 833
  drug-nutrient interactions and, 824t
  feeding intolerance in, 823, 825–833
  formulas for, 823t
  free water in formulas, 823t

Pneumonia, 220
Pneumothorax, 166
 iatrogenic, 166–167
 in central venous catheter insertion, 773–776t, 774t
 open, 166
 tension, 167
 transvenous temporary pacing and, 389
Portable oxygen tank, 77–79, *79*
Portable x-ray, 908–909
Portal venous pressure, 541
Portex tracheostomy tube, *56*
Positive end-expiratory pressure (PEEP), 97, *98*, 102t
 central venous catheter insertion and, 779
 high-frequency jet ventilation and, 160
 in auto-PEEP, 138–141, *139*
 intrinsic or inadvertent, 138, *139*
  high-frequency jet ventilation and, 160
 manual self-inflating resuscitation bag in, 120
 pulse oximetry and, 202
Positive-pressure ventilation (PPV), cardiac function and, 97, *98*
 complications of, 144
 defined, 96
 high-frequency ventilation versus, 154t
 initiation and management of, 97–117, *100, 104, 108*
  assessment for, 98–100, *99, 100*
  intermittent, 82–86, *85*
  weaning from, 144–154
Postpyloric placement, of feeding tube, 816–817
Postural drainage, 87–91, *88–89*
Potassium, bolus administration of, 839
 in drug-nutrient interactions, 824t
 in stored blood, 697
Pouches, 569t
 colostomy, *565*. See also Colostomy.
Power-isolation transformer, 898
PR interval, in twelve-lead electrocardiograph, 245
 monitoring of, 237
Precordial shock, 251–266
 cardioversion and, 252–257, *255, 256*
 defibrillation and, external, 248t, 257–262
  internal, 262–266, 263t, *265*
 defined, 251
Pregnancy, radiation exposure in, 908
Preload, cardiac output and, 353
 pulmonary artery wedge pressure and, 318
Premature infant oxygen therapy, 66
Preoperative skin preparation, for central venous catheter, *778*
Pressure, in closed chest drainage systems, 175
 in hyperbaric oxygen chamber, 224–225
 pleural, 165
 skin, from body weight on mattress, 624
Pressure-preset ventilators, 96
Pressure-relieving and pressure-reducing devices, 624–643
 air fluidized therapy in, 626–630
 foam and air mattresses in, 639–642
 indications, contraindications, advantages, and disadvantages of, 625t
 low air loss therapy in, 630–633
 oscillating support therapy in, 633–639
Pressure sores, 738–749
 casts and, 653, 656
 debridement in, 739t
 enzyme preparations in, 746–749
 pressure-reducing devices and products for, 740, 742t
 pressure-relieving and pressure-reducing de-

vices for. See Pressure-relieving and pressure-reducing devices.
 prevention of, 738–743, 739t, 740t, 742t
 risk factors for, 739, 740t
 semipermeable occlusive dressings in, 743–746
 sites of, 739, 740
 stages of, 739t
Pressure support (PS), 102t
Pressure transducer systems, 282–284, 282–295, *286–294*
 assessment and, 283–284
 leveling and, 283, 288–291, *290–292*
 multiple, 282, 287–288, *288–290*
 single, disposable, *284*, 287
  indications for, 283–284
  reusable, 282, *282–284*, 287, *287*
 zeroing and, 283, 291
Proliferation, in wound healing, 718
Proportioning system, for dialyzer, 592
Protein, in cerebrospinal fluid, 502t
 nutritional deficit and, 801, 819, 820
 total parenteral nutrition and, 805, 806t
Protein-calorie malnutrition, 819, 820
Proteolytic enzymes, 746
Pulmonary. See also Lung.
Pulmonary arterial waveform. See also Arterial pressure waveform.
 absent, troubleshooting for, 337, 342–343
 continuously wedged, troubleshooting for, 338, 343
 dampened, 298, *299*
  in pulmonary artery pressure and pulmonary artery wedge pressure measurements, 334, *335*
  troubleshooting for, 337–338, 343
 in child, 301, 302t
 visible or absent, with balloon inflation, 339, 343–344
Pulmonary artery catheter, 314, *315*
 ambulation and, 333
 blood backup in, 340, 344
 blood sampling from, *345*, 345–348
 care and troubleshooting of, 333–344, *334, 335*
 electrical safety precautions for, 901
 gate valve in open position on, *324*
 in atrial pressure measurement, 303
 in mixed venous oxygen saturation monitoring, 212–213
 in right ventricle, troubleshooting for, *330*, 338–339, 343
 in transvenous temporary pacing, 375, *376*, 385–386
 migration of, 333, *335*
 removal of, 348–352
 rupture of artery and, 318, *324*, 341
 site care for, 337, 342
Pulmonary artery pressure, 314–332, *315*, 316t, *317, 320, 322–330*, 327t. See also Pulmonary artery wedge pressure.
 assessment for, 318
 changes in, 316t
  to pulmonary artery wedge pressure waveform, *324–325*
 control-mode ventilation and, 328, *328*
 intermittent mandatory ventilation and, 329, *329*
 mitral regurgitation and, 329–330
 reading from paper printout in, 319, *320*
 synchronized intermittent mandatory ventilation and, 328–329
 respiratory fluctuations of, *320*
 unexpected changes in, 340, 344
 variations in, *322–323*

Pulmonary artery wedge pressure, 314–332, *315*, 316t, *317, 320, 322–330*, 327t. See also Pulmonary artery pressure.
 a, c, and *v* waves in, 314, *316*
 a and *v* waves in, elevated, 327, *327*
 assessment for, 318
 balloon inflation and, 339–340, 344
 blood or fluid warming devices and, 447
 changes in, 317t
  to pulmonary artery pressure waveform, *324–325*
 control-mode ventilation and, 328, *328*
 intermittent mandatory ventilation and, 329, *329*
 interpretation of waveforms in, 327t
 mitral regurgitation and, 329–330
 procedure and precautions for, 319–324, *322–325*
 reading from paper printout in, 324–327, *326–330*
 synchronized intermittent mandatory ventilation and, 328–329
 in transvenous temporary pacing, 376
 mechanical ventilation and, 328, *328*
 microwaved solutions and, 451
 normal, 314, *316*
 pressure transducer systems and, 282–283
 respiratory variations in, *326*
 without respiratory variations, *326*
Pulmonary compromise. See Respiratory compromise.
Pulmonary disorders, chronic obstructive, 66, 819
 enteral feedings in, 819
 oscillating support therapy for, 633
Pulmonary edema, 429, 430
Pulmonary embolism, 776t, 791, 794, 808, 810–811
Pulmonary infarction, 341
Pulmonary pleura, 165
Pulmonary procedures, special, 199–231
 bronchoscopy in, 219–224
 continuous end-tidal carbon dioxide monitoring in, 206–210, 206–212
 continuous mixed venous oxygen saturation monitoring in, 212t, 212–219, *213, 214*
 hyperbaric oxygen therapy in, 224–230, *225*, 226t
 oxygen saturation monitoring by pulse oximetry in, *200*, 200–206, *201*, 201t, *204*
Pulmonary vascular resistance (PVR), *98*
Pulsatile waveform generation, 296, *296*
Pulse, assessment of, 650, *651*
 pulse oximetry and, 200–205
Pulse generators, 368
 battery function in, 381
 external, *371*
 in asynchronous atrial pacing, *378*
 in overdrive atrial pacing, 391, *391*
 in permanent pacing, 401, *401*
 positive and negative connectives of, 383
 sequential atrioventricular, *378*
 temporary, 378, *378, 384*
Pulse oximetry, *200*, 200–206, *201*, 201t, *204*
 sensor types and sensor sites for, 203, *204*
Pulse pressure, 296, *296*
Pump, blood, 704–707
 intraaortic balloon. See Intraaortic balloon pump.
Puncture, arterial, in central venous catheter insertion, 774t
 lumbar or cisternal, 505–511, *506, 508*
Purdue column-disc catheter, *610*
Pylorus, feeding tube and, 816–817
Pyothorax, 166